P9-APG-618

WITHDRAWN FROM LIBRARY

CARDIOPULMONARY RESUSCITATION

WITHDRAWN FROM LIBRARY

CONTEMPORARY CARDIOLOGY

CHRISTOPHER P. CANNON, MD
SERIES EDITOR

MONTGOMERY COLLEGE
ROCKVILLE CAMPUS LIBRARY
ROCKVILLE, MARYLAND

CARDIOPULMONARY RESUSCITATION

Edited by

JOSEPH P. ORNATO, MD, FACP, FACC, FACEP
MARY ANN PEBERDY, MD, FACC

Departments of Emergency Medicine and Internal Medicine (Cardiology), Virginia Commonwealth University Health System, Richmond, VA

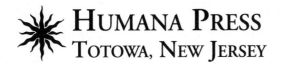

HUMANA PRESS
TOTOWA, NEW JERSEY

319984

MAR 2 8 2006

© 2005 Humana Press Inc.
999 Riverview Drive, Suite 208
Totowa, New Jersey 07512

humanapress.com

All rights reserved. No part of this book may be reproduced, stored in a retrieval system, or transmitted in any form or by any means, electronic, mechanical, photocopying, microfilming, recording, or otherwise without written permission from the Publisher.

The content and opinions expressed in this book are the sole work of the authors and editors, who have warranted due diligence in the creation and issuance of their work. The publisher, editors, and authors are not responsible for errors or omissions or for any consequences arising from the information or opinions presented in this book and make no warranty, express or implied, with respect to its contents.

Due diligence has been taken by the publishers, editors, and authors of this book to assure the accuracy of the information published and to describe generally accepted practices. The contributors herein have carefully checked to ensure that the drug selections and dosages set forth in this text are accurate and in accord with the standards accepted at the time of publication. Notwithstanding, as new research, changes in government regulations, and knowledge from clinical experience relating to drug therapy and drug reactions constantly occurs, the reader is advised to check the product information provided by the manufacturer of each drug for any change in dosages or for additional warnings and contraindications. This is of utmost importance when the recommended drug herein is a new or infrequently used drug. It is the responsibility of the treating physician to determine dosages and treatment strategies for individual patients. Further it is the responsibility of the health care provider to ascertain the Food and Drug Administration status of each drug or device used in their clinical practice. The publisher, editors, and authors are not responsible for errors or omissions or for any consequences from the application of the information presented in this book and make no warranty, express or implied, with respect to the contents in this publication.

Production Editor: Robin B. Weisberg
Cover design by Patricia F. Cleary

For additional copies, pricing for bulk purchases, and/or information about other Humana titles, contact Humana at the above address or at any of the following numbers: Tel.: 973-256-1699; Fax: 973-256-8341, E-mail: humana@humanapr.com; or visit our Website: www.humanapress.com

This publication is printed on acid-free paper. ∞
ANSI Z39.48-1984 (American National Standards Institute) Permanence of Paper for Printed Library Materials.

Photocopy Authorization Policy:
Authorization to photocopy items for internal or personal use, or the internal or personal use of specific clients, is granted by Humana Press Inc., provided that the base fee of US $25.00 is paid directly to the Copyright Clearance Center at 222 Rosewood Drive, Danvers, MA 01923. For those organizations that have been granted a photocopy license from the CCC, a separate system of payment has been arranged and is acceptable to Humana Press Inc. The fee code for users of the Transactional Reporting Service is: [1-58829-283-5/05 $25.00].

Printed in the United States of America.   10 9 8 7 6 5 4 3 2 1

eISBN 1-59259-814-5

Library of Congress Cataloging-in-Publication Data

Cardiopulmonary resuscitation / edited by Joseph P. Ornato, Mary Ann Peberdy.
   p. ; cm. -- (Contemporary cardiology)
 Includes bibliographical references and index.
 ISBN 1-58829-283-5 (alk. paper)
 1. CPR (First aid)
 [DNLM: 1. Cardiopulmonary Resuscitation. WG 205 C2677 2005] I. Ornato, Joseph P.
II. Peberdy, Mary Ann. III. Series: Contemporary cardiology (Totowa, N.J. : Unnumbered)
 RC87.9.C3732 2005
 616.1'025--dc22

                                                                              2004002774

PREFACE

More than 460,000 Americans die each year from sudden, unexpected cardiac arrest. Despite the fact that there have been more than 50 years of scientific, experimental, and clinical studies since the introduction of modern cardiopulmonary resuscitation (CPR) by researchers at Johns Hopkins University in the 1950s, survival remains dismal. Only 1 out of 5 adults survive in-hospital, and less than 1 in 10 survive out-of-hospital, cardiac arrest. Thus, there is ample room for further discovery and enhancement of resuscitative interventions.

CPR is at best an inexact science spanning many different specialties and medical disciplines. Organizations such as the American Heart Association, the Canadian Heart and Stroke Foundation, the European Resuscitation Council, and the International Liaison Committee on Resuscitation develop and publish guidelines for resuscitation approximately every 5 years. Many of the authors in this book are active members of these organizations and contribute regularly to these international guidelines documents. The purpose of *Cardiopulmonary Resuscitation* is to provide physicians, nurses, paramedics, and other members of the in- or out-of-hospital emergency response team with the latest information on the science and practice of CPR. Unlike the *American Heart Association Guidelines in Cardiopulmonary Resuscitation and Emergency Cardiovascular Care* or the *Advanced Cardiac Life Support* textbook, *Cardiopulmonary Resuscitation* explores the physiology behind current state-of-the-art clinical resuscitation in depth.

Generous portions of this book translate resuscitation physiology and principles into practical bedside recommendations, clinical tips, and expert techniques. The collective wisdom of the authors—an international, stellar group of resuscitation thought leaders— on how best to approach difficult resuscitation decisions should be of great benefit to in- or out-of-hospital resuscitation team members. The book reviews major ongoing research in resuscitation science that will likely affect the next set of international resuscitation guidelines. Finally, there is an extensive discussion of ethical issues surrounding resuscitation of both children and adults.

Cardiopulmonary Resuscitation is dedicated to the countless victims of sudden, unexpected cardiac arrest, and to their families, friends, and loved ones. If our readers can learn from this book even one new, practical technique that can save a life, our efforts will not have been in vain.

Joseph P. Ornato, MD, FACP, FACC, FACEP
Mary Ann Peberdy, MD, FACC

CONTENTS

CONTRIBUTORS

BENJAMIN S. ABELLA, MD, MPhil • *Section of Emergency Medicine, Department of Medicine, University of Chicago, Chicago, IL*

TOM P. AUFDERHEIDE, MD • *Department of Emergency Medicine, Medical College of Wisconsin, Milwaukee, WI*

CHARLES F. BABBS, MD, PhD • *Department of Basic Medical Sciences, Purdue University, West Lafayette, IN*

R. WAYNE BARBEE, PhD • *Department of Emergency Medicine, VCU Reanimation Engineering Shock Center, Virginia Commonwealth University Medical Center, Richmond, VA*

LANCE B. BECKER, MD, FAHA • *Section of Emergency Medicine, Department of Medicine, University of Chicago, Chicago, IL*

ROBERT A. BERG, MD FAAP, FCCM • *Department of Pediatrics, University of Arizona College of Medicine, Tucson, AZ*

CHARLES E. CADY, MD • *Department of Emergency Medicine, Medical College of Wisconsin, Milwaukee, WI*

LEONARD A. COBB, MD, FACP • *Department of Medicine (Cardiology), University of Washington School of Medicine; Medic One Support Group, Harborview Medical Center, Seattle, WA*

CATHERINE COOPER, MD • *Department of Anesthesiology, Virginia Commonwealth University Medical Center, Richmond, VA*

MARY ANN COOPER, MD • *Departments of Bioengineering and Emergency Medicine, University of Illinois, Chicago, IL*

MARSH CUTTINO, MD • *Department of Emergency Medicine, Virginia Commonwealth University Medical Center, Richmond, VA*

DANIEL F. DANZL, MD • *Department of Emergency Medicine, University of Louisville, Louisville, KY*

GARY A. DILDY, III, MD • *Department of Obstetrics and Gynecology, Louisiana State University Health Sciences Center, New Orleans, LA*

ALIDENE DOHERTY, RN, BSN • *University of Washington Medical Center, Seattle, WA*

MICKEY S. EISENBERG, MD, PhD • *Department of Medicine, University of Washington, Seattle, WA*

JOHN M. FIELD, MD • *Division of Cardiology, Penn State Milton S. Hershey Medical Center, Hershey, PA*

ANDREA GABRIELLI, MD • *Division of Critical Care Medicine, Department of Anesthesiology, University of Florida College of Medicine, Gainesville, FL*

EDGAR R. GONZALEZ, PharmD, FASHP • *Nevada College of Pharmacy, Henderson, NV*

JOSEPH A. GRILLO, PharmD • *Center for Drug Evaluation and Research, US Food and Drug Administration, Rockville, MD*

ALFRED HALLSTROM, PhD • *Department of Biostatistics, University of Washington, Seattle, WA*

HENRY HALPERIN, MD, MA • *Departments of Medicine, Radiology, and Biomedical Engineering, Johns Hopkins University, Baltimore, MD*

KRISTIN R. HANSON, BA, EMT • *National Center for Early Defibrillation, Department of Emergency Medicine, University of Pittsburgh School of Medicine, Pittsburgh, PA*

RAYMOND E. IDEKER, MD, PhD • *Division of Cardiovascular Disease, University of Alabama at Birmingham, Birmingham, AL*

AHAMED H. IDRIS, MD • *Division of Emergency Medicine, Department of Surgery, University of Texas Southwestern Medical Center at Dallas, Dallas, TX*

RAO R. IVATURY, MD • *Division of Trauma and Critical Care Surgery, Departments of Surgery, Emergency Medicine, and Physiology, VCU Reanimation Engineering Shock Center, Virginia Commonwealth University Medical Center, Richmond, VA*

ALLAN S. JAFFE, MD • *Cardiovascular Division, Departments of Medicine, Laboratory Medicine, and Pathology, Mayo Medical School, Rochester, MN*

SARA ASHLEY JOHNSON, MD • *Department of Emergency Medicine, MacNeal Hospital, Berwin, IL*

RICHARD E. KERBER, MD • *Cardiology Division, University of Iowa College of Medicine; Department of Medicine, University of Iowa Hospitals and Clinics, Iowa City, IA*

KARL B. KERN, MD • *Department of Medicine, Sarver Heart Center, University of Arizona, Tucson, AZ*

CHERYL R. KILLINGSWORTH, DVM, PhD • *Division of Cardiovascular Disease, University of Alabama at Birmingham, Birmingham, AL*

ANETTE C. KRISMER, MD • *Department of Anesthesiology and Critical Care Medicine, Leopold-Franzens-University, Innsbruck, Austria*

A. JOSEPH LAYON, MD, FACP • *Division of Critical Care Medicine, Departments of Anesthesiology, Surgery, and Medicine, University of Florida College of Medicine, Gainesville Fire Rescue Service, Gainesville, FL*

KARL H. LINDNER • *Department of Anesthesiology and Critical Care Medicine, Medical University of Innsbruck, Innsbruck, Austria*

RUSSELL V. LUEPKER, MD, MS • *Division of Epidemiology, School of Public Health, University of Minnesota, Minneapolis, MN*

JOSEPH E. MARINE, MD • *Cardiology Division, Johns Hopkins Bayview Medical Center, Baltimore, MD*

JEROME H. MODELL, MD • *Department of Anesthesiology, University of Florida College of Medicine and University of Florida College of Veterinary Medicine, Gainesville, FL*

VINCENT N. MOSESSO, JR., MD, FACEP • *National Center for Early Defibrillation, Department of Emergency Medicine, University of Pittsburgh School of Medicine, Pittsburgh, PA*

ANTONIO E. MUÑIZ, MD, FACEP, FAAP, FAAEM • *Departments of Emergency Medicine and Pediatrics, Virginia Commonwealth University Medical Center, Richmond, VA*

VINAY M. NADKARNI, MD, FAAP, FCCM • *Department of Anesthesia and Critical Care Medicine, The Children's Hospital of Philadelphia, University of Pennsylvania School of Medicine, Philadelphia, PA*

PAMELA NERHEIM, MD • *Division of Cardiology, University of Iowa Hospitals, Iowa City, IA*

MARY M. NEWMAN, BS • *National Center for Early Defibrillation, Department of Emergency Medicine, University of Pittsburgh School of Medicine, Pittsburgh, PA*

BRIAN OLSHANSKY, MD • *Division of Cardiac Electrophysiology, University of Iowa Hospitals, Iowa City, IA*

JOSEPH P. ORNATO, MD, FACP, FACC, FACEP • *Departments of Emergency Medicine and Internal Medicine (Cardiology), Virginia Commonwealth University Medical Center, Richmond, VA*

UTPAL H. PANDYA • *Department of Medicine, Mayo Clinic and College of Medicine, Rochester, MN*

NORMAN A. PARADIS, MD • *Departments of Emergency Medicine, Surgery, and Medicine, University of Colorado Health Sciences Center, Denver, CO*

MARY ANN PEBERDY, MD, FACC • *Departments of Emergency Medicine and Internal Medicine (Cardiology), Virginia Commonwealth University Medical Center, Richmond, VA*

PAUL E. PEPE, MD, FACEP, FACP, FCCM • *Emergency Medicine, Internal Medicine, Surgery and Public Health, University of Texas Southwestern Medical Center; The Parkland Health and Hospital System; and Dallas Metropolitan BioTel (EMS) System, Dallas, TX*

BARRY K. RAYBURN, MD • *Division of Cardiovascular Disease, University of Alabama at Birmingham, Birmingham, AL*

BARBARA RIEGEL, DNSc, RN, CS, FAAN • *School of Nursing, University of Pennsylvania, Philadelphia, PA; Sharp HealthCare, San Diego, CA*

ALISON A. RODRIGUEZ, MD • *Department of Obstetrics and Gynecology, Louisiana State University Health Sciences Center, New Orleans, LA*

LYNN P. ROPPOLO, MD • *Department of Emergency Medicine, University of Texas Southwestern Medical Center and The Parkland Health and Hospital System; Dispatch Operations, Dallas, TX*

JEFFREY ROSENBLATT, PharmD • *Nevada College of Pharmacy, Henderson, NV*

MICHAEL R. SAYRE, MD • *Department of Emergency Medicine, Good Samaritan Hospital, Cincinnati, OH*

DOMENIC A. SICA, MD • *Section of Clinical Pharmacology and Hypertension, Division of Nephrology, Virginia Commonwealth University, Richmond, VA*

JOHN SOUTHALL, MD • *Department of Emergency Medicine, Maine Medical Center, Portland, ME*

BRUCE D. SPIESS, MD, FAHA • *Department of Anesthesiology, VCU Reanimation Engineering Shock Center, Virginia Commonwealth University Medical Center, Richmond, VA*

SHIJIE SUN, MD, FCCM • *Institute of Critical Care Medicine, Palm Springs, CA; and Keck School of Medicine, University of Southern California, Los Angeles, CA*

WANCHUN TANG, MD, FCCP, FCCM • *Institute of Critical Care Medicine, Palm Springs; and Keck School of Medicine, University of Southern California, Los Angeles, CA*

TERRY L. VANDEN HOEK, MD • *Department of Emergency Medicine, University of Chicago, Chicago, IL*

ALEJANDRO VASQUEZ, MD • *Department of Medicine, Sarver Heart Center, University of Arizona, Tucson, AZ*

MARTIN VON PLANTA, MD • *University of Basel, Basel, Switzerland*

GREGORY P. WALCOTT, MD • *Division of Cardiovascular Disease, University of Alabama at Birmingham, Birmingham, AL*

LIH-JEN WANG, MS, PharmD, BCPS • *Columbus Regional Medical Center, Columbus, GA*

KEVIN R. WARD, MD • *Departments of Emergency Medicine and Physiology, VCU Reanimation Engineering Shock Center, Virginia Commonwealth University Medical Center, Richmond, VA*

MAX HARRY WEIL, MD, PhD, MACP, FACC, MasterFCCP, FCCM • *Institute of Critical Care Medicine, Palm Springs, CA; and Keck School of Medicine, University of Southern California, Los Angeles, CA*

VOLKER WENZEL • *Department of Anesthesiology and Critical Care Medicine, Leopold-Franzens-University, Innsbruck, Austria*

LARS WIK, MD • *Norwegian Competence Center for Emergency Medicine, Institute for Experimental Medical Research, Ulleval University Hospital, Oslo, Norway*

VALUE-ADDED eBOOK/PDA

This book is accompanied by a value-added CD-ROM that contains an eBook version of the volume you have just purchased. This eBook can be viewed on your computer, and you can synchronize it to your PDA for viewing on your handheld device. The eBook enables you to view this volume on only one computer and PDA. Once the eBook is installed on your computer, you cannot download, install, or e-mail it to another computer; it resides solely with the computer to which it is installed. The license provided is for only one computer. The eBook can only be read using Adobe® Reader® 6.0 software, which is available free from Adobe Systems Incorporated at www.Adobe.com. You may also view the eBook on your PDA using the Adobe® PDA Reader® software that is also available free from Adobe.com.

You must follow a simple procedure when you install the eBook/PDA that will require you to connect to the Humana Press website in order to receive your license. Please read and follow the instructions below:

1. Download and install Adobe® Reader® 6.0 software
   You can obtain a free copy of the Adobe® Reader® 6.0 software at www.adobe.com
   *Note: If you already have the Adobe® Reader® 6.0 software installed, you do not need to reinstall it.
2. Launch Adobe® Reader® 6.0 software
3. Install eBook: Insert your eBook CD into your CD-ROM drive
   PC: Click on the "Start" button, then click on "Run"
   At the prompt, type "d:\ebookinstall.pdf" and click "OK"
   *Note: If your CD-ROM drive letter is something other than d: change the above command accordingly.
   MAC: Double click on the "eBook CD" that you will see mounted on your desktop. Double click "ebookinstall.pdf"
4. Adobe® Reader® 6.0 software will open and you will receive the message "This document is protected by Adobe DRM" Click "OK"
   *Note: If you have not already activated the Adobe® Reader® 6.0 software, you will be prompted to do so. Simply follow the directions to activate and continue installation.

Your web browser will open and you will be taken to the Humana Press eBook registration page. Follow the instructions on that page to complete installation. You will need the serial number located on the sticker sealing the envelope containing the CD-ROM.

If you require assistance during the installation, or you would like more information regarding your eBook and PDA installation, please refer to the eBookManual.pdf located on your CD. If you need further assistance, contact Humana Press eBook Support by e-mail at ebooksupport@humanapr.com or by phone at 973-256-1699.

*Adobe and Reader are either registered trademarks or trademarks of Adobe Systems Incorporated in the United States and/or other countries.

1   History of the Science
of Cardiopulmonary Resuscitation

Mickey S. Eisenberg, MD, PhD

CONTENTS

THE WILL OF RESUSCITATION

Through much of recorded history, resuscitation was forbidden. Although written accounts of resuscitation can be found, it is clear that successful reversal of death was thought to have been performed directly by God or through appointed agents. For example, stories of resuscitation in the Bible involve prophets acting clearly as vessels through which God's power restores life *(1,2)*. In these and other resuscitation accounts, reversal of death was considered the province of God and not something mere mortals should undertake. This "prohibition" against resuscitation was challenged during the Enlightenment, an amazing period of scientific discovery. Starting around 1750, scientists and philosophers questioned the dogma of the past and came to believe that humans could understand and control their own destinies. They wished to discover the workings of the universe as well as the ticking of life itself. To speak of the science of resuscitation one must begin where science begins. And there is no more crucial ingredient to science than the scientific method—a key achievement of the Enlightenment. The intellectual giants of the Enlightenment claimed that the world could best be understood through scientific discovery, and the means to achieve this was the scientific method.

From the experiments and swirling discoveries of the Enlightenment came the belief that if life could be understood, then death itself could be reversed. The will to resuscitate manifested itself in the first organized effort to deal with the problem of sudden death.

From: *Contemporary Cardiology: Cardiopulmonary Resuscitation*
Edited by: J. P. Ornato and M. A. Peberdy © Humana Press Inc., Totowa, NJ

In the 1700s, drowning, particularly in the large European port cities, was the leading cause of sudden death. In response, Amsterdam founded the first organized resuscitation effort—there were as many as 400 deaths per year in that city *(3)*. The establishment of the Amsterdam Rescue Society in 1767 represents humanity's collective desire to attempt resuscitation of the suddenly dead. No longer was religion invoked as the sole life-saving force, instead humankind empowered itself to deal with matters of life and death. Within 4 years of its founding, the Amsterdam Rescue claimed to have saved 150 persons from watery deaths. The Royal Humane Society in London began a few years later in 1774 *(4)*. The Society's emblem shows an angel blowing on an ember with a Latin inscription that translates "A little spark may yet lie hid." This emblem is a wonderful metaphor of the prevailing belief that as long as there was warmth in the body, life could be reignited. The will to resuscitate began with the Enlightenment. It would take approx 200 years for the way to be found *(5)*.

THE SEARCH FOR THE WAY OF RESUSCITATION

Rescue societies were formed in many European and American cities after the Enlightenment, and all of these societies recommended techniques to deal with drowning victims *(6)*. For example, one technique advocated placing the victim over a barrel and rolling him or her back and forth while holding the legs. This technique allowed the abdomen to be alternatively squeezed and to perhaps allow a small amount of air to reach the lungs. Another recommended procedure was to use bellows to directly blow air into the victim's mouth. Clearly, most of the air would go into the stomach or out the nose. There were even recommendations to use tobacco smoke inserted rectally in the drowning victim *(7,8)*. Tobacco was a stimulant, and there were animal experiments suggesting that smoke in the rectum could revive unconscious individuals. These techniques relied on common sense. It seemed logical to stimulate the body to restart breathing. With these and many other fanciful methods it is tempting to ridicule the science of the 18th century. What is important, however, is not the success of these early methods, but rather their very existence as emblematic of the quest to reverse sudden death.

From 1767 to 1949, there were literally hundreds of techniques and procedures recommended for artificial ventilation *(9)*. Most relied on direct pressure to the abdomen, chest, or back. The inventors of these techniques thought, wrongly, that passive entrainment of air into the lungs was sufficient to maintain adequate oxygenation. Hundreds of thousands of individuals in Europe and the United States learned these techniques, although none of the methods were very effective *(10)*. Perhaps it is surprising that no scientist recommended direct mouth-to-mouth respiration, but it must be remembered that for many years it was considered loathsome for a rescuer to place his or her lips on another person's mouth. And then there was the belief, strongly held for many decades, that expired air did not contain enough oxygen to sustain life.

THE WAY IS FOUND

It wasn't until James Elam, an anesthesiologist, entered the scene that mouth-to-mouth resuscitation was rediscovered. I say "rediscovered" because it had been known for many centuries that it could be useful in newborn resuscitation. Elam's discovery occurred in the middle of a polio outbreak in 1949 in Minneapolis. Here is how Elam describes the event.

I was browsing around to get acquainted with the ward when along the corridor came a gurney racing—a nurse pulling it and two orderlies pushing it, and the kid on it was blue. I went into total reflex behavior. I stepped out in the middle of the corridor, stopped the gurney, grabbed the sheet, wiped the copious mucous off his mouth and face, . . . sealed my lips around his nose and inflated his lungs. In four breaths he was pink (5).

The evening before this rediscovery, Elam read a chapter on the history of resuscitation in which mouth-to-mouth ventilation for newborns was described. He credits this chapter for his "reflex behavior." It is comforting to think that historians played a crucial role in scientific discoveries. Elam's passion led to his proselytizing about the merits of mouth-to-nose ventilation. He set out to prove that exhaled air was adequate to oxygenate non-breathing persons. To accomplish this he obtained permission from his chief of surgery to do studies on postoperative patients before the ether anesthesia wore off. He demonstrated that expired air blown into the endotracheal tube maintained normal oxygen saturation *(11)*.

Several years later, Elam met Peter Safar, and Safar joined the effort to convince the world that mouth-to-mouth ventilation was effective. Safar set out on a series of experiments using paralyzed individuals to show that the technique could maintain adequate oxygenation *(12)*. Safar describes the experiments.

Thirty-one physicians and medical students, and one nurse volunteered. . . . Consent was very informed. All volunteers had to observe me ventilate anesthetized and curarized patients without a tracheal tube. I sedated the volunteers and paralyzed them for several hours each. Blood O_2 and CO_2 were analyzed. I demonstrated the method to over 100 lay persons who were then asked to perform the method on the curarized volunteers (5).

Within a year of these experiments, Safar and Elam convinced the world to switch from manual to mouth-to-mouth ventilation. The US military accepted and endorsed the method in 1957 and the American Medical Association (AMA) followed suit in 1958. *The Journal of the American Medical Association (JAMA)* stated the following endorsement, "Information about expired air breathing should be disseminated as widely as possible" *(13)*.

Unlike cessation of respiration, an obvious sign of sudden death, the cessation of circulation, and particularly the rhythm of the heart, was invisible to an observer. Perhaps as a result, the appreciation of artificial circulation lagged considerably behind the obvious need for artificial respirations. Plus, even if scientists in the post-Enlightenment period appreciated the need to circulate blood there was simply no effective means to do so. Even though closed chest massage was described in 1904 *(14)*, its benefit was not appreciated and anecdotal case reports did little to promote the benefit of closed chest massage. The prevailing belief was described in a physician's quote from 1890, "We are powerless against paralysis of the circulation."

Here's where serendipity plays a role. It would be nice to believe that all scientific discoveries are the result of the painstaking accumulation of small facts leading to a grand synthesis, yet, the role of accident cannot be discounted. Chest compression was really an accidental discovery made by William Kouwenhoven, Guy Knickerbocker, and James Jude. They were studying defibrillation in dogs and they noticed that by forcefully applying the paddles to the chest of the dog with a fair amount of force, they could achieve a pulse in the femoral artery. This was the key observation that led them eventually to try it on humans. The first person saved with this technique was recalled by Jude as ". . . rather an obese female who . . . went into cardiac arrest as a result of flurothane anesthetic. . . . This woman had no blood pressure, no pulse, and ordinarily we would have opened up her chest. . . . Instead, since we weren't in the operating room, we applied external cardiac massage. . . . Her blood pressure and pulse came back at once. We didn't have to open her chest. They went ahead and did the operation on her, and she recovered completely" *(5)*. They published their findings on 20 cases on in-hospital cardiac arrest (CA) in a 1960 *JAMA* article *(15)*. Of the 20 patients, 14 (70%) were discharged from the hospital. Chest compression ranged from 1 to 65 minutes in the patients. The authors write in their landmark article, "Now anyone, anytime, can institute life saving measures." Later that year, mouth-to-mouth ventilation was combined with chest compression and cardiopulmonary resuscitation (CPR), as we practice it today, was developed. The American Heart Association (AHA) formally endorsed CPR in 1963 *(5)*.

THE SEARCH FOR DEFIBRILLATION

The discovery of electricity was another product of the Enlightenment. In the late 1700s, many scientists began experimenting with this "newly discovered" force called electricity. There were early descriptions of possible defibrillation *(16)*. For example, in this account from 1780 there is a report of "Sophia Greenhill who fell from a window and was taken up, by all appearances, dead." The report goes on to say that "Mr. Squires tried the effects of electricity, and upon transmitting a few shocks to the thorax, perceived a small pulsation" *(17)*. Protodefibrillators had two electrodes and glass rods to protect the operator. They even had a capacitor and a means to dial in a variable amount of current.

Ventricular fibrillation (VF) was first appreciated in animals 150 years ago when two German scientists noticed that strong electric currents applied directly to the ventricles of a dog's heart caused VF. It was considered a medical curiosity with no relevance for humans. John McWilliam made the first detailed descriptions of VF in animals and he was the first to postulate an importance for humans in a series of articles from 1887 to 1889 published in the *British Medical Journal (BMJ) (18,19)*. In McWilliam's day it was assumed that sudden cardiac collapse took the form of a sudden standstill—in other words, no electrical activity. Experiments performed by McWilliam on dogs disproved this idea. McWilliam's descriptions of VF, written more than 100 years ago, are classic:

> *The normal beat is at once abolished, and the ventricles are thrown into a tumultuous state of quick, irregular, twitching action. . . . The cardiac pump is thrown out of gear, and the last of its vital energy is dissipated in a violent and prolonged turmoil of fruitless activity in the ventricular walls. . . . It seems to me in the highest degree probable that a similar phenomenon occurs in the human heart, and is the direct and immediate cause of death in many cases of sudden dissolution (18).*

In addition to studying dogs, McWilliam performed experiments on both young and adult cats, rabbits, rats, mice, hedgehogs, eels, and chickens. He noted that the lower and smaller mammals, and the fetal hearts of larger animals, could not sustain VF. The hearts were simply too small to sustain the rhythm. His delineation of heart size and its ability to maintain VF were major factors in his speculation that fibrillation is an important cause of sudden death in humans. At the time McWilliam was writing, VF had never been observed directly in humans, as the electrocardiogram (ECG) wasn't invented until 1930.

Although McWilliam used an electric current to induce the fibrillation, he never tried electricity to stop the fibrillations of a heart muscle. One would not intuitively assume that the electrical stimulation that caused the fibrillation could not also defibrillate the heart. Nevertheless, McWilliam deserves recognition for his landmark studies in fibrillation and for being the first scientist to defibrillate animals.

MODERN CURRENTS

The connection between electricity and defibrillation was picked up again in the 1920s. The Edison Electric Institute, concerned about fatal electrical shocks suffered by its utility workers, funded research to prevent fatalities. The researchers were Hooker, Langworthy, and Kouwenhoven (20). This is the same Kouwenhoven who later was one of the codiscoverers of CPR—he was working on defibrillation involving dogs and noticed how the pressure of the paddles on the dogs' chest led to a pulse. This accidental observation led to modern CPR. Throughout the early 1930s, Hooker et al. showed that even small electric shocks could induce VF in the heart and that more powerful shocks could erase the fibrillation. These investigators induced VF in dogs and then were able to defibrillate the heart without opening the chest. But their closed-chest defibrillation was successful only if the fibrillatory contractions were vigorous and the period of no circulation or breathing did not exceed several minutes. If the period was longer than several minutes, open-heart massage was necessary before the electric shock could defibrillate the heart. The term "countershock" was derived from their research. Because an initial shock was required to place the heart in VF, it was only logical to call the subsequent shock, which defibrillated the heart, the countershock. The term countershock for many years was used synonymously to mean defibrillation.

Hooker et al.'s research was well on its way toward developing effective defibrillation in humans; unfortunately, however, their work had to be halted because of World War II.

Claude Beck, professor of surgery at Western Reserve University (later to become Case Western Reserve) in Cleveland, worked for years on a technique for defibrillation of the human heart. Beck probably witnessed his first CA during his internship in 1922, while on the surgery service at the Johns Hopkins Hospital. During a urological operation, the anesthetist announced that the patient's heart had stopped. To Beck's amazement, the surgical resident removed his gloves and went to a telephone in a corner of the room and called the fire department. Beck remained in total bewilderment as the fire department rescue squad rushed into the operating room 15 minutes later and applied oxygen-powered resuscitators to the patient's face. The patient died, but the episode left an indelible impression on Beck. Twenty years later, Beck wrote, "surgeons should not turn these emergencies over to the care of the fire department." Recalling the same event, he remarked to medical students in typically understated fashion, "The experience left me with a conviction that we were not doing our best for the patient" (21). Beck ultimately developed techniques to take back the management of CA from the fire department and place it in the hands of surgeons. Ironically, 20 years after his accomplishment, CA management was utilized by emergency medical technicians (EMTs), thus returned to the fire department.

Beck realized that VF often occurred in hearts that were basically sound and he coined the phrase "Hearts Too Good to Die." In 1947, Beck accomplished his first successful resuscitation of a 14-year-old boy using open-chest massage and internal defibrillation with alternating current. The boy was being operated on for a severe congenital funnel chest. In all other respects, the boy was normal. During the closure of the large incision in the boy's chest, his pulse suddenly stopped and his blood pressure (BP) fell to zero.

Seeing the boy was in CA, Beck immediately reopened his chest and began manual heart massage. As Beck looked at and felt the heart, he realized that VF was present. Massage continued for 35 minutes, then an ECG was taken that confirmed the presence of VF. Another 10 minutes passed before the defibrillator was brought to the operating room. The first shock, using electrode paddles placed directly on the sides of the heart, was unsuccessful. Beck administered procainamide and then gave a second shock that wiped out the fibrillation. Within a very few seconds a feeble, regular, and fast contraction of the heart occurred. The boy's BP rose from 0 to 50 mmHg. Beck noted that the heartbeat remained regular and that the pressure slowly began to rise. Twenty minutes after the successful defibrillation, the chest wound was closed. Three hours later, the BP rose to a normal level, and the child awoke and was able to answer questions. The boy made a full recovery, with no neurological damage *(22)*.

The defibrillators used by Beck were individually made. Ever the scientist, Beck kept experimenting with different models in order to improve the efficiency of the machine. Because these models were intended for open-heart defibrillation, Beck designed a model that would both shock and perform heart massage. Suction cups were attached to the walls of the heart and alternating suction would expand and allow the heart to relax. According to Beck, the machine could massage at the rate of 120 beats per minute, and relieved the surgeon of performing cardiac massage. The suction cups doubled as defibrillator electrodes. It was an ingenious device, but closed-chest compression and closed-chest defibrillation ultimately turned Beck's defibrillator machine into an historical curiosity.

For Paul Zoll, the development of an external defibrillator was a natural extension of his earlier work with an external cardiac pacemaker. Zoll was also quite aware of open-heart defibrillation. He worked in a hospital where that procedure was used to resuscitate people whose hearts went into fibrillation during operations. The standard procedure would then be to crack open the patient's chest and massage the heart by hand to restore blood circulation. Then, the doctors would apply an electrical alternating current (AC) countershock directly to the heart.

The decision to develop an external defibrillator using AC rather than direct current (DC) was a practical one. DC batteries and capacitor technology that were both powerful and portable for practical use simply did not exist in the early 1950s. In 1955, a 67-year-old man survived several episodes of VF, thanks to Zoll's external defibrillator, and went home from the hospital after 1 month. Over a period of 4 months, Zoll had successfully stopped VF 11 times in four different patients. The energy required for defibrillation ranged from 240 to 720 volts (V). Zoll's findings were published in the *New England Journal of Medicine (NEJM)* in 1956 *(23)*.

The defibrillator designed by Zoll, as well as earlier versions invented by Kouwen-hoven and Beck, utilized AC and were run off the electricity from any wall socket, or line current. These AC defibrillators were very large and heavy, primarily because they contained a transformer to step up the line current from 110 V to 500 or 1000 V. Not many lives would be saved unless the inherent nonportability of AC defibrillators could be solved.

The portability problem was finally solved by Bernard Lown. Lown devised a defibrillator that utilized DC instead of AC. With DC it was possible to use power, supplied by a battery, to charge a capacitor over a few seconds. The capacitor stored the energy until it was released in one massive jolt to the chest wall. The availability of new, small capacitors considerably reduced the size and weight of the device. No longer would defibrillators require bulky transformers and no longer would they be tied to line current. The cord was cut—the defibrillator could travel to the patient.

In 1960, little was known about the effect of DC current on the heart. Lown divided the problem into two parts: What is safe? What is effective? A series of animal experiments on dogs in 1960 and 1961 established that DC shocks were extremely effective in shocking the heart. What's more, it was clear that DC would be many times safer than AC when applied through the chest wall.

In a 1962 article in the *American Journal of Cardiology (24),* Lown noted that the incidence of VF was 10 times more frequent after AC than DC cardioversion. Lown did discover one short period of time during the procedure when a DC shock could induce VF. Thus, the trick was simply to build a device that would shock the heart while avoiding this so called "vulnerable period" of a few milliseconds. It was his breakthrough to DC that eventually made the portable defibrillator practical.

The development of small but powerful DC batteries and small capacitors would be the next technological link. At that point, the need to carry a 50-pound step-up transformer to the patient and the need to find an electrical outlet in which to plug an AC-based defibrillator vanished.

PRESENT CURRENTS

With DC defibrillation proved, all the elements were in place for widespread dissemination of the procedure. Defibrillation spread quickly into hospital coronary care units, emergency departments, and, then, in the late 1960s and early 1970s the first paramedic programs began. Now the defibrillator traveled directly to a patient in VF. The first programs began almost simultaneously in Seattle, Portland, Columbus, Ohio, Miami, and Los Angeles *(5).* By the 1980s, studies to demonstrate successful defibrillation by EMTs were conducted in King County, Washington. The first study demonstrated an improvement in VF survival from 7 to 26%. Slowly, other communities began EMT defibrillation programs *(25).*

The idea for an automatic defibrillator was first conceived by Dr. Arch Diack, a surgeon in Portland *(26).* Diack's prototype, literally assembled in a basement, utilized a unique defibrillation pathway—tongue to chest. There was a breath detector that was a safeguard to prevent shocking breathing persons. The electrode was essentially a rate counter, far more crude than today's sophisticated VF detectors. The production model weighed 35 pounds and gave verbal instructions. It was an idea ahead of its time. Most people viewed it as a curiosity. By the late 1980s, however, other manufacturers entered the field leading to the crop of automated external defibrillators (AEDs) we have today. AEDs, with ease of training and use, allowed EMT defibrillation programs to expand rapidly. The first program to demonstrate the safety and effectiveness of EMT defibrillation with AEDs was also conducted in King County (by Richard Cummins) *(27).* From EMT defibrillation with AEDs, there was a natural and logical progression to the early First Responder defibrillation and finally the current situation of widespread public access defibrillation. Perhaps the future will witness AEDs in homes, and they will be thought of as personal safety devices.

FUTURE CURRENTS

Future AEDs will likely interact more with the victim of CA and provide feedback to the rescuer. For example, a device may obtain information from the heart's ECG, or wall motion or internal sound that could be fed back to tell the rescuer to perform CPR prior to defibrillation. In other words, the ECG signal may be a surrogate for downtime that in turn can better advise how to proceed with the resuscitation. Back in the early 1970s, it was dogma that CPR should precede defibrillation to "prime the pump" and rid the heart of lactic acid. By the 1980s, there was a growing body of information to suggest that time to shock was the best predictor of outcome. Thus, defibrillation became the priority and defibrillatory shocks were to be given as rapidly as possible. The mantra became, "CPR until the defibrillator arrives." Now with recent studies from Seattle and Oslo, some are once again questioning whether CPR should be given prior to defibrillation. It may well turn out that both are correct, namely immediate shock for witnessed VF or VF of short duration and CPR prior to shock for VF of longer duration.

We now appreciate that there is an interaction between CPR and defibrillation. Each procedure is not independent of the other. It is possible to learn much from the VF signal that can be used to provide feedback regarding whether CPR or immediate defibrillation is the procedure of choice. Recent studies coming from the world of engineering demonstrate that the probability of return of spontaneous circulation (P_{ROSC}) based on the VF signal can be calculated. This probability is determined from calculations of spectral densities, frequency, amplitude, and other electrical terms. This information is translated into a probability. And because it can be calculated every second, it will be possible to determine if the P_{ROSC} is rising or falling. This in turn can guide the resuscitation. For example, if the P_{ROSC} is 20% after attaching the pads, then CPR is indicated and perhaps medication. Once the P_{ROSC} reaches 60% then, a shock is indicated. Shocking for low P_{ROSC} are not indicated because they are likely to damage the heart with low likelihood of success and deprive the heart of CPR during the pause for defibrillatory shock. It is possible to gain the information from the VF signal even in the presence of chest compressions and ventilation.

THE SCIENCE OF RESUSCITATION CONTINUES

The will to resuscitate, as exemplified by rescue societies, emerged during the Enlightenment. It took approx 200 years for the way of resuscitation to be found. The elements of mouth-to-mouth ventilation, chest compression, and defibrillation each had to be discovered separately and integrated for reversal of sudden death to become a reality. The science of resuscitation is founded on the scientific method of experimentation. Many false starts, particularly in ventilation and defibrillation, happened before new understandings led to effective techniques. We now can reverse sudden death reliably and numerous scientists and investigators can take pride in this accomplishment. But the real challenge remains for the future. The real challenge is to fully understand the causes and triggers of VF and to develop preventive measures. Whether this will require 20 or 200 years, one thing is certain—future chapters in the science of resuscitation are still to be told.

REFERENCES

1. Hebrew Bible (Kings:1)
2. Hebrew Bible (Kings:2)
3. Johnson A. An account of some societies at Amsterdam and Hamburg for the recovery of drowned persons. London, UK: 1773.
4. Bishop PJ. A short history of the Royal Humane Society. Royal Humane Society, LondonUK: 1974.
5. Eisenberg MS. Life in the balance: emergency medicine and the quest to reverse sudden death. Oxford, NY: 1997.
6. Thompson EH. The role of physicians in humane societies of the eighteenth century. Bulletin of the History of Medicine 1963; 37:43–51.

7. Lee RV. Cardiopulmonary resuscitation in the eighteenth century. Journal of the History of Medicine 1972:October:418–433.
8. Cary RJ. A brief history of the methods of resuscitation of the apparently drowned. Journal of the Johns Hopkins Hospital Bulletin 1918; 270:243–251.
9. Karpovich P. Adventures in artificial respiration. New York, NY: Associated Press, 1953, p. 32
10. Gordon AS, Sadove MS, Raymon F, Ivy AC. Critical survey of manual artificial respiration. Journal of the American Medical Association 1951; 147:1444–1453.
11. Elam JO. Rediscovery of expired air methods for emergency ventilation. In: Safar P, ed. Advances in Cardiopulmonary Resuscitation. New York, NY: Springer-Verlag, 1977, pp. 263–265.
12. Safar P. History of cardiopulmonary-cerebral resuscitation. In: Kaye W, Bircher N, ed. Cardiopulmonary Resuscitation. New York, NY: Churchill Livingston, 1989, pp. 1–53.
13. Dill DB. Symposium on mouth to mouth resuscitation (expired air inflation), Council on Medical Physics. Journal of the American Medical Association 1958; 167:317–319.
14. Jude JR, Kouwenhoven WB, Knickerbocker GG. External cardiac resuscitation. Monographs in Surgical Science 1964; I:65.
15. Kouwenhoven WB, Jude JR, Knickerbocker GG. Closed-chest cardiac massage. Journal of the American Medical Association 1960; 173:94–97.
16. Schechter DC. Exploring the Origins of Electrical Cardiac Stimulation. Minneapolis, MN: Medtronic, 1983, p. 15.
17. Kite C. An Essay on the Recovery of the Apparently Dead. London, UK: C. Dilly, 1788, p. 166.
18. McWilliam JA. Cardiac failure and sudden death. British Medical Journal 1889; 5:6–8.
19. McWilliam JA. Electrical stimulation of the heart in man. British Medical Journal 1899; 16:348–350.
20. Hooker DR, Kouwenhoven WB, Langworthy OR. The effect of alternating electrical currents on the heart. American Journal of Physiology 1933; 103:444–454.
21. Meyer JA. Claude Beck and cardiac resuscitation. Annals of Thoracic Surgery 1988; 45:103–105.
22. Beck CS, Pritchard WH, Feil HS. Ventricular fibrillation of long duration abolished by electric shock. Journal of the American Medical Association 1947; 135:985, 986.
23. Zoll PM, Linenthal AJ, Gibson W, Paul MH, Norman LR. Termination of ventricular fibrillation in man by externally applied electric countershock. New England Journal of Medicine 1956; 254:727–732.
24. Lown B. "Cardioversion" of arrhythmias (I). Modern concepts of cardiovascular diseases. American Heart Association 1964; 33:863–868.
25. Eisenberg M, Copass M, Hallstrom A et al. Treatment of out-of-hospital cardiac arrest with rapid defibrillation by emergency medical technicians. New England Journal of Medicine 1980; 302:1379–1383.
26. Diack AW, Wellborn WS, Rullman RG et al. An automatic cardiac resuscitator for emergency treatment of cardiac arrest. Medical Instruments 1979; 13:78–81.
27. Cummins RO, Eisenberg MS, Litwin PE, Graves JR, Hearne TR, Hallstrom A. Automatic external defibrillation used by emergency technicians: a controlled clinical trial. JAMA 1987; 257:1605–1610.

2 Epidemiology of Sudden Death

Russell V. Luepker, MD, MS

CONTENTS

INTRODUCTION

Sudden death, mainly out-of-hospital death, is a major public health burden throughout the world. It accounts for 50 to 75% of all fatal cardiovascular disease (CVD) events in countries where data are collected. It is usually unexpected, affecting all age, gender, and ethnic groups (1). The immediate mechanism of death is ventricular fibrillation or ventricular standstill, but the underlying cause is commonly ischemic coronary heart disease (CHD). However, other causes including different forms of cardiac pathology, genetic and environmentally induced, are also well recognized.

Classification of out-of-hospital death is deficient because of its sudden onset and lack of information from the victim. This lack of information limits the accuracy and extent of possible classification, as well as our understanding. Prospective epidemiological studies do provide more pre-event information but still face limited data on the circumstances surrounding the fatality and its causes. Although patients who undergo resuscitation from fatal events provide information, these events are uncommon and patients may be amnestic for the event. At the community or national level, the main sources of information are death certificates with their inherent limitations, and postmortem examination to confirm cause of death is infrequent in most areas.

This chapter will describe the population patterns, trends, and risk factors for out-of-hospital death in CVD. It will discuss the underlying pathophysiology in the population and ongoing attempts to better understand this common problem.

From: *Contemporary Cardiology: Cardiopulmonary Resuscitation*
Edited by: J. P. Ornato and M. A. Peberdy © Humana Press Inc., Totowa, NJ

INCIDENCE/PREVALENCE

Out-of-hospital CVD is the most common cause of death in much of the industrialized world. In the United States, almost 50% of deaths result from CVD and 60–70% of all cardiovascular deaths occur outside of hospitals (1,2). Similar data are observed in the international MONICA study, which includes populations in Europe and Asia as well as North America (3).

The age-adjusted annual rate for out-of-hospital death in the United States in 1998 was 410.6 per 100,000 for men and 274.6 per 100,000 for women (1). These figures differed only modestly from those in the early 1980s as described by Gillum (4).

The determination of rates of out-of-hospital death is based on death certificates. Site of death is a required part of this data collection. Although there may be some misclassification of those who are pronounced dead in the emergency room as in-hospital death, this proportion is thought to be modest at best (5). Data on site of death from death certificates is felt to be of generally high quality.

The age-adjusted rates of out-of-hospital death differ for men and women and by race (1). As shown in Fig. 1 for men, African Americans have the highest rates of out-of-hospital death. They are followed by white Americans and, at a much lower level, Native Americans and Asian Americans. Similar patterns are shown in Fig. 2 for women. However, the age-adjusted rates for women are much lower. This is a function of age-adjustment as out-of-hospital death is common in women but occurs at older ages. Again, African Americans have the highest rate of out-of-hospital death, followed by whites, Native Americans, and Asians.

The difference in out-of-hospital death and in-hospital fatality are shown in Fig. 3. At all the age levels in Scotland, out-of-hospital death exceeds rates of in-hospital death among both men and women (6). Also observed in this study are slightly higher rates of out-of-hospital death for men. This is compensated by somewhat higher in-hospital rates of death for women. Women are more likely to reach the hospital with severe CVD, whereas men are more likely to die at home.

TRENDS

Overall age-adjusted CVD mortality has fallen steadily since the mid-1960s at 1–2% per year (Fig. 4; 7). Out-of-hospital death rates are also falling in the United States as shown in Figs. 2 and 3. Over the past 30 years, there is a decline in age-adjusted rates of approx 1–2% per year for men and women in all major race and ethnic groups (1).

Although the steady decline indicates progress is being made, it is significantly slower than the improvement of in-hospital mortality. In Fig. 5, data from Minnesota finds in-hospital mortality is falling much more rapidly (2–3% per year) than out-of-hospital death. These data suggest that much greater progress in improving survival is being made once people reach the hospital. The result is that out-of-hospital death constitutes a growing proportion of the burden. This shift is particularly evident among women (Fig. 5).

DEFINITIONS

Although the fact and site of out-of-hospital death are based on reliable data, other information surrounding the event is less available and reliable. Other potentially important data are shown in Table 1. The victim cannot supply much of this data. The data relate

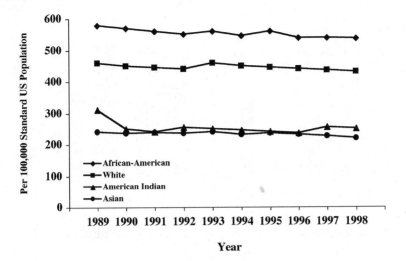

Fig. 1. Men and sudden death trends.

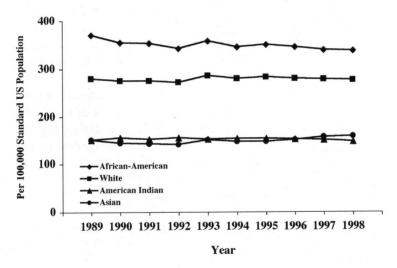

Fig. 2. Women and sudden death trends.

to the circumstances surrounding the event and medical history. Among the most important factors has been timing. Although the classic popular version of out-of-hospital death is sudden and dramatic without early symptoms, such circumstances are probably uncommon. Determining the onset of symptoms to demise is difficult even when the person is under observation. The definition of *sudden*—commonly viewed as less than 1 hour since last seen alive—obscures the nature of the problem.

Many epidemiologists now suggest that a 24-hour window from onset of symptoms or when the victim was last seen alive should define sudden out-of-hospital death.

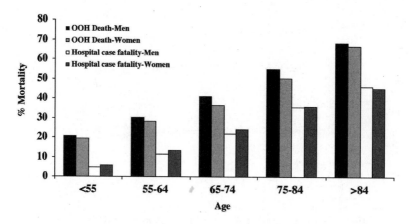

Fig. 3. Survival in acute myocardial infarction, Scotland 1986–1995.

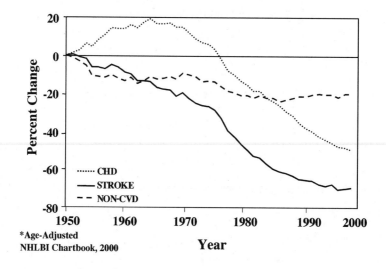

Fig. 4. Percent change in death rates (age adjusted) since 1950.

SITE OF SUDDEN DEATH

The site of sudden death is available on death certificates. In a study by Kuller et al., 70% of out-of-hospital deaths occurred at home *(8)*. A much smaller proportion occurred while the victim was at work (12%) and while traveling (7%). Only 1% occurred while participating in recreational activities and 2% while observing recreational activities. This distribution by site roughly approximates the amount of time an individual spends at each of these places. It is skewed toward events at home and not at work partly because many of the victims are retired. The Kuller study also observed that women (84%) were more likely than men (65%) to die at home, which may be a function of the earlier presentation and work status of this disease among males. Also observed in this study is a similar distribution of sites for whites and African Americans. A more recent study by Tunstall-Pedoe et al. in Scotland showed a similar distribution of site of death *(9)*.

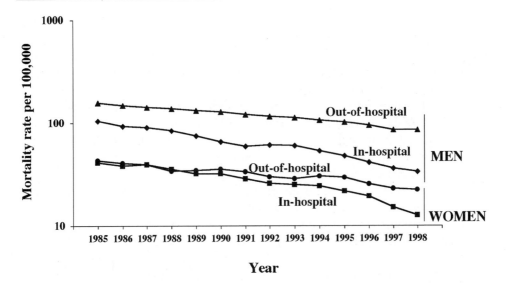

Fig. 5. Time trends (1985–1998) in congestive heart disease mortality rates in Twin Cities residents, ages 30–74. Years, by location of death.

Table 1
Definitions

- Observed or unobserved
- Symptomatic or not
- CPR or not
- Timing
  - 15 minutes
  - 1 hour
  - 6 hours
  - 24 hours

As one considers acute interventions for out-of-hospital death, the preponderance of events at home, as opposed to public places, should influence planning.

PATHOLOGY

Postmortem examination at autopsy is the well-accepted arbiter of underlying cause of death pathology. Unfortunately, sudden out-of-hospital death is usually an electral event resulting in ventricular tachycardia and fibrillation. The process is quite sudden and may leave no macro- or microscopic clues for the examining pathologist. Additionally, the autopsy rate in the United States and internationally has fallen to very low levels. This is particularly true in the older adult population because the cause of death is not of forensic interest, and families will not give permission.

Nonetheless, there are studies of sudden out-of-hospital deaths attributed to cardiac causes based on postmortem autopsy findings. They tend to be highly selected in cases in which the cause of death is not suspected from prior medical history. A recent study by Chugh et al. found that a group of hearts referred for specialized examination in the setting of sudden out-of-hospital death resulted in the discovery of a number of common findings *(10)*. In that select group of hearts, approximately two-thirds (65%) had anatomical evidence of CHD. A second subgroup (23%) had congenital conditions including arrhythmogenic right ventricular dysplasia and hypertrophic obstructive cardiomyopathy. Myocarditis was found in 11%. There were a number of other much less common abnormalities and some hearts had more than one pathology.

In a group of 76 hearts referred for specialized examination because they were apparently normal on gross examination, 79% had cardiac pathology when examined microscopically. This included local myocarditis and conduction system disease in most cases. Only a small proportion had a structurally normal heart without any evidence of pathology *(11)*.

It is apparent from these and other postmortem studies that most out-of-hospital deaths have evidence of CHD either clinically manifest or unknown to the victim.

The current thinking about the pathophysiology of acute coronary syndrome implicates thrombosis formation in the setting of a disrupted plaque. Pathologists have begun to look more systematically for this phenomenon in sudden out-of-hospital death. The work of Davies demonstrated 81% of postmortem cases with disrupted plaque and/or active thrombosis *(12)*. Others have found lower rates. Farb et al. described 57% active lesions in their study *(13)*. These differences are not surprising given the differences in selection factors for those hearts available for examination by cardiac pathologists. Atherosclerotic plaque rupture with resultant ischemia appears to be a common underlying event.

ETIOLOGY

Although the death certificate and autopsy provide clues to the causes of sudden out-of-hospital death, there are additional epidemiologic data providing substantial information. It is clear that most cases are associated with CHD. Congestive heart failure, an increasingly prevalent condition associated with out-of-hospital death, is most commonly the result of chronic ischemic CHD as well. Other factors are less common but some are well studied. For example, congenital heart disease including hypertrophic cardiomyopathy, arrhythmic right ventricular dysplasia, and other malformations of the heart and blood vessels are associated with sudden out-of-hospital death, particularly among younger individuals. Cardiomyopathies of congenital, infectious, and other etiology are also more commonly associated. Other genetic abnormalities that are increasingly studied are those of the conduction system.

It is also apparent that there are factors that provoke sudden out-of-hospital death particularly in the population in which atherosclerotic CHD is common as in industrialized societies. These factors include environmental issues such as air pollution and a wide variety of medications known to cause long QT abnormality. Recently, more attention has been paid to acute risk factors such as stress, anger, physical activity, and others as triggers of acute myocardial infarction and out-of-hospital death.

The growing body of observational data based on prospective epidemiologic studies, patient histories, and medical records allows a better picture of out-of-hospital sudden cardiac death (CD).

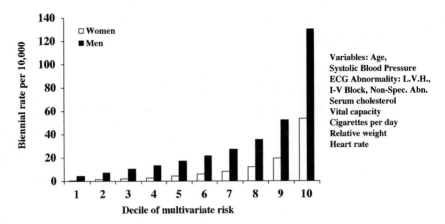

Fig. 6. Risk of sudden cardiac death by decile of multivariate risk: 26-year follow-up: Framingham Study.

Atherosclerotic CHD

A growing number of prospective epidemiologic studies have evaluated the predictive power of risk factors for atherosclerosis and sudden out-of-hospital CD. Among these is the Framingham study, which demonstrated increasing multivariate risk of out-of-hospital death is associated with age, systolic blood pressure, ECG abnormalities, serum cholesterol, vital capacity, cigarettes, relative weight, and heart rate *(14)*. A relative risk of 25 or more is found for men and women between the lowest and highest declines of risk (Fig. 6). The Pooling Project showed similar relationships using serum cholesterol, diastolic blood pressure, and cigarette smoking *(15)*. The more recent Paris Prospective Study of middle-aged men found that those who suffered sudden out-of-hospital death had significantly higher body mass index, tobacco consumption, diabetes, systolic and diastolic blood pressure, blood cholesterol, and blood triglycerides than the controls. These levels were also somewhat, although not always, significantly higher than men who suffered fatal myocardial infarctions in the hospital *(16)*. It is clear that traditional cardiovascular risk factors are associated with sudden out-of-hospital death in large prospective studies just as they are for other forms of atherosclerotic CHD.

Medications and Food Intake

Medications have the ability to affect the QT interval, prolonging it. A long QT is associated with fatal arrhythmias. This acquired long QT syndrome has been associated with numerous agents including antihistamines, antimicrobials, psychotropic agents, food supplements, and anti-arrhythmic agents *(14)*. The well-described association of a high-protein diet with sudden out-of-hospital death is another example. Antipsychotic drugs, particularly in high doses have also been associated with an increased rate ratio (2.39) of sudden out-of-hospital CD *(17)*. This effect was particularly high in those with known prior CVD *(17)*.

Most recently, usual diet has been suspected as an etiologic factor. Intake of n-3 polyunsaturated fatty acids from seafood was observed to be protective in cardiac arrest

(18). However, studies such as this require significantly more exploration and confounding factors may play an important role in explaining the results.

Acute Risk Factors

The observation that out-of-hospital sudden death had an increased incidence in the morning has increased our understanding of the role of a number of acute risk factors or triggers *(19)*. Key factors include time of day, strenuous physical activity, anger, stress, alcohol excess, and sexual intercourse *(20–23)*. There is evidence that commonly used medications such as aspirin and β-blockers blunt this effect. Acute risk factors present an intriguing new approach to out-of-hospital sudden CD. However, it must be remembered that this phenomenon occurs in the context of widespread atherosclerotic CVD in the population.

GENETIC FACTORS

Genetic abnormalities leading to sudden CD are an area of increased interest and speculation as methods to explore genes improve *(24,25)*. Much interest has centered on inherited electrical abnormalities rather than traditional structural abnormalities of congenital heart disease. The long QT syndrome, Brugada syndrome and Lev's syndrome are among the best known. There are currently ten identifiable genetic variants of long QT syndrome associated with out-of-hospital sudden CD. It is anticipated that more will be discovered as the human genome is further understood *(26)*. These and the recently described Brugada syndrome affect potassium and sodium regulation mechanisms in the heart. Most of the genetic variances are thought to be rare although there is growing interest and debate about their prevalence.

In addition to the identification of genetic conduction abnormalities, there is also growing interest on the interaction of these factors with environmental characteristics. It appears intuitive that a lethal conduction system defect would be manifest early and fatally. However, interaction between the environment and genes may provide some insight into their effects among mature adults. For example, studies of long QT syndrome show that exercise, emotion, sleep, and other circumstances are variably associated with long QT-1, long QT-2, and long QT-3 *(27)*. For example, long QT-1 is associated with cardiac events during exercise, whereas association is much less common with other variants. These observations suggest that more will be learned on gene–environment interactions.

CONCLUSION

Out-of-hospital sudden CD is a common and major public health problem accounting for approx 25% of all mortality in the United States. Although overall age-adjusted CVD mortality is falling in most industrialized countries, the rate of improvement is less for out-of-hospital sudden CD. Patients are more likely to survive a cardiovascular event including sudden death once they reach the hospital and the many therapies it provides. Atherosclerotic CHD is the underlying substrate for the overwhelming majority of cases. Given its ubiquity in the adult population, it is not surprising that primary prevention through risk factor modification is an important strategy as the traditional risk characteristics predict out-of-hospital sudden death. However, there is also an interest in identifying the portion of the adult population that has atherosclerosis and is at higher risk.

Methods for identifying these victims are still lacking as approximately half of the out-of-hospital sudden death have no diagnosed CVD.

Acute risk factors are emerging and may provide an insight into prevention. More will be learned about this along with the emergence of genetic factors and their interaction with environmental stressors.

We do know something about the pathophysiology of sudden CD. It is based on diseased tissue either acquired or genetic with local electrical instability. Treatments are emerging as we learn about the effects of aspirin and β-blockers. Additionally, for the most severe identifiable cases, intracardiac defibrillators are becoming more widely used. These may provide insights into the events preceding sudden death as their discharge may be lifesaving. Unfortunately, many of these devices and treatments are too late for most. Primary prevention of CVD remains the best population-wide approach to confront this difficult health problem.

REFERENCES

1. Zheng Z-J, Croft JB, Giles WH, Mensah GA. Sudden cardiac death in the United States, 1989 to 1998. Circulation 2001; 104:2158–2163.
2. American Heart Association. 2002 Heart and Stroke Statistical Update. Dallas, TX: American Heart Association, 2001.
3. Chambless L, Keil U, Dobson A, et al. Population versus clinical view of case fatality from acute coronary heart disease: results from the WHO MONICA Project 1985–1990. Circulation 1997; 96:3849–3859.
4. Gillum RF. Sudden coronary death in the United States: 1980–1985. Circulation 1989; 79:756–765.
5. Iribarren C, Crow RS, Hannan PJ, Jacobs DR Jr., Luepker RV. Validation of death certificate diagnosis of out-of-hospital sudden cardiac death. Am J Cardiol 1998; 82:50–53.
6. MacIntyre K, Stewart S, Capewell S, et al. Gender and survival: a population-based study of 201,114 men and women following a first acute myocardial infarction. J Am Coll Cardiol 2001; 38:729–735.
7. National Institutes of Health. NHLBI Morbidity and Mortality 2000 Chartbook on Cardiovascular, Lung, and Blood Diseases, 2000, p. 8.
8. Kuller LH, Cooper M, Perper J, Fisher R. Myocardial infarction and sudden death in an urban community. Bull NY Acad Med 1973; 49:532–543.
9. Tunstall-Pedoe H, Morrison C, Woodward M, Fitzpatrick B, Watt G. Sex differences in myocardial infarction and coronary deaths in the Scottish MONICA population of Glasgow 1985 to 1991: presentation, diagnosis, treatment, and 28-day case fatality of 3991 events in men and 1551 in women. Circulation 1996; 93:1981–1992.
10. Chugh SS, Kelly KL, Titus JL. Sudden cardiac death with apparently normal heart. Circulation 2000; 102:649–654.
11. Corrado D, Basso C, Thiene G. Sudden cardiac death in young people with apparently normal heart. Cardiovasc Res 2001; 50:399–408.
12. Davies MJ. Anatomic features in victims of sudden coronary death: coronary artery pathology. Circulation 1992; 85(1 Suppl):119–124.
13. Farb A, Tang AL, Burke AP, Sessums L, Liang Y, Virmani R. Sudden coronary death: frequency of active coronary lesions, inactive coronary lesions, and myocardial infarction. Circulation 1995; 92:1701–1709.
14. Zipes DP, Wellens HJJ. Sudden cardiac death. Circulation 1998; 98:2334–2351.
15. Stamler J. Primary prevention of sudden coronary death. Circulation 1975; 52(6 Suppl):258–279.
16. Jouven X, Desnos M, Guerot C, Ducimetière P. Predicting sudden death in the population: the Paris Prospective Study I. Circulation 1999; 99:1978–1983.
17. Ray WA, Meredith S, Thapa PB, Meador KG, Hall K, Murray KT. Arch Gen Psych 2001; 58:1161–1167.
18. Siscovick DS, Raghunathan T, King I, Weinmann S, Bovbjerg VE, Kushi L, et al. Dietary intake of long-chain n-3 polyunsaturated fatty acids and the risk of primary cardiac arrest. Am J Clin Nutr 2000; 71(1 Suppl):208S–212S.
19. Willich SN, Levy D, Rocco MB, Tofler GH, Stone PH, Muller JE. Circadian variation in the incidence of sudden cardiac death in the Framingham Heart Study population. Am J Cardiol 1987; 60:801–806.
20. Kauhanen J, Kaplan GA, Goldberg DE, Salonen JT. Beer binging and mortality: results from the Kuopio ischemic heart disease risk factor study, a prospective population based study. BMJ 1997; 315:846–851.

21. Mittleman MA, Maclure M, Tofler GH, Sherwood JB, Goldberg RJ, Muller JE. Triggering of acute myocardial infarction by heavy physical exertion: protection against triggering by regular exertion. New Engl J Med 1993; 329:1677–1683.
22. Maron BJ, Poliac LC, Roberts WO. Risk for sudden cardiac death associated with marathon running. J Am Coll Cardiol 1996; 28:428–431.
23. Peckova M, Fahrenbruch CE, Cobb LA, Hallstrom AP. Circadian variations in the occurrence of cardiac arrests: initial and repeat episodes. Circulation 1998; 98:31–39.
24. Spooner PM, Albert C, Benjamin EJ, et al. Sudden cardiac death, genes, and arrhythmogenesis: consideration of new population and mechanistic approaches from a National Heart, Lung, and Blood Institute Workshop, Part I. Circulation 2001; 103:2361–2364.
25. Spooner PM, Albert C, Benjamin EJ, et al. Sudden cardiac death, genes, and arrhythmogenesis: consideration of new population and mechanistic approaches from a National Heart, Lung, and Blood Institute Workshop, Part II. Circulation 2001; 103:2447–2452.
26. Chiang C-E, Roden DM. The long QT syndromes: genetic basis and clinical implications. J Am Coll Cardiol 2000; 36:1–12.
27. Schwartz PJ, Priori SG, Spazzolini C, et al. Genotype-phenotype correlation in the long QT syndrome: gene-specific triggers for life-threatening arrhythmias. Circulation 2001; 103:89–95.

3

Prevention of Sudden Cardiac Death

Joseph E. Marine, MD

CONTENTS

INTRODUCTION

Since the 1960s, important advances have been made in resuscitation of patients from sudden cardiac death (SCD). Despite these advances, rates of survival to hospital discharge range from only 2 to 30% (generally 5–10%); rates of survival with intact neurological status are even lower *(1)*. Approximately 400,000 out-of-hospital sudden deaths occur in the United States each year *(2)*. These grim statistics point to the importance of prevention in approaching the problem of SCD from a public health standpoint.

It has been estimated that one-half to two-thirds of out-of-hospital sudden death is caused by ventricular arrhythmias (VA) (ventricular tachycardia [VT] and ventricular fibrillation [VF]) *(3)*. Bradyarrhythmias, such as complete atrioventricular block and asystole, are a less frequent cause of arrhythmic sudden death. A substantial minority of cases of apparent SCD may be because of nonarrhythmic causes, such as massive pulmonary embolus, ruptured aortic aneurysm or dissection, or stroke *(4)*. Because most research into prevention of SCD has focused on VA, this subject will form the basis for this chapter. Preventive strategies will be considered according to the etiology of cardiac disease.

CORONARY ARTERY DISEASE

Coronary artery disease (CAD) is the leading cause of death in Western countries and the most common cardiac substrate for SCD. It is now recognized that CAD is a systemic disease of the cardiovascular system that is often far advanced by the time it is clinically manifest. The first signs of atheroma formation may begin in adolescence. As CAD progresses, atheromas may encroach on the coronary artery lumen, causing flow-limiting stenosis. At this stage, patients may develop ischemia in the absence of infarction, often with exertion or stress. Ischemia in turn may lead to arrhythmias, particularly polymorphic VT and VF. Ischemic VA may also occur in the absence of significant atherosclerosis, usually associated with coronary artery spasm or congenital coronary anomalies.

From: *Contemporary Cardiology: Cardiopulmonary Resuscitation*
Edited by: J. P. Ornato and M. A. Peberdy © Humana Press Inc., Totowa, NJ

Coronary atherosclerotic plaques of any size may rupture, triggering platelet adhesion, thrombus formation, and acute myocardial infarction (AMI). Serious VAs, especially VFs, are common in this setting, and they account for a substantial proportion of deaths from AMI, particularly in the prehospital setting. Later in the course of infarction, the infarct zone undergoes cellular and tissue remodeling with the laying of collagen scar and ventricular dilatation. This process creates the anatomic substrate for future VAs, particular sustained monomorphic VT.

Primary Prevention of CAD

Approximately 12.6 million people in the United States have CAD and about 1 million suffer AMIs annually (2). Given the scope of the problem, effective primary prevention of CAD could have a substantial impact on prevention of SCD. Particularly important is changing modifiable risk factors, especially cigarette smoking, dyslipidemia, atherogenic diet, obesity, and physical inactivity (5). Optimal control of predisposing medical conditions, such as systemic hypertension and diabetes mellitus, may also reduce the incidence of coronary disease and related SCD. Hopefully, improved public education regarding primary prevention of CAD will ultimately translate into reduction of SCD rates as well as CAD incidence.

There is evidence that improvements in treatment of AMI are also reducing rates of SCD. Both fibrinolytic therapy and primary percutaneous coronary intervention reduce all-cause mortality as well as SCD. Moreover, by reducing infarct size, acute revascularization in AMI likely reduces late risk of SCD by modifying the substrate for arrhythmogenesis. Modification of the arrhythmic substrate may also account for some of the mortality benefit of angiotensin-converting enzyme (ACE) inhibitors in treatment of AMI. The Coronary Artery Surgery Study showed that coronary artery bypass grafting (CABG) leads to improved survival in selected high-risk patients with CAD. Further analysis of this trial has shown reduction in SCD in high-risk patients who underwent surgery (6).

Medical Therapy for Prevention of SCD After Myocardial Infarction

Table 1 summarizes the outcomes of nine large trials of antiarrhythmic therapy after AMI. Probably the most important aspect of medical treatment of AMI survivors for prevention of SCD is β-blocker therapy. These agents block the β-1 adrenergic receptor in the heart, blunting the pro-arrhythmic effects of the sympathetic nervous system and circulating cathecholamines, and reducing myocardial oxygen consumption and ischemia. In addition to reducing incidence of late coronary events, β-blockers have been shown in several trials to reduce all-cause mortality as well as life-threatening VAs (7–10). The antiarrhythmic action of β-blockers was also demonstrated in a recent small trial, which showed that sympathetic blockade was superior to standard antiarrhythmic drugs for treatment of recurrent VF in AMI (11).

Prospective observational studies published in the early 1980s established that frequent isolated ventricular premature contractions and nonsustained VT are markers of increased mortality risk after MI, particularly in patients with left ventricular (LV) systolic dysfunction (12). Further studies showed that type I antiarrhythmic drugs effectively suppressed these VAs in this setting, leading to the organization of the Cardiac Arrhythmia Suppression Trial (CAST). Publication of the results of this trial, which showed a doubling of mortality rates in patients receiving flecainide, encainide, or

Table 1. Randomized Trials of Anti-Arrhythmic Medications After MI

Trial	Year of publication	Result
BHAT (7)	1981	Improved survival with propranolol
ISIS-1 (8)	1986	Improved survival with atenolol
CAPRICORN (9)	2001	Improved survival with carvedilol
CAST-I (13)	1989, 1991	Increased mortality with flecainide or encainide
CAST-II (14)	1992	Increased mortality with moricizine
SWORD (15)	1996	Increased mortality with D-sotalol
DIAMOND (16)	2000	No effect of dofetilide on mortality
EMIAT (19)	1997	No effect of amiodarone on mortality
CAMIAT (20)	1997	No effect of amiodarone on mortality

moricizine, led to a re-examination of the use of these agents in patients with CAD and other forms of structural heart disease (13,14). There is now general agreement that type I antiarrhythmic drugs, particularly type Ic agents, should be avoided in patients with CAD because of the pro-arrhythmic effects demonstrated in CAST.

A similar increased risk of death was seen in a trial of the class III antiarrhythmic D-sotalol in postinfarction patients (15). The Survival With Oral D-Sotalol trial recruited 3121 patients with LV ejection fraction (EF) of 0.40 or less and prior MI. Patients were randomly assigned to long-term treatment with D-sotalol (a pure type III anti-arrhythmic agent with no β-blocking activity) or matching placebo. After a mean follow-up period of 150 days and halfway into recruitment, the trial was stopped early because of a 65% increased relative risk of mortality in the D-sotalol treatment arm (5 vs 3.1% in placebo group, $p=0.006$). The excess mortality was felt to be because of an increase in arrhythmic deaths.

In contrast, a large trial of dofetilide, another pure class III antiarrhythmic drug, found no increase in mortality on survivors of MI (16). The Danish Investigations of Arrhythmia and Mortality on Dofetilide (DIAMOND) Study Group randomized 1510 patients with recent MI and LVEF of 0.35 or less to treatment with dofetilide (dose based on creatinine clearance) or matching placebo. After a median follow-up of 456 days, mortality was nearly identical in the two groups (31 vs 32%, respectively, $p = 0.61$).

Amiodarone, a unique antiarrhythmic drug that exhibits actions of all four Vaughn-Williams drug classes, was originally developed as an anti-anginal medication. On the basis of its efficacy in the treatment of recurrent VA and its safety compared with other antiarrhythmic drugs in survivors of cardiac arrest (CA), two large trials were organized to test its efficacy in high-risk survivors of AMI (17,18). The European Myocardial Infarction Amiodarone Trial (EMIAT) enrolled 1486 patients 5 or more days after MI only on the basis of depressed LVEF of 0.40 or less (19). Patients were treated with amiodarone (200 mg per day after loading) or placebo. After a median follow-up period of 21 months, overall mortality was identical in the two groups (14% in each, $p = 0.96$).

The Canadian Amiodarone Myocardial Infarction Arrhythmia Trial (CAMIAT) studied 1202 patients enrolled 6–42 days after AMI, who had frequent ventricular premature contractions or nonsustained VT; LV systolic dysfunction was not required for entry into the trial (20). Patients were treated with amiodarone (200 mg per day after loading) or placebo and followed for a mean of 1.8 years. No significant difference in overall mortality was found (9.4% in the amiodarone group vs 11.4% in the placebo group, $p = 0.129$).

Both EMIAT and CAMIAT did find a reduction in death ascribed to arrhythmia, but the significance of this finding in the absence of overall mortality benefit has been questioned. A posthoc analysis of both trials suggested a possible synergistic benefit of amiodarone and β-blockers, but this remains to be demonstrated prospectively.

In summary, proven medical therapy for primary prevention of sudden death in patients with CAD is limited to β-blocker use. Type I antiarrhythmic drugs and D-sotalol have been shown to be harmful in this population. Amiodarone and dofetilide had a neutral effect on all-cause mortality and are relatively safe to use for treatment of symptomatic arrhythmias in patients with CAD.

Role of the Implantable Cardioverter Defibrillator in CAD

The implantable cardioverter defibrillator (ICD) has had a major impact on clinical approach to prevention of SCD. Conceived by Morton Mower and Michel Mirowski and introduced after a decade of preclinical development, the ICD was first used in humans in the late 1970s *(21)*. Implantation initially required thoracotomy to place epicardial patches and rate-sensing electrodes. First generations of pulse generators were large (>250 g) and required implantation in an abdominal pocket. Pacing function and programmability were extremely limited. Rapid evolution of the ICD ensued, leading to a succession of improved lead systems and smaller generators with greater functionality *(22)*.

Current ICD systems can be implanted transvenously via subclavian or cephalic vein access, similar to pacemakers, using a single 8–10 French lead and a pectorally implanted generator as small as 75 g. They are capable of all bradycardia-pacing functions, including, with addition of one or more leads, dual-chamber and biventricular pacing. They are also capable of detecting arrhythmias in several different programmable rate zones and delivering a different series of programmable therapies for each zone (Fig. 1). They have capacity to store large amounts of information regarding each arrhythmia episode for later analysis. Finally, they incorporate increasingly sophisticated algorithms for distinguishing supraventricular from VAs.

ICDs detect VAs from the tip electrode of the lead, usually implanted at the right ventricular apex. When a ventricular rate is detected that exceeds the programmed detection rate (usually 150–200 beats per minute [bpm]) for the programmed number of beats (usually 10–20), the ICD begins charging the capacitors. This generally takes between 1 and 5 seconds, after which the device confirms continuation of tachycardia before delivering the programmed energy (anywhere from 1–40 J) between the metal shell of the generator and one or more coils on the ICD lead (Fig. 2A). The ICD then re-analyzes the ventricular rate to determine if therapy was successful. If the rate has not fallen below the arrhythmia detection limit, the ICD proceeds to deliver the next therapy. This process continues until the arrhythmia is terminated or all programmed therapies (usually a maximum of six to eight) are exhausted.

In addition to delivering shock therapies, ICDs may be programmed to deliver sequences of antitachycardia pacing (ATP), usually 8–12 beats, to terminate sustained monomorphic (regular) VT (Fig. 2B). This therapy has the advantage of being delivered more rapidly and being entirely painless. Potential disadvantages of ATP include possibility of accelerating the tachycardia to a more unstable type and delaying delivery of shock therapy if ATP is unsuccessful. ATP is not useful for treating VF or polymorphic VT.

When first released for clinical use in the early 1980s, ICDs were targeted toward patients who had survived multiple CAs with recurrent VAs that were refractory to conventional anti-arrhythmic drug treatment. As the design of ICDs improved over the

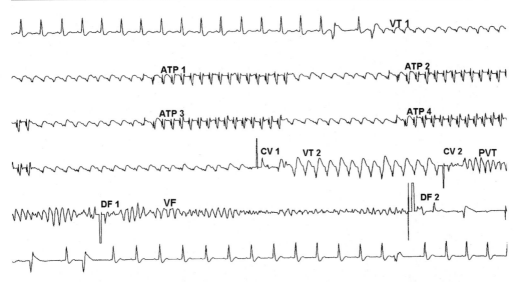

Fig. 1. Tiered therapy of VAs by the ICD. The figure shows stored single-channel telemetry strip during an episode of ventricular tachyarrhythmia in a patient with an implantable cardioverter defibrillator who was hospitalized. A ventricular premature beat initiates sustained monomorphic ventricular tachycardia (VT 1). Four cycles of antitachycardia pacing (ATP 1-4) fail to terminate the arrhythmia. A low-energy cardioversion (CV 1) results in a different morphology of monomorphic VT (VT 2). A second low-energy cardioversion (CV 2) results in polymorphic VT (PVT). After the first high-energy defibrillation (DF 1), the rhythm degenerates into ventricular fibrillation (VF). A second high-energy defibrillation (DF 2), results in restoration of sinus rhythm.

next decade, and the limitations of anti-arrhythmic drugs were exposed through randomized clinical trials, the ICD gained increasing favor for treatment of CA survivors. In this setting, several clinical trials were organized to test the efficacy of the ICD in secondary prevention (for patients who had survived a sustained life-threatening VA) and primary prevention (for high-risk patients without history of sustained arrhythmia) of SCD (Tables 2 and 3).

ICD FOR SECONDARY PREVENTION IN CAD

The first published trial comparing the ICD and conventional medical therapy for secondary prevention of SCD was the Anti-arrhythmics Versus Implantable Defibrillator (AVID) trial *(23)*. This National Institutes of Health (NIH)-sponsored multicenter study enrolled 1016 patients in 56 North American centers who were resuscitated from VF or sustained VT between 1993 and 1997. The mean age of enrolled patients was 65 years and the mean LVEF was 0.32. Eighty-one percent of patients had CAD and 67% had a history of MI. Patients were randomly assigned to receive an ICD or to treatment with anti-arrhythmic drug therapy, predominantly amiodarone (96% of assigned patients). Over a mean follow-up period of 18 months, 122 of 509 patients (24%) in the anti-arrhythmic drug therapy group died vs only 80 of 507 patients (16%) assigned to receive an ICD. This difference corresponds to a 33% relative risk reduction and an 8% absolute risk reduction in total mortality in favor of the ICD ($p < 0.02$). Of note, this treatment effect was demonstrated despite a significant crossover to ICD therapy in the drug therapy arm, reaching 25% at 3 years.

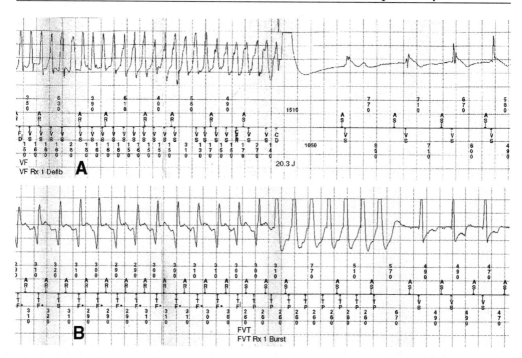

Fig. 2. Treatment of different ventricular arrhythmias in the same patients with an implantable cardioverter defibrillator (ICD). The figure shows stored internal electrograms and marker channels of two episodes of sustained monomorphic ventricular arrhythmia in a 38-year-old man with cardiac sarcoidosis. The first event shown in **A** is an episode of ventricular fibrillation that was successfully treated with a single 20-J internal defibrillation by the ICD, restoring the patient to sinus rhythm. The second event shown in **B** is an episode of sustained monomorphic ventricular tachycardia with a rate of 200 bpm successfully treated with a single sequence of 8 beats of antitachycardia pacing.

Strengths of the AVID trial include its relatively large size, NIH sponsorship, and its use of total mortality as an unambiguous and unquestionably important primary endpoint. Because the trial included only a small proportion of patients without CAD, it is difficult to draw conclusions about benefit of ICD in other subgroups. No placebo group was used, raising the question of whether the some of the apparent benefit of the ICD was because of a detrimental effect of amiodarone; other trials, however, have demonstrated the safety of amiodarone in patients with structural heart disease. Finally, β-blocker use was much greater in the ICD arm (about 40%) compared to the drug therapy arm (10–15%), probably because of the bradycardic effects of amiodarone; this discrepancy might account for some of the apparent benefit of the ICD. Despite these criticisms, the AVID trial has led to the ICD becoming the treatment of choice for survivors of CA without contraindications to its use.

Two smaller trials of ICD therapy in secondary prevention of SCD have been reported since the AVID trial was published. The first, the Canadian Implantable Defibrillator Study (CIDS), enrolled 659 patients with an episode of unstable sustained VA in 24 centers in Canada, Australia, and the United States between 1990 and 1997 (24). Baseline patient characteristics were similar to those of the AVID population, with a mean age of 63.5 years, mean LVEF of 0.34, and an 82% prevalence of CAD. After a mean follow-

Table 2
ICD Trials for Primary and Secondary Prevention of SCD

Trial	Primary or secondary prevention	Year of publication	Number of patients	Mean follow-up (months)	Relative risk reduction	Absolute risk reduction	p-value
AVID (23)	Secondary	1997	1016	18	33%	8%	p < 0.02
CIDS (24)	Secondary	2000	659	36	28%	4.3%	p = 0.14
CASH (25)	Secondary	2000	288	57	18%	8%	p = 0.08
MADIT (26)	Primary	1996	196	27	59%	23%	p = 0.009
MUSST (27)	Primary	1999	704	39	60%	31%	p < 0.001
CABG-Patch (28)	Primary	1997	900	32	–8%	–1.7%	p = NS
MADIT-II (29)	Primary	2002	1232	20	28%	5.6%	p = 0.016

Table 3
Nonischemic Cardiomyopathies Associated With Sudden CA

Dilated cardiomyopathies
   Idiopathic
   Postviral
   Alcohol-related
   Valvular heart disease
   Postpartum
   Familial
   Chagas' disease
Hypertrophic cardiomyopathy
Arrhythmogenic right ventricular cardiomyopathy
Cardiac sarcoidosis
Cardiac amyloidosis

up period of 3 years, 98 of 331 patients (29.6%) assigned to amiodarone had died vs 83 of 328 patients assigned to ICD therapy (25.3%). On an annualized basis, the absolute risk reduction for death was 1.9% per year in favor of the ICD arm, with a relative risk reduction of 19.7% ($p = 0.142$).

The Cardiac Arrest Study Hamburg (CASH) enrolled 288 CA survivors (84% with VF) in eight centers in northern Germany between 1987 and 1996 and randomly assigned them to ICD implantation, amiodarone therapy, or metoprolol treatment in a 1:1:1 fashion (25). The trial had originally included a propafenone treatment arm, which was discontinued in 1992 because of the 61% higher all-cause mortality in that group. Over a mean follow-up period of 57 months, the crude death rates were 36.4% in the ICD arm and 44.4% in the two drug treatment arms, an absolute reduction of 8% and a relative risk reduction of 18% ($p = 0.081$). The relative risk reduction was 42% at 1 year and 28% at 3 years. Secondary analysis showed that this nonsignificant reduction in total mortality appeared to be due entirely to a significant reduction in sudden death ($p = 0.005$). As in CIDS, there was a trend toward increased efficacy of the ICD in higher risk subgroups with lower LVEF and higher New York Heart Association (NYHA) heart failure class. Although neither CIDS nor CASH reached statistical significance, the degree of treatment effect was similar to that seen in AVID and these trials are generally viewed a supportive for ICD treatment in secondary prevention of SCD.

ICD FOR PRIMARY PREVENTION IN CAD

With the rapid evolution of the ICD and its clear effectiveness in treating VAs, it was reasonable to presume that the ICD might be effective in primary prevention of SCD in high-risk patients. Several trials were designed to test this hypothesis. The first to be published was the Multicenter Automatic Defibrillator Implantation Trial (MADIT) *(26)*. This device industry-sponsored study enrolled 196 high-risk CAD patients in 32 US and European centers from 1990 to 1996 and randomly assigned them to implantation of ICD or to conventional therapy (determined by treating physician, with amiodarone in 74%). Eligible patients had a documented MI greater than 3 weeks prior to enrollment and an episode of asymptomatic nonsustained VT of 3 to 30 beats with a rate of at least 120 bpm. Patients with NYHA class IV symptoms were excluded because of a known high mortality from pump failure. Eligible patients then underwent invasive electro-physiologic study, with delivery of one, two, and three-paced ventricular premature beats at increasingly close coupling intervals. If sustained VT or VF was induced, stimulation was repeated after giving intravenous procainamide. If the arrhythmia remained inducible, then the patient became eligible for randomization. The mean age of randomized patients was 64 years, the mean LVEF was 0.26, and 65% had NYHA class II or III symptoms.

After a mean follow-up of 27 months, the trial was stopped early because of a marked treatment effect in favor of the ICD. Over the follow-up period, 39 of 101 patients (39%) in conventional treatment group died vs only 15 of 95 patients (16%) assigned to ICD, an absolute risk reduction of 23% and a relative risk reduction of 59%. The relative hazard for overall mortality was 0.46 in the ICD arm ($p = 0.009$).

Despite the results, MADIT initially met with skepticism owing to its small sample size, ICD industry-sponsorship, and low use of β-blockers (5–8%) in the conventional therapy arm. These criticisms were largely answered with the publication of the Multicenter Unsustained Tachycardia Trial (MUSTT) 3 years later *(27)*. This study involved 704 patients with CAD enrolled at 85 centers in the United States and Canada between 1990 and 1996, and was sponsored by the NIH, with additional grant support from several drug and ICD manufacturers. Similar to MADIT, eligible patients had CAD with depressed LVEF (0.40 or less), and a qualifying episode of nonsustained VT of three or more beats at least 96 hours after a MI or revascularization procedure. Potential patients underwent invasive electrophysiologic (EP) study and, if inducible for sustained VA, were eligible for randomization to either electrophysiologically guided anti-arrhythmic therapy or to no anti-arrhythmic therapy. Patients in the therapy arm were then randomly assigned to a Food and Drug Administration-approved class I or class III anti-arrhythmic drug followed by repeat EP testing. If no effective anti-arrhythmic drug was found, an ICD was implanted. ICD therapy was permitted, at investigator discretion, after one to three failed drug trials. Out of 351 patients, 202 in this arm (58%) ultimately received an ICD. β-Blocker and ACE inhibitor treatment was encouraged in all patients, and 40% of all were receiving β-blockers at hospital discharge. The median age of enrolled patients was 66 years and the median LVEF was 0.30.

After a median follow-up period of 39 months, the 2- and 5-year rates of overall mortality were 28% and 48% in the group assigned to no anti-arrhythmic therapy and 22% and 42% in the EP-guided therapy arm (relative risk 0.80 at 5 years, $p = 0.06$). Subsequent analysis of the data showed that this treatment effect was entirely attributable to treatment with the ICD; the overall mortality rate at 5 years was 24% in patients receiving an ICD and 55% in those who did not (adjusted relative risk of overall mortality 0.40, $p < 0.001$). In fact, patients treated with anti-arrhythmic drugs without an ICD had a trend toward higher mortality than the control arm of the study, possibly because of a high use of type I anti-arrhythmic agents in the drug-therapy group (26% at initial hospital discharge). Thus, although MUSTT had a complex design, which was not primarily intended to test the efficacy of the ICD, its results supported the apparent benefit of the ICD for primary prophylaxis demonstrated in MADIT and led to widespread use of the ICD in high-risk coronary patients for this indication.

In contrast to MADIT and MUSST, the Coronary Artery Bypass Graft (CABG) Patch trial used a different test (signal-averaged ECG) to identify high-risk CAD patients and found no benefit to prophylactic epicardial ICD implantation in the population studied *(28)*. This NIH-sponsored study screened patients less than 80 years old with LVEF of 0.35 or less who were scheduled for CABG surgery at 37 centers in the United States and Germany between 1990 and 1996. Patients were screened with signal-averaged electro-cardiography (SAECG), a variation of the standard surface ECG used to analyze QRS complexes for prolongation or the presence of late potentials, which reflect myocardial scarring and substrate for VAs. A pilot study had shown that patients with abnormal SAECG had a mortality rate in the 2 years after CABG surgery twice as high as patients with normal SAECG, which is in line with previous studies of this technique. Neither nonsustained VT nor invasive EP study was required for study entry.

After screening, 900 patients were assigned randomly to receive an epicardial ICD system at the time of CABG surgery (446 patients) or to CABG surgery alone (454 patients). Baseline characteristics were similar to MADIT patients, with a mean age of 64 years, mean LVEF of 0.27, and 73% with NYHA class II or III heart failure symptoms. Ninety-one percent of patients had two- (36%) or three- (55%) vessel CAD. After an average follow-up of 32 months, the trial was terminated because of a lack of efficacy, at which point 101 of 446 (22.6%) patients in the ICD arm had died vs 95 of 454 (20.9%) patients in the control arm. No subgroups were identified that appeared to benefit from the ICD.

There are several possible explanations for the difference in outcome between the CABG-Patch Trial and other trials, which demonstrate efficacy of the ICD for primary prophylaxis. These include relatively low mortality rate in the control arm, an independent anti-arrhythmic effect of complete revascularization, use of epicardial devices, and potential harmful effect of prolonging operative time with ICD implant and testing.

The Multicenter Automatic Defibrillator Implantation Trial II (MADIT-II) was recently published and may significantly expand the population eligible for primary prophylaxis of SCD with the ICD *(29)*. This industry-sponsored trial randomized 1232 patients in 76 US and European centers with prior MI (1 month or more before entry) and LVEF of 0.30 or less to receive a transvenous ICD or usual medical therapy. Patients were not required to have any spontaneous or induced arrhythmias for entry. Enrolled patients had a mean age of 64 years and a mean LVEF of 0.23. In contrast to MADIT, β-blocker use was high (70% in each arm). After a mean follow-up of 20 months, 19.8% of patients in the usual therapy group had died, and 14.2% of patients in the ICD arm ($p = 0.016$), indicating a hazard ratio of 0.69 in favor of the ICD arm, and an absolute risk reduction of 5.6%. There were no statistically significant interactions with baseline characteristics, but patients with lower LVEFs and those with wider QRS duration showed trend toward greater benefit from the ICD. An unexplained trend toward higher rates of hospitalization for heart failure was also present in the ICD arm.

ECONOMIC IMPACT OF ICD USE IN CAD

The MADIT-II trial, for the first time, demonstrated efficacy of the ICD in reducing all-cause mortality in a population defined solely by cardiac substrate (prior MI and reduced LVEF) and not by presence of any arrhythmia. Other ongoing trials are testing the ability of the ICD to reduce SCD mortality in other populations, including all patients with heart failure and reduced EF from any cause, and in other lower risk populations with CAD. The health care cost implications of such expansion of ICD indications are substantial. The MADIT-II authors estimated that up to 4 million patients in the United States might qualify for ICD therapy under the new indication, with addition of up to 400,000 new patients annually (29). At a conservative estimate of $25,000 per ICD implant, it would cost $100 billion to implant all current MADIT-II eligible patients in the United States, and $10 billion to implant newly eligible cases each year. There would be additional costs associated with follow-up, generator replacements, and management of late complications and device/lead malfunction.

Cost-effectiveness analysis of ICD therapy has been performed based on MADIT and AVID data. Analysis of MADIT results, which had initial ICD implantation cost of $18,000–$27,000, showed a cost-effectiveness ratio of $27,000 per year of life saved, based on a survival advantage of 0.8 years in the ICD group (30). Patients in the ICD arm had higher initial costs, which were later balanced by higher medication costs in the medically treated group after 4 years. Total net health care costs over follow-up were about $98,000 in the ICD group and $76,000 in the control group; the difference was largely because of a longer survival in the ICD group. Corresponding economic analysis of the AVID study showed estimated 3-year medical costs of $87,000 in the ICD group and $73,000 in the anti-arrhythmic drug group (31). As in MADIT, initial hospital costs were higher in the ICD arm and medication costs were higher in the drug arm. Because the mortality difference was smaller in AVID (about 0.21 years advantage for ICD), the cost-effectiveness ratio was higher—about $67,000 per year of life saved. These cost-effectiveness ratios, although high, are comparable to other accepted health care interventions.

Economic analysis of MADIT-II is currently in progress. Review of currently published data suggests that the cost-effectiveness ratio may be higher than in MADIT, because of a smaller absolute survival advantage, higher costs for heart failure hospitalizations in the ICD group, and lower costs for anti-arrhythmic drugs in the control arm. Regardless of the ratio, the absolute cost of expanding ICD indications will have to be considered by health care payers. Some investigators have expressed hope that market competition will reduce costs of ICD therapy and that expanding indications for the ICD will spur manufacturers to design and market a lower cost model for primary prophylaxis in lower risk patients (32).

DILATED CARDIOMYOPATHY

Although not as common as CAD, several other forms of cardiomyopathy (listed in Table 2) are associated with an elevated risk of SCD. The most prevalent of these is dilated cardiomyopathy (DCM). Numerous studies have shown that patients with DCM have significantly elevated risk of all-cause mortality and SCD, and that degree of risk correlates with heart failure class (33). Interestingly, although patients with the most severe heart failure symptoms have the highest mortality rates, the proportion of deaths classified as because of SCD is lower than in those with lower heart failure class; the proportion of deaths because of pump failure rises accordingly. Other important risk factors for arrhythmic mortality in DCM include degree of LV dilatation, impairment of LV systolic function, and increased QRS duration, especially with left bundle branch block. Frequency of nonsustained VT has also been shown to increase risk of mortality in one study *(34)*, but another failed to show this association *(35)*. Syncope, regardless of etiology, was shown in one study to increase risk of mortality nearly fourfold *(36)*. Although recognized as an insensitive marker, inducibility of sustained VAs at invasive EP study also seems to confer elevated risk of death *(37)*.

Medical Therapy of DCM

Several medications without anti-arrhythmic action have been shown to improve all-cause mortality in DCM, and also may reduce SCD because of a modification of the underlying arrhythmic substrate. These medications include ACE inhibitors, hydralazine-isosorbide, metoprolol, carvedilol, and spironolactone. Digoxin use, even though improving heart failure symptoms and modestly reducing hospitalization, does not appear to significantly affect survival *(38)*. In contrast, several positive inotropic drugs, including enoximone, amrinone, and high-dose vesnarinone, have been shown to increase mortality in heart failure patients, possibly through ventricular proarrhythmic effects. Several studies of type I (sodium-channel blocking) anti-arrhythmic drugs have shown that these agents are associated with excess mortality in patients with heart failure and structural heart disease *(13,14,39)*. Sodium-channel blocking drugs have both negative-inotropic and proarrhythmic side effects in this population. On the basis of these trials, these drugs should generally be avoided in patients with DCM.

AMIODARONE FOR DCM

There have been two large trials of amiodarone for primary prophylaxis of SCD in heart failure patients. The GESICA trial was conducted in 26 hospitals in Argentina between 1989 and 1993. Patients ($N = 516$, mean age 59 years) with stable chronic class II, III, and IV congestive heart failure on appropriate medical treatment with LVEF of 0.35 or less (mean = 0.20) were randomized to receive amiodarone (300 mg/day chronically) or usual treatment *(40)*. Forty percent of patients had prior MI and 10% had Chagas' disease. After a mean 13 months of follow-up, 87 of 260 patients (33.5%) treated with amiodarone died vs 106 of 256 control patients (41.4%), a relative risk reduction of 28% and an absolute risk reduction of 7.9% ($p = 0.024$). Subsequent substudies of GESICA showed particular benefit in patients with baseline heart rate above 90 bpm.

The STAT-CHF trial was a US-based trial conducted in Veteran's Affairs medical centers enrolling 674 patients (99% men) with LVEF of 0.40 or less, class II, III, or IV congestive heart failure symptoms, and 10 or more ventricular premature contractions per hour on Holter monitor *(41)*. Patients were randomized to amiodarone (300 mg per day) or placebo and were followed for a mean of 4 years. In contrast to GESICA, this trial showed no significant difference in outcome between the two groups, either in total mortality or in sudden death.

The explanation for the discrepancy between the two trials has been attributed to the difference in populations studied. GESICA included a higher proportion of patients with nonischemic cardiomyopathy, including Chagas' disease in 10%. In CHF-STAT, there was also a trend toward improved survival with amiodarone in the smaller subgroup without CAD. Additionally, mortality in the placebo group at 2 years was higher in GESICA (50%) than in CHF-STAT (30%), suggesting that amiodarone may only benefit those at very high risk. Alternatively, CHF-STAT included a much longer follow-up period, and hence GESICA might have shown less benefit for amiodarone if patients had been followed longer. No clear consensus exists for utility of amiodarone for primary prevention of SCD in the heart failure population because of the conflicting results of these two trials. Preliminary results of the Sudden Cardiac Death in Heart Rate Failure Trial (SCD-HeFT; *see* below) also suggest that amiodarone does not prolong survival in heart failure patients.

ICD FOR DCM

Patients with DCM who are resuscitated from sustained VT or VF warrant strong consideration for ICD therapy based on AVID and the other secondary prevention studies discussed above. ICDs are also appropriate for patients with symptoms consistent with VA (such as syncope) who have inducible VAs at EP study. Based on natural history studies, unexplained syncope is considered by some to constitute an indication for an ICD in patients with DCM. Other indications for ICD implantation in this group need to be defined.

To date, there have been no completed large-scale randomized trials of the ICD for primary prevention of SCD in patients with DCM. One small pilot trial conducted in Germany randomized 104 patients with DCM and LV ejection of 0.30 or less to ICD or usual therapy *(42)*. After 5 years of follow-up, there was no significant difference in mortality between the two groups. Lack of efficacy of the ICD was ascribed to lower-than-expected mortality in this group. The Amiovert trial, recently reported in abstract form, compared ICD therapy with amiodarone in 178 patients with nonischemic cardiomyopathy and nonsustained VT *(43)*. This trial also appeared to be underpowered to detect a treatment effect of the ICD, and was terminated prematurely having shown no significant difference in outcome between the two groups.

The SCD-HeFT is a multicenter study that has enrolled approx 2500 patients with DCM because of any cause with LVEF of 0.35 or less and class II or III heart failure symptoms *(44)*. Patients were randomly assigned to ICD implantation, amiodarone therapy, or placebo in a 1:1:1 fashion. Follow-up was completed in 2003 and preliminary results were presented at the annual Scientific Sessions of the American College of Cardiology in March 2004 (available at www.sicr.org). After a mean follow-up period of 45 months, there was a statistically significant 23% relative reduction in all-cause mortality in the patients assigned to ICD therapy. Patients with ischemic and non-ischemic etiologies of heart failure appeared to benefit equally. There was no significant mortality difference in patients assigned to amiodarone treatment. Assuming these results are confirmed in the final published report, SCD-HeFT may result in significant expansion in patients eligible for ICD therapy for primary prevention of SCD.

OTHER FORMS OF CARDIOMYOPATHY

Several forms of cardiomyopathy expose individuals to elevated risk of SCD in the absence of significant LV systolic dysfunction. These less common diseases include hypertrophic cardiomyopathy (HCM), arrhythmogenic right ventricular cardiomyopathy, cardiac sarcoidosis, and cardiac amyloidosis.

Hypertrophic Cardiomyopathy

HCM is a group of diseases caused by inherited mutations in genes encoding protein components of the cardiac sarcomere *(45)*. To date, 11 different HCM-associated genes have been identified; others likely remain to be discovered. The disease results in myocyte disorganization, progressive myocardial wall thickening, and diastolic dysfunction. Increased LV wall thickening develops during childhood and adolescence and is usually present by young adulthood in affected individuals. Some forms may develop systolic dysfunction late in the course of disease. The disease was first characterized in patients that had disproportionate thickening of the interventricular septum with dynamic LV outflow tract gradient (idiopathic hypertrophic subaortic stenosis [IHSS]). Further studies have demonstrated that neither septal hypertrophy nor outflow tract gradient is a requirement for the disease, and numerous different patterns of LV wall thickening have been identified.

SCD as a result of VAs is believed to be the most common cause of death in HCM, with annual incidence ranging from 1% per year in all patients and up to 5% per year in high-risk subgroups. The highest risk is present in patients who have survived a CA or episode of sustained VT. These patients generally warrant ICD therapy for secondary prophylaxis. Other proposed markers of risk include extreme LVH with wall thickness greater than 30 mm, frequent runs of nonsustained VT on Holter monitoring, history of unexplained syncope, hypotensive response to exercise, and malignant family history. Preliminary data suggest that some genotypes, particular certain mutations in β-myosin heavy chain and cardiac troponin T, confer increased risk of SCD. Genotyping, however, is not widely available and not currently practical for risk stratification. Younger patients appear to be at higher risk, although a cut-off age indicating low risk has not been defined.

Resulting from the relative rarity of the disease and the overall low mortality rate, it has been difficult to define effective therapies for prevention of SCD in HCM. Vigorous physical exertion and participation in competitive sports should be proscribed. β-Blockers have been used based on their efficacy in other cardiac substrates; a retrospective study also suggests effectiveness (46). Amiodarone has been used to treat nonsustained and sustained VAs, but the potential for extracardiac adverse effects with lifelong treatment in relatively young patients is substantial (47). There are no controlled trials of ICD use in patients with HCM. Criteria for secondary prevention are applied generally as with other AVID-eligible patients. There are no prospectively defined criteria for ICD implantation for primary prophylaxis in this disease.

A retrospective cohort study of 128 patients with HCM who had ICDs implanted for perceived high risk of SCD was recently reported (48). This study found that, over a mean follow-up period of 3 years, 19 of 43 patients (44%) implanted for secondary prophylaxis had appropriate ICD discharges for VT or VF, and 10 of 85 patients (12%) implanted for primary prophylaxis did as well. This percentage is lower than that seen in primary prophylaxis trials in patients with CAD or DCM. Because the ICD cannot distinguish between truly life-threatening arrhythmias and VT which would terminate spontaneously without treatment, it is difficult to draw conclusions regarding mortality reduction in this study. Moreover, 18 of 128 patients (14%) had device-related complications in the 3-year follow-up period, including 12 ICD lead failures. Thirty-two patients (25%) had inappropriate ICD discharges for sinus tachycardia, atrial fibrillation, or ICD lead failure; 25 of these patients did not receive an appropriate discharge from the device. These data underscore the potential complications of ICD therapy, particularly applied to young people with long life expectancy. Thus, while this study suggests that some HCM patients may benefit from ICD therapy, definitive data to guide patient selection for primary prophylaxis are not currently available.

Arrhythmogenic Right Ventricular Cardiomyopathy

Arrhythmogenic right ventricular cardiomyopathy (ARVC) is a rare entity first described in 1977, which appears to be more common in Italy *(49)*. The pathologic hallmark of the disease is progressive replacement of the free wall of RV with fibrofatty tissue, often with discrete aneurysm formation. The interventricular septum and LV may be involved later in the disease. Clinically, patients typically present with nonsustained or sustained VT with a left bundle branch block pattern originating in the right ventricle and may later develop heart failure symptoms. Resulting from the rarity of the disease and its diverse clinical presentation and challenging diagnosis, the natural history of ARVC and risk factors for SCD have not been well-defined. Sotalol was shown in one study to be the most effective drug in suppressing inducibility of VT *(50)*. AVID-eligible patients with ARVC are generally treated with an ICD. Primary prevention with an ICD can be considered for patients with unexplained syncope, a malignant family history, or nonsustained VT with inducible VT at invasive EP study. Efficacy data for ICD therapy in this disease are limited. One cohort study of 12 patients found that 8 (66%) had appropriate ICD discharges in follow-up *(51)*. Another study of nine patients implanted for sustained VT also showed high rate of appropriate ICD therapies *(52)*.

Cardiac Sarcoidosis and Amyloidosis

Cardiac sarcoidosis (CS) and amyloidosis are infiltrative heart diseases that may cause conduction disturbances, including complete AV block, and VAs in the absence of LV dysfunction. CS has a wide clinical spectrum and the natural history regarding risk of SCD is not well-defined. Anti-arrhythmic drug and ICD therapy is generally prescribed as with other forms of cardiomyopathy *(53)*. Patients with cardiac amyloidosis and VAs generally have a very poor prognosis in the absence of organ transplantation and/or high-dose chemotherapy. One small cohort study of ICD use in this disease found a high mortality rate and low ICD efficacy because of rapid progression of heart failure, pulseless electrical activity, and failure of other organ systems *(54)*.

Long QT Syndrome

The long QT syndrome (LQTS) is the most common of the cardiac ion channel diseases that cause SCD. The acquired form is most commonly caused by medications, which prolong cardiac repolarization. For a complete updated list of medications associated with LQTS, the reader is referred to www.torsades.org. Other causes of acquired LQTS include hypokalemia and hypomagnesemia; severe bradycardia, such as during complete AV block; and neurological insults, such as subarachnoid hemorrhage and stroke. The congenital form of the disease is associated with mutations in one of at least six identified gene loci (LQT 1–6) *(55)*. LQT1, LQT2, LQT5, and LQT6 are all caused by mutations in different genes encoding for components of cardiac potassium channels, but LQT3 is caused by mutations in the cardiac sodium channel. All result in prolonged repolarization of the cardiac action potential with resulting prolongation of the QT interval and predisposition to torsades de pointes, which may in turn degenerate into VF.

Recognition of the ECG pattern in patients presenting with symptoms is an important component of sudden death prevention in this disorder *(56)*. The ECG in LQTS is highly variable in degree of QT prolongation and morphology of the T wave, which may make recognition difficult. Detection of LQTS is an important reason for careful review of the ECG in any patient presenting with palpitations or syncope. Occasionally, the syndrome presents as a seizure disorder in young children. Once an affected individual has been identified, family members should be screened for the disease.

The most important medical component of treatment for congenital LQTS is β-blocker therapy. This medication has been shown to reduce incidence of syncope and sudden death in congenital LQTS patients *(57)*. Other treatments that have been shown to reduce symptoms include left cardiac sympathectomy and permanent atrial pacing. Preliminary data suggest that sodium channel blockade may be beneficial in the LQT3 subtype. Criteria for ICD implantation are controversial, and the decision is difficult in young patients with long life expectancy. Patients resuscitated from CA and those with recurrent syncope because of torsade de pointes despite β-blockade are the most obvious candidates. Patients with syncope of undetermined etiology and patients with malignant family history are often considered as well.

Brugada Syndrome

The Brugada syndrome is a recently described inherited disease consisting of an abnormal ECG pattern (incomplete right bundle branch block with coved ST segment elevation in leads V_1–V_3) and idiopathic VF *(58)*. In some cases, the ECG pattern is elicited only after sodium-channel blockade. Patients usually present after resuscitation from CA or, less commonly, with recurrent syncope. ICD implantation is currently the only effective therapy for symptomatic individuals. Evaluation and treatment of asymptomatic patients and affected family members is controversial. One report suggests that VT or VF inducibility at EP study has prognostic value *(59)*. Although another report reached the opposite conclusion *(60)*.

Commotio Cordis

Commotio cordis has received attention as a cause of SCD in children and young adults during sporting activities, particularly baseball and hockey *(61)*. The mechanism is believed to be VF induced by a blow to the precordium during the vulnerable period of the cardiac cycle (just prior to the peak of the T-wave). Most affected individuals have structurally normal hearts. Although very rare, events have a high mortality rate and wider impact on affected families and communities. Preventive efforts have focused on use of softer baseballs and improved chest protection equipment.

FUTURE DIRECTIONS

Recent efforts to reduce the public health burden of SCD have focused on expansion of indications for ICD therapy. These trials have clearly shown efficacy of the ICD in the high-risk groups in which it has been studied. It has been noted that the majority of victims of SCD do not have risk factors that would currently make them eligible for an ICD *(62)*. Although further reduction in implant-related complications may make the ICD effective in lower risk patients, the cost-effectiveness ratios associated with this approach would be prohibitively high without a reduction in ICD costs. Additionally, the long-term economic, psychological, and health effects of chronic ICD therapy in low-risk populations are not yet well-understood, and it is unclear to what degree low-risk populations would accept ICD therapy.

The disappointing history of anti-arrhythmic drug trials for prevention of SCD make these agents unattractive for primary prophylaxis of SCD in lower risk groups. To be useful for this purpose, an agent should have low cost and side-effect profile and negligible proarrhythmic risk. Preliminary studies of ω-3 polyunsaturated fatty acids ("fish oils") have shown marked protective effect against VF in animal models of ischemia and infarction, possibly because of stabilizing effects on the membrane of the cardiomyocyte *(63)*. Further trials in humans will be required to demonstrate clinical efficacy.

In order to better target preventive therapies, others have worked on identifying novel markers of high risk of SCD. A recent report has observed that patients with congestive heart failure and depressed LVEF who had elevated brain natriuretic peptide levels (>130 pg/mL) had more than 10-fold higher risk of sudden death than those with lower values *(64)*. Other noninvasive electrocardiographic markers of risk include microvolt T-wave alternans, heart rate variability, and heart rate turbulence. Whether any of these markers can predict benefit of ICD or other preventive strategies remains to be proven *(65)*.

REFERENCES

1. Eisenberg MS, Horwood BT, Cummins RO, Reynolds-Haertle R, Hearne TR. Cardiac arrest and resuscitation: a tale of 29 cities. Ann Emerg Med 1990; 19:179–86.
2. Centers for Disease Control and Prevention (CDC). State-Specific Mortality From Sudden Cardiac Death—United States, 1999. MMWR 2002; 51(6);123–6.
3. Zipes DP, Wellens HJJ. Sudden cardiac death. Circulation 1998; 98:2334–2351.
4. Pratt CM, Greenway PS, Schoenfeld MH, Hibben ML, Reiffel JA. Exploration of the precision of classifying sudden cardiac death. Circulation 1996; 93:519–524.
5. Pearson TA, Blair SN, Daniels SR, et al. AHA Guidelines for Primary Prevention of Cardiovascular Disease and Stroke: 2002 Update. Circulation 2002; 106:388.
6. Holmes DR, Davis KB, Mock MB, et al. The effect of medical and surgical therapy on subsequent sudden cardiac death in patients with coronary artery disease: a report from the Coronary Artery Surgery Study. Circulation 1986; 73:1254–1263.
7. Goldstein S. Propranolol therapy in patients with acute myocardial infarction: the Beta-Blocker Heart Attack Trial. Circulation 1983; 67:I53–I57.
8. ISIS-1 (First International Study of Infarct Survival) Investigators. Randomised trial of intravenous atenolol among 16,027 cases of suspected acute myocardial infarction: ISIS-1. Lancet 1986; 2:57–66.
9. The CAPRICORN Investigators. Effect of carvedilol on outcome after myocardial infarction in patients with left ventricular dysfunction: the CAPRICORN randomized trial. Lancet 2001; 357: 1385–1390.
10. Norris RM, Brown MA, Clarke ED, et al. Prevention of ventricular fibrillation during acute myocardial infarction by intravenous propranolol. Lancet 1981; 2:883–886.
11. Nademanee K, Taylor R, Bailey WE, Rieders DE, Kosar EM. Treating electrical storm: sympathetic blockade versus advanced cardiac life support-guided therapy. Circulation 2000; 102:742–747
12. Bigger JT, Fleiss JL, Kleiger R, Miller JP, Rolnitzky LM. The relationships among ventricular arrhythmias, left ventricular dysfunction, and mortality in the 2 years after myocardial infarction. Circulation 1984; 69:250–258.
13. Echt DS, Liebson PR, Mitchell LB, et al. Mortality and morbidity in patients receiving encainide, flecainide, or placebo. The Cardiac Arrhythmia Suppression Trial. N Engl J Med 1991; 324:781–788.
14. The Cardiac Arrhythmia Suppression Trial II Investigators. Effect of the antiarrhythmic agent moricizine on survival after myocardial infarction. N Engl J Med 1992; 327:227–233.
15. Waldo AL, Camm AJ, deRuyter H, et al. Effect of d-sotalol on mortality in patients with left ventricular dysfunction after recent and remote myocardial infarction. Lancet 1996; 348:7–12.
16. Kober L, Bloch-Thomsen PE, Moller M, et al. Effect of dofetilide in patients with recent myocardial infarction and left-ventricular dysfunction: a randomised trial. Lancet 2000; 356:2052–2058.
17. Herre JM, Sauve MJ, Malone P, et al. Long-term results of amiodarone therapy in patients with recurrent sustained ventricular tachycardia or ventricular fibrillation. J Am Coll Cardiol 1989; 13:442–449.
18. The CASCADE Investigators. Randomized antiarrhythmic drug therapy in survivors of cardiac arrest (the CASCADE study). Am J Cardiol 1993; 72:280–287.
19. Julian DG, Cam AJ, Frangin G, et al. Randomised trial of effect of amiodarone on mortality in patients with left-ventricular dysfunction after recent myocardial infarction: EMIAT. Lancet 1997; 349: 667–674.

20. Cairns JA, Connolly SJ, Roberts R, et al. Randomised trial of outcome after myocardial infarction in patients with frequent or repetitive ventricular premature depolarisations: CAMIAT. Lancet 1997; 349: 675–682.

21. Mirowski M, Reid PR, Mower MM, et al. Termination of malignant ventricular arrhythmias with an implanted automatic defibrillator in human beings. N Engl J Med. 1980; 303:322–324.

22. Peters RW, Gold MR. Implantable cardiac defibrillators. Medical Clinics of North America 2001; 85: 343–367.

23. The AVID Investigators. A comparison of antiarrhythmic-drug therapy with implantable defibrillators in patients resuscitated from near-fatal ventricular arrhythmias. N Engl J Med 1997; 337:1576–1583.

24. Connolly SJ, Gent M, Roberts RS, et al. Canadian Implantable Defibrillator Study (CIDS): a randomized trial of the implantable cardioverter defibrillator against amiodarone. Circulation 2000; 101:1297–1302.

25. Kuck K-H, Cappato R, Siebels J, Ruppel R. Randomized comparison of antiarrhythmic drug therapy with implantable defibrillators in patients resuscitated from cardiac arrest: the Cardiac Arrest Study Hamburg (CASH). Circulation 2000; 102:748–754.

26. Moss AJ, Hall J, Cannom DS, et al. Improved survival with an implanted defibrillator in patients with coronary disease at high risk for ventricular arrhythmias. N Engl J Med 1996; 335:1933–1940.

27. Buxton AE, Lee KL, Fisher JD, Josephson ME, Prystowsky EN, Hafley G, for the Multicenter Unsustained Tachycardia Trial Investigators. A randomized study of the prevention of sudden death in patients with coronary artery disease. N Engl J Med 1999; 341:1882–1890.

28. Bigger JT, for the Coronary Artery Bypass Graft (CABG) Patch Trial Investigators. Prophylactic use of implanted cardiac defibrillators in patients at high risk for ventricular arrhythmias after coronary-artery bypass graft surgery. N Engl J Med 1997; 337:1569–1575.

29. Moss AJ, Zareba W, Hall WJ, et al. Prophylactic implantation of a defibrillator in patients with myocardial infarction and reduced ejection fraction. N Engl J Med 2002; 345:877–883.

30. Mushlin AI, Hall WJ, Zwanziger J, et al. The cost-effectiveness of automatic implantable cardiac defibrillators: results from MADIT. Multicenter Automatic Defibrillator Implantation Trial. Circulation 1998; 97:2129–2135.

31. Larsen G, Hallstrom A, McAnulty J, et al. Cost-effectiveness of the implantable cardioverter-defibrillator versus antiarrhythmic drugs in survivors of serious ventricular tachyarrhythmias: results of the Antiarrhythmics Versus Implantable Defibrillators (AVID) economic analysis substudy. Circulation 2002; 105:2049–57.

32. Exner DV, Klein GJ, Prystowsky EN. Primary prevention of sudden death with implantable defibrillator therapy in patients with cardiac disease. Circulation 2001; 104:1564–1570.

33. Dec GW, Fuster V. Medical progress: idiopathic dilated cardiomyopathy. N Engl J Med 1994; 331: 1564–1575.

34. Doval HC, Nul DR, Grancelli HO, et al. Nonsustained ventricular tachycardia in severe heart failure: independent marker of increased mortality due to sudden death. Circulation 1996; 94:3198–3203.

35. Teerlink JR, Jalaluddin M, Anderson S, et al. Ambulatory ventricular arrhythmias in patients with heart failure do not specifically predict an increased risk of sudden death. Circulation 2000; 101:40–46.

36. Middlekauff HR, Stevenson WG, Stevenson LW, Saxon LA. Syncope in advanced heart failure: high risk of sudden death regardless of origin of syncope. J Am Coll Cardiol 1993; 21:110–116.

37. Gossinger HD, Jung M, Wagner L, et al. Prognostic role of inducible ventricular tachycardia in patients with dilated cardiomyopathy and asymptomatic nonsustained ventricular tachycardia. Int J Cardiol 1990; 29:215–220.

38. The Digitalis Investigation Group. The Effect of Digoxin on Mortality and Morbidity in Patients with Heart Failure. N Engl J Med 1997; 336:525–533.

39. Coplen SE, Antman EM, Berlin JA, Hewitt P, Chalmers TC. Efficacy and safety of quinidine therapy for maintenance of sinus rhythm after cardioversion. A meta-analysis of randomized control trials. Circulation 1990; 82:1106–1116.

40. Doval HC, Nul DR, Grancelli HO, et al. Randomised trial of low-dose amiodarone in severe congestive heart failure. Lancet 1994; 344:493–498.

41. Singh BN, Fletcher RD, Fisher SG, et al. Amiodarone in patients with congestive heart failure and asymptomatic ventricular arrhythmia (CHF-STAT). N Engl J Med 1995; 333:77–82.

42. Bansch D, Antz M, Boczor S, et al. Primary prevention of sudden cardiac death in idiopathic dilated cardiomyopathy: the Cardiomyopathy Trial (CAT). Circulation 2002; 105:1453–1458.

43. Strickberger AS. Amiodarone vs implantable defibrillator in patients with nonischemic cardiomyopathy and asymptomatic nonsustained ventricular tachycardia. Circulation.2000; 102:2794

44. Klein H, Auricchio A, Reek S, Geller C. New primary prevention trials of sudden cardiac death in patients with left ventricular dysfunction: SCD-HEFT and MADIT-II. Am J Cardiol 1999; 83: 91D–97D.
45. Maron BJ. Hypertrophic cardiomyopathy: A systematic review. JAMA 2002; 287:1308–1320.
46. Ostman-Smith I, Wettrell G, Riesenfeld T. A cohort study of childhood hypertrophic cardiomyopathy: improved survival following high-dose beta-adrenoceptor antagonist treatment. J Am Coll Cardiol 1999; 34:1813–1822.
47. McKenna WJ, Oakley CM, Krikler DM, et al. Improved survival with amiodarone in patients with hypertrophic cardiomyopathy and ventricular tachycardia. Br Heart J 1985; 53:412–416.
48. Maron BJ, Shen W-K, Link MS, et al. Efficacy of implantable cardioverter-defibrillators for the prevention of sudden death in patients with hypertrophic cardiomyopathy. N Engl J Med 2000; 342:365–373.
49. Gemayel C, Pelliccia A, Thompson PD. Arrhythmogenic right ventricular cardiomyopathy. J Am Coll Cardiol 2001; 38:1773–1781.
50. Wichter T, Borggrefe M, Haverkamp W, Chen X, Breithardt G. Efficacy of antiarrhythmic drugs in patients with arrhythmogenic right ventricular disease: results in patients with inducible and non-inducible ventricular tachycardia. Circulation 1992; 86:29–37.
51. Link MS, Wang PJ, Haugh CJ, et al. Arrhythmogenic right ventricular dysplasia: Clinical results with implantable cardioverter-defibrillators. J Interventional Cardiac Electrophysiol 1997; 1:41–48.
52. Tavernier R, Gevaert S, De Sutter J, et al. Long term results of cardioverter-defibrillator implantation in patients with right ventricular dysplasia and malignant ventricular tachyarrhythmias. Heart 2001; 85:53–56.
53. Gregoratos G, Abrams J, Epstein AE, et al. ACC/AHA/NASPE 2002 Guideline update for implantation of cardiac pacemakers and antiarrhythmia devices: summary article. Circulation 2002; 106:2145–2161.
54. Falk RH, Monahan K, Smith T. Failure of implantable defibrillator to prevent sudden death in cardiac amyloidosis. Circulation 2002; 102:II–396.
55. Chiang CE, Roden DM. The long QT syndromes: genetic basis and clinical implications. J Am Coll Cardiol 2000; 36:1–12.
56. Brugada P, Geelen P. Some electrocardiographic patterns predicting sudden cardiac death that every doctor should recognize. Acta Cardiologica 1997; 52:473–484.
57. Moss AJ, Zareba W, Hall WJ, et al. Effectiveness and limitations of beta-blocker therapy in congenital long-QT syndrome. Circulation 2000; 101:616–623.
58. Gussak I, Antzelevitch C, Bjerregaard P, Towbin JA, Chaitman BR. The Brugada syndrome: clinical, electrophysiologic and genetic aspects. J Am Coll Cardiol 1999; 33:5–15.
59. Brugada P, Geelen P, Brugada R, Mont L, Brugada J. Prognostic value of electrophysiologic investigations in Brugada syndrome. J Cardiovasc Electrophysiol 2001; 12:1004–1007.
60. Priori SG, Napolitano C, Gasparini M, et al. Natural history of Brugada syndrome: insights for risk stratification and management. Circulation 2002; 105:1342–1347.
61. Maron BJ, Gohman TE, Kyle SB, Estes NA, Link MS. Clinical profile and spectrum of commotio cordis. JAMA 2002; 287:1142–1146.
62. Huikuri HV, Castellanos A, Myerburg RJ. Sudden death due to cardiac arrhythmias. N Engl J Med 2001; 345:1473–1482.
63. Billman GE, Kang JX, Leaf A. Prevention of sudden cardiac death by dietary pure omega-3 polyunsaturated fatty acids in dogs. Circulation 1999; 99:2452–2457.
64. Berger R, Huelsman M, Strecker K, et al. B-type natriuretic peptide predicts sudden death in patients with chronic heart failure. Circulation 2002; 105: 2392–2397.
65. Myerburg RJ. Scientific gaps in the prediction and prevention of sudden cardiac death. J Cardiovasc Electrophysiol 2002; 13:709–723.

4   Physiology of Ventilation During Cardiac Arrest

Andrea Gabrielli, MD, A. Joseph Layon, MD, FACP, and Ahamed H. Idris, MD

INTRODUCTION

Ventilation—the movement of fresh air or other gas from the outside into the lungs and alveoli in close proximity to blood for the efficient exchange of gases—enriches blood with oxygen (O_2) and rids the body of carbon dioxide (CO_2) by movement of alveolar gas from the lungs to the outside *(1)*.

The importance of ventilation in resuscitation is reflected in the "ABCs" (Airway, Breathing, Circulation), which is the recommended sequence of resuscitation practiced in a broad spectrum of illnesses including traumatic injury, unconsciousness, and respiratory and cardiac arrest (CA). Since the modern era of cardiopulmonary resuscitation (CPR) began in the early 1960s, ventilation of the lungs of a victim of CA has been assumed important for successful resuscitation.

From: *Contemporary Cardiology: Cardiopulmonary Resuscitation*
Edited by: J. P. Ornato and M. A. Peberdy © Humana Press Inc., Totowa, NJ

Recently, this assumption has been questioned and is currently being debated *(2)*. Several laboratory studies of CPR have shown no clear benefit to ventilation during the early stages of CA *(3–5)*. Furthermore, exhaled gas contains approx 4% CO_2 and 17% O_2, thus making mouth-to-mouth ventilation the only circumstance in which a hypoxic and hypercarbic gas mixture is given as recommended therapy *(6)*. The introduction of the American Heart Association's (AHA) Guidelines 2000 for Cardiopulmonary Resuscitation emphasizes a new, evidence-based approach to the science of ventilation during CPR. New evidence from laboratory and clinical science has led to less emphasis being placed on the role of ventilation following a dysrhythmic CA (arrest primarily resulting from a cardiovascular event, such as ventricular fibrillation [VF] or asystole). However, the classic airway patency, breathing, and circulation CPR sequence remains a fundamental factor for the immediate survival and neurological outcome of patients after asphyxial CA (CA primarily resulting from respiratory arrest).

This chapter reviews pulmonary anatomy and physiology, early studies of ventilation in respiratory and CA, the effect of ventilation on acid–base conditions and oxygenation during low blood flow states, the effect of ventilation on resuscitation from CA, manual, mouth-to-mouth, and newer techniques of ventilation, and current recommendations for ventilation during CPR.

HISTORY OF ARTIFICIAL VENTILATION AND CPR TECHNIQUES

With the onset of CA, effective spontaneous respiration quickly ceases. Attempts to provide ventilation for victims of respiratory and CA have been described throughout history. Early descriptions are found in the Bible *(7)* and in anecdotal reports in the medical literature of resuscitation of victims of accidents and illness. Early examples of mouth-to-mouth ventilation are described in the resuscitation of a coal miner in 1744 *(8)*, and in an experiment in 1796 demonstrating that expired air was safe for breathing *(9)*. In 1954, Elam and colleagues described artificial respiration with the exhaled gas of a rescuer using a mouth-to-mask ventilation method *(10,11)*. Descriptions of chest compression to provide circulation *(12)* can be found in the historical literature of more than 100 years ago. Electrical defibrillation has been applied in animal laboratory research since the early 1900s, and by Kouwenhoven in 1928 *(11)*.

The modern era of CPR began when artificial ventilation, closed-chest cardiac massage, and electrical defibrillation were combined into a set of practical techniques to initiate the reversal of death from respiratory or CA. Resuscitation is associated with hypoperfusion and consequent ischemia. Recent studies suggest dual defects of hypoxia and hypercarbia during ischemia *(13)*. Thus, the primary purpose of CPR is to bring oxygenated blood to the tissues and to remove CO_2 from the tissues until spontaneous circulation is restored. In turn, the purpose of ventilation is to oxygenate and to remove CO_2 from blood. The "gold standard" of providing ventilation during CPR is direct intubation of the trachea, which not only affords a means of getting gas to the lungs, but also protects the airway from aspiration of gastric contents and prevents insufflation of the stomach. Because this technique requires skill and can be difficult during CA, other airway adjuncts have been developed when intubation is contraindicated or impractical because of user skill.

Before the arrival of an ambulance, ventilation given by bystanders must employ techniques that do not require special equipment. Manual methods of ventilation (i.e., the Sylvester method, the Shafer prone pressure method, and so on) consisting of the rhythmic application and release of pressure to the chest or back and lifting of the arms had been in widespread use for 40 to 50 years prior to the rediscovery of mouth-to-mouth ventilation. These manual techniques were taught in Red Cross classes, to lifeguards, in the military, and in the Boy Scouts as recently as the 1960s, before being replaced by mouth-to-mouth ventilation as the standard for rescue breathing. Safar and Elam first showed that obstruction of the upper airway by the tongue and soft palate occurs commonly in victims who lose consciousness or muscle tone and that ventilation with manual techniques is markedly reduced or prevented altogether by such obstruction *(14,15)*. Subsequently, Safar and colleagues developed techniques that prevent obstruction by extending the neck and jaw and applying this in conjunction with mouth-to-mouth ventilation *(16)*. Although mouth-to-mouth ventilation has been studied extensively in human respiratory arrest and has been shown to maintain acceptable oxygenation and CO_2 levels, its evaluation in laboratory models of CA and in actual human CA has been limited.

PULMONARY PHYSIOLOGY
DURING LOW BLOOD FLOW CONDITIONS

Effects of Hypoxemia and Hypercarbia on Pulmonary Airways

During respiratory and CA, hypoxemia and hypercarbia gradually increase over time. The concentrations of both oxygen and CO_2 affect ventilation and gas exchange. Hypoxemia has variable effects on airway resistance, which is the frictional resistance of the airway to gas flow and is expressed by:

Airway resistance (cm $H_2O/L/s$) = pressure difference (cm H_2O)/flow rate (L/s)

A number of studies in animals and humans, albeit with effective circulation, have shown that hypocapnia causes bronchoconstriction resulting in increased airway resistance, although the effect of hypercapnia on the airways is inconclusive *(17–22)*. In one study, when end-tidal CO_2 was increased from between 20 and 27 mmHg to between 44 and 51mmHg, airflow resistance decreased to 29% of the initial mean *(17)*. However, other studies have shown that hypercapnia causes an increase in airflow resistance through a central nervous system (CNS) effect mediated by the vagus nerve *(18–22)*. It appears that hypocapnia causes bronchoconstriction and increased resistance to flow through a direct local effect on airways, although hypercapnia causes increased airway resistance through action on the CNS *(18–22)*.

Hypoxic Pulmonary Vasoconstriction

HPV is a physiologic mechanism that minimizes venous admixture by diverting blood from underventilated, hypoxic areas of the lung to areas that are better ventilated *(23)*. Pulmonary vessels perfusing underventilated alveoli are normally vasoconstricted. This effect is opposed by increases in the partial pressure of O_2. HPV matches local perfusion to ventilation, increasing with low airway PO_2 and low mixed venous PO_2. The greater the hypoxia, the greater the pulmonary vasoconstriction until a point is reached in which vasoconstriction becomes so intense and widespread that the response becomes pathologic and pulmonary hypertension develops *(24,25)*.

HPV is inhibited by respiratory and metabolic alkalosis and potentiated by metabolic acidosis *(26)*. Additionally, pulmonary vasoconstriction is more pronounced when pulmonary artery pressure is low and is attenuated by increased pulmonary vascular pressure

(26). Hence, a consequence of low inspired O_2 concentration, as occurs during mouth-to-mouth ventilation, could be decreased blood flow caused by increased pulmonary vascular resistance. Whether HPV occurs during CA and CPR is unknown, and warrants evaluation because hypoxemia occurs commonly.

The Ventilation/Perfusion Ratio (V/Q Ratio): The Relationship of Blood Flow and Ventilation During Low-Flow Conditions

During normal cardiac output, ventilation is closely matched with perfusion through a series of physiologic mechanisms exemplified by the maintenance of alveolar and arterial PCO_2 within a range close to 40 mmHg at rest. However, during low blood flow states, the ventilation–perfusion relationship becomes altered.

When systemic blood flow decreases, the flow of blood through the lungs decreases as well. With less venous CO_2 delivered to the lungs, less is available for elimination via exhalation and the concentration of CO_2 in exhaled gas decreases. Because CO_2 elimination is diminished, CO_2 accumulates in venous blood and in the tissues. Mixed venous PCO_2 thus reflects primarily systemic and pulmonary perfusion and is an indicator of the tissue acid–base environment. On the other hand, during low-flow conditions arterial PCO_2 and PO_2 reflect primarily the adequacy of alveolar ventilation. During low rates of blood flow, if alveolar ventilation is adequate, blood flowing through the pulmonary capillary bed is over-ventilated because of a large ventilation–perfusion mismatch. The relationship between alveolar ventilation and pulmonary blood flow is expressed in the ventilation–perfusion ratio equation *(27)*:

$$\dot{V}A/\dot{Q} = 8.63 \bullet R \bullet (CaO_2 - C\bar{v}O_2)/PACO_2$$

in which $\dot{V}A$ is alveolar ventilation; $\dot{Q}$ is the volume of blood flowing through the lungs each minute; 8.63 is a factor relating measurements made at body temperature, ambient pressure, and saturated with water vapor to measurements made at standard temperature, pressure, and dry; R is the respiratory exchange ratio (CO_2 minute production/O_2 consumption); CaO_2 is arterial oxygen content; $C\bar{v}O_2$ is mixed venous oxygen content; and $PACO_2$ is the partial pressure of alveolar CO_2.

This equation appears simple, but it can be solved only by numerical analysis with a computer because alveolar PO_2 is an implicit variable (i.e., alveolar PO_2 decreases when alveolar PCO_2 increases). The ventilation–perfusion ratio equation predicts that as pulmonary blood flow decreases (increasing VA/Q ratio), arterial PO_2 and mixed venous PCO_2 will increase and arterial PCO_2 will decrease. It predicts that as pulmonary perfusion is further reduced (VA/Q ratio approaches infinity), arterial PO_2 and PCO_2 approach the composition of inspired gas. In contrast, if blood flow is present, but alveolar ventilation is absent (VA/Q ratio is 0), arterial PO_2 and PCO_2 approach the composition of mixed venous blood. A study of ventilation during precisely controlled low blood flow conditions found that arterial and mixed venous blood gases behaved as the equation predicts: as blood flow decreased, arterial PCO_2 decreased and PO_2 increased *(28)*.

Although mixed venous gas provides more accurate information regarding flow status during resuscitation, it can be obtained during CPR only rarely, when and if a pulmonary artery catheter is already present. Animal laboratory work seems to suggest that the intraosseous blood gas analysis can be a viable alternative to venous pH and PCO_2 measurements during cardiopulmonary resuscitation. In a swine pediatric model of hypoxic CA, the intraosseous blood gas correlated closely to the mixed venous gas within 15 minutes of CPR. Beyond this time, the intraosseous blood gas reflected more local acid–base conditions or the effect of intraosseous administration of medications than mixed venous blood gas *(29)*.

Gas Exchange and the Transport of Oxygen and Carbon Dioxide in Blood

Hemoglobin is the principle protein of red blood cells (RBCs) and functions importantly in the transport of O_2 and in the elimination of CO_2 through the carbamate and bicarbonate pathways *(30)*. Although hemoglobin is usually considered solely in its role as a carrier of oxygen from the lungs to the tissues, it has an equally important role as a carrier of CO_2 from the tissues to the lungs. Deoxyhemoglobin binds about 40% more CO_2 than oxyhemoglobin and, conversely, when hemoglobin becomes oxygenated during passage through the lungs, CO_2 is actively driven off. This mechanism is referred to as the Bohr-Haldane effect and is responsible for about 50% of the total CO_2 excreted by the lungs during each circulation cycle *(31,32)*. The principle mechanism of the Bohr-Haldane effect is the binding of CO_2 as carbamate compounds to the α-amino groups of hemoglobin *(33,34)*. When oxygen is released by hemoglobin in the tissues, a change takes place in the shape of the hemoglobin molecule making binding sites available for the uptake of CO_2 *(35)*. When hemoglobin takes up O_2 in the lungs, the change in hemoglobin conformation repels CO_2 and promotes its excretion. Plasma proteins also function in the transport of CO_2, but have only one-eighth the buffering capacity of hemoglobin *(36)*.

A small amount of CO_2 dissolves in plasma (5–10% of total CO_2) and a much larger amount (60%) is converted to carbonic acid intracellularly in RBCs through catalytic hydration. Cellular membranes are extremely permeable to CO_2. As RBCs traverse the tissue capillary bed, CO_2 diffuses into RBCs and it is converted by carbonic anhydrase to carbonic acid, which then dissociates to bicarbonate and proton. The conversion of CO_2 to bicarbonate would soon stop if protons were not buffered by hemoglobin, and bicarbonate would otherwise be trapped within the RBC because of its polarity, preventing diffusion through the RBC membrane. However, a membrane transport system rapidly exchanges plasma chloride for intracellular bicarbonate and preserves the CO_2-carbonic acid-bicarbonate gradient *(36)*. Another important aspect of the interaction of proton with hemoglobin is its effect on lowering the affinity of hemoglobin for oxygen, and by the law of action and reaction, oxygenation of hemoglobin lowers its affinity for proton. When hemoglobin is exposed to higher concentrations of CO_2 from respiring tissues, the formation of protons helps unload O_2, which becomes available to tissues. When hemoglobin is oxygenated in the pulmonary capillaries, protons are released from hemoglobin and bicarbonate is converted back to water and CO_2, which then diffuses out of the blood into the alveoli. Thus, oxygenation of hemoglobin actively promotes the pulmonary excretion of CO_2, and CO_2 from tissues promotes the release of O_2 from hemoglobin at the tissue level.

In summary, hemoglobin is the principle protein responsible for lung-to-tissue transport of O_2 and tissue-to-lung transport of CO_2. Hemoglobin transports CO_2 as carbamino compounds and in the form of bicarbonate. It can be appreciated from these mechanisms of CO_2 exchange and O_2 transport that alveolar oxygenation and ventilation as well as pulmonary blood flow play crucial roles in the removal of CO_2 from the tissues. Because pH and CO_2 levels affect the affinity of hemoglobin for O_2, these issues are important during the treatment of CA.

VENTILATION DURING LOW BLOOD FLOW CONDITIONS

Effect of Ventilation on Acid–Base Conditions and Oxygenation

Acid–base conditions and oxygenation are important issues in resuscitation from low blood flow states such as shock *(37–42)* and CA *(43–48)*. Hypoxemia and hypercarbic acidosis critically reduce the force of myocardial contractions *(49–53)*, make defibrillation difficult *(54,55)*, and are associated with poor outcome *(54,55)*. It has been observed that, during CA, arterial blood gases do not reflect tissue conditions and that mixed venous blood has a level of CO_2 that is frequently twice the level of the arterial side *(51,52,58)*.

Arterial and mixed venous metabolic acidosis and mixed venous hypercarbic acidosis are associated with failure of resuscitation from CA *(43,46,48)*. Studies of both human and animal CA have shown that during CPR, the pH of blood is largely determined by the concentration of CO_2 *(56–71)* and that arterial blood is often alkalemic although mixed venous blood is acidemic because of differences in CO_2 levels. A recent Norwegian study measured arterial PCO_2 and pH in patients receiving tidal volumes of 500 mL vs 1000 mL several minutes after intubation during out-of-hospital CA (mean time of approx 15 minutes) *(72)*. The study showed that mean PCO_2 was 28 and 56 mmHg with 1000 mL and 500 mL tidal volume, respectively. These results indicate that tidal volume affects arterial PCO_2 and pH significantly: larger tidal volume is associated with respiratory alkalosis and smaller tidal volume is associated with respiratory acidosis.

The arteriovenous PCO_2 gradient increases substantially during CPR and returns to near normal when spontaneous circulation is restored *(13,38,57,62,64,73–75)*. The CO_2 gradient likely results from reduced blood flow through the lungs, decreased pulmonary elimination of CO_2 accumulation of CO_2 on the venous side of the circulatory system, and over-ventilation of blood entering the arterial side *(13,56,62,73)*. A recent study showed that changes in ventilation could affect excretion of CO_2 even when blood flow rate is as low as 12% of normal *(28)*. Additionally, with decreasing blood flow, the decrease in end-tidal CO_2 parallels the decrease in arterial PCO_2. Thus, both arterial PCO_2 and end-tidal CO_2 vary directly with blood flow, although mixed venous PCO_2 varies inversely with blood flow.

Mixed venous PCO_2 and pH can be improved with proper ventilation and becomes worse with hypoventilation. Because mixed venous blood gases reflect tissue acid–base status, intracellular hypercarbia can be altered with ventilation, which emphasizes the potential importance of ventilation during low blood flow states.

Effect of Ventilation on VF and Defibrillation

Sudden death is thought to be a primary cardiac electrical event and may not be a result of myocardial injury, although there is often underlying myocardial ischemia, which can reduce electrical stability and lead to ventricular ectopy. The event is often fatal and is probably initiated by ventricular tachycardia (VT), or VF. Investigations have shown that hypoventilation, hypoxemia, hypercarbia, and metabolic acidosis can lower the threshold for VF as well as affect the tendency of the heart to develop ventricular arrhythmias (VAs). Furthermore, arterial hypoxemia has been shown to cause arrhythmia by excitation of the autonomic nervous system and by affecting vagal tone *(76)*. Both hyperventilation and hypoventilation are associated with severe VA and supraventricular arrhythmias *(77)*. Hypoxemia and other issues such as hypoglycemia, hyper- and hypokalemia cause VF by shortening the duration of the cardiac action potential *(78)*.

Hypercarbia without hypoxemia lowers the VF threshold and respiratory alkalosis raises the VF threshold and enhances spontaneous recovery from VF *(79)*. In another study, ischemia, but not hypoxemia, lowered the VF threshold *(80)*.

The effect of ventilation on the defibrillation threshold, which is the minimum electrical energy required for defibrillation of a fibrillating ventricle, has not been studied directly. Instead, the defibrillation threshold has been investigated under conditions of hypoxemia, and metabolic and hypercarbic acidosis, either alone or in combination *(46,48,54,81)*. The findings of different studies have been somewhat contradictory, but generally show the defibrillation threshold is unaffected by acid–base conditions existing either before or during CPR. However, more recent studies using animal models of CA suggest that hypercarbia is associated with VF refractory to defibrillation *(46,52,55)*. Coronary perfusion pressure, duration of untreated VF, and duration of CPR are critical issues known to affect success of defibrillation *(82)*.

A human study of issues that influenced the success of defibrillation found that arterial hypoxemia and acidemia, and delay in defibrillation attempts were associated with failure to defibrillate *(54)*, but it was not possible to distinguish the effect of these issues independently because they tended to occur together. A canine study, in which ischemia, ventricular hypertrophy, hypoxemia, acidosis, and alkalosis were well-controlled independent variables, did not find an adverse effect of these issues on defibrillation threshold *(81)*. Surprisingly, hypoxemia was found to lower the threshold for defibrillation. Another study found that metabolic acidosis, but not metabolic alkalosis or respiratory acidosis or alkalosis lowered the threshold for VF *(83)*. More recent laboratory CPR studies of hypercarbic acidosis found a substantial reduction in rate of resuscitation. Although the defibrillation threshold was not investigated, four of six animals ventilated with 50% CO_2 had refractory VF *(46)*. In other studies of acid–base conditions, most animals with sufficient coronary perfusion pressure during CPR were defibrillated, but only animals without substantial hypercarbia recovered adequate cardiac output *(52,55,84–88)*. A recent study of human CPR also found that return of spontaneous circulation was associated with improved levels of arterial and mixed venous PO_2 and PCO_2 *(44)*.

There are important differences in physiology during normal cardiac output and CPR that may not be widely appreciated. For example, high levels of arterial and mixed venous hypercarbia are usually tolerated well by humans *(89)* and animals *(46,90–93)* when there is normal spontaneous cardiac output. Nevertheless, during CA, hypercarbia substantially reduces success of resuscitation by adversely affecting myocardial contractility *(46,52,55,84–88)*. At least one laboratory study found that hypercarbia was associated with refractory VF *(55)*. In this rat model, very high levels of inspired and thus, myocardial PCO_2 were produced and may help explain the difference in findings of another study *(81)* that used more modest levels of hypercarbia and failed to find an effect on defibrillation threshold.

Among issues that can affect the likelihood of defibrillation, the duration of VF is of great importance *(94)*. In human CPR, the rate of successful defibrillation is approx 80% if administered immediately after onset of VF, but the chance of success decreases approx 5% for each additional minute of VF *(95,96)*. After 12 minutes of VF with CPR, the rate of success is only about 20%. A similar effect of duration of VF is seen in laboratory CPR models *(97–99)* and may be explained, in part, by the gradual depletion of myocardial adenosine triphosphate, which is thought to be a marker for ischemic tissue damage and the metabolic state of the myocardium *(100)*. Additionally, potassium uptake by myocardial cells is increased during VF and is related to hydrogen ion, CO_2, and lactate production *(101)*. Earlier work found that the ratio of intracellular to extracellular potassium concentration affected the defibrillation threshold *(102)*.

In summary, hypoxemia and hypercarbia decrease the threshold for VF. Hypoxemia and hypercarbia have a negligible effect on the defibrillation threshold when the duration VF is brief. Recent studies suggest that hypoxemia and hypercarbia make defibrillation more difficult when VF persists for several minutes or more.

Effect of Ventilation on Myocardial Force and Rate of Contraction

Studies using an isolated heart model demonstrated that hypoxia and hypercarbia caused a profound decrease in myocardial force of contraction independent of pH *(53,103–106)*. Studies examining the effect of hypercarbia on isolated spontaneously contracting myocytes have found that rate and force of contraction are inhibited by modestly increased concentrations of CO_2, with pH held at 7.40 and PO_2 at 142 mmHg *(107)*. The model demonstrated a rapid and profound effect of CO_2 independent of pH, PO_2, vascular tone, neuroendocrine issues, or inflammatory mediators. In contrast, isolated decreased blood or perfusate pH is not associated with reduced ventricular force of contraction *(49–53)*. The reason for these differences in myocardial response to extracellular CO_2 and hydrogen ion is that CO_2 is a nonpolar, lipid soluble molecule that is permeable to cellular membranes and diffuses rapidly into the intracellular space. Once CO_2 enters the cell, it lowers intracellular pH by dissociating to hydrogen ion and bicarbonate. In contrast, hydrogen ion is polar, diffusing at a very slow rate through cell membranes, and this may account for its lack of effect on myocardial dynamics under most experimental conditions *(108)*. There is accumulating evidence that reduced intracellular pH affects calcium ion flux, exchange, and binding and ultimately affects excitation–contraction coupling and myocardial contractility *(108)*.

During VF, the heart continues to perform work and very likely has energy utilization greater than during normal contractions; metabolites in the form of hydrogen ion, lactate, and CO_2 continue to be produced. With the onset of VF, myocardial CO_2 tension increases rapidly from a normal value of approx 50 mmHg to 350 mmHg and there is a parallel increase in hydrogen ion concentration *(74,103)*. As we have noted above, the removal of CO_2 from tissues is dependent on blood flow; thus, coronary blood flow is an important cofactor influencing levels of myocardial CO_2. A coronary perfusion pressure of less than 10 mmHg was associated with myocardial CO_2 tensions 400 mmHg or more and failure of resuscitation, although a coronary perfusion pressure of greater than 10 mmHg was associated with myocardial CO_2 tensions 400 mmHg or less and successful resuscitation *(109)*. Decreased intracellular pH is associated with changes to the structure and function of regulatory and enzyme proteins and if not corrected soon enough leads to irreversible loss of cell function and cell death *(110)*.

In summary, both isolated hypoxemia and isolated hypercarbia have a negative inotropic effect on the heart. Ischemia would be predicted to be a more injurious event than hypoxemia or hypercarbia alone, because ischemia causes both decreased delivery of O_2 and decreased elimination of tissue CO_2. To the extent that ventilation can affect the elimination of CO_2 and enhance tissue oxygenation, it can likely provide some benefit during CA and CPR. There are promising therapies that perfuse the heart with oxygen-containing fluorocarbon compounds (SAPO: selective aortic arch perfusion and oxygenation) resulting in higher rates of restoration of spontaneous circulation after prolonged CA and CPR *(111)*.

Hypoxemia, Hypercarbia, and the Vasopressor Effect of Catecholamines

The importance of the administration of such catecholamines as epinephrine during CPR cannot be overstated. Numerous studies and years of experience treating CA have shown that epinephrine is often a pivotal factor in reversing sudden death by increasing coronary perfusion pressure and the likelihood of defibrillation *(112)*. The interaction of ventilation and the vasopressor activity of epinephrine and other catecholamines need to be examined.

A number of studies have shown that increases in blood PCO_2 in animal models and in humans results in a decrement of the pressor response to epinephrine and norepinephrine by more than 50% *(113–115)*. The mechanism for the failure of blood pressure to increase is primarily decreased peripheral vasoconstriction and vascular resistance *(113–119)* with a smaller contribution caused by a cardiac arrhythmia other than tachycardia *(113–115)*. Metabolic acidosis (i.e., increased hydrogen ion concentration) has also been found to inhibit vasoconstriction, but to a much smaller degree than "respiratory" acidosis (i.e., increased PCO_2; *119)*. With return of CO_2 to normal levels, the inhibitory effect of hypercarbia on epinephrine activity is reversed completely within 10 minutes in human volunteers with normal cardiac function *(118)*.

Hypoxemia also has been found to decrease the pressor response to epinephrine *(51)*. Hypoventilation, through simultaneous hypoxemia and retention of CO_2, causes greater peripheral vasodilation and loss of the pressor effect of epinephrine than isolated hypercarbia or hypoxemia alone *(51)*. There are few studies specifically examining the effect of ventilation on the pressor response to catecholamines during CA and CPR. Successful resuscitation is associated with epinephrine-induced increases in coronary perfusion pressure, and there are data suggesting that hypoxemia and hypercarbia may modulate the increase *(120,121)*.

Hemodynamic Effects of Ventilation

Mean intrathoracic pressure is higher during positive pressure ventilation (PPV) than during spontaneous breathing. During normal heart function, increased intrathoracic pressure decreases right and left ventricular filling. If sufficient airway pressure is applied, pulmonary vascular resistance increases. The effect of lung inflation on pulmonary vessels is complex. At abnormally low lung volumes, vessels are collapsed and pulmonary vascular resistance is increased *(27)*. When the lung is inflated, collapsed vessels open and resistance decreases. Alveolar capillaries are compressed and resistance increases at high inflation volumes. Underventilation and ventilation perfusion mismatch at low lung volumes results in a progressive decrease in lung compliance and an increase in alveolar-arterial oxygen tension difference. Because blood flow is related inversely to pulmonary vascular resistance, if the lungs are poorly inflated during CPR, pulmonary blood flow may possibly decrease further. The α-adrenergic effect of epinephrine during CA specifically depresses PaO_2 absorption and CO_2 elimination of low V/Q lung units. Interestingly, vasopressin has significantly less adverse effect on pulmonary gas exchange, after CPR. It has been speculated that vasopressin could rehabilitate the pulmonary circulation through the agonist effect of the V_2 vasopressinergic receptor *(122)*. However, there are little data available in this area.

A number of studies have shown that PPV can impair cardiac output in normally functioning hearts, and that positive end-expiratory pressure can impair cardiac output further because of increased intrathoracic pressure, which reduces venous return *(123–*

125). In fact, positive end-expiratory pressure has been used to create a model of functional hypovolemia to study the effect of conventional and high frequency jet ventilation on cardiac output and blood pressure *(126)*. In this study, conventional ventilation during conditions of functional hypovolemia resulted in decreased cardiac output and arterial blood pressure, although high frequency jet ventilation did not affect hemodynamics, probably because of lower airway pressure, lower intrathoracic pressure, and improved venous return.

In contrast to the physiology of ventilation and blood flow during spontaneous cardiac circulation, the physiology of blood flow is somewhat different during CPR with external chest compression. Chandra et al. have shown convincingly that blood enters the lungs from the right heart during periods of *low intrathoracic* pressure corresponding to the release of pressure on the chest, although forward flow of blood from lungs to the left heart and then out to the systemic circulation takes place during chest compression and is associated with *increased intrathoracic* pressure *(127)*. Furthermore, intrathoracic pressure can be increased even more with high airway pressure (70–80 mmHg) ventilation simultaneous with chest compression, which is associated with increases in carotid blood flow and cerebral perfusion *(128–130)*. The application of negative airway pressure during the release phase further enhances carotid blood flow by increasing venous return to the chest. Another study showed that arterial pressure and blood flow during chest compressions is related directly to peak intrathoracic pressure up to pressures as high as 50 mmHg, beyond which no further increases in blood flow occur *(131)*. Continuous positive airway pressure ventilation (CPAP or postive end-expiratory pressure [PEEP]) given during both the compression and release phase of chest compression would be expected to interfere with venous return and to decrease blood flow just as it does during spontaneous circulation *(132)*. PEEP can also be the inadvertent result of excessive tidal volume, increased respiratory rate and reduced inspiratory time (auto-PEEP) and is associated with an increased incidence of pulseless electrical activity during resuscitation *(133)*.

An impedance threshold device that causes negative intrathoracic pressure during CPR and hemorrhagic shock has been shown to increase venous return, right myocardial preload, blood pressure, and blood flow to the heart and brain *(134–137)*. It also has been shown to improve survival from CA and hemorrhagic shock. The device is based on the physiologic principle that negative intrathoracic pressure enhances venous blood return to the chest and heart thus making increased cardiac output possible.

Another very important study was performed in the setting of hemorrhagic shock using PPV. This study showed that blood pressure decreased progressively as ventilation rate increased from 12 breaths to 30 breaths per minute (bpm; *138)*. More importantly, systolic blood pressure improved from 66 to 84 mmHg when ventilation rate was decreased from 12 breaths to 6 bpm and the lower rate was associated with a significantly improved survival. The study emphasizes the principle that the duration of increased intrathoracic pressure is proportional to the ventilation rate when PPV is used. Another principle is that blood pressure is inversely proportional to ventilation rate.

Application of CPAP without active ventilation has been recently studied in CPR. In a pig model of CA, CPAP titrated to achieve 75% of a baseline end-tidal CO_2 was compared with intermittent PPV *(139)*. A significant difference in both airway pressure and diastolic blood pressure could be detected between the two techniques (27 ± 58 mmHg in CPR vs 13 ± 11 mmHg in CPR_{CPAP}), and there was an improvement in arterial and mixed venous pH, O_2 saturation, and CO_2 in the CPR_{CPAP} animals. Cardiac output did not change significantly between the two methods. This technique has the potential advantage of simplifying CPR, decreasing pulmonary atelectasis, and improving both oxygenation and ventilation. However, it can also have a negative effect on diastolic blood pressure and, thus, on both coronary and cerebral blood flow.

Despite the potential for decreased venous return, it is possible that very small amounts of positive airway pressure may decrease intrapulmonary shunting, pulmonary vascular collapse, and atelectasis without adverse hemodynamic effects. In fact, recent use of a multislice CT scanner to allow dynamic imaging of tridimensional volume of the lung during CPR suggested that CPAP was superior to simple volume controlled ventilations or no ventilations CPR in maintaining better lung distension and preventing atelectasis *(140)*.

In conclusion, movement of venous blood into the lungs takes place during the release phase of external chest compression when intrathoracic pressure is low. When the chest is compressed, intrathoracic pressure rises and blood moves out of the lungs and heart and into the systemic circulation. Negative airway pressure enhances blood flow and venous return to the chest, although CPAP ventilation inhibits venous return and blood flow but decreases lung atelectasis. These studies emphasize the crucial relationship between ventilation mechanics and circulation.

The Effect of Ventilation on Outcome From Resuscitation

For more than 30 years, emergency ventilation has been considered an essential component of CPR. There are few studies and little direct evidence that ventilation affects outcome from CA, although it has been assumed crucial for resuscitation. Recommendations for ventilation were based on studies performed in the 1950s and 1960s in living humans with normal cardiac output *(14–16)*. These studies presumed that the goal of ventilation during CPR was to achieve near "normal" tidal volumes and minute ventilation. However, substantially less ventilation may be sufficient for gas exchange during CPR because cardiac output and pulmonary blood flow are only 10%–15% of normal during manual chest compression *(130)*. As a consequence, the amount of hemoglobin passing through the pulmonary bed is reduced and the amount of oxygen necessary to saturate hemoglobin is also reduced if there is not a large ventilation/perfusion mismatch. Because venous return and thus the quantity of CO_2 delivered to the lungs are decreased, the amount of ventilation necessary to remove CO_2 is presumably reduced.

The time when ventilation must be initiated during CPR to achieve satisfactory results and the ventilatory requirements during CPR is unclear. In a canine model of CA, arterial pH, PCO_2, and PO_2 had no significant change after 5 minutes of untreated VF *(141)*, although arterial PO_2 decreased from 81 to 69 mmHg under similar conditions in a swine model *(142)*. In the canine study, there was no significant change in arterial PO_2 and PCO_2 for 30 seconds after initiation of chest compressions without ventilation. At 45 seconds, arterial PO_2 was 52 mmHg, a significant decline. Another canine study showed that chest compression alone without assisted ventilation will produce a minute ventilation of 5.2 ± 1.1 L per minute and will maintain O_2 saturation at 90% or more for more than 4 minutes *(4)*. A murine study found that chest compression alone produced tidal volumes of 26% of baseline and although arterial PCO_2 increased to 80 mmHg after 9 minutes, resuscitation rate was not impaired *(5,143)*. The animals were intubated in all of these studies. It is likely that ventilation induced by chest compression would be less in nonintubated models, but the way this would affect blood gases is unknown.

Other studies have shown that ventilation has an important role in resuscitation. An early study showed that well oxygenated dogs had better carotid artery blood flow than asphyxiated dogs. This was attributed to loss of peripheral vascular tone *(144)*. Weil and colleagues showed that spontaneous gasping during CA in a swine model favored successful resuscitation and also showed that both the frequency and duration of gasps correlated with coronary perfusion pressure and predicted outcome *(145)*.

More recent studies were designed specifically to test the effect of ventilation on outcome in swine models of CPR. One study compared a group receiving mechanical ventilation during CPR with a group receiving chest compression alone and a group without chest compression or ventilation. The duration of untreated VF was 30 seconds followed by 12 minutes of CPR in the treatment groups. All animals were successfully defibrillated and entered a 2-hour intensive care period. However, after 24 hours, only two of eight animals that had no CPR survived, although all 16 animals survived in the groups receiving chest compression with and without ventilation *(3)*. Another study allocated 24 swine to groups with and without ventilation during 10 minutes of chest compression following 6 minutes of untreated VF. Nine of twelve ventilated animals and only 1 of 12 nonventilated animals had return of spontaneous circulation. The nonventilated animals died with significantly greater arterial and mixed venous hypoxemia and hypercarbia *(146)*. A follow-up study was done to test whether hypoxemia or hypercarbia independently affects survival from CA. Using a swine model of isolated arterial and mixed venous hypoxemia without hypercarbia in one group and isolated hypercarbia without hypoxemia in another group, there was only one of ten animals with return of spontaneous circulation in each group *(121)*.

Other experimental work in large animal survival and neurological outcome up to 48 hours were not different when ventilation was withheld during resuscitation. These initial studies, although clearly de-emphasizing the importance of ventilation during the first few minutes of CPR, were limited by the persistence of an "artificial" patent airway in the animal, which resulted from the presence of an endotracheal tube (ETT) allowing exchange of ventilations from gasping and chest compressions/decompressions *(147,148)*.

More recent studies eliminated the possible influence of an artificial patent airway in animal models during CPR. When standard CPR was compared with compression-only CPR in a pig model in which the airway was occluded, no difference was found in 24-hour outcome *(149)*. It is important to note that a supine, unconscious dog or pig usually has a patent airway, whereas a supine, unconscious human has an obstructed airway resulting from the kinked nature of the human airway. These model differences are rarely discerned in CPR ventilation experiments but do have fundamental clinical importance. These latest observations confirmed that ventilation for a few minutes after dysrhythmic CA was not fundamental and suggested the need to test the no-ventilation hypothesis in humans *(150)*.

There are important differences between all these studies including duration of untreated VF, the use of 100% O_2 before CA, and whether or not agonal respirations were prevented with a paralytic agent. However, taken together, these studies provide some evidence that ventilation may possibly be withheld when chest compression is initiated promptly after CA, but that ventilation is important for survival when chest compression is delayed.

There are even fewer human studies of the role of ventilation during CA. Because ventilation is such a well-accepted intervention, the ethical considerations of doing a controlled study by withholding ventilation in one group has been difficult to overcome.

Indirect evidence pointing to a less important role of ventilation immediately after CA has existed since the early 1990s. For example, in Seattle, where ambulance response time is short, patients who were seen to have spontaneous agonal respiratory efforts immediately after CA had a higher rate of successful resuscitation *(151)*. Another study found that hypoxemia and hypercarbia was associated with the use of the esophageal obturator airway in the field and also a lower resuscitation rate *(65)*. Mixed venous oxygenation saturation is associated with prognosis for survival from CA; mixed venous pH, PO_2, and PCO_2 measured during hemorrhagic shock and CA were significantly better in those with return of spontaneous circulation *(44,152)*. In the Netherlands, clinical CPR is given in the order "CAB" (Chest Compression–Airway–Breathing) with ventilation being delayed and chest compression being initiated as soon as possible. Using "CAB," CPR survival data from the Netherlands is comparable to that reported in the United States *(153)*. Human data also suggest that prompt chest compression following CA improves brain and heart perfusion and the success of defibrillation *(154)*.

Related to this, more human studies became available in the last few years. In a prospective, observational study of CPR and ventilation, chest compression-only CPR, and no CPR, survival from CPR (i.e., return of spontaneous circulation) was found to be 16%, 15%, and 6% respectively *(155)*. Although both forms of basic life support (BLS) were significantly better than no CPR, there were no differences between CPR with or without ventilation. Similar results were reported more recently in North America in a study of telephone dispatcher-assisted BLS-CPR in which survival of compression-only CPR vs ventilation CPR was 14% vs 10%, respectively, with a slight trend of survival favoring chest compression-only CPR *(156)*. Although this study emphasized that CPR without ventilation is better than nothing, it presents several limitations in design. Mouth-to-mouth ventilation performed by a bystander was assessed by emergency medicine dispatcher only and not by the investigator at the scene; the patency of the airway was unclear in some patients, and primary respiratory arrests were excluded. Additionally, if the bystander knew how to perform CPR, then the patient was excluded from the study. Nevertheless, the study suggested a need to reconsider BLS with a goal of minimizing the time to onset of CPR in the CA victim and maximizing the efficacy of chest compression. When the concept of this "simplified CPR" was tested in a mannequin, effective compression was achieved an average of 30 seconds earlier than with the standard technique, and the number of compressions per minute were approximately doubled *(157)*.

Despite the overall enthusiasm for the relatively positive results of dispatcher-assisted CPR instructions without ventilation as described by the providers *(158,159)*, it has been emphasized by independent observers that the concept of no-ventilation CPR could be a misnomer, because, provided that the airway is open, patients undergoing VF often exchange a significant amount of air through gasping *(160)*. Therefore, the term "CPR without assisted ventilation" has been suggested. Although the North American literature seems to de-emphasize the importance of ventilation in the first few minutes after CA, a recent Swedish report of 14,000 patients showed increased survival to one month for "complete CPR" (both chest compressions and ventilation) vs "incomplete CPR" (compression only; survival, 9.7% vs 5.1%; $p < 0.001$; *161*).

In this study, ventilation, and duration of less than 2 minutes between patient collapse and the beginning of lay bystander CPR, were both powerful modifying issues on survival at 30 days, emphasizing the need for better and earlier CPR. A limitation of these out-of-hospital studies is the lack of proper neurological examination during or immediately after resuscitation. Therefore, the relative influence of ventilation on cerebral perfusion is unclear. In swine models, pupillary diameter light reaction was used and found to have a reasonable correlation with cerebral perfusion pressure. However, the animal was ventilated during resuscitation with a tidal volume of 15 mL/kg at an FiO_2 of 1.0. It is unknown if these clinical findings could be used in a human prospective randomized study during CPR to evaluate the level of influence of ventilation on neurological outcome *(162)*.

In summary, the standards for ventilation during CPR are based on studies that are somewhat contradictory and inconclusive. The amount of ventilation required during CPR is still unclear. It is likely that the number of bpm needed during conventional CPR is less than currently recommended. It is logical that ventilation should be matched with perfusion of blood through the lungs and the systemic circulation. Thus, when blood flow is 0, ventilation is unnecessary because it would not affect tissue oxygenation and CO_2 removal. However, with CPR techniques that improve blood flow, such as use of device adjuncts for chest compression, more ventilation may be necessary.

The duration of VF before the start of chest compression is likely to be of significance regarding the need for ventilation, although the importance of ventilation in CPR has been de-emphasized in favor of the need for more effective chest compression and early defibrillation. In fact, it is likely that time of defibrillation is an important factor in determining whether ventilation is necessary for successful resuscitation. The etiology of CA is another very important factor related to the role of ventilation in CPR. Ventilation has primary importance when CA occurs from asphyxia, such as in drowning, and is the most frequent cause of pediatric CA.

TECHNIQUES OF VENTILATION DURING CPR

Ventilation Techniques That Can Be Used for Basic CPR by the Lay Public: Manual, Mouth-to-Mouth, and Mouth-to-Mask Ventilation

In the 1950s and early 1960s, alternative methods of artificial respiration were investigated additionally to mouth-to-mouth ventilation. A number of studies showed that the application of external pressure to the chest during manual maneuvers in normal volunteers caused substantial respiratory tidal volumes that ranged from 50 to 1114 mL *(10,14–16,163–168)*. The rate of manual ventilation was 10–12 compressions per minute and total minute ventilation (the product of tidal volume and respiratory rate per minute) provided by these techniques was 0.5–11.1 L per minute. When these techniques were applied to patients with pre-existing pulmonary disease, tidal volumes were considerably less (50–540 mL) than in healthy subjects *(168)*. These studies also noted that tidal volumes generated by actively expanding the chest with arm-lift or hip-lift techniques were 20–40% greater when compared with passive chest expansion *(166)*. Techniques that relied exclusively on passive chest expansion were ineffective for adequate ventilation and resulted in mean arterial oxygen saturations of 67% in normal volunteer subjects *(163)*. Manual techniques that included active chest expansion produced mean arterial oxygen saturations of 93% in human subjects, and thus were able to maintain acceptable gas exchange without PPV *(163)*. In contrast with the manual techniques previously mentioned, pressure applied directly over the sternum of curarized, intubated volunteers produced mean tidal volumes of only 156 mL. Furthermore, without intubation sternal pressure produced no tidal exchange because of airway obstruction by the tongue *(15)*.

However, with the head extended to prevent airway obstruction, five of six patients had tidal volumes greater than 340 mL and three of six had tidal volumes in excess of 500 mL.

Simultaneous with studies of manual ventilation techniques, mouth-to-mouth ventilation was also studied extensively. Several research projects were funded by the Department of the Army because of the urgency of problems of resuscitation in nerve gas poisoning. In one study, 29 volunteers were paralyzed with curare, and mouth-to-mask resuscitation was started before the onset of cyanosis *(169)*. The arterial oxygen saturation of the volunteers receiving artificial ventilation was never below 85% and the mean oxygen saturation was 94%. Alveolar CO_2 tensions, measured in 21 patients, were maintained at or below 50 mmHg. The mean alveolar CO_2 concentration was 5.6% before resuscitation and 3.9% during resuscitation. Expired gas resuscitation produced a fall in alveolar CO_2 concentration in all 12 patients. The authors concluded that with mild hyperventilation, the rescuer readily converted his exhaled gas to a suitable resuscitation gas. These experiments were designed to simulate a respiratory arrest and only healthy volunteers were studied. Whether exhaled gas would benefit a patient who suffers CA was not considered and has not been investigated.

Because exhaled gas contains CO_2, it may have adverse cardiovascular effects during CPR, but few investigations have addressed this issue. A study of the effect of ventilation on resuscitation during CPR using an animal model showed that both hypoxemia and hypercarbia independently have an adverse effect on outcome from CA. Swine were ventilated with experimental gas mixtures consisting of 85% oxygen in a control group, 95% O_2 and 5% CO_2 in a hypercarbic group, and 10% O_2 and 90% N_2 in a hypoxic group. The model succeeded in producing isolated hypoxemia without hypercarbia and isolated hypercarbia without hypoxemia. Only 1 of 10 (10%) animals could be resuscitated in each of the hypercarbic and hypoxic groups, although 9 of 12 (75%) animals were resuscitated in the control group *(121)*.

A study of the isolated effect of CO_2 on spontaneously contracting chick myocytes showed that myocytes perfused with 4.6% or 9.6% CO_2 had inhibition of both rate and force of contraction with both concentrations. The model demonstrated a rapid and profound effect of CO_2 independent of pH, PO_2, vascular tone, neuroendocrine issues, or inflammatory mediators *(107)*.

A study of the composition of gas given by mouth-to-mouth ventilation during simulated one- and two-rescuer CPR showed that the rescuers exhaled a mean concentration of CO_2 of 3.5% to 4.1% and a mean concentration of O_2 of 16.6% to 17.8% *(6)*. Therefore, the gas given by mouth-to-mouth ventilation has a similar concentration of CO_2 and is more hypoxic than the gas shown to be deleterious in the above-cited animal study. When compared with mouth-to-mouth ventilation, room air is a superior gas for ventilation because it contains 21% oxygen and a negligible amount of CO_2 (0.03%).

Furthermore, when these gas concentrations were used in a swine model with 6 mL/kg ventilation, profound arterial desaturation was noted and was shortly followed by hemodynamic instability *(170)*. This instability and desaturation were not observed if the tidal volume was increased to 12 mL/kg, or if a fraction of inspired oxygen of 0.70 was used with a tidal volume of 6 mL/kg. Two main features make older human studies different from more recent animal laboratory experiences: the patients described in the original case reports were typically paralyzed, and the rescuer hyperventilated to the point of feeling dizzy, an arterial partial pressure of CO_2 of about 20 mmHg *(10)*. These differences highlight the need for more controlled human studies before recommending withholding mouth-to-mouth ventilation during CA.

However an important factor might affect the feasibility of such studies: a widespread fear of acquiring contagious diseases from victims of CA that has recently resulted in reluctance among the lay public, and even some health professionals, to perform mouth-to-mouth ventilation.

Infectious disease concerns published in the literature include *Helicobacter pylori*, *Salmonella*, *Herpes simplex* virus, tuberculosis, HIV, and the hepatitides *(171–174)*. Being repulsed by the sight of a victim in agony and the fear of doing harm may also affect the decision to provide mouth-to-mouth ventilation. Recent surveys of CPR instructors reported that all would perform mouth-to-mouth ventilation on a 4-year-old drowned child, but only 54% on a college student, 35% on a hemophiliac, 18% on a stranger in a bus in San Francisco, and 10% on a person who had overdosed on heroin *(175,176)*. Awareness of new infectious disease issues, if not new infectious diseases, has resulted in the current recommendation of the AHA to use barrier devices to protect the rescuer against contamination with any infective secretions *(174)*. Effective barriers against contamination increase efficacy and effectiveness of CPR, helping the rescuer to overcome fear of contamination and to start resuscitation immediately. However, the overall willingness to perform bystander CPR is disappointingly low in the United States, Europe, and Japan, both for lay bystanders and health care providers alike. Different reasons are likely responsible for this widespread attitude. In the United States and Europe, the factor deterring performance of mouth-to-mouth ventilation by a bystander or health care provider is fear of contracting infectious diseases. This does not seem to be the case in Japan, where unwillingness to perform mouth-to-mouth ventilation is mostly a result of lack of confidence in one's ability to properly perform CPR *(177)*. The difference may be related to the 200-fold lower incidence of HIV in Japan, as compared with the United States *(178)*.

Education and increased retention of proper mouth-to-mouth ventilation technique is fundamental but difficult to apply to all populations. The use of television spots as a means of teaching basic skills of CPR in at-risk populations has been explored in Brazil. Although television spots seem to increase skill retention over 1 year, mouth-to-mouth ventilation and effective external cardiac compression are recognized as skills that are dependent on supervised practice with mannequins. Although the study is limited, it makes sense to use an alternative methodology to promote resuscitation skills in the lay population, including the use of educational clips or scenarios in entertaining and motivating television spots *(179)*.

Although recent evidence-based literature acknowledges the importance and efficacy of CPR without ventilation, the need for assisted ventilation in CA with asphyxia (CA primarily resulting from respiratory arrest) or in pediatric populations (generally younger than 8 years of age) cannot be overemphasized *(180)*. CA with asphyxia was originally illustrated in the first case of external chest compressions *(181)*. The rationale of ventilation during CPR for CA is based on the assumption that CPR delays brain death in no-flow situations, and that hypoxia and respiratory acidosis can aggravate the injury. A critical decrease of brain ATP of 25% below the normal level has been observed after 4 minutes in an animal model of decapitated normothermic dog *(182)*.

In general, arterial partial pressure of oxygen is maintained within the normal range for approx 1 minute in a dog model of chest compressions without ventilation *(183)*. Furthermore, when asphyxia is the cause of CA, oxygen consumption has proceeded to near complete exhaustion, and CO_2 and lactate have significantly accumulated just before CA. This is in contrast with VF, in which hypoxemia and acidemia become significant only several minutes after the onset of CA. In a model of resuscitation after asphyxia (clamping of the ETT in an anesthetized pig), the animal subjects were randomly selected to receive resuscitation with and without simulated mouth-to-mouth ventilation. Return of spontaneous circulation was noted only when ventilation was added to chest compression *(184)*. Successful chest compressions and mouth-to-mouth rescue breathing allowed complete neurological recovery in 90% of the animals.

The presence of a foreign body obstructing the airway is an uncommon, but important, cause of CA with asphyxia, with an incidence of 0.65 to 0.9 per 100,000 CAs *(185)*. A recent study seems to support the original investigation of Ruben and MacNaughton *(186)*, in that abdominal thrust is not necessary in foreign body choking, and that chest compressions can achieve higher airway pressure than the Heimlich maneuver *(187)*. In fact, when CPR was performed and compared with an abdominal thrust in the cadaver, median and peak airway pressure (PAP) reached a value of 30 cm H_2O vs 18 cm H_2O and 41 cm H_2O vs 26 cm H_2O, respectively. The mean airway pressure produced by the Heimlich maneuver was higher than that produced with chest compression only in a moderately obese cadaver. The European Resuscitation Council (ERC) has recently addressed acute asphyxia from airway obstruction *(188)*.

Despite recent knowledge that occurrence of VF in children may be more frequent than previously thought *(189)*, asphyxia is still the most common cause of CA in the pediatric population. The Pediatric Resuscitation Subcommittee of the Emergency Cardiovascular Care Committee of the AHA worked with the Neonatal Resuscitation Program Steering Committee (American Academic of Pediatrics) and the Pediatric Working Group of the International Liaison Committee on Resuscitation to review recommendations on oxygenation and ventilation in neonatal resuscitation *(190)*. The approach to the recommendations has been the same as that described in the AHA Guidelines 2000 for adults, which uses five classes of recommendations centered on evidence-based medical data. Up to 10% of newborn infants require resuscitation at birth. The majority, because of meconium airway obstruction/aspiration, require immediate intervention and assisted ventilation. Because of their unique physiology, the importance of ventilation/oxygenation in newborns cannot be overemphasized. Fluid-filled lungs and intracardiac as well as extracardiac shunts at birth are physiologically reversed in the first few minutes of extrauterine life with either spontaneous or assisted vigorous chest expansion. Failure to normalize this function may result in persistence of right-to-left, intracardiac and extracardiac shunt, pulmonary hypertension, and systemic cyanosis. Bradycardia usually follows, with severe hemodynamic instability and rapid deterioration to CA. Although these physiologic characteristics are typical of the newborn (minutes to hours after birth), similar events can be triggered by hypoxia in neonates (first 28 days of life) and infants (up to 12 months of age). The importance of proper ventilation/oxygenation and the small margin of safety resulting from the unique physiology and high oxygen consumption of the newborn mandate the need for immediate ventilation and the presence of skilled personnel at the bedside to perform proper basic steps of resuscitation. Clearance of meconium fluid should be the immediate maneuver performed on birth and providing PPV should be considered within 30 seconds when bradycardia or apnea is present. Tracheal intubation remains the gold standard for providing immediate ventilation/oxygenation to the newborn. European and American guidelines have essentially the same sequence of resuscitative events in neonates, recommending a chest compression-to-ventilation ratio of 3:1, with about 90 compressions and 30 bpm with emphasis on quality of ventilation and compressions *(191)*. In young patients up to 8 years of age, the airway patency, breathing, and circulation approach to CPR sequencing was not modified, reflecting a 5:2 compression-to-ventilation ratio. Moreover, the importance of immediate, aggressive management of the airway and ventilation in this group of patients has been reaffirmed ("go fast 911" instead of "call first 911").

In summary, at the time of this writing ventilation remains essential in CA with asphyxia in both adult and pediatric patients. However, the need for immediate ventilation in dysrhythmic CA in adults is less clear. Although it is clear that future studies are needed to address whether mouth-to-mouth ventilation during CA is any better than chest compression without ventilation and the best "exhaled" volume to be provided to the victim, such large-scale studies in out-of-hospital CA appear unfeasible. Nevertheless, at the end of 2001, a panel of resuscitation experts summarized current recommendations for the Action Sequence for the Layperson during Cardiopulmonary Resuscitation concluding that the current status of knowledge in CPR de-emphasizes the need for ventilation in the immediate period after adult CA *(192)*.

Positive Pressure Ventilation in an Unprotected Airway: The Problem of Gastric Insufflation and Pulmonary Aspiration

Manual techniques of ventilation used for rescue breathing were in widespread use from the early 1900s to the early 1960s, when they were replaced with mouth-to-mouth ventilation. Although manual techniques were capable of providing reasonably good tidal volume and minute ventilation in patients with patent airways, a major drawback was that prevention of upper airway obstruction was not an integral part of the technique, and airway obstruction could prevent movement of air. The principle advantage of mouth-to-mouth ventilation is that providing an open airway through backward tilt of the head and lifting of the mandible is part of the technique. Also, because the provider is immediately aware of upper airway obstruction when increased resistance to ventilation is encountered, further steps can be taken to relieve the obstruction.

Upper airway obstruction in an unconscious patient is caused by occlusion of the oropharynx by the relaxed tongue. The base of the tongue is retracted against the posterior wall of the pharynx when the head is in a flexed position and occurs whether the patient is in a supine or prone position Extension of the head can relieve obstruction in most patients and the addition of forward displacement of the mandible and/or an oropharyngeal airway opens the airway completely in 88%–98% of subjects *(193–195)*. The back-pressure-arm-lift method produces a mean tidal volume of only 126 mL when the head is allowed to remain in a natural position. Tidal volume increases to 520 mL with extension of the head and only one of six subjects studied (17%) had a tidal volume that was less than dead space *(195)*.

Unlike manual techniques of ventilation that produce negative intrathoracic pressure to move air into the lungs, mouth-to-mouth ventilation uses positive pressure to inflate the lungs. Because air under pressure can flow into the esophagus as well as the trachea, a frequent complication of mouth-to-mouth ventilation is gastric insufflation. Peak inflation pressure is directly related to the product of inspiratory flow rate and airway resistance. Delivering a large tidal volume over a brief inspiratory time results in increased peak inflation pressure and leads to gastric insufflation and hypoventilation in victims with an unprotected (not intubated) airway. Delivered volume to the lungs can be

increased by using a longer duration of inspiration and a lower inspiratory flow rate
(196). The pressure necessary to move gas into the lungs depends on airway resistance
and total thoracic compliance, which is equal to the sum of chest and lung compliance:

Compliance (L/cm H_2O) = change in volume (L)/change in pressure (cm H_2O)

Lung compliance decreases with decreasing lung volume and the tidal volume necessary to prevent decreased compliance is approx 7 mL/kg of body weight in patients with
normal lungs. Lung compliance also is decreased by pulmonary edema and atelectasis.
Chest compliance is decreased by kyphoscoliosis, scleroderma, obesity, and the supine
position.

Chest compression has been shown to affect compliance during CA and compliance
decreases with each minute of chest compression *(197)*. Compliance becomes a crucial
factor for ventilation when the upper airway is not intubated. Because the trachea,
pharynx, and esophagus are all exposed to the same positive pressure during mouth-to-
mouth ventilation, or bag-mask ventilation, air could preferentially enter the stomach
via the esophagus. During CA and CPR, chest compliance decreases and thus greater
pressure is needed to inflate the lungs adequately. At the same time, lower esophageal
sphincter tone decreases during CA and there is less resistance for air to enter the
stomach *(198)*.

Work done in anesthetized patients found that the pressure needed to produce gastric
insufflation ranged from 10 to 35 cm H_2O with a face mask technique of ventilation and
the most frequent pressure needed for insufflation was 15 cm H_2O *(199)*. Regurgitation
of gastric contents and pulmonary aspiration does not occur with chest compressions
alone, but requires inflation of the stomach *(200,201)*. Mouth-to-mouth ventilation was
shown to cause regurgitation in 48% of patients, probably because of gastric insufflation
(201). In a study of nonsurvivors of CA, 46% were found to have full stomachs and at least
29% had evidence of pulmonary aspiration of gastric contents *(202)*. Similar complications occur with the use of a bag-mask ventilation device in patients with unprotected
airways *(203)*. Aside from pulmonary aspiration of gastric contents, gastric insufflation,
if sufficient, causes elevation and splinting of the diaphragm with consequent loss of lung
volume, decreased compliance, hypoventilation, and greater risk of further gastric insufflation. Gastric insufflation can be prevented in many patients by applying pressure over
the cricoid to seal off the esophagus *(203)*. Additionally, spontaneous techniques of
ventilation would not be expected to produce gastric insufflation because inspiratory
airflow is caused by negative airway pressure and airflow during expiration is associated
with very low airway pressures of approx 0–1 cm H_2O.

Effectiveness and safety of ventilation of the unprotected airway have been studied
extensively in bench models. When a mechanical ventilator was used to provide tidal
volumes of 500 mL and 1000 mL, respectively, in an in vitro model of an unprotected
airway, significantly less stomach inflation was found when applying a smaller tidal
volume (approx 500 mL) with a mechanical ventilator compared with a tidal volume of
approx 1000 mL *(206)*. For the same reason, the use of a smaller, pediatric, self-inflating
bag delivering a maximal volume of 500 mL showed less gastric inflation in the same
model when compared with the large adult bag *(170,207)*. All of these studies suggest
that when the PAP exceeds lower esophageal sphincter pressure during ventilation of an
unprotected airway, the stomach is likely to be inflated. As a result, a tidal volume of
6 to 7 mL/kg body weight (approx 500 mL) and an inspiratory time of 1.2–2 seconds was

recommended by the ERC in 1998 and, later, by the International Guidelines 2000 for CPR and Emergency Cardiovascular Care, as long as oxygen supplementation is available *(185,208)*.

The performance of the apparatus used to deliver bag-valve mask (BVM) ventilation has recently been reviewed extensively. Seven commercially available models of ventilating bags used on an advanced cardiac life support training mannequin connected to an artificial lung in which compliance and resistance were set at normal have been evaluated regarding the tidal volume provided *(209)*. Interestingly, standard ventilations with one hand averaged a tidal volume between 450 to 600 mL in both genders despite significant differences in the size of male and female hands. When the technique was modified to open palm and total squeezing of the self-inflating bag against the flexed rescuer's knee, next to the patient's head, total volume ranged from 888 to 1192 mL. This study seems to indicate that most of the commercially available ventilating bags can provide both the 5 mL/kg and 12 mL/kg volume ventilation, as recommended by the new BLS guidelines, with and without available oxygen in a reliable manner. However, this study was performed on a mannequin with normal compliance and resistance, and gastric inflation was not measured.

When ventilation is provided to a victim of CA, proper tidal volume cannot be easily assessed. Excitement and over enthusiasm of the professional rescuer at the scene of CA can increase the chance of unnecessary gastric inflation *(210)*. In a recent, intriguing paper from Austria, it was shown that the stomach inflation of the victim, as assessed by postresuscitation chest radiograph, was minimal and statistically lower (15%) when the lay bystander provided mouth-to-mouth ventilation vs when professional paramedics ventilated the victim with a BVM device *(211)*. There are many possible explanations for these results, which are related partially to the limitation of the chest radiograph as a test to assess gastric inflation and the lack of autopsy reports from the nonsurviving victims. However, it is also possible that "extreme efficiency" of ventilation by the paramedics as compared with the bystander's mouth-to-mouth ventilation determined the difference. This finding, combined with the observation that professional rescuers tend to squeeze the bag very rapidly during the excitement of CPR (generally in <0.5 seconds and with power), suggests the need for better teaching of basic manual resuscitation skills *(207)*.

Limiting the size of the ventilating bag to a pediatric volume could theoretically decrease the danger of delivering an exaggerated tidal volume during CPR. However, if oxygen is not available at the scene of an emergency and small tidal volumes are given during BLS ventilation with a pediatric self-inflatable bag and room air (21% oxygen), insufficient oxygenation and/or inadequate ventilation may result. A recent study was done of 80 patients who were randomly allocated to receive ventilation with either an adult (maximum volume = 1500 mL) or pediatric (maximum volume = 700 mL) self-inflatable bag for 5 minutes although apneic after induction of general anesthesia and before intubation. The study used ventilation with 40% O_2 and showed no significant difference in mean arterial O_2 saturation (98% vs 97%) or $ETCO_2$ (26 vs 33 mm Hg) with the adult or pediatric bag, respectively *(212)*. The investigators did a follow-up study using the same methodology, but this time they used room air instead of 40% O_2 as the ventilating gas *(213)*. When using an adult (*N* = 20) vs pediatric (*N* = 20) self-inflatable bag, tidal volumes and tidal volumes per kilogram (mean ± standard error) were significantly larger (719 ± 22 mL/kg vs 455 ± 23 mL/kg and 10.5 ± 0.4 mL/kg vs

6.2 ± 0.4 mL/kg, respectively; $p < 0.0001$). Compared with an adult self-inflatable bag, BVM ventilation with room air using a pediatric self-inflatable bag resulted in lower arterial PO_2 values (73 ± 4 mmHg vs 87 ± 4 mmHg; $p < 0.01$) but comparable CO_2 elimination (40 ± 2 mmHg vs 37 ± 1 mmHg; not significant), indicating that smaller tidal volumes of about 6 mL/kg (approx 500 mL) given with a pediatric self-inflatable bag and room air maintain adequate CO_2 elimination but decrease oxygenation during simulated BLS ventilation. This study confirms previous observations that if small (6 mL/kg) tidal volumes are used during BLS ventilation when oxygen is not available, larger tidal volumes of about 10–12 mL/kg should be used to maintain both sufficient oxygenation and CO_2 elimination *(170)*.

Both the ERC and the AHA recommend using a smaller tidal volume during BVM ventilation to minimize stomach inflation when the airway is unprotected, provided that supplemental oxygen is available *(185,208)*.

Proper mask ventilation is a fundamental skill of resuscitation and should receive a high priority in training of both adult and pediatric providers *(214,215)*. Using recommended guidelines for tidal volume and inspiratory time, pulmonary ventilation can be maximized and gastric inflation can be minimized. However, gastric inflation and pulmonary aspiration can be totally prevented only when the airway is protected with endotracheal intubation, always regarded as the "gold standard" of providing ventilation during CPR.

Ventilation Caused by Chest Compression: Standard and Active Chest Compression–Decompression

When the chest is pressed with the hands or a mechanical device, intrathoracic pressure increases above atmospheric pressure and air flows out of the lungs if the upper airway is unobstructed. Air flows back into the lungs when pressure on the chest is released and the thorax recoils passively creating negative intrathoracic pressure. Although the tidal volume caused by chest compression usually is less than dead space, effective gas exchange can take place under certain conditions, particularly if the frequency of compression is high enough.

Knowledge of dead space is helpful in understanding high frequency ventilation. Inhaled air passes through the conducting airways to the alveoli in which gas exchange takes place. The conducting airways (the nose, mouth, pharynx, larynx, trachea, bronchi, and bronchioles) do not participate in gas exchange and have a volume, termed anatomic dead space, of about 150–180 mL in the adult human *(1)*. The total volume of alveoli not perfused with blood and thus not participating in gas exchange is called alveolar dead space. Physiologic dead space is the sum of anatomic and alveolar dead space, and is the volume of the lung that does not eliminate CO_2. Physiological dead space is a functional measurement, approx 2.2 mL/kg of lean body weight. Physiologic dead space increases during conditions of ventilation–perfusion inequality. During conventional ventilation, tidal volume must exceed physiologic dead space for effective delivery of O_2 and elimination of CO_2. During high-frequency ventilation, gas exchange can take place when tidal volume is less than physiologic dead space presumably because of enhanced diffusion and mixing of gases.

Ventilation caused by chest compression is a form of high-frequency ventilation (HFV), which is defined as lung ventilation at a frequency of at least four times the normal breathing frequency, usually with tidal volumes less than anatomical dead space *(216)*.

Gas exchange depends on several mechanisms, including bulk flow of gases, molecular diffusion, asymmetric velocity profiles in which the profile is direction dependent, cardiogenic mixing, mixing caused by turbulent airflow, and interregional "pendelluft" as a result of time-constant inequalities, which results in gas from fast-filling lung units redistributing into slow-filling units (216,217).

HFV has been produced by applying external pressure to the chest by means of a pressure cuff around the thorax. In a canine experiment, HFV using chest compression with tidal volumes of approx 50 mL and frequencies of 3–5 Hz (180–300 compressions per minute) produced better arterial oxygenation and elimination of CO_2 than conventional ventilation at standard tidal volumes and rate (218). The effectiveness of HFV depends on where compression is applied to the body. One study found that it is more effective when applied to the abdomen (219). HFV was found to have equally efficient gas exchange when applied at the trachea or the chest (220) and provided enhanced ventilation in a model of airway obstruction (221–223). Adequate gas exchange can take place with tidal volumes as low as 12% of dead space (224).

There is a striking similarity between HFV with chest compression and chest compression during CA. The recommended frequency of chest compression during CPR is approx 2 Hz (100 compressions per minute). If obstruction of the upper airway can be prevented, then tidal volume can be produced during sternal compression. In an intubated swine CA model, a study showed that sternal compression with a mechanical device-produced ventilation with a mean tidal volume of 45 mL during the first minute of resuscitation and decreased to 16 mL during the tenth minute. Because chest compressions were given at a rate of 100 per minute, minute ventilation was 4.5 L during the first minute of resuscitation and 1.6 L during the tenth minute. However, when compared with conventional ventilation, CO_2 elimination was less with chest compression ventilation resulting in significantly greater hypercarbic acidosis (204).

Active compression–decompression CPR is a recently developed technique of chest compression in which force is applied to the chest during both downward compression and upward lifting by means of a suction cup applied to the chest. Thus, the chest is re-expanded actively with this technique instead of passively recoiling as in conventional CPR. It has been shown that during CPR thorax and lung compliance gradually decrease over time and would explain, in part, why ventilation produced by conventional chest compression decreases over a 10-minute period. Active compression–decompression CPR may overcome the loss of compliance because the chest is forcibly re-expanded. In another swine study of CPR, active compression–decompression chest compression was compared with conventional chest compression (205). The tidal volume and minute ventilation caused by active compression–decompression were twice that of standard chest compression, did not decrease during 10 minutes of CPR, and produced significantly better arterial pH, PO_2, and PCO_2.

An interesting recent application has been the use of adjunct CPAP and pressure support ventilation (CPAP–PSV) during the decompression phase. In a swine model of CA CPAP-PSV showed a significantly higher PaO_2 and lower A-aDO_2, maintaining moderate hypercarbia when compared with the control animals. Remarkably, an unexplained increase of VO_2 was observed in all the animals with applied CPAP–PSV (225). Further studies are necessary to determine if ventilation with active compression–decompression CPR is as effective as preliminary results suggest and as effective as conventional ventilation in terms of survival from CA.

Current Standards for Ventilation During CPR
and Adjunct Devices for Ventilation

The AHA, in cooperation with the NRC, has developed and set training standards and guidelines for CPR and emergency cardiac care *(226)*. Control of the airway during CPR is divided into three general categories: basic airway management, advanced airway control, and postresuscitation airway management.

Basic management of the airway entails establishing unresponsiveness, calling for help, opening the airway with various maneuvers, maintenance of airway patency, determination of breathlessness, and provision of ventilation and oxygenation in conjunction with chest compression. Advanced airway control requires endotracheal intubation and use of ancillary equipment to support ventilation and oxygenation. Following successful resuscitation, the patient may remain supported by endotracheal intubation and mechanical ventilation.

BASIC AIRWAY MANAGEMENT

Basic airway management is indicated for patients who suffer respiratory and/or CA. Primary respiratory arrest may occur during drowning, foreign body obstruction, smoke inhalation, drug overdose or anaphylactic reaction, cerebrovascular accident, thermal or electrical injury, trauma, acute myocardial infarction, epiglottitis, sepsis, and coma of whatever cause. Early initiation of rescue breathing may improve survival and prevent CA.

The goal of basic airway management is to provide enough oxygen to the brain and heart until definitive medical treatment can restore normal heart and ventilatory activity *(226)*. Rescue breathing brings oxygen into the lungs although chest compression promotes oxygen transport from the lungs to vital tissues. Immediate initiation of resuscitation is necessary because the highest rate and quality of survival are achieved when BLS is started within 4 minutes from the time of arrest and when advanced cardiac life support is initiated within 8 minutes *(227)*.

Provision and Maintenance of a Patent Upper Airway

The maneuvers utilized to provide a patent upper airway in an unconscious patient are designed primarily to relieve obstruction by the tongue gravitating toward the posterior pharyngeal wall. Relaxation of the head and neck muscles supporting the mandible during loss of consciousness results in the loss of the tongue's muscular tone. When the tongue falls against the posterior pharynx, it causes upper airway obstruction. Airway obstruction is aggravated in a comatose patient by a semiflexed neck, which causes narrowing of the distance from the tongue to the posterior pharynx. The epiglottis also tends to fall back onto the glottis. Furthermore, breathing against an obstructed upper airway pulls the tongue toward the airway, worsening the obstruction. The negative pressure generated in the airway during inspiration causes a ball valve type of tracheal obstruction. Even in normal, spontaneously breathing anesthetized patients, some airway obstruction occurs in 90% when the head is in neutral position and the airway is unsupported *(193)*.

Unless contraindicated, the victim should be positioned properly, before resuscitation is initiated: a firm, flat surface, and the arms alongside the body, is preferred. The patient's head should be below the level of the thorax. If the victim is prone, the patient should be moved supine as a unit to avoid twisting the head neck or back. The rescuer should kneel beside the patient's shoulder. Spontaneous breathing should be ascertained.

Several maneuvers are utilized to open the airway. In Europe, it is taught that breathing should be ascertained in the position the victim is found. The victim is positioned supine if respirations cannot be assessed or if absent.

HEAD TILT–CHIN LIFT MANEUVER

In the absence of head and neck trauma, the head tilt–chin lift maneuver is utilized to open the airway (228). This maneuver is also referred to as the "sniffing position" and is considered to be the most effective method of opening the airway of an unconscious victim. A roll or towel may be placed under the victim's occiput to maintain this position. The victim's mouth should be examined for dentures and debris. A piece of cloth is used to wipe out fluid or semiliquid material. Solid materials are removed with a hooked index finger. Dentures may be left in place to maintain a normal facial shape, facilitating adequate lip seal and mouth-to-mouth breathing. However, if dentures obstruct the airway, they must be removed. One hand is placed on the patient's forehead and the head is tilted backward with a firm pressure. The fingers of the other hand are positioned firmly beneath the chin's bony portion, lifting it upward. This brings the chin forward and the teeth almost to occlusion, supporting the jaw and helping to tilt the head backward. Pressure on the soft tissue under the chin should be avoided because it can aggravate airway obstruction. Unless mouth-to-nose breathing is indicated, the mouth should not be completely closed. During mouth-to-nose breathing, the mouth can be closed by increasing the pressure on the hand that is already on the chin. This technique is the recommended maneuver of choice because of its simplicity, safety, effectiveness, and ease of learning. The maneuver was found to be superior in opening the airway during mouth-to-mouth resuscitation of apneic patients, achieving airway patency in 91% of cases vs 78% with the jaw thrust and 39% with simple neck lift (229). Greater tidal volume was also delivered during head tilt–chin lift maneuver when compared to other techniques.

In pediatric victims, airway patency is also established by maintaining the head in the sniffing position. However, direct pressure on the trachea or hyperextension of the head should be avoided. The pediatric trachea is not yet fully developed and does not have a well-formed rigid cartilaginous ring. Any direct or indirect pressure on this structure causes it to collapse.

JAW-THRUST MANEUVER

The angles of the mandible may be displaced anteriorly by grasping the lower jaw with both hands from one side and pulling forward, and simultaneously tilting the head backwards. The elbows of the CPR provider should rest on the surface where the patient is lying. To open the lips, the lower lip can be retracted with the thumb. Mouth-to-mouth breathing can be delivered by occluding the victim's nostrils with the rescuer's cheek pressed tightly against them. To avoid extension of the neck in patients with suspected neck injury, a modified jaw thrust maneuver is performed. Forward traction is applied on the mandible without head tilt and care must be observed to avoid moving the head from side to side. If this maneuver is unsuccessful in opening the airway, careful slight tilting of the head may be done. Although jaw-thrust maneuver is highly effective in providing upper airway patency, the technique may be technically problematic and the rescuer tires easily. It is considered as an ancillary method and is utilized as a secondary method by professional rescuers.

TRIPLE AIRWAY MANEUVER

This is a modification of the head tilt–chin lift maneuver whereby the lower lip is retracted with the thumb to open the mouth after tilting the head backward and lifting the chin upward. This maneuver is usually utilized by a more experienced rescuer.

MANDIBULAR DISPLACEMENT

Another method to open the upper airway is to pull the mandible forward by placing the rescuer's thumb in the patient's mouth and put the fingers underneath the chin to pull the lower jaw upward. Although effective in opening the airway in spontaneously breathing, edentulous patients, it can cause injury to the rescuer if the patient wakes up and suddenly bites on the rescuer's thumb.

Determination of Breathlessness

There are several recommended methods of determining the absence of spontaneous breathing in an unconscious patient. Spontaneous respiration may be difficult to observe unless the airway is opened. Once airway patency is established, the rescuer should place his or her ear over the victim's mouth and nose. The rise and fall of the chest should be noted. One must listen for breath sounds and feel for expired air. The absence of these signs is indicative of apnea. Occasionally, a gasping sound or agonal respiration may be observed during CA. This is not sustained and should not be mistaken for spontaneous respiration. In some instances, the victim may show respiratory efforts but no air exchange is observed. This indicates upper airway obstruction and opening the airway facilitates resumption of air movement.

Once spontaneous respiration and pulse are established during resuscitation, the CPR provider should continue maintaining a patent airway. To reduce the likelihood of aspiration and obstruction, the patient should be rolled on his or her side. This is called the recovery position. The victim must be rolled as a unit, moving the head, shoulders and torso simultaneously without twisting. However, if trauma is suspected, the patient should not be moved unless absolutely necessary. There are several options on how the dependent arm may be placed in the recovery position: (a) it may be bent at the elbow and placed alongside the victim and the other hand rests under the cheek of the victim; (b) the dependent arm may be alongside the victim; or (c) the dependent arm may be bent at the elbow with the hand under the face. The fundamental goal of the recovery position is to have the patient on their side so that aspiration and accidental airway obstruction is prevented.

Initiation of Respiration (Rescue Breathing)

Delivery of an adequate tidal volume is required during rescue breathing. Usually, 700–1000 mL of tidal volume is considered adequate for an adult. Of course, it is difficult for the rescuer to know exactly how much tidal volume is given during mouth-to-mouth ventilation. Therefore, it is recommended that the rescuer give enough tidal volume with each breath to make the chest rise visibly.

The oxygen concentration of expired air is approx 16%–17%. With this oxygen concentration, the maximum alveolar oxygen partial pressure is about 80 mmHg, enough to meet the victim's oxygen need. It is recommended that two initial breaths should each be delivered over 2 seconds. Sufficient time should be allowed for exhalation between breaths. Using this longer inspiratory time (2 seconds), and therefore a lower inspiratory flow rate, reduces the chances of exceeding esophageal sphincter opening pressure, thereby decreasing the chance of gastric distention, the most common major problem associated with rescue breathing. Gastric distention elevates the diaphragm, reduces lung volume, and promotes regurgitation and aspiration. Sellick's maneuver, the application of cricoid pressure against the cervical vertebra, helps prevent regurgitation against esophageal pressure of up to 100 cm of water. However, this technique requires an assistant and is only recommended to trained professionals. If regurgitation is observed during CPR, the victim's entire body should be turned to the side and the mouth wiped clean. The patient is then turned back to supine position and CPR is resumed. Additionally, excessive PAPs may be generated during exhaled oxygenation (rescue breathing), increasing the risk of barotrauma.

BLS-CPR can be performed either by one or two rescuers. During both one- and two-rescuer CPR, two slow breaths are given during a pause after every 15 chest compressions. Exhalation occurs passively after each breath and during chest compression. Rescue breathing can be delivered through mouth-to-mouth, mouth-to-nose, mouth-to-stoma, and mouth-to-barrier devices.

After opening the airway by the head tilt–chin lift maneuver, the rescuer can seal the nose by pinching it with the thumb and index finger of the hand on the victim's forehead. The rescuer breathes deeply and puts his or her lips around the patient's mouth, creating an airtight seal. Two slow breaths are delivered at a chest compression to ventilation ratio of 15:2 with one- or two-rescuer CPR; the ratio is changed to 5:1 in the pediatric victim (less than 8 years old). Upward movement of the chest and sensing the escape of air during exhalation assure the rescuer that adequate ventilation has been delivered. *The most common cause of failure to ventilate is improper positioning of the head and chin.* If attempts to ventilate fail, the patient's head and chin should be repositioned. If after repositioning, the patient cannot be ventilated, evaluation of the airway for foreign bodies should be performed. These maneuvers will be discussed later in this chapter. Also, it should be emphasized that pauses for ventilation pertain only to subjects with an unprotected airway (i.e., unintubated). Once the airway is intubated, ventilation and chest compressions are given asynchronously without interruption of chest compressions. Chest compression is given at a rate of 100 per minute with about 10–15 bpm. Recent studies suggest that fewer breaths may improve blood flow during shock or CA and provide a better ventilation to perfusion match. This is an important area of active investigation and randomized, controlled trials are currently being planned.

If it is difficult or contraindicated to deliver mouth-to-mouth breathing, mouth-to-nose breathing can be performed. It is indicated in patients with mouth trauma, trismus, or in those in which a tight mouth-to-mouth seal is impossible to achieve. After the head is properly positioned and the mouth closed (as previously described), the rescuer inhales deeply, puts his or her mouth in a tight seal around the victim's nose, and breathes out into it. The rescuer then removes his or her lips from the patient's nose and lets exhalation occur passively. The mouth may also be opened after breath delivery to allow air to escape through the mouth.

If the patient has a previous laryngectomy and has a permanent opening connecting the trachea to the front base of the neck, ventilation during CPR can be performed by delivering the breath through the stomal opening. In a similar fashion to mouth-to-mouth or mouth-to-nose breathing, the rescuer's mouth puts a tight seal around the stoma and two deep breaths are delivered. When the rescuer stops breathing into the stoma, air passively escapes from the opening.

The presence of vomitus and fear of infectious contamination may affect the willingness of rescuers to perform mouth-to-mouth resuscitation. Lawrence and Sivaneswaran showed that only 13% of 70 hospital staff members surveyed would use mouth-to-mouth ventilation and 59% would prefer to do mouth-to-mask ventilation (230). Specialized masks with a one-way valve are currently utilized during CPR. The valve prevents the exhaled air from entering the rescuer's mouth. Additionally, bacterial filters are incorporated in some of the commercially available masks to prevent contamination of the rescuer. Also, some resuscitation masks are capable of delivering as much as 50% oxygen (230). Mouth-to-mask ventilation can provide adequate tidal volume at a significantly lower airway pressure when compared to mouth-to-mouth resuscitation (9). Other barrier devices such as face shields are also available. Unlike the masks, many face shields do not have a one-way valve and air may leak around the shield. If a barrier device is used during rescue breathing, it must be placed tightly around the patient's mouth and slow, deep breaths should be delivered in a manner similar to mouth-to-mouth ventilation.

CPR occurring in the hospital setting is often managed initially with BVM ventilation. There are studies reporting this device incapable of delivering adequate tidal volume when only one person is doing pulmonary resuscitation (231–234). The basic problem arises from the need to provide an adequate seal between the face and the mask although controlling the airway by head extension at the same time. Additionally, familiarity with the use of the equipment requires special training and additional manpower. It has been shown that this technique is more effective in delivering adequate ventilation when two rescuers are supporting the airway (234,235). One rescuer effectively seals the mask to the mouth and maintains head extension and the other squeezes the bag with both hands to deliver adequate tidal volume. However, the central issue is that the individual providing BVM ventilation must be well trained in the proper use of this instrument before attempting to control the airway in an arrested patient for the first time.

Oxygen supplementation can be provided during BVM ventilation, delivering 40%–60% O_2 without and with an oxygen reservoir, respectively (236). Complications associated with the use of a BVM are primarily as a result of excessively high ventilating pressures including pneumothorax, pneumomediastinum, pneumocephalus, and gastric rupture (237). When oxygen is available, ventilation should be limited to approximately one-third of the total bag volume (about 600 mL in the 1.8 L adult bag) and delivered over 1–2 seconds; the recommended inspiratory time is a little faster because of the smaller tidal volume. Unless the rescuer is proficient in the use of anesthesia bags, it is preferable to use self-inflating hand held resuscitator bags during CPR. Anesthesia bags such as the Mapleson system (Mallinckrodt, St. Louis, MO) are not self-inflating and require a continuous oxygen source (238). Some resuscitator bags have a pressure relief valve, a safety feature designed to limit the maximum pressure that can be delivered thereby preventing gastric insufflation and hyperinflation of the lungs and subsequent pulmonary barotrauma. However, these valves may malfunction, and one must recognize that improper venting can cause inadequate ventilation. A functioning relief valve may be recognized by the sound of air escaping through the valve while squeezing the bag. Adjusting or partially occluding the valve may be lifesaving.

The basic principles governing rescue breathing of pediatric patients are the same as those of the adults. However, the pediatric airway may be flattened by excessive extension of the cervical spine during the head tilt–chin lift maneuver. In infants and smaller children, mouth-to-nose ventilation may be necessary during CPR. Smaller breaths must be used to avoid abdominal distention, regurgitation, and pulmonary barotrauma. Ventilation in the newborn needs special consideration. In fact, appropriate ventilation is essential for the survival of the newborn infant.

Although hypoxia before delivery can influence the time of successful resuscitation of a newborn, it is recommended that assessment of adequate ventilation should be done immediately and endotracheal intubation should be carried out within 30–60 seconds of birth *(239)*. This time should be reduced to 30 seconds or less in preterm babies, although no clear literature exists *(240)*. Trauma should be avoided by maintaining inflation volume at about 6 mL/kg *(241)*. Physiologic considerations in the newborn seem to confirm that this volume for resuscitation is probably adequate. It is known that a first breath using a medium tidal volume of 5 mL/kg is usually sufficient to achieve a functional residual capacity (FRC) lung volume almost immediately (reaching a total FRC volume of 28 to 30 mL/kg) *(242)*. Furthermore, it is possible that a small tidal volume would stimulate the newborn to spontaneously breathe through a reverse Hering-Breuer reflex (called head paradoxical reflex) *(243)*. This level of tidal volume and a real mask inflation pressure to less than 20 cm H_2O can usually limit gastric inflation *(244,245)*.

ADVANCED AIRWAY SUPPORT

Even if ventilation is provided during BLS, some degree of hypoxemia and hypercarbia will occur. Advanced airway management such as endotracheal intubation, provision of supplemental oxygen, and the use of adjunctive airway equipment should be instituted as soon as possible. The use of advanced airway support is designed to assure complete control of the airway, allow augmented ventilation, provide higher fraction of inspired oxygen, and isolate the trachea from the gastrointestinal tract.

Endotracheal Intubation

Endotracheal intubation is considered the gold standard against which all other means of airway control must be measured. However, the procedure requires training, familiarity, and skill to perform. Its use is limited to medical personnel who are highly trained and who either perform intubation frequently or are retrained frequently *(246)*. It is the preferred method of airway control because it isolates and maintains patency of the airway, allows optimal adjustment of tidal volume and respiratory rate, permits reliable addition of supplemental oxygen to the inspired gas, and protects the lungs from inhalation of gastric contents when the cuff is inflated with air to provide a seal around the trachea. Furthermore, it facilitates intermittent PPV, provides an alternative route for drug administration, and allows tracheal suctioning.

Intubation can either be performed by the orotracheal or nasotracheal route. Ventilation should not be interrupted more than 30 seconds during attempted intubation and adequate ventilation and oxygenation should be provided between attempts *(226)*. This procedure is indicated when the unconscious victim can not be ventilated with the initial maneuvers to control the airway, when the patient can no longer protect the airway either because of cardiopulmonary arrest, coma or areflexia, or when a conscious patient can not ventilate adequately.

OROTRACHEAL INTUBATION

Orotracheal intubation is the most commonly employed method of intubation. It can be performed easily and rapidly. Ideally, the procedure is best performed with the head of the patient at the level of the rescuer's xiphoid. The rescuer must hold the laryngoscope with the left hand. The victim's head is tilted back with the right hand. This maneuver automatically opens the victim's mouth. In some instances, the right hand may be placed inside the mouth to open the jaw using the cross finger technique. The thumb is used to depress the lower teeth and the index finger raises the upper teeth.

Once the mouth is opened, the laryngoscope blade is inserted at the right side along the groove between the tongue and the alveolar ridge. The tongue is pushed to the left side by the flange of the blade as it is gently and deliberately advanced. A curved blade is inserted up to the base of the tongue, with the tip of the blade resting on the vallecula. Gentle pressure on this structure opens the epiglottis and exposes the vocal cords. If a straight blade is used, the tip is used to lift the epiglottis. Once the particular blade is in position, the handle is pulled forward (toward the patient's feet), avoiding flexion of the wrist. This maneuver elevates the tongue, avoids teeth injury, maintains the larynx within sight, and allows for visualization of the vocal cords.

The ETT is inserted in the right side of the mouth just lateral to the laryngoscope. The tube is then advanced gently between the vocal cords. Direct visualization of the vocal cords and observing ETT passage through them is the best confirmation of proper tube placement. A stylet may be utilized to direct the tube into the larynx but should be removed as soon as the tube tip passes the cords. The tube is advanced several centimeters into the trachea beyond the disappearance of the cuff from view in the adult, and 2–4 centimeters in children. The laryngoscope blade is withdrawn and the ETT is attached to a resuscitator bag or a breathing circuit. The cuff is inflated with sufficient air to prevent an air leak. Chest movement should be observed during the delivery of the first manual breath. Observing the tube for "misting" during exhalation, bilateral auscultation for breath sounds over the axillary areas and over the epigastrium helps to confirm correct tube position. A CO_2 detection device may be of help if circulation is present. If "tube misting" is not noted, no breath sounds are heard, the chest does not move, and gurgling sounds are heard over the epigastrium, one must assume that the esophagus has been intubated and the ETT must be immediately pulled out. The victim should be adequately ventilated and oxygenated before a second attempt is made. If multiple attempts by the same operator are unsuccessful, a second, more experienced operator must take over, ensuring that the victim receives appropriate ventilation and oxygenation between attempts. Once proper tube placement has been confirmed, the tube is secured with tape to prevent accidental extubation. An oropharyngeal airway is placed in the mouth to prevent the patient from biting down on the tube. A chest x-ray should be done to confirm placement of the tube as soon as feasible and rule out any complication that may arise, such as mainstem intubation or pneumothorax (247).

Preferably, Sellick's maneuver (cricoid pressure) should be applied by an assistant during emergency intubation. Application of pressure on the anterolateral aspect of the cricoid cartilage with the thumb and the index finger provides protection against gastric regurgitation and aspiration of gastric contents. Excessive application of pressure should be avoided because it may distort the anatomy of the airway and may hinder endotracheal intubation. Pressure should be maintained until the tracheal cuff is inflated and the rescuer performing the intubation indicates that it is acceptable to release pressure.

Nasotracheal Intubation

Nasotracheal intubation is indicated in instances when oral intubation fails or is technically difficult to perform. It is also used in those with suspected cervical injury in which movement of the head may cause or aggravate spinal cord injury. The technique is more difficult to perform, takes longer, and is more traumatic. It can be performed blindly or with direct visualization in the field. It should be avoided in patients with basal skull fractures, bleeding diathesis, in anticoagulated patients, and those with nasal injuries.

If not contraindicated, the head and neck position of the victim during nasotracheal intubation by direct visualization are the same as for oral intubation. The rescuer stands immediately behind the victim's head. Preferably, the ETT should be lubricated during insertion to minimize trauma. The tube is inserted into the nostril with the bevel pointing toward the septum and then directed downward until it reaches the oropharynx. The mouth is then opened by extending the head or using the crossed-finger maneuver. A laryngoscope blade is inserted in the mouth in the same manner as described during orotracheal intubation. The ETT may be directed into the larynx and vocal cords by manipulating it from the top. Alternatively, a Magill forceps may be used to direct the tube toward the glottic opening. The forceps should be held in the right hand and the tube tip is gripped at a point just above the attachment of the cuff, so as not to damage the cuff. The tube is then gently advanced by an assistant although the operator directs the tube pass through the vocal cords. The laryngoscope blade and Magill forceps are then withdrawn. Once the tube is in place and secured, proper placement should be confirmed in the same way as with orotracheal intubation.

Blind nasotracheal intubation is utilized when direct visualization of the airway is technically difficult or impossible because the patient is unable to open the mouth, or when instrumentation of the oral cavity may result in damage to the teeth and surrounding tissues. To minimize epistaxis, the nose may be sprayed with a vasoconstrictor agent like phenylephrine or 4% cocaine, if available. With the patient in the supine position, the nose well prepared, and the tube well lubricated, the tube is placed in the nostril, gently advancing it to the oropharynx. The cervical spine may be flexed, the head extended and the mandible pulled upward with the left hand to facilitate tube insertion. If the victim has spontaneous breathing, the operator can lower his or her left ear over the ETT and listen for air movement as the ETT tip enters the upper airway as the tube is gently advanced into the trachea with the right hand. Often times, when the tube enters the airway, a breathing victim coughs and a tubular sound can be heard. This method of intubation does not always result in successful intubation during the first try and may require several attempts. The tube may be accidentally placed in the esophagus, vallecula, or either side of the piriform sinus. If the tube is not in place, it should be withdrawn back into the oropharynx and another attempt should be made. Palpation of the neck may help determine the direction of tube insertion. Evidence and confirmation of proper tube insertion should be done in the same manner as described during orotracheal intubation.

Once the trachea is successfully intubated by whatever route, the patient should be ventilated and supplemental oxygen should be provided. During CPR, it is ideal to provide a tidal volume of 10–15 mL/kg body weight, a respiratory rate of 10–12 bpm (one breath every 5–6 seconds) and 100% oxygen. A device for detecting CO_2 is often attached to the proximal part of the ETT to assure proper positioning of the tube. Absence of CO_2 indicates esophageal intubation. However, if the blood flow to the lungs is very low (as in CA), or when the alveolar dead space is great (as in massive pulmonary embolism), CO_2 may not be detectable.

It is also very important to know the appropriate tube size to use. Too large of a tube may result in a failed intubation or tracheal trauma; too small a tube may cause excessive gas leakage resulting in hypoventilation when an uncuffed tube is used, or excessive inflation pressure in a cuffed tube. Additionally, the work of breathing and airway resistance become markedly elevated if the tube size is inappropriate *(248)*. Tubes for pediatric patients are generally uncuffed and are based on age and size. Several easy formulas are used to calculate uncuffed tubes for children 6 years and younger. A tracheal tube one size above and below the calculated size should be immediately available to allow proper selection after the vocal cords are visualized. The following formula may be used:

$$Tube\ Size\ (ID\ in\ mm) = (18 + age/4)$$

The proper depth to which the tube should be inserted can also be calculated by several equations:

1. For oral intubation (the length of the tube from the alveolar ridge to the tip positioned in the midtrachea):

$$Tube\ Length\ (cm) = 12 + (age/2)$$

2. For nasal intubation (the length of the tube from the nostril to the tip positioned in the midtrachea):

$$Tube\ Length\ (cm) = 15 + (age/2)$$

The correct position of the tracheal tube tip should be approx 5 cm above the adult carina. Movement of the head may change the position of the tip. If the neck is extended from neutral position, the tube tip usually moves an average of 1.9 cm toward the pharynx. Flexion of the neck moves the tube a similar distance toward the carina. Lateral rotation moves the tube 0.7 cm away from the carina *(249)*. In pediatric patients, the length of the tracheal tube varies with age. ETT cuffs should be of the low-pressure high-volume type to prevent excessive application of pressure on the tracheal mucosa once the cuff is inflated.

Adjunctive Airway Equipment

Airway control may be facilitated with the use of adjunctive airway devices. This equipment is generally available to the rescuing paramedics or hospital personnel. It is mandatory that people using these devices are familiar with their use and potential problems. They should be regarded as a "bridge to" rather than "alternate to" endotracheal intubation.

OXYGEN SOURCE

Oxygen supplementation should be initiated as soon as possible during CPR by the trained rescuer to avoid the adverse effects of hypoxemia. If oxygen is inadequate, all other resuscitation efforts will fail; 100% oxygen should be utilized during resuscitation. If a pulse oximeter is available, it should be used to determine oxygen saturation.

Oxygen is generally stored either in liquid form or in cylinder reservoirs. A portable oxygen tank is color coded green in the United States. It is provided with a regulator and flowmeter. The regulator reduces the pressure to 50 psig for delivery to the flowmeter. Most emergency medical service (EMS) personnel carry the smaller E cylinder. This is pressurized to 1800 to 2400 psig at 70° F and 14.7 psig absolute pressure. The cylinder holds 659 liters of oxygen and lasts approx 1 hour when the flow rate is set at 10 liters per minute. Oxygen is considered a "drug," hence its use is regulated by health agencies in most states.

FACE MASKS

A pocket face mask is the simplest adjunct beyond mouth-to-mouth resuscitation. An ideal face mask should be colorless to provide direct visualization of the mouth, lips, nose, and the presence of vomitus or secretions. It should have a soft pliable edge to create an effective seal against the face. To assure proper ventilation, an airtight seal is necessary to avoid oxygen and air escaping during supportive ventilation. The mask should provide an oxygen inlet with a standard 15 mm to 22 mm coupling size. Various sizes should be available for adults and children. A reservoir bag with a one-way valve may be attached to the mask for manual ventilation of the lungs.

Face-mask placement is best achieved when the operator is positioned at the top of the patient's head. An airtight seal can be provided by single handed or double handed technique. Single-handed technique requires that the rescuer fits the mask snugly on the victim's face, using the thumb and the index finger in a pincer grip although simultaneously displacing the mandible upward and lifting the chin with the other three fingers. The middle finger should rest on the mandible, the ring finger is positioned midway between the chin and the angle of the jaw, and the little finger is on the mandibular angle. Pressure on the soft tissue should be avoided because it is uncomfortable and can lift the base of the tongue and can cause upper airway obstruction.

Mouth-to-mask ventilation can be achieved by the rescuer sealing his or her lips around the coupling adapter of the mask. If ventilation is inadequate or if airway obstruction is unrelieved, a double-handed technique should be utilized. The fingers are placed on the same position as the single handed method but applied on both sides of the face. However, a second rescuer is necessary to deliver exhaled or manual ventilation. Care must be observed to avoid pressure damage to the eyes and soft tissues.

MANUAL RESUSCITATORS (BAG-VALVE DEVICES)

Bag-valve devices of various designs are available for adults and children, but a self inflating, manually operated bag with a nonrebreathing valve is preferable because it allows ventilation even if there is no connecting oxygen supply. This device may be used in conjunction with a face-mask, ETT, or other invasive airway device.

The standard parts include a delivery port with a 15 mm to 22 mm adapter coupling size that can be connected to the mask or tracheal tube. It is provided with a one-way, nonjam valve that allows a minimum of 15 liters per minute oxygen flow rate for spontaneous and controlled ventilation. It should also have a system for delivering high oxygen concentration through an auxiliary oxygen inlet at the back of the bag or by an oxygen reservoir. A PEEP valve can also be incorporated. The bag should be a self-refilling one that can be readily cleaned and sterilized. The bag usually holds a volume of up to 1600 mL. Some pediatric resuscitator bags are provided with a 25–30 cm H_2O pop-off valve to avoid excessive CPAP. This device is expected to perform satisfactorily under all common environmental conditions and extremes of temperature.

To properly operate this equipment, the operator must be positioned at the top of the victim's head. After proper head positioning as previously described, appropriate tidal volume should be delivered (10–12 mL/kg in the intubated patient, 400–600 mL in the nonintubated patient) if oxygen is available over 1.5–2 seconds. An oropharyngeal airway may be used to open the mouth. A single rescuer may have difficulty maintaining head position and delivering adequate tidal volume at the same time. It is therefore recommended that two rescuers operate this device. One to hold an airtight seal over the face, the other to manually squeezes the bag. The proper use of this device requires training, practice and familiarity with the equipment.

ORAL AND NASAL AIRWAYS

The most common cause of airway obstruction in an unconscious victim is the falling back of the tongue into the back of the pharynx. If head positioning fails to correct the obstruction, the use of an oral or nasal airway may be indicated. These devices provide an artificial passage to airflow by separating the posterior pharyngeal wall from the tongue. An oral airway is preferred to a nasal airway in an unconscious person because it is easy to insert and less likely to cause trauma and bleeding. If the victim is conscious, it is preferable to use a nasal airway to prevent the patient from gagging vomiting or going into laryngospasm.

Oral airways are available as metallic, black rubber or plastic devices in the shape of an "S" or semicircular curve. There are various sizes suitable for pediatric and adult patients. An appropriate sized airway is one that holds the tongue in the normal anatomic position and follows its natural curvature. Its insertion is enhanced by the use of a tongue blade that depresses the tongue and moves it laterally. Improper placement may aggravate airway obstruction by pushing the tongue against the pharynx. It can also cause trauma to the teeth and surrounding structures.

Nasal airways are made of soft rubber or pliable plastic. They are uncuffed tubes approx 15 cm in length. This device is inserted via the naris into the posterior pharynx. It is tolerated better by conscious patients or when the oral route is inaccessible because of oral or lower facial fractures. Several age-appropriate sizes are available.

Insertion of a nasal airway requires a patent naris. The tube should be adequately lubricated to facilitate insertion. The use of a local vasoconstrictor is recommended to reduce the incidence of bleeding. The length of the nasal tube to be inserted can be approximated by measuring the distance from the nasal tip to the external auditory meatus. During insertion, the tip should be directed perpendicularly to the face and not upward toward the cribriform plate. The tube should be placed smoothly and deliberately; any resistance requires the tube to be gently rotated until no obstruction is felt. The ideal tip position should be at a point just above the epiglottis. The use of the nasal airway should be avoided in the presence of a coagulopathy, basal skull fracture, nasopharyngeal infection, or distorted nasopharyngeal anatomy. Problems associated with its use include epistaxis and nasopharyngeal trauma.

Two soft nasopharyngeal airways may be connected to a suitable 15-mm adapter to form a binasal-pharyngeal airway. It is inserted in both nares in a similar fashion as a single nasal airway. It should not be used in patients with a full stomach and should be used only by skilled medical personnel during difficult intubations or when more sophisticated devices are unavailable.

OXYGEN-POWERED MANUALLY TRIGGERED DEVICES

Oxygen-powered breathing devices have also been used by EMS personnel during CPR. These machines are expensive, and require high oxygen flow rates to overcome air leak *(230)*. Although they may be able to deliver adequate tidal volumes, oxygen-powered devices carry the risk of gastric distention and regurgitation. Most of these devices are time-cycled and deliver high instantaneous flow rates by a manual control button. They can be used in conjunction with a face mask, ETT, esophageal airway, or tracheostomy tube.

Parts of an oxygen-powered manually triggered device include a standard 15 mm/22 mm adapter coupling, a compact, rugged, break-resistant mechanical design that is easy to hold, and a trigger positioned so that both hands of the rescuer can remain on the face mask to hold it in position. It should also have the following characteristics: a constant flow rate of 100% oxygen at lesss than 40 liters per minute, and an inspiratory pressure relief valve that opens at approx 60 cm H_2O and vents any remaining volume to the atmosphere or ceases gas flow. Furthermore, an alarm sound system is provided to alert the rescuer that the pressure relief valve has been exceeded indicating that the patient requires high inflationary pressure and may not be receiving adequate tidal volume. It should be able to operate satisfactorily under common environmental conditions and extremes of temperature. It should be provided with a demand flow system that does not impose additional work *(226)*. These devices are contraindicated in children and spontaneously breathing patients. The potential for complications is high and its use requires training and familiarity.

Suction Devices

A suction apparatus is essential during advanced airway support. Suction may be provided by portable, battery operated or electrically powered equipment. In the hospital, wall vacuum outlets are available for suctioning. This device should be available during resuscitation prior to airway instrumentation. Vomitus, secretions, or blood may occlude the airway and can be aspirated into the lungs, compromising the ability to adequately ventilate and oxygenate the victim. In addition to a suction apparatus, a flexible catheter or a rigid tonsillar suction tip should be attached to large bore, nonkinking suction tubing that should be 14 French or greater internal diameter. A rigid tonsillar tip can rapidly suction particulate materials or large volumes of fluid from the pharynx. Flexible catheters are available in various sizes for children and adults and are used to decompress the stomach, suction the esophagus, pharynx, and ETT.

The wall suction units should provide airflow of more than 30 L per minute at the end of the delivery tube and a vacuum of more than 300 mmHg when the tube is clamped. The suction apparatus should have an adjustable knob to control the amount of suctioning power, especially in children. It must be designed for easy cleaning and subsequent decontamination. Suctioning may damage the teeth and surrounding structures. Prolonged airway suctioning can cause deoxygenation. It is recommended that the procedure be limited to less than10 seconds at a time and the patient be on 100% O_2 in the intervals between suctioning.

SPECIALIZED AIRWAY DEVICES IN CPR

Specialized airway devices in CPR include the laryngeal mask airway (LMA; Laryngeal Mask Co., San Diego, CA), the esophageal tracheal airway (Combitube; Kendall-Sheridan Catheter Corp., Argyle, NY), the pharyngotracheal lumen airway (PTL), the cuffed oropharyngeal airway (COPA; Mallinckrodt, St. Louis, MO), emergency tracheostomy and cricothyroidotomy, and endotracheal intubation. Although many of these devices have been extensively or anecdotally tested in the field during CA, only a few of them have been included in the new AHA advanced cardiac life support guidelines for ventilation.

LARYNGEAL MASK AIRWAY

Although recently introduced, the LMA already has a solid track record of "saves" in the established difficult airway and in specific unpredictable situations of the American Society of Anesthesiologists' difficult airway algorithm, such as emergency cesarean sections, airway trauma, and the newborn infant. Once placed, the LMA may be left in place to provide ventilation and oxygenation or may be exchanged for a more definitive airway. Based on the widespread experience of anesthesiologists using this device, the LMA should be considered first among the alternative airways to be used during CPR. The main limitations of the LMA are that it offers little protection against passive pulmonary aspiration of gastric contents, and its cuff limits efficacy in PPV.

The incidence of regurgitation during insertion of the LMA is controversial, and the only experience available is in patients with a difficult airway who are not in CA. A recent observation in this setting shows that the LMA can be associated with risk of aspiration through relaxation of the lower esophageal sphincter, distention of the hypopharyngeal muscles, and prevention of ejection of regurgitated food *(250)*. Experienced practitioners consider the LMA in selected difficult airway conditions only when laryngeal obstruction, tumor, tonsillar bleeding, epiglottitis, or laryngeal abscesses are absent. Although most of the literature on the LMA is available from anesthesiologists, the evidence in favor of this airway in prehospital difficult airway management and CA is rapidly accumulating.

In the United States, specially trained paramedic and/or registered nurse flight crews perform airway management in the field. Although there is controversy regarding what constitutes appropriate field airway management in the patient in CA, most paramedics would ventilate using the BVM technique or by placing an ETT *(251)*. A prospective comparison between LMA and ETT management by paramedic students showed that LMA placement was successful on the first attempt 94% of the time compared with 69% in the ETT group ($p < 0.01$) *(252)*. The insertion of the LMA was also statistically faster to detection of end-tidal CO_2. The same observation was confirmed when respiratory therapists or medical students manipulated the airway *(253,254)*.

The usual PAP limitation of the LMA is about 15–20 cm H_2O. As demonstrated in patients under an anesthetic that included neuromuscular blockade and mechanical ventilation, PPV with peak inflation pressures ranging between 15 cm H_2O and 30 cm H_2O may result in a progressive decrease in tidal volume from 13% to 27%, and an increase in gastric esophageal inflation from 2% to 35% *(255)*. In this situation, the risk of gastric insufflation is aggravated by the fact that cricoid pressure cannot be applied without further displacing the LMA *(256)*. A modification of the LMA, the LMA-ProSeal (Laryngeal Mask Co.) has been recently designed with an extra cuff and a channel that can accommodate a small nasogastric tube *(257)*. Unique advantages of this modified airway are the potential limitation of regurgitation of gastric contents in the pharynx and subsequent pulmonary aspiration and the ability to provide PPV up to a PAP of 30–35 cm H_2O, which are both desirable when attempting to ventilate a CA victim *(258)*. However, there are currently no available clinical reports of the use of this device during CPR.

COMBITUBE

The Combitube (Kendall-Sheridan Catheter Corp., Argyle, NY), an evolutionary step in the design of the esophageal obturator airway, provides a complete seal of the upper airway and, therefore, can be used in patients with a high risk of regurgitation and aspiration of gastric contents *(259)*. The main indication for the Combitube has been in the rapid establishment of an airway during CPR *(260,261)*.

The Combitube is essentially a double-lumen tube that is inserted blindly through the mouth and is more likely to pass into the esophagus (80% of the time) than into the trachea (20% of the time). Both lumens are color-coded: blue for the esophagus and clear for the trachea. A proximal latex esophageal balloon (inflated first after placement) is filled with 100 mL of air, and a distal plastic cuff is filled with 10–15 mL of air. These cuffs provide a good seal of the hypopharynx and stability in the trachea or esophagus. The esophageal lumen is closed distally and perforated at the hypopharyngeal level with several small openings. The trachea lumen is open distally. The Combitube has the same limitations as the LMA and, thus, may not be suitable in patients with hypopharyngeal pathology or preexisting esophageal pathology, such as a malignancy or esophageal varices (262).

The Combitube is available in standard adult and small adult sizes. The most common reason for failure to ventilate with this device is placement of the device too deeply, so that the perforated pharyngeal section has entirely entered the esophagus. Pulling the Combitube back 3–4 cm usually resolves the problem. To minimize this problem, use of the smaller version for patients less than 5 feet tall is recommended by the manufacturer. Although our experience with this device is limited in both difficult airway and CPR scenarios, that of others seems to suggest that the smaller version has a higher chance of success and a lower risk of damaging the hypopharynx and the esophagus (263). The Combitube can be inserted safely in patients with cervical spine injuries, because flexion of the neck is not required. However, it is not well-tolerated in patients with a persistent, strong gag reflex after resuscitation and should be exchanged with an alternative airway as soon as possible.

PHARYNGOTRACHEAL LUMEN AIRWAY

The PTL airway is essentially an improvement on the design of the esophageal obtu-rator airway and the esophageal gastric tube airway (264). Both devices are double-lumen airways that are inserted blindly, preferably into the esophagus. The PTL has an oral balloon that provides a seal for the airway. An inflatable distal cuff prevents aspiration of gastric contents. Just like the Combitube, the attendant should evaluate carefully if the device is in the esophagus or the trachea and, based on this evaluation, ventilate through the appropriate lumen.

Laryngeal Mask Airway, Combitube, Pharyngotracheal Lumen Airway, and Cuffed Oropharyngeal Airway

An in vitro and in vivo comparison of the LMA and Combitube with BVM ventilation is available. In a bench model simulating CA in which the compliance was set at approximately half of normal and resistance was doubled to simulate CA conditions, both the LMA and Combitube proved to be superior to a face mask in providing effective ventilation (265). Several issues make this study remarkable: (a) EMS training for the LMA and Combitube was brief but very successful; (b) the achievement of appropriate ventilation with BVM ventilation was the fastest, whereas the Combitube was the slowest; and (c) there was significantly greater gastric inflation with BVM ventilation than with the LMA and Combitube (PAPs, 27 ± 2 cm H_2O vs 17 ± 2 cm H_2O vs 21 ± 2 cm H_2O, respectively). EMS personnel's objective assessment during the study clearly favored both Combitube and LMA over BVM. Although short-term retention of skills was present in both LMA and Combitube placement, poor performance with the Combitube was usually noted 6 months after the initial training.

Recently, the performance of the PTL, Combitube, and the LMA were compared in 470 cases of cardiorespiratory arrest *(261)*. No significant difference was found in objective measurement of ventilatory effectiveness, as measured by arterial blood gas analysis and spirometry, between the three devices. This was a true prospective, randomized study with the patient blinded to oral airway and BVM ventilation vs alternative airway. The crossover mechanism allowed emergency medical services personnel to use BVM ventilation and to switch to an alternative airway if ventilation was unsatisfactory.

Several interesting points can be drawn from this study. Overall, there was no statistically significant difference between any of the airways used, although a slight increased trend in hospital discharges was found in the patients in whom the LMA was used. Furthermore, there was a significant increase in successful LMA insertion among EMS personnel trained in the operating room vs on mannequins. The incidence of aspiration was not statistically different for any of the devices, including BVM ventilation. Although the study was unable to demonstrate a statistically different outcome between different airways and BVM ventilation, it should be noted that in 91% of the cases the cause of arrest was cardiac, a situation in which ventilation is believed not to be fundamental to survival for the first few minutes after the arrest. Furthermore, the observation of adequacy of ventilation was performed by the EMS personnel and physicians who witnessed the arrest and not by the investigators.

The Combitube and LMA seem to have a good track record in trauma. In a randomized crossover design, 12 Navy SEALs participated in a 2-week advanced battlefield trauma course based on an instructional video and mannequin training *(266)*. In these highly specialized paramedical personnel, placement of an ETT averaged about 36.5 seconds vs 40 seconds for the Combitube. LMA insertion time was significantly shorter (22 seconds) in simulated active combat trauma during which the battlefield was covered with smoke. This scenario can be extrapolated to paramedical personnel involved with scenes in which the victim cannot be immediately extricated and/or the airway cannot be accessed for BVM ventilation or tracheal intubation. Such scenarios have been described in case reports *(267)*.

A remarkable advantage of the LMA is its rapid learning curve. Several recent studies show that minimally experienced staff on a ward can successfully use the LMA during CPR *(268–270)*. Ventilation efficiency with the LMA was also compared with BVM in personnel with no previous resuscitation experience *(271)*. The results were striking. The effectiveness of ventilation with the LMA by inexperienced paramedics was superior to the ability of anesthetists to use a face mask. Rapid insertion time is another advantage of the LMA. A number of studies seem to demonstrate that skilled and unskilled personnel can achieve control of the airway more rapidly with LMA compared with endotracheal intubation and more effectively compared with BVM ventilation *(252–254,272)*.

A relative advantage of the Combitube over the LMA in a trauma and CA situation is the decreased incidence of gastric regurgitation and pulmonary aspiration. However, a recent meta-analysis showed a very low incidence of aspiration when the LMA was used in fasting patients scheduled for elective surgery. The relevance of these findings in nonfasted trauma patients is questionable *(273)*. Several studies have described the use of the Combitube in the prehospital setting *(274–276)*. The Combitube was evaluated as a backup airway in case of failed endotracheal intubation. In a study of 52 patients in a rural prehospital system, successful ventilation was achieved in 69% (277). Although the percentage of success was limited, this study highlights the importance of alternative ventilatory devices in both rural and suburban systems in which the response to CA and the availability of highly skilled paramedical personnel trained in cardiopulmonary arrest is limited. The rate of successful attempts for the Combitube increases to 100% in an urban environment where trauma patients receive care (278).

Close attention has been paid to the use of the alternative airway during CPR in patients with suspected cervical spine injuries. The LMA has the theoretical advantage of achieving control of the airway without manipulations of the neck (279,280). However, recent studies in cadavers have shown a potential for increased posterior dislocations of the cervical spine with LMA use (281). The Combitube has the potential advantage of being placed into the esophagus with the neck in an absolutely neutral and immobilized position. This allows for rapid airway control without removing a stiff cervical spine immobilization collar that is already in place. A preliminary study in healthy, anesthetized patients showed a high rate of success in ventilating patients with a cervical spine immobilization collar when the collar was positioned after placement of the Combitube (282). However, when Combitube intubation was attempted in American Society of Anesthesiologists physical status class I and II patients with a cervical collar already in place, the rate of success decreased to only 33%. The use of gentle laryngoscopy, although not recommended by the manufacturer, improved the rate of successful insertion to 75% (282).

TRACHEOSTOMY AND CRICOTHYROIDOTOMY

When the airway is compromised by trauma or when massive oropharyngeal or hypopharyngeal pathology is present, emergency access to the airway can be obtained only through an emergency surgical airway (tracheostomy or cricothyroidotomy) or a percutaneous cricothyroidotomy. Emergency tracheostomy is usually performed via a vertical incision from the cricoid cartilage down, for approx 1 cm, in the direction of the sternal notch. A no. 11 surgical blade is preferably used. A skilled, surgically trained operator can rapidly approach the trachea via this route and insert a small, cuffed ETT. Emergency cricothyroidotomy is a valid alternative to the emergency tracheostomy for an operator who is not skilled or trained in the surgical approach to the airway. This technique requires identification of the cricothyroid membrane. The cricothyroid membrane (ligament) is directly under the skin and is composed primarily of yellow, elastic tissue (283). It covers the cricothyroid space, which averages 9 mm in height and 3 cm in width. The membrane is located in the anterior neck between the thyroid cartilage superiorly and the cricoid cartilage inferiorly and consists of a central triangular portion (conus elasticus) and two lateral portions. It is often crossed horizontally in its upper third by the superior cricothyroid arteries (109). Because the vocal cords are located a centimeter or more above the cricothyroid space, they are usually not injured, even during emergency cricothyroidotomy. The anterior jugular vein runs vertically in the lateral aspect of the neck and is usually spared injury during the procedure. There is, however, considerable variation in both the arterial and venous vessel patterns. Although the arteries are always located deep to the pretracheal fascia and are easily avoided during a skin incision, veins may be found in both the pretracheal fascia and between the pretracheal and superficial cervical fascias. To minimize the possibility of bleeding, the cricothyroid membrane should be incised at its inferior third. This technique has the relative advantage of achieving access to the airway through a relatively avascular part of the neck, especially in lean individuals. However, the cricothyroid membrane is not always easy to appreciate in obese patients or in those with a short neck. Melker and Florete have described percutaneous cricothyroidotomy using the Seldinger technique *(284)*. The main advantage of this technique is the blunt dissection of the subcutaneous tissues all the way to the cricothyroid membrane. An airway catheter is then introduced over a dilator threaded over the guide-wire. This technique allows the ultimate insertion of an airway that is considerably larger than the initial needle or catheter and often of sufficient internal diameter to allow ventilation with conventional ventilation devices, suctioning, and spontaneous ventilation.

Needle cricothyroidotomy is an alternative to the use of the more invasive cricothyroidotomy or tracheostomy, regardless of whether it is surgical or percutaneous. This can be achieved with a large-caliber angiocatheter, usually no. 12 or no. 14 gauge, or a specialized armored no. 12 gauge angiocatheter. Needle cricothyroidotomy always requires the use of a jet device to provide ventilation, and it is associated with a high incidence of complications, such as massive subcutaneous emphysema, barotrauma with pneumothorax or tension pneumothorax, and air trapping with severe hemodynamic instability. Experience with needle cricothyroidotomy in CPR is limited.

ALTERNATIVE METHODS OF VENTILATION AFTER SUCCESSFUL ENDOTRACHEAL INTUBATION

The relation between airway pressure, intrathoracic pressure, and circulation during CPR has been recently studied *(285)*. During the decompression phase of CPR, venous return is enhanced. A small inspiratory impedance valve has recently been introduced to occlude the airway selectively during the decompression phase of CPR without interfering with exhalation or active ventilation. The effect of this device on venous return, coronary perfusion pressure, and blood flow during resuscitation has been studied recently in animals and humans. A remarkable improvement in all of the physiological parameters usually associated with restoration of spontaneous circulation after defibrillation was demonstrated (end-tidal CO_2, systolic blood pressure, diastolic blood pressure). Furthermore, the beneficial effect of this valve could be seen in models of both protected and unprotected ventilation *(286,287)*. Remarkably, when the effect of PEEP was combined with negative inspiratory pressure produced with the inspiratory threshold valve (CPAP level up to 10 cm H_2O), the increase in oxygenation was still appreciated with improved respiratory system compliance but without the detrimental effect on hemodynamics expected with the use of CPAP *(288)*. Negative pressure pulmonary edema is one possible complication can occur during airway obstruction or an exaggerated Mueller maneuver *(289)*.

TRANSPORT VENTILATORS

Although the introduction of transport ventilators for prehospital and hospital care was typically aimed at providing mechanical ventilation in patients with an ETT in place, some of their features can be used to provide ventilation of the unprotected airway during and after CPR. These devices are typically compact, lightweight, time- or flow-cycled, durable, pneumatically or electronically powered, easy to operate, and low maintenance. An excellent review is available in the literature *(290)*.

During transport of artificially ventilated patients, automatic transport ventilators (ATVs) are found to be superior at maintaining constant minute ventilation and adequate arterial blood gases when compared with BVM devices *(291)*. Advantages of ATVs include allowing the rescuer to do other tasks when the patient is intubated, and it allows the rescuer to use both hands to hold the mask in patients not intubated. The rescuer can also perform the Sellick maneuver with one hand although the other hand holds the mask. ATVs can provide a specific tidal volume, respiratory rate, and minute ventilation.

The Emergency Cardiac Care Committee and Subcommittee of the AHA recommends that ATVs should function as constant inspiratory flow rate generators and should have the following features:

1. a lightweight connector with a standard 15 mm\22 mm adapter coupling for a mask, ETT, or other airway adjunct;
2. a lightweight (2–5 kg) compact, rugged design;
3. capability of operating under all common environmental conditions and extremes of temperatures;
4. a peak inspiratory pressure limiting valve set at 60 cm H_2O with an option of an 80 cm H_2O pressure that is easily accessible to the user;
5. an audible alarm that sounds when the peak inspiratory limiting pressure is generated to alert the rescuer that low compliance or high airway resistance is resulting in a diminished tidal volume delivery;
6. minimal gas consumption allowing the device to run for a minimum of 45 minutes on an E cylinder;
7. minimal gas compression volume in the breathing circuit;
8. ability to deliver 100% oxygen;
9. an inspiratory time of 2 seconds in adults and 1 second in children, and maximal inspiratory flow rates of approx 30 L per minute in adults and 15 L per minute in children;
10. at least two rates, 10 bpm for adults and 20 bpm in children.

If a demand flow valve is incorporated, it should deliver a peak inspiratory flow rate on demand of at least 100 L/minute at –2 cm H_2O triggering pressure to minimize the work of breathing *(225)*. Additional desirable features include a pressure gauge, provision for CPAP, controls for rate and tidal volume, and low pressure alarms to indicate low oxygen pressure either from disconnection or depletion of the gas source. Theoretically, both time or flow cycle transport ventilators can replace BVM ventilation during CPR. However, one particular model, the Ohmeda HARV or pneuPAC 2-R (Ohmeda Emergency Care, Orchard Park, NY), is commercially available for either transport ventilation or assisted mask ventilation. HARV produces a rectangular flow waveform that is time-triggered, flow- or pressure-limited, and time-cycled. A single control sets one of seven rate to tidal volume combinations *(290)*.

Mechanically operated mask ventilation undoubtedly presents advantages during CPR, because it frees the resuscitator's hand that typically is involved in squeezing the bag. However, the use of this pressure-powered machine that operates from an external pneumatic source (wall-pressured oxygen or portable oxygen tank) presents the hidden danger of providing exaggerated tidal volume and/or excessive flow rate with short inspiratory time. Nevertheless, such a device could be helpful as an addition to the CPR health provider airway armamentarium, provided that the provider has the skill and knowledge necessary to operate it safely.

MONITORING VENTILATION DURING CPR

End-Tidal Carbon Dioxide As a Tool for Monitoring the Progress of CPR

A number of studies have shown that end-tidal CO_2 varies directly with cardiac output during CA *(47,292–294)* and provides a useful indicator of the efficacy of resuscitation efforts *(295–303)*. The presence of end-tidal CO_2 has been investigated as a guide to correct placement of endotracheal intubation *(304–307)*. Additionally, capnography has been used in resuscitation research as an indication of pulmonary blood flow, which serves as a proxy for the direct measurement of cardiac output *(308–311)*.

Aerobic and anaerobic cellular metabolism generate CO_2, which diffuses out of the cell into tissue capillaries, and is transported to the lungs, exhaled, and can be measured as end-tidal CO_2 *(312,313)*. Under normal conditions, end-tidal CO_2 is 2–5 mmHg less than the $PaCO_2$. Systemic metabolism changes little during CPR, which is usually relatively brief, although ischemic hypoxia can alter the respiratory quotient *(312,314)*. The concentration of exhaled CO_2 changes when blood flow to the lungs changes and is an indirect indicator of cardiac output and systemic blood flow. Under conditions of constant minute ventilation, end-tidal CO_2 is linearly related to cardiac output, even during extremely low blood flow rates *(315)*. The decrease in end-tidal CO_2 parallels closely the decrease in $PaCO_2$ that occurs when blood flow decreases, and is therefore useful clinically as a monitor of perfusion during shock and CPR. End-tidal CO_2 changes rapidly with changes in flow, changing one breath after a change in perfusion and almost reaching a new steady state within 30 seconds. However, following the administration of epinephrine, the prior relationships of end-tidal CO_2 may be altered as a result of the changes in pulmonary and peripheral vascular resistance and preferential redirection of blood flow *(302)*. In some instances, epinephrine may cause decreased pulmonary blood flow and end-tidal CO_2, although at the same time coronary perfusion pressure increases because of increased peripheral vascular resistance *(316)*.

During the past two decades, there has been great interest in the physiology of end-tidal CO_2, especially in low blood flow states. The primary reason for this interest is the difficulty in directly measuring low rates of blood flow, particularly during human CA. Because it is much easier to measure, end-tidal CO_2 has been used as an indicator of pulmonary blood flow that serves as a proxy or substitute for the direct measurement of cardiac output.

In animal models of CA and resuscitation, end-tidal CO_2 has been shown to vary directly with cardiac output *(47,292,293)*. Coronary artery perfusion pressure, one of the best prognostic indicators of survival in CA *(317)*, correlates closely with end-tidal CO_2 *(299,300)*. For example, end-tidal CO_2 was higher during CPR in 17 animals that survived when compared to five animals that failed resuscitation *(294)*. Thus, end-tidal CO_2 is correlated with blood flow and successful resuscitation from CA.

Investigators have used end-tidal CO_2 as a substitute for the measurement of blood flow in studies of CPR techniques *(308–311)*. End-tidal CO_2 levels were found to increase when greater force was applied during external chest compression force in humans *(308)*, although changes in compression rate had little effect on end-tidal CO_2 *(309)*. Because end-tidal CO_2 is related directly to cardiac output when minute ventilation is held constant, it is a useful tool in CPR research as a substitute for the direct measurement of cardiac output. However, because lack of end tidal CO_2 may simply represent inefficient chest compression during CPR, new devices have been introduced to confirm endotracheal intubation in a setting of CA. A suction bulb and a large syringe, both with standard fitting for an ETT adaptor have been used to recognize the tracheal vs a "virtual and collapsible lumen" represented by the esophagus. At the time of this writing, the sensitivity and specificity of these devices during CPR has not been well established *(318)*.

Several studies of end-tidal CO_2 during low blood flow states found that levels changed significantly with changes in minute ventilation *(28,319)*. When minute ventilation doubled, end-tidal CO_2 decreased 50% and when minute ventilation decreased 50%, end-tidal CO_2 doubled. Thus, end-tidal CO_2 varies inversely with minute ventilation and can be used to monitor ventilation during low-flow conditions. If both perfusion and ventilation are not constant, end-tidal CO_2 levels can be difficult to interpret.

The Use of Arterial and Central Venous Blood Gases During CPR

It has been a longstanding practice to use arterial blood pH, PO_2, PCO_2, and HCO_3 to monitor ventilation and to guide therapeutic interventions for abnormalities in acid–base conditions during CPR *(226)*. Although $PaCO_2$ and PaO_2 are useful for monitoring pulmonary ventilation, there is mounting evidence that arterial blood may not reliably reflect tissue acid–base conditions during low blood flow states and that central venous blood more accurately reflects conditions at the tissue level.

One study showed that after 5 minutes of untreated VF, arterial and mixed venous blood gases remained nearly unchanged from baseline pre-arrest values *(142)*. Only the PaO_2 decreased by 10 mmHg, but it was still within the normal range. This demonstrates an important relationship between blood flow, tissue perfusion, and acid–base conditions. Blood that is contained within the large arteries under no-flow conditions is static and does not reflect ongoing intracellular metabolism until some perfusion is restored so that blood at the tissue level is mobilized back into circulation. Thus, if blood flow is sufficiently low, pHa, PaO_2, and $PaCO_2$ might remain "normal" for a prolonged period of time. Moreover, if ventilation is held constant, pHa and PaO_2 will increase and $PaCO_2$ will decrease as perfusion becomes worse *(56)*.

A number of investigations support the view that pHa and $PaCO_2$ can be used for monitoring the effectiveness of resuscitation efforts during CA *(28,56,320,321)*. Arterial PCO_2 has been shown to correlate closely with cardiac output and coronary perfusion pressure, which is known to be a good predictor of success of resuscitation. However, changes must be interpreted differently compared to conventional practice: when perfusion improves, arterial blood becomes more acidemic, $PaCO_2$ increases, and PaO_2 may decrease; when perfusion becomes worse, arterial blood becomes more alkalemic, $PaCO_2$ decreases and PaO_2 increases *(28,66,320)*.

Additionally, the timing of blood sampling is another variable that must be considered. If arterial blood gases are measured during CPR within 8 minutes of CA, pH is usually normal or alkaline because significant MA has not yet developed and $PaCO_2$ is lower than normal. As the duration of CPR progresses, increasing blood lactate and decreasing bicarbonate concentrations ultimately cause an acidemic arterial pH *(67)*. Administration of sodium bicarbonate, which has been shown to cause an increased pHa and $PaCO_2$, must also be considered when interpreting blood gases *(59,68)*.

Another important consideration when using arterial blood gases is that $PaCO_2$ and PaO_2 values respond quickly to changes in minute ventilation. In one study, $PaCO_2$ increased by approx 85% when minute ventilation was decreased to 25% of the previous setting; similar changes were observed with blood flow rates as low as 12% of normal *(28)*. Therefore, arterial blood gas analysis can be used to assess perfusion when minute ventilation is held constant, or to assess minute ventilation when perfusion is held constant. When both perfusion and minute ventilation are uncontrolled, it is difficult to interpret arterial blood gases.

Mixed venous pH, PO_2, and PCO_2 are more useful than arterial gases for assessing acid-base status and perfusion during low-flow states because they more closely reflect the tissue environment *(13,46,55,56,62,64,70,322)*. One study of hemorrhagic shock showed that mixed venous oxygen saturation averaged 46% in survivors and only 25% in nonsurvivors *(152)*; others have found a similar relationship *(323,324)*. A study of human CA found that mixed venous oxygen saturation was associated with prognosis for survival and mixed venous pH, PO_2, and PCO_2 measured during CA was substantially better in those that ultimately had return of spontaneous circulation *(44)*. Additionally, mixed venous blood gases are more useful than arterial blood gases for assessing perfusion during CPR, because they are much less affected than arterial gases by changes in minute ventilation *(28)*. Because of the great difficulty in obtaining mixed venous blood samples during CPR other venous sites may be used as a substitute. Evidence exists that central, femoral, intraosseous, and mixed venous blood gas values are very similar to each other even during prolonged CA and CPR *(325–327)*.

Both hyperventilation and hypoventilation change pHa, $PaCO_2$, and PaO_2. Additionally, mixed venous PCO_2 and pH can be improved with hyperventilation and become worse with hypoventilation. Because mixed venous blood gases reflect tissue acid-base conditions, intracellular hypercarbia can be altered with ventilation.

In summary, $PaCO_2$, mixed venous pH and PO_2, and end-tidal CO_2 vary directly with blood flow, although mixed venous PCO_2 varies inversely with blood flow. Arterial PO_2 and pH vary directly with minute ventilation, although arterial and mixed venous PCO_2 vary inversely with minute ventilation. Both arterial and mixed venous blood gases are useful for assessing the efficacy of resuscitation efforts. Arterial PO_2 and PCO_2 are most useful for assessing the adequacy of ventilation, although mixed venous PO_2 and PCO_2 are most useful for assessing the adequacy of circulation. At the present time, there are no conclusive data that allow one to recommend how frequently arterial or venous gases should be monitored during resuscitation.

CONCLUSION

During normal cardiac activity, ventilation serves to remove CO_2 from and provide oxygen to tissues. The effect of ventilation on tissues continues even during low-flow states, although its ability to provide oxygen and remove CO_2 is diminished and limited by blood flow. Ventilation during the first few minutes of dysrhythmic adult CA has been somewhat de-emphasized in favor of more effective chest compression. Manual techniques of ventilation have a number of advantages over mouth-to-mouth ventilation including safety from transmission of infectious diseases and a superior ventilation gas (i.e., room air). If obstruction of the airway could be prevented, manual ventilation may be a useful alternative and should be studied. Additionally, chest compression alone can provide some ventilation, and tidal volume and minute ventilation are enhanced by active compression–decompression CPR. The relationship between ventilation mechanics and circulation has been studied recently in CA and hemorrhagic shock. Studies have found that PPV may decrease blood flow by decreasing venous return to the heart. Additional studies are necessary to confirm that fewer breaths per minute are better than current recommendations.

Chest compression alone may be effective for the first few minutes of CA. This would certainly be an advantage because chest compression without ventilation could be more easily mastered by lay CPR providers and there would be less hesitation to provide bystander chest compression without mouth-to-mouth ventilation. Although the few studies of ventilation and its effect on outcome from CA in humans are inconclusive, legal restrictions are increasingly limiting the opportunities for research in this unique study population, always unable to give informed consent. The issues surrounding ventilation in resuscitation are critical and involve more than 500,000 patients per year in United States. The scientific community must respond to this challenge with a targeted, multidisciplinary research effort involving animal and human research.

REFERENCES

1. Hlastala MP. Ventilation. In: Crystal RG, West JB, eds.The Lung: Scientific Foundations, New York, NY: Raven Press, 1991, pp. 1209–1214.
2. Cobb LA, Eliastam M, Kerber RE, et al. Report of the American Heart Association task force on the future of cardiopulmonary resuscitation. Circulation 1992; 85:2346–2355.
3. Berg RA, Kern KB, Sanders AB, Otto CW, Hilwig RW, Ewy GA. Bystander cardiopulmonary resuscitation: Is ventilation necessary? Circulation 1993; 88:1907–1915.
4. Chandra NC, Gruben KG, Tsitlik JE, Guerci AD, Permutt S, Weisfeldt ML. Observations of ventilation during resuscitation in a canine model. Circulation 1994; 90:3070–3075..
5. Weil MH, Sun S, Bisera J, Tang W, Gazmuri RJ. Challenge to the ABC's of cardiopulmonary resuscitation. Chest 1992; 102:127S.
6. Wenzel V, Idris AH, Banner MJ, Fuerst RS, Tucker KJ. The composition of gas given by mouth-to-mouth ventilation during CPR. Chest 1994; 106:1806–1810.
7. The Bible, II Kings 4:32–35.
8. DeBard ML. The history of cardiopulmonary resuscitation. Ann Emerg Med 1980; 9:273–275.
9. Hermreck AS. The history of CPR. Am J Surg 1988; 156:430–436.
10. Elam JO, Brown ES, Elder JD, Jr. Artificial respiration by mouth-to-mask method: a study of the respiratory gas exchange of paralyzed patients ventilated by operator's expired air. New Engl J Med 1954; 250:749–754.
11. Safar P. History of cardiopulmonary-cerebral resuscitation. In: Kaye W, Bircher N, eds. Cardiopulmonary resuscitation. New York, NY: Churchill Livingston, 1989, pp. 1–53.
12. Boehm R. Ueber wiederbelebung nach vergiftungen and asphyxie. Arch Exp Pathol Pharmakol 1878; 8:68–101.
13. Johnson BA, Weil MH. Redefining ischemia due to circulatory failure as dual defects of oxygen deficits and of carbon dioxide excesses. Crit Care Med 1991; 19:1432–1438.
14. Safar P. Failure of manual respiration. J Appl Physiol 1959; 14:84–88.
15. Safar P, Brown TC, Holtey WJ, Wilder RJ. Ventilation and circulation with closed-chest cardiac massage in man. JAMA 1961; 176:574–576.
16. Safar P, Escarraga LA, Elam JO. A comparison of the mouth-to-mouth and mouth-to-airway methods of artificial respiration with the chest-pressure arm-lift methods. New Engl J Med 1958; 258: 671–677.
17. Don HF, Robson JG. The mechanics of the respiratory system during anesthesia: the effects of atropine and carbon dioxide. Anesth 1965; 26:168–178.
18. Severinghaus JW, Swenson EW, Finley TN, Lategola MT, Williams J. Unilateral hypoventilation produced in dogs by occluding one pulmonary artery. J Appl Physiol 1961; 16:53–60.
19. Nadel JA, Widdicombe JG. Effect of changes in blood gas tensions and carotid sinus pressure on tracheal volume and total lung resistance to airflow. J Physiol (Lond) 1962; 163:13–33.
20. Severinghaus JW, Stupfel M. Respiratory dead space increase following atropine in man, and atropine, vagal or ganglionic blockade and hypothermia in dogs. J Appl Physiol 1955; 8:81–87.
21. Daly M de Burgh, Lambertsen CJ, Schweitzer A. The effects upon the bronchial musculature of altering the O_2 and CO_2 tension in the blood perfusing the brain. J Physiol (Lond) 1953; 119:292–314.
22. Parker JC, Peters RM, Barnett TB. Carbon dioxide and the work of breathing. J Clin Invest 1963; 42: 1362–1372.

23. Scanlon TS, Benumof JL, Wahrenbrock EA, Nelson WL. Hypoxic pulmonary vasoconstriction and the ratio of hypoxic lung to perfused normoxic lung. Anesth 1978; 49:177–181.
24. Rodman DM, Voelkel NF. Regulation of vascular tone. In: Crystal RG, West JB, eds. The Lung: Scientific Foundations. New York, NY: Raven Press, 1991, pp. 1105–1119.
25. Marshall BE, Marshall C. Pulmonary hypertension. In: Crystal RG, West JB, eds. The Lung: Scientific Foundations. New York, NY: Raven Press, 1991, pp. 1177–1187.
26. Benumof JL, Wahrenbrock EA. Blunted hypoxic pulmonary vasoconstriction by increased lung vascular pressures. J Appl Physiol 1975; 38:846–850.
27. West JB. Respiratory Physiology. The Essentials. Baltimore, MD: Williams and Wilkins, 1974, pp. 57–60.
28. Idris AH, Staples E, O'Brian DJ, et al. The effect of ventilation on acid-base balance and oxygenation in low blood-flow states. Crit Care Med 1994; 22:1827–34.
29. Abdelmoneim T, Kissoon N, Johnson L, et al. Acid-base status of blood from intraosseous and mixed venous sites during prolonged cardiopulmonary resuscitation and drug infusions. Crit Care Med 1999; 27:1923–1928.
30. Perutz MF. Hemoglobin structure and respiratory transport. Scientific American. 1978; 92–125.
31. Christiansen J, Douglas CG, Haldane JS. The absorption of carbon dioxide by human blood. J Physiol 1914; 48:244–277.
32. Klocke RA. Mechanisms and kinetics of the Haldane effect in human erythrocytes. J Appl Physiol 1973; 35:673–681.
33. Perella M, Kilmartin JV, Fogg J, Rossi-Bernardi L. Identification of the high and low affinity CO_2-binding sites of human hemoglobin. Nature 1975; 256:759–761.
34. Arnone A. X-ray studies of the interaction of CO_2 with human deoxyhaemoglobin. Nature 1974; 247: 143–145.
35. Kilmartin JV, Rossi-Bernardi L. Interaction of hemoglobin with hydrogen ions, carbon dioxide, and organic phosphates. Physiol Rev 1973; 53:836–890.
36. Klocke RA. Carbon Dioxide, In: Crystal RG, West JB, eds. The Lung: Scientific Foundations. New York, NY: Raven Press, 1991, pp. 1233–1239.
37. Bersin RM, Arieff AI. Improved hemodynamic function during hypoxia with carbicarb, a new agent for the management of acidosis. Circulation 1988; 77:227–233.
38. Ducey JP, Lamiell JM, Gueller GE. Arterial-venous carbon dioxide tension difference during severe hemorrhage and resuscitation. Crit Care Med 1992; 20:518–522.
39. Dunham CM, Siegal JH, Weireter L, et al. Oxygen debt and metabolic acidemia as quantitative predictors of mortality and the severity of the ischemic insult in hemorrhagic shock. Crit Care Med 1991; 19: 231–243.
40. Graf H, Leach W, Arieff AI. Evidence for a detrimental effect of bicarbonate therapy in hypoxic lactic acidosis. Science 1984; 227:754–756.
41. Graf H, Leach W, Arieff AI. Effects of dichloroacetate in the treatment of hypoxic lactic acidosis in dogs. J Clin Invest. 1985; 76:919–923.
42. Romeh SA, Tannen RL. Therapeutic benefit of dichloroacetate in experimentally induced hypoxic lactic acidosis. J Lab Clin Med 1986; 107:378–383.
43. Niemann JT, Criley JM, Rosborough JP, Niskanen RA, Alferness C. Predictive indices of successful cardiac resuscitation after prolonged arrest and experimental cardiopulmonary resuscitation. Ann Emerg Med 1985; 14:521–528.
44. Rivers EP, Martin GB, Smithline H, et al. The clinical implications of continuous central venous oxygen saturation during human CPR. Ann Emerg Med 1992; 21:1094–1101.
45. Steinhart CR, Permutt S, Gurtner GH, Traystman RJ. B-Adrenergic activity and cardiovascular response to severe respiratory acidosis. Am J Physiol 1983; 244(Heart Circ Physiol 13):H46–H54.
46. von Planta I, Weil MH, von Planta M, Gazmuri RJ, Duggal C. Hypercarbic acidosis reduces cardiac resuscitability. Crit Care Med 1991; 19:1177–1182.
47. Weil MH, Ruiz CE, Michaels S, Rackow EC. Acid-base determinants of survival after cardiopulmonary resuscitation. Crit Care Med 1985; 13:888–892.
48. Yakaitis RW, Thomas JD, Mahaffey JE. Influence of pH and hypoxia on the success of defibrillation. Crit Care Med 1975; 3:139–142.
49. Cingolani HF, Faulkner SL, Mattiazzi AR, Bender HW, Graham TP, Jr. Depression of human myocardial contractility with "respiratory" and "metabolic" acidosis. Surgery 1975; 77:427–432.
50. Downing SE, Talner NS, Gardner TH. Cardiovascular responses to metabolic acidosis. Am J Physiol 1965; 208:237–242.

51. Poole-Wilson PA. Is early decline of cardiac function in ischaemia due to carbon dioxide retention? Lancet 1975; ii:1285–1287.

52. Tang W, Weil MH, Gazmuri RJ, Bisera J, Rackow EC. Reversible impairment of myocardial contractility due to hypercarbic acidosis in the isolated perfused rat heart. Crit Care Med 1991; 19:218–224.

53. Weisfeldt ML, Bishop RL, Greene HL. Effects of pH and pCO_2 on performance of ischemic myocardium. In: Roy PE, Rona G, eds. The Metabolism of Contraction. Recent Advances in Studies on Cardiac Structure and Metabolism, vol 10. Baltimore, MD: University Park Press, 1975, 355–364.

54. Kerber RE, Sarnat W. Factors influencing the success of ventricular defibrillation in man. Circulation 1979; 60:226–230.

55. Tang W, Weil MH, Maldonado FA, Gazmuri RJ, Bisera J. Hypercarbia decreases the effectiveness of electrical defibrillation during CPR. Crit Care Med 1992; 20(Suppl):S24.

56. Angelos MG, DeBehnke DJ, Leasure JE. Arterial pH and carbon dioxide tension as indicators of tissue perfusion during cardiac arrest in a canine model. Crit Care Med 1992; 20:1302–1308.

57. Benjamin E, Paluch TA, Berger SR, Premus G, Wu C, Iberti TJ. Venous hypercarbia in canine hemorrhagic shock. Crit Care Med 1987; 15:516–518.

58. Beyar R, Kishon Y, Kimmel E, Sideman S, Dinnar U. Blood gas and acid-base balance during cardiopulmonary resuscitation by intrathoracic and abdominal pressure variations. Basic Res Cardiol 1986; 81: 326–333.

59. Bishop RL, Weisfeldt ML. Sodium bicarbonate administration during cardiac arrest. JAMA 1976; 235: 506–509.

60. Fillmore SJ, Shapiro M, Killip T. Serial blood gas studies during cardiopulmonary resuscitation. Ann Intern Med 1970; 72:465–469.

61. Greenwood PV, Rossall RE, Kappagoda CT. Acid-base changes aftercardiorespiratory arrest in the dog. Clin Sci 1980; 58:127–133.

62. Grundler W, Weil MH, Rackow EC. Arteriovenous carbon dioxide and pH gradients during cardiac arrest. Circulation 1986; 74:1071–1074.

63. Martin GB, Carden DL, Nowak RM, Tomlanovich MC. Comparison of central venous and arterial pH and PCO_2 during open-chest CPR in the canine model. Ann Emerg Med 1985; 14:529–533.

64. Nowak RM, Martin GB, Carden DL, Tomlanovich MC. Selective venous hypercarbia during CPR. Implications regarding blood flow. Ann Emerg Med 1987; 16:527–530.

65. Ornato JP, Gonzalez ER, Coyne MR, Beck CL, Collins CL. Arterial pH in out-of-hospital cardiac arrest. Response time as a determinant of acidosis. Am J Emerg Med 1985; 3:498–501.

66. Ralston SH, Voorhees WD, Showen L, Schmitz P, Kougias C, Tacker WA. Venous and arterial blood gases during and after cardiopulmonary resuscitation in dogs. Am J Emerg Med 1985; 3:132–136.

67. Sanders AB, Ewy GA, Taft TV. Resuscitation and arterial blood gas abnormalities during prolonged cardiopulmonary resuscitation. Ann Emerg Med 1984; 13 (Part 1):676–679.

68. Sanders AB, Otto CW, Kern KB, Rogers JN, Perrault P, Ewy GA. Acid-base balance in a canine model of cardiac arrest. Ann Emerg Med 1988; 17:667–671.

69. Weil MH, Grundler W, Yamaguchi M, Michaels S, Rackow EC. Arterial blood gases fail to reflect acid-base status during cardiopulmonary resuscitation. A Preliminary report. Crit Care Med 1985; 13:884,885.

70. Weil MH, Rackow EC, Trevino R, Grundler W, Falk JL, Griffel MI. Difference in acid-base state between venous and arterial blood during cardiopulmonary resuscitation. N Engl J Med 1986; 315:153–156.

71. Weil MH, von Planta M, Gazmuri RJ, Rackow EC. Incomplete global ischemia during cardiac arrest and resuscitation. Crit Care Med 1988; 16:997–1001.

72. Langhelle A, Sunde K, Wik L, et al. Arterial blood gases with 500-versus 1000-mL tidal volumes during out-of-hospital CPR. Resus 2000; 45:27–33.

73. Johnson BA, Maldonado F, Weil MH, Tang W. Venoarterial carbon dioxide gradients during shock obey a modified Fick relationship. Crit Care Med 1992; 20(Suppl):S91.

74. von Planta M, Weil MH, Gazmuri RJ, Bisera J, Rackow EC. Myocardial acidosis associated with CO_2 production during cardiac arrest and resuscitation. Circulation 1989; 80:684–692.

75. Weil MH, Grundler W, Rackow EC, Bisera J, Miller JM, Michaels S. Blood gas measurements in human patients during CPR. Chest 1984; 86:282.

76. Szekeres L, Papp GY. Effect of arterial hypoxia on the susceptibility to arrhythmia of the heart. Acta Physiol Academ Scientiarum Hungaricae 1967; 32:143–161.

77. Ayres SM, Grace WJ. Inappropriate ventilation and hypoxemia as causes of cardiac arrhythmias. Am J Med 1969; 46:495–505.

78. Burn JH, Hukovic S. Anoxia and ventricular fibrillation; with a summary of evidence on the cause of fibrillation. Brit J Pharmacol 1960; 15:67–70.

79. Dong, Jr. E, Stinson EB, Shumway NE. The ventricular fibrillation threshold in respiratory acidosis and alkalosis. Surgery 1967; 61:602–607.
80. Turnbull AD, MacLean LD, Dobell ARC, Demers R. The influence of hyperbaric oxygen and of hypoxia on the ventricular fibrillation threshold. J Thoracic Cardiovasc Surg 1965; 6:842–848.
81. Kerber RE, Pandian NG, Hoyt R, et al. Effect of ischemia, hypertrophy, hypoxia, acidosis, and alkalosis on canine defibrillation. Am J Physiol 1983; 244(Heart Circ Physiol 13):H825–H831.
82. Guerci AD, Chandra N, Johnson E, et al. Failure of sodium bicarbonate to improve resuscitation from ventricular fibrillation in dogs. Circulation 1986; 74(Suppl IV):75–79.
83. Gerst PH, Fleming WH, Malm JR. Increased susceptibility of the heart to ventricular fibrillation during metabolic acidosis. Circulation Research 1966; 19:63–70.
84. von Planta M, Gudipati C, Weil MH, Kraus LJ, Rackow EC. Effects of tromethamine and sodium bicarbonate buffers during cardiac resuscitation. J Clin Pharmacol 1988; 28:594–599.
85. Gazmuri RJ, von Planta M, Weil MH, Rackow EC. Cardiac effects of carbon dioxide-consuming and carbon dioxide-generating buffers during cardiac resuscitation. J Am Coll Cardiol 1990; 15:482–490.
86. Kette F, Weil MH, von Planta M, Gazmuri RJ, Rackow EC. Buffer agents do not reverse intramyocardial acidosis during cardiac resuscitation. Circulation 1990; 81:1660–1666.
87. Federiuk CS, Sanders AB, Kern KB, Nelson J, Ewy GA. The effect of bicarbonate on resuscitation from cardiac arrest. Ann Emerg Med 1991; 20:1173–1177.
88. Kette F, Weil MH, Gazmuri RJ. Buffer solutions may compromise cardiac resuscitation by reducing coronary perfusion pressure. JAMA 1991; 266:2121–2126.
89. Goldstein B, Shannon DC, Todres ID. Supercarbia in children: clinical course and outcome. Crit Care Med 1990; 18:166–168.
90. Holmdahl MH. Pulmonary uptake of oxygen, acid-base metabolism, and circulation during prolonged apnea. Acta Chir Scand 1956; 212(Suppl):108.
91. Graham GR, Hill DW, Nunn SF. Supercarbia in the anesthetized dog. Nature 1959; 184:1071–1072.
92. Clowes GHA, Hopkins AL, Simeone FA. A comparison of the physiological effects of hypercapnia and hypoxia in the production of cardiac arrest. Ann Surg 1955; 142–466.
93. Litt LO, Gonzalez-Mendez R, Severinghaus JW, et al. Cerebral intracellular changes during supercarbia: an in vivo 31P nuclear magnetic resonance study in rats. J Cereb Blood Flow Metab 1985; 5:537–544.
94. Winkle RA, Mead RH, Ruder MA, Smith NA, Buch WS, Gaudiani VA. Effect of duration of ventricular fibrillation on defibrillation efficacy in humans. Circulation 1990; 81:1477–1481.
95. Eisenberg M, Hallstrom A, Bergner L. The ACLS score. JAMA 1981; 246:50–52.
96. Weaver WD, Cobb LA, Hallstrom AP, Fahrenbruch C, Copass MK, Ray R. Factors influencing survival after out-of-hospital cardiac arrest. J Am Coll Cardiol 1986; 7:752–757.
97. Sanders AB, Kern KB, Atlas M, Bragg S, Ewy GA. Importance of the duration of inadequate coronary perfusion pressure on resuscitation from cardiac arrest. J Am Coll Cardiol 1985; 6:113–118.
98. Yakaitis RW, Ewy GA, Otto CW, Taren DL, Moon TE. Influence of time and therapy on ventricular defibrillation in dogs. Crit Care Med 1980; 8:157–163.
99. Brown CG, Dzwonczyk R, Werman HA, Hamlin RL. Estimating the duration of ventricular fibrillation. Ann Emerg Med 1989; 18:1181–1185.
100. Kern KB, Garewal HS, Sanders AB, et al. Depletion of myocardial adenosine triphosphate during prolonged untreated ventricular fibrillation: effect on defibrillation success. Resus 1990; 20:221–229.
101. von Planta M, Weil MH, Gazmuri RJ, Rackow EC. Myocardial potassium uptake during experimental cardiopulmonary resuscitation. Crit Care Med 1989; 17:895–899.
102. Babbs CF, Whistler SJ, Yim GKW, Tacker WA, Geddes LA. Dependence of defibrillation threshold upon extracellular/intracellular K+ concentrations. J Electrocardiology 1980; 13:73–78.
103. Gremels H, Starling EH. On the influence of hydrogen ion concentration and of anoxaemia upon the heart volume. J Physiol London 1926; 61:297–304.
104. Jacobus WE, Pores IH, Lucas SK, Weisfeldt ML, Flaherty JT. Intracellular acidosis and contractility in the normal and ischemic heart as examined by 31PNMR. J Mol Cell Cardiol 1982; 14(Supp 3):13–20.
105. Monroe RG, French G, Whittenberger JL. Effects of hypocapnia and hypercapnia on myocardial contractility. Am J Physiol 1960; 199:1121–1124.
106. Tyberg JV, Yeatman LA, Parmley WW, Urschel CW, Sonnenblick EH. Effects of hypoxia on mechanics of cardiac contraction. Amer J Physiol 1970; 218:1780–1788.
107. Becker LB, Idris AH, Shao Z, Schorer S, Art J, Zak R. Inhibition of cardiomyocyte contractions by carbon dioxide. Circulation 1993; 88(Suppl 1):I–225.

108. Orchard CH, Kentish KC. Effects of changes of pH on the contractile function of cardiac muscle. Am J Physiol 1990; 258(Cell Physiol 27);C967–C981.
109. Kette F, Weil MH, Gazmuri RJ, Bisera J, Rackow EC. Intramyocardial hypercarbic acidosis during cardiac arrest and resuscitation. Crit Care Med 1993; 21:901–906.
110. Grum CM. Tissue oxygenation in low flow states and during hypoxemia. Crit Care Med 1993; 21(2 Suppl): S44–49.
111. Paradis NA, Rose MI, Gawryl MS. Selective aortic arch perfusion and oxygenation: an effective adjunct to external chest compression-based cardiopulmonary resuscitation. J Am Coll Cardiol 1994; 23:497–504.
112. Paradis N, Martin GB, Rivers EP, et al. Coronary perfusion pressure and the return of spontaneous circulation in human cardiopulmonary resuscitation. JAMA 1990; 263:1106–1113.
113. Weil MH, Houle DB, Brown, EB, Jr, Campbell GS, Heath C. Influence of acidosis on the effectiveness of vasopressor agents. Circulation 1957; 16:949.
114. Houle DB, Weil MH, Brown, EB, Jr, Campbell GS. Influence of respiratory acidosis on ECG and pressor responses to epinephrine, norepinephrine and metaraminol. Proc Soc Exp Biol Med 1957; 94: 561–564.
115. Campbell GS, Houle DB, Crisp, NW, Jr, Weil MH, Brown, EB, Jr. Depressed response to intravenous sympathicomimetic agents in human acidosis. Dis Chest 1958; 33:18–22.
116. Köhler E, Noack E, Strobach H, Wirth K. Effect of acidosis on heart and circulation in cats, pigs, dogs and rabbits. Res Exp Med 1972; 158:308–320.
117. Bendixen HH, Laver MB, Flacke WE. Influence of respiratory acidosis on circulatory effect of epinephrine in dogs. Circulation Res 1963; 13:64–70.
118. Sechzer PH, Egbert LD, Linde HW, Cooper DY, Dripps RD, Price HL. Effect of CO_2 inhalation on arterial pressure, ECG and plasma catecholamines and 17-OH corticosteroids in normal man. J Appl Physiol 1960; 15:454–458.
119. Anderson MN, Mouritzen C. Effect of respiratory and metabolic acidosis on cardiac output and peripheral vascular resistance. Ann Surg 1966; 163:161–168.
120. Kern KB, Elchisak MA, Sanders AB, Badylak SF, Tacker WA, Ewy GA. Plasma catecholamines and resuscitation from prolonged cardiac arrest. Crit Care Med 1989; 17:786–791.
121. Idris A, Fuerst R, Wenzel V, Becker L, Orban D, Banner M. Does hypoxia or hypercarbic acidosis independently affect survival from cardiac arrest? Circulation 1993; 88(Suppl):I–225.
122. Lockinger A., Kleinsasser A, Wenzeo V, et al. Pulmonary gas exchange of the cardiopulmonary resuscitation with either vasopressin or epinephrine. Crit Care Med 2002; 30:2059–2062.
123. Cournand A, Motley HL, Werko L, Richards DW. Physiological studies of the effects of intermittent positive pressure breathing on cardiac output. Am J Physiol 1948; 152:162–74.
124. Sykes MK, Adams AP, Finley WE, McCormick PW, Economides A. The effects of variations in end expiratory inflation pressure on cardiorespiratory function in normo, hypo, and hypervolemic dogs. Br J Anaesth 1970; 42:669–677.
125. Qvist J, Pontoppidan H, Wilson RS, Lowenstein E, Laver MB. Hemodynamic responses to mechanical ventilation with PEEP: The effect of hypovolemia. Anesth 1975; 42:45–55.
126. Otto CW, Quan SF, Conahan TJ, Calkins JM, Waterson CK, Hameroff SR. Hemodynamic effects of high-frequency jet ventilation. Anesth Analg 1983; 62:298–304.
127. Cohen JM, Chandra N, Alderson PO, Van Aswegen A, Tsitlik JE, Weisfeldt ML. Timing of pulmonary and systemic blood flow during intermittent high intrathoracic pressure cardiopulmonary resuscitation in the dog. Am J Cardiol 1982; 49:1883–1889.
128. Chandra N, Weisfeldt ML, Tsitlik J, et al. Augmentation of carotid flow during cardiopulmonary resuscitation by ventilation at high airway pressure simultaneous with chest compression. Am J Cardiol 1981; 48:1053–1063.
129. Chandra N, Rudikoff M, Weisfeldt ML. Simultaneous chest compression and ventilation at high airway pressure during cardiopulmonary resuscitation. Lancet 1980; 26;1(8161):175–178.
130. Koehler RC, Chandra N, Guerci AD, et al. Augmentation of cerebral perfusion by simultaneous chest compression and lung inflation with abdominal binding after cardiac arrest in dogs. Circulation 1983; 67:266–275.
131. Babbs CF, Voorhees WD, Fitzgerald KR, Holmes HR, Geddes LA. Influence of interposed ventilation pressure upon artificial cardiac output during cardiopulmonary resuscitation in dogs. Crit Care Med 1980; 8:127–130.
132. Hodgkin BC, Lambrew CT, Lawrence FH, Angelakos ET. Effects of PEEP and of increased frequency of ventilation during CPR. Crit Care Med 1980; 8:123–126.

133. Woda RP, Dzwonczyk R, Bernacki BL, et al. The ventilatory effects of auto-positive end-expiratory pressure development during cardiopulmonary resuscitation. Crit Care Med 1999; 27:2212–2217.
134. Sigurdsson G, Yannopoulos D, McKnite SH, Lurie KG. Cardiorespiratory interactions and blood flow generation during cardiac arrest and other states of low blood flow. Curr Opin Crit Care. 2003; 9:183–188. Review.
135. Samniah N, Voelckel WG, Zielinski TM, et al. Feasibility and effects of transcutaneous phrenic nerve stimulation combined with an inspiratory impedance threshold in a pig model of hemorrhagic shock. Crit Care Med. 2003; 31:1197–202.
136. Lurie KG, Zielinski T, Voelckel W, McKnite S, Plaisance P. Augmentation of ventricular preload during treatment of cardiovascular collapse and cardiac arrest. Crit Care Med. 2002; 30(4 Suppl): S162–S165. Review.
137. Lurie KG, Zielinski T, McKnite S, Aufderheide T, Voelckel W. Use of an inspiratory impedance valve improves neurologically intact survival in a porcine model of ventricular fibrillation. Circulation. 2002; 105:124–129.
138. Pepe PE, Raedler C, Lurie KG, Wigginton JG. Emergency ventilatory management in hemorrhagic states: elemental or detrimental? J Trauma. 2003; 54:1048–55; discussion 1055–1057.
139. Hevesi CG, Thrush DN, Downs JB, et al. Cardiopulmonary resuscitation effect of CPAP on gas exchange during chest compressions. Anesth 1999; 90:1078–1083.
140. Markstaller K, Karmrodt J, Doebrich M, et al. Dynamic computed tomography: A novel technique to study lung aeration and atelectasis formation during experimental CPR. Resuscitation 2002; 53:307–313.
141. Meursing BTJ, Zimmerman ANE, van Heyst ANP. Experimental evidence in favor of a reversed sequence in cardiopulmonary resuscitation. J Am Coll Cardiol 1983; 1:610 (Abstract).
142. Tucker KJ, Idris AH, Wenzel V, Orban DJ. Changes in arterial and mixed venous blood gases during untreated ventricular fibrillation and cardiopulmonary resuscitation. Resuscitation 1994; 28:137–141.
143. Tang W, Weil MH, Sun S, et al. Myocardial function after CPR by precordial compression without mechanical ventilation. Chest 1991; 100(Suppl):132S.
144. Pearson JW, Redding JS. Influence of peripheral vascular tone on cardiac resuscitation. Anesth Analg 1965; 44:746–752.
145. Yang L, Weil MH, Noc M, Tang W, Turner T, Gazmuri RJ. Spontaneous gasping increases the ability to resuscitate during experimental cardiopulmonary resuscitation. Crit Care Med 1994; 22:879–883.
146. Idris AH, Becker LB, Fuerst RS, et al. The effect of ventilation on resuscitation in an animal model of cardiac arrest. Circulation 1994; 90:3063–3069.
147. Noc M, Weil MH, Tang W, et al. Mechanical ventilation may not be essential for initial cardiopulmonary resuscitation. Chest 1995; 108:821–827.
148. Berg RA, Kern KB, Hilwig RW, et al. Assisted ventilation during 'bystanders' CPR in a swine acute myocardial infarction model does not improve outcome. Circulation 1997; 96:4364–4371.
149. Kern KB, Hilwig RW, Berg RA, et al. Efficacy of chest compression-only BLS CPR in the presence of an occluded airway. Resuscitation 1998; 39:179–188.
150. Kern KB. Cardiopulmonary resuscitation without ventilation. Crit Care Med 2000; 28(11 Suppl): N186–N189.
151. Clark JJ, Larsen MP, Culley LL, Graves JR, Eisenberg MS. Incidence of agonal respirations in sudden cardiac arrest. Ann Emerg Med 1992; 21:1464–1467.
152. Kazarian KK, Del Guercio LRM. The use of mixed venous blood gas determinations in traumatic shock. Ann Emerg Med 1980; 9:179–180.
153. Simoons ML, Kimman GP, Ivens EMA, Hartman JAM, Hart HN. Follow up after out of hospital resuscitation. European Heart J 1990; 11(Abstract Suppl):92.
154. Thompson RG, Hallstrom AP, Cobb LA. Bystander-initiated cardiopulmonary resuscitation in the management of ventricular fibrillation. Ann Emerg Med 1979; 9:737–740.
155. Van Hoeyweghen RJ, Bossaert L, Mullie A, et al. Quality and efficiency of bystander CPR. Belgian Cerebral Resuscitation Study Group. Resuscitation 1993; 26:47–52.
156. Hallstrom A, Cobb L, Johnson E, et al. Cardiopulmonary resuscitation by chest compression alone or with mouth-to-mouth ventilation. N Engl J Med 2000; 342:1546–1553.
157. Assar D, Chamberlain D, Colquhoun M, et al. A rational stage of teaching basic life support. Resuscitation 1998; 39:137–143.
158. Van Hoeyweghen RJ, Bossaert L, Mullie A, et al. Quality and efficiency of bystander CPR. Belgian Cerebral Resuscitation Study Group. Resuscitation 1993; 26:47–52.
159. Hallstrom A, Cobb L, Johnson E, et al. Cardiopulmonary resuscitation by chest compression alone or with mouth-to-mouth ventilation. N Engl J Med 2000; 342:1546–1553.

160. Becker LB, Berg RA, Pepe PE, et al. A reappraisal of mouth-to-mouth ventilation during bystander-initiated cardiopulmonary resuscitation: A statement for the Healthcare Professionals from the Ventilation Working Group of Basic Life Support and Pediatric Life Support Subcommittees, American Heart Association. Ann Emerg Med 1997; 30:654–666.

161. Holmberg M, Holmberg S, Herlitz J. Factors modifying the effect of bystander cardiopulmonary resuscitation on survival in out-of-hospital cardiac arrest patients in Sweden. Eur Heart J 2001; 22: 511–519.

162. Shao D, Weil MH, Tang W, et al. Pupil diameter and light reaction during cardiac arrest and resuscitation. Crit Care Med 2001; 29(4):825–828.

163. Waters RM, Bennett JH. Artificial respiration: comparison of manual maneuvers. Anesth Analg 1936; 15:151–154.

164. Gordon AS, Fainer DC, Ivy AC. Artificial respiration: A new method and a comparative study of different methods in adults. JAMA 1950; 144:1455–1464.

165. Gordon AS, Sadove MS, Raymon F, Ivy AC. Critical survey of manual artificial respiration. JAMA 1951; 147:1444–1453.

166. Gordon AS, Affeldt JE, Sadove M, Raymon F, Whittenberger JL, Ivy AC. Air-flow patterns and pulmonary ventilation during manual artificial respiration on apneic normal adults II. J Appl Physiol 1951; 4:408–420.

167. Gordon AS, Frye CW, Gittelson L, Sadove MS, Beattie EJ. Mouth-to-mouth versus manual artificial respiration for children and adults. JAMA 1958; 167:320–328.

168. Nims RG, Conner EH, Botelho SY, Comroe, Jr. JH. Comparison of methods for performing manual artificial respiration on apneic patients. J Appl Physiol 1951; 4:486–495.

169. Elam JO, Greene DG, Brown ES, Clements JA. Oxygen and carbon dioxide exchange and energy cost of expired air resuscitation. JAMA 1958; 167:328–341.

170. Idris AH, Gabrielli A, Caruso LJ, et al. Tidal volume for bag-valve mask (BVM) ventilations: Less is more. Circulation 1999; 100(Suppl):1664 (Abstract).

171. Kofler J, Sterz F, Hofbauer R, et al. Epinephrine application via an endotracheal airway and via the Combitube in esophageal position. Crit Care Med 2000; 28:1445–1449.

172. Saviteer SM, White GC, Cohen MS, et al. HTLV-III exposure during cardiopulmonary resuscitation. N Engl J Med 1985; 313:1606–1607.

173. Kline SE, Hedemark LL, Davies SF. Outbreak of tuberculosis among regular patrons of a neighborhood bar. N Engl J Med 1995; 333:222–227.

174. Lufkin KC, Ruiz E. Mouth-to-mouth ventilation of cardiac arrested humans using a barrier mask. Prehosp Disaster Med 1993; 8:333–335.

175. Hew P, Brenner B, Kauffman J. Reluctance of paramedics and emergency technicians to perform mouth-to-mouth resuscitation. J Emerg Med 1997; 15:279–284.

176. Ornato JP, Hallagan LF, McMahan SB, et al. Attitudes of BCLS instructors about mouth-to-mouth resuscitation during the AIDS epidemic. Ann Emerg Med 1990; 19:151–156.

177. Shibata K, Taniguchi T, Yoshida M, et al. Obstacles to bystander cardiopulmonary resuscitation in Japan. Resuscitation 2000; 44:187–193.

178. Tajima K, Soda K. Epidemiology of AIDS/HIV in Japan. J Epidemiol 1996; 6(3 Suppl):S67–S74.

179. Capone PL, Lane JC, Kerr CS, et al. Life supporting first aid (LSFA) teaching to Brazilians by television spots. Resuscitation 2000; 47:259–265.

180. Pepe PE, Gay M, Cobb LA, et al. Action sequence for layperson cardiopulmonary resuscitation. Ann Emerg Med 2001; 37(4 Suppl):S17–S25.

181. Kouwenhoven WB, Jude JR, Knickerbocker GG. Landmark article July 9, 1960: Closed-chest massage. JAMA 1984; 251:3133–3136.

182. Michenfelder JD, Theye RA. The effect of anesthesia and hypothermia on canine cerebral ATP and lactate during anoxia produced by decapitation. Anesth 1970; 33:430–439.

183. Meursing BTJ, Zimmerman ANE, Van Huyst ANP. Experimental evidence in favor of reverted sequence in cardiopulmonary resuscitations. J Am Cardiol 1983; 1:610 (Abstract).

184. Berg RA, Hilwig RW, Kern KB, et al. "Bystander" chest compression and assisted ventilation independently improved outcome from piglet asphyxia pulseless "cardiac arrest". Circulation 2000; 101: 1743–1748.

185. Guidelines 2000 for cardiopulmonary resuscitation and emergency cardiovascular care: international consensus on science. Circulation 2000; 102:I-1–I-384.

186. Ruben H, MacNaughton FI. The treatment of food choking. Practitioner 1978; 221:725–729.

187. Langhelle A, Sunde K, Wik L, et al. Airway pressure with chest compression vs Heimlich maneuver in recently dead adults with complete airway obstruction. Resuscitation 2000; 44:105–108.
188. Handley AJ, Monsieurs KG, Bossaert LL. European resuscitation council guidelines 2000 for adult basic life support. A statement from the Basic Life Support and Automated External Defibrillation Working Group (1) and approved by the Executive Committee of the European Resuscitation Council. Resuscitation 2001; 48:199–205.
189. Mogayzel C, Quan L, Graves JR, et al. Out-of-hospital ventricular fibrillation in children and adolescents: Causes and outcomes. Ann Emerg Med 1995; 25:484–491.
190. Niermeyer S, Kattwinkel J, Van Reempts P, et al. International guidelines for neonatal resuscitations: An excerpt from the Guidelines 2000 for Cardiopulmonary Resuscitation and Emergency Cardiovascular Care: international Consensus on Science. Contributors and Reviewers for the Neonatal Resuscitation Guidelines. Pediatrics 2000; 106:1–16.
191. Phillips B, Zideman D, Garcia-Castrillo L, et al. European Resuscitation Council Guidelines 2000 for Advanced Paediatric Life Support. A statement from Paediatric Life Support Working Group and approved by the Executive Committee of the European Resuscitation Council. Resuscitation 2001; 48:235–239.
192. Pepe PE, Gay M, Cobb LA, et al. Action sequence for layperson cardiopulmonary resuscitation. Ann Emerg Med 2001; 37(4 Suppl):S17–S25.
193. Safar P, Escarraga LA, Chang F. Upper airway obstruction in the unconscious patient. J Appl Physiol 1959; 14:760–764.
194. Morikawa S, Safar P, DeCarlo J. Influence of the head-jaw position upon upper airway patency. Anesth 1961; 22:265–270.
195. Safar P. Ventilatory efficacy of mouth-to-mouth artificial respiration: Airway obstruction during manual and mouth-to-mouth artificial respiration. JAMA 1958; 167:335–341.
196. Melker RJ, Banner MJ. Ventilation during CPR. Two-rescuer standards reappraised. Ann Emerg Med 1985; 14:397–402.
197. Fuerst R, Idris A, Banner M, Wenzel V, Orban D. Changes in respiratory system compliance during cardiopulmonary arrest with and without closed chest compressions. Ann Emerg Med 1993; 22:931.
198. Bowman FP, Duckett T, Check B, Menegazzi J. Lower esophageal sphincter pressure during prolonged cardiac arrest and resuscitation. Acad Emerg Med 1994; 1:A18.
199. Ruben H, Knudsen EJ, Carugati G. Gastric inflation in relation to airway pressure. Acta Anaesth Scand 1961; 5:107–114.
200. Ruben A, Ruben H. Artificial respiration: Flow of water from the lung and the stomach. Lancet April 14, 1962; 780–781.
201. Ruben H. The immediate treatment of respiratory failure. Br J Anaesth 1964; 36:542–549.
202. Lawes EG, Baskett PJF. Pulmonary aspiration during unsuccessful cardiopulmonary resuscitation. Intensive Care Med 1987; 13:379–382.
203. Petito SP, Russell WJ. The prevention of gastric insufflation - A neglected benefit of cricoid pressure. Anaesth Intens Care 1988; 16:139–143.
204. Idris AH, Banner MJ, Fuerst R, Becker LB, Wenzel V, Melker RJ. Ventilation caused by external chest compression is unable to sustain effective gas exchange during CPR: a comparison with mechanical ventilation. Resuscitation 1994; 28:143–150.
205. Idris AH, Wenzel V, Tucker KJ, Orban DJ. Chest compression ventilation: A comparison of standard CPR and active-compression/decompression CPR. Acad Emerg Med 1994; 1:A17.
206. Idris AH, Wenzel V, Banner MJ, et al. Smaller tidal volumes minimize gastric inflation during CPR with an unprotected airway. Circulation 1995; 92:I–759 (Abstract).
207. Wenzel V, Idris AH, Banner MJ, et al. The influence of tidal volume on the distribution of gas between the lungs and stomach in the unintubated patient receiving positive pressure ventilation. Crit Care Med 1998; 26:364–368.
208. Guidelines for the basic management of the airway and ventilation during resuscitation. A statement by the Airway and Ventilation Management Working Group of the European Resuscitation Council. Resuscitation 1996; 31:187–200.
209. Wolcke B, Schneider T, Mauer D, et al. Ventilation volumes with different self-inflating bags with reference to ERC guidelines for airway management: comparison of two compression techniques. Resuscitation 2000; 47:175–178.
210. Wenzel V, Dorges V, Lindner KH, et al. Mouth-to-mouth ventilation during cardiopulmonary resuscitation: word of mouth in the street versus science. Anesth Analg 2001; 93:4–6.

211. Oschatz E, Wunderbaldinger P, Sterz F, et al. Cardiopulmonary resuscitation performed by bystanders does not increase adverse effects as assessed by chest radiography. Anesth Analg 2001; 93:128–133.
212. Wenzel V, Keller C, Idris AH, Doerges V, Lindner KH, Brimacombe JR. Effects of smaller tidal volumes during basic life support ventilation in patients with respiratory arrest: Good ventilation, Less risk? Resuscitation 1999; 43:25–29.
213. Dorges V, Ocker H, Hagelberg S, et al. Smaller tidal volumes with room air are not sufficient to ensure adequate oxygenation during bag-valve-mask ventilation Resuscitation 2000; 44:37–41.
214. Cummins RO, Hazinski MF. The most important changes in the international ECC and CPR guidelines 2000. Resuscitation 2000; 46:431–437.
215. Gausche M, Lewis RJ, Stratton SJ, et al. Effect of out of hospital pediatric endotracheal intubations on survival and psychological outcome: A controlled clinical trial. JAMA 2000; 283:783–790.
216. Froese AB, Bryan AC. High frequency ventilation. Am Rev Respir Dis 1987; 135:1363–1374.
217. Slutsky AS. Nonconventional methods of ventilation. Am Rev Respir Dis 1988; 138:175–183.
218. Zidulka A, Gross D, Minami H, Vartian V, Chang HK. Ventilation by high-frequency chest wall compression in dogs with normal lungs. Am Rev Respir Dis 1983; 127:709–713.
219. Fuyuki T, Suzuki S, Sakurai M, Sasaki H, Butler JP, Takashima T. Ventilatory effectiveness of high-frequency oscillation applied to the body surface. J Appl Physiol 1987; 62:2410–2415.
220. Harf A, Bertrand C, Chang HK. Ventilation by high-frequency oscillation of thorax or at trachea in rats. J Appl Physiol 1984; 56:155–60.
221. Gross D, Vartian V, Minami H, Chang HK, Zidulka A. High frequency chest wall compression and carbon dioxide elimination in obstructed dogs. Bull Eur Physiopathol Respir 1984; 20:507–511.
222. George RJD, Winter RJD, Flockton SJ, Geddes DM. Ventilatory saving by external chest wall compression or oral high-frequency oscillation in normal subjects and those with chronic airflow obstruction. Clin Sci 1985; 69:349–359.
223. Piquet J, Isabey D, Chang HK, Harf A. High frequency transthoracic ventilation improves gas exchange during experimental bronchoconstriction in rabbits. Am Rev Respir Dis 1986; 133:605–608.
224. Ward HE, Power JHT, Nicholas TE. High-frequency oscillations via the pleural surface: an alternative mode of ventilation? J Appl Physiol: Respirat Environ Exercise Physiol 1983; 54:427–433.
225. Kleinsasser A, Lindner KH, Schaefer A, et al. Decompression-triggered positive-pressure ventilation during cardiopulmonary resuscitation improves pulmonary gas exchange and oxygen uptake. Circulation 2002; 106:373–378.
226. Guidelines for cardiopulmonary resuscitation and emergency cardiac care. Emergency Cardiac Care Committee and Subcommittees, American Heart Association. JAMA 1992; 268:2171–2302.
227. Cobb LA, Hallstrom AP. Community based cardiopulmonary resuscitation: What have we learned? Ann NY Acad Sci 1982; 382:330–342.
228. Finucane TB, Santora AH. Basic airway management and cardiopulmonary resuscitation (CPR). In: Principles of Airway Management. Philadelphia, PA: FA Davis, 1988, p. 16.
229. Guildner CW. Resuscitation - opening the airway. A comparative study of techniques for opening an airway obstructed by the tongue. JACEP 1976; 5:588–590.
230. Lawrence PJ, Sivaneswaran N. Ventilation during cardiopulmonary resuscitation: which method? Med J Austr 1985; 143:443–446.
231. Johannigman JA, Branson RD, Davis K Jr, Hurst JM. Techniques of emergency ventilation: A model to evaluate tidal volume, airway pressure, and gastric insufflation. J Trauma 1991; 31:93–98.
232. McSwain GR, Garrison WB, Artz CP. Evaluation of resuscitation from cardiopulmonary arrest by paramedics. Ann Emerg Med 1980; 9:341–345.
233. Harrison RR, Maull KI. Pocket mask ventilation: a superior method of acute airway management. Ann Emerg Med 1982; 11:74–76.
234. Hess D, Baran C. Ventilatory volumes using mouth-to-mouth, mouth-to-mask, and bag-valve-mask techniques. Am J Emerg Med 1985; 3: 292–296.
235. Jesudian MC, Harrison RR, Keenan RL, Maull KI. Bag-valve mask ventilation; two rescuers are better than one: Preliminary report. Crit Care Med 1985; 13:122–123.
236. Hodgkin JE, Foster GL, Nicolay LI. Cardiopulmonary resuscitation: development of an organized protocol. Crit Care Med 1977; 5:93–100.
237. Hirschman AM, Kravath RE. Venting vs ventilating. A danger of manual resuscitation bags. Chest 1982; 82:369–370.
238. Florete OG Jr. Airway devices and their application. In: Kirby RR, Gravenstein N, eds. Clinical Anesthesia Practice. Philadelphia, PA: WB Saunders, 1994, 303.

239. Milner A. The importance of ventilation to effective resuscitation in the term and preterm infant. Semin Neonatol 2001; 6:219–224.

240. Vyas H, Field D, Milner AD, Hopkin IE. Determinants of the first inspiratory volume and functional residual capacity at birth. Pediatr Pulmonol 1986; 2:189–193.

241. Ikegami M, Kallapur S, Michna J, et al. Lung injury and surfactant metabolism after hyperventilation of premature lambs. Pediatr Res 2000; 47:398–404.

242. Milner AD, Saunders RA. Pressure and volume changes during the first breath of human neonates. Arch Dis Child 1977; 52:918–924.

243. Head H. On the regulation of respiration. J Physiol 1889; 10:1–70.

244. Vyas H, Milner AD, Hopkin IE. Efficacy of face mask resuscitation at birth. BMJ 1984; 289:1563–1565.

245. Vyas H, Milner AD, Hopkin IE. Face mask resuscitation: Does it lead to gastric distension? Arch Dis Child 1983; 58:373–375.

246. Pepe PE, Copass MK, Joyce TH. Prehospital endotracheal intubation: Rationale for training emergency medical personnel. Ann Emerg Med 1985; 14:1085–1092.

247. Florete Jr, OG. Airway Management. In: Civetta JM, Taylor RW, Kirby RR, eds. Critical care, 2nd Ed. Philadelphia, PA: JB Lippincott, 1991, p. 1427.

248. Bolder PM, Healey TE, Bolder AR Beatty PC, Kay B. The extra work of breathing through adult endotracheal tubes. Anesth Analg 1986; 65:853–859.

249. Conrardy PA, Goodman LR, Lainge F, Singer MM. Alteration of endotracheal tube position: Flexion and extension of the neck. Crit Care Med 1976; 4:8–12.

250. Rabey PG, Murphy PJ, Langton JA, et al. Effect of laryngeal mask airway on lower oesophageal sphincter pressure in patients during general anaesthesia. Brit J Anaesth 1992; 69:346–348.

251. Rhee KJ, O'Malley RJ, Turner JE, et al. Field airway management of the trauma patient: The efficacy of bag mask ventilation. Am J Emerg Med 1988; 6:333–336.

252. Pennant JH, Walker MB. Comparison of the endotracheal tube and the laryngeal mask in airway management by paramedical personnel. Anesth Analg 1992; 74:531–534.

253. Reinhart DJ, Simmons G. Comparison of placement of the laryngeal mask airway with endotracheal tube by paramedics and respiratory therapists. Ann Emerg Med 1994; 24:260–263.

254. Davies PRF, Tighe SQM, Greenslade GL, et al. Laryngeal mask airway and tracheal tube insertion by unskilled personnel. Lancet 1990; 336:977–979.

255. Devitt JH, Wenstone R, Noel AG, et al. The laryngeal mask airway and positive-pressure ventilation. Anesth 1994; 80:550–555.

256. Brimacombe J, White A, Berry A. Effect of cricoid pressure on ease of insertion of the laryngeal mask airway. Br J Anaesth 1993; 71:800–802.

257. Brain AIJ, Verghese C, Strube PJ. The LMA 'ProSeal'—a laryngeal mask with an esophageal vent. Br J Anaesth 2000; 84:650–654.

258. Keller C, Brimacombe J. Mucosal pressure and oropharyngeal leak pressure with the ProSeal vs laryngeal mask airway in anaesthetized paralyzed patients. Br J Anaesth 2000; 85:262–266.

259. Schofferman J, Oill P, Lewis AJ. The esophageal obturator airway: A clinical evaluation. Chest 1976; 69:67–71.

260. Shea SR, MacDonald JR, Gruzinski G. Prehospital endotracheal tube airway or esophageal gastric tube airway: A critical comparison. Ann Emerg Med 1985; 14:102–112.

261. Rumball CJ, McDonald D. The PTL, Combitube, laryngeal mask and oral airway: A randomized prehospital comparative study of ventilatory device effectiveness and cost-effectiveness in 470 cases of cardiorespiratory arrest. Prehosp Emerg Care 1997; 1:1–10.

262. Vézina D, Lessard MR, Bussières J, et al. Complications associated with the use of the esophageal-tracheal Combitube. Can J Anaesth 1998; 45:76–80.

263. Walz R, Davis S, Panning B. Is the Combitube a useful emergency airway device for anesthesiologists? [letter]. Anesth Analg 1999; 88:233.

264. Niemann JT, Rosboough JP, Myers R, et al. The pharyngotracheal lumen airway: preliminary investigation of a new adjunct. Ann Emerg Med 1984; 13:591–596.

265. Ocker H, Wenzel B, Schmucker P, et al. Effectiveness of various airway management techniques in a bench model simulating a cardiac arrest. J Emerg Med 2001; 20:7–12.

266. Calkins MD, Robinson TD: Combat trauma airway management: Endotracheal intubation versus a laryngeal mask airway versus Combitube. Use by Navy SEAL and reconnaissance combat corpsmen. J Trauma 1999; 46:927–932.

267. Greene MK, Roden R, Hinchley G. The laryngeal mask airway: Two cases of pre-hospital care. Anaesth 1992; 47:688–689.
268. Kokkinis K. The use of the laryngeal mask airway in CPR. Resuscitation 1994; 27:9–12.
269. Martens P. The use of laryngeal mask airway by nurses during cardiopulmonary resuscitation. Anaesth 1994; 49:731–773.
270. Leach A, Alexander CA, Stone B. The laryngeal mask in cardiopulmonary resuscitation in a district general hospital: A preliminary communication. Resuscitation 1993; 25:245–248.
271. Alexander R, Hodgson P, Lomax D, et al. A comparison of the laryngeal mask airway and Guedel airway, bag and facemask for manual ventilation formal training. Anaesth 1993; 48:231–234.
272. Martin PD, Cyna AM, Hunter WA, et al. Training nursing staff in airway management of resuscitations: a clinical comparison of the facemask and laryngeal mask. Anaesth 1993; 48:33–37.
273. Brimacombe JR, Berry A. The incidence of aspiration associated with laryngeal mask airway: Meta-analysis of published literature. J Clin Anesth 1995; 7:297–305.
274. Frass M, Frenzer R, Zdrahal F, et al. The esophageal tracheal Combitube: Preliminary results with a new airway for CPR. Ann Emerg Med 1987; 16:768–772.
275. Frass M, Frenzer R, Zdrahal F, et al. Ventilation with the esophageal tracheal Combitube in cardiopulmonary resuscitations. Promptness and effectiveness. Chest 1988; 93:781–784.
276. Staudinger T, Brugger S, Watschinger B, et al. Emergency intubation with a Combitube: Comparison with the endotracheal airway. Ann Emerg Med 1993; 22:1573–1575.
277. Atherton GL, Johnson GC. Ability of paramedics to use the Combitube in prehospital cardiac arrest. Ann Emerg Med 1993; 22:1263–1268.
278. Blostein PA, Koestner AJ, Hoak S. Failed rapid sequence intubation in trauma patients: Esophageal tracheal Combitube is a useful adjunct. J Trauma 1998; 44:534–537.
279. Gabbott DA, Sasada MP. Orotracheal intubations in trauma patients with cervical fractures. Arch Surg 1994; 129:1104–1105.
280. Pennant JH, Jajraj NM, Pace NA. Laryngeal mask airway in cervical spine injuries. Anesth Analg 1992; 74:1074–1075.
281. Keller C, Brimacombe J, Kleinsasser A. Does the ProSeal laryngeal mask airway prevent aspiration of regurgitated fluid? Anesth Analg 2000; 91:1017–1020.
282. Mercer MH, Gabbott DA. Insertion of the Combitube airway with a cervical spine immobilized in the rigid cervical collar. Anaesth 1998; 53:971–974.
283. Caparosa RJ, Zavatsky AR. Practical aspects of the cricothyroid space. Laryngoscope 1957; 67:577–591.
284. Melker RJ, Florete OG. Percutaneous cricothyroidotomy and tracheostomy. In: Benumof JL, ed. Airway management: principles and practice. St. Louis, MO: Mosby, 1996, pp. 484–512.
285. Laurie K, Zielinski T, McKnit S, et al. Improving the efficiency of cardiopulmonary resuscitation with an inspiratory impedance threshold valve. Crit Care Med 2000; 28(11 Suppl):207–209.
286. Lurie KG, Mulligan KA, McKnite S, et al. Optimizing standards of cardiopulmonary resuscitation with an inspiratory impedance threshold valve. Chest 1998; 113:1084–1090.
287. Plaisance P, Lurie KG, Payen D. Inspiratory impedance during active compression-decompression cardiopulmonary resuscitation: a randomized evaluation in patients in cardiac arrest. Circulation 2000; 101:989–994.
288. Voelckel WG, Lurie KG, Zielinski T, et al. The effect of positive end-expiratory pressure during active compression decompression cardiopulmonary resuscitation with the inspiratory threshold valve. Anesth Analg 2001; 92:967–974.
289. Sulek CA, Kirby RR. The recurring problem of negative-pressure pulmonary edema. Curr Rev Anesth 1998; 18:243–250.
290. Branson RD. Transport ventilators. In: Branson, RD, Hess DR, Chatburn RL, eds. Respiratory Care Equipment, 2 nd Ed. Philadelphia, PA: Lippincott Williams & Wilkins 1999, pp. 527–565.
291. Gervais HW, Eberle B, Konietzke D, et al. Comparison of blood gases of ventilated patients during transport. Crit Care Med 1987; 15:761.
292. Gazmuri RJ, Weil MH, Bisera J, Rackow EC. End-tidal carbon dioxide tension as a monitor of native blood flow during resuscitation by extracorporeal circulation. J Thorac Cardiovasc Surg 1991; 101: 984–988.
293. Gudipati CV, Weil MH, Bisera J, Deshmukh HG, Rackow EC. Expired carbon dioxide: A noninvasive monitor of cardiopulmonary resuscitation. Circulation 1988; 77:234–239.
294. Sanders AB, Atlas M, Ewy GA, Kern KB, Bragg S. Expired CO_2 as an index of coronary perfusion pressure. Am J Emerg Med 1985; 3:147–149.
295. Kalenda Z. The capnogram as a guide to the efficacy of cardiac massage. Resuscitation 1978; 6:259–263.

296. Falk JL, Rackow EC, Weil MH. End-tidal carbon dioxide concentration during cardiopulmonary resuscitation. N Eng J Med 1988; 318:607–611.

297. Garnett AR, Ornato JP, Gonzalez ER, Johnson EB. End-tidal carbon dioxide monitoring during cardiopulmonary resuscitation. JAMA 1987; 257:512–515.

298. Grundler WG, Weil MH, Bisera J, Rackow EC. Observations on end-tidal carbon dioxide during experimental cardiopulmonary arrest. J Clin Res 1984; 32:672A.

299. Sanders AB, Ewy GA, Bragg S, Atlas M, Kern KB. Expired PCO_2 as a prognostic indicator of successful resuscitation from cardiac arrest. Ann Emerg Med 1985; 14:948–952.

300. Sanders AB, Kern KB, Otto CW, Milander MM, Ewy GA. End-tidal carbon dioxide monitoring during cardiopulmonary resuscitation: A prognostic indicator for survival. JAMA 1989; 262:1347–1351.

301. Trevino RP, Bisera J, Weil MH, Rackow EC, Grundler WG. End-tidal CO_2 as a guide to successful cardiopulmonary resuscitation: a preliminary report. Crit Care Med 1985; 13:910–911.

302. Wiklund L, Söderberg D, Henneberg S, Rubertsson S, Stjernström H, Groth T. Kinetics of carbon dioxide during cardiopulmonary resuscitation. Crit Care Med 1986; 14:1015–1022.

303. Callaham M, Barton C. Prediction of outcome of cardiopulmonary resuscitation from end-tidal carbon dioxide concentration. Crit Care Med 1990; 18:358–362.

304. Bhende MS, Thompson AE, Cook DR. Validity of a disposable end-tidal CO_2 detector in verifying endotracheal tube position in infants and children. Ann Emerg Med 1990; 19:483.

305. Mickelson KS, Sterner SP, Ruiz E. Exhaled PCO_2 as a predictor of endotracheal tube placement. Ann Emerg Med 1986; 15:657.

306. Ornato JP, Shipley JB, Racht EM, et al. Multicenter study of end-tidal carbon dioxide in the prehospital setting. Ann Emerg Med 1992; 21:518–523.

307. Vukmir RB, Heller MB, Stein KL. Confirmation of endotracheal tube placement: A miniaturized qualitative CO_2 detector. Ann Emerg Med 1991; 20:726–729.

308. Ornato JP, Levine RL, Young DS, Racht EM, Garnett AR, Gonzalez ER. Effect of applied chest compression on systemic arterial pressure and end-tidal carbon dioxide concentration during CPR in human beings. Ann Emerg Med 1989; 18:732–737.

309. Ornato JP, Gonzalez ER, Garnett AR, Levine RL, McClung BK. Effect of cardiopulmonary resuscitation compression rate on end-tidal carbon dioxide concentration and arterial pressure in man. Crit Care Med 1988; 16:241–245.

310. Ward KR, Menegazzi JJ, Zelenak RR. A comparison of mechanical CPR and manual CPR by monitoring end-tidal PCO_2 in human cardiac arrest. Ann Emerg Med 1990; 19:456.

311. Ward KR, Sullivan RJ, Zelenak RR, Summer WR. A comparison of interposed abdominal compression CPR and standard CPR by monitoring end-tidal PCO_2. Ann Emerg Med 1989; 18:831–837.

312. Bircher NG. Acidosis of cardiopulmonary resuscitation: carbon dioxide transport and anaerobiosis. Crit Care Med 1992; 20:1203–1205.

313. Gravenstein JS, Paulus DA, Hayes TJ. Capnography in Clinical Practice. Boston, MA: Butterworth Publishers, 1989, 65–70.

314. Lambertsen CJ. Transport of oxygen and carbon dioxide by the blood. In: Mountcastle VB, Ed. Medical Physiology. St. Louis, MO: Mosby, 1974, pp. 1399–1422.

315. Idris A, Staples E, O'Brien D, et al. End-tidal carbon dioxide during extremely low cardiac output. Ann Emerg Med 1994; 23:568–572.

316. Martin GB, Gentile NT, Paradis NA, Moeggenberg, Appleton TJ, Nowak RM. Effect of epinephrine on end-tidal carbon dioxide monitoring during CPR. Ann Emerg Med 1990; 19:396–398.

317. Niemann JT, Rosborough JP, Ung S, Criley JM. Coronary perfusion pressure during experimental cardiopulmonary resuscitation. Ann Emerg Med 1982; 11:127–131.

318. Falk JL, Sayre MR. Confirmation of airway placement. Prehosp Emerg Care 1999; 3:273–278.

319. Barton CW, Callaham ML. Possible confounding effect of minute ventilation on $ETCO_2$ in cardiac arrest. Ann Emerg Med 1991; 20:445–446.

320. Gazmuri RJ, von Planta M, Weil MH, Rackow EC. Arterial PCO_2 as an indicator of systemic perfusion during cardiopulmonary resuscitation. Crit Care Med 1989; 17:237–240.

321. Angelos MG, DeBehnke DJ, Leasure JE. Arterial blood gases during cardiac arrest: markers of blood flow in a canine model. Resuscitation 1992; 23:101–111.

322. Tenney SM. A theoretical analysis of the relationship between venous blood and mean tissue oxygen pressures. Resp Phys 1974; 20:283–296.

323. Lee J, Wright F, Barber R, et al. Central venous oxygen saturation in shock. Anesth 1972; 36:472–478.

324. Kasnitz P, Druger GL, Yorra F, et al. Mixed venous oxygen tension and hyperlactemia. JAMA 1976; 236:570–574.

325. Emerman CL, Pinchak AC, Hagen JF, Hancock D. A comparison of venous blood gases during cardiac arrest. Am J Emerg Med 1988; 6:580–583.

326. Kissoon N, Rosenberg H, Gloor J, Vidal R. Comparison of the acid-base status of blood obtained from intraosseous and central venous sites during steady- and low-flowstates. Crit Care Med 1993; 21: 1765–1769.

327. Kissoon N, Idris A, Wenzel V, Peterson R, Murphy S, Rush W. Comparison of the acid-base balance of intraosseous and mixed venous blood gases during cardiopulmonary resuscitation. Pediatric Research 1994; 35(Part 2):54A.

5 Management of Ventilation During Resuscitation

Marsh Cuttino, MD

INTRODUCTION

The decision to control a patient's airway during cardiopulmonary resuscitation (CPR) is straightforward. Patients in cardiopulmonary arrest generally are totally unresponsive, and airway techniques can be used without the need for pharmacological adjuncts. Much of the decision making relates to timing and the type of ventilation method to use. These decisions are influenced by the patient's oxygenation status, duration of arrest, expected difficulties with airway control, and operator experience and training.

VENTILATION

Establishing a secure patent airway is one of the primary tasks of the emergency care provider during resuscitation. Adequate ventilation can reduce hypoxia and hypercapnea. The airway should be obtained as soon as possible during resuscitation. Failure to control the airway can have ominous consequences.

Endotracheal intubation is considered the optimal method for securing the airway currently because it allows adequate ventilation, oxygenation, and airway protection. The Combitube (Kendall Healthcare Products, Mansfield, MA) and laryngeal mask airway (LMA North America, San Diego, CA) are acceptable and possibly helpful alternative airway devices.

The main advantages of alternative airway devices is that they (a) are generally easier to insert than an endotracheal tube (ETT); (b) may provide ventilation results similar to

From: *Contemporary Cardiology: Cardiopulmonary Resuscitation*
Edited by: J. P. Ornato and M. A. Peberdy © Humana Press Inc., Totowa, NJ

that provided by endotracheal intubation and superior to bag-valve-mask ventilation; and (c) have similar complication rates to endotracheal intubation. Additionally, alternative airway devices can sometimes be used when tracheal intubation is not possible *(1)*.

The amount of ventilation required during resuscitation is not well established. Although the minute ventilation requirements may be decreased by a low cardiac output, the excess load of carbon dioxide returning from ischemic tissue beds must be cleared by ventilation. Chest compressions alone do not generate adequate or consistent ventilation in humans, even after intubation *(2)*. In the resuscitation patient, 100% oxygen should be started immediately using a bag-valve-mask. This should be followed rapidly by endotracheal intubation once skilled individuals arrive on scene. If intubation is unsuccessful, then an alternative airway should be employed.

When a nonintubated patient is ventilated, the distribution of gas between the lungs and stomach depends on the patient's lower esophageal sphincter pressure, respiratory mechanics (the respiratory system compliance and degree of airway obstruction), and the technique of the rescuer performing basic life support (BLS; inspiratory flow rate, peak airway pressure, and tidal volume). Accidental stomach inflation during CPR can elevate intragastric pressure and lead to the cascade of regurgitation, aspiration, pneumonia, and death even in the successfully resuscitated patient *(3)*.

Ventilation has an impact on blood gases even at very low cardiac output states *(4)*. Hypoxia and hypercarbia have an independent adverse effect on resuscitation, and can be corrected with appropriate ventilation. Adequate ventilation is important for return of spontaneous circulation *(5)*. Successful ventilation with rapid and uninterrupted chest compressions significantly improves coronary perfusion during CPR *(6)* and this makes successful defibrillation more likely *(7)*.

In cardiac arrest (CA) there is generally sufficient oxygenation in the blood that a reasonable oxygen saturation persists for approx 5 minutes when there is adequate chest compression *(8)*. Bystander CPR for the first 5 minutes has equivalent outcomes with or without mouth-to-mouth ventilation *(9)*. This suggests that airway control is most useful when achieved in the first 5–6 minutes of CA.

INDICATIONS FOR ASSISTED VENTILATION

Rapid assessment of the patient allows for appropriate decision on airway management. Important considerations include adequacy of ventilation, airway patency, need for neuromuscular blockade, cervical spine stability, safety of the technique, and the skill of the operator *(10)*.

Some patients are intubated for airway protection and others are intubated specifically for failure of ventilation or oxygenation. Objective indicators of ventilatory status include arterial blood gas, pulse oximetry, capnography, chest radiography, and spirometry. Methods to maintain an open airway range from BLS measures (e.g., head tilt–chin lift) to advanced airway techniques (e.g., endotracheal intubation). Medical providers should be proficient in several techniques at each level of airway control. This allows the operator to be flexible in the management of the airway as the situation demands.

Once a patient has been found to be unresponsive, and the emergency response system has been activated, the airway needs to be assessed. First, the patient should be placed in the supine position. If trauma is suspected, the cervical spine must be protected, and the patient should be log rolled. The rescuer should open the airway and assess breathing by looking for a chest rise, listening for exhaled breath, and feeling for air exchange at the nose and mouth. If the airway and breathing are inadequate, the airway should be opened. In the unresponsive patient, the tongue and epiglottis may be obstructing the pharynx.

There are two techniques for opening an airway manually: the head tilt–chin lift and the jaw thrust maneuver. In some patients, spontaneous breathing returns after the airway becomes patent. These patients should then be placed in a recovery position to reduce the risk of aspiration. The American Heart Association (AHA) Guidelines released in 2000 for the recovery position include the following *(11)*:

- Use a lateral position, with the head dependent to allow free fluid drainage.
- Make sure position is stable.
- Avoid pressure on the chest that impairs breathing.
- Good observation and access to the airway should be possible.
- The position should not give rise to injury to the patient.
- It should be possible to return the patient to the supine position quickly and easily, and maintain cervical stability.
- Repositioning should occur to prevent prolonged time in one position.
- Patient should be monitored until airway is definitively secured.

Head Tilt–Chin Lift

Placing one hand on the patient's forehead and the index and middle finger of the other hand on the bony part of the chin performs the head tilt–chin lift. The patient's head is rotated as the chin is lifted. This lifts the jaw and elevates the tongue off the back of the pharynx, opening the airway.

Jaw Thrust

Grasping the angles of the jaw with the index and middle fingers and lifting with both hands performs the jaw thrust. The head is maintained in the neutral position without any flexion or extension. As the jaw is lifted, the patient's mouth is opened with the thumbs. This is the preferred method when there is a possibility of cervical spine injury.

Basic Life Support Techniques

The first step is to open the airway, then look, listen, and feel for breathing. If the patient is not breathing adequately, rescue breathing must be performed. The AHA recommends that lay rescuers check for "signs of circulation" (e.g., normal breathing, coughing, or normal movement in response to stimulation) rather than perform a pulse check to determine if chest compression's should be administered. Trained health care providers are encouraged to check for a pulse. Rescue breathing for both single rescuer CPR and multiple rescuer CPR with an unprotected airway is at a 15:2 ratio of chest compression to breathing with a rate of 100 compressions per minute *(11)*.

Mouth-to-Mouth Ventilation and Variants

Rescue breathing through mouth-to-mouth ventilation has been an important part of CPR for more than 30 years. Concern about transmission of infectious disease has made both professional medical providers and lay people reluctant to provide mouth-to-mouth ventilation to adult strangers *(12)*. This has led to consideration of removing mouth-to-mouth ventilation guidelines from CPR *(9)*. Current guidelines still recommend mouth-to-mouth ventilation in out-of-hospital arrest, but recognize that basic CPR with chest compression alone is still better than no CPR *(13)*. All out of hospital pediatric arrest victims should receive mouth-to-mouth ventilation, since most pediatric CA have a large respiratory component *(14)*.

TECHNIQUE

Mouth-to-mouth ventilation is the most basic form of positive pressure ventilation. The rescuer positions him or herself at the patient's side. After opening the airway, the rescuer takes a deep breath, pinches the patient's nose, and seals his or her mouth around the patient's mouth. Slow deep breaths are delivered, and after each breath the mouth is removed to allow passive exhalation. Using slow breaths helps prevent gastric inflation and aspiration from reflux and regurgitation.

Mouth-to-Nose Rescue Breathing

Mouth-to-nose rescue breathing can be used when there are contraindications to mouth-to-mouth breathing. Conditions such as anatomic abnormalities, trismus, or severe trauma could prevent formation of an appropriate seal. The rescuer positions the patient's head in extension. One hand is placed on the forehead and the other lifts the mandible and closes the mouth. The rescuer's mouth is placed over the patient's nose and a seal is formed with the lips. The appropriate breaths are delivered, and the mouth is removed from the patient's nose to allow passive exhalation. It may be necessary to open the mouth intermittently to allow complete exhalation.

Mouth-to-Shield Ventilation

Face shields are small, disposable, plastic barrier devices that can be used during mouth-to-mouth ventilation. This removes any concern over infectious disease transmission. Shields may have enhancements such as one-way valves. The rescuer positions the shield on the patient, pinches the nose and seals his or her mouth around the center opening of the face shield. After the appropriate breaths are delivered, the rescuer lifts his or her mouth from the shield and allows the patient to exhale. Figure 1 shows an example of a pocket shield device. There are numerous other examples available on the market with similar function.

Mouth-to-Mask Method

Another technique designed to isolate the rescuer from the patient is the mouth-to-mask method. A standard face mask is used and fitted over the mouth using the same position as used for the bag-valve-mask (Fig. 2). The rescuer can provide rescue breaths either into the mask directly or indirectly using a one-way valve adapter. When the adapter is used the face mask must be released to allow exhalation.

VENTILATION VOLUME

Mouth-to-mouth ventilation with a tidal volume of 1000 mL contains about 17% oxygen and about 4% carbon dioxide *(15)*. The gas composition can be improved to about 19% oxygen and 2–3% carbon dioxide by taking a deep breath and exhaling only about 500 mL *(16)*. With normal cardiac output, tidal volumes of 800–1000 mL are required to maintain adequate oxygenation *(17,18)*. Some authors have suggested that because

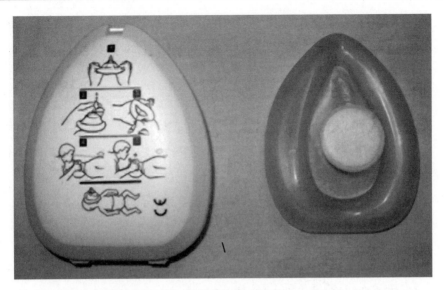

Fig. 1. Example of a pocket shield device.

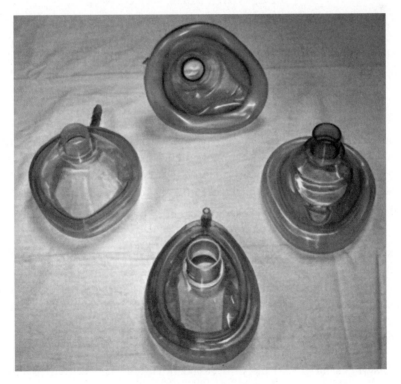

Fig. 2. Ventilation masks.

cardiac output is reduced to at best 20–30% of normal during CPR there is a reduced requirement for ventilation *(19,20)*. It appears that a tidal volume of 500 mL may be adequate during CPR when supplemental oxygen is added *(21)*. Current guidelines recommend a tidal volume of 10 mL/kg or 700 to 1000 mL over 2 seconds *(13)*.

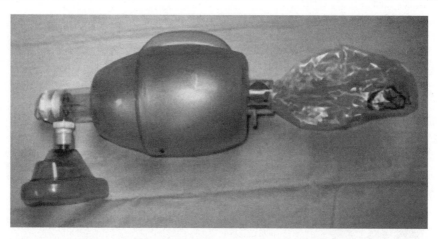

Fig. 3. Example of a typical bag-valve-mask assembly.

INTERMEDIATE AIRWAY TECHNIQUES AND DEVICES

Bag-Valve-Mask Device

The bag-valve-mask is a common device for delivering positive pressure ventilation in the initial stages of resuscitation (Fig. 3). The key to proper use of the bag-valve-mask is to maintain a tight seal. There are different techniques depending on whether there is a single operator or two operators.

Techniques

SINGLE OPERATOR

The rescuer stands at the head of the patient. The mask is applied to the patient's face with one hand. The thumb and index fingers secure the mask, and the remaining fingers are placed over the bony portion of the mandible. As the rescuer ventilates the patient, the fingers on the mandible maintain the head tilt and jaw thrust to keep the airway patent and the mask snug against the face.

DUAL OPERATORS

The first rescuer stands at the head of the patient. The mask is applied to the patient's face, and the thumb and index fingers of both hands secure the mask and maintain a good seal. The remaining fingers are used on the bony portion of the mandible to maintain the head tilt and jaw thrust. The second rescuer stands to the right of the patient, and provides two-handed compression of the bag to ventilate the patient (Fig. 4).

Oropharyngeal Airway Device

An oropharyngeal airway is a plastic or rubber device that can be inserted into a victim's mouth to elevate the tongue and create a path between the tongue and palate (Fig. 5). This device should not be used on a patient who has an intact gag reflex. It is indicated in the unresponsive or obtunded patient and can be used in conjunction with a bag-valve-mask device.

To size an oropharyngeal airway, choose one that fits from the middle of the mouth to the angle of the jaw. The airway is inserted by turning it 90° and inserting it halfway into the mouth. Then rotate back 90° so that the bottom wraps around the back of the tongue.

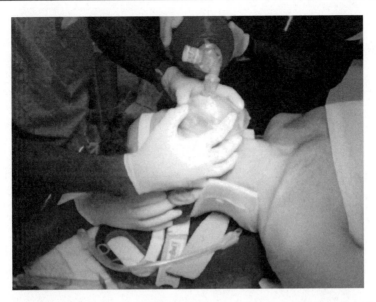

Fig. 4. Two-person bag-valve-mask technique. Note the set of hands on the bottom left maintaining in-line cervical stabilization.

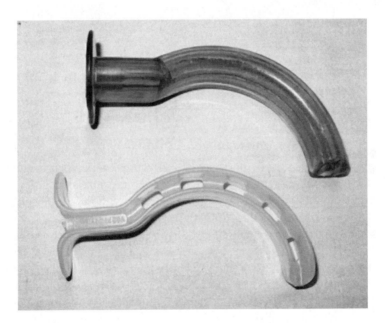

Fig. 5. Oropharyngeal airways.

The distal portion of the airway should remain outside of the mouth to ensure that it does not become an airway obstruction.

If the patient begins to gag, the oropharyngeal airway should be pulled out. The oropharyngeal airway may be contraindicated in facial or mandibular trauma patients. This airway will not maintain a patent airway if the patient has incorrect head placement.

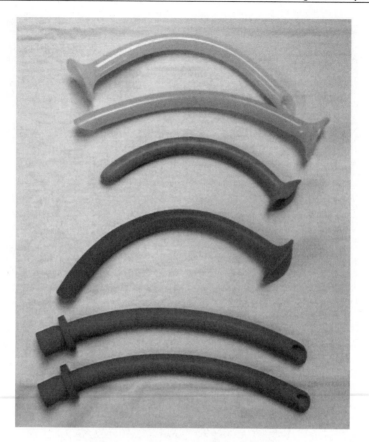

Fig. 6. Nasopharyngeal airways.

Nasopharyngeal Airway Device

A flexible tube designed to be inserted into the nares and extend to the base of the tongue (Fig. 6). A nasopharyngeal airway can help maintain airway patency in an unconscious or obtunded patient but does not ensure patency without good head positioning. This airway adjunct can be used in conjunction with a bag-valve-mask to facilitate ventilation. Nasopharyngeal airways can be used with patients that still have an intact gag reflex.

To size a nasopharyngeal airway, choose a tube that extends from the tip of the nose to the angle of the patient's mandible. The diameter of the tube should approximate the diameter of the nares. The tube is lubricated and inserted into the nares so that the beveled tip is midline, and the curve of the tube follows the curvature of the patient's airway.

ADVANCED AIRWAYS

Orotracheal Intubation

The most common technique of advanced airway control is orotracheal intubation with direct visualization laryngoscopy. Laryngoscopes are used to provide a direct view of the vocal cords and facilitate placement of the ETT. Most intubations during CPR are "crash" airways and do not require pharmacologic adjuncts such as rapid sequence induction.

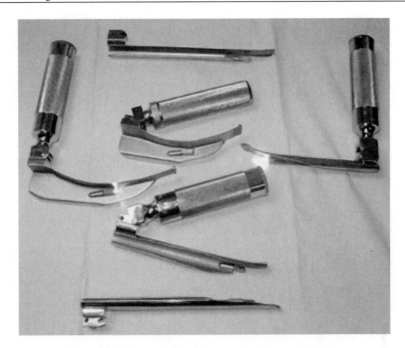

Fig. 7. Examples of laryngoscope handles and blades.

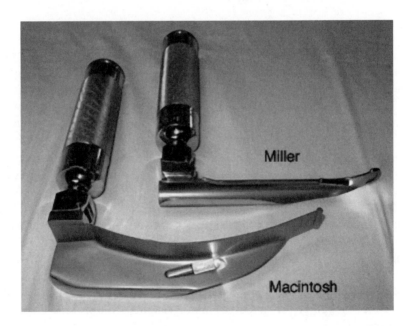

Fig. 8. Miller and MacIntosh laryngoscope blades.

The laryngoscope is an apparatus designed to permit direct visualization of the larynx and facilitate endotracheal intubation through direct laryngoscopy (Figs. 7 and 8). There are two basic blade designs. The first is the curved blade, typified by the MacIntosh blade. The second type is the straight blade such as the Miller or Wisconsin blades (Welch Allyn, Skaneateles Falls, NY). Various sizes are available for adult and pediatric use. The main

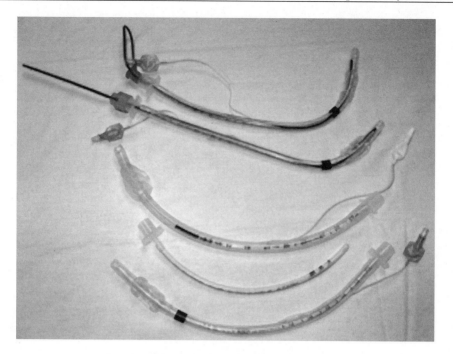

Fig. 9. Endotracheal tubes.

difference in the usage of the blades regards the epiglottis. A straight blade lifts the epiglottis directly, but the curved blade tip fits in the vallecula and indirectly lifts the epiglottis.

The choice of which blade to use should be based on the patient's clinical history. Straight blades are better for pediatric patients, patients with an anterior larynx, patients with a long floppy epiglottis, or patients with a scarred epiglottis. Straight blades allow for more control of the airway in trauma patients, and may offer some advantages when there is debris in the airway. There are several disadvantages with straight blades. They are hard to use with large teeth, and may be more likely to break teeth than their curved counterparts. Straight blades can stimulate the superior laryngeal nerve and lead to laryngospasm. These blades can be inserted inadvertently into the esophagus and lead to esophageal intubation. Curved blades offer better control of the tongue can allow more room in the hypopharynx to pass the endotracheal tube. Curved blades possibly require less forearm strength to use. Medical providers with less experience frequently prefer curved blades as they can provide a superior view with less provider effort.

Endotracheal Tubes

The standard endotracheal tube is plastic and about 30 cm in length (Fig. 9). The tube size is measured based on the internal diameter in millimeters. An adult male usually requires a 7.5–9.0 mm ETT, however women can usually be intubated with a 7.0–8.0 mm tube. The best time to intubate a patient during resuscitation is often described as "as soon as physically possible." Animal models of out-of-hospital arrest suggest that the definitive airway can be delayed for 5–6 minutes without decreasing the likelihood of spontaneous return of circulation *(5)*.

Technique

PREPARE EQUIPMENT

1. Check suctioning equipment.
2. Inflate and deflate the endotracheal tube balloon to check for leaks.
3. Connect laryngoscope blade to the handle to check bulb function.

POSITION

1. Place the patient's head in the sniffing position if no evidence of trauma.
2. If trauma is suspected, maintain in-line cervical stabilization in the neutral position.
3. Preoxygenate.
4. Maximize oxygen saturation by administering 100% O_2 preferably by face mask or bag-valve-mask.
5. Pass the tube.
6. Holding the laryngoscope in the left hand, insert the laryngoscope into the right side of the mouth and sweep the tongue to the left. Advance the blade and visualize the epiglottis and vocal cords. Insert the endotracheal tube through the vocal cords. Inflate the balloon.

PLACEMENT

Check for tube placement by auscultating over the chest and abdomen. If capnometry or capnography is available, it can be used to confirm placement. Capnometry (colorimetric, analog, or digital) can yield false negative results during low-flow states such as during resuscitation. Capnography remains accurate in determining endotracheal tube placement even in the presence of a low-flow state. An alternate method to confirm ETT placement is to use an esophageal detector suction device. When time allows, obtain a chest x-ray to confirm endotracheal tube location.

DEVICES FOR CONFIRMATION OF ENDOTRACHEAL TUBE PLACEMENT

There are numerous devices that can be utilized to confirm the proper placement of an ETT. A detailed examination of placement confirmation devices is beyond the scope of this chapter.

Capnography uses a chemical paper to rapidly determine the presence of carbon dioxide in exhaled air. This is a qualitative, not quantitative device. A change in color suggests tracheal intubation (Fig. 10).

To use the bulb suction device, first deflate the bulb with the thumb and then place the device securely on the ETT connector (Fig. 11). The bulb is released, and if the endotracheal tube is inserted in the esophagus the suction of the bulb collapses the flexible tissue of the esophagus and the bulb does not inflate. With proper placement the rigid structures of the trachea do not collapse and the bulb rapidly inflates. Rapid bulb inflation confirms tracheal intubation.

A similar technique is used with the syringe aspiration test (Fig. 12). Instead of bulb inflation, the syringe is attached and the plunger rapidly drawn back by the provider. Increased resistance suggests esophageal intubation.

These confirmation techniques have the advantage that they can be utilized in high noise environments or in situations in which stethoscopes are unavailable or unusable, such as during a disaster.

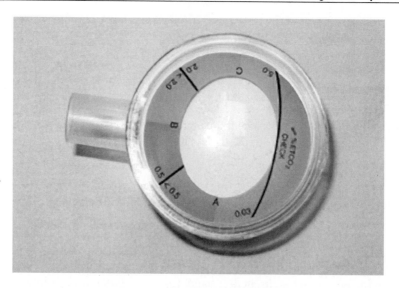

Fig. 10. Example of a capnograph.

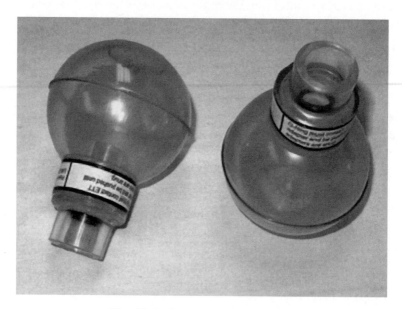

Fig. 11. Bulb esophageal detector.

Endotrol Endotracheal Tube

Nasotracheal intubation is an alternative technique in which the ETT or Endotrol tube (Mallinckrodt Critical Care Inc., St. Louis, MO) is inserted through the nares down into the trachea. The Endotrol tube is an ETT with a loop attached that increases the curvature of the tip when pulled. The Endotrol is used during nasogastric intubation. Usually the tube size chosen is slightly smaller (by 0.5–1.0 mm) than would be used for endotracheal intubation. As nasotracheal intubation requires that the patient be spontaneously breathing, it will not be considered further in this chapter.

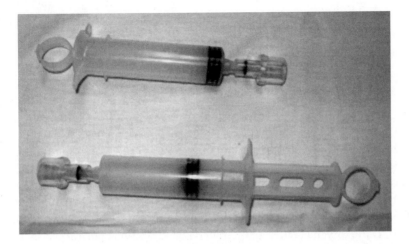

Fig. 12. Syringe aspirator.

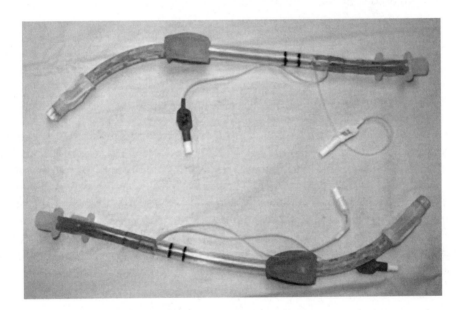

Fig. 13. Combitubes.

Combitube

The Combitube is a double lumen tube with two balloons (Fig. 13). It is designed for blind insertion during emergency situations and difficult airways. The esophageal obturator tube is sealed at the distal end, and has perforations at the pharyngeal level. The tracheal tube has a clear distal opening. The large upper oropharyngeal balloon serves to seal off the mouth and nose. The distal cuff balloon seals off either the trachea or the esophagus.

One advantage of the Combitube is that insertion requires less skill than direct laryngoscopy. Because it can be inserted blindly, it can be used under difficult lighting and space restrictions. It is very useful when visualization of the vocal cords is impossible.

Contraindications include patients with intact gag reflexes, patient height less than 4 feet, a history of known esophageal pathology, a recent history of ingestion of caustic substances, or central airway obstruction.

TECHNIQUE

To insert a Combitube, grasp the back of the tongue and jaw between the thumb and index finger and lift. Insert the Combitube in a curved downward motion. Insertion should not require any force by the operator. Inflate the oropharyngeal balloon first with between 85 and 100 cc of air (depending on the size of the Combitube) then inflate the distal balloon with 5–15 cc of air.

The most likely result of a blind intubation is esophageal intubation. Attempt ventilation through the longer blue tube. If breath sounds are present then the tip of the Combitube is in the esophagus. If breath sounds are absent, then the tip of the tube is in the trachea. If the tube has entered the trachea, ventilation is performed using the distal lumen just like a standard endotracheal tube. Tracheal intubation can be achieved by using a laryngoscope in conjunction with a Combitube.

Laryngeal Mask Airway

The LMA was introduced into clinical practice in 1988. The LMA is a triangular shaped inflatable pink silicon laryngeal mask (Fig. 14). The mask has an opening in the middle that prevents accidental obstruction of the tube by the tip of the epiglottis. Gastric distention is minimized because excess pressure is vented upward around the LMA instead of into the esophagus.

The LMA can be used when the patient is unresponsive or the protective reflexes have been sufficiently depressed. The mask is deflated to form a flat wedge that will pass behind the tongue and behind the epiglottis. The LMA is blindly inserted into the pharynx with the point of the triangle in the esophagus and the mask over the laryngeal inlet. The mask is then inflated and seals off the laryngeal inlet. The LMA is not a definitive airway, and provides almost no prevention of aspiration of stomach contents from below or blood and secretions from above. The LMA is best for providers not trained in endotracheal intubation. It can be used as an adjunct in the difficult airway when primary endotracheal intubation has been attempted unsuccessfully.

TECHNIQUE

Completely deflate the LMA until the cuff forms a smooth spoon shape without any wrinkles. Hold the LMA like a pen, with the mask facing forward and the black line on the tube oriented toward the upper lip. Insert the mask with the tip of the cuff up toward the hard palate. The index finger can be used to assist in guiding the LMA behind the tongue. Advance the LMA into the hypopharynx until resistance is felt. Inflate the cuff with enough air to obtain a seal. Normal intracuff pressures are around 60 cm H_2O.

CONCLUSION

Providers should be familiar with BLS techniques in addition to advanced airway techniques. The patient's airway should be secured definitively within the first 5–6 minutes of CPR. This allows for adequate ventilation, and increases the possibility of return of spontaneous circulation. Endotracheal intubation is the method most commonly used to secure the airway. Alternative methods include the Combitube and LMA. The position of an advanced airway should be confirmed with capnography or an esophageal detector device.

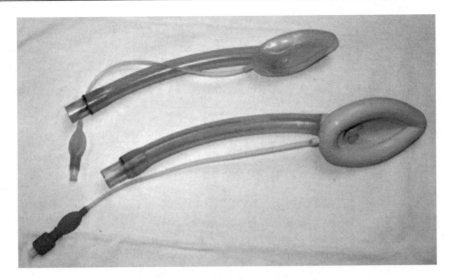

Fig. 14. Laryngeal mask airway.

REFERENCES

1. Barnes T, Macdonald D, Nolan J, et al. Cardiopulmonary resuscitation and emergency cardiovascular care. Airway devices. Ann Emerg Med 2001; 37:S145–S151.
2. Neumar R, Ward K. Adult Resuscitation. In: Rosen's Emergency Medicine: Concepts and Clinical Practice, J. Marx, ed. St. Louis, MO: Mosby, 2002.
3. Wenzel V, Idris AH, Montgomery WH, et al. Rescue breathing and bag-mask ventilation. Ann Emerg Med 2001; 37:S36–S40.
4. Idris AH, Banner MJ, Wenzel V, Fuerst RS, Becker LB, Melker RJ. Effect of ventilation on acid-base balance and oxygenation in low blood-flow states. Crit Care Med 1994; 22:1827–1834.
5. Idris A. Does hypoxia or hypercarbia independently affect resuscitation from cardiac arrest? Chest 1995; 108:522–8.
6. Feneley M, Maier GW, Kern KB, et al. Influence of compression rate on initial success of resuscitation and 24 hour survival after prolonged manual cardiopulmonary resuscitation in dogs. Circulation 1988; 77:240–250.
7. Sato Y, Weil MH, Sun S, et al. Adverse effects of interrupting precordial compression during cardiopulmonary resuscitation. Crit Care Med 1997; 25:733–736.
8. Chandra N. Observations of Ventilation during resuscitation in a canine model. Circulation 1994; 90:3070–5.
9. Kern K. Cardiopulmonary resuscitation without ventilation. Crit Care Med 2000; 28(Suppl):N186–9.
10. Clinton J, McGill J. Basic Airway Management and Decision Making, in Clinical Procedures in Emergency Medicine, Roberts JR, Hedges JR, Eds. Philadelphia: W.B. Saunders Co., 1998.
11. Pepe P, Gay M, Cobb LA, et al. Action sequence for layperson cardiopulmonary resuscitation. Ann Emerg Med 2001; 374 (Suppl):S17–25 (suppl).
12. Ornato J, Hallagan LF, McMahan SB, Peeples EH, Rostafinski AG. Attitudes of BCLS instructors about mouth-to-mouth resuscitation during the AIDS epidemic. Ann Emerg Med 1990; 19:151–156.
13. Stapleton E. Basic life support cardiopulmonary resuscitation. Cardiol Clin 2002; 20:1–12.
14. Berg R, Hilwig RW, Kern KB, Babar I, Ewy GA. Simulated mouth-to-mouth ventilation and chest compression (bystander cardiopulmonary resuscitation) improves outcome in a swine model of out-of-hospital pediatric asphyxial cardiac arrest. Crit Care Med 1999; 27:1893–1899.
15. Wenzel V, Idris A, Banner M. The composition of gas given by mouth-to-mouth ventilation during CPR. Chest 1994; 106:1806–1810.
16. Htin K, Birenbeaum DS, Idris AH, Banner MJ, Gravenstein N. Rescuer breathing pattern significantly affects O2 and CO2 received by the patient during mouth-to-mouth ventilation. Crit Care Med 1998; 26(Suppl 1):A56.

17. Dorges V, Ocker H, Hagelberg S, Wenzel V, Schumucker P. Optimisation of tidal volumes given with self-inflatable bags without additional oxygen. Resuscitation 2000; 43:195–199.
18. Stallinger A, Wenzel V, Oroszy S, et al. The effects of different mouth-to-mouth ventilation tidal volumes on gas exchange during simulated rescue breathing. Anesth Analg 2001; 93(5):1265–9.
19. Weil MH, Rackow EC, Trevino R, Grundler W, Falk JL, Griffel MI. Differences in acid-base state between venous and arterial blood during cardiopulmonary resuscitation. N Engl J Med 1986; 315:153–156.
20. Sanders A, Otto CW, Kern KB, Rogers JN, Perrault P, Ewy GA. Acid-base balance in a canine model of cardiac arrest. Ann Emerg Med 1988; 17:667–671.
21. Idris A. Effects of inspired gas content during respiratory arrest and cardiopulmonary resuscitation. Crit Care Med 2000; 28(11 Suppl):N196–198.

6 Management of Airway Obstruction

Michael R. Sayre, MD

INTRODUCTION

Death by acute airway obstruction has been recognized for centuries. George Washington is thought to have died in 1799 from upper airway obstruction caused by acute bacterial epiglottitis *(1)*. Although letting of more than 2 L of blood out of their patient, President Washington's physicians apparently discussed performing a tracheotomy, a procedure that had been described in detail only the year before. However, they did not have the courage to carry out the new procedure on the retired president of the United States. Dr. R. K. Haugen wrote a now-classic description of the problem of choking in 1963 *(2)*. He described what he termed the café coronary:

> *A middle-aged or elderly person, at a fashionable restaurant, is partaking of filet mignon, or perhaps broiled lobster or prime rib of beef. At the same time, he is conversing with companions at dinner. Suddenly, he ceases to eat and talk. The dinner companions are perplexed but not alarmed for there is no indication of distress. Then, the person suddenly collapses at the table.*

Dr. Haugen then described an unsuccessful attempt at resuscitation. In his article, he detailed nine similar cases. The food found in the airway was steak in four cases, beef in two, ham fat in one, kippered herring in one, and broiled lobster in the last *(2)*. In his conclusion, he noted "the only effective means of treatment is an emergency, on the scene, tracheotomy." Acute airway obstruction is an uncommon cause of sudden cardiac

From: *Contemporary Cardiology: Cardiopulmonary Resuscitation*
Edited by: J. P. Ornato and M. A. Peberdy © Humana Press Inc., Totowa, NJ

Table 1
Deaths From Choking in the United States: 1999

Age range (years)	Deaths	Death rate per 100,000
Under 1	46	1.2
1–4	76	0.5
5–9	23	0.1
10–14	16	0.1
15–19	12	0.1
20–24	23	0.1
25–34	61	0.2
35–44	123	0.3
45–54	202	0.6
55–64	239	1.0
65–74	506	2.8
75–84	984	8.1
Over 85	1157	27.7
All ages	**3468**	**1.2**

From the CDC and Prevention WONDER search tool of deaths in 1999 from ICD-10 code W79 (inhalation and ingestion of food causing obstruction of respiratory tract) and W80 (inhalation and ingestion of other objects causing obstruction of respiratory tract) [3]).

arrest (CA). However, it is frequently treatable, if recognized in time. Accidental choking killed 3468 persons in the United States in 1999. The problem primarily affects the young and the elderly. There were about 1.2 deaths per 100,000 infants from acute airway obstruction recorded annually in the United States; but after dropping in childhood and young adulthood, the rate rises dramatically in old age reaching 27.7 per 100,000 adults aged greater than 85 (*see* Table 1 [3]). Despite widespread education on the use of the Heimlich maneuver and other techniques for treatment of acute airway obstruction, the death rate remains stable.

ETIOLOGY

Acute airway obstruction can be caused by either an intrinsic or extrinsic blockage to airflow. A wide variety of objects, both living and inanimate, have been identified as the cause acute airway obstruction. Intrinsic blockage can be caused by the tongue, the epiglottis, blood, tumors, or stomach contents. The most common extrinsic object is improperly chewed food, usually meat in adults. Adults with pre-existing dysphagia are at an increased risk of death by choking.

Adults often choke during a meal that includes the consumption of alcohol. They do not chew the food into pieces small enough to prevent obstruction of the glottic opening. They often talk and chew during the process of swallowing or inhaling; the food becomes lodged in the glottis completely obstructing airflow. If the blockage is not removed in a few minutes, the reservoir of oxygen present in the lungs from the last good breath will be depleted. Once the individual becomes hypoxic, loss of consciousness will ensue, and death will soon follow. Children also choke on pieces of food and on small objects found in their immediate environment such as coins, small balls, balloons, and small pieces of larger toys.

In 1994, Drs. Andazola and Sapien conducted an epidemiological survey of pediatric choking episodes in Albuquerque, New Mexico. There were 103 emergency medical services (EMS) calls for obstructed airway in children less than 15 years of age *(5)*. Forty percent occurred in children less than 1 year old, 50% in children between 1 and 5 years of age, and 10% in children older than 5. Seventy-eight percent of the children under the age of 1 self-cleared their airway or had their airway cleared prior to EMS arrival, compared with 89% of those between 1 and 5, and 100% of those older than 5. Because 52% of the patients whose obstructions resolved were not transported to the hospital, the incidence of choking may be underestimated as frequently only patients who present at the emergency department are included in choking estimates.

PREVENTION

Prevention of choking begins at home. Children should be taught to chew food thoroughly so that the habit becomes ingrained by adulthood. Chewing food with the mouth closed is not only polite but also inhibits inhalation through the mouth thereby preventing food from being pulled into and obstructing the glottis. Consumption of alcohol in excess during meals also increases the chances of choking and should be avoided. Improperly fitted dentures inhibit effective chewing and may also detach and obstruct the glottis.

PEDIATRIC ISSUES

More than 17,000 children 15 years of age or younger were treated for choking episodes in emergency departments in the United States during the year 2000. This translates to a rate of 29 per 100,000 people *(4)*. Less than 1% died. More than half were choking on food, including hard candy and gum, and about 13% were choking on coins. The Centers for Disease Control (CDC) maintains a web site devoted to choking prevention at www.cdc.gov/ncipc/duip/spotlite/choking.htm.

Toddlers should not be fed peanuts, grapes, raw carrots, whole or large sections of hot dogs, meat sticks, or hard candies *(5)*. Additionally, young children should not be permitted to run with food in their mouths. Rather, they should be seated with an adult present during meals.

Although anyone who has supervised a toddler knows the challenges involved with monitoring their activities, adults need to work to keep the environment around the small child clear of objects such as coins, small balls, and rubber balloons that can cause choking *(6)*. In general, toys that can fit through a toilet paper tube should be kept away from young children *(7)*. The US Consumer Product Safety Commission has established standards for labeling toys to prevent choking episodes. Toys with parts smaller than 1.75 inches in diameter must be labeled with the phrase "WARNING: CHOKING HAZARD—Small parts. Not for children under 3 yrs."

Toy rubber balloons and similar conforming objects represent a significant risk for choking in older children *(6,8)*. The caps and other parts of inexpensive ballpoint pens are also a well-recognized choking hazard in older children who may walk about school and home with the pens in their mouths *(9)*.

RECOGNITION

At times, choking is easy to recognize. However, at other times it can be confused with simple fainting, sudden CA, stroke, seizure, or drug overdose. Educating the public in using the universal sign of choking should be encouraged. The universal choking sign is displayed by clutching the neck with both thumbs and fingers.

During choking, obstruction to airflow may be partial or complete. Partial airflow obstruction can be subdivided further into having good air exchange or poor air exchange. Partial obstruction with good air exchange can be recognized by the presence of a vigorous cough and sometimes wheezing. Patients with good air exchange should initially be left alone and allowed to cough out the offending object. Partial obstruction with poor air exchange is present when he or she has only a weak cough, stridor, or cyanosis. Partial obstruction with poor air exchange is a medical emergency demanding immediate action and should be treated as a complete obstruction.

When obstruction to airflow is complete, he or she is unable to cough or breathe. There is no air movement. The diagnosis can be confirmed by asking if he or she is choking. If choking is present, then he or she should be asked to speak. A lack of speech indicates that a complete airway obstruction is present and requires immediate action.

EVIDENCE-BASED TREATMENT OF CHOKING

Unfortunately, the level of evidence guiding therapy for acute airway obstruction is weak. There are no randomized clinical trials, but this lack of evidence may be consistent with the relative rarity of the problem.

Controversy About Treatment

One of the more interesting aspects of the medical treatment of choking has been the approach to changing treatment recommendations by those who favor abdomenominal thrusts as the primary method of treatment for choking. Traditionally, new medical therapy is introduced by providing convincing evidence of its efficacy and then using a variety of educational methods to promote the new treatment. This process takes years to implement and sometimes does not produce the desired change in physician behavior (10).

Henry Heimlich published his description of the abdominal thrust for the treatment of choking in the magazine *Emergency Medicine* in 1974 (11). In the article, he described the use of subdiaphragmatic pressure to relieve foreign body airway obstruction in four dogs. He had not tried the procedure on humans, but asked that those who did send him information about the results of their use of the technique. In 1975, Heimlich published the results of this request for information in the *Journal of the American Medical Association (JAMA [12])*. The *JAMA* article described 162 cases in which abdominal thrusts reportedly dislodged foreign objects obstructing the airway. The author encouraged others to use abdominal thrusts on choking victims.

Rather than publish additional research in peer-reviewed medical journals to convince other physicians to teach the procedure, Dr. Heimlich used the data from his case series to appeal directly to the public, discounting previous recommendations by the American Heart Association (AHA), the American Red Cross (ARC), and the American Academy of Pediatrics (13). In December 1978, Dr. Heimlich submitted a letter to the *New England Journal of Medicine* in which he defended the use of abdominal thrusts as the primary technique for the treatment of choking *(14)*. In 1979, Dr. Heimlich appealed directly to EMS professionals with an editorial entitled *Back Blows are Death Blows*. In the article he castigated professional organizations for not adopting abdominal thrusts as the primary treatment for choking *(15)*.

Today, there is some physiological evidence to guide decision making. It is clear that abdominal thrusts have saved many lives among victims of choking. Questions remain about whether other techniques, such as chest compression, are as effective or possibly more effective.

One of the principal obstacles of determining effective treatment for acute airway obstruction is the anecdotal nature of the case reports. There is surely a positive reporting bias in which authors attribute success to the procedure used although unsuccessful attempts are ascribed to issues other than the technique such as the type and location of the foreign material or the inexperience of the rescuer. Additionally, the last technique tried before revival of the victim is likely to be given full credit for success, although perhaps a combination of different techniques was in fact responsible for removing the offending object.

Certainly, there is no shortage of medical interventions advocated as useful and desirable based on anecdotal evidence. One of the most famous of these was the practice of bleeding ill patients in an attempt to restore appropriate balance among the "four body humors." One of the major medical journals, *Lancet*, is named for one of the tools of this practice, widespread at the time of the journal's founding. Because of the lack of rigorous scientific support for any individual technique, it is important to keep an open mind about the subject of the effectiveness of all different techniques.

CASE REPORTS

Most of the available evidence regarding treatment for choking is in the form of case reports. In 1975, Heimlich described 162 communications he received reporting successful application of the abdominal thrust technique to resolve choking *(12)*. A wide variety of objects were expelled from victims including food, pills, and candy. Five of the reports described the use of the method on drowning victims, a use Heimlich did not anticipate. Two rib fractures were the only complications reported.

Others have reported on the results of different techniques for treatment of choking. In 1979, Dr. Ingalls, a survivor of a café coronary in 1973 *(16)*, described how a well-timed slap on the back removed a piece of food from a physician attending a Board of Directors meeting of the Philadelphia County Medical Society *(17)*. Dr. Richard Westfal reported on two patients who were found by paramedics to be cyanotic with complete airway obstructions as a result of food impaction that had not responded to repeated Heimlich maneuvers. In both cases, paramedics were successfully able to retrieve the offending food using Magill forceps with laryngoscopy *(18)*. In 2002, Brown et al. reported on the use of 60% oxygen and 40% helium gas (Heliox) administration to temporarily ease the work of breathing in a 22-month-old child with partial airway obstruction as a result of the aspiration of a sunflower seed into the right mainstem bronchus *(19)*. This technique might also be useful with partial obstruction of the trachea or pharynx.

CADAVER STUDIES

The recently dead human body provides an excellent model of the unresponsive person with choking, although it may not be a good model of choking in the responsive person because the muscle tone in the pharynx, chest, and abdomen probably influence the effectiveness of various methods to remove foreign material from the trachea and glottis. Twelve unsuccessfully resuscitated victims of out-of-hospital CA were studied in Oslo to determine whether chest compression or abdominal thrusts generated higher peak airway pressure *(20)*. The investigators found that chest compression generated a peak airway pressure of 40.8 ± 16.4, which was significantly higher than the 26.4 ± 19.8 cm H_2O pressure generated with abdominal thrusts. In 2 of the 12 patients, no tracheal air pressure whatsoever was generated by abdominal thrusts. Dr. Heimlich responded with a letter to the editor of *Resuscitation* in which he promoted the use of the Heimlich maneuver over chest compression based on the duration and amount of airflow and not just the peak pressure generated *(21)*. Additionally, Dr. Heimlich suggested that the term subdiaphragmatic pressure was a more accurate description than abdominal thrust of the method used. Dr. Steen and his colleagues *(22)* responded to Dr. Heimlich's analysis by pointing out that their study of chest compression was congruent with results obtained by Ruben and MacNaughton that chest compression was more effective than subdiaphragmatic pressure *(23)*.

MECHANICAL MODELS

Dr. Day and colleagues performed a series of experiments to measure the forces induced by back blows applied to young adult volunteers *(24)*. Two adults had accelerometers taped to the anterior neck at the level of the thyroid cartilage. Vigorous blows, insufficient to cause pain or bruising, applied on the backs of the subjects developed acceleration forces ranging from 0.8 to 1.8 g. The accelerometer was moved to measure the upward force the range was 1.5 to 3.3 g. The authors pointed out that these forces might tend to propel an object above the vocal cords down into the trachea. Day et al. also performed experiments in which airflow was measured when the Heimlich maneuver was applied and compared those measurements with those taken when back blows were applied. Day et al. consistently found much higher airflow with the Heimlich maneuver. Others have found deficiencies in the design of the experiment and note that the accelerometer measurements were not conducted with the Heimlich maneuver *(13)*. Better models need to be developed.

LIVING MODELS

In his 1975 account of the abdominal thrust, Heimlich described an experiment involving four dogs *(12)*. After receiving general anesthesia, the animals had raw hamburger inserted into the larynx until the airway was occluded totally. In each case, after one or two firm thrusts were made on the abdomen a short distance inferior to the rib cage, the bolus was expelled.

Heimlich briefly described the use of the abdominal thrust method on 10 healthy human volunteers and noted a peak expiratory flow rate of 205 L per minute with 940 mL of air expelled in one-fourth of a second *(25)*. There are no other published human experiments.

TECHNIQUE

ABDOMINAL THRUSTS

Abdominal thrusts are performed using the following procedure. The rescuer stands behind the choking person and wraps his or her arms around the victim's waist. Making a fist with one hand, the rescuer places the thumb side of fist against the abdomen in the midline just above the umbilicus and well below the xiphoid process. The fist is grasped with the other hand and the rescuer quickly pulls inward and upward.

The procedure can be repeated several times until the object is expelled *(26)*. Abdominal thrusts can be self-administered using ones hands or by forcefully bending over an object such as back of a chair or porch railing *(27)*.

Abdominal thrusts may be performed on unresponsive choking victims by placing the victim supine on the floor. Then the rescuer straddles the victim and places one hand on the abdomen in the midline just above the umbilicus. The other hand is placed on top of the first, and firm inward and upward thrusts are applied.

CHEST THRUSTS

Chest thrusts are performed when a female victim is pregnant or the victim is too large for the rescuer to get his or her arms around the abdomen. Again, the rescuer should stand behind the responsive victim and wrap his or her arms around the victim's chest just below the axillae. After making a fist, the rescuer places the thumb side of the fist against lower sternum while avoiding the xiphoid process and lower costal margin so as not to injure the abdominal organs. Then the fist is grasped with the other hand. Finally, the rescuer should pull hard in a repeated thrusting motion until the obstruction is relieved or consciousness is lost *(26)*.

If the rescuer's arms are too short to encircle the chest or if the victim is unresponsive, the victim is placed supine on the floor; and the rescuer kneels close to the victim's side. Using a hand position similar to that used for chest compressions during CPR, the rescuer pushes hard on the chest to relieve the obstruction.

ADVANCED METHODS

Properly trained rescuers can use more advanced techniques to remove or bypass the obstruction. Unfortunately, these will often not be helpful because most victims cannot be brought together with a well-trained rescuer within the short window of time before hypoxia causes irreversible brain injury or death. Both the Magill forceps and the Kelly clamp have been used to retrieve foreign bodies from the pharynx using direct vision *(18)*. The object can be visualized using a laryngoscope or, in some cases, a tongue blade and a flashlight.

Emergency cricothyrotomy or tracheotomy can also be lifesaving. These surgical techniques require more skill than the use of the Magill forceps. Many paramedics are taught techniques for transtracheal administration of oxygen using a small catheter attached to a high-pressure jet ventilation valve. Use of high-pressure oxygen in the setting of a complete tracheal obstruction might result in expelling the object from the trachea. It might also lead to pneumothorax or pneumomediastinum. However, when the patient is in a high-risk situation in which all other techniques such as repeated abdominal thrusts and attempted removal of the foreign body using the direct visualization technique have failed to open the airway, doing nothing will certainly result in death. In such cases, the benefits of using high-pressure jet ventilation outweigh the risk and are justified.

MANAGEMENT RECOMMENDATIONS

The AHA, in conjunction with international organizations, issued revised management guidelines for foreign body airway obstruction in 2000 *(26)*. However, unlike most other domains of emergency management of resuscitation, there is not international agreement on the best methods for clearing a foreign body airway obstruction. For example, the AHA recommends the use of abdominal thrusts as the initial maneuver in responsive adults although the European Resuscitation Council recommends five back blows or slaps initially *(28)*. The back blows are given with the heel of the rescuer's hand between the victim's shoulder blades. In Australia, back blows with the patient in a lateral recumbent position are the first treatment followed by lateral chest thrusts. The Australian resuscitation organization recommends that abdominal thrusts be avoided as too dangerous and likely to injure internal organs.

ADULT (AGE 8 OR OLDER)

Responsive. If the victim is responsive, then the AHA guidelines recommend that abdominal thrusts be used until the airway is cleared as judged by the individual's ability to cough or speak or consciousness is lost *(26)*.

Unresponsive. In the 2000 AHA guidelines, the lay-rescuer is not taught the complete skills for treatment of foreign body airway obstruction *(26)*. Because the likelihood of encountering an unresponsive person whose problem is airway obstruction is small and the amount of time to teach skills is limited, the instruction time should be spent on more commonly used procedures such as reinforcing chest compression skills for unconscious victims of ventricular fibrillation. Should the victim become unresponsive, the lay rescuer is urged to activate EMS or send someone else to do it; and then begin standard CPR. The guidelines point out that the chest compressions of CPR may themselves dislodge the foreign body.

The 2000 guidelines recommend that health care providers who treat an unresponsive victim be taught additional skills *(26)*. If the health care provider witnesses the victim's collapse and knows that the problem is foreign body airway obstruction, then the rescuer should activate the emergency response system and begin a systematic approach to restoring airflow. First, the rescuer is to perform a tongue–jaw lift, followed by a finger sweep to remove the offending object if present. Next, ventilation is attempted. If effective breaths cannot be given (determined by observing chest rise), then the Heimlich maneuver with the victim supine is recommended and may be repeated up to five times as needed. The cycle of jaw lift, finger sweep, attempt ventilation, and Heimlich maneuver is repeated until the airway is cleared or advanced equipment is available. When Magill forceps, Kelly clamp, or cricothyrotomy kit is available and the airway remains obstructed, then they should be used by persons properly trained in the techniques of removal of foreign bodies using direct visualization or surgical cricothyrotomy.

If the individual is found to be unresponsive, then the rescuer has to determine whether foreign body airway obstruction or primary CA or some other reason for the apparent unresponsiveness is present. Foreign body airway obstruction may be diagnosed when the rescuer follows the CPR sequence and attempts to ventilate an unresponsive person who is not breathing spontaneously and finds that the chest does not rise. The most likely cause is obstruction as a result of soft tissues in the pharynx. So the first treatment is to reposition the head and attempt ventilation again. If that does not work, then the Heimlich maneuver is tried up to five times with the individual supine. The same sequence of steps is followed as described in the section on the witnessed collapse of the choking victim.

PREGNANT WOMEN OR VERY OBESE INDIVIDUALS

The 2000 AHA guidelines recommend the use of chest thrusts on lieu of abdominal thrusts for pregnant women or the extremely obese when the rescuer's arms cannot encircle the individual's abdomen.

CHILD (AGE 1–8)

Responsive. The 2000 AHA guidelines recommend repeated abdominal thrusts in the child 1 year of age or older until the airway is successfully opened, as judged by the ability of the child to cough or speak, or until consciousness is lost.

Unresponsive. When an unresponsive child with a suspected foreign body airway obstruction is found, the lay-rescuer is advised to perform standard CPR with one addition. The added step is to look for the obstructing object in the back of the pharynx each time the airway is opened. If the object is visible, the rescuer should remove it. This sequence of steps is intended to simplify the teaching of CPR, and the chest compressions provided during CPR may dislodge the foreign body.

When a health care provider encounters an unresponsive child between 1 and 8 years old with suspected foreign body airway obstruction, the 2000 AHA guidelines suggest first opening the airway and looking for the object (29). If the object is visible, it should be removed. Blind finger sweeps are not recommended. Then the airway is opened and rescue breathing attempted. If air does not make the chest rise, then the airway is repositioned and rescue breathing attempted a second time. If the chest still does not rise, then up to five abdominal thrusts are performed with the child in a supine position. The steps are repeated until the foreign object is removed, rescue breathing is effective, or signs of circulation are lost. If signs of circulation are lost, then standard CPR is begun.

Once advanced equipment is available, the removal of the foreign object using Magill forceps under direct vision provided by a laryngoscope can be attempted. As a last resort, an effort to perform an emergency tracheotomy can be made provided that the rescuer has been trained in the technique.

INFANT

The 2000 AHA Guidelines recommend using a combination of back blows and chest thrusts to treat complete foreign body airway obstruction in a responsive infant less than 1 year old (29). The Heimlich maneuver is not recommended in this age group because of the relatively large and unprotected liver in the infant. The infant is held with the head lower than the trunk and the rescuer strikes the infant's back between the scapulae with the heel of the hand.

If the infant becomes unconscious, the lay-rescuer is advised to perform 1 minute of standard CPR in the hope that the chest compressions will dislodge the offending object. If the problem is not resolved after 1 minute in a single-rescuer situation, the rescuer should suspend efforts to resuscitate and contact the emergency response system. Then CPR is resumed.

If the rescuer is a health care provider who is treating an unresponsive infant with suspected foreign body airway obstruction, then the first step is to open the airway and attempt rescue breathing. If air is not moving, then the head is repositioned; and rescue breathing attempted again. If that does not work, then five back blows followed by five chest thrusts are administered. The airway is reopened and rescue breathing is attempted again. This sequence is repeated until the object is removed or up to about 1 minute. Then in the single-rescuer situation, the rescuer stops resuscitation and activates EMS. Following EMS activation, the rescuer should check for signs of circulation and begin chest compressions if necessary. If circulation is present, then the sequence of opening the airway, attempting breathing, administering back blows, administering chest thrusts, and rechecking the airway is continued until the foreign body is removed or signs of circulation are lost.

COMPLICATIONS

All of the procedures used to treat acute airway obstruction may lead to complications. Perhaps the most important complication is delay in the use of effective treatment when hypoxia is present. However, because the most effective treatment is not known, it is challenging to measure incidence of this adverse event.

Back blows may lodge the foreign body more tightly in the trachea. As a result, Dr. Heimlich renamed back blows "death blows" *(15)*. Dr. Heimlich wrote about a case in which a teenager who was choking on a sandwich and had a partial airway obstruction developed a complete obstruction after administration of back blows. In many cases in which back blows seemed harmful, it appears that the back blows were applied to victims with only partial airway obstruction *(30)*. This serves to emphasize that there is no reason to apply any technique of artificial cough when victims can move air and cough, as a natural cough is many times more forceful than an artificial cough whether induced by back blow, Heimlich maneuver, or chest compression.

The use of the Heimlich maneuver has been associated with rupture of internal organs and laceration of viscera *(31–34)*. Chest compressions are well known to cause rib and sternal fractures. Although usually benign, these fractures can lead to additional morbidity such as pneumonia or even death from respiratory insufficiency. Nonetheless, given the large number of people worldwide who have multiple chest compressions during CPR, it would appear that the incidence of serious complications following only a few chest compressions is very small and may in fact be less than that associated with the Heimlich maneuver *(21)*.

In the past, rescue organizations such as the ARC and the AHA recommended the use of blind finger sweeps to attempt to remove foreign bodies. Given evidence that this technique may result in the further impaction of the object against the larynx as well as injury to the pharynx, the use of blind finger probing of the pharynx is to be avoided *(35)*. It is probably reasonable to have victims undergo a medical evaluation to exclude complications after use of any abdominal thrust or chest compression to relieve choking.

SUMMARY

There is little evidence with which to guide the best treatment of choking. A strong body of anecdotal evidence favors the use of subdiaphragmatic pressure, the Heimlich maneuver, as the first treatment in complete airway obstruction for most victims. Chest thrusts and back blows are helpful in some victims. A combination of procedures may be better than continued use of one procedure that has failed. Thus, the current AHA recommendations seem to be a reasonable guide to the practicing physician and the public, although not a guide based on strong evidence. Addition information is needed, and good epidemiological studies are desirable to identify ways to reduce the more than 3000 deaths that occur annually from choking in the United States.

REFERENCES

1. Morens DM. Death of a president. N Engl J Med 1999; 341:1845–1849.
2. Haugen RK. The café coronary: sudden death in restaurants. JAMA 1963; 186:142–143.
3. Centers for Disease Control. 1999 Mortality for Choking (ICD-10 Codes W79-W80) in the United States. http://wonder.cdc.gov. 2002. Centers for Disease Control and Prevention WONDER Search Tool. Accessed: 1-3-2003.

4. Nonfatal choking-related episodes among children—United States, 2001. MMWR Morb Mortal Wkly Rep 2002; 51:945–948.
5. American Academy of Pediatrics. Toddler's diet: Understanding your toddler's diet. http://www.medem.com/search/article_display.cfm?path=n:&mstr=/ZZZ61B4NH4C.html&soc=AAP&srch_typ=NAV_SERCH. 2000. American Academy of Pediatrics. Accessed: 12-16-2002.
6. Rimell FL, Thome A, Jr., Stool S, et al. Characteristics of objects that cause choking in children. JAMA 1995; 274:1763–1766.
7. Tarrago SB. Prevention of choking, strangulation, and suffocation in childhood. WMJ 2000; 99: 43–6, 42.
8. Ryan CA, Yacoub W, Paton T, Avard D. Childhood deaths from toy balloons. Am J Dis Child 1990; 144:1221–1224.
9. Bhana BD, Gunaselvam JG, Dada MA. Mechanical airway obstruction caused by accidental aspiration of part of a ballpoint pen. Am J Forensic Med Pathol 2000; 21:362–365.
10. Lundberg GD. Changing physician behavior in ordering diagnostic tests. JAMA 1998; 280:2036.
11. Heimlich HJ. Pop goes the café coronary. Emerg Med 1974; 6:154–155.
12. Heimlich HJ. A life-saving maneuver to prevent food-choking. JAMA 1975; 234:398–401.
13. Sternbach G, Kiskaddon RT. Henry Heimlich: a life-saving maneuver for food choking. J Emerg Med 1985; 3:143–148.
14. Heimlich HJ. Heimlich defends his maneuver. N Engl J Med 1978; 299:1415.
15. Heimlich HJ. Back blows or death blows. Emerg Med Serv 1979; 8:88–95.
16. Ingalls TH. Death comes to dinner: the hazards of high living. Arch Environ Health 1973; 27:342–343.
17. Ingalls TH. Heimlich versus a slap on the back. N Engl J Med 1979; 300:990.
18. Westfal R. Foreign body airway obstruction: when the Heimlich maneuver fails. Am J Emerg Med 1997; 15:103–105.
19. Brown L, Sherwin T, Perez JE, Perez DU. Heliox as a temporizing measure for pediatric foreign body aspiration. Acad Emerg Med 2002; 9:346–347.
20. Langhelle A, Sunde K, Wik L, Steen PA. Airway pressure with chest compressions versus Heimlich manoeuvre in recently dead adults with complete airway obstruction. Resuscitation 2000; 44:105–108.
21. Heimlich HJ, Spletzer EG. Chest compressions yielded higher airway pressures than Heimlich maneuvers when the airway was obstructed. Resuscitation 2001; 48:185–187.
22. Langhelle A, Wik L, Sunde K. Correspondence. Resuscitation 2001; 48:186–187.
23. Ruben H, MacNaughton FI. The treatment of food-choking. Practitioner 1978; 221:725–729.
24. Day RL, Crelin ES, DuBois AB. Choking: the Heimlich abdominal thrust vs back blows: an approach to measurement of inertial and aerodynamic forces. Pediatrics 1982; 70:113–119.
25. Heimlich HJ, Hoffmann KA, Canestri FR. Food-choking and drowning deaths prevented by external subdiaphragmatic compression: physiological basis. Ann Thorac Surg 1975; 20:188–195.
26. Guidelines 2000 for Cardiopulmonary Resuscitation and Emergency Cardiovascular Care. Part 3: adult basic life support. The American Heart Association in collaboration with the International Liaison Committee on Resuscitation. Circulation 2000; 102:I22–I59.
27. Heimlich HJ. Self-application of the Heimlich maneuver. N Engl J Med 1988; 318:714–715.
28. Handley AJ, Monsieurs KG, Bossaert LL. European Resuscitation Council Guidelines 2000 for Adult Basic Life Support. A statement from the Basic Life Support and Automated External Defibrillation Working Group and approved by the Executive Committee of the European Resuscitation Council. Resuscitation 2001; 48:199–205.
29. Guidelines 2000 for Cardiopulmonary Resuscitation and Emergency Cardiovascular Care. Part 9: pediatric basic life support. The American Heart Association in collaboration with the International Liaison Committee on Resuscitation. Circulation 2000; 102:I253–I290.
30. Hoffman JR. Treatment of foreign body obstruction of the upper airway. West J Med 1982; 11–22.
31. Ayerdi J, Gupta SK, Sampson LN, Deshmukh N. Acute abdominal aortic thrombosis following the Heimlich maneuver. Cardiovasc Surg 2002; 10:154–156.
32. Bintz M, Cogbill TH. Gastric rupture after the Heimlich maneuver. J Trauma 1996; 40:159–160.
33. Valero V. Mesenteric laceration complicating a Heimlich maneuver. Ann Emerg Med 1986; 15:105–106.
34. Wolf DA. Heimlich trauma: a violent maneuver. Am J Forensic Med Pathol 2001; 22:65–67.
35. Hartrey R, Bingham RM. Pharyngeal trauma as a result of blind finger sweeps in the choking child. J Accid Emerg Med 1995; 12:52–54.

7 Etiology, Electrophysiology, Myocardial Energy Mechanics, and Treatment of Bradyasystole

Charles E. Cady, MD and Tom P. Aufderheide, MD

INTRODUCTION

Definition

Bradyasystole is a term encompassing many different types of rhythms meeting the following definition: any electrical rhythm that has a ventricular rate below 60 beats per minute (bpm) in adults and/or periods of absent heart rhythm (asystole). A bradyasystolic state is a clinical condition in which the predominant cardiac rhythm can be classified as bradyasystole. Bradyasystolic rhythms other than asystole may be accompanied by a pulse. A bradyasystolic rhythm even with a pulse is frequently a precursor to cardiac arrest (CA) and requires prompt intervention. Some of the causes of bradyasystole are the same whether or not a pulse is present. More commonly bradyasystole occurs without a pulse. Bradycardic rhythms without a pulse are one group of many different types of rhythms described as pulseless electrical activity (PEA).

Incidence

As with any pre-arrest or initial arrest rhythm, the incidence is difficult to determine. Many CAs are unwitnessed by medical personnel and immediate rhythm monitoring is not available. The initial rhythm identified may or may not represent the actual rhythm antecedent to or present at the time of collapse. Many studies have been performed to determine the incidence of particular rhythms at the time of CA *(1–20)*.

There are four basic ways the incidence of rhythms at the time of CA have been estimated: (a) ambulatory electrocardiogram (ECG) monitor recordings at the time of

From: *Contemporary Cardiology: Cardiopulmonary Resuscitation*
Edited by: J. P. Ornato and M. A. Peberdy © Humana Press Inc., Totowa, NJ

cardiac arrest, (b) telemetry recordings on inpatients at the time of CA, (c) initial rhythms recorded on emergency medical services (EMS) arrival, and (d) rhythms recorded at the time of arrests witnessed by EMS providers. All of these methods have limitations.

It was once thought that more than 90% of children who suffer CA have an initial bradyasystolic rhythm (20,21). Now more episodes of ventricular tachycardia (VT) and ventricular fibrillation (VF) are being recognized in the pediatric population (up to an incidence of 15% [1,10]). VF was once thought to be the initial rhythm in as many as 83% of adult CA victims (3,6–9,14–17,22,23). These data, however, only reflect patients on ambulatory ECG monitors or those admitted to cardiac care units who are more likely to have a VT thus leading to their monitoring. It does not accurately reflect the thousands of unselected sudden cardiac death victims without a prior history or complaint.

Bradyasystole has been reported as the initial rhythm in 25 to 56% of adult out-of-hospital CAs (11,24,25). Because these arrests are frequently not witnessed, it is uncertain if bradyasystole represents the arresting rhythm, or represents rhythmic deterioration from prolonged arrest. Survival to hospital discharge in bradyasystolic patients ranges from 0 to 4% (11,24,25). It is unclear whether this dismal survival rate is related directly to the rhythm, or indirectly to prolonged arrest time. Iseri et al. (26) found that bradyasystole was the initial rhythm in 46% of EMS-witnessed arrests.

Thus, the collective data suggests that bradyasystole may account for CA in up to 50% of sudden cardiac death patients.

ETIOLOGY (TABLE 1)

Primary

In primary bradyasystole, the cardiac conduction system fails intrinsically. It can either fail to initiate or propagate an adequate rhythm leading to inadequate ventricular contraction or cardiac output. Sick sinus syndrome is one example (27,28).

This syndrome encompasses a variety of disorders that affect the heart's pacemaker. Some of the presentations include persistent or intermittent unexplained sinus bradycardia, sinus arrest without any escape pacemaker functioning, atrial fibrillation with a slow ventricular response, predominant bradycardia with episodes of atrial tachycardia, relative bradycardia (inability to mount a physiologic tachycardic response), and an inability to resume normal sinus rhythm after cardioversion. Although seen most frequently in the elderly, people of all ages can have a sick sinus syndrome.

Histologic degeneration of the cells of the sinoatrial (SA) node and conduction tissue between the SA and atrioventricular (AV) nodes has been associated with sick sinus syndrome (27,28). Lenegre's disease (29) is an idiopathic sclerodegeneration of the AV node and the bundle branches. Lev's disease (30,31) involves invasion of the conduction system by fibrosis or calcification from adjacent cardiac structures.

Direct ischemic injury to the pacemaker and conduction cells can also cause primary bradyasystole. This occurs with occlusion of the right coronary artery, which frequently supplies the SA and AV nodes.

Secondary

In secondary bradyasystole, the cardiac conduction system fails as a result of the effects of other pathologic processes.

HYPOXIA

Hypoxia, resulting in pacemaker and conduction system ischemia, frequently causes secondary bradyasystole. Hypoxia has a direct depressant effect on pacemaker cells. Hypoxia also causes an increase in parasympathetic discharge resulting in vagal stimulation of the heart. Examples of common clinical conditions that often cause bradyasystole by hypoxia include suffocation, near drowning, stroke, and heroin overdose. Pulmonary embolus (PE) can cause bradyasystole as a result of hypoxia and an acute increase in pulmonary vascular pressure. Tension pneumothorax and asthma can lead to bradyasystole through increased intrathoracic pressures causing decreased venous return and inadequate cardiac output.

DRUGS

Many drugs affect the cardiac conduction system. Digoxin acts by inhibiting the sodium/potassium pump causing an influx of calcium, which results in its therapeutic action of increasing myocardial contractility. This same mechanism may also contribute to slowing electrical conduction in the atria and AV node. Digoxin also has some direct parasympathetic effect.

β-Adrenergic blockers are competitive inhibitors of catecholamines at the β-receptor. The cardiac effects are related to binding of the β-1 receptors, which are responsible for increasing cardiac contractility, electrical conduction, and heart rate. With β-blocker toxicity, there is slowing of the heart rate either through depression of the SA node and/or AV nodal conduction. Some β-blockers have direct central nervous system (CNS) effects at toxic levels, which may cause respiratory depression and hypoxia.

Calcium-channel blockers antagonize the slow calcium channels causing a decrease in cardiac contractility, depression of SA node activity, and slowing of conduction through the AV node. At toxic levels, this can lead to AV blocks, junctional rhythms, sinus arrest, and asystole.

Anti-arrhythmics may cause bradyasystole. Class IA agents (e.g., procainamide, quinidine) slow atrial automaticity, AV conduction, and conduction through the His-Purkinje system. Class IB agents (e.g., lidocaine, phenytoin) also slow cardiac conduction. Intravenous phenytoin is of particular concern because its carrier, propylene glycol, can cause myocardial depression and sudden asystole if it is infused too quickly (>40 mg per minute [32]). The class III agents (bretylium, ibutilide, sotalol, and amiodarone) also slow automaticity and AV nodal conduction. These effects are more prominent than in the class IB agents. The most common side effects or toxicity of intravenous amiodarone are hypotension and bradycardia.

Methyldopa and clonidine, both α-2 receptor agonists, can cause bradycardia and AV block *(33)*. Nitroglycerin has been implicated in bradyasystole by triggering the Bezold-Jarisch reflex through venodilation and its resultant hypotension *(34,35)*. Severe chloroquine overdoses may cause quinidine like cardiotoxicity leading to sinus arrest, bradycardia, AV blocks, and asystole *(36)*. Lithium can cause heart block and sinus arrest. Sinus node dysfunction can occur with therapeutic and toxic levels *(37,38)*.

Physostigmine increases the levels of acetylcholine causing increased vagal stimulation. This can lead to bradycardia, but may progress to complete heart block and asystole. Tricyclic antidepressants cause conduction abnormalities that may lead to bradyasystole *(39)*.

Table 1
Causes of Bradyasystole

Primary
    Intrinsic failure
        Sick sinus syndrome
        Direct ischemic injury
Secondary
    Hypoxia
    Drugs/medications
        Digoxin
        β-adrenergic blockers
        Calcium-channel blockers
        Anti-arrhythmics
            Procainamide
            Quinidine
            Lidocaine
            Flecainide
            Encainide
            Bretyllium
            Ibutilide
            Sotalol
            Amiodarone
    Methyldopa
    Clonidine
    Nitrates
    Chloroquine
    Lithium
    Physostigmine
    Tricyclic antidepressants
    Toxins
        Antimony
        Lead
        Diphtheria toxin
        Carbon monoxide
        Snake venom
        Plants
            Christmas rose
            Be-still tree
            Dogbane
            Foxglove
            Lily of the valley
            Oleander
            Pheasant's eye
            Squill
            Star of Bethlehem
            Rhododendrons
            Azaleas
            Mountain laurel
            Labrador tea
            Rusty leaf
            Ivy bush (sheepkill)
            Black snakeroot

Table 1 *(Continued)*

False hellebore
Skunk cabbage
Andromedotoxin contaminated honey
Neurologic and neuromuscular
    Spinal cord injury
    Reflexes
        Oculocardiac
        Maxillofacial
        Hypersensitive carotid sinus syndrome
        Deglutition reflex
        Prostatic massage reflex
    Cerebral vascular accident
        Thrombotic stroke
        Hemorrhagic stroke
        Subarachnoid hemorrhage
            Traumatic and spontaneous
    Guillain-barre syndrome
    Becker's dystrophy
    Limb-girdle dystrophy of Erb
    Landouzy-dejerine dystrophy
    Emery-Dreifuss disease
    Myotonic dystrophy
    Kearns-Sayre syndrome
    Nemaline myopathy
    McArdle syndrome
    Poliomyelitis
Hormonal and Metabolic
    Hyperkalemia
    Hypothyroidism
    Acromegaly
    Adrenal insufficiency
    Hyperbilirubinemia
    Hyperparathyroidism
Hypothermia
Infectious disease
    Influenza
    Mumps
    Mononucleosis
    Viral hepatitis
    Rubella
    Rubeola
    RSV
    Tuberculosis
    Streptococcal infections
    Meningococcal infections
    Syphilis
    Leptospirosis
    Relapsing fever
    Lyme disease
        Chagas' disease

continued

Table 1
Causes of Bradyasystole *(Continued)*

Myocardial and pericardial disorders
    Myocardial contusion
    Pericarditis
    Pericardial tamponade
    Infiltrative disease
        Malignancies and tumor
        Amyloid
        Hemochromatosis
Rheumatic diseases
    Rheumatic fever
    Ankylosing spondylitis
    Reiter's syndrome
    Rheumatoid arthritis
    Systemic lupus erythematosis
    Wegener's granulomatosis
    Polymyositis
    Dermatomyositis
Iatrogenic
    Surgical removal of tumors
    Valve replacement
    Congenital defect repair
    Transplant
    Ablation

TOXINS

Antimony, which has a variety of industrial uses, can cause AV block and bradycardia *(40)*. Lead, which is one of the most common environmental toxins, typically presents with GI, nervous system, hematologic, and constitutional symptoms, but it has also been implicated in AV nodal conduction disturbances *(41)*. Diphtheria toxin can lead to myocarditis. Often this results in tachycardia and congestive heart failure, but conduction disturbances and heart blocks are not uncommon *(42)*.

Carbon monoxide poisoning can lead to bradyasystole through its anoxic effects.

Venomous snake bites are a very uncommon cause of bradyasystole, although direct cardiotoxic effects resulting in CA have occurred *(43)*. Cardiotoxic plants contain substances similar to digoxin. Cardiac glycosides are found in Christmas rose, be-still tree, dogbane, foxglove, lily of the valley, oleander, pheasant's eye, squill, and star of Bethlehem.

Andromedotoxin, also known as acetylandromedol or grayanotoxin, is a glycoside typically found in rhododendrons and azaleas, which causes bradyasystole. It is also found in mountain laurel, lily of the valley shrub, Labrador tea, rusty leaf, and ivy bush *(44,45)*. Veratramine is another toxin that causes direct SA node suppression leading to periodic rhythm (normal sinus rhythm interposed between episodes of asystole *[46]*). Veratramine and related substances are found in black snakeroot, false hellebore, and skunk cabbage. Bees can ingest andromedotoxin as they feed on flowers and then they incorporate this toxin into their honey. Ingestion of affected honey may cause symptomatic bradycardia *(47,48)*.

SPINAL CORD INJURY

Patients with spinal cord injuries often have significant fluctuations in heart rate with cardiovascular instability. Cervical and upper thoracic spinal cord injuries cause profound bradycardia (49). The sympathetic nerves are disrupted as they exit the spinal cord at the low cervical and upper thoracic levels, although the parasympathetic system (mediated by the uninvolved vagus nerve, which runs outside of the spinal column) remains unopposed. The risk of hemodynamically significant bradycardia usually peaks at 3–5 days after the acute injury, and then stabilizes in 2–8 weeks. Ten percent of quadriplegics have significant bradycardia, which can be resistant to atropine (50). Any mild visceral stimulus such as suctioning or urinary retention can initiate severe symptoms.

REFLEXES

There are several reflexes that can cause bradycardia.

Oculocardiac Reflex

This is the reflex that occurs when applying ocular pressure to terminate supraventricular tachycardia. The short ciliary nerve and the ophthalmic division of the trigeminal nerve carry afferent stimulus as they terminate at the fourth ventricle in the trigeminal nucleus. The efferent portion of the reflex is carried by the vagus nerve. This reflex can occur with a retrobulbar block, eye trauma, orbital hematomas, traction on the extraocular muscles, or pressure on the globe from any other source and cause bradyasystole (51).

Maxillofacial Reflex/Diving Reflex

The maxillofacial reflex occurs with stimulation of the afferent parasympathetic fibers of the maxillary and mandibular divisions of the trigeminal nerve during maxillofacial trauma or surgery (52,53). The efferent limb of this reflex is carried through the vagus nerve. Similarly, the diving reflex causes bradycardia as sensory branches of the trigeminal nerve are stimulated by immersion of the face in cold water (employed to terminate SVT VF [54–57]). This reflex is most pronounced in children and young adults. Its basis relates to its benefit in aquatic mammals, which allow them to remain under water for prolonged periods of time as it slows cardiac oxygen consumption and creates a low metabolic state.

Other Reflexes

Hypersensitive carotid sinus syndrome (58) is caused by increased and sensitized afferent nerve stimulation leading to profound bradycardia and sudden but transient episodes of syncope or presyncope. Many other causes of reflex mediated bradycardia have been described. Bradycardia with hemodynamic compromise can occur with severe pain, particularly in the ear, nasal and oropharynx, and larynx. Thoracentesis and paracentesis have also been shown to cause bradycardic syncope. Deglutition syncope (59) occurs through stimulation of afferents in the esophagus during swallowing. Prostatic massage has caused bradycardia and syncope. Micturation syncope is a reflex-mediated phenomenon in men that occurs during or just after urination (60–63).

SYSTEMIC NEUROLOGIC AND NEUROMUSCULAR DISEASES

Thrombotic stroke, hemorrhagic stroke, and subarachnoid hemorrhage can be accompanied by bradyasystole. Traumatic intracranial hemorrhage, cerebral edema, or seizures can cause bradycardia and/or asystole *(64–69)*. These intracranial pathologies interfere with the normal balance of parasympathetic and sympathetic tone as directed by the normally functioning brain.

Guillain-Barre syndrome (ascending spinal cord paralysis) can cause bradycardia, through unopposed parasympathetic activity similar to that seen in cervical spine injuries *(70)*. Degenerative neuromuscular diseases often directly affect the heart interfering with cell-to-cell electrical conduction. These include Becker's dystrophy, limb-girdle dystrophy of Erb, fascioscapulohumeral dystrophy (Landouzy-Dejerine), Emery-Dreifuss disease, myotonic dystrophy, Kearns-Sayre syndrome, Nemaline myopathy, McArdle syndrome, and adult poliomyelitis *(71–78)*.

Hormonal and Metabolic Abnormalities

Hyperkalemia causes slowing of the electrical conduction system, resulting in tented and peaked T waves, increased P-R interval, widened QRS complex, then absent P-waves on the electrocardiogram. Further progression of hyperkalemia can lead to bradyasystole (79). Severe hypothyroidism frequently causes bradycardia. Myxedema patients frequently have atrioventricular and intraventricular blocks leading to bradyasystole *(80)*. Acromegaly patients, with an excess of growth hormone production, have an increased risk of sudden death secondary to intraventricular conduction defects related to degenerative disease of the SA node and AV node *(81)*. Adrenal insufficiency, often marked by orthostatic hypotension, can cause sinus bradycardia, atrioventricular conduction delays, and prolonged QT intervals *(82,83)*. Hyperparathyroidism causes increased calcium levels, decreased QT interval, and complete heart block *(84)*.

Hyperbilirubinemia has been associated with bradyasystole. Bradycardia and asystole has occurred in patients with obstructive jaundice as bilirubin levels rise above 15% *(85)*. It is unclear whether the bilirubin itself causes the bradycardia, or perhaps more plausibly there is an increase in parasympathetic tone as bile ducts are distended and obstructed.

Hypothermia

Mild hypothermia (30–35°C) increases heart rate and cardiac output. Severe hypothermia (<30°C) can cause bradycardia, asystole, and VF *(86)*. These rhythms are resistant to standard therapy and treatment should be initially directed at rewarming.

Infectious Disease

Many infections can cause subclinical myocarditis, resulting in cardiac conduction disorders and bradycardia. Influenza, mumps, mononucleosis, viral hepatitis, rubeola, arboviruses, and respiratory syncytial virus have been associated with symptomatic bradycardia and complete heart block *(87–93)*. Tuberculosis can invade the heart and cause complete heart block and sudden death *(94)*. Streptococcal and meningococcal disease has also been reported to cause conduction disturbances leading to bradycardia and sudden death *(95,96)*. Congenital rubella can cause malformations such as patent ductus arteriosis, pulmonary artery anomalies, and abnormalities of the conduction system *(97)*.

Spirochete disease including syphilis, leptospirosis, and relapsing fever also can affect the conduction system *(98–100)*. Lyme disease can cause both transient and permanent AV blocks *(101,102)*. Chagas' disease, one of the most frequent causes of heart failure in the world, causes bradyarrhythmias. Often the bradycardia is caused by autonomic dysfunction. Although right bundle branch blocks and left anterior fascicular blocks are most common, AV block also occurs. Even in the absence of symptoms, most people with Chagas' disease have an AV conduction abnormality *(103)*.

Systemic candidiasis frequently causes endocarditis, and microabscesses can invade the conduction system causing bradyasystole *(104)*.

Myocardial and Pericardial Disorders

Because the interventricular septum and right bundle branch are located beneath the sternum, myocardial contusion following blunt trauma can result in bundle branch blocks and bradyarrhythmias *(105)*. Pericarditis can also cause bradycardias. Inflamed pericardium induces vagal stimulation. Rapidly accumulated pericardial effusions can result in cardiac tamponade, characterized by vagally mediated bradycardia and rapid cardiovascular collapse *(106,107)*.

Infiltrative Disease

Metastatic malignancies can affect the heart *(108,109)*. Most common are breast, colon, bronchogenic, esophageal, prostatic, ovarian, and gastric carcinomas, melanoma, sarcoma, Hodgkin's disease, and leukemia as they invade the myocardium and interfere with propagation of electrical impulses. Primary tumors, originating within the myocardium and also interfering with propagation of electrical impulses, include: myxoma, rhabdomyoma, fibroma, lipoma, hemangioma, hamartoma, and papillary fibroelastoma. Mesotheliomas and angiomas have a predilection for the AV node and lead to conduction disturbances *(110)*. Amyloid (amyloidosis *[111,112]*) and iron (hemochromatosis) infiltration of the cardiac conduction system causes heart block *(113,114)*.

Rheumatic Diseases

Rheumatic diseases have been implicated in conduction disturbances leading to bradyasystole. These diseases include: rheumatic fever, ankylosing spondylitis, Reiter's syndrome, rheumatoid arthritis, systemic lupus erythematosis, Wegener's granulomatosis, polymyositis, and dermatomyositis *(115–118)*.

Iatrogenic Causes

Surgical removal of tumors can damage the conduction system of the heart. Other surgeries such as valve replacement or congenital defect repairs can also lead to conduction abnormalities predisposing to bradycardia, asystole, and sudden death. Radiation treatment can cause endocardial fibrosis resulting in conduction defects. Radio-frequency ablation can result in anything from mild intraventricular conduction delays to complete heart block.

ELECTROPHYSIOLOGY

The heart contains specialized structures that initiate and/or propagate electrical activity efficiently. These structures are the SA node, specialized atrial fibers, the AV node, bundle of His, and Purkinje fibers. Cells that make up these structures have the ability to spontaneously generate an electrical impulse called automaticity. This is accomplished through spontaneous phase-4 depolarization.

To elicit spontaneous phase-4 depolarization, a time-dependent potassium current increases the transmembrane voltage toward 0 until a threshold is reached and depolarization in phase 0 occurs. This electrical impulse generated by these specialized cells is then transmitted cell to cell throughout the myocardium to cause normal depolarization and systole of the entire heart.

All cells of the heart function as a result of depolarization. Active ion pumping normally maintains a transmembrane voltage of –90 mV during diastole or relaxation. Activation of the myocardial cells causes movement of sodium ions into the cell causing a rapid change of transmembrane voltage to +90 mV. This is called depolarization. This depolarization causes excitation and contraction of the myocyte. The myocardial cell then goes through a series of phases *(1–3)* to repolarize and return the resting potential to –90 mV. Pacemaker cells, however, typically have a resting potential of about –60 mV. Whereas in the myocardial muscle cells sodium currents are predominant in the depolarization of the cell, calcium is the key molecule in depolarization of the specialized myocardial cells that are characterized by automaticity *(119)*.

The SA node normally fires at a rate faster than the other structures and is the dominant pacemaker for impulse generation. If the SA node fails to spontaneously fire, or if its depolarization is not appropriately transmitted through the specialized tracts to initiate normal depolarization and contraction throughout the heart, cells from the other structures can take over with their own normal automaticity and provide escape pacing. Although the SA node normally fires at a rate of 60–100 bpm, AV node cells have a normal escape rate of 40–60 bpm. The ventricular structures with normal automaticity will fire 30 to 40 times per minute. The atrial and ventricular myocardial cells do not have normal automaticity, but they can generate arrhythmias through a variety of abnormal automatic mechanisms including sustained depolarization, delayed repolarization, afterdepolarization, and a host of membrane oscillatory mechanisms.

If the firing rate of the SA node is depressed or fails to fire completely, bradycardia will occur. Bradycardia can also occur if problems transmitting the SA node's impulse exist such as SA exit block, AV block, or bilateral bundle branch block. The escape pacemakers however should temper the bradycardia as they take over control of the heart's rhythm. For severe bradycardia or asystole to occur, there must be further failure of the backup pacemakers.

There are many factors that affect the electrophysiology of the heart. For the pacemaker and conducting tissue cells to initiate and propagate impulses, the cellular metabolic functions must be intact. Ischemia will directly disable cellular metabolism and disable the cells from actively transporting ions to initiate action potentials. Occlusion of the proximal right coronary artery can cause ischemia and infarction of the SA and AV nodes. The SA node receives its blood supply from a branch of the proximal right coronary artery 55% of the time *(120)*. The AV node receives its blood supply from a branch of the distal right coronary artery 90% of the time *(120)*. The bundle branches typically have multiple blood supplies, but may be affected in severe three-vessel coronary artery disease (CAD) and lead to significant bradycardia and/or asystole with extensive myocardial infarction (MI).

Many endogenous chemicals will also alter the ability of the SA node as well as the remainder of the electrical system to function. Endogenous adenosine, for example, is released during myocardial ischemia *(121)*. Not only does adenosine impair AV conduction and pacemaker automaticity, it also relaxes smooth muscle and decreases myocardial contractility *(122,123)*. Adenosine stimulates outward potassium current as does the parasympathetic chemical acetylcholine *(124,125)*. This leads to hyperpolarized atrial and nodal cells, decreased duration of the action potential, and decreased spontaneous phase-4 depolarization of the SA node cells (126). It also slows AV conduction by depressing the AV nodal cells' action potentials in the same manner (127). During myocardial ischemia, adenosine is formed by dephosphorylation of adenosine monophosphate (128,129).

Pacemaker cells are also influenced by a variety of hormonal, pharmacological, and toxicological effects. The parasympathetic mediator acetylcholine will suppress SA node automaticity and AV node conduction in the same manner as adenosine. Catecholamines, thyroid hormone, methylxanthines, and other stimulants will increase automaticity of the SA node through an increase in calcium influx as well as potentially enhance the pacing capabilities of the other cells within the heart's conduction system. β-Adrenergic blocking agents, calcium-channel blockers, parasympathomimetics, as well as hypercapnea will decrease automaticity. Exogenous adenosine will work much like endogenous adenosine.

The autonomic nervous system also plays a key role in the function of the conduction system of the heart. The parasympathetic system is mediated through the vagus nerve. The right vagus innervates the SA node and when stimulated will slow its firing rate. The left vagus retards AV conduction as its innervation of the AV node is stimulated. The sympathetic system increases automaticity and shortens the refractory period of the myocytes. The left sympathetic nerve innervates the SA node and the right nerve innervates the AV node area.

The sympathetic and parasympathetic systems are normally balanced. Any interference with this balance can lead to an arrhythmia. CNS damage, damage to the stellate ganglia, or neuropathy of the nerves supplying the heart from viral infections, diabetes, degenerative disorders, or infiltrative disease can all disrupt this delicate balance.

Vagal denervation such as in cardiac transplant will make the heart unusually sensitive to acetylcholine (130). Likewise, transplanted hearts are very sensitive to endogenous or exogenous adenosine (131). Adenosine appears to be the primary mediator of sinus node dysfunction in postoperative cardiac transplant patients.

Myocardial ischemia also leads to autonomic dysfunction. One would think that the heart would always be in a sympathetic state in the face of ischemia as hypoxic states lead to a release of endogenous epinephrine and norepinephrine. During resuscitation from CA, the exogenous administration of epinephrine is also common. This unresponsiveness to sympathetic stimulation during bradyasystolic CA suggests there is a primary or secondary failure of cardiac pacemaker generation or propagation.

Ischemia can excite both vagal and sympathetic afferents leading to vagally mediated depression or sympathetic excitation, or sometimes a certain level of both (132–135). Furthermore, ischemia can disrupt neural transmissions interfering with the normal autonomic response (136,137). When these neural transmissions remain intact, ischemia may also affect the CNS control of the autonomic nervous system (138–142).

MYOCARDIAL ENERGY MECHANICS

The energy mechanics in bradyasystole are poorly understood. A lower heart rate requires less myocardial oxygen demand, as represented in the efficacy of β-blocker use in acute ischemia. In animal models, during bradyasystole, there is very little myocardial oxygen consumption (143). It would seem that ongoing hypoxic injury would be reduced when there is little oxygen demand. If intracellular energy stores of adenosine triphosphate are adequate, one would expect a high incidence of spontaneous return of circulation. Nonetheless, return of spontaneous circulation is infrequent in bradyasystole. This suggests that the energy mechanics of bradyasystole are more complex involving ongoing hypoxic insult, energy consumption and possibly intracellular depletion of key electrolyte balance and energy stores.

TREATMENT
General

Patients with bradyasystole require immediate airway, ventilatory, and circulatory support. A rapid search for reversible causes should be undertaken while these basic initial resuscitative efforts are started. Prehospital providers, family, medical records if immediately available, and the patient's family physician are all potential sources of information for the emergency physician caring for a patient with bradyasystole. An estimate of time from onset of CA and whether it was witnessed or unwitnessed may assist clinical decision making. Witnesses or family may be able to relate the patient's symptoms prior to onset of arrest, such as an extended period of shortness of breath possibly indicating a pulmonary etiology. The patient's past medical history may be helpful in determining the cause of bradyasystole. A prior history of CAD may indicate myocardial ischemia or possible MI. Renal dialysis patients are at risk to develop severe hyperkalemia. Patients who have undergone prolonged immobilization, such as casting following an orthopedic procedure, are at risk for a PE. A history of chronic obstructive pulmonary disease or smoking may lead the clinician to consider tension pneumothorax. A prior history of psychiatric illness or depression may lead one to consider the possibility of a drug overdose. Current medications should be determined and assessed for potential cardiac toxicity, including tricyclic antidepressants, β-blockers, calcium-channel blockers, and digitalis.

Specific Treatments (Table 2)

SICK SINUS SYNDROME

Sick sinus syndrome is a constellation of pathologies affecting sinus node function. Some treatments will be more effective than others depending on the specific disorder. Atropine, dopamine, epinephrine, or isoproterenol can be effective temporizing measures. Emergent pacing constitutes definitive stabilizing intervention. Transcutaneous pacing should be initiated as preparations are made for transvenous pacing. Definitive treatment usually requires insertion of a permanent pacemaker.

ISCHEMIA

Symptoms of ischemia include substernal, crushing chest pain that may radiate to the arm or jaw associated with diaphoresis, nausea, or dyspnea. However, bradycardia may be the only presenting sign and an electrocardiogram should be obtained to identify any evidence of ischemia. Acute coronary syndromes should be identified and treated quickly with supplemental oxygen, morphine, aspirin, nitrates, β-blockers, and heparin as appropriate. Patients who meet appropriate criteria should receive rapid definitive intervention with cardiac catheterization or thrombolytic therapy.

HYPOXIA

All efforts should be made to maximize oxygenation and ventilation. The presence of acute airway obstruction should be considered and immediately corrected if identified. Continuous positive airway pressure or bilevel positive airway pressure may be very

Table 2
Specific Treatments

Etiology	Treatment
Sick sinus syndrome	Atropine, dopamine, epinephrine, emergent pacing
Ischemia	Thrombolytics/emergent cardiac catheterization
Hypoxia	Oxygen and airway support
Toxins/medications	
Digoxin overdose	Atropine, pacing, digoxin-binding antibodies
β-Blocker overdose	Dopamine, atropine, epinephrine, glucagon
Calcium-channel blocker overdose	Calcium
Lithium	Atropine, pacing, dialysis
Tricyclic antidepressants	Bicarbonate
Carbon monoxide	Oxygen/consider hyperbaric
Snake venoms	Antivenom
Hormonal and metabolic	
Hyperkalemia	Calcium, bicarbonate, insulin and glucose, sodium polystyrenesulfonate, dialysis
Adrenal insufficiency	Glucocorticoid replacement
Hypothermia	Aggressive rewarming
Pericardial tamponade	Pericardiocentesis
Tension Pneumothorax	Emergent decompression, thoracostomy tube

beneficial in patients with acute pulmonary edema from congestive heart failure, in some cases obviating the need for endotracheal intubation.

Tension pneumothorax, with hypotension, decreased breath sounds on the affected side, and a deviated trachea, requires emergent decompression. This can be accomplished by inserting a 14-gauge angiocatheter through the second intercostal space of the anterior chest wall. The needle should be removed with the plastic catheter left in place until definitive treatment with a thoracostomy tube is complete.

If a PE is causing clinically significant hemodynamic compromise, thrombolytic therapy should be empirically and immediately instituted (rt-PA, 1 mg per minute, 100 mg total). Fibrinolytic therapy has replaced surgical intervention in almost all cases. Surgery is reserved for those that have absolute contraindications to fibrinolytic therapy.

DIGOXIN

Successful treatment of digoxin toxicity requires initial stabilization, decontamination, and administration of digoxin binding antibody. Atropine and pacing should be initially used in patients with hemodynamic compromise. Hyperkalemia, often seen with digoxin toxicity, should be emergently treated (as described below) with the important exception of intravenous calcium, which, if administered, can result in lethal arrhythmias or tetanic contraction of left ventricular myocardium, resulting in death of the patient *(144)*. Airway stabilization, gastric decontamination, and administration of repeat-dose activated charcoal to enhance elimination of digoxin should be performed. Because serum levels of digoxin do not correlate with toxicity, criteria for administration of digoxin-specific antibodies are based on clinical presentation. In both acute and chronic overdose digoxin-specific antibodies should be given for severe hyperkalemia or life-threatening arrhythmias. Dosing is often empiric with 10 vials typically needed for acute ingestion and 5 vials for chronic toxicity. Response should be seen within 30 to 60 minutes of administration. The dose should be increased, as appropriate, for continued toxicity. Digoxin-specific antibodies have some usefulness in the treatment of related cardiac glycoside ingestions such as from plants *(145)*.

β-ADRENERGIC BLOCKERS

Bradycardia associated with hemodynamic compromise can respond to volume replacement, dopamine, other vasopressor support, atropine, isoproterenol, and cardiac pacing. For bradycardia not responsive to these measures, intravenous glucagon bolus (2–5 mg followed by an infusion at 2–5 mg per hour *[146]*) as well as the administration of epinephrine by bolus or continuous infusion may be lifesaving.

Hemodialysis may be necessary or helpful in overdose cases with β-blockers that have a small volume of distribution such as atenolol *(147)*.

CALCIUM-CHANNEL ANTAGONISTS

Intravenous calcium gluconate or calcium chloride should be administered to reverse depression of cardiac contractility. Calcium administration will not affect sinus node dysfunction or AV node conduction delays. Cardiac pacing should be instituted for those with hemodynamically significant bradycardia. For refractory hypotension, glucagon, and epinephrine are the agents of choice.

TRICYCLIC ANTIDEPRESSANTS

Because serious cardiac toxicity may present without any antecedent toxidrome and can progress rapidly, patients with suspected tricyclic antidepressant overdose should be monitored closely. A QRS duration of 0.16 seconds or longer is highly correlated with serious cardiotoxicity *(148)*. Any increase in QRS duration compared with the patient's normal baseline should be treated with intravenous sodium bicarbonate. Pacing may be needed for significant AV block. Physostigmine is contraindicated as its use may further aggravate conductions disturbances and cause irreversible asystole *(39)*.

LITHIUM

Cardiac conduction abnormalities and bradycardia caused by lithium toxicity should be treated with atropine and pacing. Activated charcoal is not indicated because it will not absorb lithium. Lithium is eliminated from the body exclusively by the kidneys. Patients that have renal failure as well as those that have toxicity not responding to supportive care should undergo hemodialysis *(149)*.

HYPERKALEMIA

If a patient is at risk for hyperkalemia and the electrocardiogram is diagnostic for hyperkalemic changes, treatment should begin empirically without waiting for laboratory potassium levels. Calcium chloride or calcium gluconate should be administered intravenously, with the important exception of patients on digoxin. Intravenous calcium has immediate cardioprotective effects, stabilizing myocardial membranes. Intravenous sodium bicarbonate increases serum pH, driving potassium into the cell, within 5 minutes of administration. Intravenous administration of 10 units of regular insulin and 1 ampule of intravenous glucose also drives potassium into the cell with an onset of action of 30 minutes. These emergent interventions, although lifesaving are only temporizing. For definitive treatment, the total body concentration of potassium must be decreased to normal levels, either through the administration of an exchange resin, sodium polystyrenesulfonate (onset of action about 6 hours) or hemodialysis.

PERICARDIAL TAMPONADE

Patients at risk for pericardial tamponade are those with end-stage renal disease, pericarditis, postinfarction, and trauma. Physical exam findings are unreliable and include a narrow pulse pressure, distended neck veins, and distant heart sounds. Hemodynamic compromise is related to the speed of accumulation of pericardial fluid rather than the absolute amount. The chest x-ray may not reveal a large cardiac silhouette. Echocardiography is, therefore, the diagnostic procedure of choice. Emergent intervention for patients with hemodynamic compromise consists of pericardiocentesis via the subxiphoid or parasternal approach.

Anticholinergic Therapy

Unopposed parasympathetic stimulation is involved in many instances of bradyasystole and antagonism with intravenous atropine is the chemical agent of choice. Atropine functions as a competitive inhibitor of acetylcholine (the chemical messenger of the parasympathetic nervous system) at the muscarinic receptor. Atropine-mediated parasympathetic blockade can therapeutically reverse symptomatic bradycardia. At low doses (<0.5 mg IV), atropine can cause a paradoxical bradycardia because of its centrally acting parasympathetic stimulant properties. For this reason, the minimal appropriate adult dose is 0.5 mg intravenously. Atropine is an American Heart Association (AHA) Class I intervention for symptomatic sinus bradycardia. It is Class IIa for AV blocks at the nodal level (Mobitz type I). Its use may cause further bradycardia and is rarely beneficial in blocks below the nodal level (Mobitz type II and third degree [150]). Atropine remains in the AHA's algorithm for asystole based on anecdotal case reports (25,151,152). The current recommended dose for atropine in asystole is 0.04 mg/kg IV. If atropine is administered through an endotracheal tube, doubling the dose is recommended (150). High-dose atropine has been reported to be detrimental (153,154).

Adrenergic Therapy

Adrenergic agents improve coronary perfusion pressure by augmenting systemic vascular resistance. Increased coronary perfusion pressure has been shown experimentally and clinically to be predictive of return of spontaneous circulation (155,156). Epinephrine is the adrenergic agent of choice in asystole (157). The recommended dose is 0.01 mg/kg up to 1 mg IV (157). If epinephrine is given through the endotracheal tube, the dose should be doubled (150). The efficacy of varying doses and types of adrenergic agents has been studied extensively in VF CA (158–169) but not in bradyasystole.

β-1-stimulation with agents such as isoproterenol improves chronotropism (150). However, β-stimulation also causes vasodilatation, which may decrease cerebral and myocardial blood flow (170). Isoproterenol may be useful as an adjunct to epinephrine in treating bradyasystole related to β-blocker toxicity (171).

Calcium and Glucagon

When bradyasystole is caused by hyperkalemia, hypocalcemia (such as following massive blood transfusion), or calcium-channel blocker overdose, intravenous calcium administration may be lifesaving (172). Glucagon has been shown to be beneficial in cases of β-blocker overdose (146).

Acid–Base Therapy

Maintaining adequate alveolar ventilation is the basis for controlling acid–base balance during CA. Bicarbonate administration may compromise coronary perfusion pressure, may cause adverse effects as a result of extracellular alkalosis, including shifting the oxyhemoglobin saturation curve, inhibiting the release of oxygen, may induce hyperosmolarity and hypernatremia, produces carbon dioxide, which is freely diffusible into myocardial and cerebral cells and paradoxically contributes to intracellular acidosis, possibly decreases coronary perfusion pressure, and may inactivate simultaneously administered catecholamines *(173–176)*.

The use of bicarbonate is indicated in treating cardiotoxicity of tricyclic antidepressant overdose, and hyperkalemia *(84,176,177)*. The bicarbonate should be titrated to normalize the rhythm in a tricyclic antidepressant overdose patient. After protracted arrest or long resuscitative efforts, intravenous bicarbonate may be beneficial *(176)*.

Electrical Therapy—Pacing

Pacing has been shown to be effective in treating bradyasystolic patients who still have a pulse *(157)*. Its use in pulseless patients, particularly asystole, does not improve patient outcome *(178,179)*. Electrical therapy, when indicated or considered, should be instituted as soon as possible.

TRANSCUTANEOUS PACING

Transcutaneous pacing can be applied rapidly and serves as a bridge to transvenous pacing. Because of discomfort from chest wall muscle contraction, conscious patients require intravenous anxiolytic and/or analgesic agents.

TRANSVENOUS PACING

Transvenous pacing can be instituted quickly in the emergency setting by a physician skilled in its use. Central venous access is first obtained with a no. 8 French catheter in the right internal jugular vein, left subclavian vein, or femoral vein. The balloon-tipped bipolar pacing catheter is then advanced, allowing flow-guided placement in the right ventricle. The current threshold usually required to attain consistent ventricular capture has been reported to be less than 1.0–1.5 mA in emergency situations and the final current recommended to be two to three times the threshold current *(180)*. Higher currents are likely to be required in the setting of CA. Electrical capture and mechanical activity must be assessed and confirmed separately following placement.

REFERENCES

1. Atkins DL, Hartley LL, York DK. Accurate recognition and effective treatment of ventricular fibrillation by automated external defibrillators in adolescents. Pediatrics 1998; 101(Pt 1):393–397.
2. Cummins RO, Eisenberg MS, Hallstrom AP, Litwin PE. Survival of out-of-hospital cardiac arrest with early initiation of cardiopulmonary resuscitation. Am J Emerg Med 1985; 3:114–119.
3. Denes P, Gabster A, Huang SK. Clinical, electrocardiographic and follow-up observations in patients having ventricular fibrillation during Holter monitoring. Role of quinidine therapy. Am J Cardiol 1981; 48:9–16.
4. Edgren E, Kelsey S, Sutton K, Safar P. The presenting ECG pattern in survivors of cardiac arrest and its relation to the subsequent long-term survival. Brain Resuscitation Clinical Trial I Study Group. Acta Anaesthesiol Scand 1989; 33:265–271.

5. Eisenberg MS, Horwood BT, Cummins RO, Reynolds-Haertle R, Hearne TR. Cardiac arrest and resuscitation: a tale of 29 cities. Ann Emerg Med 1990; 19:179–186.

6. Gradman AH, Bell PA, DeBusk RF. Sudden death during ambulatory monitoring. Clinical and electrocardiographic correlations. Report of a case. Circulation 1977; 55:210–211.

7. Hinkle LE, Jr., Argyros DC, Hayes JC, et al. Pathogenesis of an unexpected sudden death: role of early cycle ventricular premature contractions. Am J Cardiol 1977; 39:873–879.

8. Kempf FC, Jr., Josephson ME. Cardiac arrest recorded on ambulatory electrocardiograms. Am J Cardiol 1984; 53:1577–1582.

9. Lahiri A, Balasubramanian V, Raftery EB. Sudden death during ambulatory monitoring. Br Med J 1979; 1:1676–1678.

10. Mogayzel C, Quan L, Graves JR, Tiedeman D, Fahrenbruch C, Herndon P. Out-of-hospital ventricular fibrillation in children and adolescents: causes and outcomes. Ann Emerg Med 1995; 25:484–491.

11. Myerburg RJ, Conde CA, Sung RJ, et al. Clinical, electrophysiologic and hemodynamic profile of patients resuscitated from prehospital cardiac arrest. Am J Med 1980; 68:568–576.

12. Myerburg RJ, Estes D, Zaman L, et al. Outcome of resuscitation from bradyarrhythmic or asystolic prehospital cardiac arrest. J Am Coll Cardiol 1984; 4:1118–1122.

13. Myerburg RJ. Sudden cardiac death: epidemiology, causes, and mechanisms. Cardiology 1987; 74 (Suppl 2):2–9.

14. Nikolic G, Bishop RL, Singh JB. Sudden death recorded during Holter monitoring. Circulation 1982; 66:218–225.

15. Panidis IP, Morganroth J. Sudden death in hospitalized patients: cardiac rhythm disturbances detected by ambulatory electrocardiographic monitoring. J Am Coll Cardiol 1983; 2:798–805.

16. Salerno D, Hodges M, Graham E, Asinger RW, Mikell FL. Fatal cardiac arrest during continuous ambulatory monitoring. N Engl J Med 1981; 305:700.

17. Savage DD, Castelli WP, Anderson SJ, Kannel WB. Sudden unexpected death during ambulatory electrocardiographic monitoring. The Framingham Study. Am J Med 1983; 74:148–152.

18. Scott RP. Cardiopulmonary resuscitation in a teaching hospital. A survey of cardiac arrests occurring outside intensive care units and emergency rooms. Anaesthesia 1981; 36:526–530.

19. Stueven HA, Waite EM, Troiano P, Mateer JR. Prehospital cardiac arrest—a critical analysis of factors affecting survival. Resuscitation 1989; 17:251–259.

20. Walsh CK, Krongrad E. Terminal cardiac electrical activity in pediatric patients. Am J Cardiol 1983; 51:557–561.

21. Guidelines for cardiopulmonary resuscitation and emergency cardiac care. Emergency Cardiac Care Committee and Subcommittees, American Heart Association. Part I. Introduction. JAMA 1992; 268:2171–2183.

22. Bayes dL, Coumel P, Leclercq JF. Ambulatory sudden cardiac death: mechanisms of production of fatal arrhythmia on the basis of data from 157 cases. Am Heart J 1989; 117:151–159.

23. Pool J, Kunst K, van Wermeskerken JL. Two monitored cases of sudden death outside hospital. Br Heart J 1978; 40:627–629.

24. Eisenberg MS, Hadas E, Nuri I, et al. Sudden cardiac arrest in Israel: factors associated with successful resuscitation. Am J Emerg Med 1988; 6:319–323.

25. Iseri LT, Humphrey SB, Siner EJ. Prehospital brady-asystolic cardiac arrest. Ann Intern Med 1978; 88:741–745.

26. Iseri LT, Siner EJ, Humphrey SB, Mann S. Prehospital cardiac arrest after arrival of the Paramedic Unit. JACEP 1977; 6:530–535.

27. Chiche P, Lellouch A, Denizeau JP. Autonomic influences and cardiac conduction in patients with sinus node disease. Cardiology 1976; 61(Suppl 1):98–112.

28. Rosen KM, Loeb HS, Sinno MZ, Rahimtoola SH, Gunnar RM. Cardiac conduction in patients with symptomatic sinus node disease. Circulation 1971; 43:836–844.

29. Lenegre J. Etiology and pathology of bilateral bundle branch block in relation to complete heart block. Prog Cardiovasc Dis 1964; 6:409.

30. Lev M. The pathology of complete atrioventricular block. Prog Cardiovasc Dis 1964; 6:317.

31. Lev M. Anatomic basis for atrioventricular block. Am J Med 1964; 37:742.

32. York RC, Coleridge ST. Cardiopulmonary arrest following intravenous phenytoin loading. Am J Emerg Med 1988; 6:255–259.

33. Sadjadi SA, Leghari RU, Berger AR. Prolongation of the PR interval induced by methyldopa. Am J Cardiol 1984; 54:675–676.

34. Antonelli D, Barzilay J. Complete atrioventricular block after sublingual isosorbide dinitrate. Int J Cardiol 1986; 10:71–73.
35. Brandes W, Santiago T, Limacher M. Nitroglycerin-induced hypotension, bradycardia, and asystole: report of a case and review of the literature. Clin Cardiol 1990; 13:741–744.
36. Michael TA, Arivazzadek S. The effects of acute chloroquine poisoning with special reference to the heart. Am Heart J 1970; 79:831.
37. Montalescot G, Levy Y, Farge D, et al. Lithium causing a serious sinus-node dysfunction at therapeutic doses. Clin Cardiol 1984; 7:617–620.
38. Ong AC, Handler CE. Sinus arrest and asystole due to severe lithium intoxication. Int J Cardiol 1991; 30:364–366.
39. Pentel P, Peterson CD. Asystole complicating physostigmine treatment of tricyclic antidepressant overdose. Ann Emerg Med 1980; 9:588–590.
40. Honey M. The effects of sodium antimony tartrate on the myocardium. Br Heart J 1960; 22:601.
41. Henretig FM. Lead. In: Goldrank LR, ed. Goldfrank's Toxicologic Emergencies, sixth edition. New York, NY: McGraw-Hill, 1998, pp. 1277–1309.
42. Ledbetter MK, Cannon AB, Costa AF. The electrocardiogram in diphtheritic myocarditis. Am Heart J 1964; 68:599.
43. Weiser E, Wollberg Z, Kochva E, Lee SY. Cardiotoxic effects of the venom of the burrowing asp. Toxicology 1984; 22:767.
44. Shih RD, Goldfrank LR. Plants. In: Goldfrank LR, ed. Goldfrank's Toxicologic Emergencies, sixth edition. McGraw-Hill, New York, 1998, pp. 1243–1259.
45. Woo OF. Plants and herbal medicines. In: Olson KR, ed. Poisoning and drug overdose, third edition. Stamford: Appleton and Lange, 1999, pp. 265–274.
46. Thron CD, McCann FV. Studies on the bradycardia and periodic rhythm caused by veratramine in the sinoatrial node of the guinea pig. J Electrocardiol 1998; 31:257–268.
47. Lampe KF. Rhododendrons, mountain laurel, and mad honey. JAMA 1988; 259:2009.
48. von Malottki K, Wiechmann HW. [Acute life-threatening bradycardia: food poisoning by Turkish wild honey]. Dtsch Med Wochenschr 1996; 121:936–938.
48. Lehmann KG, Lane JG, Piepmeier JM, Batsford WP. Cardiovascular abnormalities accompanying acute spinal cord injury in humans: incidence, time course and severity. J Am Coll Cardiol 1987; 10:46–52.
49. Kewalramani LS. Autonomic dysreflexia in traumatic myelopathy. Am J Phys Med 1980; 59:1–21.
50. Gold RS, Pollard Z, Buchwald IP. Asystole due to the oculocardiac reflex during strabismus surgery: a report of two cases. Ann Ophthalmol 1988; 20:473–475, 477.
51. Lang S, Lanigan DT, Van der WM. Trigeminocardiac reflexes: maxillary and mandibular variants of the oculocardiac reflex. Can J Anaesth 1991; 38:757–760.
52. Precious DS, Skulsky FG. Cardiac dysrhythmias complicating maxillofacial surgery. Int J Oral Maxillofac Surg 1990; 19:279–282.
53. Valladares BK, Lemberg L. Use of the "diving reflex" in paroxysmal atrial tachycardia. Heart Lung 1983; 12:202–205.
54. Whitman V, Sakeosian GM. The diving reflex in termination of supraventricular tachycardia in childhood. J Pediatr 1976; 89:1032–1033.
55. Wildenthal K, Leshin SJ, Atkins JM, Skelton CL. The diving reflex used to treat paroxysmal atrial tachycardia. Lancet 1975; 1:12–14.
56. Wildenthal K. Treatment of paroxysmal atrial tachycardia by diving reflex. Lancet 1978; 1:1042.
57. Weiss S., Baker J.P. The carotid sinus reflex in health and disease: its role in the causation of fainting and convulsions. Medicine 1933; 12:297.
58. Antonelli D, Rosenfeld T. Deglutition syncope associated with carotid sinus hypersensitivity. Pacing Clin Electrophysiol 1997; 20(Pt 1):2282–2283.
59. Bilbro RH. Syncope after prostatic examination. N Engl J Med 1970; 282:167–168.
60. Klotz PG. Syncope during prostatic examination. N Engl J Med 1970; 282:1046.
61. Lieberman A. Syncope after prostatic massage. N Engl J Med 1970; 282:515.
62. Sakakibara R, Hattori T, Kita K, Yamanishi T, Yasuda K. Urodynamic and cardiovascular measurements in patients with micturition syncope. Clin Auton Res 1997; 7:219–221.
63. Bhatnagar HN, Shah DR, Gupta RC. Sick sinus syndrome associated with cerebrovascular accident. J Indian Med Assoc 1978; 70:158–160.
64. Boggs JG, Painter JA, DeLorenzo RJ. Analysis of electrocardiographic changes in status epilepticus. Epilepsy Res 1993; 14:87–94.
65. Kiok MC, Terrence CF, Fromm GH, Lavine S. Sinus arrest in epilepsy. Neurology 1986; 36:115–116.

66. Kushner M, Peters RW. Prolonged sinus arrest complicating a thrombotic stroke. Pacing Clin Electrophysiol 1986; 9:248–249.

67. Myers MG, Norris JW, Hachinski VC, Weingert ME, Sole MJ. Cardiac sequelae of acute stroke. Stroke 1982; 13:838–842.

68. Weintraub BM, McHenry LC, Jr. Cardiac abnormalities in subarachnoid hemorrhage: a resume. Stroke 1974; 5:384–392.

69. Greenland P, Griggs RC. Arrhythmic complications in the Guillain-Barre syndrome. Arch Intern Med 1980; 140:1053–1055.

70. Dickey RP, Ziter FA, Smith RA. Emery-Dreifuss muscular dystrophy. J Pediatr 1984; 104:555–559.

71. Fairfax AJ, Lambert CD. Neurological aspects of sinoatrial heart block. J Neurol Neurosurg Psychiatry 1976; 39:576–580.

72. Gottdiener JS, Sherber HS, Hawley RJ, Engel WK. Cardiac manifestations in polymyositis. Am J Cardiol 1978; 41:1141–1149.

73. Griggs RC, Davis RJ, Anderson DC, Dove JT. Cardiac conduction in myotonic dystrophy. Am J Med 1975; 59:37–42.

74. Hassan Z., Fastabend CP, Mohanty PK, Isaacs ER. Atrioventricular block and supraventricular arrhythmias with X-linked muscular dystrophy. Circulation 1979; 60:1365–1369.

75. Meier C, Gertsch M, Zimmerman A, Voellmy W, Geissbuhler J. Nemaline myopathy presenting as cardiomyopathy. N Engl J Med 1983; 308:1536–1537.

76. Roberts NK, Perloff JK, Kark RA. Cardiac conduction in the Kearns-Sayre syndrome (a neuromuscular disorder associated with progressive external ophthalmoplegia and pigmentary retinopathy). Report of 2 cases and review of 17 published cases. Am J Cardiol 1979; 44:1396–1400.

77. Rtinov G, Baker WP, Swaiman KF. McArdle's syndrome with previously unreported electrocardiographic and serum enzyme abnormalities. Ann Intern Med 1965; 62:328.

78. Bashour T, Hsu I, Gorfinkel HJ, Wickramesekaran R, Rios JC. Atrioventricular and intraventricular conduction in hyperkalemia. Am J Cardiol 1975; 35:199–203.

79. Vanhaelst L, Neve P, Chailly P, Bastenie PA. Coronary-artery disease in hypothyroidism. Observations in clinical myxoedema. Lancet 1967; 2:800–802.

80. Rossi L, Thiene G, Caragaro L, Giordano R, Lauro S. Dysrhythmias and sudden death in acromegalic heart disease. A clinicopathologic study. Chest 1977; 72:495–498.

81. Krug JJ. Cardiac arrest secondary to Addison's disease. Ann Emerg Med 1986; 15:735–737.

82. Walker C, Butt W. A case of cardiovascular collapse due to adrenal insufficiency. Aust Paediatr J 1988; 24:197–198.

83. Gibbs MA, Wolfson AB, Tayal VS. Electrolyte disturbances. In: Emergency Medicine Concepts and Clinical Practice. 4th edition. Rosen P, Ed. St Louis, MO: Mosby, 1998, pp. 2432–2456.

84. Bashour TT, Antonini C, Sr., Fisher J. Severe sinus node dysfunction in obstructive jaundice. Ann Intern Med 1985; 103:384–385.

85. Ornato JP. Special resuscitation situations: near drowning, traumatic injury, electric shock, and hypothermia. Circulation 1986; 74(Pt 2):IV23–IV26.

86. Anzi M, Ippoliti B, Zamperetti N. [Inter-atrial dissociation. Description of a case]. Folia Cardiol 1968; 27:113–119.

87. Arita M, Ueno Y, Masuyama Y. Complete heart block in mumps myocarditis. Br Heart J 1981; 46: 342–344.

88. Bairan AC, Cherry JD, Fagan LF, Codd JE, Jr. Complete heart block and respiratory syncytial virus infection. Am J Dis Child 1974; 127:264–265.

89. Bell H. Cardiac manifestations of viral hepatitis. JAMA 1971; 218:387–391.

90. Marc MO, Anconina J, Dodinot B, et al. [Irreversible auriculo-ventricular block of viral origin]. Ann Cardiol Angeiol (Paris) 1993; 42:23–24.

91. Verel D, Warrack AJ, Potter CW, Ward C, Rickards DF. Observations on the A2 England influenza epidemic: a clinicopathological study. Am Heart J 1976; 92:290–296.

92. Obeyesekere I, Hermon Y. Myocarditis and cardiomyopathy after arbovirus infections (dengue and chikungunya fever). Br Heart J 1972; 34:821–827.

93. Wallis PJ, Branfoot AC, Emerson PA. Sudden death due to myocardial tuberculosis. Thorax 1984; 39:155–156.

94. Caraco J, Arnon R, Raz I. Atrioventricular block complicating acute streptococcal tonsillitis. Br Heart J 1988; 59:389–390.

95. Sandler MA, Pincus PS, Weltman MD, et al. Meningococcaemia complicated by myocarditis. A report of 2 cases. S Afr Med J 1989; 75:391–393.

96. Thanopoulos BD, Rokas S, Frimas CA, Mantagos SP, Beratis NG. Cardiac involvement in postnatal rubella. Acta Paediatr Scand 1989; 78:141–144.

97. Kirchner GI, Krug N, Bleck JS, Fliser D, Manns MP, Wagner S. [Fulminant course of leptospirosis complicated by multiple organ failure]. Z Gastroenterol 2001; 39:587–592.

98. Nicolas G, Leborgne P, Menuet JC, Bouhour JB, Pony JC, Godin JF. [A case of complete atrioventricular block caused by syphilitic gumma of the interventricular septum]. Arch Mal Coeur Vaiss 1973; 66:925–933.

99. Wengrower D, Knobler H, Gillis S, Chajek-Shaul T. Myocarditis in tick-borne relapsing fever. J Infect Dis 1984; 149:1033.

100. Steere AC, Batsford WP, Weinberg M, et al. Lyme carditis: cardiac abnormalities of Lyme disease. Ann Intern Med 1980; 93:8–16.

101. Veyssier P, Davous N, Kaloustian E, Maitre B, Lallement PY, Serret A. [Cardiac involvement in Lyme disease. 2 cases]. Rev Med Interne 1987; 8:357–360.

102. Pimenta J, Miranda M, Pereira CB. Electrophysiologic findings in long-term asymptomatic chagasic individuals. Am Heart J 1983; 106:374–380.

103. Hall JC, Giltman LI. Candida myocarditis in a patient with chronic active hepatitis and macronodular cirrhosis. J Tenn Med Assoc 1986; 79:473–476.

104. Bognolo DA, Rabow FI, Vijayanagar RR, Eckstein PF. Traumatic sinus node dysfunction. Ann Emerg Med 1982; 11:319–321.

105. Friedman HS, Gomes JA, Tardio AR, Haft JI. The electrocardiographic features of acute cardiac tamponade. Circulation 1974; 50:260–265.

106. Vestri A, D'Intino S, Mazzacurati G. [Electrophysiological repercussions of pericardial effusion on the activity of the artificial pacemaker]. Policlinico [Med] 1966; 73:246–256.

107. Applefeld M.M., Pollock S.H. Cardiac disease in patients who have malignancies. Curr Prob Cardiol 1980; 4:5.

108. Cole TO, Attah EB, Onyemelukwe. Burkitt's lymphoma presenting with heart block. Br Heart J 1975; 37:94–97.

109. Nishida K, Kamijima G, Nagayama T. Mesothelioma of the atrioventricular node. Br Heart J 1985; 53:468–470.

110. Anzai N, Akiyama K, Tsuchida K, Yamada M, Kito S, Yamamura Y. Treatment by pacemaker in familial amyloid polyneuropathy. Chest 1989; 96:80–84.

111. Bharati S, Lev M, Denes P, et al. Infiltrative cardiomyopathy with conduction disease and ventricular arrhythmia: electrophysiologic and pathologic correlations. Am J Cardiol 1980; 45:163–173.

112. Aronow WS, Meister L, Kent JR. Atrioventricular block in familial hemochromatosis treated by permanent synchronous pacemaker. Arch Intern Med 1969; 123:433–435.

113. Rosenqvist M, Hultcrantz R. Prevalence of a haemochromatosis among men with clinically significant bradyarrhythmias. Eur Heart J 1989; 10:473–478.

114. Ahern M, Lever JV, Cosh J. Complete heart block in rheumatoid arthritis. Ann Rheum Dis 1983; 42: 389–397.

115. Maisch B, Lotze U, Schneider J, Kochsiek K. Antibodies to human sinus node in sick sinus syndrome. Pacing Clin Electrophysiol 1986; 9(Pt 2):1101–1109.

116. Ohkawa S, Miyao M, Chida K, et al. Extensive involvement of the myocardium and the cardiac conduction system in a case of Wegener's granulomatosis. Jpn Heart J 1999; 40:509–515.

117. Sairanen E, Paronen I, Mahonen H. Reiter's syndrome: a follow-up study. Acta Med Scand 1969; 185:57–63.

118. Zipes DP. Genesis of cardia arrhythmias: electrophysiological considerations. In: Heart Disease, 5th edition. Braunwald E, ed. Philadelphia, PA: W. B. Saunders Company, 1997, pp. 548–592.

119. James TN. The coronary circulation and conduction system in acute myocardial infarction. Prog Cardiovasc Dis 1968; 10:410–449.

120. Wesley RC, Jr., Belardinelli L. Role of endogenous adenosine in postdefibrillation bradyarrhythmia and hemodynamic depression. Circulation 1989; 80:128–137.

121. Belardinelli L, Linden J, Berne RM. The cardiac effects of adenosine. Prog Cardiovasc Dis 1989; 32: 73–97.

122. Schrader J, Baumann G, Gerlach E. Adenosine as inhibitor of myocardial effects of catecholamines. Pflugers Arch 1977; 372:29–35.

123. Belardinelli L, Isenberg G. Isolated atrial myocytes: adenosine and acetylcholine increase potassium conductance. Am J Physiol 1983; 244:H734–H737.

124. Belardinelli L, Giles WR, West A. Ionic mechanisms of adenosine actions in pacemaker cells from rabbit heart. J Physiol 1988; 405:615–633.

125. West GA, Belardinelli L. Correlation of sinus slowing and hyperpolarization caused by adenosine in sinus node. Pflugers Arch 1985; 403:75–81.

126. Clemo HF, Belardinelli L. Effect of adenosine on atrioventricular conduction. I: Site and characterization of adenosine action in the guinea pig atrioventricular node. Circ Res 1986; 59:427–436.

127. Lloyd HG, Deussen A, Wuppermann H, Schrader J. The transmethylation pathway as a source for adenosine in the isolated guinea-pig heart. Biochem J 1988; 252:489–494.

128. Olsson RA, Gentry MK, Townsend RS. Adenosine metabolism: properties of dog heart microsomal 5'-nucleotidase. Adv Exp Med Biol 1973; 39:27–39.

129. Kaseda S, Zipes DP. Supersensitivity to acetylcholine of canine sinus and AV nodes after parasympathetic denervation. Am J Physiol 1988; 255(Pt 2):H534–H539.

130. Ellenbogen KA, Thames MD, DiMarco JP, Sheehan H, Lerman BB. Electrophysiological effects of adenosine in the transplanted human heart. Evidence of supersensitivity. Circulation 1990; 81:821–828.

131. Malliani A, Schwartz PJ, Zanchetti A. A sympathetic reflex elicited by experimental coronary occlusion. Am J Physiol 1969; 217:703–709.

132. Malliani A, Recordati G, Schwartz PJ. Nervous activity of afferent cardiac sympathetic fibres with atrial and ventricular endings. J Physiol 1973; 229:457–469.

133. Recordati G, Schwartz PJ, Pagani M, Malliani A, Brown AM. Activation of cardiac vagal receptors during myocardial ischemia. Experientia 1971; 27:1423–1424.

134. Thoren PN. Activation of left ventricular receptors with nonmedullated vagal afferent fibers during occlusion of a coronary artery in the cat. Am J Cardiol 1976; 37:1046–1051.

135. Herre JM, Wetstein L, Lin YL, Mills AS, Dae M, Thames MD. Effect of transmural versus nontransmural myocardial infarction on inducibility of ventricular arrhythmias during sympathetic stimulation in dogs. J Am Coll Cardiol 1988; 11:414–421.

136. Inoue H, Skale BT, Zipes DP. Effects of ischemia on cardiac afferent sympathetic and vagal reflexes in dog. Am J Physiol 1988; 255(Pt 2):H26–H35.

137. Engel GL. Sudden and rapid death during psychological stress. Folklore or folk wisdom? Ann Intern Med 1971; 74:771–782.

138. Lown B, Verrier RL. Neural activity and ventricular fibrillation. N Engl J Med 1976; 294:1165–1170.

139. Lown B, Verrier RL, Rabinowitz SH. Neural and psychologic mechanisms and the problem of sudden cardiac death. Am J Cardiol 1977; 39:890–902.

140. Lown B. Sudden cardiac death—1978. Circulation 1979; 60:1593–1599.

141. Wolf S. The end of the rope: the role of the brain in cardiac death. Can Med Assoc J 1967; 97:1022–1025.

142. Brown CG, Werman HA. Adrenergic agonists during cardiopulmonary resuscitation. Resuscitation 1990; 19:1–16.

143. Lewin NA. Cardiac glycosides. In: Goldfrank's Toxicologic Emergencies, sixth edition. Goldfrank LR, ed. New York, NY: McGraw Hill, 1998, pp. 801–807.

144. Howland MA. Cardiac glycosides: digoxin-specific antibody fragments. In: Goldfrank's Toxicologic Emergencies. 6th edition. Goldfrank LR, ed. New York, NY: McGraw Hill, 1998, pp. 801–807.

145. Brubacher JR, Howland MA. Beta-adrenergic antagonists. In: Goldfrank's Toxicologic Emergencies, sixth edition. Goldfrank LR, ed. New York, NY: McGraw Hill, 1998, pp. 809–828.

146. Saitz R, Williams BW, Farber HW. Atenolol-induced cardiovascular collapse treated with hemodialysis. Crit Care Med 1991; 19:116–118.

147. Boehnert MT, Lovejoy FH, Jr. Value of the QRS duration versus the serum drug level in predicting seizures and ventricular arrhythmias after an acute overdose of tricyclic antidepressants. N Engl J Med 1985; 313:474–479.

148. Benowitz NL. Lithium. In: Poisoning and Drug Overdose, third edition. Olson KR, ed. Stamford: Appleton and Lange, 1999, pp. 204–206.

149. Part 6: Advanced cardiovascular life support, section 5: Pharmacology I: Agents for arrhythmias. Guidelines 2000 for cardiopulmonary resuscitation and emergency cardiovascular care. Circulation 2000; 102:I-112–I-128.

150. Brown DC, Lewis AJ, Criley JM. Asystole and its treatment: the possible role of the parasympathetic nervous system in cardiac arrest. JACEP 1979; 8:448–452.

151. Gupta K, Lichstein E, Chadda KD. Transient atrioventricular standstill. Etiology and management. JAMA 1975; 234:1038–1042.

152. DeBehnke DJ, Swart G, Spreng D, Aufderheide T. Effects of atropine on resuscitation from pulseless electrical activity. Crit Care Med 1995; 23:A175 (abstract).

153. Engdahl J, Bang A, Lindqvist J, Herlitz J. Can we define patients with no and those with some chance of survival when found in asystole out of hospital? Am J Cardiol 2000; 86:610–614.

154. Paradis NA, Martin GB, Rivers EP, et al. Coronary perfusion pressure and the return of spontaneous circulation in human cardiopulmonary resuscitation. JAMA 1990; 263:1106–1113.

155. Sanders AB, Ogle M, Ewy GA. Coronary perfusion pressure during cardiopulmonary resuscitation. Am J Emerg Med 1985; 3:11–14.

156. Part 6: Advanced cardiovascular life support, section 7C: A guide to the international ACLS algorithms. Guidelines 2000 for cardiopulmonary resuscitation and emergency cardiovascular care. Circulation 2000; 102:I-142–I-157.

157. Brown CG, Werman HA, Davis EA, Hamlin R, Hobson J, Ashton JA. Comparative effect of graded doses of epinephrine on regional brain blood flow during CPR in a swine model. Ann Emerg Med 1986; 15:1138–1144.

158. Brown CG, Werman HA, Davis EA, Hobson J, Hamlin RL. The effects of graded doses of epinephrine on regional myocardial blood flow during cardiopulmonary resuscitation in swine. Circulation 1987; 75:491–497.

159. Brunette DD, Jameson SJ. Comparison of standard versus high-dose epinephrine in the resuscitation of cardiac arrest in dogs. Ann Emerg Med 1990; 19:8–11.

160. Kosnik JW, Jackson RE, Keats S, Tworek RM, Freeman SB. Dose-related response of centrally administered epinephrine on the change in aortic diastolic pressure during closed-chest massage in dogs. Ann Emerg Med 1985; 14:204–4208.

161. Lindner KH, Ahnefeld FW, Prengel AW. Comparison of standard and high-dose adrenaline in the resuscitation of asystole and electromechanical dissociation. Acta Anaesthesiol Scand 1991; 35: 253–256.

162. Paradis NA, Martin GB, Rosenberg J, et al. The effect of standard- and high-dose epinephrine on coronary perfusion pressure during prolonged cardiopulmonary resuscitation. JAMA 1991; 265:1139–1144.

163. Brown CG, Katz SE, Werman HA, Luu T, Davis EA, Hamlin RL. The effect of epinephrine versus methoxamine on regional myocardial blood flow and defibrillation rates following a prolonged cardiorespiratory arrest in a swine model. Am J Emerg Med 1987; 5:362–369.

164. Brown CG, Werman HA, Davis EA, Katz S, Hamlin RL. The effect of high-dose phenylephrine versus epinephrine on regional cerebral blood flow during CPR. Ann Emerg Med 1987; 16:743–748.

165. Brown CG, Davis EA, Werman HA, Hamlin RL. Methoxamine versus epinephrine on regional cerebral blood flow during cardiopulmonary resuscitation. Crit Care Med 1987; 15:682–686.

166. Brown CG, Taylor RB, Werman HA, Luu T, Ashton J, Hamlin RL. Myocardial oxygen delivery/consumption during cardiopulmonary resuscitation: a comparison of epinephrine and phenylephrine. Ann Emerg Med 1988; 17:302–308.

167. Robinson LA, Brown CG, Jenkins J, et al. The effect of norepinephrine versus epinephrine on myocardial hemodynamics during CPR. Ann Emerg Med 1989; 18:336–340.

168. Silfvast T, Saarnivaara L, Kinnunen A, et al. Comparison of adrenaline and phenylephrine in out-of-hospital cardiopulmonary resuscitation. A double-blind study. Acta Anaesthesiol Scand 1985; 29: 610–613.

169. Hoffman BB. Adrenoceptro-Activating and Other Sympathomimetic Drugs. In: Basic and Clinical Pharmacology, sixth edition. Katzungl BG, ed. Norwalk: Appleton and Lange, 1995, pp. 115–131.

170. Jaffe R, Weiss AT, Rosenheck S. Combined isoproterenol and epinephrine for the resuscitation of patients with cardiac asystole secondary to coronary artery disease. Am J Cardiol 1996; 77:194–195.

171. Part 8: Advanced challenges in resuscitation, section 1: Life threatening electrolyte abnormalities. Guidelines 2000 for cardiopulmonary resuscitation and emergency cardiovascular care. Circulation 2000; 102:I-217–I-222.

172. Berenyi KJ, Wolk M, Killip T. Cerebrospinal fluid acidosis complicating therapy of experimental cardiopulmonary arrest. Circulation 1975; 52:319–324.

173. Kette F, Weil MH, von Planta M, Gazmuri RJ, Rackow EC. Buffer agents do not reverse intramyocardial acidosis during cardiac resuscitation. Circulation 1990; 81:1660–1666.

174. Kette F, Weil MH, Gazmuri RJ. Buffer solutions may compromise cardiac resuscitation by reducing coronary perfusion presssure. JAMA 1991; 266:2121–2126.

175. Part 6: Advanced cardiovascular life support, section 6: Pharmacology II: Agents to optimize cardiac output and blood pressure. Guidelines 2000 for cardiopulmonary resuscitation and emergency cardiovascular care. Circulation 2000; 102:I-129–I-135.

176. Benowitz NL. Tricyclic Antidepressants. In: Poisoning and Drug Overdose, third edition. Olson KR, ed. Stamford: Appleton and Lange, 1999, pp. 310–312.

177. Barthell E, Troiano P, Olson D, Stueven HA, Hendley G. Prehospital external cardiac pacing: a prospective, controlled clinical trial. Ann Emerg Med 1988; 17:1221–1226.
178. Cummins RO, Graves JR, Larsen MP, et al. Out-of-hospital transcutaneous pacing by emergency medical technicians in patients with asystolic cardiac arrest. N Engl J Med 1993; 328:1377–1382.
179. Manning JE, Zoll P.M. Therapy of bradyasystolic arrest. In: Cardiac Arrest: The Science and Practice of Resuscitation Medicine. Paradis NA, Halperin HR, Nowak RM, eds. Baltimore: Williams and Wilkins, 1996, p. 627.

8 Pulseless Electrical Activity

John M. Field, MD

A small group of patients with acute myocardial infarction who die suddenly present with a most unusual sequence of events: there is loss of consciousness, pulse and blood pressure; heart sounds are inaudible; respiration is gasping; and yet the electrocardiogram is seemingly unaltered.

Eugene Braunwald in The Heart, 1980

INTRODUCTION

In the early resuscitation guidelines, electrical mechanical dissociation (EMD) referred to the prescence of organized electrical activity in the absence of synchronous myocardial contraction *(1–3)*. As such, electrical activity was detected on the surface electrocardiogram but no effective cardiac output was present owing to the absence of coupled mechanical activity. The clinical result was the absence of pulse, blood pressure, and heart tones. EMD was observed in a variety of resuscitation situations and was felt to be secondary to prolonged global cardiac ischemia. The organized rhythm varied from sinus tachycardia with a normal duration QRS complex to brady-dysrhythmias with wide aberrant or idioventricular ventricular morphologies. A poor resuscitation outcome and dismal prognosis was a common shared observation. Collectively, this ominous rhythm was found to have a resuscitation rate of only about 20% and a hospital discharge rate of 4 to 5% *(4,5)*.

Early animal studies and resuscitation attempts with inotropic and chronotropic drugs, calcium chloride, and electrical pacing proved ineffective *(5–11)*. Recent evaluations of clinical predictors and prognosis have found that pulseless electrical activity (PEA) continues to be poor predictor of survival. Only 15% of victims of prehospital cardiac arrest (CA) are admitted alive to hospital and only 2.4% were discharged alive *(12)*. PEA

From: *Contemporary Cardiology: Cardiopulmonary Resuscitation*
Edited by: J. P. Ornato and M. A. Peberdy © Humana Press Inc., Totowa, NJ

as the presenting CA for inhospital resuscitation attempts has the lowest survival rate. If PEA was unwitnessed, no patient survived to hospital discharge *(13)*.

The term electromechanical dissociation poorly characterized the heterogeneous group of clinical rhythms confronting rescuers and presenting with some form of organized electrical activity and no detectable pulse. In the early 1990s, the resuscitation community began to refer to this clinical presentation of CA as PEA. A dismal prognosis reflects the fact that PEA is a preterminal rhythm and not a specific entity. As such, PEA is observed in a broad spectrum of clinical disorders that have global severe cardiac ischemia or myocyte dysfunction as a final common pathway yet diverse inciting etiologies.

PATHOBIOLOGY

An improved understanding of the mechanisms responsible for PEA has provided a refined pathophysiology of this disorder. As described originally, PEA was perceived as subcellular myocyte failure occurring in the presence of electrical excitation. Working myocytes have a centrally located nucleus and abundant contractile protein elements organized into myofibrils. The flux and interaction of calcium with myofibrillar elements initiates and terminates contraction by concentration characteristics at regulatory sites. This interaction is very complex and excitation–contraction coupling involves cell components called the plasma membrane, sarcoplasmic reticulum, and myofilaments.

An envelope called the plasma membrane surrounds and penetrates the working myocardial cell. The surrounding plasma membrane is called the sarcolemma. Plasma membrane that penetrates into the cells interior and internally transmits the action potential is called the transverse-tubular (t-tubular) system. Physiologists have also identified an intracellular transfer system in addition to the plasma membrane separating the extracellular space from myocyte. This system is called the sarcoplasmic reticulum. After electrical excitation, calcium ions are released from storage compartments of the sarcoplasmic reticulum, called cisternae, and flood the cytosol initiating systolic contraction. Another compartment of the sarcoplasmic reticulum surrounds the contractile proteins and is called the sarcotubular network and contains adenosine triphosphate (ATP)ase-dependent proteins that actively pump calcium back into the cisternae, ready for the next excitatory stimulus.

The Energy of Heart Muscle Contraction

A heart muscle cell must convert chemical or stored energy into kinetic energy for effective cardiac contraction. The heart stores energy as ATP. When ATP is cleaved into adenosine diphosphate (ADP), inorganic phosphate and a proton (H^+) are released generating energy. A terminal pyrophosphate bond (P-O-P) releases this energy as it is split by a muscle enzyme called myosin ATPase. Myosin ATPase is only active when interacting with another muscle protein called actin.

$$ATP + H_2O \rightarrow ADP + Phosphate (Pi) + H^+ + energy$$

However, an effective cardiac contraction requires synchronized myocyte contraction. The coupling of an electrical signal to myocyte shortening is referred to as excitation–contraction coupling. Specialized cardiac myocytes initiate and propagate an electrical signal called an action potential (nodal cells and His-Purkinje cells). The specialized and working myocytes form a functional syncytium with cells linked electrically and mechanically. Transitional cells, intermediate between His-Purkinje and working myocytes, are found in ventricular locations where the Purkinje network of fibers communicates with the working myocytes. In addition to electrical coupling of the specialized Purkinje fibers with working myocytes, myocyte to myocyte coupling is effected by proteins called connexins located in low resistance gap junctions between cells.

The Biomechanics of Heart Muscle Contraction

The heart muscle thickens prior to contraction when observed by echocardiography or gated nuclear studies. In fact, the absence of this event is evidence of myocardial ischemia or necrosis. The swelling of myocardial sarcomeres causes this gross cardiac muscle observation during contraction. Swelling occurs since myocyte (and sarcomere) volume is constant.

Cardiac contraction occurs as interlacing myosin thick filaments slide over actin thin filaments causing myocardial sarcomere shortening and swelling. The contractile biomechanics of the heart involve two sets of proteins. The first set, myosin and actin, are involved with the mechanics of contraction. The second, tropomyosin and the troponins (troponin I, troponin T, and troponin C) are regulatory in nature and allow interaction with calcium for coupling of electrical to mechanical events.

Critical to actin and myosin interaction are crossbridges extending from myosin toward the actin thin filament. Each myosin filament ends in a bilobed structure that acts like an oar and pulls the thin actin filament longitudinally along its length. Each thick filament of myosin is composed of approx 100 myosin molecules. Fifty are oriented to each end of the sarcomere. In the crossbridges, ATP is hydrolyzed and provides the energy necessary for shortening. The interaction of the bilobed myosin heads is however controlled by cytosolic calcium. During a very short period, cytosolic calcium occupies receptor sites on troponin C (TnC). This interaction increases the amount of actin available for interaction with myosin heads through complex mechanisms. During diastole, calcium uptake occurs and troponin-I (TnI) inhibits calcium interaction with binding sites on the myosin heads.

MYOCARDIAL STUNNING, ISCHEMIA, AND CELL DEATH

Ineffective cardiac contraction in clinical situations of PEA is poorly understood. In part, this is because PEA has diverse etiologies and the clinical presentation represents a pathological outcome and not a resuscitation rhythm disorder. The most likely common final mechanism and injury is global MI caused by a severe reduction in coronary flow. The situation may be compounded if accompanying hypoxemia or demand conditions that increase myocardial oxygen consumption are present. The degree and duration of ischemia determine the amount of residual myocardial function available to "recover" the patient from an insult resulting in decreased coronary perfusion. Global ischemia is potentially reversible. At some point, however, the myocardium is incapable of the burden of recovery owing to a phenomenon called myocardial stunning.

Regional ischemia occurs in the presence of a flow limiting epicardial stenosis when downstream myocardium is placed under an increased workload. Typically, this results in effort angina pectoris. When a thrombus occludes an artery, ischemia develops and cell death occurs unless reperfusion is established. Global ischemia develops when the entire heart is deprived of coronary flow and oxygen supply. The reasons for this are diverse. Experimentally, global ischemia can be produced in 30 seconds with aortic cross-clamping impeding left ventricular ejection.

Three mechanisms are currently thought to contribute to contractile dysfunction and left ventricular myocardial impairment. First, regardless the pathological etiology, failure of adequate oxygen delivery to myocyte mitochondria reduces energy supplies for cytoplasmic processes. As such, ischemic metabolites accumulate and ATP stores are depleted. Originally, loss of high-energy phosphates was felt to be responsible for contractile failure. Next, current evidence also supports an effect of oxidative metabolites, such as phosphates and protons that accumulate, as cellular transport and efflux are impaired. Protons can compete with calcium for activator sites on the contractile proteins. Finally, residual CO_2 generation from mitochondria and generation from bicarbonate lower myocyte pH and further impairs contractility. The effects of increased cytosolic calcium in ischemia are unclear, but decreased muscle function is observed. Proposed mechanisms include mitochondrial damage, activation of phospholipases, increased depolarization, and ischemic contracture *(14)*.

The above mechanisms cause either contractile (systolic) failure of the myocardium or (diastolic) ischemic contracture and demise of the heart. The majority of clinical situations likely result in initial systolic failure as ischemia begins a continuum of electrical and contractile failure (*see* below). The low and rapidly decreasing availability of oxygen results in increasing levels of toxic metabolites and an acidic myocyte environment leading to systolic contractile failure. During this brief window of time, these changes are reversible depending on the ability to correct a precipitating cause and the amount of myocardium available to meet coronary flow and systemic recovery requirements. In anoxic arrest and following severe and prolonged ischemia, total ATP falls to very low levels. This results in higher intracellular calcium levels as membrane pumps lack energy to reestablish ionic concentration gradients. Also, insufficient ATP is present to resupply the contractile proteins resulting in a state of rigor and ischemic contracture. Pioneer cardiac surgeons feared this postoperative infrequent but catastrophic cardiac condition and coined the term "stone heart" recognizing the irreversibility and demise of the patient (Fig. 1).

PEA most likely represents a continuum initially presenting with organized rhythm that deteriorates to true PEA. In the intermediate stage, no clinical pulse is detected but patients may have ineffective low amplitude waveforms (low cardiac output) detectable in the central aorta. This finding has been referred to as pseudo-PEA. Finally, as the electrical cells fail and QRS widens, true PEA/EMD occurs as the myocardium is mechanically incapable of responding to any action potential delivered. This sequence of events accounts for the poor prognosis observed when a wide complex rhythm is associated with unwitnessed arrest or long arrest times. An attempt to resuscitate these functionally impaired hearts is unsuccessful, or only transiently so, as the amount of stunned myocardium is excessive or the stone heart has arrived *(15)*.

TREATMENT

Identification of Underlying Cause

A patient's small chance for survival lies in the rapid identification of a correctable cause, obvious within minutes of presentation, amenable to a specific rapid intervention. No resuscitation methodology, including early cardiopulmonary resuscitation (CPR), has been shown to be effective. Unfortunately, discernible causes amenable to favorable clinical intervention are present in a small minority of patients. The Guidelines 2000 for Cardiopulmonary Resuscitation and Emergency Cardiovascular Care recognize this fact,

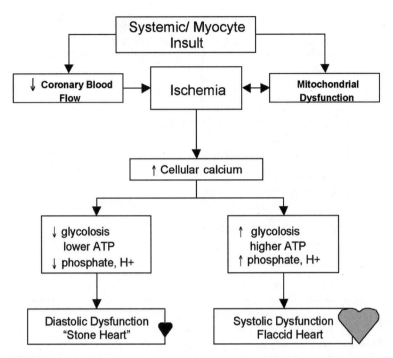

Fig. 1. Contractile failure occurring in the setting of ischemia. A decrease in oxygen supply results in a rise in intracellular calcium. When adenosine triphosphate (ATP) stores remain high or the high calcium is opposed by inorganic phosphate and cellular acidosis, systolic contractile failure occurs with a flaccid, poorly contracting heart. This situation is observed most often in clinical pulseless electrical activity (PEA) or pseudo-PEA. If there is prolonged ischemia or when glycolysis is impaired and ATP levels are low, diastolic tension increases and an ischemic contracture occurs that is irreversible. (Modified from ref. *15a*.)

but have organized the most common causes for PEA and listed the five "Hs" and the five "Ts" for rapid recall and review *(16)*. These conditions include hypovolemia, hypoxia, severe acidosis (hydrogen ion), severe electrolyte abnormalities (hypo/hyperkalemia), and hypothermia. Other causes include cardiac tamponade, tension pneumothorax, toxicological emergencies, pulmonary embolism (PE), and acute coronary syndromes.

THE FIVE Hs and THE FIVE Ts of PEA

- Hypovolemia
- Hypoxia (oxygen, ventilation)
- Hydrogen Ion (buffer, ventilation)
- Hyper/Hypokalemia
- Hypothermia

- Tablets (drug OD)
- Tamponade, Cardiac
- Tension Pneumothorax
- Thrombosis, Cardiac
- Thrombosis, Pulmonary

Using the available history, clinical presentation, and electrocardiogram if available, a possible etiology may be identified. The clinical differential and initial treatment often occur concurrently due to the brief window of treatment opportunity. Success or failure of the resuscitation is determined by the opportunity and ability to identify and correct the underlying cause of PEA. In this regard also, survival is often linked to the prognosis of the inciting pathological condition.

Pulseless Electrical Activity
(**PEA** = rhythm on monitor, without detectable pulse)

Primary ABCD Survey
Focus: basic CPR and defibrillation
- **Check** responsiveness
- **Activate** emergency response system
- **Call** for defibrillator
A **Airway:** open the airway
B **Breathing:** provide positive-pressure ventilations
C **Circulation:** give chest compressions
D **Defibrillation:** assess for and shock VF/pulseless VT

Secondary ABCD Survey
Focus: more advanced assessments and treatments
A **Airway:** place airway device as soon as possible
B **Breathing:** confirm airway device placement by exam plus confirmation device
B **Breathing:** secure airway device; purpose-made tube holders preferred
B **Breathing:** confirm effective oxygenation and ventilation
C **Circulation:** establish IV access
C **Circulation:** identify rhythm → monitor
C **Circulation:** administer drugs appropriate for rhythm and condition
C **Circulation:** assess for occult blood flow ("pseudo-EMT")
D **Differential Diagnosis:** search for and treat identified reversible causes

Review for most frequent causes [1]
- **Hypovolemia**
- **Hypoxia**
- **Hydrogen ion** — acidosis
- **Hyper-/hypokalemia**
- **Hypothermia**
- **"Tablets"** (drug OD, accidents)
- **Tamponade,** cardiac
- **Tension** pneumothorax
- **Thrombosis,** coronary (ACS)
- **Thrombosis,** pulmonary (embolism)

Epinephrine 1 mg IV push, [2]
repeat every 3 to 5 minutes

Atropine 1 mg IV (if PEA rate is *slow*), [3]
repeat every 3 to 5 minutes as needed, to a total
dose of 0.04 mg/kg

Special mention should be made of PEA occurring after electrical defibrillation. PEA can be seen after defibrillation and may be a recovery rhythm in a small percentage of patients. Suggesting survival is PEA with a narrow QRS complex, short resuscitation times, and a relatively rapid return to a supraventricular mechanism with detectable pulses. A wide complex, long resuscitation times, transient recovery of a supraventricular mechanism and subsequent deterioration suggest a poor prognosis. Likely, in the later, global ischemia with myocardial stunning, accumulation of free radicals and ATP depletion preclude effective institution of a recovery hemodynamic situation leading to sustained coronary perfusion and some degree of myocardial function. Recently, this phenomenon has been studied in patients with automatic implantable cardiac defibrillators (AICDs). Approximately 30% of patients with AICDs still suffer from sudden death. The most common mechanism of death in these patients is postshock EMD after an appropriate shock for ventricular fibrillation and ventricular tachycardia. The largest subgroup of patients was younger with poor New York Heart Association functional classification (III–IV), lower ejection fraction, and higher energy defibrillation requirements. The authors have referred to this phenomenon as cardiac annihilation *(17)*.

Advanced Cardiac Life Support Treatment Algorithm: Epinephrine and Atropine

The advanced cardiac life support treatment algorithm shares similarities with asystole, another highly fatal rhythm and calls for CPR and epinephrine, as well as atropine for slower rates. Calcium was recommended in earlier resuscitation strategies. As discussed above, the calcium interaction with troponin C is crucial to effective contraction. In normal states, only one-half of the contractile sites are occupied by calcium. A reasonable strategy assumed that supplemental calcium administered intravenously would increase intracellular calcium available to interact with contractile proteins or increase available calcium in the sarcoplasmic reticulum.

Another potential treatment involved the use of epinephrine as a cytosolic catecholamine stimulant. Myocardial generation of force (dP/dt, or the developed pressure over a period of time) increases with catecholamine β-adrenergic stimulation. Cytosolic-free calcium is both released and lowered more quickly in the presence of catecholamines. Theoretically, the increased calcium released by epinephrine would be available to bind with troponin C and increase effective cardiac force generation.

Unfortunately, both experimental trials and clinical data found these interventions to be ineffective. The reasons are likely multifactorial but may be related to the observation that calcium desensitization occurs in the presence of ischemia owing to the accumulation of inorganic phosphate and acidification of the cytosol.

Fig. 2. *(opposite page)* The International Guidelines Treatment Algorithm for Pulseless Electrical Activity. The algorithm was modified to emphasize the need to immediately consider and search for a correctable cause in this usually fatal clinical situation. The five "Hs" and five "Ts" should be recalled in the context of available clinical history and scenario, searching for an underlying abnormality amenable to targeted intervention.

SUMMARY

Standard CPR, epinephrine, calcium, buffer therapy, atropine, and cardiac pacing have not been shown to improve survival in PEA. As such, these therapies addressing electrocardiographic and clinical patterns are only temporizing measures while conducting a rapid search and identifying a specific treatment for a correctable precipitating disorder. Sometimes, the presenting clinical scenario will suggest a cause leading to a targeted intervention. More often, the diagnosis is arrived at postmortem and an intervention would have produced little chance of success even had the diagnosis been identified at the bedside, e.g., saddle PE, left ventricular rupture and tamponade following myocardial ischemia, aortic dissection with hemopericardium, hypovolemia, and blunt trauma. Caregivers need to recognize the futility of a prolonged resuscitation and prepare the family for compassionate counseling.

REFERENCES

1. American Heart Association. Standards for cardiopulmonary resuscitation (CPR) and emergency cardiac care (ECC). J Amer Med Assoc 1974; 227:833–868.
2. American Heart Association. Standards and guidelines for cardiopulmonary resuscitation (CPR) and emergency cardiac care (ECC). JAMA 1986; 255:2841–3044.
3. American Heart Association Emergency Cardiac Care Committee. Guidelines for cardiopulmonary resuscitation (CPR) and emergency cardiac care (ECC). JAMA 1992; 268:2171–2295.
4. Aufderheide TP, Thakur RK, Stueven HA, et al. Electrocardiographic characteristics in EMD. Resuscitation 1989; 17:183–193.
5. Vincent JL, Thijs L, Weil MH, Michaels S, Silverberg RA. Clinical and experimental studies on electromechanical dissociation. Circulation 1981; 64:18–27.
6. Redding JS. Drowning and near drowning. Can the victim be saved? Postgrad Med 1983; 74:85–97.
7. Tintinalli JE, White BC. Transthoracic pacing during CPR. Ann Emerg Med 1981; 10:113–116.
8. Hazard PB, Benton C, Milnor JP. Transvenous cardiac pacing in cardiopulmonary resuscitation. Crit Care Med 1981; 9:666–668.
9. Niemann JT, Garner D, Pelikan PC, Jagels G. Predictive value of the ECG in determining cardiac resuscitation outcome in a canine model of postcountershock electromechanical dissociation after prolonged ventricular fibrillation. Ann Emerg Med 1988; 17:567–571.
10. Best R, Martin GB, Carden DL, Tomlanovich MC, Foreback C, Nowak RM. Ionized calcium during CPR in the canine model. Ann Emerg Med 1985; 14:633–635.
11. Blecic S, De Backer D, Huynh CH, et al. Calcium chloride in experimental electromechanical dissociation: a placebo-controlled trial in dogs. Crit Care Med 1987; 15:324–327.
12. Engdahl J, Bang A, Lindqvist J, Herlitz J. Factors affecting short- and long-term prognosis among 1069 patients with out-of-hospital cardiac arrest and pulseless electrical activity. Resuscitation 2001; 51:17–25.
13. Brindley PG, Markland DM, Mayers I, Kutsogiannis DJ. Predictors of survival following in-hospital adult cardiopulmonary resuscitation. Cmaj 2002; 167:343–348.
14. Owen P, Dennis S, Opie LH. Glucose flux rate regulates onset of ischemic contracture in globally underperfused rat hearts. Circ Res 1990; 66:344–354.
15. Opie JC, Taylor G, Ashmore PG, Kalousek D. "Stone heart" in a neonate. J Thorac Cardiovasc Surg 1981; 81:459–463.
15a. Opie LH. The Heart: Physiology and Metabolism (2nd ed.). New York, NY: Raven Press, 1991.
16. The American Heart Association in collaboration with the International Liaison Committee on Resuscitation. Guidelines 2000 for Cardiopulmonary Resuscitation and Emergency Cardiovascular Care. Part 6: advanced cardiovascular life support: 7B: understanding the algorithm approach to ACLS. Circulation 2000; 102(Suppl):I140–I141.
17. Mitchell LB, Pineda EA, Titus JL, Bartosch PM, Benditt DG. Sudden death in patients with implantable cardioverter defibrillators: the importance of post-shock electromechanical dissociation. J Am Coll Cardiol 2002; 39:1323–1328.

9

Chest Compression Technique

*A Neglected Key to Success
in Cardiopulmonary Resuscitation*

Charles F. Babbs, MD, PhD

CONTENTS

INTRODUCTION

The concept of "external cardiac massage," first introduced in the early 1960s by Kouwenhoven, Jude, and Knickerbocker *(1)*, includes chest compressions at a rate of 60 to 100 per minute in conjunction with mouth-to-mouth rescue breathing *(2)*. Refinements of standard cardiopulmonary resuscitation (CPR) since its introduction in the 1960s have included increasing the rate of chest compression from 60 per minute to 100 per minute, which research makes little difference in blood flow *(3)*, and recently decreasing the tidal volume of the positive pressure ventilations under certain circumstances *(2,4)*. Elimination of the carotid artery pulse check in the year 2000 guidelines has abolished an unnecessary delay in starting chest compressions by lay rescuers. Yet for many of us, chest compression remains the centerpiece of resuscitation from full cardiopulmonary arrest, and there has been precious little investigation of how to do it properly.

Today, the optimization of chest compressions in CPR remains a grossly neglected area of research and practical training. The definition of proper chest compression technique is open to question, regarding such basic aspects as depth, rate, and the ventilation to compression ratio. Only one systematic study of compression depth has been published *(5)*. The importance of a particular compression rate is generally over emphasized, and overrated, despite research evidence showing that rates in the range of 60 per minute to 100 per minute are about equally effective. Several thoughtful investigators have suggested and demonstrated in practice that chest compression only CPR—without any ventilations—can be equally effective or more effective than standard CPR *(6–12)*.

From: *Contemporary Cardiology: Cardiopulmonary Resuscitation*
Edited by: J. P. Ornato and M. A. Peberdy © Humana Press Inc., Totowa, NJ

Even if one accepts that current guidelines describe correct chest compression technique, several studies have shown that chest compressions are improperly performed by most lay rescuers and many health care workers as well *(13–15)*.

The time has come for serious efforts to optimize guidelines for chest compression and to implement those guidelines effectively in the field. This chapter reviews the mechanisms by which chest compressions generate blood flow in CPR, the scientific basis for effective techniques of chest compression, the issue of unnecessary interruptions of chest compressions, and the optimal ventilation to compression ratio in CPR.

PHYSIOLOGY OF CHEST COMPRESSION IN CPR

Chest compressions can move blood during cardiac arrest (CA) and CPR by two different mechanisms. These are known as the cardiac pump and the thoracic pump. The cardiac pump mechanism was the first to be recognized by the original discoverers of closed-chest CPR *(1)*. This pump mechanism is operative to the extent that external chest compression squeezes the cardiac ventricles between the sternum and the spine. As a result, forward blood flow occurs through the aortic and pulmonic valves without mitral or tricuspid incompetence. In particular, when the cardiac pump mechanism is operative in CPR, the aortic valve is open and the mitral valve is closed during chest compression *(16)*. The cardiac pump mechanism is also operative during open-chest cardiac massage.

The thoracic pump mechanism was discovered in the 1980s as a result of Criley's clinical observation of cough CPR *(17,18)* and extensive laboratory studies at Johns Hopkins University, led by Myron Weisfeldt and coworkers *(19,20)*. This pump is operative to the extent that chest compression causes a global rise in intrathoracic pressure sufficient to force blood from the pulmonary vasculature, through the heart, and into the periphery. When the thoracic pump mechanism is operative both the mitral valve and the aortic valve are open simultaneously during chest compression *(21–23)*. In this situation, the left heart acts as a conduit, and the collective pulmonary vasculature constitutes the main pumping chamber that fills and empties.

A hybrid pump mechanism can also occur in which the global intrathoracic pressure within the pulmonary capillaries, venae cavae, and aorta is intermediate between the values that would appear during thoracic pump CPR and those that would appear during cardiac pump or open chest CPR. Indeed current dogma suggests that such a combined pump mechanism is operative in most persons. In adults, the hybrid pump is predominantly thoracic and in children the hybrid pump is predominantly cardiac *(24)*.

The reasons why these pumps work are not rocket science. They can be demonstrated in relatively simple mathematical models that represent the essential features of the human cardiovascular system *(25–30)*. Understanding of the relevant physiology has led to inventiveness. Over the past 20 years a variety of ways of enhancing pump function have been explored and are discussed elsewhere in this volume. High impulse CPR, for example *(31–33)*, aims to enhance the action of the cardiac pump mechanism. Vest CPR *(34,35)* aims to enhance the action of the thoracic pump mechanism through the action of a pneumatic vest that is rapidly inflated and deflated at a rate of 60 to 150 times per minute. Active compression–decompression CPR *(36,37)* aims to improve filling of the either the cardiac pump or the thoracic pump by creating negative pressure in the thorax during decompression. Interposed abdominal compression CPR *(38–42)* aims to improve priming of either chest pump through active abdominal counterpulsation. These methods have been called "CPR adjuncts," because they usually require the

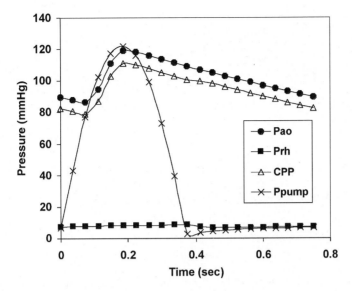

Fig. 1. Pressures in a mathematical model of the normal adult human circulation with the cardiac ventricles beating. The heart rate is 80 per minute. Pressures are plotted as a function of cycle time in the thoracic aorta, Pao; the right atrium, Prh; the intrathoracic pump, Ppump, here the left ventricle. Mean coronary perfusion pressure (CPP) is calculated as Pao minus Prh. CPP is 95 mmHg. Forward flow is 5.0 L per minute.

deployment of an extra rescuer or device, with the hope of improving perfusion during CPR. The focus of the present chapter, however, is on ordinary, conventional chest compression, which is often done poorly at best.

One easy way to demonstrate and study the physiology of blood flow during chest compression is through a mathematical model of the circulation that includes both cardiac and thoracic pumps *(30)*. In such a model, only a small number of assumptions is required to obtain realistic results *(30)*. These are limited to (a) the existence of compliant vessels and resistive vascular beds; (b) the definition of compliance ($\Delta V/\Delta P$); (c) normal anatomy, that is the arrangement of connected vessels and cardiac chambers; and (d) a linear relation between flow and pressure (i.e., "Ohm's Law" flow = pressure/resistance). Although much more complex models of the circulation can be created, only these basic assumptions are needed to demonstrate the mechanisms of blood flow during CPR. Circulatory systems that have these properties will behave similarly, including those of large and small people and experimental animals. The exact values of vascular compliances and resistances, as well as other technical details of a working model, which can be implemented in a Microsoft Excel spreadsheet, are fully described elsewhere *(30)*.

As a point of reference and calibration, Fig. 1 illustrates pressures in a simplified cardiovascular system for a nonarrested circulation of a hypothetical 70 kg man. Here a cardiac pump generates left ventricular pressures (P_{pump}) of 122/2 mmHg at a heart rate of 80 per minute. Systemic arterial blood pressure is 119/82, mean arterial pressure is 95 mmHg, and cardiac output is 5.0 L per minute. These are classical textbook values for the normal human circulatory system *(30)*. Note the essentially normal arterial pulse waveforms and low systemic venous pressures. The data point representing the exact minimum, diastolic pressure at 82 mmHg is not plotted on the chart.

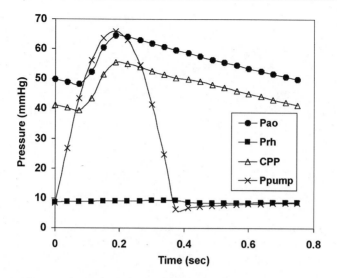

Fig. 2. Pressures in a mathematical model of the normal adult human circulation during CA and CPR with a pure cardiac pump mechanism. The compression rate is 80 per minute. Intrathoracic pressure acting on the cardiac ventricles ranges from 0 to +60 mmHg with a half sinusoidal waveform. Other pressures are defined as in Fig. 1. Forward flow is 2.5 L per minute, and CPP is 47 mmHg.

Cardiac Pump CPR

Figure 2 illustrates the action of a pure cardiac pump CPR in the same circulatory model during CA. Steady-state conditions are shown after stable pressures have been achieved by 20 prior compressions. In this simulation only the right and left ventricles of the heart are compressed at a rate of 80 per minute with a half sinusoidal waveform having a peak pressure of 60 mmHg, a typical value reported in the literature of standard CPR (28). There is no intrinsic myocardial contractility in this system, and there is no pump priming effect of atrial contractions (which in some circumstances could exist for a few minutes in witnessed arrests). The cardiac pump produces reasonable aortic pressures and very small venous pulsations. These are pressures that the CPR pioneers of the 1960s had in mind when they conceived of "external cardiac massage." Note especially the low right-sided central venous pressures. There is substantial coronary perfusion pressure (aortic to right atrial gradient) throughout the compression cycle. Forward flow is 2.5 L per min, and systemic perfusion pressure is 47 mmHg. This state of affairs represents idealized classical external CPR in which "the heart is squeezed between the sternum and the spine" as reported in 1965 by DelGuercio (43). It is also a reasonable representation of open chest CPR with manual cardiac compression (44–47), which obviously works by a pure "cardiac pump" mechanism. A similar state of affairs can occur in children (and young pigs [48,49]), who have small compliant chest walls.

Figures 1 and 2 were generated using positive applied extravascular pressures during the compression phase and extravascular pressure during the relaxation phase. A relatively recent concept in the physiology of CPR is the use of active decompression, rather than simple relaxation, between chest compressions. Decompression can be accomplished by the use of "plunger-like" devices (discovered accidentally using a real toilet plunger! [36,50]) or by sticky adhesive pads that make contact with the skin of the anterior chest or abdomen such as those incorporated into the Lifestick device (51). This

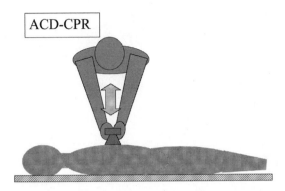

Fig. 3. Sketch of active compression–decompression cardiopulmonary resuscitation using a plunger-like device. Active decompression at a minimum ensures full chest wall recoil and promotes blood return to the chest.

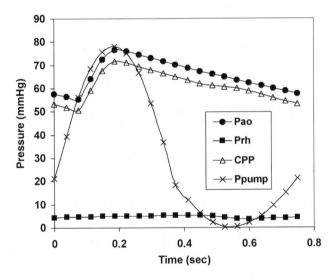

Fig. 4. Pressures in a mathematical model of an adult human during cardiac arrest and active compression–decompression cardiopulmonary resuscitation with a pure cardiac pump mechanism. The compression rate is 80 per minute. Intrathoracic pressure acting on the cardiac ventricles ranges from 0 to +60 mmHg with a half sinusoidal waveform. Maximal decompression pressure is –20 mmHg. Other pressures are defined as in Fig. 1. Forward flow is 3.2 L per minute and coronary perfusion pressure is 61 mmHg.

approach is known as active compression–decompression CPR (ACD-CPR; Fig. 3). Today, active decompression of the chest during CPR can be accomplished using a specially designed plunger applied to the human sternum *(47,52–54)*, which is sold commercially in Europe as the Ambu Cardiopump®.

Figure 4 illustrates the steady-state effect of active decompression of the chest to negative 20 mmHg, the maximum reported in the literature *(52,55,56)*. This particular simulation is for cardiac pump CPR. Combining both positive and negative chest pressures has a salubrious effect on hemodynamics. Cardiac filling is enhanced during the negative pressure phase, so that greater stroke output can be achieved on the next positive pressure phase.

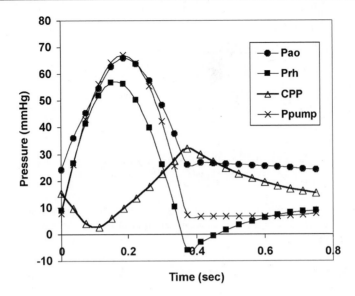

Fig. 5. Pressures in a mathematical model of the normal adult human circulation during cardiac arrest and cardiopulmonary resuscitation with a pure thoracic pump mechanism. The compression rate is 80 per minute. Global intrathoracic pressure acting on the cardiac ventricles, right heart, venae cavae, and thoracic aorta ranges from 0 to +60 mmHg with a half sinusoidal waveform. Other pressures are defined as in Fig. 1. Forward flow is 0.93 L per minute; CPP is 18 mmHg.

Note in Fig. 4 the particular times near 0.55 seconds in the cycle when pump pressure is substantially less than right heart pressure. At this stage enhanced pump filling occurs. The result of enhanced pump filling is greater forward flow and greater perfusion pressures—3.2 vs 2.5 L per minute and 61 vs 47 mmHg.

An effect similar to active decompression may be obtained with conventional CPR, properly performed with no leaning on the chest. Especially in a younger individual there is natural recoil of the ribs after compression (in the absence of chest wall breakdown or broken ribs). This recoil helps to create transient negative pressure in the chest that promotes pump filling. Poorly performed external CPR with leaning on the chest inhibits this normal passive decompression. One can also regard Fig. 4 as a model of ordinary chest compression in a young adult, performed by a rescuer who allows full chest recoil between down strokes. Only when filling is unimpeded can chest compression be effective. Otherwise, compression of pumping chambers that are already empty produces little flow.

Thoracic Pump CPR

When it works, the cardiac pump mechanism is the most effective and natural of the three pumps in CPR (cardiac, thoracic, and abdominal [27]). Its operation in external CPR, however, depends on good mechanical coupling between the sternum and the heart. In most adults the coupling of chest compression to the heart is indirect, and a thoracic pump mechanism tends to predominate (23,24,34).

Thoracic pump CPR has a quite different set of pressure profiles. Figure 5 illustrates the action of a pure thoracic pump. In this simulation all intrathoracic blood containing

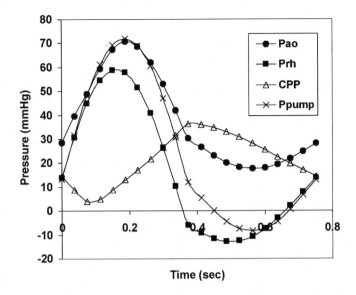

Fig. 6. Active decompression with thoracic pump cardiopulmonary resuscitation. The compression rate is 80/min. Intrathoracic pressure acting on the cardiac ventricles ranges from 0 to +60 mmHg with a half sinusoidal waveform. Other pressures are defined as in Fig. 1. Maximal chest compression pressure is +60 mmHg. Maximal decompression pressure is –20 mmHg. Here forward flow is 1.1 L per minute and CPP is 22 mmHg.

chambers are pressurized equally at a rate of 80 per minute with a peak pressure of 60 mmHg, as before. This state of affairs happens in broad chested older individuals. It also happens during vest CPR, in which a pneumatic vest encircles the chest to produce pulses of compression from all sides simultaneously.

In thoracic pump CPR forward flow occurs even though the heart is not being squeezed between the sternum and the spine. Coronary blood flow and systemic blood flow occur when aortic pressure is greater than systemic venous or right heart pressure. As shown in Fig. 5, positive coronary and systemic perfusion pressures occur mostly during "diastole," between compressions, rather than during "systole" (i.e., during compressions). Phase differences in central arterial and venous pressure waveforms may allow limited systolic perfusion as well. Because of the tendency toward equalization of aortic and venous pressures during systole, forward flow with the thoracic pump mechanism tends to be less than with the cardiac pump mechanism, other factors being equal. In the thoracic pump model of Fig. 5 forward flow is only 0.94 L per minute and systemic perfusion pressure is 18 mmHg.

If an active decompression phase is added (Fig. 6), perfusion pressures are somewhat increased, but to a lesser extent than with cardiac pump CPR. Now forward flow is 1.14 L per minute and systemic perfusion pressure is 22 mmHg. Herein lies the challenge of performing external chest compressions in adults. One must generate not only pressure pulses, but also forward flow of blood. The chances of doing this are improved by using a thoughtful technique based on research findings from the animal laboratory and the clinic.

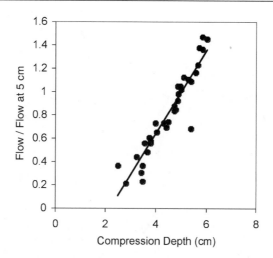

Fig. 7. Relative forward flow in cardiopulmonary resuscitation (CPR) as a function of compression depth, as reported in the animal studies of Fitzgerald et al. *(3)*. As compression depth during Thumper® CPR increased, flow increased in each animal. However, no flow was obtained at compression depths less than 2 cm. The solid line is a least squares linear regression to data from eight anesthetized dogs.

TECHNIQUE OF CHEST COMPRESSION IN CPR

Amplitude or Depth of Compression

Current guidelines for CPR state that chest compressions be performed "to a depth of 1.5 to 2 inches"—approx 4 to 5 cm. This recommendation is based on the experience of early pioneers of CPR. There are no clinical data in humans that describe what happens to blood flow when chest compressions are between 0 and 1.5 inches (how bad is too little), when chest compressions are between 1.5 and 2 inches (how stable is the target region), or when chest compressions are greater than 2 inches (how much more can be squeezed out of the system and at what cost in complications). The vigor of manual chest compression may vary widely among rescuers and may progressively diminish as a given rescuer tires. The effects of these variations are unknown, but would be inconsequential only if the function relating blood flow to chest compression depth showed a broad plateau in the neighborhood of 1 to 2 inches.

In the only existing study of the relationship of blood pressure and flow during CPR to chest compression amplitude, small (6–12 kg) anesthetized dogs were resuscitated during 2-minute periods of electrically induced ventricular fibrillation (VF) and Thumper® CPR *(3)*. Cardiac output was measured using a special indicator dilution method designed for accuracy during the low-flow conditions of CPR. The results (Fig. 7) showed anything but a plateau. Chest compressions exceeding a threshold value (x_0) between 1.5 and 3.0 cm were required in each animal to produce measurable cardiac output. Cardiac output increased as a linear function of compression depth beyond the compression threshold. That is $CO = a(x - x_0)$ if $x > x_0$ for chest displacement, x, and constant, a. However, if $x < x_0$ $CO = 0$.

The mean value of x_0 was 2.3 cm, a value very close to 1 inch (2.54 cm). A similar threshold of 1.8 cm was found for measurable blood pressure in response to chest compression. For chest compression depths greater than 2.5 cm relatively modest increases

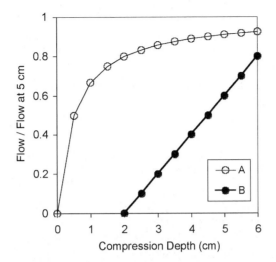

Fig. 8. Conceptual models of forward flow in cardiopulmonary resuscitation as a function of compression depth. A = plateau function implied in the guidelines. B = actual function from laboratory studies, including the effective compression threshold at 2 cm.

in chest compression caused relatively large increases in cardiac output (Fig. 7). These observations are supported by clinical experience, as well *(57)*. Experienced rescuers have learned that in some persons 1 to 2 inches of sternal compression may be inadequate and a slightly greater degree of chest compression may be needed to generate an adequate carotid or femoral pulse. Authorities suggest in the guidelines for basic life support that optimal sternal compression is best gauged by using the compression force that generates a palpable carotid or femoral pulse. Yet we know from physiology and from tracings such as Fig. 5 that pressure pulses do not guarantee blood flow if the venous and arterial pulses are the same.

Current guidelines for compressions to a depth of 1.5 to 2 inches or 4 to 5 cm are supported by limited research data. However, the guidelines and associated teaching materials do not emphasize the depth of compression as a critical variable. Rather, they seem to imply that any degree of chest compression within the prescribed range of 1.5 to 2 inches is satisfactory. Such an interpretation would be rational if the true function relating cardiac output and compression depth were as shown in Fig. 8, curve A. This hypothetical function rises to a plateau, such that any degree of compression in the plateau region would be close to maximally effective.

Research data (Fig. 7) however, argue strongly that the actual functional relationship is more like that of line B in Fig. 8. In this situation flow is quite sensitive to small changes in sternal displacement, and for some displacements below a critical threshold value, cardiac output is virtually nil.

Under field conditions in which the force and depth of chest compression may vary, it is unlikely that a given victim receives optimal CPR for the duration of the resuscitation effort. Chest compression may drift below the effective compression threshold as rescuer fatigue sets in. The steepness of the slope of the actual flow vs compression depth line, cries out for a more effective monitor of chest compression during CPR—either a monitor of compression depth itself, or better still, a monitor of blood flow or organ perfusion, so that professional rescuers could use biofeedback to maintain effective chest compression throughout the duration of a resuscitation effort.

Of course, there is potential harm form more forceful chest compressions that must be balanced against the hemodynamic benefit. In a previous study Redding and Cozine *(44)* found that during closed chest massage in dogs, mediastinal hemorrhage, fractured ribs, and lacerations of the liver were frequently encountered when maximal force was applied to the chest sufficient to produce the greatest possible blood pressure. However, Redding and Cozine quickly developed a moderately forceful technique that generally avoided these complications.

Current CPR has been likened to "flying a 747 aircraft without instruments." The existence of an effective chest compression threshold is a powerful reason for more effective monitoring of circulation during CPR on a routine basis. One simple expedient, in lieu of future high tech monitors is placement of a long soft rubber tube, filled with water, in the esophagus for pressure monitoring. This system can be completely safe if a cuffed endotracheal tube is in place. When pressure pulses generated in the esophageal tube are 50 mmHg or greater, nearly maximal cardiac output is obtained in laboratory experiments *(5)*. Greater forces are ineffective in generating greater flow; hence the 50-mmHg esophageal pressure rule provides a convenient yardstick for optimal chest compression. Unfortunately, this simple and low cost approach has yet to be implemented clinically.

A new and interesting twist on monitoring of chest compressions is a device incorporated into the chest compression pad of the Zoll AED-Plus automatic external defibrillator. The sternal chest compression pad, located between stick-on defibrillating electrodes includes a miniature accelerometer. The signal from this electronic device is doubly integrated to produce a measure of compression depth that is monitored by the device. Auditory feedback can be provided to the rescuer if chest compression depth, so monitored, falls outside the recommended range. Technical aids such as this one may improve the quality of external chest compressions in the future. Although not a physiologic end point, compression depth, accurately displayed to the rescuer on a push-by-push basis would at least improve consistency and control over an important independent variable in the physiologic equation of CPR.

Compression Rate

Kevin Fitzgerand et al. conducted an extensive laboratory study in anesthetized dogs of compression rate using a specially designed, computer-controlled Thumper® (a piston for chest compression driven by compressed gas). Fitzgerald et al. measured cardiac output during electrically induced VF and CPR as the major dependent variable, using a technique adapted to low-flow conditions. Chest compression rates ranging from 60 to 120 per minute were equally effective in this model. A mathematical curve fit to the data yielded a function beginning appropriately with 0 flow at 0 compression rate and rising to a plateau between 60 and 120 compressions per minute. In the plateau region there was about a plus or minus 20% variation in flow, with little evidence suggesting that one compression rate was better than another (Fig. 9).

This empirical result has also been demonstrated in analog computer models of the circulation *(27)*. In the plateau region stroke volume of the chest pump diminishes with increasing chest compression rate, much as that of the natural heart. The reason is prob-

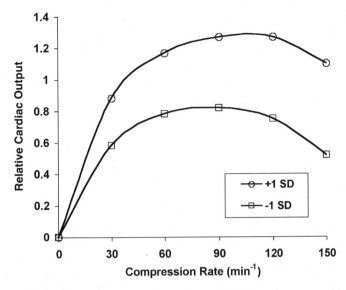

Fig. 9. Relative cardiac output as a function of compression rate after Fitzgerald et al. Range of relative flows based on 20 to 30 determinations in 10 animals is plotted in terms of the ± 1 SD values, where SD denotes 1 standard deviation from the mean. 1.0 on the ordinate represents 42 mL per minute per kg body weight. In the range of 60 to 120 compressions per minute there is little effect of compression rate.

ably the same—reduced pump filling with shorter cycle times. When it comes to compression rate, unlike compression amplitude, the functional curve really does have a plateau. Hence one could say that current teaching of basic life support has it backwards regarding which variable is critical. We should not be stressing that trainees achieve a particular target rate in doing chest compressions, although any compression depth in the range of 1.5 to 2 inches is acceptable. We should be stressing that compression depth is the critical variable, and any rate between 60 and 100 per minute is acceptable.

Duty Cycle or Compression Duration

It was my mentor, Dr. Leslie Geddes, an award winning biomedical engineer, who introduced the term "duty cycle" into the literature of CPR. Duty cycle is defined as the ratio of compression duration to total cycle time. For example, the recommended duty cycle for standard CPR is 50%—half compression, half relaxation. In the animal laboratory Fitzgerald et al. also studied the effects of changes in duty cycle at a variety of compression rates with the programmable Thumper®. For anesthetized dogs in electrically induced VF Fitzgerald et al. found inverted U-shaped functions at all rates (Fig. 10). Peak flow occurred between 30 and 50 and duty cycle—that is 30 to 50 and compression duration. Other investigators using other models have confirmed these results. For example, Babbs and Thelander *(58)*, using a mathematical computer model of the human circulation, found that total pulmonary artery flow and coronary artery flow peaked at 30 to 40% duty cycle for standard CPR. Interestingly, cranial flow to the brain, unlike that to other organs, peaked at near 60% duty cycle, in keeping with the observation of Taylor, Weisfeldt, and coworkers *(59)*, who measured ultrasonic doppler flow velocity index in carotid arteries of anesthetized dogs and in carotid arteries of humans during CPR.

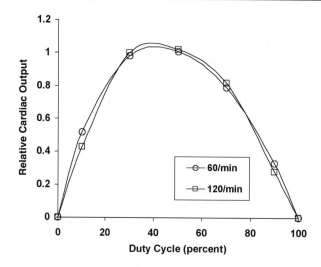

Fig. 10. Average values of relative cardiac output as a function of duty cycle of compression at 60 per minute and 120 per minute compression rate. Data are from Fitzgerald et al. Here each animal served as its own control. The effects of duty cycle are independent of rate in the range of 60 to 120 compressions per minute.

Taylor's study proved to be historically influential in standards writing. In response to the evidence that increased duty cycle created better brain flow, standards writers decided to increase the recommended rate of compression, because practical rescuers tended to compress the chest with a fixed duration of about one-third of a second. Increasing rate, assuming the compression duration is constant, automatically increases the duty cycle without requiring learns to alter two different aspects of their technique. Unfortunately this change, together with subsequent rate increases in the year 2000 guidelines, failed to account for the effect of faster compression rates on total cardiac output when compression-to-ventilation ratios are kept the same. This interesting and controversial subject is discussed fully in the final section of this chapter.

HAND POSITION ON THE CHEST

Proper hand placement for chest compression has been established through clinical experience rather than through systematic research. The compression point has become accepted as the middle of the lower half of the sternum. In studies of cardiac angiography during CPR *(60)* this location appeared to be most effective. However, if compression is centered too high, that is too far cranial, in the upper half of the sternum, the aortic and pulmonary artery roots are squeezed and kinked at the base of the heart, actually obstructing outflow. In this situation forward flow is close to 0. If compression is centered too low, the xiphoid process may be driven into the left lobe of the liver, resulting in liver laceration. If the compression point is shifted laterally the costochondral junctions may be subluxed or ribs may be broken.*

---

*I have become aware of anecdotal reports of more effective CPR when the compression point is shifted left of midline to a position "over the left ventricle." The method is said to produce a "facial flush," indicative of dramatically improved blood flow, and to have achieved a handful of dramatic rescues. However, reports of the technique, known as the Williams' maneuver after its inventor, have not yet appeared in the peer-reviewed literature.

Typically, the long axis of the heel of the rescuer's hand is placed on the long axis of the lower half of the sternum. This alignment helps to keep the main force of compression on the sternum and to decrease the chance of rib fracture. The fingers may be either extended or interlaced but should be kept off the chest, again to reduce chances of rib fracture. An acceptable alternative hand position is to grasp the wrist of the hand on the chest with the opposite hand. This technique is helpful for rescuers with arthritic hands and wrists *(57)*.

It is important not to lift the hands from the chest or change position frequently, otherwise correct hand position may be lost. However, it is also important not to lean on the chest, maintaining forceful contact during the release phase, because this action limits venous return to the pump. Bouncing compressions, jerky movements, improper hand position, and leaning on the chest can decrease the effectiveness of resuscitation and are more likely to cause injuries. To ease fatigue of the triceps muscles, the elbows should be locked into position, with arms straightened, and shoulders positioned as directly over the hands as possible, so that the thrust for each chest compression is straight down on the sternum. If the thrust is not vertical, the torso has a tendency to roll; part of the downward force is displaced, and the chest compression may be less effective.

BIOMECHANICS OF RESCUER ACTION

After all this positioning, which mercifully takes much longer to read than to perform in actual practice, it is now time to begin chest compressions. Classically *(57)* rescuers have been taught to lean forward with the shoulders until they are directly over the outstretched hands. That is to lean forward until the body reaches "natural imbalance"— a point at which there would be a sensation of falling forward if the hands and arms were not providing support. With this technique the weight of the trunk creates the necessary force to depress the sternum; arm strength is not required.

The approach just described works well for the down stroke. However, an up stroke or recovery phase is also important and is needed to complete the full cycle. Unfortunately, a fatigue-generating problem can easily occur during the recovery phase of rescuer action. The problem is that when one leans forward from the waist, the obvious recovery stroke is to lift up the torso from the waist using the back muscles (erector spinae complex), which in humans are relatively weak and prone to fatigue, as well as prone to painful spasm at the most unfortunate of times.

A LEARNING ACTIVITY, PART 1

To understand the importance of this point deeply, try standing up and bending forward enough to touch your knees with your hands and then lifting your shoulders back to a standing position at the recommended rate of 100 times in 60 seconds. Do not be shy. Try this right now; it is part of the book chapter. Notice that you had difficulty doing all 100 bends in the time allowed. Notice the feeling of fatigue, if not pain in your back muscles. Notice your feeling of anger at my making you do this. Indeed people who use this approach on a chest or manikin find it so difficult that they soon tend to allow the chest recoil push their own torso weight upward to save energy. That is they "lean on the chest" to compensate for the imbalance. Unfortunately for the patient this action results in greater "diastolic" (recovery phase) force on the chest than is needed. This extra force impedes chest pump filling and reduces the effectiveness of CPR. Some of the effectiveness of active compression-decompression-CPR may simply be a result of its allowing natural chest recoil to occur, rather than allowing the individual's chest recoil to "rescue the rescuer" from fatigue!

A LEARNING ACTIVITY, PART 2

Now try the following experiment, which is much more pleasant than the first one. Although standing, bend your knees slightly to lower your hips and torso as a unit through a distance of 5 cm toward the floor and return to a standing posture. Repeat this cycle 100 times in 60 seconds. Keep your back straight, head up, and shoulders back. Look forward and just bounce up and down 5 cm each time. You probably noticed how much easier this exercise is than bending over. It is certainly no more tiring than jogging or running in place or dancing. It is also much easier to do at a faster rate approaching 100 per minute. There is even some energy return from the legs during upward motion, because of natural recoil of tendons and muscles of the legs. Here the muscles that are doing the work are the quadriceps femoris muscles of the anterior thighs—the largest and most powerful muscles in the human body. This is a better way to do CPR.

Now consider the following biomechanically efficient approach to chest compression. This technique produces reduced back fatigue for the rescuer and greater effectiveness for the individual. The rescuer either kneels beside the thorax of the individual—as close as possible—or works astride the individual on his or her knees. If the patient is raised on a table, a stool may be needed by the rescuer to provide the necessary elevation. The arms should be straight and as vertical as possible, and the elbows should be locked, as before. In this position the rescuer can work effectively by raising and lowering the hips (not the shoulders) against gravity, *using the anterior thigh muscles, NOT the back.*

As the rescuer's hips are lowered in the kneeling position with the back straight and firm, the weight of the rescuer's body can be used to apply compression. As the rescuer's hips are raised the quadriceps muscles of the anterior thigh can work to complete the cycle, although the rescuer's arms remain straight. As a final exercise the reader is encouraged to try this motion in the kneeling position while palpating the quadriceps and hamstring muscles. Note that when the hips are raised when kneeling, the leg is extended at the knee joint by the quadriceps and the thigh is extended at the hip joint by the hamstrings. Posterior compartment (hamstring) muscles are active as well in the kneeling position. Reliance on the strong anterior and posterior thigh muscles minimizes fatigue and keeps the exercise aerobic for either male or female rescuers. These same muscles should be used as much as possible in the standing position as well. Upper body strength is not required, once rescuers learn to use leg muscles and NOT back muscles. Even with this more biomechanically efficient technique, adequate personnel need to be available, whenever possible, so that frequent changes can occur every 3–5 minutes to avoid fatigue. As fatigue sets in, rescuers tend to revert to former habitual methods of chest compression, which are less effective.

A FINAL NOTE REGARDING THE RELEASE PHASE

The release phase of chest compression is just as important as compression itself. Release chest compression pressure between each compression to allow blood to flow into the chest and heart. The pressure must be released and the chest must be permitted to return to its normal position after each and every compression. Chest recoil is considered by thoughtful students of CPR physiology to be critical in promoting venous return to the chest pump and proper filling for the next cycle.

CPR Performed on a Soft Surface Such as a Mattress

Because the effectiveness of chest compression during standard CPR may be seriously degraded on soft supporting surfaces such as hospital beds; it is standard practice to place a backboard under the patient to provide a more unyielding surface. According to guidelines for basic life support *(4)*: "If the individual is in bed, a board, preferably the full width of the bed, should be placed under the patient's back to avoid the diminished effectiveness of chest compression." For those patients who are large or who are connected to many monitoring and life support devices, the placement of a backboard can be difficult and time consuming. Sometimes the patient is moved to the floor, requiring interruption of CPR. Sometimes backboards are not immediately available, or there is a delay in finding one. Under these circumstances rescuers must make do with a modified technique.

One approach is to use a modified compression technique for soft surfaces developed by Boe and Babbs, who conducted a systematic mechanical analysis of the effects of substrate stiffness on chest compression in CPR *(61)*. Their modified technique is called the constant peak force technique. With this approach the rescuer concentrates on the force applied, rather than the distance moved by the compressing hands. The rescuer compresses the sternum using the same maximum force regardless of any patient motion. This mode is similar to that applied by the Thumper® mechanical resuscitator, and also by smaller adult rescuers who focus on using body weight to apply chest compressions.

The constant peak force technique helps to compensate for underlying bed softness vs chest stiffness. In Boe and Babbs' analysis if the rescuer used a conventional constant 5 cm peak displacement, sternum-to-spine compression fell from 4.3 to 1.0 cm, as underlying bed stiffness decreased from 50,000 to 5000 N per meter. At a typical bed stiffness of 10,000 N per meter less than 35% of intended chest compression occurred. At the same time peak power exerted by the rescuer fell to about half that for a hard surface, because it is easier to compress a mattress than an adult human chest. However, if a constant peak force of 400 N was applied, regardless of the observed displacement of the chest and bed, greater than 85% of maximal chest compression was obtained at a typical bed stiffness of 10,000 N per meter. The cost of the increased effectiveness was that the power exerted by the rescuer was approximately double that required on a hard surface. That is, the rescuer had to work harder because he or she was compressing both the mattress and the patient.

The good news is if necessary, CPR can be performed effectively on a softer surface using a constant peak force technique. Although a firm surface is most desirable, the constant peak force technique is capable of maintaining a significant degree of chest compression on all but the softest surfaces, albeit at the expense of greatly increased work by the rescuer. This approach may be quite useful in coronary care unit settings, for example, when arrests are brief, lines and cables are numerous, and electrical defibrillation is readily available.

INTERRUPTON OF CHEST COMPRESSIONS FOR VENTILATION

Current adult CPR by one or two rescuers is based on the traditional ABCs—airway, breathing, circulation—with a 15:2 compression to ventilation ratio *(2)*. That is, the rescuer compresses the chest 15 times, pauses to give two mouth-to-mouth ventilations, and then continues with chest compressions. The former convention of 5:1 compression ventilation ratio for two-rescuer CPR has been dropped in the most recent guidelines for the sake of simplification and coordination between North American and European practice.

The 15:2 ratio is essentially the same as the normal ratio of heart rate to breathing in a quietly resting adult with a heart rate of 75 beats per minute and a respiratory rate of 10 breaths per minute, namely 7.5:1 or 15:2. Recently, the issue of the most desirable compression to ventilation ratio has been reopened because of the reluctance of many rescuers, both lay and professional, to perform mouth-to-mouth rescue breathing, owing to the fear of contracting serious communicable diseases such as AIDS *(62–64)*. Moreover, the relatively long pauses in chest compression required for ventilation lead to disturbingly long interruptions in chest compressions and associated blood flow. In turn, the average systemic perfusion pressure over a complete compression/ventilation cycle may be much lower than is generally appreciated.

Consider, for example, a set of 15 compressions at a compression rate of 100 per minute *(2)*, which requires 9 seconds to deliver. If a rescuer takes 5 seconds to administer two slow, deep rescue breaths of 700 to 1000 mL each, as specified in current guidelines *(2)*, then chest compressions are only being delivered 9/14ths of the time. The 5-second pause for ventilation following every 15 chest compressions has been shown in experimental models to reduce coronary perfusion pressure by 50% *(10)*. This loss of perfusion pressure must be rebuilt during each subsequent set of compressions, and typically requires about 5 to 10 compressions before the previous level is achieved *(10)*. In some cases the 5-second pause for ventilation may reduce overall mean systemic perfusion below the value of approx 25 mmHg required for effective resuscitation *(65–67)*.

In the real world, interruptions of chest compressions get worse. Recent videotape analysis of lay rescuers in action shows that the interruption of chest compression for rescue breathing consistently requires about 16 seconds to perform *(68,69)*. The act of delivering two slow, deep rescue breaths is not just blowing into the mouth of the individual, but the physical task of stopping compressions, leaving the chest, moving to the head, performing a head tilt–chin lift maneuver to open the airway, taking in a breath, bending over, getting a good mouth to mouth seal, blowing in the breath, rising up, taking in a second breath, bending over again, recreating a good seal, blowing in the second breath, watching the chest rise, leaving the head and returning to the chest, finding the proper hand position, and finally beginning to compress the chest again! This kinesthetically complex set of tasks is much more difficult for the once trained, but unpracticed, rescuer than is the rhythmic repetition of chest compression.

Hence in a practical, real-world setting, with a compression rate of 100 per minute (the new value specified in the year 2000 international guidelines *[2]*), chest compressions would be interrupted for ventilations a majority of the time (9 seconds for 15 compressions, 16 seconds for 2 ventilations). In this case chest compressions would be delivered during only 36% of the total resuscitation time.

The consequences of interruptions of chest compressions for ventilation in adults have recently been studied by the author and Karl B. Kern using mathematical modeling *(70)*. We developed equations describing oxygen delivery and blood flow during CPR as functions of the number of compressions and the number of ventilations delivered over time from principles of classical physiology. These equations were solved explicitly in terms of the compression/ventilation ratio and evaluated for a wide range of conditions using Monte Carlo simulations.

We found that as the compression to ventilation ratio is increased from 0 to 50 (that is from 0:2 to 100:2) oxygen delivery to peripheral tissues increases to a maximum value and then gradually declines. For parameters typical of standard CPR as taught and speci-

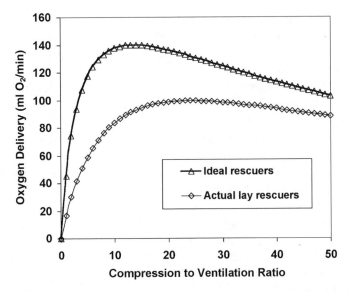

Fig. 11. Oxygen delivery as a function of compression to ventilation ratio in the theoretical study of Babbs and Kern *(70)*. The compression to ventilation ratio is normalized to one ventilation. Hence, a value of 20 represents 40:2, if two ventilations are given. Ideal professional rescuers are assumed to deliver two rescue breaths in 5 seconds, as specified in guidelines. Lay rescuers are assumed to deliver two breaths in 16 seconds, as observed in the field. Maximal oxygen delivery occurs at ratios near 25:2 for ideal rescuers and 50:2 for lay rescuers.

fied in international guidelines (that is, 5 seconds to deliver two rescue breaths) maximum oxygen delivery occurs at compression/ventilation ratios near 30:2. For parameters typical of actual lay rescuer performance in the field (that is, 16 seconds to deliver two rescue breaths) maximum oxygen delivery occurs at compression to ventilation ratios near 60:2. The complete curves are shown in Fig. 11. If these theoretical results are true in the real world, current guidelines overestimate the need for ventilation during standard CPR by two- to fourfold. In turn, blood flow and oxygen delivery to the periphery can be improved by eliminating interruptions of chest compression for these unnecessary ventilations.

Unnecessary interruptions of chest compression have actually become a greater problem with successive refinements of the guidelines. Historically, the problem was compounded when compression rate was increased from 60 per minute to 90 per minute, and most recently in the year 2000, to 100 per minute. As shown in detail in reference *(70)*, the optimum ventilation to compression ratio for maximizing oxygen delivery to peripheral tissues is directly proportional to the compression rate. This means that if one increases the rate of chest compression by a certain percentage, it is prudent to increase the recommended compression to ventilation ratio by the same percentage also. For example, suppose that 15:2 had been the optimum compression to ventilation ratio with 60 per minute compressions under the original CPR guidelines. Suppose further that the guidelines changed to recommend a 120 per minute compression rate, just to keep the arithmetic simple. Under the "new" guidelines, it would take exactly half the time to deliver 15 compressions than it did previously, because the compression rate is doubled.

The time for ventilations, however, would remain constant. Thus, the duration of interruptions of chest compression for ventilation must become a larger percentage of total resuscitation time whenever the compression rate is increased without changing the ventilation to compression ratio.

When the recommended compression rate was in fact increased from 60 per minute to 90 per minute, the compression to ventilation ratio should have been automatically increased from 15:2 to 23:2, simply by virtue of the fact that the compression rate had increased. When the recommended compression rate was further increased to 100 per minute, the compression to ventilation ratio should have been automatically increased to 25:2. Actually 15:2 never was optimal for standard CPR in adults, but failure to adjust ventilation as the compression rate was increased has further compounded the problem.

The ultimate extension of the concept of increasing the number of chest compressions between ventilation ventilations is "continuous chest compression CPR" without any ventilations at all. Such a strategy, crazy as it may seem, has been extensively studied in a swine model of resuscitation and has shown identical outcome results to standard 15:2 compression to ventilation CPR (6–8,11,12,71,72). Recently, Hallstrom et al. (73) have reported a clinical study of simplified, dispatcher assisted CPR, in which no ventilations are given. In this study, persons who called 911 for help with an adult, nontraumatic CA and did not know CPR were coached by the 911 dispatcher to perform either traditional CPR or compression-only CPR without any ventilations. The results of CPR without ventilations were no worse than those of standard CPR. In particular, survival to hospital discharge was greater among patients assigned to chest compression alone than among those assigned to chest compression plus mouth-to-mouth ventilation (14.6 vs 10.4%, using intention-to-treat analysis). There was no statistically significant difference in favor of either standard CPR or chest compression-only CPR in this study of 303 randomized patients. Evidently, ventilation provided no added benefit. Importantly, Hallstrom's results were obtained for adult nontraumatic CA and are not necessarily indicative of those that would be obtained in pediatric asphyxial arrest. This study highlights how little we really know about the basic ABCs of CPR.

CONCLUSIONS

Principles of cardiovascular physiology tell us that during CA and CPR forward flow of blood can be generated by external compression of the chest. Enough has been learned in the last 25 years to suggest that most persons perform chest compressions suboptimally. Much more emphasis needs to be placed on compression depth and technique rather than on compression rate. Routine clinical monitors of effective chest compression need to be developed and used widely. Still, the exact details of chest compression including such fundamental variables as rate, duty cycle, amplitude, rescuer technique, and ventilation to compression ratio remain suboptimal, under-investigated, and newly controversial after all these years.

The original 1960s style CPR was developed on the basis of limited research and educated guesswork—some of it brilliant and insightful. The CPR pioneers like Kouwenhoven, Jude, Knickerbocker, Elam, Safar, and Redding had no government grants. They were not supported by multinational drug companies. With limited resources, these investigators made enormous progress. Nevertheless, the early standards for chest compression, which we have inherited today, were based on only partial understanding of the underlying physiology and biomechanics. Several plausible assumptions of the 1960s, such as the mechanism of external cardiac massage and the required ventilation to perfusion ratio have proved to be oversimplifications in light of subsequent research.

Today at the dawn of the 21st century the topic of chest compression in CPR is ripe for reassessment and renewed investigation. We need to know more about flow mechanisms with chest/abdominal compression and decompression. In order to optimize CPR in children it would help to know about age related differences in chest size, chest compliance, and CPR pump mechanisms. With more research we might discover entirely new ways to apply force, create flow or raise coronary perfusion pressure. We urgently need better sensors—beyond $ETCO_2$ and pulse-ox—so that CPR on individuals becomes less like flying a 747 without instruments and more like adjusting an anesthesia machine or a mechanical ventilator. There need to be clinical evaluations of alternative ventilation to compression ratios for lay CPR, and means of training individuals to perform simpler, biomechanically easier, less complex series of steps with fewer interruptions of chest compressions. It is time for a renaissance of interest, research, and teaching in the simple act of compressing the chest in CPR, which is, on closer inspection, anything but "standard."

REFERENCES

1. Kouwenhoven WB, Jude JR, Knickerbocker GG. Closed-chest cardiac massage. JAMA 1960; 173: 1064–1067.
2. Cummins RO. American Heart Association in collaboration with the International Liaison Committee on Resuscitation. Guidelines 2000 for cardiopulmonary resuscitation and emergency cardiovascular care: international consensus on science. Circulation 2000; 102(suppl I):I-1–I-384.
3. Fitzgerald KR, Babbs CF, Frissora HA, Davis RW, Silver DI. Cardiac output during cardiopulmonary resuscitation at various compression rates and durations. American Journal of Physiology 1981; 241: H442–H448.
4. Idris AH. Reassessing the need for ventilation during CPR. Ann Emerg Med 1996; 27:569–75.
5. Babbs CF, Voorhees WD, Fitzgerald KR, Holmes HR, Geddes LA. Relationship of artificial cardiac output to chest compression amplitude—evidence for an effective compression threshold. Annals of Emergency Medicine 1983; 12:527–532.
6. Berg RA, Kern KB, Sanders AB, Otto CW, Hilwig RW, Ewy GA. Bystander cardiopulmonary resuscitation. Is ventilation necessary? Circulation 1993; 88:1907–15.
7. Berg RA, Wilcoxson D, Hilwig RW, et al. The need for ventilatory support during bystander CPR. Ann Emerg Med 1995; 26:342–50.
8. Berg RA, Kern KB, Hilwig RW, et al. Assisted ventilation does not improve outcome in a porcine model of single-rescuer bystander cardiopulmonary resuscitation. Circulation 1997; 95:1635–41.
9. Berg RA, Kern KB, Hilwig RW, Ewy GA. Assisted ventilation during 'bystander' CPR in a swine acute myocardial infarction model does not improve outcome. Circulation 1997; 96:4364–71.
10. Berg RA, Sanders AB, Kern KB, et al. Adverse hemodynamic effects of rescue breathing during CPR for VF cardiac arrest. Circulation 2001; 104:2465–2470.
11. Kern KB, Hilwig RW, Berg RA, Ewy GA. Efficacy of chest compression-only BLS CPR in the presence of an occluded airway. Resuscitation 1998; 39:179–88.
12. Kern KB. Cardiopulmonary resuscitation without ventilation. Crit Care Med 2000; 28:N186–9.
13. Wilson E, Brooks B, Tweed WA. CPR skills retention of lay basic rescuers. Ann Emerg Med 1983; 12:482–4.
14. Bircher N, Otto C, Babbs C, et al. Future directions for resuscitation research. II. External cardiopulmonary resuscitation basic life support. Resuscitation 1996; 32:63–75.
15. Handley JA, Handley AJ. Four-step CPR—improving skill retention. Resuscitation 1998; 36:3–8.
16. Mair P, Furtwaengler W, Baubin M. Aortic-valve function during cardiopulmonary resuscitation. New England Journal of Medicine 1993; 329:1965–1966.
17. Criley JM, Blaufuss AH, Kissel GL. Cough-induced cardiac compression—a self-administered form of cardiopulmonary resuscitation. JAMA 1976; 236:1246–1250.

18. Criley JM, Niemann JT, Rosborough JP, Ung S, Suzuki J. The heart is a conduit in CPR. Crit Care Med 1981; 9:373–374.
19. Rudikoff MT, Maughan WL, Effron M, Freund P, Weisfeldt ML. Mechanisms of blood flow during cardiopulmonary resuscitation. Circulation 1980; 61:345–352.
20. Weisfeldt ML. Physiology of cardiopulmonary resuscitation. Ann Rev Med 1981;435–442.
21. Feneley MP, Maier GW, Gaynor JW, et al. Sequence of mitral valve motion and transmitral blood flow during manual cardiopulmonary resuscitation in dogs. Circulation 1987; 76:363–375.
22. Gall F. Incompetence of the atrioventricular valves during cardiac massage, J Cardiovasc Surg 6, 1965.
23. Paradis NA, Martin GB, Goetting MG, et al. Simultaneous aortic, jugular bulb, and right atrial pressures during cardiopulmonary resuscitation in humans: Insights into mechanisms. Circulation 1989; 80: 361–368.
24. Chandra NC. Mechanisms of blood flow during CPR. Ann Emerg Med 1993; 22:281–288.
25. Beyar R, Kishon Y, Sideman S, Dinnar U. Computer studies of systemic and regional blood flow during cardiopulmonary resuscitation. Medical & Biological Engineering and Computing 1984; 22:499–506.
26. Babbs CF, Geddes LA. Effects of abdominal counterpulsation in CPR as demonstrated in a simple electrical model of the circulation. Annals of Emergency Medicine 1983; 12:247.
27. Babbs CF, Weaver JC, Ralston SH, Geddes LA. Cardiac, thoracic, and abdominal pump mechanisms in CPR: studies in an electrical model of the circulation. American Journal of Emergency Medicine 1984; 2:299–308.
28. Babbs CF, Ralston SH, Geddes LA. Theoretical advantages of abdominal counterpulsation in CPR as demonstrated in a simple electrical model of the circulation. Annals of Emergency Medicine 1984; 13:660–671.
29. Babbs CF, Thelander K. Theoretically optimal duty cycles for chest and abdominal compression during external cardiopulmonary resuscitation. Acad Emerg Med 1995; 2:698–707.
30. Babbs CF. CPR techniques that combine chest and abdominal compression and decompression: hemo-dynamic insights from a spreadsheet model. Circulation 1999; 100:2146–2152.
31. Maier GW, Newton JR, Wolfe JA, et al. The influence of manual chest compression rate on hemody-namic support during cardiac arrest: high-impulse cardiopulmonary resuscitation. Circulation 1986; 74(Suppl IV):IV-51–IV-59.
32. Maier GW, Tyson GS, Olsen CO, et al. The physiology of external cardiac massage: high-impulse cardiopulmonary resuscitation. Circulation 1984; 70:86–101.
33. Babbs CF. High-impulse compression CPR: simple mathematics points to future research. Academic Emergency Medicine 1994; 1:418–422.
34. Halperin HR, Tsitlik JE, Guerci AD, et al. Determinants of blood flow to vital organs during cardiop-ulmonary resuscitation in dogs. Circulation 1986; 73:539–550.
35. Halperin HR, Tsitlik JE, Beyar R, Chandra N, Guerci AD. Intrathoracic pressure fluctuations move blood during CPR: comparison of hemodynamic data with predictions from a mathematical model. Ann Biomed Eng 1987; 15:385–403.
36. Tucker KJ, Idris A. Clinical and laboratory investigations of active compression- decompression car-diopulmonary resuscitation. Resuscitation 1994; 28:1–7.
37. Tucker KJ, Khan JH, Savitt MA. Active compression-decompression resuscitation: effects on pulmo-nary ventilation. Resuscitation 1993; 26:125–31.
38. Babbs CF, Tacker WA. Cardiopulmonary resuscitation with interposed abdominal compression. Circu-lation 1986; 74(Suppl IV):37–41.
39. Babbs CF. Interposed abdominal compression-CPR: a case study in cardiac arrest research. Ann Emerg Med 1993; 22:24–32.
40. Einagle V, Bertrand F, Wise RA, Roussos C, Magder S. Interposed abdominal compressions and carotid blood flow during cardiopulmonary resuscitation. Support for a thoracoabdominal unit. Chest 1988; 93:1206–1212.
41. Sack JB, Kesselbrenner MB, Bregman D. Survival from in-hospital cardiac arrest with interposed abdominal counterpulsation during cardiopulmonary resuscitation. JAMA 1992; 267:379–385.
42. Sack JB, Kesselbrenner MB. Hemodynamics, survival benefits, and complications of interposed abdomi-nal compression during cardiopulmonary resuscitation. Acad Emerg Med 1994; 1:490–497.
43. DelGuercio L, Feins NR, Cohn JD, Coomaraswamy RP, Wollman SB, State D. Comparison of blood flow during external and internal cardiac massage in man. Circulation 1965; 31(Suppl I).
44. Redding JS, Cozine RA. A comparison of open chest and closed chest cardiac massage in dogs. Anes-thesiology 1961; 22:280–285.

45. Babbs CF. Hemodynamic mechanisms in CPR: a theoretical rationale for resuscitative thoracotomy in non-traumatic cardiac arrest. Resuscitation 1987; 15:37–50.
46. Weiser FM, Adler LN, Kuhn LA. Hemodynamic effects of closed and open chest cardiac resuscitation in normal dogs and those with acute myocardial infarction. Am J Cardiol 1962; 10:555–561.
47. Sanders AB, Kern KB, Ewy GA, Atlas M, Bailey L. Improved resuscitation from cardiac arrest with open chest massage. Annal Emerg Med 1984; 13:672–675.
48. Lurie KG, Coffeen P, Shultz J, McKnite S, Detloff B, Mulligan K. Improving active compression-decompression cardiopulmonary resuscitation with an inspiratory impedance valve. Circulation 1995; 91:1629–1632.
49. Lindner KH, Pfenninger EG, Lurie KG, Schurmann W, Lindner IM, Ahnefeld FW. Effects of active compression-decompression resuscitation on myocardial and cerebral blood flow in pigs. Circulation 1993; 88:1254–1263.
50. Lurie KG, Lindo C, Chin J. CPR: The P stands for plumber's helper. JAMA 1990; 264:1661.
51. Tang W, Weil MH, Schock RB, et al. Phased chest and abdominal compression-decompression. A new option for cardiopulmonary resuscitation. Circulation 1997; 95:1335–1340.
52. Cohen TJ, Tucker KJ, Lurie KG, et al. Active compression-decompression. A new method of cardiopulmonary resuscitation. JAMA 1992; 267:2916–2923.
53. Chang MW, Coffeen P, Lurie KG, Shultz J, Bache RJ, White CW. Active compression-decompression CPR improves vital organ perfusion in a dog model of ventricular fibrillation. Chest 1994; 106: 1250–1259.
54. Plaisance P, Lurie KG, Payen D. Inspiratory impedance during active compression-decompression cardiopulmonary resuscitation: a randomized evaluation in patients in cardiac arrest. Circulation 2000; 101:989–994.
55. Wik L, Naess PA, Ilebekk A, Nicolaysen G, Steen PA. Effects of various degrees of compression and active decompression on haemodynamics, end-tidal CO2, and ventilation during cardiopulmonary resuscitation of pigs. Resuscitation 1996; 31:45–57.
56. Sunde K, Wik L, Naess PA, Ilebekk A, Nicolaysen G, Steen PA. Effect of different compression—decompression cycles on haemodynamics during ACD-CPR in pigs. Resuscitation 1998; 36:123–131.
57. Cummins RO. Advanced Cardiac Life Support. Emergency Cardiovascular Care Programs. Dallas: American Heart Association, 1997.
58. Babbs CF, Thelander K. Theoretically optimal duty cycles for chest and abdominal compression during external cardiopulmonary resuscitation [see comments]. Acad Emerg Med 1995; 2:698–707.
59. Taylor GJ, Tucker WM, Greene HL, Rudikoff MT, Weisfeldt ML. Medical Intelligence—Importance of prolonged compression during cardiopulmonary resuscitation in man. N Engl J Med 1977; 296: 1515–1517.
60. Babbs CF, Blevins WE. Abdominal binding and counterpulsation in cardiopulmonary resuscitation. Critical Care Clinics 1986; 2:319–332.
61. Boe JM, Babbs CF. Mechanics of cardiopulmonary resuscitation performed with the patient on a soft bed vs a hard surface. Acad Emerg Med 1999; 6:754–757.
62. Locke CJ, Berg RA, Sanders AB, et al. Bystander cardiopulmonary resuscitation. Concerns about mouth-to-mouth contact. Arch Intern Med 1995; 155:938–943.
63. Becker LB, Berg RA, Pepe PE, et al. A reappraisal of mouth-to-mouth ventilation during bystander-initiated cardiopulmonary resuscitation. A statement for healthcare professionals from the Ventilation Working Group of the Basic Life Support and Pediatric Life Support Subcommittees, American Heart Association. Resuscitation 1997; 35:189–201.
64. Kern KB, Paraskos JA. 31st Bethesda Conference—Emergency Cardiac Care (1999). Journal of the American College of Cardiology 2000; 35:825–880.
65. Pearson JW, Redding JS. Influence of peripheral vascular tone on cardiac resuscitation. Anesth Analg 1965; 44:746–752.
66. Ralston SH, Voorhees WD, Babbs CF, Tacker WA. Regional blood flow and short term survival following prolonged CPR. Medical Instrumentation 1981; 15:326.
67. Redding JS. Abdominal compression in cardiopulmonary resuscitation. Anesthesia and Analgesia 1971; 50:668–675.
68. Chamberlain D, Smith A, Colquhoun M, Handley AJ, Kern KB, Wollard M. Randomized controlled trials of staged teaching for basic life support. 2. Comparison of CPR performance and skill retention using either staged instruction or conventional teaching. Resuscitation 2001; 50:27–37.
69. Assar D, Chamberlain D, Colquhoun M, et al. Randomised controlled trials of staged teaching for basic life support. 1. Skill acquisition at bronze stage. Resuscitation 2000; 45:7–15.

70. Babbs CF, Kern KB. Optimum compression to ventilation ratios in CPR under realistic, practical conditions: a physiological and mathematical analysis. Resuscitation 2002; 54:147–157.
71. Berg RA, Hilwig RW, Kern KB, Ewy GA. "Bystander" chest compressions and assisted ventilation independently improve outcome from piglet asphyxial pulseless "cardiac arrest." Circulation 2000; 101:1743–1748.
72. Noc M, Weil MH, Tang W, Turner T, Fukui M. Mechanical ventilation may not be essential for initial cardiopulmonary resuscitation. Chest 1995; 108:821–827.
73. Hallstrom A, Cobb L, Johnson E, Copass M. Cardiopulmonary resuscitation by chest compression alone or with mouth- to-mouth ventilation. N Engl J Med 2000; 342:1546–1553.

10   Alternate Cardiopulmonary Resuscitation Devices and Techniques

Henry Halperin, MD, MA
and Barry K. Rayburn, MD

INTRODUCTION

The standard technique of external chest compression in cardiopulmonary resuscitation (CPR) has changed little since the landmark paper of Kouwenhoven et al. in 1960 *(1)*. The rhythmic application of force to the body of the patient is fundamental to the process of generating blood flow in CPR, but there is little agreement regarding the optimal technique for applying that force. There is a great need for improved external chest compression techniques, because only an average of 15% of patients treated with standard CPR survive cardiac arrest (CA *[2,3]*), and it is widely agreed that increasing the blood flow generated by chest compression will improve survival. Given the potential importance of newer devices and techniques that may augment blood flow, this chapter will explore several alternate devices and techniques that have been studied.

PISTON CHEST COMPRESSION

According to the most recently published guidelines of the Emergency Cardiac Care Committee of the American Heart Association (AHA *[4]*), external chest compressions are applied by the rescuer who places the hands over the individual's sternum. Force is applied straight down with the elbows locked and the shoulders in line with the hands.

From: *Contemporary Cardiology: Cardiopulmonary Resuscitation*
Edited by: J. P. Ornato and M. A. Peberdy © Humana Press Inc., Totowa, NJ

The goal is to displace the sternum 1.5 to 2 inches for an average-sized adult, 100 times per minute, with compression maintained for 50% of each cycle. Unfortunately, compressions are often done incorrectly *(5,6)*, and incorrect chest compression can compromise survival *(7,8)*. One way of potentially improving the quality of chest compression is with mechanical devices, which can potentially apply compression more consistently than manually.

One such type of mechanical device uses a pneumatic piston (Fig. 1) to administer external chest compressions at a specified rate, compression depth, and duty cycle (percent of time compression is held during each cycle). The piston is located at the end of an arm that extends over the patient's chest, and is based on a board, which provides a firm surface under the patient's back. Additionally, a ventilation circuit is integrated into the device, which allows for continuous CPR with minimal operator input once the device is set up. Specific instructions for applying these devices are provided by the manufacturers and should be carefully followed. Although there are some differences between mechanical and manual external chest compression in the time course of application of force that may affect hemodynamics *(9,10)*, one small study showed no difference in survival using the two techniques *(10)*. Two additional small studies suggested a slight hemodynamic benefit to CPR performed by the pneumatic piston, one using end-tidal CO_2 as a surrogate measure for cardiac output *(11)* and the other showing a slight improvement in mean arterial pressure (25 vs 31 mmHg), although no statistical analysis was provided *(10)*. Despite these slight differences in hemodynamics, chest compression performed by a pneumatic device probably has the same physiology as manual chest compression and is generally considered an extension of the standard technique.

Trauma is the major complication from piston CPR. The reported incidence of trauma, as the result of piston CPR, can be as high as 65% *(12,13)*. The most frequent thoracic injuries, occurring more than 20% of the time, include chest abrasions or contusions, defibrillator burns, sternal and rib fractures, gastric dilation, and pulmonary edema. Even properly executed CPR can lead to injury.

Despite the substantial amount of trauma, however, the detrimental effects of trauma are unclear, because most research on the incidence of CPR-related trauma has focused on nonsurvivors of CPR, who might have died even if no trauma had occurred. Improvements in outcome may be achieved by external CPR techniques that improve blood flow; but such improvement has not been convincingly demonstrated for piston type devices. These devices do, however, allow CPR to be preformed in situations in which standard manual CPR would be difficult, such as in moving ambulances, and were personnel are limited.

SIMULTANEOUS COMPRESSION AND VENTILATION

Simultaneous compression and ventilation (SCV), as originally described, requires the subject to be intubated endotracheally or to have a tracheostomy *(14–16)*. Compressions are administered as with standard external chest compression, but at a slower rate (typically 40 compressions per minute). Instead of interposed ventilation between every fifth and sixth compression, ventilation to a high airway pressure (typically 60–100 mmHg) is performed synchronously with each compression. Some authors have modified this technique slightly, compressing at faster rates or adding an abdominal binder *(14,16,17)*. Most studies of this technique in both animal models and humans were performed using a mechanical compression device with an integrated system to deliver ventilation to the endotracheal tube.

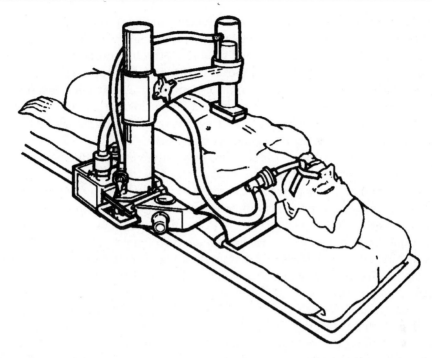

Fig. 1. Thumper PCR System (Model 1007), a piston device used for performing mechanical external chest compressions. (Courtesy of Michigan Instruments, Grand Rapids, MI.)

In 1967, Wilder et al. reported an increase in blood flow in dogs by using SVC and external chest compression at low airway pressures *(18)*. This phenomenon was left unexplained and largely unexplored, however, until the late 1970s when it was studied by a group of investigators at Johns Hopkins *(14,15)*, and subsequently by other groups *(17,19–21)*.

Physiology

SCV-CPR was a direct by-product of the theory that intrathoracic pressure fluctuations are responsible for blood movement during CPR. The assumption was that if blood flow is a result of fluctuations in intrathoracic pressure, then anything that makes those fluctuations larger should increase blood flow. Many authors went a step beyond this and added abdominal binding to the technique, assuming that binding the abdomen would restrict the motion of the diaphragm, and thus result in higher intrathoracic pressure for a given applied force.

Animal studies of the hemodynamics of SCV-CPR resulted in a number of observations that were unanticipated by the investigators, but ultimately led to an increased understanding of the determinants of blood flow during chest compressions. For example, when electromagnetic flow probes around the carotid artery were used as an estimate of cerebral blood flow *(16)*, administration of epinephrine resulted in a paradoxical decrease in carotid flow, despite an increase in cerebral perfusion pressure. This observation led investigators to seek alternative techniques for measuring cerebral blood flow and resulted in the routine use of radioactive microspheres during animal studies of CPR.

Such studies showed that carotid flow measurements in dogs estimate blood flow to the facial muscles and tongue, and not to the brain *(14)*. Brain flow was actually augmented by epinephrine, as was myocardial blood flow *(22)*. Another observation that resulted from animal studies of SCV-CPR was that excessively high airway pressures (100 mmHg) could cause carotid collapse, which can reduce blood flow *(22)*, and that negative airway pressure in between compressions, can augment blood flow *(16)*. Although not recognized at the time, this latter mechanism may be operative in other forms of CPR that induce negative intrathoracic pressure in between compressions.

Another somewhat surprising observation was that abdominal binding can actually reduce coronary perfusion pressure. The mechanism of this phenomenon remains incompletely understood, but it is probably the result of an alteration of the distribution of vascular compliance. During the compression phase of CPR, blood moves out of the thorax into a relatively compliant set of vessels, mostly in the abdomen. This blood is then readily available for redistribution to the thoracic vasculature to provide for coronary blood flow during the release phase. Abdominal binding seems to reduce this extrathoracic arterial compliance, thus reducing the amount of blood available for coronary perfusion.

In human studies of SCV-CPR, Chandra et al. reported an increase in radial artery pressure and carotid flow velocity in a hemodynamic study of 11 patients at the end of failed conventional resuscitation *(5)*. Martin et al. examined hemodynamics in five patients and found a decrease in coronary perfusion pressure with SCV-CPR *(21)*. These patients were very late in resuscitation, which may have adversely affected the outcome. A major clinical trial of SCV-CPR was reported by Krischer et al., in which 994 patients with out-of-hospital CA were treated with either SCV-CPR or standard CPR *(23)*. The ambulance crews, rather than the patients, were randomized, so that the crews knew which form of CPR was going to be administered prior to arrival at the scene of the arrest. The survival (to hospital admission) was greater with standard CPR than with SCV-CPR (26 vs 19%). Examination of a wide variety of variables failed to reveal any difference between the groups other than the CPR technique that was used. This study did utilize abdominal binding with the SCV-CPR. Abdominal binding was subsequently shown to have a deleterious effect on coronary perfusion. Because of the lack of significant resuscitation survival benefit in any study, there is little active research on this technique.

HIGH-IMPULSE EXTERNAL CHEST COMPRESSION

High-impulse external chest compression is performed by placing the hands in a position identical with that of standard external chest compression. The compression itself, however, is done at a higher rate (typically 120–150 per minute) and with a very quick, jabbing onset and offset. Ventilation is provided as with standard CPR, at a rate of 12 per minute.

Investigators at Duke University first proposed high-impulse chest compression as a replacement for standard external chest compressions in 1984 *(24)*. Despite one reference cited for rapid compressions from the 1890s, these authors were clearly the major force that brought this technique into the modern era of CPR research. High-impulse CPR became one of the focal points of the debate between the two schools of thought (direct cardiac compression vs intrathoracic pressure fluctuations) on the mechanism of blood flow in CPR *(9,24–32)*. Those investigations led to a significantly improved understanding of the physiology of blood movement during chest compression.

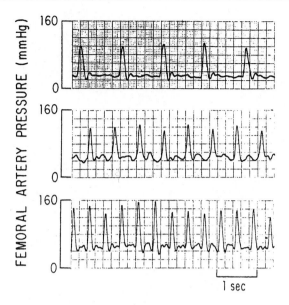

Fig. 2. Femoral artery pressure tracings from a patient undergoing CPR. The top tracing shows CPR at a rate of 60 per minute, the middle at 100 per minute, and the bottom at a rate of 150 per minute (high-impulse cardiopulmonary resuscitation). On each tracing, the amount of time spent in compression is comparable, so that there is a high percentage of the cycle in compression at the higher rates. (Reproduced from ref. *24*. Copyright 1984 American Heart Association.)

Physiology of Blood Flow During External Chest Compression

In studies of the physiology of blood flow during external chest compression in dogs, Maier et al. noted that increasing the rate of compressions resulted in increased cardiac output and increased coronary flow compared with slower rates *(24)*. Maier et al. showed that stroke volume stayed constant and cardiac output rose. Coronary blood flow tended to be higher, although not significantly, at a compression rate of 150 per minute vs 60 per minute *(24)*. These data were interpreted as showing that direct cardiac compression was the predominant mechanism of blood flow, because stroke volume was constant for each compression, and cardiac output rose at higher rates as more stroke volumes were delivered per unit time. The investigators attempted to control compression force by measuring intrapleural pressure with micromanometers in the intrapleural space. This was one of the two major criticisms of the work because measurements of intrapleural pressure are difficult and often inaccurate. Nevertheless, Maier et al. did achieve the same reading in a given animal for each compression rate.

The second major criticism is illustrated in Fig. 2; a variable not controlled by the investigators in these initial studies was the compression duration, or the percent of the compression–decompression cycle during which compression occurs. At low compression rates, the duration of compression appeared to be approx 20% of the cycle; at high rates, it was much closer to 50%, the currently recommended standard. This provided a potential mechanism for the increase in cardiac output, even if an intrathoracic pump mechanism was operative, because compression duration does affect blood flow in the intrathoracic pump model. Subsequent animal studies examined survival differences

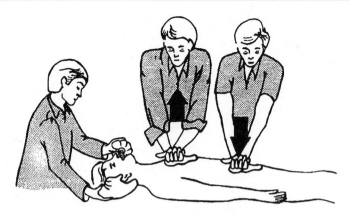

Fig. 3. Interposed abdominal compression cardiopulmonary resuscitation with three rescuers. The arrows depict how one rescuer pushes as the other relaxes. (From ref. *53*. Copyright 1992, American Medical Association.)

between high-impulse external chest compression and standard CPR. Kern et al. found no difference in 24-hour survival between a group receiving standard external chest compression and a group receiving high-impulse CPR *(33)*. A later study by Feneley et al. did show improved survival in a group of animals receiving high-impulse CPR compared with standard manual CPR *(32)*. In this latter study, the authors attempted to control for duty cycle between the two groups. Compression force was not quantitatively reported, however, and pressures generated in the control group were substantially lower than in other studies of standard external compression done by the same research group *(24)*.

A number of case-report type studies of high-impulse CPR have been published *(24,34)*. Minimal quantitative analysis of these data are available, however, and no controlled trials of standard vs high-impulse CPR in humans have been reported.

Applicability of High-Impulse CPR

High-impulse CPR requires little more than an alteration in training from that in standard external chest compression. None of the data reported for high-impulse CPR, however, provide convincing evidence that this technique would provide substantial benefit over standard CPR in the general population. There may be subsets of patients in whom the jabbing chest compressions of high-impulse CPR are beneficial. These chest compressions may alter airway mechanics in these patients to produce higher intrathoracic pressure, or alternatively, may enhance cardiac compression. If these groups can be identified, it is conceivable that high-impulse CPR could provide a hemodynamic benefit over standard external chest compression.

INTERPOSED ABDOMINAL COMPRESSION

Interposed abdominal compression (IAC)-CPR (or abdominal counterpulsation CPR) includes an additional rescuer (for a total of two or three) positioned alongside or opposite the rescuer applying chest compressions in the standard fashion. This additional rescuer places his or her hands on the abdomen, usually near the umbilicus, and compresses the abdomen during the relaxation phase of chest compression (Fig. 3).

The ratio of abdominal-to-chest compressions is one to one, so the rate of abdominal compressions is is also 100 per minute. Some authors place a blood pressure cuff or another measuring device between the hands and the abdominal wall in order to measure the amount of force applied to the abdomen. Exact guidelines regarding how much to compress the abdomen, or how much force to apply if measured, have not been proposed. In studies of this technique, the forces measured from air-filled measuring devices have ranged from 20 to 150 mmHg. Most authors describe abdominal compression as lasting through the entire release phase of chest compression, resulting in a 50% compression duration for each.

Ohomoto et al. first published a description of interposed abdominal compression using a mechanical device with two pistons (one for the chest, one for the abdomen) in 1976 *(35)*. Since that time, there has been ongoing and extensive research into this method *(33,36–59)*.

Physiology of IAC-CPR

IAC-CPR may improve blood flow in CPR by a number of mechanisms. First and foremost, IAC-CPR may act in a fashion analogous with intra-aortic balloon pumping, in which abdominal and aortic compressions would result in greater retrograde aortic flow into the chest and greater aortic pressure between chest compressions, with greater coronary flow and survival. Second, abdominal pressure by itself increases intrathoracic pressure, even without chest compression. Interposed abdominal compression could therefore either (a) optimize the duration of the rise in intrathoracic pressure, because durations of compression longer than those usually present during manual CPR are known to improve flow or (b) increase the rise of intrathoracic pressure as a result of moving the diaphragm and abdominal contents upward. Additionally, during the diastolic phase (i.e., relaxation of chest compression), compression of the abdomen "charges" the intrathoracic compliance in preparation for the next chest-compression cycle. This coincides with work in our laboratory that shows, in a model of the canine circulation, that an intrathoracic pump would be optimized by minimizing the compliance of the vessels inside the thorax and maximizing the compliance of vessels in the abdomen during compression. During the relaxation phase, this extrathoracic compliance would then discharge into the intrathoracic vessels, thus maintaining myocardial blood flow during diastole. Of potential concern is that compression of the abdomen during the relaxation phase of chest compression can raise the pressure inside the thorax, because the abdominal and thoracic compartments are contiguous. This rise in intrathoracic pressure could raise right atrial and aortic pressures to an equal extent, which could actually decrease coronary perfusion pressure *(22)*. A pressure waveform during IAC-CPR is shown in Fig. 4.

Ralston et al. compared standard CPR with mechanical (Piston) external chest compression, with and without the addition of IAC *(20)*. Ralston et al. showed that with no other changes in the technique, the addition of IAC increased cardiac output, and systolic and diastolic arterial pressures in 10 dogs. Eight of the 10 dogs had an increase in the arteriovenous difference (myocardial perfusion pressure). Walker et al. *(60)*, Voorhees et al. *(61)*, and Einagle et al. *(58)* all demonstrated an increase in either brain or carotid blood flow with IAC-CPR. Despite the similarity of conclusions among these studies, however, these data are somewhat difficult to interpret. Studies by Walker and Voorhees and colleagues do show a statistically significant increase in brain blood flow vs standard CPR, but in the study by Voorhees et al., this difference is physiologically trivial (0.03 mL per minute per gram).

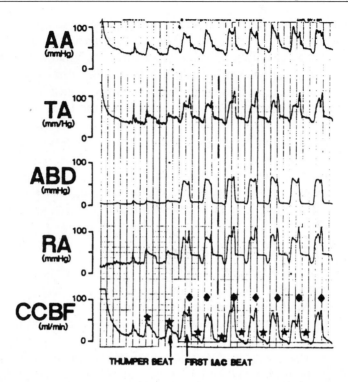

Fig. 4. Hemodynamic tracings in a dog undergoing cardiopulmonary resuscitation (CPR). Beginning at the second arrow on the bottom, mechanical CPR was augmented by interposed abdominal compression-CPR. Abdominal aorta (AA), thoracic aorta (TA), intra-abdominal (ABD), and right atrial (RA) pressures, along with carotid blood flow (CCBF) are shown. (From ref. *58*.)

Alternatively, the study by Walker et al. showed a substantial increase in brain blood flow (0.21 mL per minute per gram), but had extremely low brain blood flow in the standard CPR group, raising concern about the quality of the standard CPR. Of note, no study looking at myocardial blood flow showed a statistically significant difference between standard CPR and IAC-CPR. Kern et al. studied 24-hour survival in a dog model of CA comparing standard external chest compression, IAC-CPR, and high-impulse CPR and found no difference among the groups.

Several trials have looked at human hemodynamics or survival with IAC-CPR. Studies by Berryman and Phillips *(57)* and Howard et al. *(62)* at the end of conventional resuscitation showed an increase in mean arterial pressure with the addition of IAC-CPR. Despite these increases, Howard et al. did not find a significant difference in the myocardial perfusion pressure. Berryman and Phillips reported this information in only a single patient in whom it was increased. McDonald *(63)* reported on six patients, also late in resuscitation, in whom there was no difference in any measured variable with the addition of IAC. Mateer et al. *(56)* described a large field trial of IAC-CPR conducted by paramedics in Milwaukee: no difference in initial resuscitation was found after randomizing medical arrest patients to either standard external chest compression or IAC-CPR after intubation. In an in-hospital trial of IAC-CPR, Sack et al. *(53)* reported the results of 135 resuscitation attempts in 103 patients who had been randomized on admission to the hospital to receive either IAC-CPR or standard CPR should they arrest. In this study, Mateer et al. reported an increase in initial resuscitation (51 vs 27%), discharge from the hospital (25 vs 7%), and discharge neurologically intact (17 vs 6%) with IAC-CPR. Conducting this type of randomized trial in a hospitalized setting is in itself a considerable accomplishment. Obviously, a CPR trial cannot be a blind study, and this is one of the self-criticisms mentioned by the investigators. Additionally, no attempt was made to control for the force of sternal compression used in either group, which may account in part for the rather marked difference seen in this study. Of greater concern is the relatively low survival rate of the standard CPR group. Only 7% of these patients survived to hospital discharge, which is roughly half the survival-to-discharge rate typically reported by large studies of CPR in hospitalized patients. Again this may reflect a subtle difference in the standard CPR technique utilized during the study, or may reflect some bias in the group of patients included in the study. In a follow-up study of 143 hospitalized patients with either pulseless electrical activity or asystole, the same group demonstrated improved initial resuscitation and 24-hour survival with IAC-CPR compared with standard CPR *(52)*. Survival-to-hospital discharge was not an endpoint in this study, although the investigators noted that no patients survived to discharge neurologically intact. These results from a technique that is easy to apply should encourage ongoing investigation.

Although the incidence of abdominal trauma could be increased with IAC-CPR, specific data are limited. Kern et al. in one trial compared three methods of manually applied CPR, including IAC-CPR, and noted no difference in the incidence of trauma with the addition of abdominal counterpulsations *(33)*. In their most recent study, Sack et al. noted no clinically obvious difference in abdominal trauma between the groups, and none of the five IAC-CPR patients who underwent autopsy had any abdominal trauma *(52)*.

Applicability of IAC-CPR

IAC-CPR requires at least two rescuers. Beyond this requirement, it is a manually applied technique that requires no specialized equipment. The ability of rescuers in general to perform the technique correctly has not been determined. Hemodynamic data in humans are less convincing than those in animals, although this may reflect a limited ability to look at brain blood flow in humans. If IAC-CPR does improve brain perfusion as suggested by animal models, then it may well have clinical utility. Provided that it does not adversely affect the myocardial perfusion and therefore the chances of establishing return of spontaneous circulation, additional brain blood flow may improve the neurologic outcome of those patients who do survive resuscitation. The study reported by Sack et al., despite its limitations, may address these facts *(53)*. They showed a survival-to-hospital discharge of 25%, which is higher than historical controls, suggesting a benefit over standard CPR. Larger trials of IAC-CPR will be needed, however, before its true clinical utility can be determined.

ACTIVE COMPRESSION–DECOMPRESSION CPR

In this technique, CPR is applied by using a compression device (either manual or mechanical) with an integral suction cup (Fig. 5). The suction cup allows for active decompression of the chest between compressions. Investigators studying this technique have used standard guidelines for the rate and duration of compressions. The decompression phase actively returns the chest wall to its expanded position without breaking contact. In human studies, ventilation has been performed according to the usual guidelines,

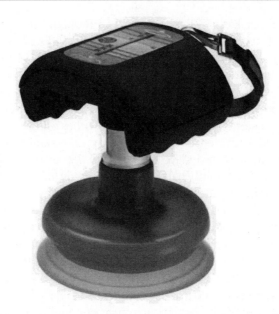

Fig. 5. Device for performing active compression–decompression cardiopulmonary resuscitation. The upper part is a hand and the lower part is a suction cup. (Courtesy of AMBU corporation.)

but some animal studies have omitted ventilation except that caused by the compression–decompression itself.

Active compression–decompression (ACD)-CPR research began with a report of an elderly man resuscitated by his uninitiated son with a bathroom plunger *(64)*. Lurie et al. at the University of California at San Francisco then began active research into the technique in both humans and an animal model. A device to perform ACD-CPR was developed by Ambu International (Copenhagen, Denmark) and other investigators have now begun to study this technique.

Physiology of ACD-CPR

ACD-CPR likely works in a fashion not dissimilar from IAC-CPR in which the active decompressions serve to prime the intrathoracic pump mechanism *(49,50,65,66)*. The active decompressions could result in greater chest expansion and filling with air between compressions, so that the next compression results in a greater rise in intrathoracic pressure and greater flow. A greater rise in intrathoracic pressure could be mediated through increased trapping of air in the lungs *(28)*, or simply increased application of force. Of note, chest compression force has not been measured in control groups undergoing standard manual CPR. Even if the peak compression forces used during active-decompression CPR and standard CPR were comparable, it would still not be known whether the reported benefit for active-decompression CPR results from the active decompressions, or from the increased force change (peak compression-to-peak decompression force) applied. For example, if 400 N compression force and 100 N decompression force were applied to the chest, is it equivalent simply to applying 500 N of compression force, or does the decompression force have unique physiological effects that improve blood flow?

The active decompressions could produce negative intrathoracic pressure between compressions and greater venous return, even without increasing the right atrial pressure relative to aortic pressure, which would impede coronary flow. Alternatively, there may be better right heart flow into the pulmonary bed between compressions. Additionally, the design of the device used for ACD-CPR results in the potential for a mechanism in the application of compression force that is slightly different from that in conventional CPR. In standard external chest compression, the hands never lose contact with the thorax, and therefore the onset of application of force is gradual. The ACD-CPR device provides an air space of a few inches between the location of the hands and the chest wall. This allows some acceleration to take place before the force of compression actually reaches the chest, resulting in a slight impact on the chest wall. The significance of this regarding the physiology of ACD-CPR is unknown. Studies reported to date have not resolved these issues. One study in pigs showed, in the absence of vasoconstrictors, increased coronary blood flow for active-decompression CPR for a standardized amount of chest compression from a mechanical chest compressor (67). Nevertheless, that same study showed no difference in coronary flow when vasoconstrictors were used.

A number of clinical trials have been reported with ACD-CPR. In the first clinical study, it was reported that 18 of 29 (62%) patients treated with active-decompression CPR had return of spontaneous circulation, compared with 10 of 33 (30%) patients treated with standard CPR. A number of larger clinical trials have been reported since that time. Most of the trials have shown no difference in survival for patients treated with standard CPR or ACD-CPR (68–72).

In one trial in Paris, France of 512 patients (73), there was an improvement is survival (ACD vs standard CPR) at 1 hour (36.6 vs 24.8%, $p = 0.003$, 24 hours (26 vs 13.6%, $p = 0.002$), and at hospital discharge (5.5 vs 1.9%, $p = 0.03$). Mean times from collapse to basic cardiac life support CPR was 9 minutes and from collapse to ACLS CPR was 21 minutes. A more recent report of 750 patients from that latter group showed that survival was also improved at 1 year (5 vs 2%, $p = 0.03$ [74]). All patients who survived to 1 year had CAs that were witnessed.

It is unclear why most trials showed no benefit for ACD-CPR over standard CPR, and that there was a statistically significant, albeit small, benefit in Paris. It has been speculated that ACD-CPR may be of more benefit if administered relatively late in the course of CA, as was done in Paris, and that the level of training and retraining is important.

There is a possibility that the high velocity of impact of the device at the start of chest compression could cause additional trauma as compared to conventional chest compressions (75,76). Additionally, the increased chest excursions produced by the active decompressions could cause increased flexing of the ribs, and increased trauma.

Applicability of ACD-CPR

ACD-CPR shares the advantages of all manual techniques in that it is readily applied in a wide variety of circumstances. The device required to perform this technique could be made widely available should it prove significantly beneficial. The technique itself is not appreciably more difficult than standard external chest compression, although it may prove substantially more tiring, given that the rescuer is required to be active during both phases (compression and decompression) of each cycle (77). The disadvantages of manual devices, however, are that an operator can perform the compressions incorrectly and chest compression must be interrupted for defibrillation.

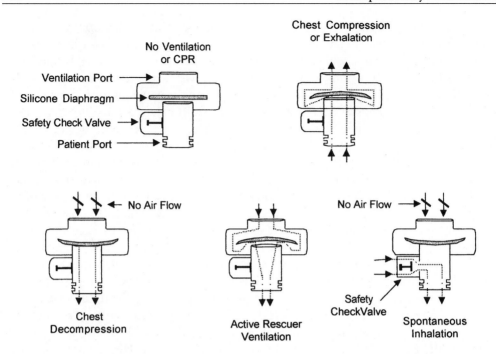

Fig. 6. Schematic diagram of impedance threshold valve. The components of the valve are shown on the upper left panel. During chest compression or exhalation(upper right panel) air moves freely through the valve. During chest decompression (lower left panel) airflow is impeded by the valve to increase the level of negative intrathoracic pressure generated. During rescuer ventilation or spontaneous inhalation (lower middle and right panels) air also moves freely through the valve. (From ref. *78.*)

IMPEDANCE THRESHOLD VALVE

The impedance threshold valve is a device placed in the airway circuit to impede the flow of air into the chest during chest decompression (Fig. 6). Its goal is to increase the level of negative intrathoracic pressure generated during chest decompression, and thereby augment the beneficial effects of that negative intrathoracic pressure.

The impedance threshold valve has been studied with standard CPR *(78)* in a porcine model of CA. Microsphere-measured myocardiac blood flow was higher with the use of the impedance threshold valve (0.32 ± 0.04 vs 0.23 ± 0.03 mL per minute per gram, $p < 0.05$), as was cerebral blood flow (0.23 ± 0.02 vs 0.19 ± 0.02; $p < 0.05$).

The impedance threshold valve has been studied most in conjunction with active compression decompression cardiopulmonary resuscitation *(79–81)*. In a prospective, randomized, blinded trial performed in Paris, France, patients in nontraumatic CA received ACD-CPR plus the valve or ACD-CPR alone for 30 minutes during advanced cardiac life support *(80)*. With the use of the impedance threshold valve there were increases in end-tidal carbon dioxide pressure (19.1 ± 1.0 vs 13.1 ± 0.9 mmHg, $p < 0.001$), diastolic blood pressure (56.4 ± 1.7 vs 36.5 ± 1.5 mmHg, $p < 0.001$), and coronary perfusion pressure (43.3 ± 1.6 vs 25.0 ± 1.4 mmHg, $p < 0.001$). Blood pressure results are shown in Fig. 7. Additionally, return of spontaneous circulation was observed in 2 of 10 patients with ACD-CPR alone after 26.5 ± 0.7 minutes vs 4 of 11 patients with ACD-CPR plus the impedance threshold valve after 19.8 ± 2.8 minutes ($p < 0.05$).

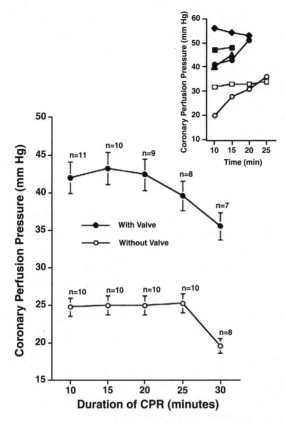

Fig. 7. Coronary perfusion pressures in patients during active compression–decompression cardiopulmonary resuscitation without (lower tracing) and with (upper tracing) the use of the impedance threshold valve. (From ref. *80.*)

The results with the impedance threshold valve are very promising. Further studies are needed to determine if the valve can be used successfully in larger studies of CA, and if the time needed to apply the valve does not seriously impact on its efficacy in general CA patients.

PHASED CHEST AND ABDOMINAL COMPRESSION

A mechanical device is being developed that allows for active compression and decompression of the chest as well as for active compression and decompression of the abdomen. The device consists of two adhesive pads that are connected to a mechanical linkage. The pads are attached to the chest and abdomen, respective. The linkage has two handles that are held by the rescuer. The rescuer pushes or pulls on the chest handle to compress or decompress the chest, and alternately pushes or pulls on the abdominal handle to compress or decompress the abdomen.

Laboratory studies of phased chest and abdominal compression has shown an increase in coronary perfusion pressure, as well as an increase in the number of animal resuscitated over that with standard CPR *(82)*. Kern studied different types of ventilation, and showed that the type of ventilation could seriously impact on the hemodynamics produced by this type of resuscitation *(83)*.

In a clinical study of phased chest and abdominal compression CPR, 54 patients were studied *(84)*. More patients treated with standard CPR survived to hospital discharge (7 vs 0), but fewer patient treated with phased chest and abdominal compression has significant trauma at autopsy.

Because there are only small studies of phased chest and abdominal compression, further studies are needed to determine if this devices will be useful in the treatment of CA victims.

VEST CARDIOPULMONARY RESUSCITATION

With vest CPR, a bladder-containing vest (analogous to a large blood pressure cuff) is placed circumferentially around the patient's chest (Fig. 8) and cyclically inflated and deflated by an automated pneumatic system. In this manner, the chest is compressed cyclically. The device permits control of rate, compression duration, and inflation pressure. The vest also maintains a small amount of positive pressure on the chest between compressions to keep the vest snugly against the chest, except during the built-in pause for ventilation, at which time the vest completely deflates. The vest is generally inflated to a pressure of approx 250 mmHg, 60 times per minute, with 40 to 50% of each cycle in compression. Adherent defibrillation pads are placed on the chest before applying the vest to allow for defibrillation without having to remove the vest or interrupt CPR.

As with SCV-CPR, vest CPR was developed as a means for augmenting intrathoracic pressure over that which could be produced by standard CPR. Vest CPR was largely developed by a group of investigators at Johns Hopkins University *(25,28,85–94)*, although other groups also made contributions *(34,95–103)*.

Physiology of Vest CPR

Vest CPR is designed to maximize the intrathoracic pressure rises generated for a given force applied to the chest. By encircling the chest (Fig. 8), force can be applied evenly, thus resulting in a large decrement in the volume of the chest with minimal displacement of an individual point on the chest wall. This circumferential compression allows for large increases in intrathoracic pressure without the trauma inherent in applying force to a single point, as with standard chest compression.

Many generations of vest CPR systems have been developed and tested. Studies with an early vest device reported by Luce et al. in 1983 and 1984 showed that hemodynamics in a dog model of CPR were only minimally if at all improved with vest CPR compared with mechanically performed standard external chest compression *(102,103)*. Niemann et al. *(100)* and Halperin et al. *(85)* used an improved system and showed augmentation of perfusion pressures and blood flows with vest CPR either with or without simultaneous ventilation. In the study by Halperin's group, survival was also better in the group of dogs receiving vest CPR. At high vest pressures, they produced myocardial and brain blood flows equivalent to that in control animals, although they noted some trauma. At somewhat lower vest pressures, myocardial blood flow was 40% of pre-arrest flow, and cerebral blood flow was essentially equal to pre-arrest flow, with no trauma. These latter flows were greater than had been reported previously with standard external chest compression by any author.

Swenson et al. reported a study of vest CPR in 10 patients late in CA *(34)*; they found no improvement in coronary perfusion pressure produced with that vest CPR system.

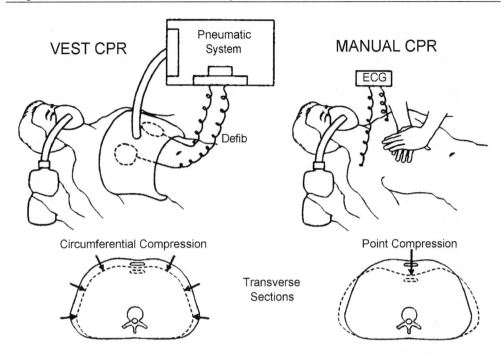

Fig. 8. Comparison of vest cardiopulmonary resuscitation (CPR) and manual CPR. The vest is like a large blood pressure cuff that encircles the chest. A pneumatic system inflates and deflates the vest to compress and release the chest. Flat defibrillator (defib) pads can be placed beneath the vest so that defibrillation can be performed during compressions. The vest compresses most of the circumference of the chest (lower panels), compared with a point compression of standard CPR. (From ref. *88*. Copyright 1993, *New England Journal of Medicine*.)

Halperin et al. subsequently reported a two-phase study of vest CPR using an improved vest CPR system, which incorporated a vest that covered more of the chest than previous systems *(88)*. This system also included a small positive pressure on the chest in between compressions to keep the vest tight against the chest. With the improved vest CPR system, hemodynamics in humans were significantly improved over those of standard external chest compression. Peak aortic pressure was nearly doubled (up to an average of 138 mmHg), and coronary perfusion pressure increased by 50%. A hemodynamic tracing during manual and vest CPR in a patient is shown in Fig. 9. Additionally, 4 of the 29 patients had return of spontaneous circulation during vest CPR despite being late (50 ± 22 minutes) in resuscitation. The second phase of the study randomized patients to either vest CPR or standard external chest compression after initial (11 ± 4 minutes) advanced cardiac life support failed to resuscitate the patients. There was a trend toward improved initial resuscitation in the vest CPR group, but the trial was too small to show a statistically significant benefit. These data formed the basis for a large-scale randomized trial of vest CPR immediately after CA, which is ongoing.

If the vest is applied below the desired thoracic region, increased abdominal trauma could be expected. The vest does not, however, appear to increase the incidence of trauma over that of manual CPR *(88)*, although only limited data are available.

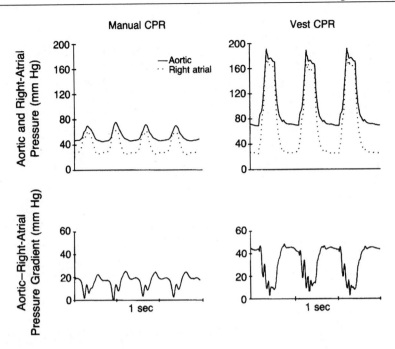

Fig. 9. Hemodynamic tracing during vest and manual cardiopulmonary resuscitation. Aortic, right atrial, and aortic minus right atrial pressures are shown. (From ref. *88.* Copyright 1993, *New England Journal of Medicine.*)

Applicability of Vest CPR

Vest CPR requires a sophisticated device for its administration, which limits its use to locations in which the device would be readily available, although a portable device may be developed. Application of the vest itself is not difficult and can be performed successfully by nurses, given only a few minutes instruction in its use. It is likely that if vest CPR proves successful in improving survival from CA, it will remain predominantly in the hands of health care professionals. It will serve as a supplement, therefore, to the best form of standard CPR available for out-of-hospital arrests. Both animal and human data show rather dramatic improvements in hemodynamics with vest CPR. If vest CPR can routinely raise the coronary perfusion gradient above the threshold required for late defibrillation to be successful, then it could make a measurable impact on the ability to achieve return of spontaneous circulation. Until sufficient human studies are done, however, we will not know whether or not this will result in improved long-term survival and neurologic recovery.

THE FUTURE

Research aimed at improving survival from CA both in- and out-of-hospital continues. The first 40 years of external chest compression have been marked by enthusiasm, disappointment, innovation, and speculation, but to date no technique has convincingly positioned itself to replace standard CPR as we now know it. Research has contributed a great deal to the science of CPR and set the stage for real advancement in the resuscitation of CA victims. The critical importance of early defibrillation is now clearly recognized. Likewise, the criteria used to judge a new CPR method have been defined.

These measures—coronary perfusion pressure (important in predicting return of spontaneous circulation), systolic arterial pressure (predictive of cerebral blood flow and likely of neurologic recovery), and ultimately survival-to-hospital discharge—will drive the search for the best method or methods of applying force to the human body over the next several years. The future may not lie so much in a replacement of current CPR as in evolution to differing types of CPR under different circumstances. Resuscitation initiated by lay persons will by necessity remain a manual technique, but some other form of CPR may be used once qualified rescuers are on the scene. Currently, the distinction between basic and advanced life support involves the availability of drugs, mechanical airways, and defibrillation. It is very possible that the form of CPR utilized may also become part of this distinction.

NOTE

The authors and the Johns Hopkins University hold equity in a commercial entity that has licensed vest and band CPR technology. Under the University Equity Policy, the equity is being held in escrow until a trigger date occurs.

REFERENCES

1. Kouwenhoven WB, Jude JR, Knickerbocker GG. Closed chest cardiac massage. JAMA 1960; 173: 1064–1067.
2. Schneider AP, II, Nelson DJ, Brown DD. In-hospital cardiopulmonary resuscitation: a 30-year review. J Am Board Fam Pract 1993; 6:91–101.
3. Tunstall-Pedoe H, Bailey L, Chamberlain DA, Marsden AK, Ward ME, Zideman DA. Survey of 3765 cardiopulmonary resuscitations in British hospitals (the BRESUS Study): methods and overall results. BMJ 1992; 304:1347–1351.
4. Guidelines 2000 for Cardiopulmonary Resuscitation and Emergency Cardiovascular Care. Part 3: adult basic life support. The American Heart Association in collaboration with the International Liaison Committee on Resuscitation. Circulation. 2000; 102:I22–I59.
5. Ochoa FJ, Ramalle-Gomara E, Lisa V, Saralegui I. The effect of rescuer fatigue on the quality of chest compressions. Resuscitation 1998; 37:149–152.
6. Hightower D, Thomas SH, Stone CK, Dunn K, March JA. Decay in quality of closed-chest compressions over time. Ann Emerg Med 1995; 26:300–303.
7. Gallagher EJ, Lombardi G, Gennis P. Effectiveness of bystander cardiopulmonary resuscitation and survival following out-of-hospital cardiac arrest. JAMA 1995; 274:1922–1925.
8. Van Hoeyweghen RJ, Bossaert LL, Mullie A, et al. Quality and efficiency of bystander CPR. Belgian Cerebral Resuscitation Study Group. Resuscitation 1993; 26:47–52.
9. Newton JR, Jr., Glower DD, Wolfe JA, et al. A physiologic comparison of external cardiac massage techniques. J Thorac Cardiovasc Surg 1988; 95:892–901.
10. McDonald JL. Systolic and mean arterial pressures during manual and mechanical CPR in humans. Ann Emerg Med 1982; 11:292–295.
11. Ward KR, Menegazzi JJ, Zelenak RR, Sullivan RJ, McSwain NE, Jr. A comparison of chest compressions between mechanical and manual CPR by monitoring end-tidal PCO_2 during human cardiac arrest. Ann Emerg Med 1993; 22:669–674.
12. Nagel EL, Fine EG, Krischer JP, Davis JH. Complications of CPR. Crit Care Med 1981; 9:424.
13. Krischer JP, Fine EG, Davis JH, Nagel EL. Complications of cardiac resuscitation. Chest 1987; 92:287–291.
14. Koehler RC, Chandra N, Guerci AD, et al. Augmentation of cerebral perfusion by simultaneous chest compression and lung inflation with abdominal binding after cardiac arrest in dogs. Circulation 1983; 67:266–275.
15. Chandra N, Rudikoff M, Weisfeldt ML. Simultaneous chest compression and ventilation at high airway pressure during cardiopulmonary resuscitation. Lancet 1980; 1:175–178.
16. Chandra N, Weisfeldt ML, Tsitlik J, et al. Augmentation of carotid flow during cardiopulmonary resuscitation by ventilation at high airway pressure simultaneous with chest compression. Am J Cardiol 1981; 48:1053–1063.

17. Sanders AB, Ewy GA, Alferness CA, Taft T, Zimmerman M. Failure of one method of simultaneous chest compression, ventilation, and abdominal binding during CPR. Crit Care Med 1982; 10:509–513.

18. Wilder R, Weir D, Rush BF, Ravitch MM. Method of coordinating ventilation and closed chest massage in the dog. Surgery 1963; 53:186–194.

19. Kern KB, Carter AB, Showen RL, et al. Comparison of mechanical techniques of cardiopulmonary resuscitation: survival and neurologic outcome in dogs. Am J Emerg Med 1987; 5:190–195.

20. Ralston SH, Babbs CF, Niebauer MJ. Cardiopulmonary resuscitation with interposed abdominal compression in dogs. Anesth Analg 1982; 61:645–651.

21. Martin GB, Carden DL, Nowak RM, Lewinter JR, Johnston W, Tomlanovich MC. Aortic and right atrial pressures during standard and simultaneous compression and ventilation CPR in human beings. Ann Emerg Med 1986; 15:125–130.

22. Michael JR, Guerci AD, Koehler RC, et al. Mechanisms by which epinephrine augments cerebral and myocardial perfusion during cardiopulmonary resuscitation in dogs. Circulation 1984; 69:822–835.

23. Krischer JP, Fine EG, Weisfeldt ML, Guerci AD, Nagel E, Chandra N. Comparison of prehospital conventional and simultaneous compression-ventilation cardiopulmonary resuscitation. Crit Care Med 1989; 17:1263–1269.

24. Maier GW, Tyson GS, Jr., Olsen CO, et al. The physiology of external cardiac massage: high-impulse cardiopulmonary resuscitation. Circulation 1984; 70:86–101.

25. Halperin HR, Tsitlik JE, Guerci AD, et al. Determinants of blood flow to vital organs during cardiopulmonary resuscitation in dogs. Circulation 1986; 73:539–550.

26. Halperin HR, Tsitlik JE, Beyar R, Chandra N, Guerci AD. Intrathoracic pressure fluctuations move blood during CPR: comparison of hemodynamic data with predictions from a mathematical model. Ann Biomed Eng 1987; 15:385–403.

27. Halperin HR, Weiss JL, Guerci AD, et al. Cyclic elevation of intrathoracic pressure can close the mitral valve during cardiac arrest in dogs. Circulation 1988; 78:754–760.

28. Halperin HR, Brower R, Weisfeldt ML, et al. Air trapping in the lungs during cardiopulmonary resuscitation in dogs. A mechanism for generating changes in intrathoracic pressure. Circ Res 1989; 65:946–954.

29. Maier GW, Newton JR, Jr., Wolfe JA, et al. The influence of manual chest compression rate on hemodynamic support during cardiac arrest: high-impulse cardiopulmonary resuscitation. Circulation 1986; 74:IV51–IV59.

30. Feneley MP, Maier GW, Gaynor JW, et al. Sequence of mitral valve motion and transmitral blood flow during manual cardiopulmonary resuscitation in dogs. Circulation 1987; 76:363–375.

31. Wolfe JA, Maier GW, Newton JR, Jr., et al. Physiologic determinants of coronary blood flow during external cardiac massage. J Thorac Cardiovasc Surg 1988; 95:523–532.

32. Feneley MP, Maier GW, Kern KB, et al. Influence of compression rate on initial success of resuscitation and 24 hour survival after prolonged manual cardiopulmonary resuscitation in dogs. Circulation 1988; 77:240–250.

33. Kern KB, Carter AB, Showen RL, et al. CPR-induced trauma: comparison of three manual methods in an experimental model. Ann Emerg Med 1986; 15:674–679.

34. Swenson RD, Weaver WD, Niskanen RA, Martin J, Dahlberg S. Hemodynamics in humans during conventional and experimental methods of cardiopulmonary resuscitation. Circulation 1988; 78:630–639.

35. Ohomoto T, Miura I, Konno S. A new method of external cardiac massage to improve diastolic augmentation and prolong survival time. Ann Thorac Surg 1976; 21:284–290.

36. Badylak SF, Kern KB, Tacker WA, Ewy GA, Janas W, Carter A. The comparative pathology of open chest vs. mechanical closed chest cardiopulmonary resuscitation in dogs. Resuscitation 1986; 13:249–264.

37. Babbs CF, Ralston SH, Geddes LA. Theoretical advantages of abdominal counterpulsation in CPR as demonstrated in a simple electrical model of the circulation. Ann Emerg Med 1984; 13:660–671.

38. Babbs CF, Weaver JC, Ralston SH, Geddes LA. Cardiac, thoracic, and abdominal pump mechanisms in cardiopulmonary resuscitation: studies in an electrical model of the circulation. Am J Emerg Med 1984; 2:299–308.

39. Babbs CF. Abdominal counterpulsation in cardiopulmonary resuscitation: animal models and theoretical considerations. Am J Emerg Med 1985; 3:165–170.

40. Babbs CF. Preclinical studies of abdominal counterpulsation in CPR. Ann Emerg Med 1984; 13:761–763.

41. Babbs CF, Tacker WA, Jr. Cardiopulmonary resuscitation with interposed abdominal compression. Circulation 1986; 74:IV37–IV41.

42. Babbs CF, Blevins WE. Abdominal binding and counterpulsation in cardiopulmonary resuscitation. Crit Care Clin 1986; 2:319–32.

43. Babbs CF. Hemodynamic mechanisms in CPR: a theoretical rationale for resuscitative thoracotomy in non-traumatic cardiac arrest. Resuscitation 1987; 15:37–50.

44. Babbs CF. Interposed abdominal compression-CPR. Low technology for the clinical armamentarium. Circulation 1992; 86:2011,2012.

45. Babbs CF. Interposed abdominal compression-cardiopulmonary resuscitation: are we missing the mark in clinical trials? Am Heart J 1993; 126:1035–1041.

46. Babbs CF. Interposed abdominal compression-CPR: a case study in cardiac arrest research. Ann Emerg Med 1993; 22:24–32.

47. Babbs CF. The evolution of abdominal compression in cardiopulmonary resuscitation. Acad Emerg Med 1994; 1:469–477.

48. Babbs CF, Sack JB, Kern KB. Interposed abdominal compression as an adjunct to cardiopulmonary resuscitation. Am Heart J 1994; 127:412–421.

49. Babbs CF. CPR techniques that combine chest and abdominal compression and decompression: hemodynamic insights from a spreadsheet model. Circulation 1999; 100:2146–2152.

50. Babbs CF, Thelander K. Theoretically optimal duty cycles for chest and abdominal compression during external cardiopulmonary resuscitation. Acad Emerg Med 1995; 2:698–707.

51. Babbs CF. Efficacy of interposed abdominal compression-cardiopulmonary resuscitation (CPR), active compression and decompression-CPR and Lifestick CPR: basic physiology in a spreadsheet model. Crit Care Med 2000; 28:N199–N202.

52. Sack JB, Kesselbrenner MB, Jarrad A. Interposed abdominal compression-cardiopulmonary resuscitation and resuscitation outcome during asystole and electromechanical dissociation. Circulation 1992; 86:1692–1700.

53. Sack JB, Kesselbrenner MB, Bregman D. Survival from in-hospital cardiac arrest with interposed abdominal counterpulsation during cardiopulmonary resuscitation. JAMA 1992; 267:379–385.

54. Sack JB, Kesselbrenner MB. Hemodynamics, survival benefits, and complications of interposed abdominal compression during cardiopulmonary resuscitation. Acad Emerg Med 1994; 1:490–497.

55. Mateer JR, Stueven HA, Thompson BM, Aprahamian C, Darin JC. Interposed abdominal compression CPR versus standard CPR in prehospital cardiopulmonary arrest: preliminary results. Ann Emerg Med 1984; 13:764–766.

56. Mateer JR, Stueven HA, Thompson BM, Aprahamian C, Darin JC. Pre-hospital IAC-CPR versus standard CPR: paramedic resuscitation of cardiac arrests. Am J Emerg Med 1985; 3:143–146.

57. Berryman CR, Phillips GM. Interposed abdominal compression-CPR in human subjects. Ann Emerg Med 1984; 13:226–229.

58. Einagle V, Bertrand F, Wise RA, Roussos C, Magder S. Interposed abdominal compressions and carotid blood flow during cardiopulmonary resuscitation. Support for a thoracoabdominal unit. Chest 1988; 93:1206–1212.

59. Voorhees WD, III, Ralston SH, Babbs CF. Regional blood flow during cardiopulmonary resuscitation with abdominal counterpulsation in dogs. Am J Emerg Med. 1984; 2:123–128.

60. Walker JW, Bruestle JC, White BC, Evans AT, Indreri R, Bialek H. Perfusion of the cerebral cortex by use of abdominal counterpulsation during cardiopulmonary resuscitation. Am J Emerg Med 1984; 2: 391–393.

61. Voorhees WD, Niebauer MJ, Babbs CF. Improved oxygen delivery during cardiopulmonary resuscitation with interposed abdominal compressions. Ann Emerg Med 1983; 12:128–135.

62. Howard M, Carrubba C, Foss F, Janiak B, Hogan B, Guinness M. Interposed abdominal compression-CPR: its effects on parameters of coronary perfusion in human subjects. Ann Emerg Med 1987; 16:253–259.

63. McDonald JL. Effect of interposed abdominal compression during CPR on central arterial and venous pressures. Am J Emerg Med 1985; 3:156–159.

64. Lurie KG, Lindo C, Chin J. CPR: the P stands for plumber's helper. JAMA 1990; 264:1661.

65. Lurie KG, Shultz JJ, Callaham ML, Schwab TM, Gisch T, Rector T, Frascone RJ, Long L. Evaluation of active compression-decompression CPR in victims of out-of-hospital cardiac arrest. JAMA 1994; 271:1405–1411.

66. Babbs CF. Circulatory adjuncts. Newer methods of cardiopulmonary resuscitation. Cardiol Clin 2002; 20:37–59.

67. Lindner KH, Pfenninger EG, Lurie KG, Schurmann W, Lindner IM, Ahnefeld FW. Effects of active compression-decompression resuscitation on myocardial and cerebral blood flow in pigs. Circulation 1993; 88:1254–1263.

68. Nolan J, Smith G, Evans R, et al. The United Kingdom pre-hospital study of active compression-decompression resuscitation. Resuscitation 1998; 37:119–125.

69. Panzer W, Bretthauer M, Klingler H, Bahr J, Rathgeber J, Kettler D. ACD versus standard CPR in a prehospital setting. Resuscitation 1996; 33:117–124.
70. Wik L, Mauer D, Robertson C. The first European pre-hospital active compression-decompression (ACD) cardiopulmonary resuscitation workshop: a report and a review of ACD-CPR. Resuscitation 1995; 30:191–202.
71. Stiell IG, Hebert PC, Wells GA, et al. The Ontario trial of active compression-decompression cardiopulmonary resuscitation for in-hospital and prehospital cardiac arrest. JAMA 1996; 275:1417–1423.
72. Luiz T, Ellinger K, Denz C. Active compression-decompression cardiopulmonary resuscitation does not improve survival in patients with prehospital cardiac arrest in a physician-manned emergency medical system. J Cardiothorac Vasc Anesth 1996; 10:178–186.
73. Plaisance P, Adnet F, Vicaut E, et al. Benefit of active compression-decompression cardiopulmonary resuscitation as a prehospital advanced cardiac life support. A randomized multicenter study. Circulation 1997; 95:955–961.
74. Plaisance P, Lurie KG, Vicaut E, et al. A comparison of standard cardiopulmonary resuscitation and active compression-decompression resuscitation for out-of-hospital cardiac arrest. French Active Compression-Decompression Cardiopulmonary Resuscitation Study Group. N Engl J Med 1999; 341:569–575.
75. Rabl W, Baubin M, Broinger G, Scheithauer R. Serious complications from active compression-decompression cardiopulmonary resuscitation. Int J Legal Med 1996; 109:84–89.
76. Baubin M, Rabl W, Pfeiffer KP, Benzer A, Gilly H. Chest injuries after active compression-decompression cardiopulmonary resuscitation (ACD-CPR) in cadavers. Resuscitation 1999; 43:9–15.
77. Shultz JJ, Mianulli MJ, Gisch TM, Coffeen PR, Haidet GC, Lurie KG. Comparison of exertion required to perform standard and active compression-decompression cardiopulmonary resuscitation. Resuscitation 1995; 29:23–31.
78. Lurie KG, Mulligan KA, McKnite S, Detloff B, Lindstrom P, Lindner KH. Optimizing standard cardiopulmonary resuscitation with an inspiratory impedance threshold valve. Chest 1998; 113:1084–1090.
79. Lurie KG, Zielinski T, McKnite S, Aufderheide T, Voelckel W. Use of an inspiratory impedance valve improves neurologically intact survival in a porcine model of ventricular fibrillation. Circulation 2002; 105:124–129.
80. Plaisance P, Lurie KG, Payen D. Inspiratory impedance during active compression-decompression cardiopulmonary resuscitation: a randomized evaluation in patients in cardiac arrest. Circulation 2000; 101:989–994.
81. Lurie K, Voelckel W, Plaisance P, et al. Use of an inspiratory impedance threshold valve during cardiopulmonary resuscitation: a progress report. Resuscitation 2000; 44:219–230.
82. Tang W, Weil MH, Schock RB, et al. Phased chest and abdominal compression-decompression. A new option for cardiopulmonary resuscitation. Circulation 1997; 95:1335–1340.
83. Kern KB, Hilwig RW, Berg RA, Schock RB, Ewy GA. Optimizing ventilation in conjunction with phased chest and abdominal compression-decompression (Lifestick) resuscitation. Resuscitation 2002; 52:91–100.
84. Arntz HR, Agrawal R, Richter H, et al. Phased chest and abdominal compression-decompression versus conventional cardiopulmonary resuscitation in out-of-hospital cardiac arrest. Circulation 2001; 104:768–772.
85. Halperin HR, Guerci AD, Chandra N, et al. Vest inflation without simultaneous ventilation during cardiac arrest in dogs: improved survival from prolonged cardiopulmonary resuscitation. Circulation 1986; 74:1407–1415.
86. Beattie C, Guerci AD, Hall T, et al. Mechanisms of blood flow during pneumatic vest cardiopulmonary resuscitation. J Appl Physiol 1991; 70:454–465.
87. Eleff SM, Schleien CL, Koehler RC, et al. Brain bioenergetics during cardiopulmonary resuscitation in dogs. Anesthesiology 1992; 76:77–84.
88. Halperin HR, Tsitlik JE, Gelfand M, et al. A preliminary study of cardiopulmonary resuscitation by circumferential compression of the chest with use of a pneumatic vest. N Engl J Med 1993; 329:762–768.
89. Rudikoff MT, Maughan WL, Effron M, Freund P, Weisfeldt ML. Mechanisms of blood flow during cardiopulmonary resuscitation. Circulation 1980; 61:345–352.
90. Weisfeldt ML, Chandra N. Physiology of cardiopulmonary resuscitation. Annu Rev Med 1981; 32:435–442.
91. Weisfeldt ML. Recent advances in cardiopulmonary resuscitation. Jpn Circ J 1985; 49:13–24.
92. Weisfeldt ML, Halperin HR. Cardiopulmonary resuscitation: beyond cardiac massage. Circulation 1986; 74:443–448.

93. Halperin HR, Weisfeldt ML. New approaches to CPR. Four hands, a plunger, or a vest. JAMA 1992; 267:2940,2941.

94. Weisfeldt ML. Challenges in cardiac arrest research. Ann Emerg Med. 1993; 22:4–5.

95. Ben-Haim SA, Anuchnik CL, Dinnar U. A computer controller for vest cardiopulmonary resuscitation (CPR). IEEE Trans Biomed Eng 1988; 35:413–416.

96. Ben-Haim SA, Shofti R, Ostrow B, Dinnar U. Effect of vest cardiopulmonary resuscitation rate on cardiac output and coronary blood flow. Crit Care Med 1989; 17:768–771.

97. Raessler KL, Kern KB, Sanders AB, Tacker WA, Jr., Ewy GA. Aortic and right atrial systolic pressures during cardiopulmonary resuscitation: a potential indicator of the mechanism of blood flow. Am Heart J 1988; 115:1021–1029.

98. Criley JM, Niemann JT, Rosborough JP, Hausknecht M. Modifications of cardiopulmonary resuscitation based on the cough. Circulation 1986; 74:IV42–IV50.

99. Criley JM. The thoracic pump provides a mechanism for coronary perfusion. Arch Intern Med 1995; 155:1236.

100. Niemann JT, Rosborough JP, Niskanen RA, Criley JM. Circulatory support during cardiac arrest using a pneumatic vest and abdominal binder with simultaneous high-pressure airway inflation. Ann Emerg Med 1984; 13:767–770.

101. Niemann JT, Rosborough JP, Ung S, Criley JM. Coronary perfusion pressure during experimental cardiopulmonary resuscitation. Ann Emerg Med 1982; 11:127–131.

102. Luce JM, Ross BK, O'Quin RJ, et al. Regional blood flow during cardiopulmonary resuscitation in dogs using simultaneous and nonsimultaneous compression and ventilation. Circulation 1983; 67:258–265.

103. Luce JM, Rizk NA, Niskanen RA. Regional blood flow during cardiopulmonary resuscitation in dogs. Crit Care Med 1984; 12:874–878.

11 Training Adults to Perform Cardiopulmonary Resuscitation

What Works?

Barbara Riegel, DNSC, RN, CS, FAAN,
Lars Wik, MD, and Alidene Doherty, RN, BSN

CONTENTS

INTRODUCTION

Cardiopulmonary resuscitation (CPR) is first-line therapy for sudden, unexpected, cardiac arrest (CA). Laypersons are most likely to administer CPR because most CAs occur in the home or in the community. Training laypersons to adminster CPR has become a routine activity but some would argue that it is not an activity that we do particularly well. Out-of-hospital resuscitation attempts have led to very low survival rates *(1–13)*—less than 10% survival in Europe *(2,3,6–8)* and the majority of urban areas in the United States *(1,9–13)*. Densely populated urban areas such as Chicago and New York City have a particularly low rate of sudden CA survival *(13)* as do rural areas.

One reason for the universally low survival rates is that the frequency of CPR initiation by bystanders remains extremely low *(10,12–17)*. Initiation of resuscitation by bystanders clearly increases survival *(1,6,17–19)* but the rate of basic life support (BLS) initiation by bystanders in the United States is typically less than 30% *(9–16)* and rarely greater than 50% in Europe *(6,8,17)*.

Our ultimate challenge is to increase the number of bystanders initiating CPR. How to manage this is not known for certain, but it is the thesis of these authors that low rates

From: *Contemporary Cardiology: Cardiopulmonary Resuscitation*
Edited by: J. P. Ornato and M. A. Peberdy © Humana Press Inc., Totowa, NJ

of CPR are a direct consequence of our ineffective teaching methods. Much is known about how to teach adults and traditional approaches violate most principles of adult learning. Perhaps current approaches to CPR training should be largely abandoned in favor of new methods. Many of the nationally recognized CPR training organizations have modified their programs to emphasize student practice time and minimize instructor lecture, a tactic consistent with adult learning principles. However, other, more radical methods should be considered. In this chapter we discuss approaches to training adults in CPR that work.

HOW DO ADULTS LEARN BEST?

Maximizing the acquisition of BLS knowledge and skills requires changing the traditional teaching model from instructor-to student-centered. Knowles (20) is usually credited with being the first to suggest that adults learn in a manner that is different from that of children. However, others such as Rogers (21), have been influential in helping us to understand that adults learn when the information is relevant, practical, and tied to existing knowledge. Adults must feel respected and free to direct their own learning if they are to acquire new knowledge. Adults are typically busy so learning situations that are fun and directed by someone who is likeable and worthy of respect facilitates learning. Barriers to learning such as lack of time, money, and transportation must be minimized if adults are to participate in learning events. These principles are described more fully later along with practical examples of ways to address them in CPR training.

RELEVANCE

Adults learn best when they see the relevance of what they are learning. Scenario-based instruction has been recommended as a method of making CPR training relevant, practical, and useful. Scenario-based instruction involves modifying the story surrounding each simulated event to fit the student's individual situation. In this way, the instructor maximizes relevance and allows the student to practice the CA scenario most like what he or she will experience. Modification of the scenario allows the student to think through an actual situation and build on existing knowledge. Scenario-based instruction is particularly helpful for students who learn primarily through observation.

Scenario modification is most effective when it is consistent with the experience of the student. For example, if training police officers who will be responding after a call to 911, it makes little sense to ask them to notify 911. However, if the scenario is modified to have the officer update the dispatcher with information, it becomes consistent with the routine practice of the officer. It is helpful if the scenario can be made as realistic as possible. For example, continuing the police officer example, using a model phone or one that is not plugged in instead of just pretending to call 911 would make the scenario more realistic (22). Current thinking is that the "pretend" or acting surrounding many of the steps in CPR training interfere with skill demonstration and perhaps with skill learning itself.

Only common, clinically relevant situations should be included in scenarios. For example, it has been shown that when an instructor ends a class by practicing an unconscious obstructed airway scenario, students tend to confuse chest compressions and abdominal thrusts (23). Additionally, if each scenario results in a return of spontaneous circulation, the student leaves the classroom with the unrealistic expectation that all CA victims will recover.

An important element influencing perceived relevance is the message that the learner receives regarding importance of the training. In one study testing the effectiveness of CPR training by videotape, about half of the 8659 recipients of the videotape did not even view it although the tape was sent to homes of patients at risk for sudden cardiac death *(24)*. An equal number of CAs occurred in each group, but the bystander CPR rates did not differ (47% video vs 53% controls), nor did hospital discharge rates ($n = 3$ vs $n = 2$). Clearly, the video recipients were not convinced that the tape would be relevant for them.

POSITIVE REGARD FOR THE INSTRUCTOR

Positive regard for the instructor facilitates learning. In 1991, Kaye *(25)* published a paper titled "The Problem of Poor Retention of Cardiopulmonary Resuscitation Skills May Lie With the Instructor, Not the Learner or the Curriculum," making this point. Others *(26)* have found that CPR instructors had limited knowledge of the courses they taught, did not understand or follow recommended teaching practices, did not read their instructor manuals, and could not even pass a CPR provider test. If this is the case, it is not surprising that one author *(27)* found that 10% of instructors were considered by students to be incompetent, 9% of the students stated they would not perform CPR after the course, and 23% stated mistakenly that they could be legally prosecuted if they did CPR on a stranger.

Most of the information that CPR instructors teach and the style used to teach it has been passed down by tradition. Instructors typically model an instructor they admired. Few have heard how their words and stories sound to the students. Few realize how they make the students feel, and how their well-intentioned words distract the learners from the important skills that they have come to learn. When instructors provide anecdotes and depart from the script, a decrease in written test scores has been demonstrated *(28,29)*. For every 2 minutes of anecdote, cognitive scores dropped 1% overall. So, adding just 20 minutes of additional material (anecdotes and stories), as most instructors do, could lower students' test scores by 10%. Clearly, more emphasis is needed on helping instructors to be better teachers, if the traditional model of instructor-based courses continues.

FREEDOM TO DIRECT ONE'S OWN LEARNING

Another important principle of adult learning is that adults learn best when they are free to direct their own learning. Several investigators have developed and tested various methods of self-learning that maximize individuals' freedom to direct their own learning experience. In the 1970s, Berkebile and colleagues *(30,31)* compared five training methods in suburban schools in Pittsburgh. A traditional instructor-led CPR class lasting 3 hours and an untrained control group were compared to (a) self-practice on recording mannequins, coached by audiotapes and flip charts, (b) repeated (16 times) viewing of a new 10-minute CPR demonstration film over a 3-month period, and (c) viewing the new 10-minute film plus self-practice on mannequins *(32)*. The recording mannequin and flip charts demonstrating proper technique were available throughout the study period in the learning laboratory. Knowledge and skill performance at 1 and 12 months were superior in the group who viewed the film and did self-practice when compared to the traditional instructor-led course. Self-practice alone was superior to repetitive film viewing alone. Repetitive film viewing alone was superior to no training. More students passed heart compressions than ventilations. In another study,

Kaye and colleagues *(33)* demonstrated superior skill performance after interactive computerized self-training compared to those given the traditional instructor-led course. These studies demonstrate that students free to direct their own learning performed better than those sitting through the traditional, instructor-led course.

An innovative approach to self-learning was developed and tested by Braslow and associates *(23,24)* called "video self-instruction" or "watch and practice." Instead of watching a video and *then* practicing, the "watch and practice" approach was designed to include synchronous practice. That is, viewers practiced and learned along with the videotaped expert demonstration—just like a Jane Fonda exercise video. To increase learning, the video contained no lectures, no information on anatomy and physiology, no rates and ratios, and no complicated methods for locating the compression point and opening the airway—to name a few. Information on heart attack care and airway obstruction was removed. This approach allowed for more than 25 minutes of continuous CPR practice, compared with approx 2.5 minutes of practice in the traditional 4-hour CPR course. When the video self-instruction was compared to the traditional instructor-based course, it worked well, even in persons over age 50, a group that often has lower skill retention than others. Participants learned CPR in only 30 minutes—without an instructor or textbook—and outperformed students who had just completed the traditional course.

The efficacy of self-training has been known since the 1970s *(30,31,35–37)*. Courses by instructors remain the accepted method of training in CPR despite this. Instructors are not the obstacle, but a fixed time available for practice is less effective than unlimited time for self-practice.

OVERCOMING BARRIERS

Common barriers to learning CPR are lack of time and/or transportation. Standard group classes with mannequin training are 3 to 4 hours in length, a significant time commitment for adult learners with other responsibilities. Another barrier is lack of interest in learning a skill one may never use. Additionally, learning style, speed, and physical agility vary widely among adults, which can be a barrier to those concerned that they may not keep up with others in a formal class. Societal cost of training large numbers of laypersons is a major barrier as well.

Motivating the Learner

Individuals who are not interested in learning CPR may be motivated to learn CPR to help others. Research into the psychology of "helping behavior" (what makes some people act when confronted with an emergency, whereas some do not act) tells us that before someone can perform in a CA or other emergency situation, psychologically, they must feel able and ready to do so *(38)*. Yet, most people are not. Historically, this prerequisite has been ignored perhaps because CPR and other emergency cardiac care training began as training for physicians and has not been tailored to lay people. Depending on the instructor, some trainees feel badgered by instructors and others feel supported to learn. Self-efficacy, or perceived ability to perform the skill of CPR must become part of the training program if the rate of bystander CPR is to increase *(39)*.

Cost to Society

The societal cost of training is a major obstacle for widespread use of CPR. In order to lower the cost, Wik et al. *(40)* introduced peer CPR training based on the belief that a handful of lay people trained as CPR instructors could train their coworkers, who in turn would train their relatives, and so on. The effect of this approach is similar to a domino effect potentially resulting in a significant increase in the number of skilled CPR providers at a low cost. An inexpensive take-home mannequin together with a flip chart and a 20-minute videotape were used. When those trained using the peer approach were compared to those trained with the traditional method, third-generation trainees proved equally effective at CPR as those trained directly with the traditional method.

In an extension of this approach, Wik *(40)* trained people in CPR and then sent a mannequin and videotape home with them to train their family members on their own. Training of family members was accomplished in under 60 minutes. How well did they do? The family members' CPR performance was equal to, or most often better than the performance of students coming out of traditional instructor-based CPR courses. Why? We believe that peer-to-peer learning and modeling are learning methods with which laypersons feel comfortable. In fact, peer-to-peer learning and modeling reflect a natural and universal method of learning. Throughout life, important learning takes place in the home and this is the environment in which most will use CPR if they ever have to use the skill.

TRANSFERRING LEARNING TO REAL-LIFE EVENTS

CPR acquisition includes both cognitive learning and skill retention. Cognitive learning regarding the correct sequence to perform occurs by seeing (reading or mimicking) and by hearing. The learner needs to remember the algorithm at the same time as it is performed with quality and speed. No study has shown that lecturing about physiology, medicine, and risk issues—common content in traditional CPR courses—improves skill performance *(25,29,41–43)*. In fact, lecturing and reading may distract the learner and result in information overload. Braslow *(23)* found that when the "heart-healthy" information was eliminated from the class, practice time increased and skill improved.

Clarity of the message (i.e., focus on essential information only) is important but controversy continues regarding what to teach the lay public about CPR. Should we teach abdominal thrusts *(44)* or back blows for suspected foreign body obstruction *(45,46)*? Is moderate backward tilt of the head plus jaw thrust and separation of the lips (the triple airway maneuver) the best airway control measure for comatose trauma victims *(47–49)*? How should we position patients in coma with spontaneous breathing (horizontal supine vs stable side position, both with head tilted backward *[45]*)? What should we teach about when the lone rescuer is justified to leave the individual temporarily to call for help?

Pathophysiology must guide instructional content. Complete airway obstruction (as in drowning, brain trauma, intoxication) results in CA within 5 to 10 minutes *(50–52)*. In many situations, complete recovery can be achieved with CPR steps A and B alone *(50–54)*, which reinforce the teaching of steps A, B, and C together. For normothermic sudden CA, we know the time limits for preventing permanent damage to the brain (4 minutes *[55–57]*) and the heart (20 minutes *[57,58]*). Therefore, teaching must stress that only resuscitation initiated within seconds of collapse can provide the necessary oxygen delivery to maintain viability of the individual until arrival of advanced life support personnel. Teaching the importance of continuous chest compression and ventilation with a minimum of pauses (no-flow periods) is essential.

Practice Time

Practice time has been shown to be the most important factor in acquisition of BLS for adult learners *(23)*. Maximizing the practice time for the students is currently the responsibility of the instructor. However, instructors vary greatly in how they set up courses and the use of videotapes, work books, and information provided. Kaye et al. *(25)* observed that in 3-hour courses, the actual mannequin practice time ranged between 2 and 16 minutes per student. Additionally, Brennan and colleagues *(29)* noted that most trainees are not even minimally competent following training; most instructors simply pass or coach students to pass. Testing by an independent instructor on a fully computerized system resulted in failure of all students whom the instructor earlier had considered competent. Kaye *(33)* suggests that lack of skill retention may reflect lack of initial skill acquisition.

Minimizing nonessential information that uses up practice time is essential. If the instructor has had personal experience in prehospital resuscitation it can add credibility to the training course but the sharing of personal experience also uses valuable time needed for skill practice. Actual personal experience relayed to students often results in students remembering the story and missing the underlying message.

Electronic devices such as CPR skill-prompting devices are effective in encouraging students to practice more effectively during the available time and for longer periods of time *(59)*. If a prompting device is used at the point in the class when the students are beginning to loose interest in skill practice, even the most experienced adult students will be willing to practice for longer periods of time. Patterns (i.e., linked content) are retained and more easily accessed in memory than isolated facts or complex algorithms, even under stress. The prompting device will help to cement the pattern by consistently repeating phrases such as, "head tilt–chin lift." Students retrained at 2 years will report remembering the phrases repeated by the prompting device.

Positive Reinforcement

Positive reinforcement is essential if individuals are to develop self-efficacy, a key predictor of performance, as discussed above. According to psychological research on "helping" behavior *(60–67)*, issues inherent in the decision to act arise from the initial response to threatening, unfamiliar and/or complex situations. The decision to act depends on acknowledging that the situation exists and having confidence in one's ability to handle the emergency (self-efficacy). Helping behavior research has focused on laypersons' response to public assault, medical emergencies such as heart attack, and trauma such as uncontrolled bleeding, involving strangers. Research on laypersons' response to CA in a family member is nearly nonexistent.

Skill Retention

Skill retention is directly affected by the amount of practice available during the learning process because the acquisition of psychomotor skills greatly depends on repetition *(68)*. Overtraining has shown to improve retention *(69–71)*. Overtraining is defined as continuing to practice a task after having achieved the performance criterion *(72)*. Overtraining has been claimed to be of particular value in the retention of skills in which the individual has no chance to "warm up" *(71)*, as is indeed the case during clinical CPR.

Other strategies recommended for improving retention include sensory input or feedback *(73)*. Feedback received at the end of skill performance appears to be less effective than that occurring during performance *(74)*. Qualitative is not as effective as quantitative feedback *(72)*. Improvement in performance depends on the frequency of feedback *(72)*. The person giving the feedback can be important as well. Feedback from a peer may be less threatening than correction from the instructor. If the observer is given a written checklist with the steps outlined, he or she can provide feedback and learn while observing his or her peers.

Why do learners not perform CPR correctly after an interval when most people have no difficulty riding a bicycle several years after initial training? The answer is feedback. When riding a bicycle, you receive instant feedback on how you are bicycling and consequently wrong performance is corrected. When performing CPR, little feedback is received. Feedback was more salient in the early training efforts. In the early training performed by Safar et al. *(47)* curarized nonintubated human volunteers would lie supine on the floor to demonstrate open airway and mouth-to-mouth ventilation. If the learners did CPR wrong, the "patient" would turn blue in a few seconds. That feedback changed their behavior and performance so that their technique created pink patients. In 1960, Lind *(75)* of Norway introduced the use of mannequins (instead of curarized patients) in the training of B-CPR steps A and B—a safer approach but one with little feedback *(68)*. Could we create a CPR "bicycle" or could an instructor play that role? Later, we propose the potential uses of technology to address these issues.

RETRAINING

Retraining of students 3 to 6 months following the initial CPR/automated external defibrillator (AED) course will result in better retention of skills. Review of skills can be as simple as asking students to demonstrate what they remember from their training class and then providing reinforcement for skill mastery and instruction in areas not mastered. This approach was used in the Public Access Defibrillation (PAD) Trial and found to require only 5.3 ± 0.1 minutes for CPR and 7.8 ± 0.1 minutes for CPR + AED to test and retrain lay volunteers *(75a)*. If the skill review is done individually with the instructor, the student is given individualized attention and peer pressure is eliminated. The skill review session also gives the instructor the opportunity to debrief students if any medical emergencies have occurred since the original training session.

Retention of CPR skills decreases significantly in a short period after training, even in medical personnel who are not routinely involved in resuscitation *(33)*. Although skill decrement may reaches low levels, it is still above pretraining levels for most at 6–12 months *(30,31,33,69,72,76–83)*. After initial training and early reinforcement, it is helpful if repeat remedial mannequin practice is made available every 6–12 months *(31,33,69,72,76–80)*.

FUTURE DIRECTIONS

One night, a friend of Dr. Wik's experienced a CA in an atypical patient—his mother—lying on the bathroom floor, looking "dead." His emergency medical technician mind was not with him that summer evening. He was too preoccupied, too nervous just like any other lone layperson facing such a situation. He did not think about details. Instead, he thought, "call 911, bend the head back, grab the chin, pinch the nose, blow." Then "hands in the middle of the chest, and start pumping and blowing." No rates or numbers were in his mind. No complex and time-consuming steps regarding where to place his hands crossed his mind. He just thought "pump and blow."

Dr. Wik's friend later realized that little of the real experience of people witnessing and acting during a CA is represented in our CPR education programs. This observation also was made by the lay bystanders surveyed regarding their thoughts, feelings, and motivations when attempting to resuscitate a stranger *(84)*. He came to recognize from his experience that CPR training has to be more readily accessible. It has to get to the right people, the people most likely to use it. It must to be perceived as being so easy that the actual learning of CPR is not even thought about or contemplated.

Technology and state of the art teaching methods are needed if we are going to achieve these goals. CPR practice that is routinely scenario-based to include professionals such as 911 dispatchers who will coach the performance will be more effective than traditional approaches. There have to be easily accessible home adjuncts such as speaker phones, a CPR prompt, and maybe someday, an even more user-friendly home AED as well as content-on-demand video instruction.

To achieve this dream, we will need to influence policy so that the government regulations of yesteryear are amended to rid our first aid and emergency cardiac care programs of superfluous content that is confusing and overwhelming to students. The data collected to date suggest strongly that this content is diffusing our message to a point that CPR learners cannot remember how to perform the most basic skills when needed.

To improve training and minimize human error, these authors believe that emergency cardiac care education must use behavior and education theory. Computer and virtual technologies like those being used in other life-essential skill domains such as pilot and physician training could be used. With simulation, expert performance can be modeled and immediate feedback obtained. With instant feedback and remediation from the simulator, CPR performance can only improve. There is technology available today—from simple clickers that give feedback when one has compressed deep enough to electronic feedback—that can give immediate feedback to students as they are learning. Earlier versions of these feedback devices were shown to improve learning, but were not used because they were misunderstood by the instructors. We now know that accurate and timely feedback is essential to learning and retention.

Technology soon to be available will provide not only immediate feedback but real-time verbal input as the student performs *(85,86)*. Using virtual reality technology, the research team of Dr. Wik of Norway has developed a system that uses a type of video self-instruction synchronous practice in which almost the entire training and testing can be supervised from central control sites thousands of miles away. Internet learning cannot teach hands-on psychomotor skills and measure skill performance directly. But, as the human eye is unable to evaluate the adequacy of ventilations and compressions—and only instrumented manikins can do so—this technology will allow immediate feedback, regardless of proximity. Additionally, simulator mannequins now available can be programmed with realistic attributes such as airways that swell, heads that are difficult to bend backwards, real lung sounds, distal pulses, agonal breaths, and so on. This technology is being used to improve the effectiveness of self-training and has been shown to increase learning and retention *(85,86)*.

Perhaps in the future, as digital bandwidth expands, would-be rescuers might be able to merely flick on their televisions to see a skills demonstration. Content-on-demand technology could allow dispatchers to send the exact demonstration needed right to the caller's television, laptop computer, or personal digital assistant, rather than trying to explain the sequence of steps verbally.

The real measure of success for CPR, AED, and other emergency cardiac care programs is *learner performance*—bystander CPR and survivor rates. Building programs and course content, methods, and administration around learner outcome is essential. We now know enough about how to teach emergency cardiac care content. Until recently, we have focused on courses that are too long and taught by instructors with lecture notes and fixed minutes for manikin practice. These courses have focused more on the acquisition of cognitive knowledge than performance skills. A new approach is needed. These authors maintain that the traditions surrounding CPR training should be respected as our history but it is time to move on and totally revise CPR training programs to emphasize simplicity, essential skills, and the use of technology to broaden the population of those trained in CPR and the use of bystander CPR in our communities.

REFERENCES

1. Eisenberg MS, Horwood BT, Cummins RO, Reynolds-Haertle R, Hearne TR. Cardiac arrest and resuscitation: a tale of 29 cities. Annals of Emergency Medicine 1990; 19:179–86.
2. Eisenburger P, List M, Schorkhuber W, Walker R, Sterz F, Laggner AN. Long-term cardiac arrest survivors of the Vienna emergency medical service. Resuscitation 1998; 38:137–43.
3. Gaul GB, Gruska M, Titscher G, et al. Prediction of survival after out-of-hospital cardiac arrest: results of a community-based study in Vienna. Resuscitation 1996; 32:169–76.
4. Sefrin P, Eilmes H. [First-aid measures in 939 fatally injured victims (author's translation)]. Anaesthesist 1975; 24:534–40.
5. Abrams JI, Pretto EA, Angus D, Safar P. Guidelines for rescue training of the lay public. Prehospital & Disaster Medicine 1993; 8:151–156.
6. Van Hoeyweghen RJ, Bossaert LL, Mullie A, et al. Quality and efficiency of bystander CPR. Belgian Cerebral Resuscitation Study Group. Resuscitation 1993; 26:47–52.
7. Mullie A, Van Hoeyweghen R, Quets A. Influence of pre-CPR conditions on EMS response times in circulatory arrest. The Cerebral Resuscitation Study Group. Resuscitation 1989; 17(Suppl):S45–S51; discussion S199–S206.
8. Lund I, Skulberg A. Cardiopulmonary resuscitation by lay people. Lancet 1976; 2:702–704.
9. Guzy PM, Pearce ML, Greenfield S. The survival benefit of bystander cardiopulmonary resuscitation in a paramedic served metropolitan area. American Journal of Public Health. 1983; 73:766–769.
10. Gallagher EJ, Lombardi G, Genis P. Effectiveness of bystander cardiopulmonary resuscitation and survival following out-of-hospital cardiac arrest. JAMA 1995; 274:1922–1925.
11. Ritter G, Wolfe RA, Goldstein S, et al. The effect of bystander CPR on survival of out-of-hospital cardiac arrest victims. American Heart Journal 1985; 110:932–937.
12. Troiano P, Masaryk J, Stueven HA, Olson D, Barthell E, Waite EM. The effect of bystander CPR on neurologic outcome in survivors of prehospital cardiac arrests. Resuscitation 1989; 17:91–98.
13. Becker LB, Ostrander MP, Barrett J, Kondos GT. Outcome of CPR in a large metropolitan area—where are the survivors? [see comments]. Annals of Emergency Medicine 1991; 20:355–361.
14. Copley DP, Mantle JA, Rogers WJ, Russell RO, Jr., Rackley CE. Improved outcome for prehospital cardiopulmonary collapse with resuscitation by bystanders. Circulation 1977; 56:901–905.
15. Cummins RO, Eisenberg MS, Hallstrom AP, Litwin PE. Survival of out-of-hospital cardiac arrest with early initiation of cardiopulmonary resuscitation. American Journal of Emergency Medicine 1985; 3: 114–119.
16. Jackson RE, Swor RA. Who gets bystander cardiopulmonary resuscitation in a witnessed arrest? Academic Emergency Medicine 1997; 4:540–544.
17. Wik L, Steen PA, Bircher NG. Quality of bystander cardiopulmonary resuscitation influences outcome after prehospital cardiac arrest. Resuscitation 1994; 28:195–203.
18. Sanders AB, Kern KB, Bragg S, Ewy GA. Neurologic benefits from the use of early cardiopulmonary resuscitation. Annals of Emergency Medicine 1987; 16:142–146.
19. Bossaert L, Van Hoeyweghen R. Bystander cardiopulmonary resuscitation (CPR) in out-of-hospital cardiac arrest. The Cerebral Resuscitation Study Group. Resuscitation 1989; 17(Suppl):S55–S69; discussion S199–S206.

20. Knowles MS. The Modern Practice of Adult Education: Andragogy Versus Pedagogy. New York: New York Association Press, 1970.
21. Rogers CR. Freedom to learn. Columbus, OH: Merrill, 1969.
22. Bilgera MC, Giesena BC, Wollanb PC, White RD. Improved retention of the EMS activation component (EMSAC) in adult CPR education. Resuscitation 1997; 35:219–224.
23. Braslow A, Brennan RT, Newman MM, Bircher NG, Batcheller AM, Kaye W. CPR training without an instructor: development and evaluation of a video self-instructional system for effective performance of cardiopulmonary resuscitation. Resuscitation 1997; 34:207–220.
24. Eisenberg M, Damon S, Mandel L, et al. CPR instruction by videotape: results of a community project. Annals of Emergency Medicine 1995; 25:198–202.
25. Kaye W, Rallis SF, Mancini ME, et al. The problem of poor retention of cardiopulmonary resuscitation skills may lie with the instructor, not the learner or the curriculum. Resuscitation 1991; 21:67–87.
26. Braslow A. An Evaluation of the Knowledge and Practices of Basic Cardiac Life Support Instructors. Urbana-Champaign, IL: University of Illinois, 1985.
27. Thell R. CPR training for driver's license applicants in Austria (in German). Rettungsdienst, in press.
28. Brennan RT. A Question of Life and Death: An Investigation of CPR Instruction Using Hierarchical Linear Modeling. Cambridge, MA: Harvard University, 1989.
29. Brennan RT. Student, instructor, and course factors predicting achievement in CPR training classes. American Journal of Emergency Medicine 1991; 9:220–224.
30. Berkebile P, Benson D, Ersoz C, Barnhill B, Safar P. Public education in heart-lung resuscitation. Evaluation of three self-training methods in teenagers. Proceedings of the National Conference on Standards for Cardiopulmonary Resuscitation and Emergency Cardiac Care. Dallas, TX: American Heart Association 1975, pp. 13–23.
31. Berkebile P. Education in cardiopulmonary-cerebral resuscitation (CPCR) using self-training methods. Prehospital & Disaster Medicine 1985; 1(Suppl 1).
32. Gordon AS. CPR training films. (a) Breath of Life (Steps A and B); (b) Pulse of Life (Steps A, B and C); (c) Prescription for Life (Steps A-D); and (d) Life in the Balance (Cardiac Care Unit). Dallas, TX: American Heart Association 1960s and 1980s; 1986.
33. Kaye W, Mancini ME. Retention of cardiopulmonary resuscitation skills by physicians, registered nurses, and the general public. Critical Care Medicine 1986; 14:620–622.
34. Braslow A, Brennan, RT, Newman NM, Kaye W. A self-instructional system for one-rescuer cardiopulmonary resuscitation. Circulation 1995; 92(Suppl):834.
35. Breivik H, Ulvik NM, Blikra G, Lind B. Life-supporting first aid self-training. Critical Care Medicine 1980; 8:654–658.
36. Esposito G, Safar P, Medsger A, Nesbitt J. Life supporting first aid self training for the lay public. Prehospital & Disaster Medicine 1985; 1(Suppl 1):91–93.
37. Safar P, Berkebile P, Scott MA, et al. Education research on life-supporting first aid (LSFA) and CPR self-training systems (STS). Critical Care Medicine 1981; 9:403–404.
38. Bierhoff H-W. Just world, social responsibility, and helping behavior. Ross, Michael 2002.
39. Bandura A. Self-efficacy mechanism in human agency. American Psychologist 1982; 37:122–147.
40. Wik L, Brennan RT, Braslow A. A peer-training model for instruction of basic cardiac life support. Resuscitation 1995; 29:119–128.
41. Bircher N, Otto C, Babbs C, et al. Future directions for resuscitation research. II. External cardiopulmonary resuscitation basic life support. Resuscitation 1996; 32:63–75.
42. Kaye W, Mancini ME. Teaching adult resuscitation in the United States—time for a rethink. Resuscitation. 1998;37:177–87.
43. Gudmundsen A. Teaching psychomotor skills. Journal of Nursing Education 1975; 14:23–27.
44. Heimlich HJ. A life-saving maneuver to prevent food-choking. Journal of the American Medical Association 1975; 234:398–401.
45. Safar P, & Bircher, N.G. Cardiopulmonary Cerebral Resuscitation. An Introduction to Resuscitation Medicine. Guidelines by the World Federation of Societies of Anaesthesiologists (WFSA), 3rd Ed. London: Saunders, 1988.
46. Gordon AS, Belton MK, Ridolpho PF. Emergency management of foreign body airway obstruction: comparison of artificial cough techniques, manual extraction maneuvers, and simple mechanical devices. In: Advances in Cardiopulmonary Resuscitation. Safar P, Elam, JO, eds. New York, NY: Springer-Verlag, 1977, pp. 39–50.
47. Safar P. Ventilatory efficacy of mouth-to-mouth artificial respiration. Airway obstruction during manual and mouth-to-mouth artificial respiration. JAMA 1958;167:335–341.

48. Safar P, Lind B. Triple airway maneuver, artificial ventilation and oxygen inhalation by mouth-to-mask and bag-valve-mask techniques. Proceedings of the National Conference on Standards for Cardiopulmonary Resuscitation and Emergency Cardiac Care, 1973. Dallas, TX: American Heart Association 1975, pp. 49–58.

49. Morikawa S, Safar P, DeCarlo J. Influence of head position upon upper airway patency. Anesthesiology 1961; 22:265–270.

50. Safar P, Paradis NA. Asphyxial cardiac arrest. In: Cardiac Arrest. The Science and Practice of Resuscitation Medicine. Paradis NA, Halperin HR, Nowak RM. eds. Philadelphia, PA: Williams and Wilkins; 1996, pp. 702–726.

51. Redding J, Voigt C, Safar P. Drowning treated with IPPB! Journal of Applied Physiology 1960; 15: 849–854.

52. Kristoffersen MB, Rattenborg CC, Holaday DA. Asphyxial death: the roles of acute anoxia, hypercarbia and acidosis. Anesthesiology 1967; 28:488–97.

53. Lind B, Stovner J. Mouth-to-mouth resuscitation in Norway. JAMA 1963; 185:933–935.

54. Elam JO, Greene DG. Mission accomplished: successful mouth-to-mouth resuscitation. Anesthesia Analgesia 1961; 40:578–80.

55. Cole SC, Four minute limit for cardiac resuscitation. JAMA 1956; 161:1454–1458.

56. Radovsky A, Safar P, Sterz F, Leonov Y, Reich H, Kuboyama K. Regional prevalence and distribution of ischemic neurons in dog brains 96 hours after cardiac arrest of 0 to 20 minutes. Stroke 1995; 26: 2127–2133; discussion 33–34.

57. Safar P, Abramson NS, Angelos M, et al. Emergency cardiopulmonary bypass for resuscitation from prolonged cardiac arrest. American Journal of Emergency Medicine 1990; 8:55–67.

58. Reich H, Angelos M, Safar P, Sterz F, Leonov Y. Cardiac resuscitability with cardiopulmonary bypass after increasing ventricular fibrillation times in dogs. Annals of Emergency Medicine 1990; 19:887–890.

59. Boyle AJ, Wilson AM, Connelly K, McGuigan L, Wilson J, Whitbourn R. Improvement in timing and effectiveness of external cardiac compressions with a new non-invasive device: the CPR-Ezy. Resuscitation. 2002; 54:63–67.

60. Latane B, Darley JM. Group inhibition of bystander intervention in emergencies. Journal of Personality & Social Psychology 1968; 10:215–221.

61. Latane B, Darley JM. Bystanders "apathy". American Scientist 1969; 57:244–268.

62. Latane B, Nida S. Ten years of research on group size and helping. Psychological Bulletin 1981; 89: 308–324.

63. Shotland RL, Stebbins CA. Emergency and cost as determinants of helping behavior and the slow accumulation of social psychological knowledge. Sociology & Psychological Quarterly 1983; 46:3646.

64. Piliavin IM, Rodin J. Good samaritanism: an underground phenomenon? Journal of Personality & Social Psychology 1969; 13:289–299.

65. Piliavin JAP, IM. Effect of blood on reactions to a victim. Journal of Personality & Social Psychology 1972; 23:353–361.

66. Darley JM, Latane B. Bystander intervention in emergencies: diffusion of responsibility. Journal of Personality & Social Psychology 1968; 8:377–383.

67. Mogielnicki RP, Stevenson KA, Willemain TR. Patient and bystander response to medical emergencies. Medical Care 1975; 13:753–762.

68. Poulsen H. Proceedings of the International Symposium on Emergency Resuscitation. Acta Anaesthesiologica Scandinavica 1961; Suppl 9.

69. Tweed WA, Wilson E, Isfeld B. Retention of cardiopulmonary resuscitation skills after initial overtraining. Critical Care Medicine 1980; 8:651–653.

70. Oxendine JB. Effect of mental and physical practice on the learning of three motor skills. Research Quarterly 1969; 40:755–763.

71. Melnick MJ. Effects of overlearning on the retention of a gross motor skill. Research Quarterly 1971; 42:60–69.

72. Vanderschmidt H, Burnap TK, Thwaites JK. Evaluation of a cardiopulmonary resuscitation course for secondary schools retention study. Medical Care 1976; 14:181–184.

73. Lovel RB. Adult Learning. New York, NY: Wiley, 1980.

74. Robb M. Feedback and skill learning. Research Quarterly 1968; 39:175–184.

75. Lind B. Teaching mouth-to-mouth resuscitation in primary schools. Acta Anaesthesiologica Scandinavica 1961; (Suppl 9):63–69.

75a. Nafziger SD, Riegel B, Sehra R, et al. Are CPR and AED skills retained over time?: results from the Public Access Defibrillation (PAD) Trial. Submitted.

76. Wilson E, Brooks B, Tweed WA. CPR skills retention of lay basic rescuers. Annals of Emergency Medicine 1983; 12:482–484.

77. Mandel LP, Cobb LA. Reinforcing CPR skills without mannequin practice. Annals of Emergency Medicine 1987; 16:1117–1120.

78. Weaver FJ, Ramirez AG, Dorfman SB, Raizner AE. Trainees' retention of cardiopulmonary resuscitation. How quickly they forget. Journal of the American Medical Association 1979; 241:901–903.

79. Berden HJ, Willems FF, Hendrick JM, Pijls NH, Knape JT. How frequently should basic cardiopulmonary resuscitation training be repeated to maintain adequate skills? [see comments.] [erratum appears in BMJ 1993 Sep 18;307:706.]. British Medical Journal 1993; 306:1576,1577.

80. Fossel M, Kiskaddon RT, Sternbach GL. Retention of cardiopulmonary resuscitation skills by medical students. Journal of Medical Education 1983; 58:568–575.

81. Grogono AW, Jastremski MS, Johnson MM, Russell RF. Education graffiti: better use of the lavatory wall. Lancet 1982; 1:1175,1176.

82. Wenzel V, Lehmkuhl P, Kubilis PS, Idris AH, Pichlmayr I. Poor correlation of mouth-to-mouth ventilation skills after basic life support training and 6 months later. Resuscitation 1997; 35:129–134.

83. Huhnigk P, Sefrin P, Paulus T. Skills and self-assessment in cardiopulmonary resuscitation of the hospital nursing staff. European Journal of Emergency Medicine 1994; 1:193–198.

84. Skora J, Riegel B. Thoughts, feelings, and motivations of bystanders who attempt to resuscitate a stranger: A pilot study. American Journal of Critical Care 2001; 10:408–416.

85. Wik L, Myklebust H, Auestad BH, Steen PA. Retention of basic life support skills 6 months after training with an automated voice advisory manikin system without instructor involvement. Resuscitation 2002; 52:273–2739.

86. Thowsen J, Steen PA. An automated voice advisory manikin system for training in basic life support without an instructor. A novel approach to CPR training. Resuscitation 2001; 50:167–172.

12 External Defibrillation

Gregory P. Walcott, MD,
Cheryl R. Killingsworth, DVM, PhD,
and Raymond E. Ideker, MD, PhD

INTRODUCTION

The history of applying electrical shocks to the heart began in the 1700s with direct current derived from a Leyden jar. In 1775, Abildgard described having shocked a chicken into lifelessness and on repeating the shock, bringing the bird back to life *(1)*. Transthoracic defibrillation was first performed clinically in the mid-1950s when Zoll introduced the alternating current (AC) defibrillator *(2)*. Several years later, Lown introduced the direct current (DC) defibrillator as an improvement on Zoll's device in several important areas, specifically that it caused less damage to the patient and that it could be made portable *(3)*. Today, internal cardioverter defibrillators are the size of a small bar of soap and can monitor and correct a patient's rhythm for several years between replacements. Likewise, the external defibrillator has been made smaller and so much simpler to operate that sixth graders can use the device successfully.

MECHANISM OF DEFIBRILLATION

The study of external defibrillation can build on much of what has been learned about internal defibrillation. A large amount of work has been done to understand the mechanisms of defibrillation following short durations of electrically induced ventricular fibrillation (VF) using internal defibrillation electrodes *(4–7)*. VF is maintained by multiple

From: *Contemporary Cardiology: Cardiopulmonary Resuscitation*
Edited by: J. P. Ornato and M. A. Peberdy © Humana Press Inc., Totowa, NJ

activation fronts that are constantly moving in a pattern of re-entry. Defibrillation can be broken down into two parts: halting fibrillation wavefronts and not restarting fibrillation.

Fundamentally, defibrillation is thought to be realized through the electrical pulse causing an alteration in the transmembrane potential of the myocyte. It most likely requires a rapid induction of changes in the transmembrane potential of the myocytes in a critical mass of myocardium (75–90% of the myocardium in dogs [8–10]). As this represents a large mass of tissue, these alterations must be achieved at a considerable distance from the stimulating electrode.

One-dimensional cable models cannot explain how the transmembrane potential changes at points distant from the shock electrodes. The cable equations predict hyperpolarization of the transmembrane potential adjacent to an extracellular anode and depolarization adjacent to an extracellular cathode with the change in transmembrane potential decreasing exponentially with distance from the electrodes. According to this model, a majority of the heart will see no change in the transmembrane potential as a result of the shock.

Changes in the transmembrane potential across the heart caused by the shock are predicted by the bidomain model of cardiac tissue. The bidomain model extends the one-dimensional cable model into two or three dimensions (11); the extracellular and intracellular spaces are represented as single continuous domains that are separated by the highly resistive cell membrane. When realistic tissue resistive anisotropies (changes in conductivity with direction) are included in the model, the bidomain formulation begins to give new insights into how shocks change the transmembrane potential. Similar to the one-dimensional cable model, the bidomain predicts that hyperpolarization of the transmembrane potential occurs under the extracellular anodal electrode and depolarization of the transmembrane potential occurs under the extracellular cathodal electrode. Additionally, the bidomain model hypothesizes that there should be changes in the transmembrane potential, either hyperpolarization or depolarization, across much of the entire heart (12). The change in transmembrane potential elicited by the shock depends on the distribution of intracellular and extracellular current that is affected by the change in the potential gradient with distance, the distance from the electrode, and the orientation of the myocardial fibers (13). Experimental studies have shown that there is a complex pattern of transmembrane potential change during the delivery of a defibrillation shock, similar to those predicted by the bidomain model (14–16). This change in the transmembrane potential by the shock leads to changes in VF wavefront propagation and initiation of postshock activation fronts that determine whether or not a shock is successful.

In order to be successful, a defibrillation shock must stop most or all of the fibrillation wavefronts (10,16–18). The extension of refractoriness hypothesis is one proposed explanation of how a shock stops fibrillation (19,20). If a shock only slightly alters the transmembrane potential in a region, then activation fronts in the region may continue to propagate, relatively unaltered, after the shock. If the shock is large enough, then it can have one of three effects on the myocardium depending on the local shock strength and its timing with respect to the local action potential. If the shock is delivered just after local activation, then there may be little or no change in the action potential duration. If the shock is large enough and delivered relatively late during the action potential, then it will initiate a new action potential. A shock that is large enough but delivered during the plateau of the action potential will modify an ongoing action potential without initiating a new action potential *(21,22)*. If the first activation front that forms after a defibrillation shock encounters tissue with an extended refractory period, the front will be stopped because it cannot propagate into the region of refractory tissue *(23)*.

Much of our understanding about the mechanism of postdefibrillation arrhythmia induction comes from studying the simpler process of induction of fibrillation by shocks during paced rhythms. This idea has been formalized in the upper limit of vulnerability hypothesis for defibrillation that states that failed defibrillation by a shock that is near the defibrillation threshold occurs by the same mechanism as VF induction caused by a premature stimulus of the same strength delivered during the vulnerable period *(24,25)*. One mechanism for the induction of these postshock arrhythmias is described by the critical point hypothesis. The critical point hypothesis postulates that functional reentry is initiated in myocardium in which a dispersion of shock potential gradients intersects a dispersion of refractoriness *(26)*. In adjacent regions, direct excitation of recovered tissue and refractory period extension in relatively refractory tissue occur. Excitation blocks in the direction of the tissue with refractory period extension and propagates away from and around it. By the time the wavefront re-encounters the tissue that was previously refractory, it has recovered and the wavefront re-enters. Using video-imaging techniques, Banville et al. have shown in isolated rabbit hearts that the centers of re-entrant wavefronts induced by shocks delivered in paced rhythms can be moved by changing the shock strength that is delivered and the coupling interval at which it is delivered *(27)*.

Focal activation is also frequently observed following defibrillation shocks, in which activation is first observed at one site followed by propagation away from this site in all directions *(28)*. Focal origins of activation fronts were first observed with recordings confined to the epicardial surface *(28)*. In these cases, it is possible that the activation front arose from the border of a directly excited region that is located intramurally. This activation front could appear to be focal when it is conducted to the epicardium. Three-dimensional mapping with plunge needles has demonstrated that foci following a shock can arise intramurally at sites in which foci were not present during VF before the shock *(29)*. Foci have also been observed with the electrical induction of VF during the vulnerable period *(30)*. The cause of the foci is unknown although it has been observed that foci during defibrillation can occur in myocardial regions exposed to shock fields of 2 to 6 V/cm, raising the possibility of early or delayed after depolarizations as the source of the foci *(28,31)*.

For successful shocks near the defibrillation threshold, the first few beats following the shock are not sinus beats *(32)*. Ectopic activations following a shock, whether they are focal or re-entrant, do not always lead to fibrillation. Chattipakorn et al. have suggested that whether or not a shock near the defibrillation threshold will defibrillate depends on the number and timing of activations that occur following the shock *(33)*. Chattipakorn et al. paced the heart after delivering a shock that was 50 to 100 V greater than the defibrillation threshold and that, when given by itself without pacing, always defibrillated. At least three rapidly paced cycles after this shock were necessary for induction of VF. Cao et al. examined the induction of fibrillation by rapid pacing in dogs *(34)*. Cato et al. showed that as pacing rate increases, a spatial heterogeneity of conduction velocities occurs, which leads to functional re-entry and VF. Understanding how postshock arrhythmias progress is important to understanding how shocks ultimately succeed or fail.

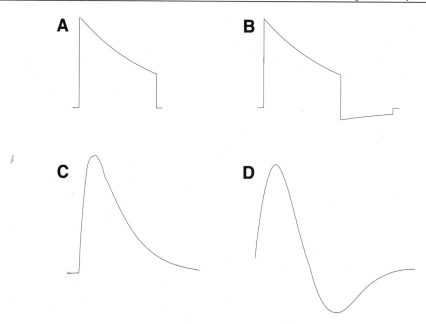

Fig. 1. (A) Truncated exponential monophasic waveform. **(B)** Truncated exponential biphasic waveform. **(C)** Damped sinusoidal monophasic waveform. **(D)** Quasi-sinusoidal biphasic waveform.

DEFIBRILLATION METHODOLOGY

Defibrillators consist of two parts: (a) a mechanism for determining whether or not it is necessary to deliver a shock to the patient, and (b) a mechanism to actually deliver that shock. The electric shock that is delivered is called the waveform. The two most common waveform shapes used clinically are monophasic and biphasic waveforms (Fig. 1). In monophasic waveforms, the polarity of the shock does not change at each electrode throughout the entire duration of the shock. In biphasic waveforms, the polarity of the shock reverses at each electrode part way through the shock. Many studies, both animal and human, have shown that biphasic waveforms can defibrillate with less current and energy than monophasic waveforms *(35–38)*. Within each type, waveforms can be described as truncated exponential or damped sinusoidal shapes. Most implantable cardioverter defibrillators use truncated exponential biphasic waveforms. In contrast, most external defibrillators until recently have used damped sinusoidal waveforms. Because of the inductor necessary to shape the damped sinusoidal waveform, these defibrillators tend to be large and heavy. More recently, lighter external defibrillators have been developed that use truncated exponential biphasic waveforms, similar those used in internal defibrillators. Quasi-sinusoidal biphasic waveforms are used in external defibrillators in Russia and similar to truncated exponential biphasic waveforms, have been shown to have an improved efficacy over monophasic waveforms *(39,40)*.

Not all biphasic waveforms are superior to monophasic waveforms. For example, if the second phase of the biphasic waveform becomes much longer than the first phase, then the energy required for defibrillation increases and can eventually rise to a level above the energy required to defibrillate with a monophasic waveform equal in duration to the first phase of the biphasic waveform *(38,41,42)*. The optimum durations of the two phases of the biphasic waveform depend on electrode impedance and defibrillator capacitance (43–46).

Several groups have shown that for square waveforms of duration less than 20 to 30 ms, defibrillation efficacy follows a strength-duration relationship similar to cardiac stimulation (47,48); as the waveform gets longer, the average current necessary to successfully defibrillate 50% of the time becomes progressively less, approaching a minimum called the rheobase (49). Unlike stimulation, at very long waveform durations, the average current necessary to defibrillate rises. On the basis of this observation, several groups have suggested that cardiac defibrillation can be mathematically modeled using a parallel resistor-capacitor (RC) network (Fig. 2 [44,46,50,52]). Empirically, it has been determined that the time constant for the parallel RC network is in the range of 2.5 to 5 ms (44–46). In one version of the model, a current waveform is applied to the RC network (46). The voltage across the network is then calculated for each time point during the defibrillation pulse. The relative defibrillation efficacy of different waveform shapes and durations can be compared by holding the peak current of the waveform constant and comparing the maximum voltage values achieved by each waveform; the higher the voltage, the lower the defibrillation threshold.

There is some evidence that this RC network is a reasonable if simplified model of the heart during defibrillation. Zhou et al. recorded the transmembrane potential of cells in a rabbit papillary muscle during delivery of a defibrillation sizes shock using a double-barrel micro-electrode technique (52). Zhou et al. showed that the transmembrane potential changed with a time constant varying from 1.6 to 6 ms depending on shock size and polarity (Fig. 3). Likewise, Mowrey et al. measured the transmembrane potential response to shocks in an isolated rabbit heart model using optical techniques (53). Mowrey et al. showed that the time constant for the transmembrane response varied from 1.6 to 14.2 ms depending on the size of the shock, its polarity and the time during the action potential that it is delivered. Both of these studies show that the cells of the heart respond to a shock with a time constant on the order of a few milliseconds, although choosing a single time constant may be too simplistic.

Several observations can be made from this model. First, for square waveforms of the same current, as the waveform duration gets longer, the voltage across the network gets progressively higher and approaches an asymptote or rheobase. For truncated exponential waveforms, however, the model voltage rises, reaches a peak and then, if the waveform is long enough, begins to decrease. Therefore, the model predicts that monophasic exponential waveforms should be truncated at a time when the peak voltage across the RC network is reached, because current or energy delivered after that point is wasted. In supporting this prediction, strength-duration relationships for waveform leading edge voltage at the defibrillation threshold for truncated exponential waveforms in both animals (46) and humans (54) do not approach an asymptote but rather reach a minimum and remain constant over a range of waveform durations. This minimum does not extend indefinitely. Schuder and colleagues showed that if the duration of the waveform gets too long, then it is no longer capable of defibrillating (55). However, this condition only occurs for waveforms more than 30 seconds in duration.

Second, the model predicts that the heart acts as a low-pass filter (51). Therefore, waveforms that rise gradually should have an improved efficacy over waveforms that reach their maximum value immediately. This prediction has been shown to hold true for both internal and external defibrillation (56,57). Ascending ramps defibrillate with a greater efficacy than do descending ramps (56,58).

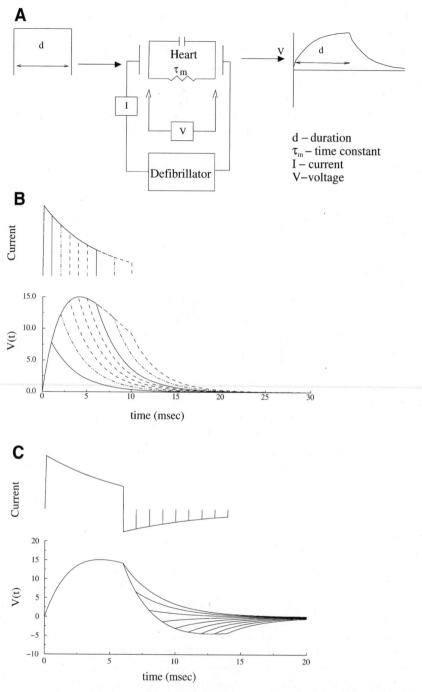

Fig. 2. Model responses to a monophasic and biphasic truncated exponential waveform with a time constant of 7 ms. Leading edge current of the input waveforms was 10A. **(A)** A schematic of the parallel RC circuit. The input is a square wave. The model response approaches a maximum assymptotically. **(B)** The model response to a monophasic waveform. Waveforms were truncated at 1, 2, 3, 4, 5, 6, 8, and 10 ms. The model response reaches a peak at 4 ms and then begins to decrease despite continued current delivery. **(C)** The model response to a biphasic waveform. Phase 1 was truncated at 6 ms. Phase 2 was truncated after 1, 2, 3, 4, 5, 6, 7, and 8 ms. The model response does not change polarity until phase-2 duration is longer than 2 ms.

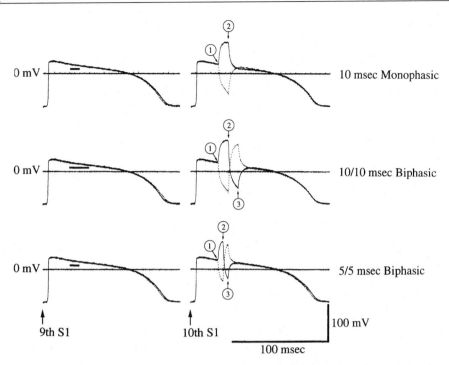

Fig. 3. Measurements of shock-induced transmembrane potential change (δ Vm). Each tracing includes recordings of 9th S1-induced action potential and 10th S1-induced action potential during which a 10-ms monophasic (top) or 10/10-ms (middle) or 5/5 ms (bottom) biphasic shock was applied. Shock strength was 11 V/cm. Tracings for the same shock waveform but opposite polarity are superimposed. One shock polarity caused depolarization (solid lines), whereas opposite polarity caused hyperpolarization (dotted lines). Arrows indicate timing of a shock: interval between arrows 1 and 2 represents duration of a monophasic shock or first phase of a biphasic shock, and interval between arrows 2 and 3 represents duration of second phase of a biphasic shock. Horizontal dark bars in 9th action potential indicate time interval during which shocks were actually given in 10th S1-induced action potential. Each action potential tracing is accompanied with an extracellular recording during which no shock artifact was recorded when both double-barrel microelectrode tips were outside the cell membrane. Voltage and time scales are given at bottom right.

Third, the model predicts that the most appropriate measure of a defibrillation waveform is current rather than energy. Studies in both animals and humans support this prediction. Kerber et al. showed in 347 patients who received 1009 shocks using a damped sinusoidal monophasic waveform that there was a clear relationship between peak current and shock success *(59)*.

Several groups have suggested that the optimal first phase of a biphasic waveform is the optimal monophasic waveform *(43,46)*. If this is true, then what does the model predict as the "best" second phase of a biphasic waveform? Empirically, it appears that the role of the second phase is to return the model voltage response to 0 as quickly as possible to maximize the increased efficacy of the biphasic waveform over that of the monophasic waveform with the same duration as phase one of the biphasic waveform. If the network voltage does not reach 0 or if it greatly overshoots 0, efficacy is lost. Swerdlow and colleagues have shown in humans that the "best" second phase of a biphasic waveform is one that returns the model response close to 0 *(46)*.

The location of the defibrillation electrodes affects the magnitude of the shock necessary to defibrillate the heart. Typically, 200 to 360 J of energy is necessary for successful defibrillation when the defibrillation electrodes are located on the body surface, as occurs in transthoracic defibrillation with a damped sinusoidal monophasic waveform. Less energy is required for a truncated exponential biphasic waveform. However, only 4 to 20% of the current that is delivered to transthoracic defibrillation electrodes ever reaches the heart. Most of the current is shunted around the heart through the muscles of the chest wall *(60)*. Moving the location of electrodes on the chest wall can also affect defibrillation efficacy. The probability of 200 to 360 J monophasic shocks converting atrial fibrillation to sinus rhythm is higher if the electrodes are on the anterior and posterior chest walls than if they are on the anterior and lateral chest walls *(61)*.

EFFECT OF HIGH-SHOCK FIELDS ON THE MYOCARDIUM

What happens if a defibrillation shock gets very large? At high-shock strengths, the probability of defibrillation success begins to drop *(62)*. It is thought that at large strengths, defibrillation shocks can have detrimental effects on the heart. Increasing the shock strength to very high levels (>1000 V with transvenous electrodes) can result in activation fronts arising from regions of high potential gradient that re-induce VF *(63)*. Cates et al. showed that for both monophasic and biphasic shocks, increasing shock strength does not always improve the probability of successful defibrillation and may in fact increase the incidence of postshock arrhythmias *(64)*.

The shape of the waveform alters the strength of the shock at which these detrimental effects occur. Use of a 10-ms truncated exponential monophasic waveform for VF in dogs resulted in temporary conduction block in regions in which the potential gradient was greater than 64 ± 4 V/cm *(65)*. Shocks that created even higher potential gradients in the myocardium prolonged the duration of this conduction block. In contrast, a potential gradient in the myocardium of 71 ± 6 V/cm was required for conduction block when a 5-ms/5-ms truncated exponential biphasic shock was used. Addition of a second phase to a monophasic waveform—making it a biphasic waveform—reduced the damage sustained by cultured chick myocytes compared to that induced by the monophasic waveform alone *(66)*. Reddy et al. showed that transthoracic defibrillation with biphasic shocks resulted in less postshock electrocardiogram evidence of myocardial dysfunction than standard monophasic damped sinusoidal waveforms, without compromise of defibrillation efficacy *(67)*. Thus, biphasic waveforms are less apt to cause electro-physiologic damage or dysfunction in high potential gradient regions than monophasic waveforms.

One mechanism that has been implicated for the mechanism of shocks causing damage to the myocardium is electroporation, the formation of holes or pores in the cell membrane. Electroporation may occur in regions in which the shock potential gradient is high (>50–70 V/cm) and had been hypothesized to occur in regions in which the potential gradient is much less than 50 V/cm *(68)*. The very high voltage can result in disruption of the phospholipid membrane bilayer and the formation of pores that permit the free influx and efflux of ions and macromolecules. Electroporation can cause massive ion exchange across the cell membrane. The transmembrane potential changes temporarily to a value almost equal to that of the plateau of a normal action potential. During this period, the cell is paralyzed electrically being both unresponsive and unable to conduct an action potential. Exposure of the myocardium to yet higher potential gradients, probably greater than 150 V/cm, results in arrhythmic beating and at very high potential gradients necrosis may occur *(69)*.

Two clinical trials have been performed comparing the effect of shock energies on survival after prehospital sudden CA. Weaver et al. compared the effect of two shock strengths on survival *(70)*. A total of 249 patients were randomized to receive either one or two (as necessary) monophasic damped sinusoidal shocks of 175 J or 320 J (2.5 or 4.6 J/kg for a 70 kg individual). If three or more shocks were required, all subsequent shocks were 320 J. In a three-way analysis of variance, both return of spontaneous circulation and survival were inversely related to the total number of shocks delivered but neither of these outcomes was related to the level of energy used for the initial two defibrillation shocks. The higher energy shocks were more likely to leave the patient in atrioventricular block following multiple shocks, but this difference did not influence survival.

Schneider et al. compared the effect of a protocol using a constant 150 J shock strength vs a protocol using an escalating 200 to 360 J shock strength *(71)*. The 150 J shock was always biphasic. Of the escalating 200 to 360 J shocks, 80% were monophasic truncated exponential shocks and 20% were monophasic damped sinusoidal shocks. In 115 patients with prehospital sudden arrest secondary to VF, there was no difference in survival in patients receiving monophasic or biphasic shocks. An increased proportion of patients did have return of spontaneous circulation in the 150 J group compared to the 200 to 360 J group but this difference can be explained by the increased defibrillation efficacy of the biphasic waveform compared to the monophasic waveforms. If the comparison is limited to patients who were successfully defibrillated, 41 of 54 patients (75%) had return of spontaneous circulation in the 150 J group compared to 33 of 49 patients (67%) in the 200 to 360 J group ($p = NS$). Both the Weaver study and the Schneider study suggest that there is neither increased survival nor decreased survival with the larger monophasic shocks. A comparison of low and high energy biphasic shocks has yet to be performed in the prehospital setting but is crucial for determining whether a constant low-strength or an escalating shock strength protocol is preferred with biphasic waveforms.

Beyond survival, it is desirable that the heart not be damaged by a defibrillation shock. Grubb et al. measured cardiac enzymes in patients resuscitated from out-of-hospital cardiac arrest (CA) including patients who received no shocks *(72)*. A rise in CK-MB and cardiac troponin T occurred in almost all cases. Patients received from 0 to no less than 2000 J of total defibrillation energy. There was a modest correlation between enzyme release for both troponin T and CK-MB and the total defibrillation energy delivered among patients without electrocardiographic evidence of acute myocardial infarction (AMI). The total amount of delivered defibrillation energy was also positively correlated with the duration of CPR. Both the mechanical trauma and the hypoperfusion associated with CPR are possible explanations for the correlation between enzyme release and total defibrillation energy.

A similar study performed by Müllner et al. examined the influence of chest compressions and external defibrillation on the release of cardiac enzymes in patients resuscitated from out-of-hospital CA *(73)*. Using a multivariate stepwise linear regression model, they showed that CK-MB concentrations 12 hours after CPR were positively associated with the presence of AMI, the duration of CPR, and the presence of cardiogenic shock in the postresuscitation period, but were not significantly associated either with the number of defibrillation shocks delivered (mean = 3, range = 1–6) or with the amount of epinephrine administered. Likewise, a similar model was constructed for troponin T concentrations 12 hours after resuscitation and again, the number of defibrillation shocks administered was not significant in the model. These studies suggest that damage caused by defibrillation during CPR is either small or nonexistent compared with the damage and dysfunction caused by the underlying pathology and period of no-flow ischemia.

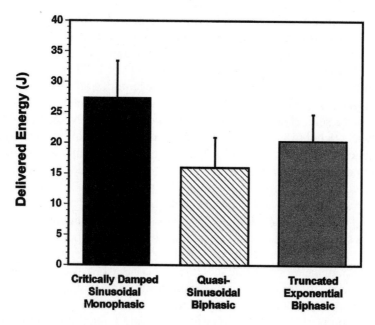

Fig. 4. Defibrillation thresholds in terms of energy for quasi-sinusoidal biphasic waveform and critically damped sinusoidal monophasic waveform after 15 seconds and after 5 minutes of fibrillation. Defibrillation threshold for biphasic waveform did not change significantly with duration of fibrillation, whereas defibrillation threshold for monophasic waveform was significantly different after 5 minutes of fibrillation vs after 15 seconds of fibrillation. In both cases, defibrillation threshold for biphasic waveform was significantly different from that of monophasic waveform.

EFFECT OF THE DURATION OF VF ON DEFIBRILLATION EFFICACY

Most defibrillation studies have been performed on healthy hearts after short periods of electrically induced VF, usually 15 to 45 seconds in duration. Yet most patients who suffer sudden CA are away from immediate medical care and fibrillate for 5 to 7 minutes before defibrillation. Jones et al. compared the efficacy of a monophasic waveform (5 ms rectangular) and an asymmetrical biphasic waveform (5 ms each pulse, V2 = 50% V1) at 5, 15, and 30 seconds using a working rabbit heart model of defibrillation *(74)*. Results showed that biphasic waveforms had significantly lower voltage and energy thresholds at all fibrillation durations and that their relative efficacy improved with increasing fibrillation duration. The biphasic waveform energy threshold was 0.67 that for the monophasic waveform after 5 seconds of fibrillation. The ratio between the biphasic waveform threshold and the monophasic waveform threshold (B/M) decreased to 0.62 at 15 seconds. At 30 seconds, B/M was 0.52.

Walcott et al. compared the relative efficacy of a damped sinusoidal monophasic and damped sinusoidal biphasic waveform after 15 seconds and 5 minutes of VF (3 minutes of unsupported VF followed by 2 minutes of femoral–femoral venous–arterial circulation at 1 L per minute) in a canine model *(40)*. The defibrillation threshold increased by 40% for the damped sinusoidal monophasic waveform ($p < 0.05$ compared to the defibrillation threshold at 15 seconds). In contrast, the defibrillation threshold increased by 10% for a damped sinusoidal biphasic waveform (p = NS defibrillation threshold at 5 minutes compared to the threshold at 15 seconds) (Fig. 4).

It is not possible to perform a paired comparison of defibrillation shock efficacy in humans but we can compare the results from different studies to estimate how shock efficacy changes with VF duration. Higgins et al. showed that 96% of patients were defibrillated with a 200 J damped sinusoidal monophasic waveform in patients in the electrophysiology laboratory following a failed internal defibrillation test shock *(75)*. Weaver et al. showed that 61% of patients were defibrillated with a 175 J damped sinusoidal monophasic waveform in patients suffering *(70)* VF outside the hospital. Furthermore, defibrillation success was not improved when the shock strength was increased to 320 J. These studies suggest that there is a decrease in defibrillation efficacy with VF duration for the monophasic damped sinusoidal waveform in humans.

The same comparison can be made for biphasic waveforms. Bardy et al. showed that 86% of patients were defibrillated with the first shock using a 130 J biphasic truncated exponential waveform following a failed internal defibrillation shock *(76)*. VF lasted for about 15 seconds before shock delivery. Schneider et al. showed that 96% of patients were defibrillated with the first shock using the same biphasic truncated exponential waveform except for shock strength, which was 150 J *(71)*. VF lasted for 9.2 ± 2.9 minutes. Thus, mirroring the animal data presented above, defibrillation efficacy does not appear to decrease with VF duration for biphasic waveforms.

EFFECT OF ISCHEMIA ON DEFIBRILLATION EFFICACY

Whether or not acute regional ischemia affects defibrillation efficacy of electrically induced VF is controversial. Occlusion or embolization of a coronary artery has been reported to increase defibrillation current and energy thresholds during the 30 to 60 minutes following the onset of myocardial ischemia in dogs *(77,78)*. Other reports either did not find increases in defibrillation thresholds after coronary artery occlusion *(79,80)* or found a lower threshold *(81)*.

More important than the effect of ischemia on defibrillation is whether the arrhythmia starts spontaneously during acute ischemia or is induced electrically. Ouyang et al. determined the defibrillation threshold for spontaneous arrhythmias induced by acute ischemia using a monophasic waveform and electrodes directly on the heart *(82)*. The lowest energy threshold for defibrillation was determined in 10 open chest dogs with reversible 10-minute coronary occlusions at various sites for each of 44 VF events. Despite similar masses of ischemia, two times as much energy was required for defibrillation of spontaneous VF (whether after occlusion or reperfusion) as for electrically induced VF.

More recently, Walcott et al. measured the defibrillation threshold for a biphasic waveform with both electrically induced VF and spontaneous VF secondary to acute ischemia *(83)*. They showed that the defibrillation threshold for electrically induced VF was 65 ± 28 J but was 228 ± 97 J for spontaneous VF secondary to acute ischemia in a dog model. Similar results were seen in swine. Of note, there appeared to be two populations of spontaneous arrhythmias, one that was defibrillated with relatively low strength shocks and a second that was defibrillated with much higher shock strengths or not at all (Fig. 5).

One possible explanation for why the defibrillation threshold is higher for spontaneous VF secondary to acute ischemia is that the shock actually does defibrillate but that the heart refibrillates before the electrocardiogram amplifiers have recovered from the shock. Qin et al. measured the defibrillation threshold for electrically induced VF in 15

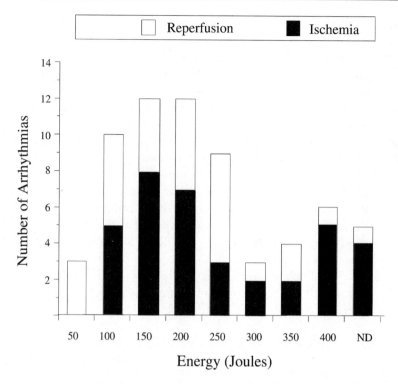

Fig. 5. Histogram of the number of arrhythmic episodes that were successfully defibrillated as a function of energy level. It appears that there are two populations of arrhythmias, one that is defibrillated at a relatively low energy level and one that is defibrillated at a much higher energy level. Open bar = reperfusion; solid bar = occlusion. ND = the VF could not be defibrillated and the animal died.

pigs before ischemia and then the efficacy of a shock 1.5 times the measured threshold during acute regional ischemia although recording a fast recovering electrogram and blood pressure trace (84). If VF was not induced during 20 minutes of ischemia, fibrillation was induced electrically. Defibrillation efficacy at 1.5 times the electrically induced VF defibrillation threshold was significantly higher for electrically induced ischemic VF (76%) than for spontaneous VF (31%). The incidence of delayed recurrence (at least one organized electrical beat before VF recurrence) after electrically induced nonischemic (3%) or ischemic (20%) VF was significantly lower than after spontaneous VF (75%). Mean VF recurrence time after spontaneous VF was 4.6 ± 5.3 seconds. These data suggest that shocks often stop spontaneous fibrillation but that fibrillation quickly recurs and that if the first two to three shocks fail then drug therapy might be more appropriate than continued shock delivery

EFFECT OF INFARCTION ON DEFIBRILLATION EFFICACY

It does not appear that previous MI has an effect on defibrillation efficacy. Human studies stratifying patient characteristics as a function of defibrillation threshold have shown that heart dimensions and body dimensions but not underlying heart disease are correlated with the defibrillation threshold of electrically induced VF for internal electrodes in the electrophysiology laboratory *(54)*. In a study of 26 patients, the defibrillation threshold was not different for patients with previous MI when compared to patients with structurally normal hearts *(85)*. Animal studies have not shown any change in defibrillation threshold when comparing animals with previous MIs to those animals with normal hearts *(78,86,87)*.

Previous MI does increase the probability of a sudden CA. Animal studies have shown that a previous myocardial infarction makes it much more likely that an episode of acute ischemia will cause a tachyarrhythmia, both when the acute ischemia is in a different perfusion bed from the infarct, and in the same perfusion bed as the infarct *(88)*.

PEDIATRIC DEFIBRILLATION

VF is a less common reason for VA in pediatric patients than in adult patients. Survival in pediatric CA patients in more likely, although, if VF is present at the time of resuscitation. Therefore there is growing interest in defibrillation for pediatric patients. Several investigators have shown that defibrillation shock success is directly related to body weight. Geddes et al. showed that the energy and current necessary to defibrillate using a damped sinusoidal monophasic waveform is related to body weight across different animal species *(89)*. Tacker et al. in a retrospective human clinical study, showed a reverse correlation between body weight and the percentage of patients successfully defibrillated by a given shock strength *(90)*. More recently, Zhang et al. have shown that the percent success for 70 J and 100 J biphasic defibrillation shocks is inversely correlated with animal size *(91)*. Killingsworth et al. showed that the energy dose at the defibrillation threshold is proportional to the weight of the animal across a group of young swine ranging from 3.8 to 20 kg *(92)*.

If automatic external defibrillators are to be used on pediatric patients, then shock strengths must be sufficient to defibrillate the larger pediatric patients although not damaging the hearts of the smallest patients. Gutgesell et al. reviewed 71 transthoracic monophasic defibrillations in 27 children *(93)* and showed that the appropriate defibrillation dose for a monophasic waveform is 2–4 J/kg. Eight-year-old patients weigh 25 kg on average. Therefore, a dose of 50 to 100 J should be adequate to treat pediatric patients.

A shock of 50 to 100 J is equivalent to 12 to 25 J/kg for newborn children. A pediatric case report describes a 150 J (9 J/kg) shock that resulted in transient ST segment changes; however both creatine kinase and troponin I were within normal limits and echocardiography showed no left ventricular (LV) dysfunction *(94)*. Animal data with monophasic waveforms suggest a wide margin of safety before myocardial injury is induced *(95–97)*. Increasing myocardial damage with increasing external monophasic shock strength has been reported at doses greater than 150 J/kg in pigs *(96)* and 30 J/kg in dogs *(98)*. A recent study indicated that there was no indication of persistent myocardial injury based on the time to return of sinus rhythm, ST segment deviation, LV dP/dt, or cardiac output in piglets weighing between 3.8 and 20.1 kg and receiving individual external biphasic shocks of up to 90 J/kg *(92)*. Nonetheless, a recent panel of experts concluded that a first shock of 150 to 200 J, with a possibility of even higher escalating energy shocks, exceeds the recommended dose of 2 to 4 J/kg for defibrillation of VF/pulseless ventricular tachycardia (VT) and is inappropriate for children less than 8 years old with a median weight less than 25 kg. Manufacturers of automatic external defibrillators (AEDs) are currently addressing the need for early defibrillation of pediatric patients with different biphasic waveforms as well as impedance compensating, nonescalating external shocks *(99)*.

An additional approach to early pediatric defibrillation is the development of a disposable attenuating pediatric electrode system that allows adult AEDs to be used for treatment of either adult or pediatric CA without modification or additional complication of the existing device *(100)*.

REFERENCES

1. Lown B. Defibrillation and cardioversion. Cardiovasc Res 2002; 55:220–224.
2. Zoll P, Linenthal AJ, Gibson W, Paul MH, Norman LR. Termination of ventricular fibrillation in man by externally applied countershock. NEJM YEAR 1956; 254:727.
3. Lown B, Amarasingham R, Neuman J, Berkovits B. Comparison of alternating current with direct current electroshock across the closed chest. JACC 1962; 10:223.
4. Chattipakorn N, KenKnight BH, Smith WM, Ideker RE. The isoelectric window after defibrillation shocks: Is it truly electrically quiescent? JACC 1997; 29(Suppl A):195A.
5. Dillon SM, Kwaku KF. Progressive depolarization: a unified hypothesis for defibrillation and fibrillation induction by shocks [in process citation]. J Cardiovasc Electrophysiol 1998; 9:529–552.
6. Efimov IR, Cheng YN, Biermann M, Van Wagoner DR, Mazgalev TN, Tchou PJ. Transmembrane voltage changes produced by real and virtual electrodes during monophasic defibrillation shocks delivered by an implantable electrode. JCELEP 1997; 8:1031–1045.
7. Usui M, Walcott GP, Strickberger SA, Rollins DL, Smith WM, Ideker RE. Effects of polarity for monophasic and biphasic shocks on defibrillation efficacy with an endocardial system. PACE 1996; 19: 65–71.
8. Chen P-S, Wolf PD, Claydon FJ, III, et al. The potential gradient field created by epicardial defibrillation electrodes in dogs. CIRC 1986; 74:626–636.
9. Zhou X, Daubert JP, Wolf PD, Smith WM, Ideker RE. Epicardial mapping of ventricular defibrillation with monophasic and biphasic shocks in dogs. CIRCRES 1993; 72:145–160.
10. Zipes DP, Fischer J, King RM, Nicoll A, Jolly WW. Termination of ventricular fibrillation in dogs by depolarizing a critical amount of myocardium. AJC 1975; 36:37–44.
11. Tung L. A bidomain model for describing ischemic myocardial DC potentials. Phd, Cambridge, MA: MIT, 1978.
12. Trayanova N, Skouibine K, Aguel F. The role of cardiac tissue structure in defibrillation. Chaos 1998; 8:221–233.
13. Eason J, Trayanova N. The effects of fiber curvature in a bidomain tissue with irregular boundaries. Proc. 15th Annu. Int. Conf. IEEE Eng. Med Biol. Soc, 1993, pp. 744–745.
14. Clark DM, Pollard AE, Ideker RE, Knisley SB. Optical transmembrane potential recordings during intracardiac defibrillation-strength shocks. JICE 1999; 3:109–120.
15. Efimov IR, Cheng Y, Van Wagoner DR, Mazgalev T, Tchou PJ. Virtual electrode-induced phase singularity: a basic mechanism of defibrillation failure. Circulation Research 1998; 82:918–25. English.
16. Chen P-S, Shibata N, Wolf PD, et al. Epicardial activation during successful and unsuccessful ventricular defibrillation in open chest dogs. CRP 1986; 7:625–648.
17. Mower MM, Mirowski M, Spear JF, Moore EN. Patterns of ventricular activity during catheter defibrillation. CIRC 1974; 49:858–861.
18. Wiggers CJ. The physiologic basis for cardiac resuscitation from ventricular fibrillation: Method for serial defibrillation. AHJ 1940; 20:413–422.
19. Dillon SM, Mehra R. Prolongation of ventricular refractoriness by defibrillation shocks may be due to additional depolarization of the action potential. JCELEP 1992; 3:442–456.
20. Tovar OH, Jones JL. Relationship between "extension of refractoriness" and probability of successful defibrillation. AJP 1997; 272(Heart Circ Physiol 41):H1011–H1019.
21. Dillon SM, Mehra R. Prolongation of ventricular refractoriness by defibrillation shocks may be due to additional depolarization of the action potential. JCELEP 1992; 3:442–456.
22. Knisley SB. Transmembrane voltage changes during unipolar stimulation of rabbit ventricle. Circ Res 1995; 77:1229–1239.
23. Kwaku KF, Dillon SM. Shock-induced depolarization of refractory myocardium prevents wave-front propagation in defibrillation. CIRCRES 1996; 79:957–973.
24. Chen PS, Shibata N, Dixon EG, et al. Activation during ventricular defibrillation in open-chest dogs. evidence of complete cessation and regeneration of ventricular fibrillation after unsuccessful shocks. Journal of Clinical Investigation 1986; 77:810–23. English.

25. Shibata N, Chen PS, Dixon EG, et al. Epicardial activation after unsuccessful defibrillation shocks in dogs. American Journal of Physiology 1988; 255(Pt 2):H902–H909. English.
26. Frazier DW, Wolf PD, Wharton JM, et al. Stimulus-induced critical point: Mechanism for electrical initiation of reentry in normal canine myocardium. JCI 1989; 83:1039–1052.
27. Banville I, Gray RA, Ideker RE, Smith WM. Shock-induced figure-of-eight reentry in the isolated rabbit heart. Circ Res 1999; 85:742–752.
28. Witkowski FX, Penkoske PA, Plonsey R. Mechanism of cardiac defibrillation in open-chest dogs with unipolar dc-coupled simultaneous activation and shock potential recordings. CIRC 1990; 82:244–260.
29. Chen P-S, Wolf PD, Melnick SD, Danieley ND, Smith WM, Ideker RE. Comparison of activation during ventricular fibrillation and following unsuccessful defibrillation shocks in open chest dogs. CIRCRES 1990; 66:1544–1560.
30. Wiggers CJ, Wégria R. Ventricular fibrillation due to single, localized induction and condenser shocks applied during the vulnerable phase of ventricular systole. AJP 1940; 128:500–505.
31. Zhou X, Daubert JP, Wolf PD, Smith WM, Ideker RE. Epicardial mapping of ventricular defibrillation with monophasic and biphasic shocks in dogs. Circ Res 1993; 72:145–60.
32. Usui M, Callihan RL, Walker RG, et al. Early activation sites after monophasic and biphasic shocks of equal voltage with an endocardial lead system. PACE 1995; 18(Part II):904.
33. Chattipakorn N, Rogers JM, Ideker RE. Influence of postshock epicardial activation patterns on the initiation of ventricular fibrillation by shocks near the upper limit of vulnerability. CIRCRES 1998; submitted.
34. Cao JM, Qu Z, Kim YH, et al. Spatiotemporal heterogeneity in the induction of ventricular fibrillation by rapid pacing: importance of cardiac restitution properties. Circulation Research 1999; 84:1318–1331. English.
35. Bardy GH, Ivey TD, Allen M, Johnson G, Mehra R, Green HL. A prospective, randomized evaluation of biphasic vs monophasic pulses on epicardial defibrillation efficacy in man. CIRC 1988; 78:II–219.
36. Block M, Hammel D, Böcker D, et al. A prospective randomized cross-over comparison on mono- and biphasic defibrillation using nonthoracotomy lead configurations in humans. J Cardiovasc Electrophysiol 1994; 5:581–590.
37. Chapman PD, Vetter JW, Souza JJ, Wetherbee JN, Troup PJ. Comparison of monophasic with single and dual capacitor biphasic waveforms for nonthoracotomy canine internal defibrillation. JACC 1989; 14:242–245.
38. Dixon EG, Tang ASL, Wolf PD, et al. Improved defibrillation thresholds with large contoured epicardial electrodes and biphasic waveforms. CIRC 1987; 76:1176–1184.
39. Gurvich NL, Markarychev VA. Defibrillation of the heart with biphasic electrical impulses. Kardiologiia 1967; 7:109–112.
40. Walcott GP, Melnick SB, Chapman FW, Jones JL, Smith WM, Ideker RE. The relative efficacy of monophasic and biphasic waveforms for transthoracic defibrillation after short and long durations of ventricular fibrillation. CIRC 1998; 98:2210–2215.
41. Feeser SA, Tang AS, Kavanagh KM, et al. Strength-duration and probability of success curves for defibrillation with biphasic waveforms. Circulation 1990; 82:2128–2141.
42. Tang AS, Yabe S, Wharton JM, Dolker M, Smith WM, Ideker RE. Ventricular defibrillation using biphasic waveforms: the importance of phasic duration. J Am Coll Cardiol 1989; 13:207–214.
43. Kroll MW. A minimal model of the single capacitor biphasic defibrillation waveform. PACE 1994; 17(Part 1):1782–1792.
44. Kroll MW. A minimal model of the monophasic defibrillation pulse. PACE 1993; 16:769–777.
45. Swerdlow CD, Fan W, Brewer JE. Charge-burping theory correctly predicts optimal ratios of phase duration for biphasic defibrillation waveforms. CIRC 1996; 94:2278–2284.
46. Walcott GP, Walker RG, Cates AW, Krassowska W, Smith WM, Ideker RE. Choosing the optimal monophasic and biphasic waveforms for ventricular defibrillation. JCELEP 1995; 6:737–750.
47. Blair HA. On the intensity-time relations for stimulation by electric currents. ii. JGENPH 1932; 15:731–755.
48. Lapicque L. L'Excitabilite en Fonction du Temps. Paris, France: Libraire J. Gilbert, 1926.
49. Mouchawar GA, Geddes LA, Bourland JD, Pearce JA. Ability of the lapicque and blair strength-duration curves to fit experimentally obtained data from the dog heart. TBME 1989; 36:971–974.
50. Irnich W. The fundamental law of electrostimulation and its application to defibrillation. PACE 1990; 13:1433–1447.
51. Sweeney RJ, Gill RM, Jones JL, Reid PR. Defibrillation using a high-frequency series of monophasic rectangular pulses: observations and model predictions. JCELEP 1996; 7:134–143.

52. Zhou X, Smith WM, Justice RK, Wayland JL, Ideker RE. Transmembrane potential changes caused by monophasic and biphasic shocks. Am J Physiol 1998; 275(Pt 2):H1798–H1807.
53. Mowrey KA, Cheng Y, Tchou PJ, Efimov R. Kinetics of defibrillation shock-induced response: design implications for the optimal defibrillation waveform. Europace 2002; 4:27–39.
54. Gold MR, Khalighi K, Kavesh MG, Daly D, Peters RW, Shorofsky SR. Clinical predictors of transvenous biphasic defibrillation thresholds. American Journal of Cardiology 1997; 79:1623–1627. English.
55. Schuder JC, Stoeckle H, West JA, Keskar PY. Transthoracic ventricular defibrillation in the dog with truncated and untruncated exponential stimuli. TBME 1971; 18:410–415.
56. Hillsley RE, Walker RG, Swanson DK, Rollins DL, Wolf PD, Smith WM, Ideker RE. Is the second phase of a biphasic defibrillation waveform the defibrillating phase? PACE 1993; 16:1401–1411.
57. Walcott GP, Melnick SB, Chapman FW, Smith WM, Ideker RE. Comparison of damped sinusoidal and truncated exponential waveforms for external defibrillation. JACC 1996; 27(2[Suppl A]):237A.
58. Schuder JC, Rahmoeller GA, Stoeckle H. Transthoracic ventricular defibrillation with triangular and trapezoidal waveforms. CIRCRES 1966; 19:689–694.
59. Kerber RE, Martins JB, Kienzle MB, et al. Energy, current, and success in defibrillation and cardioversion: clinical studies using an automated impedance-based method of energy adjustment. Circulation 1988; 77:1038–1046.
60. Lerman BB, Deale OC. Relation between transcardiac and transthoracic current during defibrillation in humans. Circ Res 1990; 67:1420–1426.
61. Kirchhof P, Eckardt L, Loh P, et al. Anterior-posterior versus anterior-lateral electrode positions for external cardioversion of atrial fibrillation: a randomised trial. Lancet 2002; 360:1275–1279.
62. Schuder JC, McDaniel WC, Stoeckle H. Defibrillation of 100-kg calves with asymmetrical, bidirectional, rectangular pulses. CARDRES 1984; 18:419–426.
63. Walker RG, Walcott GP, Smith WM, Ideker RE. Sites of earliest activation following transvenous defibrillation. CIRC 1994; 90(Part 2):I–447.
64. Cates AW, Wolf PD, Hillsley RE, Souza JJ, Smith WM, Ideker RE. The probability of defibrillation success and the incidence of postshock arrhythmia as a function of shock strength. PACE 1994; 17: 1208–1217.
65. Yabe S, Smith WM, Daubert JP, Wolf PD, Rollins DL, Ideker RE. Conduction disturbances caused by high current density electric fields. Circ Res 1990; 66:1190–1203.
66. Jones JL, Jones RE. Decreased defibrillator-induced dysfunction with biphasic rectangular waveforms. AJP 1984; 247:H792–H796.
67. Reddy RK, Gleva MJ, Gliner BE, et al. Biphasic transthoracic defibrillation causes fewer ecg st-segment changes after shock. Annals of Emergency Medicine 1997; 30:127–34.
68. DeBruin KA, Krassowska W. Electroporation and shock-induced transmembrane potential in a cardiac fiber during defibrillation strength shocks. ANBE 1998; 26:584–596.
69. Schuder JC, Gold JH, Stoeckle H, McDaniel WC, Cheung KN. Transthoracic ventricular defibrillation in the 100 kg calf with symmetrical one-cycle bidirectional rectangular wave stimuli. TBME 1983; 30: 415–422.
70. Weaver WD, Cobb LA, Copass MK, Hallstrom AP. Ventricular defibrillation – a comparative trial using 175-J and 320-J shocks. N Engl J Med 1982; 307:1101–1106.
71. Schneider T, Martens PR, Paschen H, et al. Multicenter, randomized, controlled trial of 150-J biphasic shocks compared with 200- to 360-J monophasic shocks in the resuscitation of out-of-hospital cardiac arrest victims. Optimized Response to Cardiac Arrest (ORCA) Investigators. Circulation 2000; 102: 1780–1787.
72. Grubb NR, Fox KA, Cawood P. Resuscitation from out-of-hospital cardiac arrest: implications for cardiac enzyme estimation. Resuscitation 1996; 33:35–41.
73. Mullner M, Oschatz E, Sterz F, et al. The influence of chest compressions and external defibrillation on the release of creatine kinase-mb and cardiac troponin t in patients resuscitated from out-of-hospital cardiac arrest. Resuscitation 1998; 38:99–105.
74. Jones JL, Swartz JF, Jones RE, Fletcher R. Increasing fibrillation duration enhances relative asymmetrical biphasic versus monophasic defibrillator waveform efficacy. Circ Res 1990; 67:376–384.
75. Higgins SL, Herre JM, Epstein AM, et al. A comparison of biphasic and monophasic shocks for external defibrillation. physio-control biphasic investigators. Prehosp Emerg Care 2000; 4:305–313.
76. Bardy GH, Marchlinski FE, Sharma AD, et al. Multicenter comparison of truncated biphasic shocks and standard damped sine wave monophasic shocks for transthoracic ventricular defibrillation. transthoracic investigators. Circulation 1996; 94:2507–2514.

77. Babbs CF, Paris RL, Tacker, WA, Jr., Bourland JD. Effects of myocardial infarction on catheter defibrillation threshold. Medical Instrumentation 1983; 17:18–20. English.

78. Tacker WA, Jr., Geddes LA, Cabler PS, Moore AG. Electrical threshold for defibrillation of canine ventricles following myocardial infarction. American Heart Journal 1974; 88:476–481. English.

79. Kerber RE, Pandian NG, Hoyt R, et al. Effect of ischemia, hypertrophy, hypoxia, acidosis, and alkalosis on canine defibrillation. American Journal of Physiology 1983; 244:H825–H831. English.

80. Ruffy R, Schwartz DJ, Hieb BR. Influence of acute coronary artery occlusion on direct ventricular defibrillation in dogs. Medical Instrumentation 1980; 14:23–26. English.

81. Jones DL, Sohla A, Klein GJ. Internal cardiac defibrillation threshold: effects of acute ischemia. Pacing annd Clinical Electrophysiology 1986; 9:322–331. English.

82. Ouyang P, Brinker JA, Bulkley BH, Jugdutt BI, Varghese PJ. Ischemic ventricular fibrillation: the importance of being spontaneous. American Journal of Cardiology 1981; 48:455–9. English.

83. Walcott GP, Killingsworth CR, Smith WM, Ideker RE. Biphasic waveform external defibrillation thresholds for spontaneous ventricular fibrillation secondary to acute ischemia. J Am Coll Cardiol 2002; 39:359–65.

84. Qin H, Walcott GP, Killingsworth CR, Rollins DL, Smith WM, Ideker RE. Impact of myocardial ischemia and reperfusion on ventricular defibrillation patterns, energy requirements, and detection of recovery. Circulation 2002; 105:2537–2542.

85. Jones DL, Klein GJ, Guiraudon GM, et al. Sequential pulse defibrillation in man: comparison of thresholds in normal subjects and those with cardiac disease. Medical Instrumentation 1987; 21:166–169. English.

86. Chang MS, Inoue H, Kallok MJ, Zipes DP. Double and triple sequential shocks reduce ventricular defibrillation threshold in dogs with and without myocardial infarction. Journal of the American College of Cardiology 1986; 8:1393–1405. English.

87. Wharton JM, Richard VJ, Murry CE, et al. Electrophysiological effects of monophasic and biphasic stimuli in normal and infarcted dogs. Pacing and Clinical Electrophysiology 1990; 13:1158–1172. English.

88. Cinca J, Blanch P, Carreño A, Mont L, García-Burillo A, Soler-Soler J. Acute ischemic ventricular arrhythmias in pigs with healed myocardial infarction - comparative effects of ischemia at a distance and ischemia at the infarct zone. Circ 1997; 96:653–658.

89. Geddes LA, Tacker WA, Rosborough JP, Moore AG, Cabler PS. Electrical dose for ventricular defibrillation of large and small animals using precordial electrodes. J Clin Invest 1974; 53:310–319.

90. Tacker WA, Jr., Galioto FM, Jr., Giuliani E, Geddes LA, McNamara DG. Energy dosage for human trans-chest electrical ventricular defibrillation. N Engl J Med 1974; 290:214,215.

91. Zhang Y, Clark C, Davies L, Karlsson G, Zimmerman M, Kerber R. Body weight is a predictor of biphasic shock success for low energy transthoracic defibrillation. Resuscitation 2002; 54:281.

92. Killingsworth CR, Melnick SB, Chapman FW, et al. Defibrillation threshold and cardiac responses using an external biphasic defibrillator with pediatric and adult adhesive patches in pediatric-sized piglets. Resuscitation 2002; 55:177–85.

93. Gutgesell HP, Tacker WA, Geddes LA, Davis S, Lie JT, and McNamara DG. Energy dose for ventricular defibrillation of children. Pediatrics 1976; 58:898–901.

94. Gurnett CA, Atkins DL. Successful use of a biphasic waveform automated external defibrillator in a high-risk child. Am J Cardiol 2000; 86:1051–1053.

95. Van Vleet JF, Tacker WA, Jr., Geddes LA, Ferrans VF. Sequential cardiac morphologic alterations induced in dogs by single transthoracic damped sinusoidal waveform defibrillator shocks. Am J Vet Res 1978; 39:271–278.

96. Gaba DM, Talner NS. Myocardial damage following transthoracic direct current countershock in newborn piglets. Pediatr Cardiol 1982; 2:281–288.

97. Babbs CF, Paris RL, Tacker WA, Jr., Bourland JD. Effects of myocardial infarction on catheter defibrillation threshold. Med Instrum 1983; 17:18–20.

98. Babbs CF, Tacker WA, VanVleet JF, Bourland JD, Geddes LA. Therapeutic indices for transchest defibrillator shocks: effective, damaging, and lethal electrical doses. Am Heart J 1980; 99:734–738.

99. Atkins DL, Chameides L, Fallat ME, et al. Resuscitation science of pediatrics. Ann Emerg Med 2001; 37(4 Suppl):S41–S48.

100. Jorgenson D, Morgan C, Snyder D, et al. Energy attenuator for pediatric application of an automated external defibrillator. Crit Care Med 2002; 30(4 Suppl):S145–147.

13   Public Access Defibrillation

Vincent N. Mosesso, Jr., MD, FACEP,
Mary M. Newman, BS,
and Kristin R. Hanson, BA, EMT

CONTENTS

INTRODUCTION

The value of early intervention in critically ill patients has long been recognized. As early as the 1700s, scientists recognized the value of mouth-to-mouth respiration and the medical benefits of electricity *(1)*. In the modern era, advances in resuscitation began to proliferate. In 1947, Claude Beck successfully resuscitated a 14-year-old boy through the use of *open* chest massage and an alternating current (AC) defibrillator, the kind that is used in wall outlets. In 1956, Paul Zoll demonstrated the effectiveness of *closed* chest massage with the use of an AC defibrillator. In the late 1950s, Peter Safar, William Kouwenhoven, James Jude and others began to study sudden cardiac arrest (CA) and in 1960, they demonstrated the efficacy of mouth-to-mouth ventilation and closed chest cardiac massage *(2)*. In 1961, Bernard Lown demonstrated the superiority of direct current (DC) defibrillators, the kind provided by batteries. In 1966, J. Frank Pantridge and John Geddes developed the world's first mobile intensive care unit (MICU) in Belfast, Northern Ireland, as a way to bring early advanced medical care to patients with cardiac emergencies *(3)*. In 1969, William Grace established the first MICU in the United States in New York City *(4)*. Subsequently, there were efforts in the United States and throughout the world to emulate and build on this concept. In the late 1960s and early 1970s, paramedic programs were developed by Eugene Nagel in Miami, Leonard Cobb in Seattle, Leonard Rose in Portland, Michael Criley in Los Angeles, and James Warren and Richard Lewis in Columbus. In the 1980s, Mickey Eisenberg, Richard Cummins,

From: *Contemporary Cardiology: Cardiopulmonary Resuscitation*
Edited by: J. P. Ornato and M. A. Peberdy © Humana Press Inc., Totowa, NJ

and colleagues demonstrated the effectiveness of rapid defibrillation in Seattle, Washington *(5)*, while Kenneth Stults demonstrated the same in rural Iowa *(6)*. This growing body of research demonstrated the importance of rapid care for victims of sudden CA by showing that survival improved when basic life support (mouth-to-mouth ventilation and closed chest compressions) was provided within 4 minutes and advanced life support (defibrillation, intravenous medications and fluids, and advanced airway management) within 8 minutes. Subsequent studies found that the benefits of advanced life support were primarily the result of electrical countershock for patients in ventricular fibrillation (VF). From these findings, a model of care called the "Chain of Survival," was first described by Mary Newman *(7)*, and then by Cummins et al. *(8)*, and eventually adopted by the Citizen CPR Foundation, the American Heart Association (AHA) and others. The Chain of Survival consists of four action steps that must occur in rapid succession to provide the patient the greatest likelihood for resuscitation: early access (call 911 or the local emergency number to notify the emergency medical services [EMS] system and summon on-site help); early cardiopulmonary resuscitation (CPR; begin immediately); early defibrillation; and early advanced care (transfer care to EMS professionals upon their arrival at the scene).

THE CHALLENGE OF PROVIDING EARLY DEFIBRILLATION

Growing appreciation of the value of early defibrillation prior to hospital arrival and of the need for improved care of trauma victims led to the development of EMS systems in most nonrural communities throughout the United States. Through the efforts of dedicated individuals who underwent training as emergency medical technicians and paramedics, along with government funding of well-equipped ambulances designed specifically for providing emergency medical care outside the hospital, great strides were made in improving the initial care provided to persons with out-of-hospital emergencies. Despite these advances, decades later, the death toll from sudden CA remains as high as 98 to 99% *(9,10)*, with a national average of 93% *(11)*.

The reason for the dismal survival rate from sudden CA became profoundly evident—time to intervention. Although the development of EMS systems is perhaps one of the greatest improvements in US health care this century, expecting such systems to effectively treat victims of sudden CA within our current medical understanding and the limitations of EMS response intervals clearly is fallacious. Spaite et al. developed a useful description of the time intervals between patient collapse and provision of care (Fig. 1; *[12]*). There have been many efforts made to shorten each of these time intervals. Additionally, significant advances in each phase of out-of-hospital emergency response have lead to significant improvements over the years. There is clearly a limit, however, to minimizing response-time intervals. Even small improvements in survival come at a high price. Nichol et al. demonstrated that an improvement in response time of 48 seconds would cost an estimated $40,000 to $368,000 per quality adjusted life year gained dependent on system configuration *(13)*. Thus, traditional EMS systems should not be expected to provide the first few minutes of emergency cardiovascular care, because it often is not deliverable at a reasonable cost.

AUTOMATED EXTERNAL DEFIBRILLATORS

Fortunately, medical technology has now provided a solution to this dilemma. The advent of automated external defibrillators (AEDs) now allows persons with very little

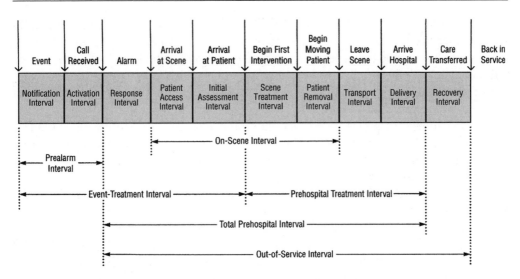

Fig. 1. Emergency medical services time-interval model.

training and no formal medical background to provide the lifesaving intervention of early defibrillation. AEDs are essential weapons in the current battle against sudden CA, and so a brief review of their characteristics is in order.

The key components of an AED are as follow:

- computer to perform ECG analysis,
- battery,
- capacitor,
- defibrillation pads and connector cable, and
- external shell with control buttons.

Although each manufacturer's device varies slightly, they are relatively consistent in their operation. Turning the device on typically initiates a series of verbal instructions. The device prompts the user to attach the defibrillation pads to the patient's chest. By detecting a change in impedance, the AED knows when the pads have been attached. (In devices in which the pads are not pre-attached, the device will prompt the user to attach the connector cable to the AED.) Once the pads are placed on the chest, the device initiates an electrocardiogram (ECG) analysis, typically evaluating two short segments of ECG strip for morphology, rate, and nonphysiologic signals (artifact and interference). If analysis of both of these segments agrees that a shock is indicated, the device charges the capacitor and advises the user of the finding. When the capacitor is charged, the device prompts the user to push the "shock" button. Some devices currently on the market will warn the user to "clear" the patient, that is, make sure no one is touching the patient, and then automatically deliver the shock, without requiring the user to push any buttons. The AED automatically initiates reanalysis after a shock to determine if another shock is needed; it will repeat this process for up to three consecutive shocks. After a third consecutive shock, the device will withhold analysis for 1 minute and prompt the user to do CPR during that interval. In all cases, users are guided by voice prompts that transfer decision making from the user to the computerized device.

The algorithms used to define shockable rhythms in AEDs have been continually refined over the last 20 years and are now quite sophisticated and accurate. Several evaluations have found their specificity to be close to 100%, which means that the device will not shock ECG rhythms that would not be shocked by an advanced care provider performing manual defibrillation. The sensitivity typically is 90 to 95% with most "misses" being very fine VF (14,15).

Multiple models of AEDs are now available and new ones are entering the market on a regular basis (Fig. 2). They include both new brands and upgraded models of existing brands. To see the current models on the market, visit the National Center for Early Defibrillation website (www.early-defib.org) (16).

A variety of AED improvements have been proposed recently. One concern is the need to shorten the "hands-off interval," during which chest compressions are withheld (17).This interval consists of listening to prompts, applying defibrillation pads, AED rhythm analysis, capacitor charging, and shock delivery and typically takes 60 to 90 seconds, even for proficient users. Another consideration is whether or not AEDs should incorporate communication capabilities to automatically alert the local 911 center when and where a device is activated and/or allow the telecommunication officer to speak with the user directly. Both options add additional cost, size, and weight to the device. Thus, the dilemma is whether it is better to have the smallest, most portable, lowest priced devices or to ensure rapid 911 notification and real-time user assistance. A lower priced device could mean wider distribution of AEDs and hopefully more rapid availability of a device, whereas an automatic connection would assist users in proper use of the device and care for the individual and the additional benefit of ensuring immediate dispatch of EMS.

An intriguing potential development is the incorporation of defibrillation success prediction guidance. Callaway has demonstrated the ability of the scaling exponent, a measure of the VF tracing's geometric characteristics, to predict likelihood of conversion to an organized rhythm (18). Others are evaluating the utility of frequency and amplitude-based analyses (19). The clinical relevance is that the AED could base the decision to shock not just on the presence of VF but also on the likelihood of successful conversion. For patients with low likelihood of conversion, basic and advanced life support could be provided prior to defibrillation.

The most optimal defibrillation waveform remains unknown. Most new devices on the market use biphasic waveforms rather than the previous standard, monophasic wave-form. The biphasic waveform at a lower energy level seems to be at least as effective as the higher energy monophasic and thus can decrease the size, weight, and cost of the device. Whether a low-energy biphasic waveform or an escalating biphasic waveform is more effective remains to be determined.

In summary, AEDs have become very simple and easy to use. A minimal amount of training is required to become familiar with the device In fact, a study comparing untrained, sixth-grade children and EMTs in the use of an AED illustrates just how easy these devices are to use: untrained children were able to operate the AED successfully in a time that was only 27 seconds longer than it took the EMTs to use the device (20).

STRATEGIES FOR EARLY DEFIBRILLATION

Today, the best known strategy for resuscitating persons in sudden CA is to provide defibrillation as soon as possible for those in ventricular tachycardia (VT) and VF,

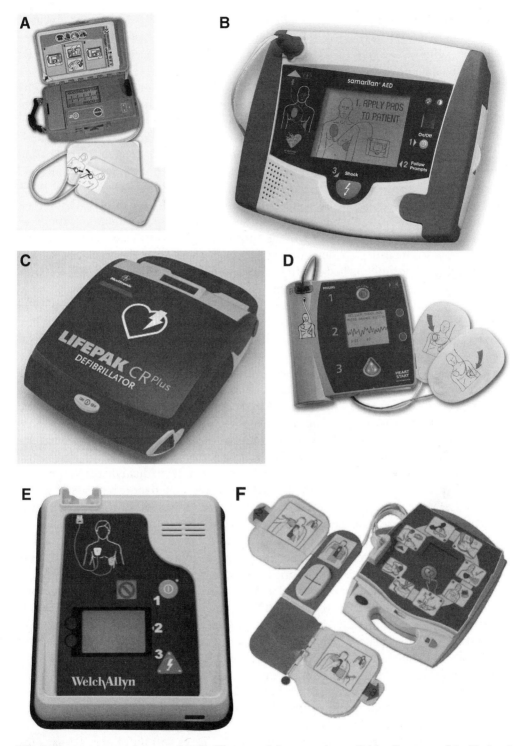

Fig. 2. Some automated external defibrillator models currently available. Courtesy of the National Center for Early Defibrillation, University of Pittsburg (www.early-defib.org). **(A)** AccessAED (Access CardioSystems); **(B)** Samaritan® AED (HeartSine Technologies Inc.); **(C)** LIFEPAK CR^Plus (Medtronic Physiocontrol Corp.); **(D)** Fr2+ (Philips Medical Systems); **(E)** AED 10 (Welch Allyn Inc.); **(F)** AED Plus (Zoll Medical Corp.).

perform closed chest compressions, and provide ventilation and oxygenation. Because victims in VF and VT have a much higher likelihood of survival than those with other rhythms, reaching these victims and delivering defibrillation has been emphasized. AEDs have provided an important means to achieve this goal.

The earliest clinical report of these devices is from Bellingham, Washington, by Diack and Wayne et al. in 1979 *(21)*. The device was designed to conduct current between a combination oral airway/metallic electrode in the orophanynx and an electrode on the mid-anterior chest. The device underwent further development and modifications including the transition to more traditional electrode placement on the left and right anterior chest. Soon thereafter, Cummins, Stults and others demonstrated safe and effective use of these devices by Emergency Medical Technicians *(7,22)*. In 1989, Weaver reported that equipping firefighter/first responders in King County, Washington with these devices would achieve a calculated survival improvement among patients in VF from 19 to 30% *(23)*. This report provided not only legitimacy to the new technology, but also a call for their deployment among first responders throughout the country.

Although paid firefighters became first responders in many urban areas, this resource was not available in many suburban communities. In these locations, police officers were often the most likely first responders. White et al. in 1996 *(24)*, and Mosesso et al. in 1998 *(25),* published reports demonstrating successful use of AEDs by police officers. White found a heretofore never reported survival rate of 45% with roughly similar survival whether shock was provided by EMS or police officers in Rochester, Minnesota. Mosesso's study in a suburban area near Pittsburgh, Pennsylvania, demonstrated a marked improvement in survival if police attempted to defibrillate sudden CA victims upon their arrival rather than waiting for EMS personnel (survival to hospital discharge 26 vs 3%, $p = 0.027$). Davis et al. reported that police officers in the Pittsburgh study were able to use the device effectively with minimal errors *(26)*. These studies also demonstrated the devices were safe and rarely malfunctioned.

The evolution of excellent 911 centers and of emergency medical dispatch (i.e., prioritized dispatch and pre-arrival instructions) has also facilitated more rapid deployment to CA calls. Despite these advances, however, first responders and EMS personnel generally are unable to reach the scene and provide therapy within the very small window of opportunity afforded to victims of sudden CA.

Therefore, it has been increasingly recognized that the only way to effectively provide what might be called "immediate defibrillation" is to have the defibrillator on site and accessible to the lay bystander. Air travel is one venue in which the need for immediate defibrillation is overt and which the AED strategy has proven success. The nature of this venue creates an exceptionally long time interval before traditional EMS is able to respond. Therefore, Qantas Airlines took what at the time was a bold step to equip nonmedical personnel, such as flight attendants, with AEDs *(27)*. Subsequently, Richard Page reported the American Airline experience *(28)*. During a 2-year period, 200 (191 on aircraft and 9 in terminal) arrests occurred. The Federal Aviation Administration (FAA) has now mandated that all airlines with at least one flight attendant be equipped with an AED and that the staff had to be trained in their use.

Determination of other appropriate venues for AEDs is still unfolding. Perhaps the largest effort to address this question is the Public Access Defibrillation (PAD) Trial *(29)*, which is comparing survival at sites with teams trained in CPR only vs sites with teams trained in CPR and AED use and equipped with AEDs. The trial found survival doubled at sites with AEDs and that no patients were shocked inappropriately *(29a)*. Researchers also hope to learn important information about effective response plan strategies and retraining requirements. The PAD Trial chose locations that would have a reasonable likelihood of CA by using the criterion of at least 250 people over age 50 present at the site for 16 hours a day or 500 persons present for 8 hours per day. Response plans were designed to initiate CPR immediately and apply the defibrillator within 3 minutes of the individual's collapse.

Several studies have tracked the incidence of sudden CA by type of location. Linda Becker found in Seattle that CA occurred most frequently at the airport, county jail, large shopping malls, public sports venues, and large industrial sites. They developed a criterion of greater than 0.03 arrests per year for "high-risk" locations and found that sites that met this criterion could be expected to use each AED once every 10 years (30). At sites that did not meet these criteria, the defibrillator would be used rarely, and thus the authors question the appropriateness of employing AEDs in those locations. Frank et al. evaluated CA in Pittsburgh and found that no single location had a particularly high incidence. The most common venues at which CA occurred were dialysis centers and nursing homes (31).

Although the concept of deploying AEDs at various public locations is just beginning to unfold, there are already questions being raised regarding the potential impact of such a strategy. This is because 57 to 75% (32,33) of CAs occur in private residences. Thus, only one-quarter to one-third of CAs can even be treated by a public access defibrillation strategy. Several studies have calculated that public access defibrillation programs, even if they achieve a high survival rate, will have only minimal impact on the overall survival in communities (34). This has led some to suggest that the ultimate venue for on-site defibrillators may be the home. The concept raises a number of issues including how often arrests at home are witnessed, the feasibility of family members using the AED in the crisis situation and the cost of placing AEDs in every home (35). A study exploring these issues is the Home Access Defibrillation Trial by researchers at the University of Washington. Nevertheless, a number of successful programs and models providing on-site defibrillation have been reported and a number of important program components have been identified.

EARLY DEFIBRILLATION PROGRAMS AND MODELS

There are a variety of different models and systems for on-site defibrillation programs. We endorse the concept that the deployment of AEDs should involve, in most cases, implementation of an emergency response plan. This is especially true in locations where there is some identifiable fixed population such as a security force or office work force. In systems with on-site security officers who can quickly respond to the location of an emergency, it is often appropriate to train and equip these officers with the AEDs. Other settings may have a steady workforce such as managers, clerks, or office workers but not a designated security response force. In these instances, it may be feasible to either assign a certain group or solicit a volunteer group to receive training and to respond to medical emergencies. Often it is appropriate to deploy AEDs in such a fashion that they are available for anyone at the site to use. The Chicago airport model reported by Caffrey et al. may best exemplify this model (36). AEDs were placed within a brisk 60- to 90-second walk apart in the Chicago O'Hare, Meigs Field, and Midway Airports. The cabinets were designed to trigger an audible alarm, strobe lights, and a dispatcher alert if the cabinet door was opened. The three airports serve more than 100 million passengers each year and employ a staff of 44,000. Of this pool of employees,

3000 were trained; users of the airports were alerted to the fact that AEDs were available in multiple ways: public service videos that repeatedly played in the waiting areas, pamphlets, and news media. In the initial 2 years of the study, 21 persons experienced nontraumatic CA; 18 out of the 21 cases were in VF. Eleven of the 18 (a remarkable 61%) survived. In five of these cases, persons who had no training or experience in the use of AEDs and no official duty to respond used the AED. This study suggests that there is benefit in making AEDs available to the general public.

When designing response plans, the goal is to provide access to defibrillation as quickly as possible. All aspects of the program should be designed to facilitate this goal. How this is achieved often is based on site-specific issues, but should include the components described in the next section, which is based in large part on a comprehensive guide by Newman and Christenson (37).

ESTABLISHING A COMMUNITY-BASED AED PROGRAM

An AED program can be considered a community initiative to promote public access to defibrillation. It may involve a consortium of any combination of community leaders, emergency medical services, local chapters of national organizations dedicated to this issue, and civic groups. This program may include ensuring that public safety-first responders are trained and equipped in the use of AEDs and promoting deployment in public venues throughout the community. Based on programs that have been published in the literature, and through personal communications with many leaders of such community programs, we have found that addressing the following 10 components will often facilitate the development of a successful and effective program.

Establish an AED Task Force

Strong community AED programs often begin with a single champion who is able to mobilize community support and buy-in. To be most effective, it helps to gather all potential stakeholders up front and form a task force. At a community level, this means people like the EMS director, fire chief or training officer, police chief or training officer, corporate leaders, elected officials, and representatives of training organizations, civic groups, senior citizens organizations, and the media.

Review Laws, Regulations, and Advisories

AED use is addressed in several federal laws and advisories, state laws, and sometimes even in local ordinances. All AEDs on the market in the United States have been cleared by the Food and Drug Administration (FDA), which means they have been determined to be safe and effective. The FDA requires a prescription for the purchase of an AED. All states now have Good Samaritan AED legislation. In general, these laws provide immunity from legal liability for those who use and deploy AEDs, but the details vary from state to state. Some states require training by nationally recognized training organizations, coordination with EMS, medical direction, and record keeping.

The federal CA Survival Act, which addresses AED placement in federal building, also fills in the gaps in state Good Samaritan legislation, providing an additional measure of immunity. Other actions at a federal level that support AED deployment are the FAA ruling that requires AEDs on airlines, the Occupational Safety and Health Administration advisory that recommends AEDs at the workplace and the General Accounting Office report that addresses CA data collection.

Conduct a Needs Assessment

Evaluate the strength of each link in the chain of survival to enable strategic improvements in the response system. Determine the highest risk sites for sudden CA and identify locations that may have delayed response by public safety and/or EMS (including delayed access to patient once on site).

Cultivate Public Awareness

Strong community AED programs depend on public awareness and involvement. The task force needs to develop a public awareness campaign, particularly if funding will be needed to support the program. This involves framing the issues, developing a statement of need, promoting media coverage, lobbying local political leaders, and identifying and addressing potential obstacles.

Estimate Program Costs

Establishing an *effective* community AED program involves not only the cost of devices, but other issues including initial and refresher training, medical direction, personnel related to program management and quality assurance, maintenance, documentation, media coverage, and community-wide CPR training. Before seeking funding, task forces should understand start-up and maintenance costs.

Seek Funding

Sometimes the costs of AED programs are incorporated into agency budgets. In many cases, however, outside funding is needed. There are many sources for AED program funding. Organizations and individuals will be more likely to contribute if your task force either forms a nonprofit 501(c)3 organization or aligns with one, so that contributions are tax deductible. For funding sources, see www.early-defib.org.

Establish Medical Oversight

Medical oversight for AED programs is required in some states. It is recommended by numerous national medical organizations, including the National Center for Early Defibrillation and the American Heart Association. The role of the medical director is to champion the program in the community, prescribe devices, and ensure quality. This involves developing or approving protocols, overseeing training, reviewing cases, providing feedback to rescuers and conducting data analysis.

Select Device

Many AED models are on the market. Some issues to consider include ease of use, compatibility with other devices in use in the service area, maintenance, ongoing manufacturer support, appropriateness for specific venue and expected users, and price. For device options, see www.early-defib.org.

Conduct Training

AED training generally takes about 2 to 4 hours, including CPR training. Refresher training should be conducted periodically and is available through on-line programs. Many experienced AED program coordinators recommend brief (i.e., as little as 10 minutes) refresher training every 3 months. Several organizations provide nationally recognized quality programs in CPR and AED use. For training options, see www.early-defib.org.

Develop a Response Plan

To ensure that every person receives optimal care as quickly as possible, it's essential to develop a comprehensive, well-designed response plan. An effective plan consists of written policies and procedures developed with and reviewed by the medical director on a regular basis. The response plan should address the following:

- Identification and training of the response team
- Specific roles of team members
- AED placement (location, installation, ancillary supplies)
- Internal and external (911) notification systems
- Response system function
- Periodic AED drills
- Postevent review and feedback

Example of Community AED Program: Montgomery County, Texas

Montgomery County Hospital District (MCHD) came to the conclusion that combating CA was not something that their ambulance service could do alone. Spanning 1100 square miles of urban, suburban, and rural areas, this Texas county with a population of 300,000, faced a number of obstacles. In the rural areas, the long distances that the MICUs needed to cover to reach a patient made achieving rapid response times difficult. In the urban areas, on the other hand, MICUs were able to arrive on scene quickly, locating the patient in a large building or crowd often created a substantial delay. In either case, achieving the 3- to 5-minute response interval needed for effective defibrillation of patients in CA was not possible using only the MICU system.

MCHD contemplated methods outside the MICU system to expedite access to defibrillation for victims of out-of-hospital CA. With this objective in mind, it designed a comprehensive first-response AED program that could be implemented in three stages over a 3-year period. The first stage was a Fire Department First Response program. MCHD purchased 30 AEDs for distribution among the 17 county fire departments. Additionally, MCHD offered firefighters free EMT or Emergency Care Attendants training. Later, MCHD created a special CPR/AED training course that included instruction in post-resuscitation care for patients who were resuscitated successfully, and lessons in what to do when a shock is not advised. More than 300 firefighters participated in the training courses. Overall, the Fire Department First Response program was a great success and recorded its first save in the first month of the program.

The second stage of the AED program was Law Enforcement First Response. MCHD invited the Shenandoah Police Department and the Montgomery County Sheriff's Department to join the AED team. MCHD provided the initial training and 36 AEDs for their use.

The third stage of the AED program was Community Access Defibrillation. MCHD focused on placing AEDs in locations where large populations of people congregate: malls, county buildings, schools and golf courses. Through local presentations on the importance of AEDs and the media coverage that they received, several community associations learned about the MCHD initiative and sought to partner with them and create AED programs in their area. MCHD consulted with each group to help them design a customized AED program that would offer the fastest and most effective response to an emergency. In most of these sites, MCHD targeted security personnel and maintenance staff as designated responders and provided them with free training. Interested citizens were invited to also partake in training and many did so. The first community save was of a man in his mid-40s on the 11th fairway during a golf tournament. Responders on bikes arrived with the AED and defibrillated successfully.

All three stages of the AED program initiated by MCHD were met with great enthusiasm by the media, public, and participators, alike. Even groups that were long-standing political adversaries of MCHD supported the hospital and its use of funds for this effective, lifesaving initiative. Additional support came from a wide variety of sources including government agencies, homeowners associations, businesses, civic associations, and grants.

To ensure continued quality management of the Montgomery County Hospital Program, all participants in the program follow the single protocol designed by the EMS medical director. A full-time program coordinator was hired to oversee deployment of AEDs and the initial and ongoing training activities for 450 lay responders and 15 community sites.

A total of 134 AEDs have been deployed within Montgomery County. The success of the program is illustrated clearly in the 28 pictures of survivors that hang on the MDHD Wall of Fame.

ESTABLISHING AN ON-SITE AED PROGRAM

The 10 principles for establishing a community AED program can be applied and expanded for on-site AED programs, as follows.

Establish Program Leadership

A program coordinator, a specific individual who is empowered to lead this effort, shold be named. This individual should have backing at the highest level of the corporation or organization and should be authorized to use resources and personnel as necessary to implement an effective program.

A medical advisor should be selected and involved in the overall planning of the program from its inception. This will ensure that the primary principles of rapid response and appropriate medical interventions by various personnel are addressed.

Review Laws and Regulations

Determine any specific laws that might impact on deployment of the AEDs, including any need for registration with state or local government or EMS.

Consider whether any requirements are imposed for the protection through Good Samaritan Laws. Consider any regulations that might affect the installation of devices, such as location for wall mounting and signage.

Site Assessment

The goal should be that a responder and the AED arrive at the individual's side within 3 minutes of system activation. Thus, site assessment must evaluate time to respond to various locations at the site and potential obstructions, such as entries with restricted access that might delay response. Occupancy and visitation rates also should be evaluated.

Develop Response Plan

A written response plan should be designed to ensure the most rapid response feasible during all hours of operation. The response plan should be developed in **collaboration** with the medical advisor and approved by top management. It should address the following components:

- Identification and training of the response team
- Specific roles of team members
- AED placement
- Internal and external (911) notification systems
- Response system function during operational hours
- Periodic AED drills
- Postevent review and feedback.

Develop a Program Budget

This should include the cost of the device, ancillary equipment for the device (this could include an extra set of pads, spare batteries, pocket mask, or other barrier device for mouth-to-mouth ventilation, protective gloves, scissors), training costs, medical consultation, general awareness and education for all site occupants, signage, and installation.

Select Device

There are a variety of different AED brands and models on the market. The various models should be evaluated for a good fit in a particular setting based on site-specific issues including storage conditions and personnel who will be using the device. For device options, see www.early-defib.org.

Conduct Training

Personnel designated to respond should receive formal training in both basic CPR and use of the AED. This generally can be accomplished in 3 to 4 hours of training initially with retraining conducted in a very brief fashion every 3 to 6 months. Formal retraining is recommended every 2 years. There are a number of organizations that provide nationally recognized quality programs in CPR and AED use. Additionally, there are also private companies that provide training. (For information, see www.early-defib.org.) If resources allow, one should consider opening training to all occupants of a site even if they are not part of the formal response team.

Device Installation

Device placement depends on the response plan. If the plan provides for delivery of the AED by designated individuals, such as a security team, then deployment should enable these personnel to have immediate and direct access to the device at all times. Whenever possible, devices should be deployed in such a way that they are also readily accessible to other occupants and visitors to the building to increase the likelihood of timely use. There are a number of brackets and enclosed cases designed for wall mounting of devices. These can be armed with alarms, both audible and visual, and can be connected to either an on-site communication center or the local 911 call center. Signage indicating the location of the device should be installed to enable it to be visible down hallways from a distance. The NCED suggests using a standard symbol for AEDs (Fig. 3).

Awareness and Education

All building occupants, and in appropriate settings, visitors, should be informed of the emergency response program and all occupants should be educated on how to activate the

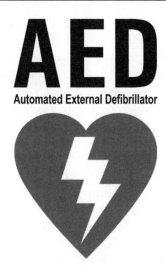

Fig. 3. Symbol for AEDs promoted by The National Center for Early Defibrillation.

response plan. One such strategy is to place signage and pamphlets at entryways and lobbies of buildings on the availability of AEDs and how to activate the on-site response team when applicable.

Continuous Evaluation

The on-site AED program should be assessed on a regular basis to ensure its effectiveness, especially the timeliness of response. After every event, the program coordinator and medical consultant should evaluate individual responses and use of the AED. Feedback should be provided both to individuals and to the entire response team. Regular reminders about when and how to activate the response team should be provided to all building occupants.

Example of Worksite AED Program: The Hillman Company

Two encounters with sudden CA brought the importance of immediate access to defibrillation to the attention of the employees at the Hillman Company. Soon after, the company decided to implement an AED program in their office in Pittsburgh, Pennsylvania.

An employee in Human Resources was selected to serve as the primary in-house AED program coordinator. The company also contracted with a medical director and AED program support specialist to assist them in designing an effective program that would ensure the best possible response to an emergency.

Creating such a response system involved several components. Placement of the AED was the first. Based on the AHA recommendations to provide defibrillation within 3 to 5 minutes of collapse, it was determined that the Hillman Company would need an AED on each floor of the building they occupy. The AEDs were placed in high-traffic areas, and supplied with ancillary items such as a razor, towel, CPR pocket mask, scissors, and alcohol wipes. All employees were alerted regarding the location of the devices.

The next order of business was determining who would be trained to use the AED. The Hillman Company already had a group of employees, called "fire marshals," that had volunteered to lead an evacuation of the building in the case of fire. The duties of the fire marshals were expanded to lead in the use of an emergency response involving the AED and their title was changed to emergency response marshals. This group, along with some additional volunteers, was trained in CPR and AED through the AHA Heartsaver AED course. They have been recertified every 2 years and receive shorter refresher training every 6 months.

The Hillman security system is used to activate the on-site response plan. Security buttons existed throughout the company under desks and near phones. Pressing one of these buttons alerts the guard at the front lobby security desk when and where an emergency occurs. The guard, in turn, calls 911, retrieves an elevator and guides the emergency medical technicians to the patient. After hours when no guard is on duty, the marshal places the call directly to 911. If alone, he or she can use a speed dial number to activate the public announcement broadcasting system and call any employee in the building to come and help.

All the components of the AED program are contained in a comprehensive policies and procedures manual. The manual includes information such as the placement of the AEDs; the names of the emergency response marshals; the procedures for calling for help; an explanation of how to perform CPR and use the AED that they had purchased for the company; checklists for the maintenance of the device, procedures for the reporting any event involving the AED to the medical director; and answers to frequently asked questions about AEDs.

The program was registered with the State of Pennsylvania's Emergency Medical Services Institute, and coordinated with the local ambulance service to help ensure seamless transfer of care. It was established that if the AED is ever used, the medical director will be contacted within 24 hours to review the response, together with the data stored in the AED, for the purpose of quality improvement. Although tested in a successful mock drill, the program has, fortunately, not been put to the test in a real situation. Hillman Company employees can rest assured, however, that if a CA event does occur, the on-site emergency response plan should ensure rapid and effective treatment.

SUMMARY

Although sudden CA remains a leading cause of death in the Western world, the advent of AEDs is allowing a new assault on this stealth, silent killer. These devices allow lay bystanders and nonmedical emergency responders to provide defibrillation—the only known effective therapy for VF. AEDs are safe and effective, easy to use and difficult to misuse, require low maintenance, and are becoming less costly. A growing number of communities and specific venues have reported successful early defibrillation programs. Public access defibrillation is a critical component of the optimal intervention strategy for combating sudden CA.

A Short History of Modern Resuscitation

1904:   George Crile performs first American case of closed-chest cardiac massage.
1933:   William Kouwenhoven et al. publish study on initiation and erasure of VF with electric shocks
1946:   James Elam performed mouth-to-nose ventilation on polio patients
1947:   Claude Beck successfully defibrillates 14-year-old boy using open-chest massage and AC defibrillator

1951:	Archer Gordon publishes study on superiority of Nielson's back-pressure arm-life method.
1954:	Elam publishes study on effectiveness of exhaled air for artificial ventilation
1956:	Paul Zoll demonstrates effectiveness of closed-chest defibrillation using AC defibrillators.
1956–1957:	Peter Safar demonstrates effectiveness of mouth-to-mouth ventilation in adults.
1957:	Archer Gordon demonstrates effectiveness of mouth-to-mouth ventilation in infants and children.
1960:	First prehospital CA patient saved with CPR and defibrillation in ED
1960:	William Kouwenhoven, James Jude and Guy Knickerbocker publish study demonstrating effectiveness of closed-chest cardiac compression.
1960:	Safar, Kouwenhoven and Jude combine mouth-to-mouth ventilation with chest compression to create modern CPR.
1961–1962:	Bernard Lown demonstrates superiority of DC over AC defibrillation.
1966–1967:	J. Frank Pantridge and John Geddes establish world's first mobile intensive care unit and publish findings.
1969:	William Grace establishes first MICU in United States (in New York City)
1969–1970:	Eugene Nagel in Miami, Leonard Cobb in Seattle, Leonard Rose in Portland, Michael Criley in Los Angeles, James Warren and Richard Lewis in Columbus establish first paramedic programs.
1972:	Leonard Cobb begins to train 100,000 citizens in CPR in Seattle *(1)*

ACKNOWLEDGMENTS

The authors would like to thank Chrysia Melnyk for her superb assistance with the preparation of this manuscript.

REFERENCES

1. Eisenberg M. Life in the Balance. Oxford: Oxford University Press, 1997.
2. Page JP. The Paramedics. Morristown, NJ: Backdraft Publications, 1979.
3. Pantridge JF, Geddes JS. A mobile intensive care unit in the management of myocardial infarction. Lancet 1967; 2:271.
4. Grace WJ, Chadborn JA. The mobile coronary care unit. Diseases of the Chest 1969; 55:452–455.
5. Eisenberg MS, Bergner L, Hallstrom A. Cardiac resuscitation in the community: importance or rapid provision and implications for program planning. JAMA 1979; 241:1905–1907.
6. Stults KR, Brown DD, Schug VL, et al. Prehospital defibrillation performed by emergency medical technicians in rural communities. N Engl J Med, 1984; 310:219–223.
7. Newman M. Chain of Survival takes hold. JEMS 1989; 14(8):11–13.
8. Cummins RO. Ornato JP. Thies WH. Pepe PE. Improving survival from sudden cardiac arrest: the "chain of survival" concept. A statement for health professionals from the Advanced Cardiac Life Support Subcommittee and the Emergency Cardiac Care Committee, American Heart Association. Circulation 1991; 83:1832–1847.
9. Lombardi G, Gallagher J, Gennis P. Outcome of out-of-hospital cardiac arrest in New York City: The Prehospital Arrest Survival Evaluation (PHASE) study. JAMA 1994; 271:678–683.
10. Becker LB, Ostrander MP, Barrett J, Kondos GT. Outcome of CPR in a large metropolitan area – where are the survivors? Ann Emerg Med 1991; 20:355–361.
11. Callaway CW. Improving neurologic outcomes after out-of-hospital cardiac arrest. Prehosp Emerg Care 1997; 1:45–47.
12. Spaite DW, Valuenzuela TD, Meislin HW, Criss EA, Hinsberg P. Prospective validation of a new model for evaluating emergency medical services systems by infield observation of specific time intervals in prehospital care. Ann Emerg Med 1993; 22:638–645.

13. Nichol G, Laupacis A, Stiell IG, et al. Cost-effectiveness analysis of potential improvements to emergency medical services for victims of out-of-hospital cardiac arrest. Ann Emerg Med 1996; 27:711–720.
14. Herlitz J, Bang A, Axelsson A, Graves JR, Lindqvist J. Experience with the use of automated external defibrillators in out of hospital cardiac arrest. Resuscitation 1998; 37:3–7.
15. Macdonald RD, Swanson JM, Mottley JL, Weinstein C. Performance and error analysis of automated external defibrillator use in the out-of-hospital setting. Ann Emerg Med 2001; 38:262–267.
16. National Center for Early Defibrillation, University of Pittsburgh, Pennsylvania. http://www.early-defib.org
17. Yu T, Weil MH, Tang W, et al. Adverse outcomes of interrupted precordial compression during automated defibrillation. Circulation 2002; 106:368–72.
18. Callaway CW, Sherman LD, Mosesso VN, Jr., Dietrich TJ, Holt E, Clarkson MC. Scaling exponent predicts defibrillation success for out-of-hospital ventricular fibrillation cardiac arrest. Circulation 2001; 103:1656–1661.
19. Jekova I, Deshanova J, Popivanov D. Method for ventricular fibrillation detectin in the external electrocardiogram using nonlinear prediction. Physiol Meas 2002; 23:337–45.
20. Gundry JW, Comess KA, DeRook FA, Jorgenson D, Bardy GH. Comparison of naïve sixth-grade children with trained professionals in the use of an automated external defibrillator. Circulation 1999; 100:1703–1707.
21. Diack AW, Welborn WS, Rullman RG, Walter CW, Wayne MA. An automatic ardiac resuscitator for emergency treatment of cardiac arrest. Medical Instrumentation 1979; 13:78–83.
22. Cummins RO, Eisenberg MS, Litwin PE, Graves JR, Hearne TR, Hallstrom AP. Automatic external defibrillators used by emergency medical technicians; a controlled clinical trial. JAMA 1987; 257: 1605–1610.
23. Weaver WD, Hill D, Fahrenbruch CE, et al. Use of the automatic external defibrillator in the management of out-of-hospital cardiac arrest. New Engl J Med 1988; 319:661–666.
24. White RD, Aspin BR, Bugiosi TF, Hankins DG. High discharge survival rate after out-of-hospital ventricular fibrillation with rapid defibrillation by police and paramedics. Ann Emerg Med 1996; 28:480–485.
25. Mosesso VN, Davis EA, Auble TE, Paris PM, Yealy DM. Use of automated external defibrillators by police officers for treatment of out-of-hospital cardiac arrest. Ann Emerg Med 1998; 32:200–207.
26. Davis EA, Mosesso VN. Performance of police first responders in utilizing automated external defibrillation on victims of sudden cardiac arrest. Preshosp Emerg Care 1998; 2:101–107.
27. O'Rourke MF, Donaldson E. The first five years of the Qantas cardiac arrest program. J Am Coll Cardio 1997; 29:404.
28. Page RL, Joglar JA, Kowal RC, et al. Use of automated external defibrillators by a US airline. N Engl J Med 2000; 343:1210–1216.
29. Public Access Defibrillation Trial Investigators. PAD Trial study design and rationale. Resuscitation 2003; 56: 135–147.
29a. Ornato JP, et al. The Public Access Defibrillation Trail. American Heart Association, Late-Breaking Clinical Trials Plenary Session VII, November 2003, Orlando, FL.
30. Becker L, Eisenberg M, Fahrenbruch C, Cobb L. Public locations of cardiac arrest: implications for public access defibrillation. Circulation 1998;97:2106–2109.
31. Frank RL, Rausch MA, Menegazzi JJ, Rickens M. The locations of nonresidential out-of-hospital cardiac arrests in the City of Pittsburgh over a three-year period: implications for automated external defibrillator placement. PEC 2001;5:247–251.
32. Cobb LA, Fahrenbruch CE, Walsh TR. Influence of cardiopulmonary resuscitation prior to defibrillation in patients with out-of-hospital ventricular fibrillation. JAMA 1999;281:1220–1222.
33. Litwin PE, Eisenberg MS, Hallstrom AP, Cummins RO. Location of collapse and its effect on survival from cardiac arrest. Ann Emerg Med 1987;16:669–672.
34. Pell JP, Sirel JM, Marsden AK, Ford I, Walker NL, Cobbe SM. Potential impact of public access defibrillators on survival after out of hospital cardiopulmonary arrest: retrospective cohort study. BMJ 2002;325:515–520.
35. Newman MM, Mosesso VN, Paris PM. "AEDs in the home: a position statement from the National Center for Early Defibrillation". National Center for Early Defibrillation website <http://www.early-defib.org> Accessed: January 2002.
36. Caffrey SL, Willoughby PJ, Pepe PE, Becker LB. Public use of automated external defibrillators. N Engl J Med 2002;347:1242–1247.
37. Newman MM, Christenson JM. Challenging sudden death: a community guide to help save lives. Carmel, IN: Catalyst Research and Communications, Inc., 1998.

14 Pacing During Cardiac Arrest

Allan S. Jaffe, MD and Utpal H. Pandya, MD

CONTENTS

INTRODUCTION
APPROACH TO TREATMENT
REFERENCES

INTRODUCTION

The incidence of sudden arrhythmic deaths continues to be a significant problem despite the fact that mortality from acute coronary syndromes continues to decrease in response to early interventions and improved secondary prevention *(1–3)*. Most patients with coronary artery disease who suffer cardiac arrest (CA) do not have acute myocardial infarction (AMI *[4–6]*). Thus, primary arrhythmic causes of CA are becoming increasingly important.

An estimated 400,000 to 460,000 people suffer CA annually. The initial rhythm noted in earlier studies was predominantly ventricular fibrillation (VF) in up to 75% of cases, with asystole at 20% and pulseless electrical activity (PEA) accounting for 5% *(1,4,6)*. Survival was directly related to the initial rhythm. Patients with VF had a 25% survival, whereas when the arrest rhythm was asystole, it was only 1%. The likelihood of the rhythm being asystole increased proportionately as the time from collapse to resuscitation increased.

Bayes de Deluna *(7)* found that the initial rhythm was frequently ventricular tachycardia (VT), which degenerated into VF (62% of cases) in a study of 157 patients with CA whose event occurred as they were being evaluated with ambulatory electrocardiographic monitoring. Bradycardia was the primary initial rhythm in only 17%. With the advent of first responder-initiated defibrillation, the success rate of resuscitation in patients with VF or VT is improving *(4,9)*. Yet, the rates of survival in asystole and/or PEA continue to be dismal *(9)*.

Unfortunately, with implantable cardioverter defibrillators and modern therapy, the percentage of patients with VT/VF as an initial rhythm is declining. In the most recent tabulation by Cobb and colleagues *(10)*, the annual incidence of CA as a result of VF had declined by approx 56% despite improved response times in most emergency medical systems. At present, VF as a first rhythm may occur in less than 50% of patients *(10)*. In Seattle at least, asystole as an initial arrest rhythm seems to increasing in women but not in men.

From: *Contemporary Cardiology: Cardiopulmonary Resuscitation*
Edited by: J. P. Ornato and M. A. Peberdy © Humana Press Inc., Totowa, NJ

Table 1
Common Causes of Bradysystolic Arrest

Drugs
    β-Blockers
    Diltiazem/verapamil
    Digoxin
    Clonidine
    Class IA, IC, and III antiarrhythmics
Autonomic
    Increased vagal output
    Vasodepressor reflex
    Carotid hypersensitivity
Hyperkalemia
Acute myocardial infarction
    Right Coronary Territory (more likely)
Hypothyroidism
Hypothermia
Sepsis
Infection—endocarditis, atrioventricular block in Lyme
disease

APPROACH TO TREATMENT

An initial rhythm of asystole has been thought to be a sign of a delay from collapse to recognition/resuscitation or a clue to the presence of a failing heart with local acidosis that precludes effective electrical-mechanical coupling. However, in some circumstances, there are reversible causes of bradyasystole (Table 1). If one can identify and treat these causes early the odds of survival may increase by preventing the initial bradyarrhythmias from disintegrating into asystole.

One of the most obvious reversible causes is AMI/myocarial ischemia with heart block. Treatment of the underlying ischemia usually reverses the bradycardia, which is often vagally mediated and may respond to atropine if the right coronary artery is involved. If the left system and particularly the left anterior descending territory is problematic, then the mechanism of bradycardia is more apt to be Mobitz Type 2 second degree atrioventricular block or complete heart block with a wide QRS escape rhythm, which requires urgent pacing. Mechanical causes such as ventricular rupture, cardiac tamponade, large pulmonary emboli, and tension pneumothorax also respond to relief of the underlying abnormality.

These observations suggest that the phases of resuscitation recently proposed by Weisfeld and Becker *(11)* may be helpful with bradyasystolic rhythms as well as VF. Weisfeld and Becker define an initial period in which they recommend electrical therapy, a period in which circulatory support is needed, and finally a metabolic phase. For bradycardia, there should be an initial phase prior to asystole in which the aggressive use of pacing and pharmacological therapy may be helpful, a second phase in which correctable abnormalities should be sought as circulatory assistance is being provided and finally a metabolic phase.

Specific Etiologies Considered During the Early Phase

A large variety of cardiac abnormalities can lead to bradycardia (Table 1). The long-standing experience with external pacemakers suggest that results are excellent when one uses the device acutely but prior to bradyasystolic arrest. The most common situation is when there is acute ischemic heart disease accompanied by drug toxicity with or without electrolyte imbalance, intrinsic conducting system disease, operative trauma (coronary artery bypass graft and or ablation), and/or acute vagal insults such as an acute intra-abdominal catastrophe. Although there are no randomized controlled trials, the most important clinical rule is that early initiation of pacing, before asystole, is the key to a good outcome. Coincident with the initiation of pacing, a thorough search for potential etiologies is mandated.

Mnemonics exist to make it facile for the physician to consider the essential diagnostic considerations in patients who present with pulseless electric activity. One mnemonic that has become popular is the "five Hs and Ts." They are also usually appropriate for patients who present with asystole. The five Hs are hypoxia, heart attack, hypovolemia, H+ (electrolyte abnormality), and hypothermia. If one thinks of hypovolemia as an acute process (e.g., cardiac or aortic rupture), although not common, this mnemonic works for bradycardia as well. The five Ts are to test for other pulses, tension pneumothorax, tamponade, toxins and therapeutic agents, and thrombo-emboli *(12)*.

Correctable Abnormalities As Circulatory Support Is Provided

Once asystole is present, the prognosis is grim. In addition to attempting to find remediable causes, pacing is worth an attempt.

The Metabolic Phase

Early intervention is critical because a variety of metabolic abnormalities develop when there is persistent and/or progressive hypoperfusion. With reduced oxygen delivery, metabolism shifts from aerobic to anaerobic pathways. Even with the subsequent initiation of cardiopulmonary resuscitation (CPR), only approx 25% of the cardiac output is restored. Because of the reduction in cardiac output and subsequent decrease in critical organ system and coronary blood flow, tissue hypoxia ensues. This leads to anaerobic metabolism and the accumulation of hydrogen ions. Acid residues are buffered by endogenous buffers, usually bicarbonate, which leads to the production of carbon dioxide. Carbon dioxide diffuses across the cell membrane and leads to tissue acidosis and cellular dysfunction, which is reflected in the venous circulation. Additionally, acidosis leads to competition for calcium ions binding to troponin. This inhibits the cross bridging between actin and mycin filaments and, hence, myocardial contractility. Hyperventilation during CPR removes the excess CO_2 but does not reverse the tissue acidosis as a result of the reduced delivery of blood back to the heart. Thus, there is an arteriovenous paradox *(13,14)* with hypercarbic venous acidemia and hypocarbic arterial alkalemia.

This is also the reason why bicarbonate is not helpful. It buffers arterial acidosis, but the increased CO_2 produced exacerbates venous and tissue acidosis. This local tissue acidosis, which is common in patients presenting with asystole whose time from collapse to resuscitation is often prolonged, is why pacing has little chance of success if applied too late (*see* Table 2). Moreover bicarbonate may have adverse effects such as depression of myocardial function, inactivation of catecholamines, and paradoxical central nervous system acidosis.. It may be that with time and better techniques to enhance blood flow in the future, local tissue acidosis may be obviated but we are not at that point presently.

Table 2
Trials of Pacing for Asystole

Primary investigator (year; reference)	Venue pacing initiated	Patient population	Results	Comments
Cummins (1993; 29)	Prehospital	112 patients with primary asystole; 46 patients with postdefibrillation asystole; a control group of 259	No statistically significant advantage in intervention group for hospital admission or survival outcomes. Technically feasible.	Pacing not occasionally initiated in the field as a result of EMT training schedule and negative No difference between primary or postshock asystole
Barthell (1988; 28)	Prehospital	103 paced for primary asystole and EMD and secondary asystole EMD 136 controls	No statistically significant difference in outcome for pacing in EMD or asystole whether 1° or 2°	5/6 patients with hemodynamically significant bradycardias survived with pacing
Vukov (1988; 27)	Prehospital	58 patients (33 primary and 25 post-shock asystole). No controls.	4/58 patients admitted to hospital, none suvived at day	Rural setting, with very high CA resuscitation rates. 32% paced within 10 minutes of collapse
Eitel (1987; 26)	Prehospital	91 paced (59 asystole, 32 PEA; 44/59 primary asystole)	85/91(93%) electrical capture 10/91 (11%) mechanical capture 1 patient admitted, 0 survived to discharge	69/91 patients pharmacologic intervention prior to pacing (epinephrine, atropine, bicarbonate), no difference in resuscitation
Syverud (1986; 19)	Prehospital	19 patients: 9 with asystole, 9 with PEA Group 1: 4/19 pacing within 5 minutes. Group 2: Pacing 5–20 minutes	2/5 in group 1 with neurologic recovery, none in group 2	Emphasizes the role of early pacing

Study	Setting	Patient Population	Results	Comments
Hedges (1987; 21)	Prehospital	101(89 actually paced) pacing group; 101 control group 28/101 pacing group with primary asystole 45/101 VT/VF degenerating into paceable rhythm	Average time from arrest to pacing; 21.8 minutes Outcome measures not statistically significant between groups	Neurologically intact patient excluded. (When paced did well) Initial rhythm of VT/VF and short time to ACLS favorable outcome
Paris (1985; 25)	Prehospital	112 patients (55 asystole, 44 PEA)	52% electrical capture, 8% mechanical capture. No survivors to discharge	Average time from arrest to pacing was 29 minutes Pharmacologic interventions implemented prior to pacing
Noe (1985; 24)	In-hospital	TCP in 23/24 patients for asystole TVP in 4/23 patients of asystole	Two of 24 patients with TCP survived	The two survivors were conscious with the arrest and had very early intervention
Dalsey (1984; 22)	ED	52 unconscious patients (30 asystole, 22 PEA)	50% with electrical capture, 15% mechanical capture. No survivors	Most paced after 20 minutes of arrest. Pacing attempted after failed drug therapy
Jaggaroa (1982; 20)	Prehospital	25 patients (16 late and 9 early arrest) Included 1° or 2° asystole/PEA	Late group no survivors Early group 3 survivors	2/3 survivors were post-defibrillation asystole. No survivors in primary asystole
Zoll (1956; 23)	In-hospital	25/34 patients with Stokes-Adams attacks	Mechanical capture with long-term survivors in the 25 with ventricular standstill	Prompt use of device after rhythm noted

Pacing Techniques

HISTORICAL PERSPECTIVE

In 1791, Galvani was the first to note that an electrical current applied across a frog heart could lead to myocardial contraction. Hyman and others in the early 1930s reported that animals who were asystolic as a result of anoxia had restoration of a perfusing rhythm after being subjected to pulsating current *(14)*. The first report of the application of transcutaneous pacing in humans was by Paul Zoll *(15)*. He applied the technique to two patients with Stokes Adams attacks (ventricular standstill) in an attempt to restore a rhythm. He used two subcutaneous external needles to deliver electrical energy across the chest wall. One patient died after 20 minutes of external pacing from cardiac tamponade as a result of previously applied intracardiac injections. The second patient survived after having been paced externally for 5 days when he developed a perfusing intrinsic idioventricular rhythm. Prior to this demonstration of the feasibility of the technique, intravenous or intracardiac epinephrine myocardial stimulation with direct massage or needles had been attempted to reverse asystolic CA with only limited success and incremental risks.

Zoll later refined the transcutaneous pacing technique with the introduction of a pair of 3-cm metal electrodes, which were designed to deliver 2-ms, 120-volt AC impulses. However, the 2-ms pulse durations resembled a short action potential of skeletal muscle rather than the longer action potentials of myocardial tissue, which led to preferential stimulation of skeletal muscle and discomfort. Also, the shorter pulse width required higher current (amperage) to reach stimulation thresholds. Finally, a smaller sized electrode meant that the current density was very high at the electrode–skin interface leading to cutaneous pain in the conscious patient. Transcutaneous pacemakers fell into disuse somewhat with the advent of implantable transvenous pacemakers. In the early 1980s, transcutaneous pacemaker and electrode pad improvements made this technique much more effective and better tolerated by patients. By increasing the pulse duration to 20 to 40 milliseconds and increasing the size of the electrodes (from 3 cm to 8 cm) to 50 to 100 cm *(2)*, the painful side effects of transcutaneous pacing were reduced, allowing the use of the technique in emergency situations.

Before transcutaneous pacemaking became safe and effective, temporary transvenous cardiac pacing was attempted in the majority of urgent circumstance. Balloon-tipped, transvenous pacing catheters are safe and expeditious and can be placed rapidly in the emergent setting by experienced operators *(16)*. However, it is clear that transcutaneous pacing seems to be both easier and more efficacious in the majority of current clinical settings.

Specific Techniques

TRANSCUTANEOUS PACING

Transcutaneous pacing is remarkably easy to apply. Two pads are applied. The larger (ground) electrode is applied posteriorly in the midline between the mid-scapula and T4 vertebra. The anterior electrode is best applied at the electrocardiographic V_3 position. When possible, body hair should be removed, but it is not recommended that it be shaved prior to electrode placement. The nicks caused by shaving have been reported to cause uneven conduction and, therefore, burns through areas of lesser resistance. Once the electrodes are applied and the pacer cable connected to its output source, one sets the generator rate to 20 to 30 beats per minute over the patient's spontaneous rate.

In general, the output is set initially at 50 milliamps. If the pacemaker does not capture, then the output is increased progressively to a maximum (usually 200 milliamps) or until capture. Once capture is achieved, one should reduce the output until capture is lost. This is called the stimulation threshold. Subsequently, one sets the output at 20% above the stimulation threshold.

Temporary Transvenous Pacing

A balloon tip, Swan pacing catheter is often used in an emergency situation because it obviates the need for fluoroscopy, which is difficult at best in the urgent circumstance. The procedure begins with gaining access percutaneously via the subclavian or internal jugular vein using the Seldinger technique. Subsequently, the distal pole of the electrode is connected to the chest lead of the electrocardiogram (ECG). Next, the balloon is inflated and the catheter electrode is advanced with monitoring of the intracavitary ECG. Once typical intraventricluar electrocardiographic complexes appear, the balloon is deflated to prevent flotation in the pulmonary artery. If a balloon tip Swan pacing catheter is used, the location of catheter can be deduced from the pressure tracings. Large ventricular ECGs showing an injury current (ST elevation) signal contact with the endothelium.

The effect of acute interventions after asystole is established have been disappointing (17,18). Efficacy is better for potentially presaging rhythms, like heart block (see above). The initial nonrandomized small pacing study by Jaggarao (19) in 1982 in the prehospital setting showed some promise. There were three survivors out of nine patients with asystole or PEA who had early pacing. Two of the survivors were asystolic postdefibrillation. Hedges defined an early period of 5 minutes or less of asystolic CA as an important factor that correlated with successful resuscitation (20). Often, he was dealing with rhythms the presaged asystole rather than asystole itself. Studies by Dalsey et al. (21) have shown that transcutaneous pacing is just as effective in the setting of CA in capturing the myocardium.

Lessons from these early studies laid the groundwork for the randomized trials in the late 1980s and 1990s. The portability of transcutaneous pacing made it possible for paramedics to use the technique in the field. Trials were designed to pace the patient in the prehospital setting, even prior to traditional pharmacologic interventions in some cases. However, without exception, these studies have been resoundingly negative once asystole has been established (Table 2). This is why early initiation of definitive therapy with either atropine, isoproterenol, or pacing prior to the onset of asystolic arrest and, subsequently, an aggressive source for underlying abnormalities is so critical.

REFERENCES

1. Myerburg RJ, Kessler KM, Castellanos A. Sudden cardiac death: epidemiology, transient risk, and intervention assessment. Ann Intern Med 1993; 119:1187–97.
2. Myerburg RJ, Interian A Jr, Mitrani RM, Kessler KM, Castellanos A. Frequency of sudden cardiac death and profiles of risk. Am J Cardiol 1997; 80:10F–19F.
3. Gordon T, Thom T. The recent decrease in CHD mortality. Prev Med 1975; 4:115–125
4. Cobb LA, Werner JA, Trobaugh GB. Sudden cardiac death: I. A decade's experience with out-of-hospital resuscitation. Mod Concepts Cardiovasc Dis 1980; 49:31–36
5. Cobb LA, Werner JA, Trobaugh GB. Sudden cardiac death: II. Outcome of resuscitation, management, and future directions. Mod Concepts Cardiovasc Dis 1980; 49:37–42
6. Cobb LA, Baum RS, Alvarez H III, Schaffer WA. Resuscitation from out-of-hospital ventricular fibrillation: 4 years follow-up. Circulation 1975; 51:III-223–III-228

7. de Luna AB, Coumel P, Leclercq JF. Ambulatory sudden cardiac death: mechanisms of production of fatal arrhythmias on the basis of data from 157 cases. Am Heart J 1989; 117:151–159

8. Thompson RG, Hallstrom AP, Cobb LA. Bystander-initiated CPR in management of ventricular fibrillation. Ann Intern Med 1979; 90:737–740.

9. Greene HL: Sudden Arrhythmic Cardiac Death—Mechanisms, Resuscitation and Classification: The Seattle Perspective. Am J Cardiol 1990; 65:4B–12B

10. Cobb LA, Fahrenbruch CE, Olsufka M, Copass M. Changing Incidence of Out-of-Hospital Ventricular Fibrillation, 1980–2000. JAMA 2002; 288:3008–3013.

11. Weisfeldt ML, Becker LB. Resuscitation after cardiac arrest-A 3-phase time-sensitive model. JAMA 2002; 288:3035–3038.

12. Grundler WG, Weil Mh, Rackow EC. Arteriovenous carbon dioxide and pH gradients during cardiac arrest. Circulation 1982; 66:297–302

13. Jaffe, AS: Cardiovascular Pharmacology I. Circulation 1986; 74S:IV-70–IV-73.

14. Weil MH, Rackow EC, Trevino R, et al. Difference in acid-base state between venous and arterial blood during cardiopulmonary resuscitation. N Engl J Med 1986; 315:153–156.

15. Hyman AS. Resuscitation of the stopped heart by intracardial therapy. Arch Int Med 1932; 50:283.

16. Zoll P. Resuscitation of the heart in ventricular standstill by external electric stimulation. N Eng J Med 1952; 247:768–771.

17. Lang R, David D, Klein HO, et al. The use of the balloon-tipped floating catheter in temporary trasvenous cardiac pacing. PACE 1981; 4:491–496.

18. Zoll PM, Zoll RH, Falk RH, Clinton JE, Eitel DR, Antman EM. External noninvasive temporary cardiac pacing: clinical trials. Circulation 1985; 71:937.

19. Syverud SA, Dalsey WC, Hedges JR. Transcutaneous and transvenous cardiac pacing for early bradysystolic cardiac arrest. Ann Emerg Med 1986; 15:121.

20. Jaggarao NSV, Heber M, Grainger R, et al. Use of an automated external defibrillator-pacemaker by ambulance staff. Lancet 1982; 2:73–75.

21. Hedges JR, Syverud SA, Dalsey WC, Feero S, Easter R, Shultz B. Prehospital trial of emergency transcutaneous cardiac pacing. Circulation 1987; 76:1337–1343.

22. Dalsey WC, Syverud SA, Hedges JR. Emergency department use of transcutaneous pacing for cardiac arrests. Crit Care Med 1985; 13:399–401.

23. Zoll PM, Linenthal AJ, Norman LR. External electric stimulation of the heart in cardiac arrest. Arch Intern Med 1956; 96:639–653.

24. Noe R, Cockrell W, Moses HW, Dove IT, Batchelder JE. Transcutaneous pacemaker use in a large hospital. PACE 1986; 9:101–104.

25. Paris PM, Stewart RD, Kaplan RM, Whipkey R. Transcutaneous pacing for bradyasystolic cardiac arrests in prehospital care. Ann Emerg Med 1985; 14:320–323.

26. Eitel DR, Guzzardi LJ, Stein SE, Drawbaugh RE, Hess DR, Walton SL. Non invasive transcutaneous cardiac pacing in prehospital cardiac arrests. Ann Emerg Med 1987; 16 531–534.

27. Vukov LF, White RD, Bachman JW, O'Brien PC. New perspectives on rural EMT defibrillation. Ann Emerg Med 1988; 17:318–321.

28. Barthell E, Troiano P, Olson D, Stueven HA, Hendley G. Prehospital external cardiac pacing: a prospective, controlled clinical trial. Ann Emerg Med 1988; 17:1221–1226.

29. Cummins RO, Graves JR, Larsen MP, Hallstrom AP, Hearne TR, Ciliberti J, Nicola RM, Horan S. Out-of-hospital transcutaneous pacing by emergency medical technicians in patients with asystolic cardiac arrest. N Engl J Med. 1993; 328:1377–1382.

15 Therapeutic Hypothermia in the Treatment of Cardiac Arrest

Benjamin S. Abella, MD, MPhil,
Terry L. Vanden Hoek, MD,
and Lance B. Becker, MD, FAHA

CONTENTS

Cold acts on the living parts by blunting the sensibility of those organs . . . the parts may remain for a longer or shorter period in state of asphyxia without losing their life; and if the cold be removed by degrees . . . the equilibrium may be easily reestablished with the function of the organs. . . .

—D.J. Baron Larrey, 1814 (1)

INTRODUCTION

Sudden cardiac death remains a major medical challenge despite the advent of defibrillation decades ago. There are few minutes to defibrillate the heart and thereby stop ongoing ischemic injury to key organs such as the heart and brain, and few therapies proven to protect against the postresuscitation phase of cardiac arrest (CA)—when up to 90% of patients go on to die despite successful defibrillation *(2)*. New approaches are desperately needed to improve CA survival, and the induction of transient hypothermia may be one of the most promising of new approaches *(2)*. Hypothermia used to protect against conditions of low blood flow has historically been induced at different times

From: *Contemporary Cardiology: Cardiopulmonary Resuscitation*
Edited by: J. P. Ornato and M. A. Peberdy © Humana Press Inc., Totowa, NJ

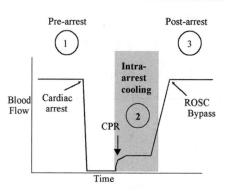

Fig. 1. Timing of hypothermia induction relative to circulatory arrest. The optimal depth of hypothermia is much lower in the pre-arrest setting than after return of spontaneous circulation (ROSC). Few studies have determined the optimal depth of intra-arrest cooling.

relative to the arrest (*see* Fig. 1): pre-arrest, intra-arrest, and postarrest. Pre-arrest cooling is typically induced to as low as 20°C for cardiac surgery and is induced before and simultaneous to the time of arrest. Postarrest cooling to 32 to 33°C was found to be protective in recent human CA trials, induced by applying cooling blankets in the subset of CA patients having return of spontaneous circulation (ROSC) who remained unresponsive *(3,4)*. The goal of this hypothermia was to prevent neurologic injury although maintaining a temperature warm enough to prevent the cardiac and numerous other side effects of more profound cooling (e.g., cardiac arrhythmias, coagulopathies, infections). This cooling was protective despite taking 8 hours to reach target temperature after ROSC *(4)*. Intra-arrest cooling, when cooling is induced after failed initial CPR, has the potential to induce a stasis state for a period of time (i.e., suspended animation) long enough for more definitive circulation (e.g., cardiac bypass) to be established and life restored. Little is known about the optimal depth or clinical potential of such hypothermia, due in large part to the technical difficulties involved in inducing profound hypothermia during the low-flow states of sudden CA.

"Suspended animation," as defined by Safar et al., is a process that allows "rapid preservation of viability of the organisms in temporarily unresuscitable CA, which allows time for transport and repair during clinical death and is followed by delayed resuscitation, hopefully to survival without brain damage" *(5)*. The most widely studied method to induce suspended animation has been induced hypothermia. In this paradigm, victims of CA may be cooled to some target temperature and maintained at this temperature for a specific period of time. With advance medical interventions, which may include cardiopulmonary bypass (CPB), metabolic correction, and controlled reperfusion, the patient is stabilized, rewarmed, and reanimation is initiated. Although many methodologies have been studied under the rubric of suspended animation, including CPB and pharmacologic interventions *(6)*, these are most often used as adjuncts to the use of hypothermia. Recently, two seminal papers were published describing the use of hypothermia to successfully treat resuscitated CA patients *(3,4)*. With these studies, hypothermia has moved from the laboratory to active clinical use.

There are many unresolved questions regarding the use of hypothermia in CA treatment. First, the optimal degree of hypothermia has yet to be established. Certainly, hypothermia can have adverse effects, including coagulation derangements, reduced immune system function, depressed pulmonary function, and other possible alterations *(7–10)*. Therefore, the therapeutic window of hypothermia must be defined to provide maximum benefit. For convenience of discussion in this review, we will define hypothermia as either mild (34–36°C), moderate (28–34°C), or deep (15–28°C *[11]*). Most clinical research has concentrated on the use of mild or moderate hypothermia. Deep hypothermia has largely been confined to studies of specific applications such as brain cooling during surgery and reduced cerebral perfusion *(12)*. Some animal investigations have directly compared different depths of cooling *(13)*. The timing of hypothermia is another crucial question. There are three general time periods in which hypothermia may be considered, although only two are realistic for clinicians. Pre-arrest hypothermia, or cooling some time before CA, is only possible in the setting of anticipated surgery, when arrest is iatrogenic and controlled (reviewed in refs. *14* and *15*). Intra-arrest hypothermia, or cooling during cardiopulmonary resuscitation (CPR), is theoretically attractive and a promising area of current research but has not been attempted clinically. Postresuscitation hypothermia, or cooling after ROSC, has been the most commonly attempted timing strategy and is certainly the most clinically convenient. Recent large-scale clinical trials have demonstrated significant benefit from induced postresuscitation hypothermia *(3,4)*. These studies raise a secondary timing question related to postresuscitation hypothermia: is the delay in hypothermia initiation clinically important? In the clinical arena, cooling to target temperatures may take several hours *(16,17)*. Some animal data, detailed in this chapter, suggests that earlier induction of hypothermia confers a greater benefit *(18,19)*.

Another question, which remains unresolved, is what duration of hypothermia is required for protection. Clinical studies to date have all maintained mild hypothermic conditions at least 12 hours *(3,4,7)*. However, animal studies have shown benefit from hypothermia lasting only 2 to 6 hours *(19,20)*. Unpublished data from our laboratory, using a mouse model of CA, show that even 1 hour of moderate hypothermia can confer a significant survival benefit after CA *(21)*. Certainly, a shorter duration of cooling would have a number of clinical advantages, including minimizing the logistical difficulties of maintaining a constant cooled state, and also minimizing the potential adverse effects from hypothermia. This question has not been directly addressed in clinical studies at this time.

Finally, a number of other aspects of hypothermic suspended animation remain to be examined. How quickly should patients be rewarmed at the end of a period of hypothermia? Would certain drugs serve as useful adjuncts to hypothermia, either to provide additional benefit or protect against certain adverse effects of a cooled state? This chapter addresses elements of the history of hypothermia, important physiology aspects to hypothermia, the laboratory data, which have developed our understanding of its use. The mechanisms by which hypothermia may protect ischemic and reperfused tissues will be introduced. Finally, after an evaluation of the various techniques used to rapidly cool patients, the future of hypothermia as therapy for sudden death will be discussed.

HISTORY OF INDUCED HYPOTHERMIA

The protective effect of hypothermia induction for resuscitation has been suggested since the time of Hippocrates, who advocated packing bleeding patients in snow *(22)*. Hypothermic protection was also noted by Napoleon's chief battlefield surgeon, Baron Larrey, during the invasion of Russia. He observed improved survival of injured soldiers left in the snow compared to those treated with warm blankets and heated drinks *(1,23)*. Induced hypothermia has been studied in a wide variety of illnesses, both ischemic and nonischemic in nature *(24–26)*. These include traumatic brain injury *(27–29)*, status epilepticus *(30)*, burns *(31)*, arrhythmia *(32)*, sepsis *(33)*, and the ischemic illnesses of myocardial infarction (MI), stroke, and CA *(5,26)*. Interestingly, the first reported use of induced hypothermia was in the setting of malignancy. In 1939, Fay and colleagues *(34)* treated patients with metastatic carcinoma, with the goal of both pain reduction and retardation of tumor growth. Although hypothermia to 32°C for 24 hours did not prove effective for the stated goals, it was considered well tolerated *(34)*.

A decade later, Bigelow studied the induction of hypothermia in the setting of cardiac surgery, with the goal of cerebral protection *(35)*. Two other studies using hypothermia as therapy for CA were also published *(36)*. Both of these early CA studies used moderate hypothermia of 30 to 34°C in patients after resuscitation from CA. One of these pioneering papers presented a series of four patients, all who were cooled and survived arrest *(37)*. In the other study, 12 patients were cooled with a survival rate of 50%, compared to 14% survival in 7 normothermic control patients *(36)*.

During the 1960s and the 1970s, the field of induced hypothermia lay relatively dormant, for reasons that remain unclear. Others have suggested that more dramatic therapies were developed that overshadowed cooling as a possible therapy, such as controlled ventilation, monitored intensive care unit management, and CPR *(24)*. Additionally, adverse effects of hypothermia were described, which may have dampened enthusiasms *(38,39)*. One scientist from the early days of induced hypothermia correctly summarized the ensuing skepticism toward hypothermia when he stated: "If a hazardous procedure such as this were mishandled, it might well fall into unwarranted disrepute before the facts and fallacies accompanying it were clearly defined" *(40)*.

Interest in "resuscitative hypothermia" was rekindled by Safar and others at the University of Pittsburgh, when it was demonstrated in a ventricular fibrillation (VF) dog model of CA that mild-to-moderate hypothermia could be induced to improve outcomes *(41,42)*. It was during this period of time that the term "suspended animation" was introduced, in the context of an exsanguination CA dog model *(43,44)*. It was understood from military combat experience that definitive therapy for penetrating trauma was often delayed for practical reasons (e.g., transportation and access to surgical care), and that measures were needed to preserve exsanguinating soldiers until appropriate care could be delivered *(45*; i.e., suspended animation). Given the animal data on exsanguination and cooling, it appeared that hypothermia might be a suitable approach *(46)*.

Since these initial observations in the 1980s and early 1990s, much of the work pertaining to hypothermia and ischemic disease has focused on focal ischemia and reperfusion (e.g., animal stroke or MI models). A variety of ischemia-reperfusion (IR) model systems have been developed over the last two decades, including cellular *(47)*, isolated organ *(48)*, and whole animal models in which arterial supply to the organ in question is temporarily occluded *(19,20)*. In this latter category are included experiences with human IR, for example during coronary vascular procedures *(49)*. Studies of hypothermia in both CA and IR models are discussed here.

INTRA-ARREST VS POSTARREST HYPOTHERMIA

Most studies of induced hypothermia have involved cooling after resuscitation (or, in the IR paradigm, after reperfusion). For example, in an isolated rat liver IR model, reactive oxygen species (ROS) production was diminished by maintaining liver tissue at 34ºC after reperfusion *(50)*. It is widely felt that ROS contribute to reperfusion injury and tissue damage after resuscitation *(51)*, and therefore the authors provide a possible link between hypothermia and prevention of reperfusion injury. Additionally, to direct protection, focal hypothermia may protect other organs via its effects on humoral issues. Patel et al. found that when rat liver is exposed to IR and then focally cooled to 25ºC, there is both decreased liver inflammation and cell death as well as reduced pulmonary injury, even though the lungs were not rendered ischemic or cooled *(52)*. This provides an important example of dissemination of pro-injury issues from a site of IR, which can only be studied easily in whole animal models. In another example of whole animal investigation, Canevari et al. produced IR injury via bilateral carotid occlusion in the gerbil, which was then reversed and allowed to reperfuse for 2 hours, either at normothermia or at 30ºC. After this time, the normothermic animals had significantly impaired mitochondrial complex IV activity compared to the animals treated with hypothermia *(53)*.

Postresuscitation hypothermia has been attempted in a number of CA models as well. In a rat asphyxia model with 8 minutes of CA, hypothermia to 34ºC and induced hypertension for 60 minutes immediately after ROSC produced improved survival compared to normothermic animals. This result was statistically significant at 4 weeks after the experiment, suggesting a lasting benefit *(54)*. A number of canine studies have also demonstrated benefit from postresuscitation hypothermia. After 15 minutes of VF, dogs that were cooled to 33ºC and maintained for 24 hours with extracorporeal lung and heart assist had better survival, improved neurologic deficit scores, and decreased heart necrosis compared to normothermic animals *(55)*. Similarly, in dogs maintained on CPB at 34ºC after 20 minutes of an exsanguination CA model, performance scores after recovery were greatly improved compared to normothermic controls, and neurologic damage was minimized on histological examination *(56)*.

There have been fewer studies of intra-arrest (or intra-ischemic) hypothermia, but what data does exist suggests that this strategy of cooling also provides significant benefit in IR injury. Two studies in focal tissue ischemic models are illustrative. Wilson et al. used a rabbit rectus femoris muscle IR model and showed that intra-ischemic hypothermia during ischemia increased muscle viability significantly *(57)*. A comparison of intra-ischemic vs postischemic cooling was tested in a peripheral nerve IR model, and intra-ischemic cooling to 28ºC showed superior benefit in a variety of parameters including electrophysiological and histological endpoints *(58)*. In a reversible global cerebral ischemia model using gerbils, Markanian et al. *(20)* compared a variety of hypothermia strategies, including early vs delayed cooling. They found that hypothermia to 32 to 33°C applied immediately after the onset of ischemia provided greater protection from infarct than equal hypothermia applied just 45 minutes later. Interestingly, in their study, cerebral ischemia was induced for 3 hours, which suggests that even a delay in cooling within the ischemic period can lead to poorer outcomes. Thus, although damage becomes most apparent in the reperfusion period, the underlying injury mechanism may begin during ischemia. A clear comparison of different cooling timing strategies was performed by Xiao et al. using a rat asphyxia model of CA *(59)*. The investigators found that cooling animals to 34ºC before arrest provided much better protection from injury than similar hypothermia induced during resuscitation.

DEPTH OF HYPOTHERMIA

Another crucial parameter of hypothermia is the depth to which cooling is applied. As described in the introduction to this chapter, there is a somewhat arbitrary convention grouping depth of cooling into several categories: mild (34–36°C), moderate (28–34°C), and deep hypothermia (15–28°C). Even 1°C of core brain cooling in the intra-arrest setting following normothermic arrest has been shown to improve outcome, however, the optimal temperature for greatest protection in this setting remains unknown (42). CA and IR experiments have focused primarily on mild and moderate hypothermia, and several studies have actually compared different temperatures in the same model. In a piglet model of brain ischemia, Laptook et al. found a clinical benefit from just 1 hour of postreperfusion hypothermia to 35.8°C compared to "normothermic" control animals at 38.3°C (60). Woods et al. performed cooling in a canine exsanguination model of CA. They found that when cooling was performed for 12 hours after arrest, better performance and histologic scores were obtained if animals were cooled to 33 to 34°C rather than 36°C (61). Note than in their animals, mean starting temperatures were 37.5°C, so 36°C did represent an average 1.5°C of cooling. Similarly, other investigations in dog exsanguination CA also found benefit of 34°C target temperature compared to 36°C (56), demonstrating that moderate hypothermia may confer more protection than mild hypothermia. Whether this logic can be extended to deeper levels of hypothermia remains an important question. Deeper levels may be protective in the intra-arrest setting, although after the heart is defibrillated and circulation reestablished more mild levels are likely best. Indeed, in some animal models, when cooling is induced after the return of blood flow following CA, mild hypothermia was better and colder temperatures possibly harmful (13,62). Possible explanations include decreased microcirculation flow (28). In human trials to date, no direct comparisons have been made regarding different depths of cooling and patient outcomes.

PHARMACOLOGICAL AUGMENTATION OF HYPOTHERMIA

A variety of drugs have also been considered in strategies for suspended animation or ischemic protection, either by themselves or in conjunction with other measures (reviewed in refs. 63 and 64). These agents have included free radical scavenging molecules, anticoagulants, glutamate receptor blocking agents, hibernation induction agents, and even thrombolytics. Certain of these agents may work by the induction of hypothermia (65). One example of this is the selective α-amino-3-hydroxy-5-methyl-4-isoxazole propionic acid receptor antagonist NBQX, which induces a mild hypothermia (66). Other drugs are thought to be helpful after ischemic insult by reduction of metabolic demands (67,68).

In a direct comparison of hypothermia with a pharmacologic treatment for IR injury, Matsumoto et al. compared thiopental burst suppression dosing vs hypothermia in a rabbit model of spinal cord IR (69). They found that hypothermia to 35°C was more protective than the barbiturate, with regards to histological and functional outcome measures. The authors did not test the two modalities in combination to see if further improvement could be generated. A drug–hypothermia combination was tested in an isolated lung IR model, and it was found that hypothermia to several depths in combination with prostaglandin E1 showed improved protection from injury than either agent alone (70). Similarly, Schwartz et al. found that in isolated rabbit hearts, function was improved when a δ-opioid agonist pentazocine was used in combination with hypothermia at 34°C (71).

There are other agents that might also confer improved survival when combined with hypothermia treatment. Antioxidants have been shown in many model systems to minimize IR injury and improve both survival and function *(72,73)*. In a cardiomyocyte model of IR, an antioxidant combination was found to dramatically reduce cell death after reperfusion *(74)*. Although these agents alone have not been shown in whole animal models to improve survival or other outcome measures after CA, it is possible that in the future they will play a supporting role to the induction of hypothermia. It is likely that oxidants play double-edged roles in both signaling and protective adaptation *(75)*, as well as injury and death *(76,77)*. Thus, future antioxidant therapies may specifically target injurious sources of oxidants although maintaining beneficial oxidant signaling *(78)*. Caspase inhibitors, a class of molecules that inhibit key components of the apoptotic pathway, may also play an important separate or adjunct role to hypothermia in treating cardiac arrest in the future. These agents are a subject of intense study *(79,80)*, and have the potential to significantly attenuate IR injury.

MECHANISMS OF HYPOTHERMIC PROTECTION

The mechanisms by which hypothermia may protect against ischemic injury are varied and incompletely understood. Given the importance of temperature in a wide range of physiologic processes, it is reasonable to conclude that multiple mechanisms might be involved, and that different mechanisms may protect in different tissues or at different times during ischemia or after reperfusion *(24,25)*. Given the multitude of possible target effects, hypothermia may represent "the ultimate neuroprotective cocktail" *(25)*. The specific targets and processes which hypothermia modulates can be crudely grouped into four categories: gross physiology, biochemistry, transcriptional/translational changes, and apoptosis. Certainly, these are not mutually exclusive categories. For example, redox changes in the cell may stimulate transcriptional/translational changes, which may in turn activate apoptotic machinery. Therefore, the groupings are somewhat arbitrary for the sake of discussion. Because brain and heart are generally understood to be the most sensitive organs to IR effects, most of the data pertaining to mechanism of injury comes from studies of these tissues in stroke or MI models.

Gross Physiology

As early as 1954, it was noted that hypothermia induced by ice-water immersion could lower cerebral oxygen consumption in dogs, by approx 7% per 1°C drop in temperature *(81)*. Other investigators have shown that mild hypothermia in rats improves postischemic cerebral blood flow disturbances *(82)*. Similarly, microsphere measurements in a dog model of CA demonstrated that hypothermia to 28°C led to better blood-flow characteristics during CPR *(83)*. Another marker of general physiologic injury after reperfusion, brain edema was also found to be reduced by hypothermia in a rat model of CA *(82,84)*, and in a gerbil brain ischemia model *(85)*. Finally, hypothermia has been shown to lessen damage to the blood–brain barrier (BBB) caused by IR *(82,86)*. Compromise of the BBB might provoke further injury by permitting blood-borne toxins to reach brain tissues *(86)*.

Biochemistry

A variety of biochemical changes provoked by IR are modified by hypothermia. In a gerbil stroke model, animals subjected to mild hypothermia were found to have decreased arachidonic acid metabolism compared with normothermic controls *(87)*. In a rat brain ischemia model, hypothermia to 32°C reduced nitric oxide (NO) production as measured in jugular blood *(88)*. Whether these aforementioned alterations are simply markers of hypothermic effects or actually issues in reperfusion injury remains to be clearly established. Other biochemical changes seem more likely to be directly linked to damage processes, such as the observation that hypothermia slows adenosine triphosphate (ATP) depletion during IR *(89)*. Free radical production also appears to be attenuated by hypothermic conditions in a rat cerebral ischemia model *(90)*. ATP depletion and free radical production might be universal mediators of IR damage, in heart, brain, and other tissues *(91)*. The release of other mediators, such as the neuron-excitatory amino acids glutamate, glycine, and aspartic acid, are reduced when neural tissues are cooled *(92–94)*. In fact, ischemic release of these neurotransmitters is quite sensitive to temperature *(95,96)*. In a gerbil brain ischemia model, glutamate release showed a direct correlation with brain temperatures from 31 to 39°C *(97)*.

Cellular Signaling Via Protein Changes

Intracellular signaling can quickly and dramatically alter the array of gene transcription activity of a cell, which in turn can trigger a variety of injury processes. In a CA mouse model, a group of signaling pathway genes known as the "immediate early genes" *(98)* were activated after resuscitation—specifically, *c-fos, c-jun,* and *krox-24 (99)*. A study of liver IR demonstrated a drop in *c-jun* terminal kinase activity at 25°C when compared to normothermic controls *(100)*. An extracellular signaling molecule thought to protect against injury, brain-derived neurotrophic factor, was increased in a rat model of CA when animals were cooled to 33°C *(101)*.

Apoptosis

Programmed cell death is a complex yet ubiquitous process by which cells actively chose, or are chosen, to die. This cellular program can be activated as part of normal physiology such as during embryonic development, or as an abnormal response in a wide variety of disease states *(102,103)*. A wide variety of evidence implicates the induction of apoptosis as a component of reperfusion injury *(91,104,105)*. To cite some human data as examples, a recent report showed that the apoptotic pathway enzyme caspase-3 was upregulated in brain tissue after resuscitation from CA, as measured on autopsy in patients who died within days of resuscitation *(106)*. Similarly, another crucial protein in the apoptotic machinery, Fas ligand, is elevated in blood after resuscitation from CA *(107)*. Fas receptor, necessary to bind Fas ligand and initiate the apoptotic pathway, is upregulated in livers harvested from donors in CA *(180)*. Widespread evidence from animals also supports the notion that apoptosis is activated after reperfusion *(48,109,110)*. Hypothermia may inhibit this process. Proteolysis of the cytoskeletal protein fodrin, a characteristic step in the apoptotic pathway, is inhibited by hypothermia to 32°C in a rat brain IR model *(111)*. The process of apoptosis is an active one, requiring protein synthesis and enzymatic activity, both of which might be inhibited by lowered temperatures. Although some suggestive data exists that the degree of apoptosis can be reduced by hypothermia, the topic certainly deserves more investigation in animal models.

METHODS FOR SUSPENDED METABOLISM AND PROTECTION FROM ISCHEMIA WITH AND WITHOUT HYPOTHERMIA

Although most methods for suspended animation use hypothermia, in theory cooling is not absolutely required to protect tissues during ischemia—as most experts believe it is the metabolic consequences of hypothermia (not temperature itself) that causes protection. If true, then it should be possible to simulate the metabolic consequences of hypothermia without necessarily decreasing the actual temperature. Experience to date with this notion is quite limited, although it is an important area of research. Most experts believe that during ischemia protective adaptive responses include: reducing energy utilization by shutting down nonessential cellular activities, reducing permeability of membranes to ion flux (thus reducing ATP required to maintain ionic gradients), and synthesis of ATP via glycolytic pathways during low oxygen states *(112)*. Similar metabolic changes are produced during hypothermia as well as during hibernation in many hibernating animal species. Natural hibernation has been suggested as an excellent model to study mechanisms of tissue protection during ischemia, because many hibernators are also hypoxia tolerant. Additionally, hibernation is an interesting model for reperfusion injury, because during arousal from hibernation, full reperfusion occurs but with no detectable injury even after prolonged periods of ischemia *(2)*.

An interesting approach to this is offered by Katz et al. who report that the neurotensin analog NT69L stimulated prolonged mild hypothermia (<35°C for nearly 300 minutes) in rats without the use of active cooling, which was in turn associated with improved outcomes after 8 minutes of asphyxial CA *(113)*. Possible mechanisms include a resetting of the hypothalamic temperature set point, with the result that mild hypothermia was produced without the need for a cooling device. Other laboratories have investigated the possibility of triggering natural hibernation pathway using a "hibernation-induction trigger," the δ-opioid receptor-binding molecules have been identified as central to this response *(114)*. Reduction of infarct size from 65 to 27% and reduction in arrhythmias have been observed using δ-opioid-receptor agonists administration *(115)*. Efforts to isolate and purify the protective proteins responsible for this protection are ongoing, a highly purified plasma fraction from hibernating woodchucks has been reported along with an α1-glycoprotein-like 88kDa "hibernation-related protein" that may contain the triggering activity *(116)*. Another approach is to consider the mechanisms of altered calcium homeostasis during ischemia and reperfusion although noting that hibernating mammals have an enhanced capacity to maintain intracellular calcium homeostasis over nonhibernating mammals (such as humans). Calcium (Ca) is a critical intracellular messenger that is tightly regulated in cells universally and dysregulation is described with ischemia and reperfusion. With low temperatures, nonhibernating hearts develop elevated intracellular Ca, reduced contraction force, and spontaneous Ca waves that have been suggested to initiate VF. By contrast hibernating animals fail to show these alterations in Ca with low temperatures and may even improve contractility at low temperatures *(117)*. Mechanisms used by hibernators to handle Ca include reducing Ca entry into the cell with channel alterations, enhancing Ca sequestration in the sarcoplasmic reticulum and increased removal *(117)*. An interesting notion is that all these mechanisms are also potentially present in nonhibernators. Although the hibernating pathways may not be active in nonhibernators, is seems likely that the full genomic/transcription/ translation machinery is potentially available in humans to use such mechanisms for ischemia tolerance.

METHODS OF HYPOTHERMIA INDUCTION

Most clinical studies of hypothermia induction have employed external means of cooling. These limited methods include use of circulating cooling blankets containing either cold air or water *(7,17,118)*, some form of direct contact with cold water or ice *(3,16,119)*, or both *(4)*. More experimental methods have also been attempted, such as an external cooling helmet which was able to cool core temperatures two to three degrees over 3 hours *(54)*. These methods are reasonably successful at inducing mild hypothermia, but to induce moderate hypothermia often takes at least several hours. External cooling of humans is difficult because of several reasons, including (a) the formidable ability of the human body to redirect blood flow away from cooled extremities or skin, preventing heat exchange, (b) the relatively compact (i.e., low surface area) nature of the human trunk, and (c) the ability to generate thermal energy to defend against cooling.

Given the limitations of external cooling described above, a number of laboratories have begun to develop novel cooling methods. Safar and colleagues have pioneered rapid blood cooling in dogs via an "aortic flush" technique *(5,56)*. This method involves the administration of cold saline via an aortic balloon catheter, which occludes the descending aorta, thus cooling the brain and heart via retrograde flow. Using aortic flush, Behringer et al. showed that 20 kg dogs could be cooled to target temperatures of 34°C within 10 to 15 minutes *(56)*. This technique grew out of experiments in the 1940s by Negovsky et al. in which retrograde arterial flush was used to treat soldiers suffering from exsanguination CA. Although the method provides robust cooling, it requires rapid aortic access, which may limit its development clinically. Another invasive technique for cooling was attempted exploiting the peritoneal space, with cold saline infusion into the peritoneum in conjunction with external ice cooling, which was able to cool dogs in VF to 34°C without significant adverse effects *(120)*. Certainly, access to the peritoneal space would be more readily achievable than aortic cannulation. Bernard has reported on a simple internal cooling technique, administration of ice-cold saline (30 mL/kg) via a peripheral intravenous line, which resulted in 1.7°C decrease in core temperature *(119)*.

Another blood cooling method under development for resuscitation involves catheters with closed cooling systems. One such commercially developed catheter has been used in swine and was able to cool 50 kg swine to a target temperature of 32°C within 60 minutes *(121)*. Clinical experiments with a similar cooling catheter are underway in Europe (F. Sterz, personal communication). It should also be noted that catheter-based cooling is being tested widely in the clinical treatment of focal ischemic processes, such as MI and stroke *(122,123)*. Several companies have developed cooling catheter systems, including Alsius (Icy catheter), Radiant (SetPoint), Innercool (Celsius Control), among others. The catheters that will prove more effective for localized cooling and for rapid induction of core hypothermia remains to be established, and will likely be a focus of intensive research over the next few years.

Other groups have pursued a pulmonary cooling strategy, exploiting the enormous surface area at the alveolar–pulmonary capillary interface. Cooling via the pulmonary route can involve a variety of media, including cold air and cold liquids. Perfluorocarbon (PFC) liquids have been under investigation for decades as possible blood substitutes and liquid ventilation media, given their ability to act as oxygen and carbon dioxide carriers. One such PFC, perflubron, has been used in a liquid ventilation protocol to cool dogs during CA *(124)*. Another PFC, perfluorodecalin, was used to successfully cool rabbits from 39 to 35°C under normal physiologic conditions *(125)*. Our laboratory has investigated the use of ice-water slurries to cool swine via the pulmonary route. In our experiments, carefully engineered microparticulate ice-water slurries with high flowability are instilled into the lungs of swine. We have demonstrated core brain-cooling rates of up to

4.8°C within 30 minutes during CPR *(126)*. Other adjunctive techniques include retrograde blood flow as in arterial perfusion of the superior vena cava during aortic arch surgery *(127)*.

FUTURE OF HYPOTHERMIA AND SUSPENDED ANIMATION

Several important enhancements are likely required before widespread hypothermia and suspended animation techniques can become a mainstream therapy. First a method for rapid cooling very early, preferably in the field, must become available to emergency medical service or even lay rescuers. Everything we know thus far about resuscitation would suggest that when earlier and faster hypothermia is accomplished, the greater is its benefit. If true, an effective method started by a lay-person on a victim of CA may result in far better outcomes than we currently see when cooling is performed slowly and relatively delayed following CA. This highlights the importance of bioengineering partnerships to advance new devices to overcome this thermodynamic challenge. An additional requirement for suspended animation is a practical method to produce improved artificial circulation although the heart is stopped. Although this is the purpose of classical chest compression CPR, we know that relatively low cardiac outputs are produced in most cases. Although these may be sufficient to restore circulation with defibrillation in the circulatory phase (approximately during arrest intervals of less than 10 minutes), chest compression alone fails to restore most victims of CA beyond this time, in the metabolic phase of CA *(128)*. However, with improved artificial circulation, as occurs with CPB, survival appears promising *(129)*. The current limitation to more widespread use of CPB is that it is currently difficult to initiate rapidly on patients (requiring often 45 minutes for establishment). Thus, another advantage of hypothermia induced during arrest (intra-arrest cooling) would be that it could allow for transport and placement of the patient on CPB support.

Suspended animation thus fits in nicely as a metabolic phase therapy with the notion of the three-phase time-sensitive model of CPR *(128)*. With the failure of defibrillation and circulation to restore a stable hemodynamic state, patients could be rapidly cooled to protect organs from ongoing ischemia and to buy time for additional therapies like establishment of CPB with controlled reperfusion. With the heart stopped and with full circulation provided by CPB, full attention could go to reversal of metabolic injury caused by free radical generation, loss of calcium homeostasis, leaky membrane integrity, overstimulation of the immune system, circulating cytokines, mediators of apoptosis, caspase activation and other biochemical pathways that lead to death if uncorrected. The limits for reversal of acute death (and how long a person can survive CA) when treated under such a suspended animation paradigm remain to be discovered.

REFERENCES

1. O'Sullivan ST, O'Shaughnessy M, O'Connor TP. Baron Larrey and cold injury during the campaigns of Napoleon. Ann Plast Surg 1995; 34:446–449.
2. Weil MH, Becker LB, Budinger T, et al. Workshop executive summary report: post-resuscitative and initial utility in life saving efforts (PULSE). Circulation 2001; 103:1182–1184.
3. Bernard SA, Gray TW, Buist MD, et al. Treatment of comatose survivors of out-of-hospital cardiac arrest with induced hypothermia. N Engl J Med 2002; 346:557–563.
4. HACA. Mild therapeutic hypothermia to improve the neurologic outcome after cardiac arrest. N Engl J Med 2002; 346:549–556.

5. Safar P, Tisherman SA, Behringer W, et al. Suspended animation for delayed resuscitation from prolonged cardiac arrest that is unresuscitable by standard cardiopulmonary-cerebral resuscitation. Crit Care Med 2000; 28:N214–N218.

6. Safar P. Cerebral resuscitation after cardiac arrest: research initiatives and future directions. Ann Emerg Med 1993; 22:324–49.

7. Yanagawa Y, Ishihara S, Norio H, et al. Preliminary clinical outcome study of mild resuscitative hypothermia after out-of-hospital cardiopulmonary arrest. Resuscitation 1998; 39:61–66.

8. Sessler DI. Complications and treatment of mild hypothermia. Anesthesiology 2001; 95:531–543.

9. Connor EL, Wren KR. Detrimental effects of hypothermia: a systems analysis. J Perianesth Nurs 2000; 15:151–155.

10. Kurz A, Sessler DI, Lenhardt R. Perioperative normothermia to reduce the incidence of surgical-wound infection and shorten hospitalization. Study of Wound Infection and Temperature Group. N Engl J Med 1996; 334:1209–1215.

11. Safar P, Klain M, Tisherman S. Selective brain cooling after cardiac arrest. Crit Care Med 1996; 24: 911–914.

12. Saccani S, Beghi C, Fragnito C, Barboso G, Fesani F. Carotid endarterectomy under hypothermic extracorporeal circulation: a method of brain protection for special patients. J Cardiovasc Surg (Torino) 1992; 33:311–314.

13. Weinrauch V, Safar P, Tisherman SA, Kuboyama K, Radovsky A. Beneficial effect of mild hypothermia and detrimental effect of deep hypothermia after cardiac arrest in dogs. Stroke 1992; 23:1454–1462.

14. Cleveland JC, Jr., Meldrum DR, Rowland RT, Banerjee A, Harken AH. Optimal myocardial preservation: cooling, cardioplegia, and conditioning. Ann Thorac Surg 1996; 61:760–768.

15. Takaba T, Inoue K. Past and present in myocardial protection. Ann Thorac Cardiovasc Surg 2000; 6:3–8.

16. Bernard SA, Jones BM, Horne MK. Clinical trial of induced hypothermia in comatose survivors of out-of-hospital cardiac arrest. Ann Emerg Med 1997; 30:146–153.

17. Zeiner A, Holzer M, Sterz F, et al. Mild resusitative hypothermia to improve neurological outcome after cardiac arrest: a clinical feasibilty trial. Stroke 2000; 31:86–94.

18. Kuboyama K, Safar P, Radovsky A, Tisherman SA, Stezoski SW, Alexander H. Delay in cooling negates the beneficial effect of mild resuscitative cerebral hypothermia after cardiac arrest in dogs: a prospective, randomized study. Crit Care Med 1993; 21:1348–1358.

19. Carroll M, Beek O. Protection against hippocampal CA1 cell loss by post-ischemic hypothermia is dependent on delay of initiation and duration. Metab Brain Dis 1992; 7:45–50.

20. Markarian GZ, Lee JH, Stein DJ, Hong SC. Mild hypothermia: therapeutic window after experimental cerebral ischemia. Neurosurgery 1996; 38:542–550; discussion 551.

21. Zhao D, Abella BS, Vanden Hoek TL, Becker LB. Intra-arrest hypothermia prior to resuscitation confers improved survival in a mouse model of cardiac arrest. Circulation 2002; 106:II-367, II-368.

22. Adams F. The genuine works of Hippocrates. New York: William Wood; 1886.

23. Bazzett HC. The effect of heat on blood volume and circulation. JAMA 1938; 111:1841–1845.

24. Bernard S. Induced hypothermia in intensive care medicine. Anaesth Intensive Care 1996; 24:382–388.

25. Colbourne F, Sutherland G, Corbett D. Postischemic hypothermia. A critical appraisal with implications for clinical treatment. Mol Neurobiol 1997; 14:171–201.

26. Eisenburger P, Sterz F, Holzer M, et al. Therapeutic hypothermia after cardiac arrest. Curr Opin Crit Care 2001; 7:184–188.

27. Resnick DK, Marion DW, Darby JM. The effect of hypothermia on the incidence of delayed traumatic intracerebral hemorrhage. Neurosurgery 1994; 34:252–5; discussion 255–256.

28. Marion DW, Leonov Y, Ginsberg M, et al. Resuscitative hypothermia. Crit Care Med 1996; 24: S81–S89.

29. Clifton GL, Miller ER, Choi SC, et al. Lack of effect of induction of hypothermia after acute brain injury. N Engl J Med 2001; 344:556–563.

30. Orlowski JP, Erenberg G, Lueders H, Cruse RP. Hypothermia and barbiturate coma for refractory status epilepticus. Crit Care Med 1984; 12:367–372.

31. Elman R, Cox WMJ, Lischer CE, Mueller AJ. Mortality in severe experimental burns as affected by environmental temperature. Proc Soc Exper Biol Med 1942; 51:350–355.

32. Balaji S, Sullivan I, Deanfield J, James I. Moderate hypothermia in the management of resistant automatic tachycardias in children. Br Heart J 1991; 66:221–224.

33. Blair E, Henning G, Hornick R. Hypothermia in bacterial shock. Arch Surg 1964; 89:619–629.

34. Fay T. Clinical report and evaluation of low temperature in treatment of cancer. Proc Inter St Post-grad Med Ass N Amer 1941; 1941:292–297.

35. Bigelow WG, Lindsay WK, Greenwood WF. Hypothermia: its possible role in cardiac surgery: an investigation of factors governing survival in dogs at low body temperature. Ann Surg. 1950; 132:849–866.
36. Benson DW, Williams GR, Spencer FC, et al. The use of hypothermia after cardiac arrest. Anesth Analg 1959; 38:423–428.
37. Williams GR, Spencer FC. The clinical use of hypothermia following cardiac arrest. Ann Surg 1958; 148:462–468.
38. Steen PA, Milde JH, Michenfelder JD. The detrimental effects of prolonged hypothermia and rewarming in the dog. Anesthesiology 1980; 52:224–30.
39. Michenfelder JD, Terry HR, Daw EF, Uihlein A. Induced hypothermia: Physiological effects, indications and techniques. Surg Clin North Am 1965; 45:889–898.
40. Talbott JH. The physiologic and therapeutic effects of hypothermia. N Engl J Med 1941; 224:281–288.
41. Leonov Y, Sterz F, Safer P, Radovsky A. Moderate hypothermia after cardiac arrest of 17 min in dogs. Effect of cerebral and cardiac outcome. A preliminary study. Stroke 1990; 21:1600–1606.
42. Leonov Y, Sterz F, Safer P, et al. Mild cerebral hypothermia during and after cardiac arrest improves neurologic outcome in dogs. Journal of Cerebral Blood Flow and Metabolism 1990; 10:57–70.
43. Tisherman SA, Safar P, Radovsky A, Peitzman A, Sterz F, Kuboyama K. Therapeutic deep hypothermic circulatory arrest in dogs: a resuscitation modality for hemorrhagic shock with 'irreparable' injury. J Trauma 1990; 30:836–847.
44. Tisherman SA, Safar P, Radovsky A, et al. Profound hypothermia (less than 10°C) compared with deep hypothermia (15°C) improves neurologic outcome in dogs after two hours' circulatory arrest induced to enable resuscitative surgery. J Trauma 1991; 31:1051–1061.
45. Bellamy RF. The causes of death in conventional land warfare: implications for combat casualty care research. Mil Med 1984; 149:55–62.
46. Bellamy R, Safar P, Tisherman SA, et al Suspended animation for delayed resuscitation. Crit Care Med 1996; 24:S24–S47.
47. Vanden Hoek TL, Shao Z, Li C, Zak R, Schumacker PT, Becker LB. Reperfusion injury in cardiac myocytes after simulated ischemia. Am J Phys 1996; 270:H1334–H1341.
48. Maulik N, Yoshida T, Das DK. Regulation of cardiomyocyte apoptosis in ischemic reperfused mouse heart by glutathione peroxidase. Mol Cell Biochem 1999; 196:13–21.
49. Ferreira R, Burgos M, Llesuy S, et al. Reduction of reperfusion injury with mannitol cardioplegia. Ann Thorac Surg 1989; 48:77-83; discussion 83–84.
50. Zar HA, Lancaster JR, Jr. Mild hypothermia protects against postischemic hepatic endothelial injury and decreases the formation of reactive oxygen species. Redox Rep 2000; 5:303–310.
51. Granger DN, Korthuis RJ. Physiologic mechanisms of postischemic tissue injury. Annu Rev Physiol 1995; 57:311–332.
52. Patel S, Pachter HL, Yee H, Schwartz JD, Marcus SG, Shamamian P. Topical hepatic hypothermia attenuates pulmonary injury after hepatic ischemia and reperfusion. J Am Coll Surg 2000; 191:650–656.
53. Canevari L, Console A, Tendi EA, Clark JB, Bates TE. Effect of postischaemic hypothermia on the mitochondrial damage induced by ischaemia and reperfusion in the gerbil. Brain Res 1999; 817:241–245.
54. Hachimi-Idrissi S, Corne L, Huyghens L. The effect of mild hypothermia and induced hypertension on long term survival rate and neurological outcome after asphyxial cardiac arrest in rats. Resuscitation 2001; 49:73–82.
55. Ao H, Tanimoto H, Yoshitake A, Moon JK, Terasaki H. Long-term mild hypothermia with extracorporeal lung and heart assist improves survival from prolonged cardiac arrest in dogs. Resuscitation 2001; 48:163–174.
56. Behringer W, Prueckner S, Kentner R, et al. Rapid hypothermic aortic flush can achieve survival without brain damage after 30 minutes cardiac arrest in dogs. Anesthesiology 2000; 93:1491–1499.
57. Wilson YT, Lepore DA, Riccio M, et al. Mild hypothermia protects against ischaemia-reperfusion injury in rabbit skeletal muscle. Br J Plast Surg 1997; 50:343–348.
58. Mitsui Y, Schmelzer JD, Zollman PJ, Kihara M, Low PA. Hypothermic neuroprotection of peripheral nerve of rats from ischaemia-reperfusion injury. Brain 1999; 122(Pt 1):161–169.
59. Xiao F, Safar P, Radovsky A. Mild protective and resuscitative hypothermia for asphyxial cardiac arrest in rats. Am J Emerg Med 1998; 16:17–25.
60. Laptook AR, Corbett RJ, Sterett R, Burns DK, Garcia D, Tollefsbol G. Modest hypothermia provides partial neuroprotection when used for immediate resuscitation after brain ischemia. Pediatr Res 1997; 42:17–23.
61. Woods R, Prueckner S, Safer P, et al. Hypothermic aortic arch flush for preservation during exsanguination cardiac arrest of 15 minutes in dogs. J Trauma 1999; 47:1028–1036.

62. Safar P, Xiao F, Radovsky A, et al. Improved cerebral resuscitation from cardiac arrest in dogs with mild hypothermia plus blood flow promotion. Stroke 1996; 27:105–113.

63. Buchan AM. Do NMDA antagonists protect against cerebral ischemia: are clinical trials warranted? Cerebrovasc Brain Metab Rev 1990; 2:1–26.

64. Koroshetz WJ, Moskowitz MA. Emerging treatments for stroke in humans. Trends Pharmacol Sci 1996; 17:227–233.

65. Menon DK, Young Y. Pharmacologically induced hypothermia for cerebral protection in humans. Stroke 1994; 25:522–523.

66. Nurse S, Corbett D. Neuroprotection after several days of mild, drug-induced hypothermia. J Cereb Blood Flow Metab 1996; 16:474–480.

67. Heros RC. Stroke: early pathophysiology and treatment. Summary of the Fifth Annual Decade of the Brain Symposium. Stroke 1994; 25:1877–1881.

68. Astrup J, Sorensen PM, Sorensen HR. Inhibition of cerebral oxygen and glucose consumption in the dog by hypothermia, pentobarbital, and lidocaine. Anesthesiology 1981; 55:263–268.

69. Matsumoto M, Iida Y, Sakabe T, Sano T, Ishikawa T, Nakakimura K. Mild and moderate hypothermia provide better protection than a burst-suppression dose of thiopental against ischemic spinal cord injury in rabbits. Anesthesiology 1997; 86:1120–1127.

70. Chiang CH, Wu K, Yu CP, Yan HC, Perng WC, Wu CP. Hypothermia and prostaglandin E(1) produce synergistic attenuation of ischemia-reperfusion lung injury. Am J Respir Crit Care Med 1999; 160: 1319–1323.

71. Schwartz CF, Georges AJ, Gallagher MA, Yu L, Kilgore KS, Bolling SF. Delta opioid receptors and low temperature myocardial protection. Ann Thorac Surg 1999; 68:2089–2092.

72. Ferrari R. Oxygen-free radicals at myocardial level: effects of ischaemia and reperfusion. Adv Exp Med Biol 1994; 366:99–111.

73. Das DK, Maulik N. Antioxidant effectiveness in ischemia-reperfusion tissue injury. Methods in Enzymology 1994; 233:601–610.

74. Vanden Hoek TL, Li C, Shao Z, Schumacker PT, Becker LB. Significant levels of oxidants are generated by isolated cardiomyocytes during ischemia prior to reperfusion. J Mol Cell Cardiol 1997; 29:2571–2583.

75. Vanden Hoek TL, Becker LB, Shao Z, Li C, Schumacker PT. Reactive oxygen species released from mitochondria during brief hypoxia induce preconditioning in cardiomyocytes. Journal of Biological Chemistry 1998; 273:18,092–18,098.

76. Vanden Hoek TL, Becker LB, Shao Z, Li C, Schumacker PT. Preconditioning in cardiomyocytes protects by attenuating oxidant stress at reperfusion. Circ Res 2000; 86:534–540.

77. Vanden Hoek TL, Qin Y, Wojcik K, et al. Reperfusion, not simulated ischemia, initiates intrinsic apoptosis injury in chick cardiomyocytes. Am J Physiol Heart Circ Physiol 2002; 284:H141–H150.

78. Vanden Hoek TL. Preconditioning and postresuscitation injury. Crit Care Med 2002; 30:S172–S175.

79. Huang JQ, Radinovic S, Rezaiefar P, Black SC. In vivo myocardial infarct size reduction by a caspase inhibitor administered after the onset of ischemia. Eur J Pharmacol 2000; 402:139–142.

80. Cursio R, Gugenheim J, Ricci JE, et al. Caspase inhibition protects from liver injury following ischemia and reperfusion in rats. Transpl Int 2000 ;13 (Suppl 1):S568–S572.

81. Rosomoff HL, Holaday DA. Cerebral blood flow and cerebral oxygen consumption during hypothermia. Am J Physiol 1954; 179:85–88.

82. Karibe H, Zarow GJ, Graham SH, Weinstein PR. Mild intraischemic hypothermia reduces postischemic hyperperfusion, delayed postischemic hypoperfusion, blood-brain barrier disruption, brain edema, and neuronal damage volume after temporary focal cerebral ischemia in rats. J Cereb Blood Flow Metab 1994; 14:620–627.

83. Shaffner DH, Eleff SM, Koehler RC, Traystman RJ. Effect of the no-flow interval and hypothermia on cerebral blood flow and metabolism during cardiopulmonary resuscitation in dogs. Stroke 1998; 29: 2607–2615.

84. Xiao F, Zhang S, Arnold TC, et al. Mild hypothermia induced before cardiac arrest reduces brain edema formation in rats. Acad Emerg Med 2002; 9:105–114.

85. Dempsey RJ, Combs DJ, Maley ME, Cowen DE, Roy MW, Donaldson DL. Moderate hypothermia reduces postischemic edema development and leukotriene production. Neurosurgery 1987; 21:177–181.

86. Dietrich WD, Busto R, Halley M, Valdes I. The importance of brain temperature in alterations of the blood-brain barrier following cerebral ischemia. J Neuropathol Exp Neurol 1990; 49:486–497.

87. Kubota M, Nakane M, Narita K, et al. Mild hypothermia reduces the rate of metabolism of arachidonic acid following postischemic reperfusion. Brain Res 1998; 779:297–300.

88. Kumura E, Yoshimine T, Takaoka M, Hayakawa T, Shiga T, Kosaka H. Hypothermia suppresses nitric oxide elevation during reperfusion after focal cerebral ischemia in rats. Neurosci Lett 1996; 220:45–48.

89. Lundberg J, Elander A, Soussi B. Effect of hypothermia on the ischemic and reperfused rat skeletal muscle, monitored by in vivo (31)P-magnetic resonance spectroscopy. Microsurgery 2001; 21: 366–373.

90. Kil HY, Zhang J, Piantadosi CA. Brain temperature alters hydroxyl radical production during cerebral ischemia/reperfusion in rats. J Cereb Blood Flow Metab 1996; 16:100–106.

91. Abella BS, Becker LB. Ischemia-Reperfusion and Acute Apoptotic Cell Death. In: Yearbook of Intensive Care and Emergency Medicine. Vincent JL, ed. Berlin: Springer, 2002, pp. 3–11.

92. Ishikawa T, Marsala M. Hypothermia prevents biphasic glutamate release and corresponding neuronal degeneration after transient spinal cord ischemia in the rat. Cell Mol Neurobiol 1999; 19:199–208.

93. Busto R, Globus MY, Dietrich WD, et al. Effect of mild hypothermia on ischemia-induced release of neurotransmitters and free fatty acids in rat brain. Stroke 1989; 20:904–910.

94. Nakashima K, Todd MM. Effects of hypothermia on the rate of excitatory amino acid release after ischemic depolarization. Stroke 1996; 27:913–918.

95. Baker AJ, Zornow MH, Grafe MR, et al. Hypothermia prevents ischemia-induced increases in hippocampal glycine concentrations in rabbits. Stroke 1991; 22:666–673.

96. Winfree CJ, Baker CJ, Connolly ES, Jr., Fiore AJ, Solomon RA. Mild hypothermia reduces penumbral glutamate levels in the rat permanent focal cerebral ischemia model. Neurosurgery 1996; 38: 1216–1222.

97. Mitani A, Kataoka K. Critical levels of extracellular glutamate mediating gerbil hippocampal delayed neuronal death during hypothermia: brain microdialysis study. Neuroscience 1991; 42:661–670.

98. Papadopoulos MC, Giffard RG, Bell BA. An introduction to the changes in gene expression that occur after cerebral ischaemia. Br J Neurosurg 2000; 14:305–312.

99. Böttiger B, Teschendorf P, Krumnikl J, et al. Global cerebral ischemia due to cardiocirculatory arrest in mice causes neuronal degeneration and early induction of transcription factor genes in the hippocampus. Mol Brain Res 1999; 65:135–142.

100. Kato A, Singh S, McLeish KR, Edwards MJ, Lentsch AB. Mechanisms of hypothermic protection against ischemic liver injury in mice. Am J Physiol Gastrointest Liver Physiol 2002; 282:G608–G616.

101. D'Cruz BJ, Fertig KC, Filiano AJ, Hicks SD, DeFranco DB, Callaway CW. Hypothermic reperfusion after cardiac arrest augments brain-derived neurotrophic factor activation. J Cereb Blood Flow Metab 2002; 22:843–851.

102. Hengartner MO. The biochemistry of apoptosis. Nature 2000; 407:770–776.

103. Jacobson MD, Weil M, Raff MC. Programmed cell death in animal development. Cell 1997; 88:347–354.

104. Collard CD, S. G. Pathophysiology, clinical manifestations, and prevention of ischemia-reperfusion injury. Anesthesiology 2001; 94:1133–1138.

105. Hearse DJ, Bolli R. Reperfusion induced injury: manifestations, mechanisms, and clinical relevance. Trends in Cardiovascular Medicine 1991; 1:233–240.

106. Love S, Barber R, Srinivasan A, Wilcock GK. Activation of caspase-3 in permanent and transient brain ischaemia in man. Neuroreport 2000; 11:2495–2499.

107. Iwama H, Tohma J, Nakamura N. High serum soluble Fas-ligand in cardiopulmonary arrest patients. Am J Emerg Med 2000; 18:348.

108. Schnurr C, Glatzel U, Tolba R, Hirner A, Minor T. Fas receptor is upregulated in livers from non-heartbeating donors. Eur Surg Res 2001; 33:327–33.

109. Loddick SA, MacKenzie A, Rothwell NJ. An ICE inhibitor, z-VAD-DCB attenuates ischaemic brain damage in the rat. Neuroreport 1996; 7:1465–1468.

110. Crack PJ, Taylor JM, Flentjar NJ, et al. Increased infarct size and exacerbated apoptosis in the glutathione peroxidase-1 (Gpx-1) knockout mouse brain in response to ischemia/reperfusion injury. J Neurochem 2001; 78:1389–1399.

111. Harada K, Maekawa T, Tsuruta R, et al. Hypothermia inhibits translocation of CaM kinase II and PKC-alpha, beta, gamma isoforms and fodrin proteolysis in rat brain synaptosome during ischemia-reperfusion. J Neurosci Res 2002; 67:664–669.

112. Hochachka PW. Defense strategies against hypoxia and hypothermia. Science 1986; 231:234–241.

113. Katz LM, Wang Y, McMahon B, Richelson E. Neurotensin analog NT69L induces rapid and prolonged hypothermia after hypoxic ischemia. Acad Emerg Med 2001; 8:1115–1121.

114. Benedict PE, Benedict MB, Su TP, Bolling SF. Opiate drugs and delta-receptor-mediated myocardial protection. Circulation 1999; 100:II357–II360.

115. Sigg DC, Coles JA, Jr., Oeltgen PR, Iaizzo PA. Role of delta-opioid receptor agonists on infarct size reduction in swine. Am J Physiol Heart Circ Physiol 2002; 282:H1953–H1960.
116. Horton ND, Kaftani DJ, Bruce DS, et al. Isolation and partial characterization of an opioid-like 88 kDa hibernation-related protein. Comp Biochem Physiol B Biochem Mol Biol 1998; 119:787–805.
117. Wang SQ, Lakatta EG, Cheng H, Zhou ZQ. Adaptive mechanisms of intracellular calcium homeostasis in mammalian hibernators. J Exp Biol 2002; 205:2957–2962.
118. Felberg RA, Krieger DW, Chuang R, et al. Hypothermia after cardiac arrest: feasibility and safety of an external cooling protocol. Circulation 2001; 104:1799–1804.
119. Bernard S, Buist M, Monteiro O, Smith K. Induced hypothermia using large volume, ice-cold intravenous fluid in comatose survivors of out-of-hospital cardiac arrest: a preliminary report. Resuscitation 2003; 56:9–13.
120. Xiao F, Safar P, Alexander H. Peritoneal cooling for mild cerebral hypothermia after cardiac arrest in dogs. Resuscitation 1995; 30:51–59.
121. Inderbitzen B, Yon S, Lasheras J, Dobak J, Perl J, Steinberg GK. Safety and performance of a novel intravascular catheter for induction and reversal of hypothermia in a porcine model. Neurosurgery 2002; 50:364–370.
122. Dae MW, Gao DW, Sessler DI, Chair K, Stillson CA. Effect of endovascular cooling on myocardial temperature, infarct size, and cardiac output in human-sized pigs. Am J Physiol Heart Circ Physiol 2002; 282:H1584–H1591.
123. Krieger DW, De Georgia MA, Abou-Chebl A, et al. Cooling for acute ischemic brain damage (cool aid): an open pilot study of induced hypothermia in acute ischemic stroke. Stroke 2001; 32:1847–1854.
124. Harris S, Darwin M, Russell S, O'Farrell J, Fletcher M, Wowk B. Rapid (0.5C/min) minimally invasive induction of hypothermia using cold perfluorochemical lung lavage in dogs. Resuscitation 2001; 50: 189–204.
125. Hong SB, Koh Y, Shim TS, et al. Physiologic characteristics of cold perfluorocarbon-induced hypothermia during partial liquid ventilation in normal rabbits. Anesth Analg 2002; 94:157–162, table of contents.
126. Becker L, Kasza K, Jayakar D, et al. Rapid induction of hypothermia using phase-change ice slurry: targeted cooling of the heart and brain during cardiac arrest. Circulation 2000:A2769.
127. Hilgenberg AD, Logan DL. Results of aortic arch repair with hypothermic circulatory arrest and retrograde cerebral perfusion. J Card Surg 2001; 16:246–251.
128. Weisfeldt ML, Becker LB. Resuscitation after cardiac arrest: a 3-phase time-sensitive model. JAMA 2002; 288:3035–3038.
129. Beyersdorf F, Kirsch M, Buckberg GG, Allen BS. Warm glutamate/aspartate-enriched blood cardioplegic solution for perioperative sudden death. J Thorac Cardiovasc Surg 1992; 104:1141–1147.

16 Percutaneous Cardiopulmonary Bypass As an Adjunctive Strategy for Resucitation

The State of the Art

Catherine Cooper, MD
and Bruce D. Spiess, MD, FAHA

CONTENTS

INTRODUCTION
PERCUTANEOUS CARDIOPULMONARY BYPASS
INDICATIONS AND CONTRAINDICTIONS FOR PCPB
PCPB TECHNIQUE
COMPLICATIONS OF PCPB
OUTCOME WITH USE OF PCPB
CONCLUSION
REFERENCES

INTRODUCTION

Cardiopulmonary bypass (CPB) is now 50 years old. Although developed originally to allow correction of congenital and valvular heart disease, CPB has affected all of medicine profoundly. As an artificial circulatory support for systemic and pulmonary functions, CPB has allowed for the development of cardiovascular surgery. Today, coronary artery bypass grafting is the most commonly performed cardiac surgery. The current trend is to perform a larger number of more complicated coronary revascularization surgeries "off pump." However, CPB supported work still accounts for the vast majority of surgeries. The CPB technology has evolved from one with large oxygenators, blood prime, and complex heating and cooling to today's smaller and less complex technologies.

CPB supports systemic blood flow, blood pressure, and tissue oxygenation when the heart and lungs are either being operated on or are unable to maintain these functions. In patients with coronary artery disease (CAD), limited flow past either a fixed obstructing lesion or an acute platelet thrombus creates a volume of myocardial tissue that is forced to switch from aerobic to anaerobic metabolism. If present for a long enough period of time, the tissue is at risk for infarction. The CPB machine physiologically

From: *Contemporary Cardiology: Cardiopulmonary Resuscitation*
Edited by: J. P. Ornato and M. A. Peberdy © Humana Press Inc., Totowa, NJ

improves the supply and demand ratios of at risk myocardium physiologically. CPB decreases demand by eliminating myocardial work, as the CPB machine takes over systemic cardiac output. Supply increases by a number of mechanisms. First, most CPB flow is nonpulsatile and with the myocardium no longer doing mechanical work and not creating left ventricular (LV) wall tension, blood flows to the left ventricle throughout the entire heart cycle. Second, the CPB machine supplies a mean blood pressure that is elevated above diastolic pressure, perfusing myocardium continuously at a higher pressure. Therefore, a luxury of perfusion occurs in a state in which metabolic oxygen demand is decreased. Cardiac surgeons realize this advantage and use the CPB machine as their "bail out" when presented with an acute ischemic emergency. It makes wonderful physiological sense to export this technology from the operating room to other hospital and potentially nonhospital environments in which CPB technology could save lives.

PERCUTANEOUS CARDIOPULMONARY BYPASS

Percutaneous cardiopulmonary bypass (PCPB) was first used in 1983 for patients with cardiac arrest (CA) and cardiogenic shock (CS [1]). The primary indication for emergent PCPB is the presence of a surgically correctible anatomic lesion causing the CA or shock state, with the highest survival rates reported in this group of patients.

PCPB is used currently in patients who fail traditional resuscitation therapies and is considered a temporary support until more definitive treatment is available. For conditions amenable to surgical intervention (e.g., coronary disease or pulmonary embolism), this temporary support may provide time for diagnostic angiography followed by emergency surgery. For conditions not readily treatable with surgery (e.g., heart failure from cardiomyopathy), PCBP is a bridge to long-term circulatory support in the form of extracorporeal membrane oxygenation (ECMO) or the implantation of a ventricular assist device (VAD).

CPB technology has evolved from bulky machines requiring complicated set up and surgical insertion of cannulae in the operating room to small, portable machines with disposable, pre-assembled circuits and percutaneously introduced cannulae. The latter allow very rapid institution of CBP throughout the hospital. PCPB systems have been studied as elective adjuncts to support high-risk cardiology interventions, particularly angioplasty and valvuloplasty. Experience with the technique used electively in the cardiac catheterization laboratory led to its use in emergency situations, including coronary dissection, ventricular failure, and ventricular rupture. The PCPB technique has been extended to other emergency cases of CA and CS unresponsive to traditional measures including acute myocardial infarction (AMI), PE, ventricular rupture, trauma, and hypothermia.

The systems utilized by centers employing PCPB are portable, fitting onto one small cart. They most often employ a centrifugal pump—often a Biomedicus (Medtronic Perfusion Systems, Anaheim, CA) system. These pumps can be run from a battery pack for transport through hospital corridors allowing movement of patients to the operating room for definitive treatment. Hollow fiber, membrane oxygenators that are heparin-bonded have been used widely in these systems. In many of the recently published series, either critical care nurses or others present in the hospital 24 hours a day were trained and primed the PCPB systems with crystalloid. Some series have utilized systemic heparinization with target activated clotting time (ACT) of 400 seconds. Often a quick 20,000 IU bolus is given to the patient and time is not taken for dosage personalization to achieve a 400 to 500 second ACT. The key difference between PCPB systems and those utilized in the operating rooms is size and portability.

For elective cardiac surgery in the operating room, arterial and venous cannulae are placed in the ascending aorta and the right atrium. Often, variations are made depending on the patient's physiology and planned operation. For PCPB, most series report the use of femoral arterial and venous cannulations. The femoral vein cannulation usually uses a long fenestrated cannula that is passed up the vena cava. Its tip is lodged in the right atrium and the fenestrations allow for drainage of blood from throughout the vena cava.

Often, the PCPB systems can be placed by a resident or attending cardiologist or surgeon. Nurses can prime the PCPB machine with crystalloid quickly. In a cardiac catheterization laboratory, vessels are already cannulated and wires are often in place, saving precious minutes. In an unwitnessed arrest or one that occurs on a hospital ward, the individual would have to undergo CPR for some time as he or she is moved to a place in which cannulation can be performed. PCPB requires a large commitment by a medical center to make teams available 24 hours a day.

INDICATIONS AND CONTRAINDICATIONS FOR PCPB

Current contraindications and indications for PCPB are based on survival data, with unwitnessed CA being a very poor prognostic indicator and probably an absolute contraindication to PCPB, except in cases of profound hypothermia. Aortic dissection and aortic regurgitation also preclude effective use of PCPB. Other relative contraindications include CA longer than 30 minutes (only rare survivors), no correctable anatomic defect, and terminal illness. Recent stroke, diabetes, and peripheral vascular disease also complicate initiation and successful weaning from PCPB *(2)*.

CA is one the most common indications for initiation of PCPB. A National Cardiopulmonary Support Registry from 17 institutions collected data on the use of PCPB and reported initial findings in 1992 *(3)*. Although published in 1992, it is still the largest series published to date on PCPB, including 187 patients from 17 major institutions. The largest number of patients had undergone CA, but significant numbers of victims had CS or hypothermia. The largest number of survivors were those who had CS but who had not gone on to CA yet. Table 1 shows the data from this study and differentiates individuals who survived less than or more than 30 days. Patients who did undergo CA were far more likely to survive if the time from witnessed arrest to institution of PCPB was short. Some patients were started on PCPB in less than 15 minutes. More than 50% of these patients survived. No patients with unwitnessed arrest survived.

Most cases of PCPB were for patients who experienced CA and on whom traditional cardiopulmonary resuscitation (CPR) had failed. AMI was the most common precipitating event. Other causes included post-pericardiotomy arrest, refractory arrhythmias, PE, rupture of aneurysm or cardiac graft, pericardial tamponade, and aortic valve lesions. CS was the second most common indication, most often as a result of AMI, myocarditis, and rupture of ventricular free wall or septum *(4)*. One series of six severe trauma patients younger than age 55 who were felt to have recoverable injuries instituted PCPB for poor oxygenation, hypothermia, hypovolemia, and coagulopathy *(5)*. Patients with pulmonary insufficiency, smoke inhalation, and status asthmaticus have also been treated with PCPB in a few cases.

Table 1
Survival After Percutaneous Cardiopulmonary Bypass

Cause	Died on bypass	Alive <30 days	Alive >30 days	Unknown outcome
Cardiac arrest	88	6	15	2
CA after cardiotomy	12	0	2	0
Cardiogenic shock	21	0	15	2
CS after cardiotomy	4	0	2	0
Hypothermia	4	0	3	0
Pulmonary insufficiency	5	1	3	0
Other	1	1	0	0
Total (N = 187)	135 (72.2%)	8 (4.3%)	40 (21.4%)	4 (2.1%)

CA, cardiac arrest; CS, cardiogenic shock. (Adapted from ref. 3.)

PCPB TECHNIQUE

The technique of implementing PCPB is similar to routine CPB, but employs a portable cart containing prepackaged circuits ready for priming; a battery-powered centrifugal pump, which actively aspirates venous blood; a membrane oxygenator with oxygen source; and percutaneously placed long, thin-walled venous and arterial cannulae. Full systemic heparinization is required with frequent monitoring of the ACT. Heparin-coated systems are being developed that may allow considerably lower levels of anticoagulation. Surgeons, cardiologists, or emergency physicians can insert PCPB cannulae with the PCPB set-up by perfusionists or ECMO-trained intensive care nurses. The time to initiation of emergency PCPB depends on the team's familiarity and experience with the procedure. Faster initiation of bypass and improved results are noted as an institution performs PCPB regularly.

COMPLICATIONS OF PCPB

Complications of PCPB are relatively rare. Bleeding at the cannulation sites is the complication reported most often. Perfusion problems include arterial or venous injury, air embolus, tubing disconnections, and embolization of arterial plaque. Ischemia of the brain, myocardium, and kidney usually result from the original CA and delay before institution of PCPB. However, femoral arterial perfusion is likely to be inadequate for adequate cerebral perfusion if used for more than 4 to 6 hours and strong consideration should be given to converting to an aortic cannula if continuing bypass support is needed. Ischemic limb complications have been reported, sometimes requiring embolectomy or amputation. Hemolysis and coagulopathy are rarely clinically significant with PCPB times of less than 6 hours. A small-sized cannula presents significant risk factor for hemolysis.

OUTCOME WITH USE OF PCPB

In 2002, Kurusz tabulated results from all case reports of PCPB use over a 10-year period in the 1990s. Long-term (>30-day) survival was better in patients with CS (40.1%

of 335 survived) vs those with CA (21.6% of 335). Other uses of PCBP were more infrequent, but had comparable survival rates to that seen in patients with CS; 5 of 12 (41.7%) patients with pulmonary causes survived, 5 of 9 (55.6%) patients with trauma survived, and 5 of 13 (38.5%) patients with hypothermia survived *(1)*. For patients with fulminant myocarditis, survival rates were as high as 70 to 100%. Patients with cardiogenic shock had the greatest benefit from PCPB, suggesting that PCPB is best applied before CA occurs and hypoxic injury begins. However, there were survivors among patients in CA who could not be resuscitated otherwise, a group with a 100% predicted mortality.

There were no survivors of PCPB in patients with unwitnessed CA, except in profound hypothermia. The duration of CPR prior to PCBP was predictive of survival, with only 5 to 14% of patients surviving who received greater than 30 minutes of CPR. In contrast, 25 to 50% of patients with less than 30 minutes of CPR survived. In one group of three pediatric patients *(6)*, two survived CPR for longer than 30 minutes, suggesting that children may tolerate CPR better than adults. Immediate application of PCPB significantly improves cardiac output, helping preserve myocardial and neurological function.

Survival is more likely in patients with correctable anatomic defects. Examples of primary correctable lesions include CAD, ventricular rupture, and PE. In patients treated with PCPB, survival was 15 to 40%, compared with 0 to 13% in patients without such an intervention.

Several authors report comparable increased survival rates in patients undergoing cardiac surgery soon after initiation of PCPB to correct anatomic defects. In 1991, Money and colleagues reported a series of 11 patients who required CPB for CA *(7)*. All of the five patients who had complications in the cardiac catheterization lab and went to the operating room survived. Of six patients on PCPB initiated outside the catheterization lab, three had lesions amenable to surgery and two of the three survived. The nonsurvivor was judged to be at a very high risk for surgery with marginally correctable anatomy. This patient required biventricular assist devices and died 4 days later. Of the three patients without surgically correctable problems, none survived. All patients were resuscitated successfully, and all seven of the patients with clearly correctable lesions survived. The authors concluded that rapid initiation of PCPB by an experienced team and rapid transport to the operating room for definitive correction allows excellent survival in desperately ill patients who would otherwise not survive.

Wittenmyer reported that 104 patients from 1987 to 1992 who received interventional therapy soon after PCBP had better survival to hospital discharge than patients who could not be so treated *(8)*. Of 74 patients receiving interventional therapy, survival was 26% for those treated in the cardiovascular lab (thrombolytics, angioplasty, and valvuloplasty) and 44% for those treated operatively (coronary bypass grafting, valve replacement, pulmonary embolectomy, ventricular septal defect repair, and cardiac perforation/rupture). Higher survival (52%) was noted in patients treated for CS than for those in CA (24%). No patient with unwitnessed CA survived. None of the three patients transferred from another hospital after PCPB initiation survived.

A more recent review of 43 patients treated with PCPB from 1992 to 1998 by Mitsui et al. examined eight patients who had cardiac surgery *(9)*. Only two of the patients survived to be discharged from the hospital, although six were weaned from CPB successfully. Three patients had coronary bypass surgery, but LV function did not recover in two of those patients. The three patients with ventricular septal defects (VSD), LV rupture, and both LV rupture and VSD, were weaned successfully but all had deterioration of LV function. Two patients had aortic valve replacement (one with a Maze procedure as well), both were weaned but both experienced postoperative ventricular arrhythmias (VAs). One survived and one died from refractory VA.

In 1999, von Segesser reviewed cardiopulmonary support (PCPB) and ECMO, highlighting both the usefulness and difficulties associated with PCPB *(10)*. PCBP is portable and rapidly available, with less technological demands for initiation. However, because of the small-bore cannulae, PCPB is a temporary measure, best used to support the circulation until a definitive anatomic repair can be performed or a more permanent circulatory support system (VAD) can be implanted. PCBP is most useful in patients with CS who have not progressed to CA.

CONCLUSION

PCPB is best used in patients with cardiogenic shock (before cardiac arrest occurs) who have anatomically correctable lesions amenable to surgical intervention. Patients with unwitnessed arrest and those with greater than 30 minutes of CPR prior to PCBP are unlikely to survive despite aggressive management of their underlying disease.

PCBP is a temporary measure designed to support the circulation until definitive diagnosis and treatment can be accomplished. In particular, cardiac deterioration as a result of CAD, ventricular rupture, ventricular septal defect, aortic stenosis, and PE has been successfully treated with PCPB. In these patients who were previously considered to have near 100% mortality, rapid initiation of PCPB, and definitive surgical correction may provide up to 35% survival to hospital discharge.

Much of the work on this technique was done in the late 1980s and early 1990s. Today, as hospital budgets get ever more trimmed it the maintenance of teams for PCPB represent a very large outlay of personnel. Technology will be ever improving for CPB and, with smaller machines, better anticoagulation and improved systems, it may be possible for survival statistics to improve further.

REFERENCES

1. Phillips SJ, Ballentine B, Slonine D, et al. Percutaneous initiation of cardiopulmonary bypass. Ann Thorac Surg 1983; 36:223–225.
2. Kurusz M, Zwischenberger. Percutaneous cardiopulmonary bypass for cardiac emergencies. Perfusion 2002; 17:269–277.
3. JG, Bruhn PS, Cohen SE et al. Emergent applications of cardiopulmonary support: A multiinstitutional experience. Ann Thorac Surg 1992; 54:699–704.
4. Willms DC, Atkins PJ, Dembitsky WP, et al. Analysis of clinical trends in a program of emergent ECLS for cardiovascular collapse. ASAIO J 1997; 43:65–68.
5. Perchinsky MJ, Long WB, Hill JG, et al. Extracorporeal cardiopulmonary life support with heparin-bonded circuitry in the resuscitation of massively injured trauma patients. Am J Surg 1995; 169:488–491.
6. Cochrane JB, Tecklenburg FW, Lau YR, et al. Emergency cardiopulmonary bypass for cardiac arrest refractory to pediatric advanced life support, Pediatr Emerg Care 1999; 15:30-32.
7. Mooney MR, Arom KV, Joyce LD, et al. Emergency cardiopulmonary bypass support in patients with cardiac arrest. J Thorac Cardiovasc Surg 1991; 101:450-454.
8. Wittenmyer BL, Pomerants BJ, Duff SB, et al. Single hospital experience with emergency cardiopulmonary bypass using the portable CPS (Bard) System. J Extra-Corpor Technol 1997; 29:73–77.
9. Mitsui N, Koyama T, Marui A, et al. Experience with emergency cardiac surgery following institution of percutaneous cardiopulmonary support. Artif Organs 1999; 23:496–499.
10. Von Segesser. Cardiopulmonary support and extracorporeal membrane oxygenation for cardiac assist. Ann Thorac Surg 1999; 68:672–677.

17 Principles of Drug Delivery During CPR

Edgar R. Gonzalez, PharmD, FASHP,
Joseph A. Grillo, PharmD,
Lih-Jen Wang, MS, PharmD, BCPS,
and Jeffrey Rosenblatt, PharmD

CONTENTS

INTRODUCTION
PHARMACOKINETIC CONSIDERATIONS IN CARDIAC ARREST
BIOAVAILABILITY AND BINDING TO THE SITE OF ACTION
ALTERATIONS IN BIOTRANSFORMATION DURING CPR
PHYSIOLOGICAL APPROACH TO OPTIMAL DRUG DELIVERY DURING CPR
SUMMARY
REFERENCES

INTRODUCTION

The time from onset of cardiopulmonary arrest until restoration of an effective, spontaneous circulation is the single most important determinant of long-term, neurologically intact survival from cardiopulmonary arrest. Prompt defibrillation of ventricular fibrillation (VF) or pulseless ventricular tachycardia (VT), when either rhythm is present, is more likely to alter patient outcome than is immediate pharmacological management *(1)*. However, treatment with pharmacological agents is frequently required in patients with VF or VT that is refractory to electrical countershocks, and in patients with asystole or pulseless electrical activity (PEA).

Because patients who require drug therapy during cardiopulmonary rsuscitation (CPR) often have a poor clinical outcome, there is some skepticism regarding the value of drug therapy during CPR *(2,3)*. The limited success observed following drug therapy during CPR may result from interventions that are administered too late or that are administered under suboptimal conditions *(4)*. The use of pharmacological agents during resuscitation must frequently proceed without adequate knowledge of the patient's history, preexisting conditions, or current medications. The interval prior to initiation of resuscitative efforts may be highly variable or may not be known with precision. Problems with vascular

From: *Contemporary Cardiology: Cardiopulmonary Resuscitation*
Edited by: J. P. Ornato and M. A. Peberdy © Humana Press Inc., Totowa, NJ

access may delay initial drug administration, and the delivery of drugs to their target end organs may be compromised by the poor blood flow generated during closed-chest compression.

The biological actions of drugs given during resuscitation may be altered by acidosis, hypoxemia, down-regulation of receptors, target end-organ damage, impaired metabolism and excretion, and drug interactions. We know that the pharmacokinetic properties and the pharmacodynamic response of drugs may be altered by the presence of hypoperfusion, hypoxia, and acidosis during cardiac arrest (CA). Although we lack concrete information describing the pharmacokinetic and pharmacodynamic profile of drugs in this setting, information obtained from animal models and clinical studies in the area of CPR has increased our understanding of the delivery and absorption of medications during CPR. Today, the theory that *corpora non agunt nisi fixata* (substances only act when they are linked to their site of action) is essential in understanding why drugs may fail to produce their desired effect during CPR and advanced cardiac life support (ACLS). This chapter discusses the link between the administration of a drug and its subsequent pharmacokinetics and pharmacodynamics during CPR.

PHARMACOKINETIC CONSIDERATIONS IN CARDIAC ARREST

After the administration of a drug, its efficacy and safety are maintained by selective interaction with the pharmacological site of action coupled with the body's normal detoxification and excretion processes to eliminate unwanted drug and its metabolites. These dose-related events define the drug's therapeutic index and recommended dosage regimen. Apart from coupling of the drug to its endogenous pharmacological receptor, the absorption, distribution, and elimination of the drug usually occur through passive diffusion. These processes are partly dependent of the molecular species of the drug, cardiac output, hepatic enzymatic activity, and glomerular filtration and secretion; and may be described by mathematical construct (i.e., pharmacokinetics) that define the agent's concentration–response curves.

The relationship between a drug and the body is described by its pharmacodynamic response (i.e., the drug's effects on the body) and its pharmacokinetic properties (i.e., the relationship between the amount of drug administered and its resultant plasma concentration over time [5]). Pharmacokinetics uses mathematical models and equations to describe the rate processing of drugs (rate of absorption, rate of distribution from the plasma compartment to tissues, rate of metabolism, and rate of excretion) by the body. In clinical practice, the pharmacokinetic parameters of ACLS drugs can be described by first-order (i.e., linear), two-compartment, pharmacokinetic models (5). Drugs enter the bloodstream directly after intravenous administration, and distribute between the central compartment (i.e., blood and highly perfused tissue) and the peripheral compartment (e.g., fat and other tissue). As plasma drug concentrations increase, the rate of drug elimination increases. Therefore, mathematical models and equations can be used to calculate "pharmacokinetic parameters," which represent the average values for the rates of absorption, distribution, metabolism, and elimination of a drug in a given sample population (i.e., normal volunteers). These estimates are used by the clinician to predict the serum drug concentration after a given dose.

However, pharmacokinetics parameters derived from "healthy volunteers" may not accurately predict the disposition of drugs during CPR (6). The absence of spontaneous circulation and subsequently a dramatic fall in myocardial and cerebral blood flow occurs during sudden cardiac death. Studies in swines show that during closed-chest CPR, myocardial blood flow is less than 5 mL per minute per 100 g (normal value = 40–100 mL per minute per 100 g *[7,8]*). Circulatory collapse causes redistribution of blood to highly perfused organs (brain and myocardium), and alters the volume of distribution *(9)*. Because of the reduced blood flow and increased circulation time, the method of drug administration also affects pharmacokinetic and pharmacodynamic profiles during CPR *(6,10)*.

BIOAVAILABILITY AND BINDING TO THE SITE OF ACTION

Bioavailability defines the fraction of the administered dose that reaches the systemic circulation. During CPR, drugs must have rapid and complete bioavailability to promptly reach their sites of action. The route of drug administration greatly influences a drug's bioavailability. In theory, an intravenously administered drug should have 100% bioavailability, whereas other routes of administration (e.g., oral, intramuscular, or endotracheal) may alter absorption of drugs and produce incomplete bioavailability. Therefore, during CPR, drugs should be given by intravenous bolus injection, to ensure the highest concentration of drug in the bloodstream. Once drugs reach the bloodstream, numerous issues affect the amount and rate of binding to the sites of action.

Lipid Solubility and Volume of Distribution

First, the lipid solubility, volume of distribution, and the size of the drug's molecular structure affect the ability of drug to diffuse passively across cell membranes to reach the intracellular site of action. Although cell membranes have a semi-permeable, phospholipid layer, drugs with high lipid solubility have an increased likelihood of penetrating into the site of action. However, drugs with increased lipid solubility and low plasma protein bindings may not reach the site of action in sufficient quantities because of a large volume of distribution throughout the body. Volume of distribution is a pharmacokinetic parameter that describes the proportionality of the amount of drug found in the plasma to the total amount of drug that enters the systemic circulation. If the volume of distribution of a given drug is 500 L, then a dose 500 mg will produce in a concentration of 1 mg per liter of blood. The 500 L exceeds the total volume of body water (i.e., 42 L); therefore, the drug distributes extensively into tissue as well as body fluids. Drugs with large volumes of distribution (e.g., digoxin, amiodarone) usually distribute into many tissue compartments.

The tissue compartment of the target organ greatly impacts the dosing regimen of a given agent. For example, lidocaine follows a two-compartment pharmacokinetic model with the heart (i.e., the site of action) located in the initial compartment *(11–13)*. Population estimates for lidocaine's distribution half-life (i.e., 8–10 minutes) suggest that in a normal patient, half the concentration of drug in the initial body compartment will redistribute to other tissues within 8 to 10 minutes after a given dose of lidocaine *(11)*. When lidocaine is administered during CPR, a second dose should be given no later than 8 minutes after the first dose to account for redistribution of drug away from the target organ to other areas.

Theoretically, if a drug is to redistribute to other tissues the rate and extent of this phenomena will depend on organ perfusion. Although organ perfusion is primarily dependent on arterial pressure, theoretically, left ventricular dysfunction or vasodilatation would limit organ perfusion and reduce the effective volume of distribution of a given drug.

Chandra et al. documented that within 1 minute after the onset of CA, perfusion to vital organs is reduced to approx 25 to 50% of pre-arrest values (12). Severe hypoperfusion explains the decrease in the volume of distribution of lidocaine into the initial compartment (0.69 ± 0.38 L/kg vs 0.06 ± 0.07 L/kg) and the tissue compartment (1.67 ± 0.49 L/kg vs 0.14 ± 0.06 L/kg) during CPR in dogs (12).

McDonald measured serum lidocaine concentrations in the peripheral blood following an intravenous dose of 1.9 mg/kg in patients undergoing CPR. The results showed that serum lidocaine concentrations within the range of 1.6–4.0 mg/L (mean value = 2.3 mg/L) could be achieved approx 23 minutes after administration (14). McDonald concluded that the clearance of lidocaine from the initial compartment was reduced during CPR in humans. McDonald suggested that a second dose of lidocaine would likely not be necessary during CPR unless spontaneous circulation was re-established (14).

Epinephrine is the classic example of a small polar molecule that rapidly equilibrates in the bloodstream where it binds to albumin (i.e., small volume of distribution) until it readily attaches to adrenergic receptors inside cell membranes. Epinephrine's small volume of distribution and wide therapeutic index, explain why weight dependent dosage adjustments are not needed during CPR. In contrast, amiodarone is a large nonpolar molecule that slowly equilibrates in the bloodstream. It is minimally protein bound and distributes widely throughout the body (large volume of distribution) until it reaches the site of action, and then redistributes away from it site of action back into peripheral organs (e.g., liver, eyes, lungs, thyroid, skin [15]). During CA, it is important to dose amiodarone on a weight-dependent basis (i.e., 5 mg/kg/dose) to sustain adequate concentrations in the myocardium during CPR. Furthermore, amiodarone's lipid solubility explains its redistribution properties and the need to administer a constant infusion to sustain adequate serum drug concentrations at the site of action.

Changes in plasma protein binding can also alter volume of distribution. Although drugs bind to blood cells and plasma proteins within the circulation, only the unbound drug can cross cell membranes to exert it's pharmacodynamic effects or undergo biotransformation. Reduced plasma protein binding via displacement or alterations in binding proteins increase the free fraction of drug and enlarge the drug's volume of distribution. Although the effect of altered plasma protein binding on the volume of distribution of lidocaine during CA has not yet been studied, patients with acute coronary syndromes have increased binding of lidocaine to plasma proteins and a subsequent reduction in volume of distribution (16,17). These changes are caused by a rise in α-1-acid glycoprotein, the primary binding protein for lidocaine. Theoretically, the total plasma lidocaine concentration may be disproportionately elevate during CA, but the concentration of free (active) lidocaine may be disproportionally low due enhanced α-1-acid glycoprotein binding. Therefore, CA patients may require plasma lidocaine concentrations in the upper range of normal to achieve a therapeutic effect.

Central vs Peripheral Intravenous Drug Administration

A second factor that affects the ability of drugs to reach sites of action during CPR is administration via central venous access or peripheral venous access. Kuhn and coworkers studied circulation time during closed-chest cardiac compression using indocyanine green injected in either the right antecubital vein or right subclavian vein during CPR in six patients (18). Blood samples were obtained via right femoral artery catheters at 30-second intervals for 5 minutes following injection. Arterial blood indocyanine green concentrations after central venous injection revealed a high concentration of the dye at 30 seconds and an emerging second peak at 5 minutes *(18)*. After peripheral injection, peak dye concentrations were not achieved during the 5-minute sampling period. The authors concluded that recovery of indocyanine green from femoral arterial blood was significantly greater after it is administered centrally vs peripherally *(18)*.

Talit and colleagues compared the pharmacokinetics of radioisotopes administered via peripheral vs central venous access during resuscitation in nine mongrel dogs *(19)*. Bolus injection of two different radioisotopes were given simultaneously through a peripheral vein and a central vein. Isotope activity was sampled through a catheter in the femoral artery at 5-second intervals for the first 90 seconds and at 30-second intervals for the remaining 210 seconds. The most prominent difference between central venous and peripheral venous injection was the difference in peak concentration of radioactive tracer. Central venous injection produced a 270% higher peak concentration ($p < 0.001$) and a significantly shorter time to peak concentration ($13 + 5$ vs $27 + 12$ seconds, $p < 0.01$ *[19]*). Because of the additional venous blood admixture for peripheral drug injection, this route of administration prolonged the time to peak concentration and significantly enlarged ($p < 0.01$) the central compartment volume of distribution of the radioisotope *(19)*. Venous admixing also explains differences in peak concentrations produced by the two methods of intravenous administration. Although the method of intravenous administration does not alter the absolute bioavailability, there were no significant differences in area under the concentration time curve, steady state volume of distribution, and total body clearance. These data show that route of administration would influence peak concentrations and time to peak concentration, but not the amount of drug ultimately available at the site of action during CPR.

Talit and colleagues' *(19)* work was confirmed by Keats *(20)* and Barsan *(21)* who used animal models of CA to demonstrate that time to peak drug concentrations, peak drug concentrations, and time to onset of biological effects for epinephrine and lidocaine were greater after central venous administration compared to peripheral venous administration. Although survival rates drop 10% for every minute that elapses between the onset of CPR and successful defibrillation, the benefits of central venous drug administration during CPR are obvious because central venous drug administration shortens the lag time to peak drug concentrations.

Reductions in total blood flow and prolonged circulatory time decrease venous return and slow the distribution of medications from the peripheral circulation into the central circulation. During CPR, central venous administration produces rapid delivery of drug to the site of action when compared with peripheral drug administration *(10,19–24)*.

Dilution of Bolus Injection

The volume of fluid used to dilute and administer the intravenous bolus dose is a third factor affecting the rate and amount of drug delivered to the central compartment during CPR. Emerman and colleagues studied the effect of a 20-mL saline bolus flush on peak indocyanine green dye peak concentration and circulation time in a canine CA model *(25)*. Circulation time and peak dye concentration were significantly improved by the administration of a 20-mL flush following peripheral injection in this animal model. In summary, when drugs are administered from a peripheral intravenous site during CPR, the extremity should be elevated and a 20-mL bolus of normal saline should be given to facilitate access of the agent to the central circulation *(25)*.

Endotracheal Drug Administration

Atropine, epinephrine, lidocaine, naloxone, and vasopressin may be administered via endotracheal route when intravenous access has not been established. However, the rate and extent of absorption of drugs following endotracheal administration offers another example of unresolved pharmacokinetic variability during CPR. Although, lidocaine, epinephrine, and atropine are agents that are administered routinely via the endotracheal route, only a few clinical studies have described the pharmacokinetic profile of drugs administered in this manner during CPR *(26–31)*. Endotracheal administration produces a lower and slightly delayed peak plasma concentration, and the onset of action may be delayed, but the magnitude of response is similar *(28–31)*. Differences in bioavailability between intravenous drug administration and endotracheal drug administration are explained by: (a) incomplete absorption of aerosolized drug, (b) metabolism of drug by lung parenchymal cells (i.e., epinephrine), and (c) poor pulmonary blood flow *(32)*.

Administration technique and dilution volume are important to assure good bioavailability following endotracheal drug administration *(33–36)*. Ralston and coworkers observed that the use of a catheter to deliver drug via an endotracheal airway enhanced the response to epinephrine *(33)*. When epinephrine (0.2 mg/kg) was administered via an endotracheal airway without a catheter, the drug did not increase blood pressure during CPR. When epinephrine (0.1 mg/kg) was administered via an endotracheal airway, with the aid of a catheter wedged deep into the bronchial tree, there was a significant increase in blood pressure *(33)*.

Mace confirmed the value of endotracheal drug delivery and documented the importance of doubling the dose of drug and the need to use a 10–20 mL volume of dilution for achieving the highest serum drug concentrations following endotracheal drug administration during CPR *(33,34)*. Drug dilution is important in the delivery of drugs via an endotracheal airway, but the question of whether sterile water (SW) or normal saline (NS) should be the preferred remains unanswered. Greenberg and coworkers compared the effects of endotracheally administered SW vs NS on arterial blood gases in dogs *(35)*. Endotracheal administration of SW significantly ($p < 0.05$) depressed arterial pH and PaO2 when compared with NS. Greenberg concluded that endotracheal administration of NS produces fewer detrimental effects on arterial blood gases when compared with endotracheal administration of SW *(35)*. However, these results were questioned by the evidence produced by Hahnel, who compared the effects of SW vs NS in 12 patients who received lidocaine via the endotracheal route *(36)*. Serum lidocaine concentrations at 5 and 10 minutes postdose were significantly higher ($p < 0.05$) in the SW group (2.35 and 2.67 mg/L) when compared with the NS group (1.59 and 1.88 mg/L). The PaO_2 dropped by 60 mmHg in the NS group and by 40 mmHg in the SW group ($p < 0.05$). Hahnel concluded that SW produced better absorption of lidocaine and less impairment of oxygenation than NS *(36)*.

In summary, the dose of drug to be administered via an endotracheal tube should be 2.5 times the recommended intravenous dose. The exception is vasopressin. This drug should be given as a 40-unit endotracheal dose (i.e., the same as the intravenous dose *[37]*). The endotracheal dose should be diluted in 10-mL to 20-mL of NS or SW and injected via a catheter that extends beyond the level of the carina. Cardiac compressions should be halted temporarily and the dose of drug should be followed by five rapid insufflations to disperse the drug throughout the pulmonary mucosa.

ALTERATIONS IN BIOTRANSFORMATION DURING CPR

Biotransformation of drugs used during CPR occurs via the liver for all drugs except epinephrine. Epinephrine is metabolized by the catechol-*o*-methyltransferase and monoamine oxidase enzymes present in the circulation and the mucosa of the lungs and the gut. Hepatic biotransformation depends the drug's intrinsic clearance rate, the fraction of unbound drug in the blood, and the rate of blood flow to the liver *(38)*. For lidocaine, the rate-limiting step in biotransformation is the rate of blood flow to the liver *(5)*. Therefore, circulatory collapse, reduces the biotransformation of lidocaine. Studies show that during CA, hepatic blood flow markedly reduced *(39)*. Chow and colleagues demonstrated that the clearance of lidocaine is reduced 10-fold during closed-chest CPR in dogs *(40)*. A series of case reports in humans show that the elimination half-life of lidocaine increased threefold to 6 hours during CA *(40)*. This observations does not affect the bolus dose of lidocaine (i.e., 1.5–3.0 mg/kg) because drug clearance does affect loading dose, but it does suggest that the maintenance dose of lidocaine should be decreased by 50–75% because of circulatory shock *(41–44)*. Furthermore, if lidocaine is used in the postresuscitation period, serum drug concentrations should be monitored to reduce the risk of lidocaine toxicity, especially in patients over 70 years of age *(41,44–45)*. In patients with renal failure, there is no need to adjust the dose of lidocaine because its clearance and volume of distribution are unchanged. However, renal failure leads to the accumulation of MEGX and GX, lidocaine's metabolites, which have little pharmacologic activity but can produce significant neurotoxicity *(42)*.

PHYSIOLOGICAL APPROACH TO OPTIMAL DRUG DELIVERY DURING CPR

As stated earlier, compartmental pharmacokinetic analysis is commonly used to describe how drugs are distributed in and eliminated from the body. This approach does not provide any information about the relationship of these kinetic compartments and rate constants to anatomic structures or physiological function; it assumes instantaneous distribution in each compartment. Compartmental analysis, typically, uses first-order differential equations or polyexponential equations containing distribution and elimination rate constants to describe the pharmacokinetic behavior of a drug. CA is a complex physiological state resulting from a hemodynamic collapse further complicated by augmentation of blood flow via chest compression and vasoactive pharmacotherapy. The assumption of instantaneous compartmental distribution may not be valid in this setting. This limits the usefulness of compartmental pharmacokinetic modeling in the CA setting.

Recently, physiologically based pharmacokinetic modeling (PBPK) has been studied as alternative approach to compartmental pharmacokinetic modeling in the CA patient *(46)*. This approach uses sets of nonlinear differential equations to provide a description of the time course of drug concentrations in any organ tissue and describes drug movement in the body based on organ blood flows and organ penetration *(47–50)*. Changes in hemodynamics or blood–tissue partitioning will thus affect the disposition kinetics of the drug under study *(47–52)*. Physiological parameters used in the model can be obtained from invasive animal studies and scaled to humans *(47–52)*.

Grillo et al. designed a flow-dependent PBPK model representing nine body tissues for lidocaine (*see* Fig. 1 *[46]*). Physiological organ flow rates, tissue volumes, and plasma–tissue partition parameters for lidocaine in humans were taken from the literature. Data

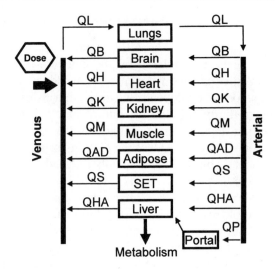

Fig. 1. PBPK model. SET, slowly equilibrating tissue (long bone, skull, spine, skin, and chest wall); Q, organ blood flow. (Used with permission from ref. *46*.)

from published animal studies were used to estimate loss of organ blood flow during CA and lidocaine tissue partition coefficients. The model assumed a 70-kg CA patient. The following five lidocaine dosing regimens were simulated: (a) 4 mg/kg IV push (IVP) (b) 1.5 mg/kg IVP then 1.5 mg/kg IVP in 4 minutes, (c) 3 mg/kg IVP, (d) 2 mg/kg IVP, and (e) 1.5 mg/kg IVP.

This PBPK model of lidocaine in CA predicted that lidocaine distribution is dramatically prolonged during resuscitation. Shunting of blood during CA results in reduced flow to muscle, adipose, and other slowly equilibrating tissues. If this model prediction is correct, relatively higher than expected lidocaine concentrations will be present in relatively well-perfused tissues (e.g., brain, heart, lungs, and so on).

A simulation of regimen 2, which at the time of the study was the current American Heart Association (AHA) recommendation, suggested that the concentration of lidocaine was suboptimal at the decision point (3–5 minutes) to administer another dose. Regimen 4 offered a slightly more rapid optimization of cardiac concentrations and more acceptable brain concentrations compared to regimens 1 through 3. The authors concluded that simulations from this PBPK model suggest that the then AHA lidocaine-dosing regimen for CA may not result in optimal lidocaine concentrations in the heart and brain. Simulations suggested that 2 mg/kg IVP may be the most acceptable lidocaine dosing regimen during CA.

Potential shortcomings of this method may involve the assumptions made and the estimates of the physiological parameters that were derived from animal studies. This is an area for future research.

SUMMARY

The ideal route of drug administration during CPR is one that combines rapid access with quick delivery of drug to the central circulation. Hemodynamic changes during CPR make central venous access the ideal route for drug delivery. The expediency required in drug administration cause peripheral venous access to be used most frequently, especially in the prehospital setting. When drugs are administered via peripheral venous access, the site of drug administration should be elevated above the level of the heart and a 20-mL bolus of NS should be administered to expedite the delivery of drug to the central compartment. If venous access cannot be readily obtained, atropine, epinephrine, lidocaine, and vasopressin may be administered via an established endotracheal airway. Except for vasopressin, which is administered at the conventional intravenous dose, the dose of drug should be increased by 2.5 times the recommended intravenous dose. The drug should be diluted to 10 to 20 mL with SW or NS, and injected via catheter that extends beyond the tip of the endotracheal tube. Cardiac compressions should be held temporarily as the drug is administered and five insufflations are delivered to aerosolize drug throughout the pulmonary mucosa. Once intravenous access is achieved, the dose should be repeated via the intravenous route.

REFERENCES

1. Kaye W, Mancini ME, Rallis SF, et al. Can better basic and advanced cardiac life support improve outcome from cardiac arrest. Crit Care Med 1985; 13:916–920.
2. Gonzalez ER: Pharmacologic controversies in CPR. Ann Emerg Med 1993; 22:317–323.
3. Guidelines for Cardiopulmonary Resuscitation and Emergency Cardiac Care. JAMA 1992; 268: 2171–2302.
4. Ornato JP, Gonzalez ER, Jaffe AS. The use of cardiovascular drugs during cardiopulmonary resuscitation. In: Cardiovascular Drug Therapy. Messerli FH, ed. Philadelphia, PA: W. B. Saunders Co., 1990, pp. 121–138.
2. Comstock TJ. Pharmacotherapeutics in the emergency department. In: Drug Therapy in Emergency Medicine. Ornato JP, Gonzalez ER, eds. New York: Churchill Livingstone, 1990, pp. 23–48.
6. Pentel P, Benowitz N. Pharmacokinetic and pharmacodynamic considerations in drug therapy of cardiac emergencies. Drugs 1984; 9:273–308.
7. Brown CG, Werman HA, Davis EA, et al. Comparative effect of graded doses of epinephrine on regional brain blood flow during CPR in a swine model. Ann Emerg Med 1986; 15:1138–1144.
8. Pharmacology I. In: Textbook of Advanced Cardiac Life Support. Jaffe AS, ed. Dallas: American Heart Association, 1987; 97–114.
9. Voorhees, WD, Babbs CF, Tacker WA. Regional blood flow during cardiopulmonary resuscitation in dogs. Crit Care Med 1980; 8:134–136.
10. Doan LA: Peripheral versus central venous delivery of medications during CPR. Ann Emerg Med 1984; 13:784–786.
11. Pieper JA, Rodman JH. Lidocaine. In: Applied Pharmacokinetics: Principles of Therapeutic Drug Monitoring, 2nd edition. Evans WE, Schentag J, Jusko WJ eds. Spokane: Applied Therapeutics Inc., 1986, pp. 639–681.
12. Chandra NC, Beyar R, Halperin HR, et al. Vital organ perfusion during assisted circulation by manipulation of intrathoracic pressure. Circulation 1991; 28:279–286.
13. Chow MSS, Ronfeld RA, Hamilton RA, et al. Effect of external cardiopulmonary resuscitation on lidocaine pharmacokinetics in dogs. J Pharmacol Exp Ther 1983; 224:531–537.
14. McDonald JL. Serum lidocaine levels during cardiopulmonary resuscitation after intravenous and endotracheal administration. Critical Care Med 1985; 13:914–915.
15. Gonzalez ER, Kannewurf BS, Ornato JP. Intravenous amiodarone for ventricular arrhythmias: overview and clinical use. Resuscitation 1998; 39:34–42.
16. Routledge PA, Shand DG, Barchowsky A, et al. Relationship between alpha 1-acid glycoprotein and lidocaine disposition in myocardial infarction. Clin Pharmacol Ther 1981;30:154–157.
17. Johansson BG, Kindmark CO, Trell EY, et al. Sequential changes of plasma proteins after myocardial infarction. Scand J Clin Lab Invest 1972;29:117–129.
18. Kuhn GJ, White BC, Swetman RE, et al. Peripheral versus central circulation time during CPR. A pilot study. Ann Emerg Med 1981;10:417–419.
19. Talit U, Braun S, Halkin H, et al. Pharmacokinetic differences between peripheral and central drug administration during cardiopulmonary resuscitation. J Am Coll Cardiol 1985;6:1073–1077.

20. Keats S, Jackson RE, Kosnik JW, et al. Effect of peripheral versus central injection of epinephrine on changes in aortic diastolic blood pressure during closed-chest massage in dogs. Ann Emerg Med 1985; 14:495 (Abstract).
21. Barsan WG, Levy RC, Weir H. Lidocaine levels during CPR. Ann Emerg Med 1981; 10:73–78.
22. Kuhn GJ, White BC, Swetman RE, et al. Peripheral versus central circulation time during CPR. A pilot study. Ann Emerg Med 1981; 10:417–419.
23. Hedges JR, Barsan WG, Doan LA, et al. Central versus peripheral intravenous routes in cardiopulmonary resuscitation. Am J Emerg Med 1984; 2:385–390.
24. Redding JS, Pearson JW. Effective routes of drug administration during cardiac arrest. Anesth Analg 1967; 46:253–258.
25. Emerman CL, Pinchak AC, Hancock D, Hagen JF. The effect of bolus injection on circulation times during cardiac arrest. Am J Emerg Med 1990; 8:190–193.
26. Hasegawa EA. The endotracheal administration of drugs. Heart Lung 1986; 15:60–63.
27. Redding JS, Asuncion JS, Pearson JW. Effective routes of drug administration during cardiac arrest. Anesth Analg 1967; 46:253–258.
28. Roberts JR, Greenberg MI, Knaub M, Baskin SI. Comparison of the pharmacological effects of epinephrine administered by intravenous and endotracheal routes. JACEP 1978; 7:260–264.
29. Roberts JR, Greenberg MI, Knaub MA, Kendrick ZV, Baskin SI. Blood levels following intravenous and endotracheal epinephrine administration. JACEP 1979; 8:53–56.
30. Scott B, Martin FG, Matchett J, Whites S. Canine cardiovascular responses to endotracheally and intravenously administered atropine, isoproterenol and propranolol. Ann Emerg Med 1987; 16:1–10.
31. Rubertsson S, Wiklund L. Hemodynamic effects of epinephrine in combination with different buffers during experimental, open chest, cardiopulmonary resuscitation. Crit Care Med 1983; 21: 1051–1057.
32. Ralston SH, Tacker WA, Showen L, et al. Endotracheal versus intravenous epinephrine during electromechanical dissociation with CPR in dogs. Ann Emerg Med. 1985; 14:1044–1048.
33. Mace SE. Effect of technique of administration on plasma lidocaine levels. Ann Emerg Med 1986; 15:552–556.
34. Mace SE. The effect of dilution on plasma lidocaine levels with endotracheal admininstration. Ann Emerg Med 1987; 16:522–526.
35. Greenberg MI, Baskin SI, Kaplan AM, et al. Effects of endotracheally administered distilled water or normal saline on the arterial blood gases in dogs. Ann Emerg Med 1982; 11:600–604.
36. Hahnel JH, Linder KH, Schurmann C, et al. Plasma lidocaine levels and PaO2 with endotracheal administration. Dilution with normal saline or distilled water. Ann Emerg Med 1990; 19:1314–1317.
37. Linder KH, Prengel AW, Brinkman A, et al. Vasopressin administration in refractory cardiac arrest. Ann Intern Med 1996; 124:1061–1064.
38. Wilkinson GR. Influence of Hepatic disease on pharmacokinetics. In: Applied Pharmacokinetics: Principles of Therapeutic Drug Monitoring, 2nd edition. Evans WE, Schentag JJ, Jusko WJ, eds. Applied Therapeutics Inc, Spokane, 1986, pp. 116–138.
39. Tabrizchi R, Lim SL, Pang CY. Possible equilibration of portal venous and central venous pressures during circulatory arrest. Am J Physiol 1993; 264:H259–H261.
40. Chow MSS, Ronfeld RA, Ruffett D, et al. Lidocaine pharmacokinetics during cardiac arrest and external cardiopulmonary resuscitation. Am Heart J 1981; 102:799–801.
41. Benowitz NL. Clinical applications of the pharmacokinetics of lidocaine. In: Cardiovascular Drug Therapy. Melmon KL, ed. Philadelphia, PA: FA Davis Co., 1976, pp. 77–101.
42. Thomson PD, Melmon KL, Richardson JA, et al. Lidocaine pharmacokinetics in advanced heart failure, liver disease, and renal failure in humans. Ann Intern Med 1973; 78:499–508.
43. Thomson PD, Rowland M, Melmon KL. The influence of heart failure, liver disease and renal failure on the disposition of lidocaine in man. Am Heart J 1971; 82:417–421.
44. Davison R, Parker M, Atkinson AJ. Excessive serum lidocaine levels during maintenance infusions: Mechanisms and prevention. Am Heart J 1982; 104:203–208.
45. Pfeifer HJ, Greenblat, DJ, Koch-Weser J. Clinical use and toxicity of intravenous lidocaine: a report from the Boston Collaborative Drug Surveillance Program. Am Heart J 1976; 92:168–173.
46. Grillo JA, Venitz J, Ornato JP. Prediction of lidocaine tissue concentrations following different dosing regimens during cardiac arrest using a physiologically based pharmacokinetic model. Resuscitation 2001; 50:331–340.
47. Leung HW. Development and utilization of physiologically based pharmacokinetic models for toxicological applications. J Toxicol Environ Health 1991; 32:247–267.

48. Gerlowski LE, Jain RK. Physiologically based pharmacokinetic modeling: principles and applications. J Pharm Sci 1983; 72:1103–27.
49. Ings RMJ. Interspecies scaling and comparisons in drug development and toxicokinetics. Xenobiotica 1990; 20:1201–1231.
50. Gibaldi M, Perrier D. Physiologic pharmacokinetic models. In: Pharmacokinetics, 2nd edition. Gibaldi M, Perrier D, eds. Drugs and the Pharmaceutical Sciences, volume 15. New York: Marcel Dekker, 1982, pp. 355–384.
51. Colburn WA. Physiologic pharmacokinetic modeling. J Clin Pharmacol 1988; 28:673–677.
52. Benowitz N, Forsyth RP, Melman KL, et al. Lidocaine Disposition in monkey and man: Prediction by a perfusion model. Clin Pharm Ther 1974; 16:87–98.

18 Pharmacological Resuscitation Interventions

Wanchun Tang, MD, FCCP, FCCM,
Shijie Sun, MD, FCCM,
and Max Harry Weil, MD, PhD, MACP, FACC,
MasterFCCP, FCCM

CONTENTS

INTRODUCTION

The primary goal of cardiopulmonary resuscitation (CPR) is to restore spontaneous circulation and manage postresuscitation myocardial dysfunction, including myocardial contractile failure and life-threatening ventricular ectopic dysrhythmias. During CPR, blood flow is determined primarily by two issues: the pump (driving force) and the peripheral vascular resistance. The mechanical interventions are intended to generate maximal cardiac output and perfusion pressure. A second issue is that of vascular tone. Accumulation of metabolic vasodilator substances, including adenosine, carbon dioxide, lactic acid, and hydrogen ions, and diminished neurovascular vasoconstriction decrease peripheral arterial resistance by causing (or allowing) arterial vasodilation. Additionally, there are variable increases in venous capacitance such that venous return to the right atrium is reduced. This has been the basis for the use of vasopressor agents, especially α-adrenergic agents. Quite distinct, however, is immediate postresuscitation management, which has as a primary goal the mitigation of postresuscitation myocardial failure. Pharmacological interventions are designed to improve myocardial systolic function by increasing stroke volume, reducing ventricular filling pressures, and controlling arrhythmias.

From: *Contemporary Cardiology: Cardiopulmonary Resuscitation*
Edited by: J. P. Ornato and M. A. Peberdy © Humana Press Inc., Totowa, NJ

Pharmacological interventions during and immediately following CPR are restrained by impaired perfusion (e.g., delivery of drugs or their metabolites to target sites is impaired) and changes in the pharmacological actions of the drugs as a result of acidosis, hypercarbia, hypoxemia, down-regulation of receptors, and altered organ functions. There is also altered drug metabolism during and following CPR. In clinical settings, the history of underlying diseases and concurrent drug treatment may not be known, thereby further thwarting the precision of pharmacological interventions.

ROUTES OF DRUG ADMINISTRATION

Most drugs are given by intravenous injection to ensure complete distribution as well as rapid pharmacological action. Alternative routes (i.e., endotracheal) are usually less predictable with respect to absorption, distribution, and pharmacologic response and their use is limited to settings in which an intravenous line cannot be established.

Intravenous

The peripheral venous route has the advantage of minimal invasiveness, technical ease, and ready physical access. However, peak blood drug concentrations and their pharmacological actions are more predictable when given by central venous injection or infusion. In a dog model of CPR, the circulation time of a dye tracer was 63 seconds after central, compared to 94 seconds after peripheral, venous injection. The peak dye concentration after central venous injection is correspondingly greater *(1)*. Central venous access may be facilitated through the femoral vein. However, the internal jugular vein and subclavian vein are appropriate alternatives but are strategically less accessible during CPR (especially during chest compression and airway manipulation). Local complications of venous cannulation include hematoma, cellulitis, thrombosis, and phlebitis. Systemic complications, including sepsis and pulmonary thromboembolism, are likely to be of little import in the CPR setting. Air embolism is best avoided with jugular or subclavian cannulation by maintaining the patient in a 10% head-down position.

Endotracheal

When an endotracheal tube is in place, drugs can be administered without the typical several minute delay to start an intravenous line. In such settings, endotracheal administration has advantages, particularly in children or in obese and/or drug abuse cardiac arrest (CA) victims in whom venous access may be difficult.

The pulmonary circulation receives the entire cardiac output and the lungs provide approx 70 square meters of capillary surface for drug absorption. A significantly prolonged pressor effect the so-called "depot-like" effect, persists for up to 30 minutes following endotracheal epinephrine administration. After intravenous injection, epinephrine's pressor effects persist for only 3 to 5 minutes. Only a single dose of epinephrine should be administered by the endotracheal route because tachycardia, hypertension, dysrhythmias, and a reduced fibrillation threshold can follow successful resuscitation as a result of its persistent effects when given by this route.

No drug other than epinephrine is approved in the United States currently for endotracheal administration during CPR. A dose of 3 mg should be diluted in 10 mL of either normal saline or sterile water. Injection is best followed by two or three forceful lung inflations. Additionally, atropine and potentially, lidocaine can be administered through the tracheal tube as well, in doses that are twice that recommended intravenously. Only

Table 1
Adrenergic Receptor

Receptors	Tissue	Responses
α_1	Myocardium	• Inotropic and chronotropic effects • Oxygen utilization
	Smooth muscles	• Contraction
α_2	Vascular smooth muscles	• Contraction
β_1	Myocardium	• Inotropic and chronotropic effects • Oxygen Utilization
β_2	Myocardium	• Inotropic and chronotropic effects • Oxygen Utilization
	Smooth muscles	• Relaxation

a minor and transient decrease in arterial PaO_2 and increased arterial $PaCO_2$ follow intratracheal injection of these drugs.

VASOPRESSOR AGENTS

Adrenergic Agents

MECHANISMS OF ADRENERGIC AGENTS

The primary effect of adrenergic agonists is to activate adrenergic receptors. In 1948, Ahlquist first hypothesized that catecholamines acted through two principal receptors (α- and β-receptors [2]). This hypothesis proved to be both correct and led to the development of selective α - and β-agonists and their corresponding antagonists. In the years that followed, subgroups of both α - and β-receptors were identified (Table 1).

α-Adrenergic receptors were subsequently classified into two subgroups. The α_1-receptors (presynaptic α-receptors) were identified in the heart, vascular, and intestinal smooth muscle and α_2-receptors (postsynaptic α-receptors) in vascular smooth muscle, pancreatic islets (β cells), and platelets. The α_1-receptors have been further subcategorized into α_{1A}-, α_{1B}-, and α_{1D}- and α_2-receptors into α_{2A}-, α_{2B}-, and α_{2C}-adrenergic receptors (3,4). Most recently, the systemic vasoconstriction effects after activation of α_2-adrenergic receptors were traced to α_{2B}-adrenergic receptors (5).

β_1-receptors were identified primarily in the heart and β_2-receptors in vascular and bronchial smooth muscle and skeletal muscle. A β_3-receptor was subsequently identified in adipose tissue (6).

Activation of α-adrenergic receptors is followed by release of intracellular Ca^{2+} from endoplasmic stores, activation of G protein-gated K^+ channel and inhibition of voltage-sensitive Ca channels. These actions account for increases in the intracellular availability of Ca^{2+}, which produce contraction of vascular smooth muscle (3,4). The number of adrenergic receptors is variable contingent on the pathophysiological condition of the organism. Global myocardial ischemia increases the number of both α_1- and β_1-adrenergic receptors at the myocyte surface. These increases in the number of adrenergic receptors account for greater arrhythmogenic effect of exogenous catecholamines during myocardial ischemia (7).

Both β_1- and β_2-agonists activate adenylate cyclase and thereby convert adenosine triphosphate (ATP) to cyclic adenosine monophosphate. This is the so-called second messenger, which activates protein kinase and voltage-sensitive calcium channels. In the heart, β-agonists induce inotropic and chronotropic effects with increases in myocardial oxygen consumption. In vascular smooth muscle, they induce relaxation and therefore reduced peripheral vascular resistance. It is not as yet clear whether β_3-receptors have cardiovascular actions (8).

EFFECTS OF ADRENERGIC AGENTS DURING CPR

The primary goal of pharmacological interventions during CPR is to increase coronary perfusion pressure by increasing peripheral vascular resistance. Optimally, an adrenergic drug would maximize arterial blood flow to the coronary and cerebral circuits by increasing arterial pressure during both compression and relaxation phases of the chest compression. In effect, there would be maximal pressor effect in the proximal aorta with reduced peripheral run-off. These benefits would be likely to accrue primarily from α-adrenergic agonists. Epinephrine, which has been the most widely used agent, however, has major β_1-effects, and to a much lesser extent, α_1-effects. Accordingly, epinephrine produces a pressor effect along with β-adrenergically induced increases in myocardial oxygen consumption. Accordingly, myocardial ischemia and postresuscitation myocardial dysfunction are increased during resuscitation. This may explain, at least in part, the disappointing outcomes after resuscitation with epinephrine (9,10).

We therefore have focused increasingly on increases in peripheral vascular resistance as the result of α_1- and α_2-mediated vasoconstriction during CPR. Theoretically, agents with predominant α-effects would be more effective. However, it is now recognized that vasoconstrictor efficacy during CPR also depends on the subtype activity of the α-receptor. During CPR, adrenergic agents with predominant α_2 effects are more effective vasoconstrictors because extrajunctional α_2-receptors are more accessible to circulating catecholamines than postjunctional α_1-receptors (11). This may explain why the predominant α_1-agonists methoxamine and phenylephrine have not replaced epinephrine as drugs of choice (12,13).

EPINEPHRINE

Epinephrine has been the preferred adrenergic agent for the treatment of human CA for more than 40 years. There is unequivocal evidence that its efficacy is as a result of its α-adrenergic vasopressor effects. Increases in ventricular fibrillation (VF) wavelet amplitude reflect α-adrenergically induced increases in coronary blood flow. Such is now known to allow for more effective defibrillation with lesser electrical power (15,16). Yet, the adverse effects of epinephrine caused by its inotropic actions, as already noted, provoke disproportionate increases in myocardial oxygen consumption. Accordingly, it increases the demand of the globally ischemic myocardium for oxygen during CA. If the heart is resuscitated, the greater ischemic injury accounts for greater postresuscitation myocardial dysfunction.

Epinephrine is a complex agent. It is a powerful agonist of α_1-, α_2-, β_1-, and β_2-adrenergic receptors and its pharmacologic effects are correspondingly complex. Its primary effects on the myocardium are the β_1- and α_1-actions that are both inotropic and chronotropic. During VF, the contractile force of the fibrillatory segments is increased and this accounts for the increases in myocardial oxygen consumption at a time when the heart is not doing any effective work *(14)*. The β-adrenergic actions also account for postresuscitation tachycardia and recurrent VF.

Epinephrine induces disproportionate increases in systolic pressure. Accordingly, the pulse pressure is increased. The effect of epinephrine on small arterioles and precapillary sphincters accounts for altered blood flow distribution to tissues and organs. Increases in cutaneous and renal vasoconstriction account for reduced blood flow to these sites. Cerebral and coronary blood flows are increased disproportionately at the expense of cutaneous and renal blood flows because neither cerebral nor coronary arterioles are constricted. High-dose epinephrine may increase pulmonary artery, pulmonary capillary, and pulmonary venous pressures. Excessive increases in pulmonary capillary filtration pressure may precipitate pulmonary edema. For the same reason, pulmonary ventilation/perfusion defects appear and these are characterized by pulmonary arteriovenous admixture with decreases in arterial oxygen tension and increases in arterial CO_2 tension with decreases in end-tidal PCO_2 *(17)*. The $β_2$-actions of epinephrine are predominantly bronchodilator. More recent studies also implicate stimulation of $β_2$-receptors in the myocardium, further increasing oxygen consumption during CPR and the severity of myocardial ischemic injury after successful resuscitation *(18)*. Although epinephrine has been recommended by the American Heart Association (AHA) as the drug of choice for CPR since 1974 and continues to be in wide use, there is as yet no confirmation that ultimate outcomes are improved, either for in-hospital or out-of-hospital CA. Understandably, a placebo-controlled clinical study is both ethically and legally problematic. Until well-designed clinical studies indicate otherwise, the authors of this chapter personally believe that the administration of epinephrine should not be routine and that it should be withheld during the initial resuscitative efforts.

The optimal dose of epinephrine for the treatment of CA was not addressed until 1974 when the Guidelines and Standards of the AHA specified a bolus injection of 0.5–1.0 mg independent of weight. In 1985, Ralston et al. *(19)* reported that higher doses of epinephrine, namely 0.01–0.1 mg/kg improved the resuscitation rate from 40 to 90%. A series of studies subsequently addressed the role of "high-dose" epinephrine. Both experimental studies and clinical reports suggested that high doses of epinephrine produced greater coronary perfusion pressure, myocardial and cerebral blood flow, and thereby improved outcomes of the initial resuscitation effort. Nevertheless, there was no proof of improved survival to hospital discharge.

These reports triggered three large randomized clinical studies to evaluate high dose epinephrine's potential benefits *(9,10,20)*. Standard and high doses of epinephrine were compared in both out-of-hospital and in-hospital CA. No statistically significant improvement was documented following high-dose epinephrine, compared to standard dose epinephrine. Most disappointing, however, was failure to confirm even benefits in terms of initial resuscitation or early neurologic outcome. Guided by these controlled human trials, current Guidelines for Advanced Cardiac Life Support call for 1 mg of intravenously injected epinephrine as an appropriate initial dose. There has also been disappointing experience with repetitive doses of epinephrine because these have but little added pressor effect *(21)*.

When epinephrine is administered during CPR the severity of myocardial ischemic injury is also caused by its $α_1$-effects. Previously, unknown was the presence of $α_1$-receptors in the myocardium which, like β-receptors, increase the myocardial inotropic state, myocardial oxygen requirements and therefore the severity of postresuscitation

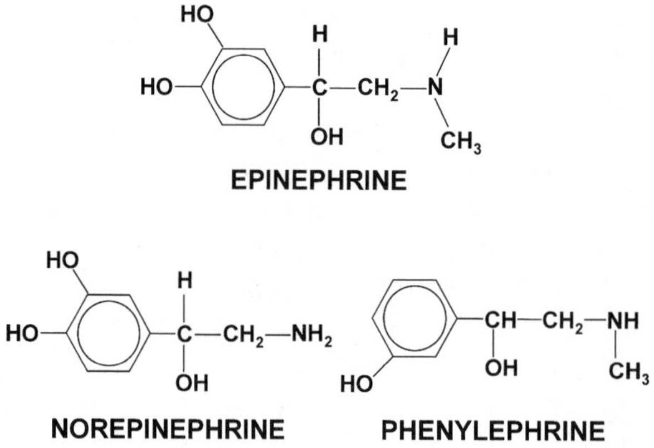

Fig. 1. Structural formulae of epinephrine, norepinephrine, and phenylephrine.

myocardial failure. Epinephrine increases myocardial lactate concentration and decreases myocardial ATP content even though coronary blood flow may be doubled (22). Epinephrine also increases the severity of postresuscitation myocardial dysfunction and decreases postresuscitation survival when compared with epinephrine combined with the β_1-blocking agent, esmolol (14). Epinephrine increased the incidence of ventricular arrhythmias, ventricular tachycardia (VT) and (recurrent) VF. These ventricular arrhythmias were significantly decreased after β-adrenergic blockade. When victims are resuscitated after a relatively short duration of CPR, a brief period of epinephrine-induced hypertension may occur, this increases afterload and further decreases cardiac output. Accordingly, the β-adrenergic actions of epinephrine increase the severity of myocardial ischemic injury and thereby the likelihood of re-entrant and ectopic ventricular dysrhythmias.

NOREPINEPHRINE

Norepinephrine is the major mediator of mammalian postganglionic adrenergic function. Its chemical structure is identical to that of epinephrine except that it lacks methyl substitution in the amino group of the phenylethylamine nucleus (Fig. 1). Between 10 and 20% of the catecholamine content of human adrenal medulla is composed of norepinephrine.

Norepinephrine is a potent α-adrenergic agonist that stimulates both α_1- and α_2-receptors. It has only minor β_2-receptor actions. Like epinephrine, norepinephrine also acts on β_1-receptors and thereby increases myocardial oxygen consumption and the risk of ischemic injury during CPR. In contrast to epinephrine, it produces greater arterial constriction than epinephrine such that total peripheral resistance is increased significantly. Both arterial systolic and diastolic pressures are increased (more the latter than the former) leading to a more narrow pulse pressure. Blood flow to skeletal muscles, liver, and kidneys is decreased disproportionately. Like epinephrine, norepinephrine produces coronary artery dilation and, together with increases in arterial blood pressure, augments coronary blood flow. The circulating blood volume is reduced after administration of norepinephrine primarily as a consequence of peripheral vascular constriction, resulting in an increased capillary hydrostatic pressure. Accordingly, there is increased filtration of protein-free fluid from the capillaries into the extravascular space. Both myocardial and cerebral blood flows are increased to a degree that is comparable to that produced by epinephrine. A major advantage may be that the inotropic and chronotropic effects are less and myocardial oxygen consumption is significantly less after norepinephrine *(23,24).* Accordingly, we would anticipate fewer myocardial dysrhythmias and recurrent VF and less postresuscitation myocardial ischemic injury.

Lindner et al. *(25)* compared the effect of equal doses of norepinephrine and epinephrine during CPR in a randomized study on 50 out-of-hospital CA victims. The initial success of resuscitation was significantly greater in the norepinephrine group. Yet, these investigators were again unable to demonstrate significant increase in neurologically intact hospital survivors. In a larger randomized study on 816 victims of out-of-hospital CA, Callaham et al. *(10)* failed to demonstrate significant differences between norepinephrine- and epinephrine-treated patients with respect to initial success of resuscitation and hospital survival. Accordingly, there are no convincing data at the time of this writing to support the routine use of norepinephrine as an alternative for epinephrine for cardiac resuscitation.

Phenylephrine

Phenylephrine is an α_1-adrenergic agonist. However, it is also a weak activator of β-adrenergic receptors. The pharmacological effects of phenylephrine are similar to those of methoxamine and, specifically, increase peripheral vascular resistance. Redding and Pearson *(26)* observed universal success with defibrillation after intracardiac administration of 10 mg phenylephrine during VF. However, no significant differences between epinephrine- or phenylephrine-treated animals were observed with respect to myocardial blood flow, myocardial oxygen delivery and consumption, the initial success of resuscitation, duration of survival, and postresuscitation neurological recovery *(27,28).*

Ditchey et al. *(29)* reinvestigated the benefits and detriments of β-adrenergic blockade. These investigators initially compared the effects of epinephrine and phenylephrine with the β-adrenergic blocking agent, propranolol, on postresuscitation myocardial ATP and lactate concentrations. They demonstrated a significantly higher myocardial ATP concentration and lower myocardial lactate concentration in animals that were resuscitated after treatment with both phenylephrine and propranolol compared to epinephrine alone. Phenylephrine with propranolol therefore improved the balance between myocardial oxygen supply and demand during CPR. After successful resuscitation from CA, our group found better systolic and diastolic myocardial function in experimental animals treated with phenylephrine together with significantly greater long-term survival. With longer durations of untreated CA, disproportionately greater myocardial contractile function and postresuscitation survival were again observed with phenylephrine *(14).* Only one randomized, double-blind study has compared the effects of epinephrine and phenylephrine on the success of clinical resuscitation. In 65 out-of-hospital CA victims no differences in the success of initial resuscitation were observed between epinephrine- and phenylephrine-treated victims *(30).*

Nonadrenergic Vasopressors

Vasopressin

The effects of vasopressin are mediated by activation of the two principal types of receptors, V_1 and V_2. The V_1-receptor has been further subclassified as V_{1a} and V_{1b}. V_{1a}-receptors are located in vascular smooth muscle, myometrium, kidney, spleen, and central nervous system. V_{1b} receptors are located only in the adenohypophysis and the V_2-receptors are predominantly located in the principal cells of the renal collecting duct system. V_1-receptors primarily mediate pressor responses and V_2-receptors primary mediate antidiuretic responses.

The cardiovascular effects of vasopressin are complex and are not defined well. Vasopressin is a potent vasoconstrictor. Vascular smooth muscle in the skin, skeletal muscle, fat, pancreas, and thyroid gland are most sensitive, with significant vasoconstriction also occurring in the gastrointestinal tract, coronary vessels, and brain. However, during spontaneous circulation, vasoconstriction is induced only after much higher concentrations of vasopressin are administered than those that produce maximal antidiuresis. During spontaneous circulation, vasopressin reduces cardiac output and heart rate. These effects are largely indirect through increases in peripheral vasoconstriction and corresponding increases in arterial pressure. A less optimal effect is coronary vasoconstriction, accounting for decreased coronary blood flow.

The effects of vasopressin as a vasopressor during CPR have been investigated extensively by Dr. Karl Lindner and his associates. Their series of studies were prompted by the observations that patients who had higher levels of endogenous vasopressin during cardiac resuscitation had better outcomes. This contrasted with endogenous levels of epinephrine and norepinephrine in which greater serum levels predicted poor outcomes (31). The effects of low (0.2 U/kg), medium (0.4 U/kg), and high (0.8 U/kg) doses of vasopressin were then compared with epinephrine (0.2 mg) on coronary perfusion pressure and myocardial blood flow during CPR in a porcine model. Medium and high doses of vasopressin produced significantly better myocardial blood flow and coronary perfusion pressure than epinephrine (32). After intravenous epinephrine and external defibrillation had failed to resuscitate eight patients, 40 U of vasopressin restored spontaneous circulation in each instance and three of the patients were discharged from the hospital with normal neurological function (33).

Unfortunately, the increases in arterial vasoconstriction produced by vasopressin also were associated with even more severe postresuscitation myocardial dysfunction than epinephrine in the early hours after restoration of spontaneous circulation (34). In pigs, postresuscitation systemic vascular resistance of the vasopressin group was twofold greater than that of the epinephrine group. This explained why there was significantly lower cardiac output and reduced myocardial contractility in the first 4 hours following successful resuscitation.

These considerations not withstanding, another study on 40 patients indicated better initial resuscitation and 24-hour survival after vasopressin compared with epinephrine. However, again no difference in survival to hospital discharge was demonstrated (35). In a just completed, large, randomized multicenter clinical study that included more than 1200 out-of-hospital cardiac arrests, Wenzel et al. (36) reported that vasopressin had no benefit on outcomes over epinephrine when used for resuscitation from VF or pulseless electrical activity. The hospital discharge rate was greater in patients who presented with asystole and who were treated with vasopressin. Yet, 40% of the patients resuscitated using vasopressin after asystole remained in coma or in vegetative states. Accordingly, the evidence that vasopressin has ultimate benefit when administered during CPR remains unconfirmed in human patients.

ANGIOTENSIN II

Angiotensin II is approx 40 times more potent than norepinephrine. Angiotensin II increases peripheral vascular resistance through its direct and indirect vasoconstrictor effects on precapillary arterioles and postcapillary venules. Vasoconstriction is induced by activation of AT_1-receptors on vascular smooth muscle cells. Angiotensin II also prompts release of endogenous catecholamines from the adrenal medulla by depolarizing chromaffin cells. When angiotensin II was injected intravenously during CPR, the already greatly increased serum concentrations of endogenous epinephrine were further increased by more than sixfold and endogenous norepinephrine by more than threefold (37).

As yet, the effectiveness of angiotensin II as a vasopressor for CPR is largely unexplored. Administration of angiotensin II to pigs doubled myocardial blood flow produced by open-chest cardiac massage (38) and during closed chest compression (39) when compared with saline placebo. At the time of this writing, however, there are no objective outcome data favoring the use of angiotensin II in settings of CPR.

ANTI-ARRHYTHMIC AGENTS

Mechanisms of Arrhythmias

When the normal sequence of cardiac impulse and propagation is disturbed, an arrhythmia occurs. Three major underlying mechanisms have been identified: enhanced automaticity, triggered automaticity, and re-entry.

Enhanced Automaticity

Enhanced automaticity usually occurs in the sinus node, AV node, and the His-Purkinje system, which normally display spontaneous diastolic depolarization. In these pacemaker systems, increases in the phase 4 slope of action potential increase pacemaker rate. Decreases in the phase 4 slope of action potential decrease pacemaker rate. Changes in automaticity may occur at sites that normally do not display spontaneous depolarization. For example, during myocardial ischemia, spontaneous depolarization of ventricular cells produces "abnormal automaticity," which is clinically manifest as ventricular arrhythmias.

TRIGGERED AUTOMATICITY

When a normal action potential is interrupted or followed by an abnormal depolarization that reaches the threshold, triggered arrhythmias occur. There are two forms of triggered arrhythmias.

1. A normal action potential is followed by a delayed after-depolarization (DAD). If this after-depolarization reaches the threshold, a triggered action potential occurs. This is usually seen under conditions of intracellular calcium overload, especially myocardial ischemia and digitalis intoxication.
2. When an action potential is significantly prolonged, its phase 3 repolarization may be interrupted by an early after-depolarization (EAD). This is commonly seen during bradycardia, after administration of anti-arrhythmic agents that prolong the action potential duration, and after depletion of extracellular potassium.

RE-ENTRY

Re-entry is the mechanism that accounts for the majority of instances of cardiac arrhythmias. When a normal impulse has traversed the ventricles, the impulse is usually terminated because ventricular muscle remains refractory to conduction. Under special conditions, however, the impulse may reenter into ventricular muscle and set up circus movement if the pathway of the initial impulse is prolonged. Both dilation and hypertrophy of the ventricle predispose to re-entry together with a decrease in the velocity of electrical conduction. In each instance, the time for the impulse to travel through the ventricles is prolonged. Conduction block through the Purkinje system, myocardial ischemia, and increases in serum potassium concentrations may be precipitating causes. Following administration of α_1- and β-adrenergic agents, and especially epinephrine, the refractory period is shortened and thereby increases the likelihood of re-entry.

Classification of Anti-Arrhythmic Agents

The classical Vaughn Williams classification of anti-arrhythmic agents *(40)* classifies the anti-arrhythmic agents into four major classes, based on the relationship between basic electrophysiological action and anti-arrhythmic effects:

Class I.   Sodium channel block: based on the rates of recovery from drug-induced block under physiological conditions; this class is further divided into three sub-classes:

   Class IA: the rate of recovery is 1–10 seconds. This subclass includes procainamide and quinidine.

   Class IB: the rate of recovery is less than 1 second. This subclass includes lidocaine and mexiletene.

   Class IC: the rate of recovery is greater than 10 seconds. This subclass includes propafenone and flecainide.

Class II.   β-Blockade: The common agents of this class include propranolol, esmolol, and sotalol.

Class III.   Action potential prolongation: Most agents produce this effect by blocking potassium channels. The common agents of this class include amiodarone, sotalol (D-L), and bretylium.

Class IV.   Calcium channel blockade: The common agents of this class include verapamil and diltiazem.

Anti-Arrhythmic Agents for CPR

In past years, during CA especially when manifested by VF or pulseless VT, anti-arrhythmic agents were routinely advised on the assumption that these agents would facilitate electrical defibrillation and minimize recurrence of VF. However, there is no secure support for such use of anti-arrhythmic drugs. Immediate defibrillation, securing the airway and breathing, and monitoring forward blood flow by chest compression have remained the principal interventions. Drugs, and most especially anti-arrhythmic drugs, have but questionable benefit *(21)*. As yet, there is also limited information but somewhat greater enthusiasm for the use of anti-arrhythmic drugs in the interval that follows successful restoration of spontaneous circulation.

LIDOCAINE

Lidocaine was developed initially as a local anesthetic. It was subsequently introduced for intravenous injection and infusion for ventricular arrhythmias. Lidocaine blocks the myocardial sodium channels, which often account for automaticity. Its effects are disproportionate in ischemic tissue *(41)*. The electrophysiological action of lidocaine is to decrease cardiac automaticity by reducing the phase-4 action potential slope and thereby the threshold for excitability. The duration of action potential is usually unaffected such that lidocaine produces no delay in conduction and therefore no significant effect on the PR or QRS duration. To the contrary, the QT duration is typically unchanged or slightly shortened.

An initial bolus of 1.0–1.5 mg/kg by intravenous injection is currently recommended for rapidly achieving therapeutic levels of lidocaine. For refractory VT/VF, an additional bolus of 0.5–0.75 mg/kg may be repeated at 5- to 10-minute intervals after the initial dose. The total recommended dose should not exceed 3 mg/kg. A continuing infusion of lidocaine in amounts of 1–4 mg per minute maintains therapeutic levels. There is no secure evidence that the administration of lidocaine, and especially its continued use after restoration of spontaneous circulation improves outcomes of CPR.

The major adverse effects of lidocaine are in the central nervous system and include seizures, tremor, dysarthria, and altered levels of consciousness in close relationship to excessive plasma levels. Nystagmus is an early sign of lidocaine toxicity.

In one prominent study in which lidocaine was administered to all patients with suspected myocardial infarction, the incidence of VF was reduced (42). However, fewer patients survived to be discharged from the hospital. A meta-analysis of eight randomized clinical studies confirmed that the in-hospital death rate was increased, probably as a result of lidocaine-exacerbated heart block or congestive heart failure (43). Lidocaine is still viewed as possibly helpful for treatment of (a) persistent VF and pulseless VT after defibrillation and epinephrine; (b) hemodynamically compromised premature ventricular beats; and (c) hemodynamically stable VT. However, current evidence would favor other anti-arrhythmic agents, and specifically amiodarone, procainamide, or sotalol (21).

BRETYLIUM

Bretylium is a quaternary ammonium compound. It prolongs cardiac action potentials and prohibits reuptake of norepinephrine by sympathetic neurons. Bretylium reduces heterogeneity of repolarization times and may therefore suppress re-entry. Although bretylium prohibits norepinephrine reuptake, it produces hypotension. Indeed, this drug was initially introduced as an antihypertensive agent. By the same mechanism, the concurrent administration of adrenergic vasopressors after administration of bretylium may induce marked hypertension.

Although bretylium has been used for the treatment of persistent VT and VF after attempted defibrillation and after administration of epinephrine, its benefits are unproven. Bretylium has been unavailable from the manufacturer since 1999, and there is no rationale for including it in the armamentarium for pharmacological management of CA (21).

AMIODARONE

Of all available agents, amiodarone remains the best single choice for management of both atrial and ventricular dysrhythmias in life-threatening settings. Amiodarone is a structural analog of thyroid hormone and has a multiplicity of pharmacological effects. Its effects on sodium and calcium channels are generally favorable. It also exerts a nonselective adrenergic blocking effect. Electropharmacological actions of amiodarone include inhibition of abnormal automaticity, prolongation of action potential duration, and decreases in conduction velocity. PR, QRS, and QT durations are prolonged and sinus bradycardia is typically induced (44).

When CA is as a result of pulseless VT or VF, an initial 300-mg rapid intravenous infusion may be administered. Alternatively, a rapid infusion of 150 mg may be followed by a continuous infusion of 1 mg per minute for 6 hours, 0.5 mg per minute thereafter, and a maximum daily dose of 2 g (21). Early conversion to oral therapy is advised. Following its intravenous administration, hypotension is induced as a result of peripheral arterial vasodilation. This may be intensified by decreases in myocardial contractility.

Side effects are less common after oral administration although corneal micro-deposits, hepatic dysfunction, hypothyroidism or hyperthyroidism, photosensitivity, and, most seriously, pulmonary fibrosis can follow prolonged administration.

After out-of-hospital CA, administration of amiodarone has been beneficial to the extent that patients survive in larger numbers up to the time of hospital admission. In a randomized clinical study on victims of sudden death as a result of VF out-of-hospital, patients received 300 mg of intravenous amiodarone (45). In comparison with patients receiving placebo, of whom only 34% were admitted alive to hospital, 44% of the individuals who received amiodarone were so admitted. Even though this difference was significant ($p = 0.03$), no significant differences in the hospital discharge rate could be documented. In another study on victims of out-of-hospital CA, Dorian et al. demonstrated that the hospital admission rate of patients receiving amiodarone was significantly greater when compared to that of patients receiving lidocaine (23 vs 12%, $p = 0.009$), yet once again no impact on ultimate survival was proven (46).

We are therefore left with limited optimism for the use of amiodarone but recognize the option of its use in settings of (a) persistent pulseless VT or VF after initial ineffective defibrillation and vasopressor therapy; and (b) hemodynamically stable VT, polymorphic VT, and wide-complex tachycardia of uncertain origin. It has potential as an adjunct to electrical cardioversion of refractory PSVTs, atrial tachycardia, and pharmacological conversion of atrial fibrillation. More remotely, amiodarone has been employed for control of rapid heart rates in settings of supraventricular tachycardia, especially when ventricular function is impaired and digitalis is contra-indicated. Finally, it may be used in settings of tachycardia as a result of aberrant atrioventricular conduction through accessory pathways (21).

PROCAINAMIDE

Procainamide is an analog of the local anesthetic, procaine. It is a sodium channel blocker with an intermediate time constant of recovery from block. It also blocks the outward potassium current so that the cardiac action potential is prolonged. Procainamide decreases automaticity, increases refractory period, and reduces conduction velocity.

The loading dose of procainamide is 1 g, administered at a rate of 20 mg per minute by intravenous injection. Its maintenance dose ranges from 1 to 4 mg per minute. Although the drug must be administered slowly, its role for life-threatening ventricular arrhythmias, including pulseless VT and VF is correspondingly limited. Procainamide is an acceptable pharmacological intervention for (a) supraventricular tachycardia, (b) reducing ventricular rate as a result of accessory pathway conduction in preexcited atrial arrhythmias, and (c) wide-complex tachycardias of unknown origin (21).

Hypotension and significant slowing of cardiac conduction, especially during rapid intravenous infusion, are major adverse effects. When plasma concentrations of procainamide exceed 30 mg/mL, there is high likelihood of torsade de pointes. Long-term oral administration also has frequent side effects, including acquired systemic lupus erythmatosis, facial and body rash, arthralgias of the small joints, and pericardial effusion with tamponade.

ATROPINE

Atropine is a muscarinic receptor antagonist. It competes with acetylcholine (Ach) and other muscarinic agonists for a common binding site on the muscarinic receptor. Atropine produces increases in heart rate by blocking the vagal effects on M_2 receptors on the SA nodal pacemaker. Its therapeutic value is in the abolishment of reflex vagal cardiac slowing or asystole, including the effects of parasympathomimetic drugs. In settings of CA and resuscitation, an initial dose in settings of asystole or pulseless electrical activity is 1 mg by intravenous injection. The same dose may be repeated at intervals of 3–5 minutes. These potential benefits notwithstanding, there is no evidence that outcomes of CA, including patients with asystole and pulseless electrical activity, are improved.

BUFFER AGENTS

Sodium bicarbonate has been administered during CPR with the assumption that reversal of metabolic and, especially lactic acidosis would favor cardiac resuscitation. In 1961, Jude et al. proposed that blood pH would best be maintained within the normal range during CPR by administration of sodium bicarbonate (47). This was intended to improve cardiac action and augment responsiveness to vasopressor agents. This practice was subsequently reinforced by anecdotal reports, which suggested that reversal of severe metabolic acidosis during CPR by the administration of sodium bicarbonate was time-coincident with return of spontaneous circulation. However, subsequent experimental and clinical studies failed to demonstrate a significant decline in arterial blood pH during the initial 10 minutes of CPR. Although the blood bicarbonate content was reduced, hyperventilation accounted for a simultaneous decline in arterial blood PCO_2 such that the pH was typically maintained within a normal range or even increased during the initial 6 minutes of CPR.

We subsequently demonstrated in pigs that neither CO_2-generating buffers nor CO_2-consuming buffers reversed myocardial hypercarbic acidosis during an 8-minute interval of CPR that followed 4 minutes of untreated CA (48,49). Each of these hypertonic solutions induced systemic vasodilation, independently of their buffer effect, and thereby decreased coronary perfusion pressure. The consequent reduction in myocardial perfusion explained, at least in part, the lesser success of resuscitation attempts after infusion of the alkaline buffer. Other unfavorable effects of hypertonic buffer agents were demonstrated, including hyperosmolal states, leftward shifts in oxyhemoglobin dissociation, and coronary and systemic venous hypercarbia. Contrary to earlier assumptions, buffer agents fail to increase the vasopressor effects of epinephrine in settings of CPR (50).

A study by Vukmir et al. (51) suggested that a combination of drugs, including sodium bicarbonate, improved outcome in dogs after CA when untreated for 15 minutes. This finding reawakened the controversy, and further stimulated the search for additional understanding of the effects of buffer agents on the postresuscitation course.

There is also evidence that buffer agents may be of benefit after resuscitation from CA by ameliorating postresuscitation myocardial dysfunction. The organic buffer, tromethamine, was especially effective, possibly related to its ability to reduce myocardial hypercarbia and its anti-inotropic effect (52). Yet, in clinical trials, no objective evidence of benefit from the use of hypertonic buffer agents has been secured. These considerations prompted the more recent CPR Guidelines of the AHA to forego routine administration of buffer agents (especially sodium bicarbonate) except when hyperkalemia or certain drug intoxications are suspected (21). The possibility that CO_2-consuming buffers and sodium bicarbonate administered during CPR may have favorable effects after restoration of spontaneous circulation was subsequently investigated by our group

(53). Tromethamine (TRIS) served as the organic CO_2-consuming buffer and Carbicarb (an equimolar concentration of Na_2CO_3 and $NaHCO_3$) served as the inorganic CO_2-consuming buffer. Postresuscitation left ventricular (LV) function was significantly decreased in all animals. However, both of the CO_2-consuming buffers Carbicarb and TRIS, significantly reduced the severity of postresuscitation myocardial dysfunction and this was associated with prolongation of postresuscitation survival. When the duration of untreated CA was increased and the severity of postresuscitation LV dysfunction was magnified, the benefits of improved postresusci-tation myocardial function and survival of the TRIS- and Carbicarb-treated animals was even more impressive. However, the applicability of these observations to human patients has not as yet been proven. We may conclude that buffer agents administered as the only pharmacological intervention during CPR do not have proven benefits with respect to return of spontaneous circulation. To the contrary, they have potential adverse effects. With respect to postresuscitation myocardial dysfunction, the "CO_2-consuming" buffers TRIS and Carbicarb may be useful in contrast to CO_2-generating sodium bicarbonate. A mixture of TRIS, acetate, sodium bicarbonate, and phosphate buffer solution, named "Tribonat" may have advantages over alkaline buffers, based on experimental studies. Nevertheless, there is no conclusive evidence that Tribonat has improved outcomes *(54)*.

NOVEL PHARMACOLOGICAL AGENTS FOR RESUSCITATION

With the recognized limitations of epinephrine for management of cardiac resuscitation, including the adverse β- and to a lesser extent α_1-adrenergic effects together with the potential limitations of vasopressin, our group has focused on more selective adrenergic agonists. This prompted our trials with selective α_2-adrenoceptor agonists. Three subtypes of α_2 receptors are now identified, namely α_{2A}, α_{2B}, and α_{2C} *(55)*. α_{2A}-Agonists, acting centrally on the medulla, mediate a tonic sympatho-inhibitory effect accounting for reductions in arterial blood pressure, myocardial contractility, and heart rate. This contrasts with a_{2B} peripheral vasoconstrictor actions. α_{2B}-Subtype receptors, which are less abundant in brain tissue, provoke a predominant peripheral vasoconstrictor response *(56,57)*. A third receptor, namely α_{2C}, has a predominant central nervous system effect like α_{2A}, but its cardiovascular actions are not as yet well-defined *(58)*. As of the time of this writing, the focus is on the α_2-receptors, which have selective peripheral vascular in contrast to central nervous actions and therefore have potential as selective non-inotropic and non-chronotropic arterial vasoconstrictors. Although α_2-adrenoceptor agonists have centrally acting vasodilator effects and peripherally acting vasoconstrictor effects, it is only the peripheral action that is of relevance in the initial management of CA. We therefore sought a selective α_2-agonist, which does not gain entry into the brain. It is in this context that we demonstrated that one selective α_2-agonist, α-methylnorepinephrine (αMNE), is as effective as epinephrine for initial cardiac resuscitation but without the α_1- or β-effects by which myocardial oxygen consumption is increased. Accordingly, adverse effects on postresuscitation myocardial function and survival are avoided *(11)*. Additionally, there is evidence that α_2-adrenergic agonists increase endothelial nitric oxide production which mitigates the α-adrenergic vasoconstrictor effects on coronary arteries and thereby potentially improve coronary blood flow *(59)*. When αMNE was compared to epinephrine in a rat model of CA and resuscitation, αMNE significantly improved the likelihood of initial resuscitation, postresuscitation myocardial function and survival. The incidence of postresuscitation ventricular arrhythmias was reduced

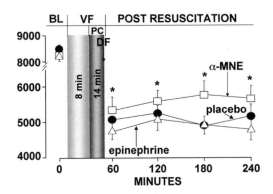

Fig. 2. Selective α_2-agonist reduces the severity of postresuscitation myocardial dysfunction (measured as dp/dt_{40} mmHg/s). BL, baseline; VF, ventricular fibrillation; αMNE, α-methylnorepinephrine. *$p < 0.05$ vs epinephrine.

strikingly (Fig. 2; *11*). We then compared the effects of αMNE on postresuscitation myocardial function with vasopressin. We again demonstrated that myocardial function was significantly better in animals treated with αMNE *(60)*. Based on these preliminary studies, we recognize that the selective α_2-adrenergic agonist has the following advantages for CPR: (a) the oxygen requirements of the fibrillating heart are not increased and therefore the severity of myocardial ischemic injury is lessened, (b) postsynaptic α_2-adrenergic receptors do not desensitize during systemic ischemia in contrast to α_1-adrenergic receptors allowing for a more persistent vasoconstrictor, (c) increases in endothelial nitric oxide production in the coronary circuit favors improved coronary blood flow. Nevertheless, the ultimate utility of these classes of agents remains to be established.

REFERENCES

1. Emerman CL, Pinchak AC, Hancock D, Hagen JF. Effect of injection site on circulation times during cardiac arrest. Crit Care Med 1988; 16:1138–1141.
2. Ahlquist RP. A study of the adrenotropic receptors. Am J Physiol 1948; 153:586–600.
3. Strader CD, Fong TM, Tota MR, Underwood D, Dixon RA. Structure and function of G protein-coupled receptors. Ann Rev Biochem 1994; 63:101–132.
4. Bylund DB: Subtypes of a_1- and a_2-adrenergic receptors. FASEB J 1992; 6:832–839.
5. Cai JJ, Morgan DA, Haynes WG, Martins JB, Lee HC. Alpha$_2$-adrenergic stimulation is protective against ischemia-reperfusion-induced ventricular arrhythmias in vivo. 2002; 283:H2606–H2611.
6. Emorine LJ, Marullo S, Briend-Sutren MM, et al. Molecular characterization of the human β_3-adrenergic receptor. Science 1989; 245:1118–1121.
7. Schoming A, Richardt G, Kurz T: Sympatho-adrenergic activation of the ischemic myocardium and its arrhythmogenic impact. Herz 1995; 20:169–186.
8. Ihl-Vahl R, Marquetant R, Bremerich J, Strasser RH. Regulation of beta-adrenergic receptors in acute myocardial ischemia: subtype-selective increase of mRNA specific for beta$_1$-adrenergic receptors. J Mol Cell Cardiol 1995; 27:437–452.
9. Brown CG, Martin DR, Pepe PE, et al. A comparison of standard-dose and high-dose epinephrine in cardiac arrest outside the hospital. N Engl J Med 1992; 327:1051–1055.
10. Callaham ML, Madsen CD, Barton CW, Saunders CR, Pointer J. A randomized clinical trial of high-dose epinephrine and norepinephrine vs standard-dose epinephrine in prehospital cardiac arrest. JAMA 1992; 268:2667–2672.
11. Sun S, Weil MH, Tang W, Kamohara T, Klouche K. Alpha-methylnorepinephrine, a selective alpha$_2$-adrenergic agonist for cardiac resuscitation. J Am Coll Cardiol 2001; 37:951–956.

12. Brown CG, Katz SE, Werman HA, Luu T, Davis EA, Hamlin RL. The effect of epinephrine versus methoxamine on regional myocardial blood flow and defibrillation rates following a prolonged cardiorespiratory arrest in a swine model. Am J Emerg Med 1987; 5:362–369.

13. Brown CG, Davis EA, Werman HA, Hamlin RL. Methoxamine versus epinephrine on regional cerebral blood flow during cardiopulmonary resuscitation. Crit Care Med 1987; 15:682–686.

14. Tang W, Weil MH, Sun SJ, Noc M, Yang L, Gazmuri RJ. Epinephrine increases the severity of postresuscitation myocardial dysfunction. Circulation 1995; 92:3089–3093.

15. Marn-Pernat A, Weil MH, Tang W, Pernat A, Bisera J. Optimizing timing of ventricular defibrillation. Crit Care Med 2001: 29:2360–2365.

16. Povoas H, Weil MH, Tang W, Bisera J, Klouche K, Barbatsis A. Predicting the success of defibrillation by electrocardiographic analysis. Resuscitation 2002; 53:77–82.

17. Tang W, Weil MH, Gazmuri RJ, Sun S, Duggal C, Bisera J. Pulmonary ventilation/perfusion defects induced by epinephrine during cardiopulmonary resuscitation. Circulation 1991; 84:2101–2107.

18. Sun S, Weil MW, Tang W, Povoas HP. Combined effects of buffer and adrenergic agents on postresuscitation myocardial function. J Pharmacol Exp Ther 1999; 291:773–777.

19. Ralston SH, Tacker WA, Showen L, Carter A, Babbs CF. Endotracheal versus intravenous epinephrine during electromechanical dissociation with CPR in dogs. Ann Emerg Med 1985; 14:1044–1048.

20. Stiell IG, Herbert PC, Weitzman BN, et al: High-dose epinephrine in adult cardiac arrest. N Engl J Med 1992; 327:1045–1050.

21. AHA Guidelines 2000 for Cardiopulmonary Resuscitation and Emergency Cardiovascular Care. Circulation 2000; 8(Suppl):I-129.

22. Ditchey RV, Lindenfeld J. Failure of epinephrine to improve the balance between myocardial oxygen supply and demand during closed-chest resuscitation in dogs. Circulation 1988; 78:382–389.

23. Lindner KH, Ahnefeld FW, Schuermann W, Bowdler IM. Epinephrine and norepinephrine in cardiopulmonary resuscitation. Effects on myocardial oxygen delivery and consumption. Chest 1990; 97: 1458–1462.

24. Lindner KH, Ahnefeld FW, Pfenninger EG, Schuermann W, Bowdler IM. Effects of epinephrine and norepinephrine on cerebral oxygen delivery and consumption during open-chest CPR. Ann Emerg Med 1990; 19:249–254.

25. Lindner KH, Ahnefeld FW, Grunert A. Epinephrine versus norepinephrine in pre-hospital ventricular fibrillation. Am J Cardiol 1991; 67:427–428.

26. Redding JS, Pearson JW. Evaluation of drugs for cardiac resuscitation. Anesthesiology 1963; 24:203–207.

27. Brillman JA, Sanders AB, Otto CW, Fahmy H, Bragg S, Ewy GA. Outcome of resuscitation from fibrillatory arrest using epinephrine and phenylephrine in dogs. Crit Care Med 1985; 13:912–913.

28. Brown CG, Taylor RB, Werman HA, Luu T, Ashton J, Hamlin RL. Myocardial oxygen delivery/consumption during cardiopulmonary resuscitation: a comparison of epinephrine and phenylephrine. Ann Emerg Med 1988; 17:302–308.

29. Ditchey RV, Rubio-Perez A, Slinker BK. Beta-adrenergic blockade reduces myocardial injury during experimental cardiopulmonary resuscitation. J Am Coll Cardiol 1994; 24:804–812.

30. Silfvast T, Saarnivaara L, Kinnunen A, et al. Comparison of adrenaline and phenylephrine in out-of-hospital cardiopulmonary resuscitation. A double-blind study. Acta Anaesthesiol Scand 1985; 29:610–613.

31. Lindner KH, Haak T, Keller A, Bothner U, Lurie KG. Release of endogenous vasopressors during and after cardiopulmonary resuscitation. Br Heart J 1996; 75:145–150.

32. Lindner KH, Prengel AW, Pfenninger EG, et al: Vasopressin improves vital organ blood flow during closed-chest cardiopulmonary resuscitation in pigs. Circulation 1995; 91:215–221.

33. Lindner KH, Prengel AW, Brinkmann A, Strohmenger HU, Lindner IM, Lurie KG. Vasopressin administration in refractory cardiac arrest. Ann Int Med 1996; 124:1061–1064.

34. Prengel AW, Lindner KH, Keller A, Lurie KG. Cardiovascular function during the post-resuscitation phase after cardiac arrest in pigs: A comparison of epinephrine versus vasopressin. Crit Care Med 1996; 24:2014–2019.

35. Lindner KH, Dirks B, Strohmenger HU. Randomized comparison of epinephrine and vasopressin in patients with out-of-hospital ventricular fibrillation. Lancet 1997; 349:535–537.

36. Wenzel V, Krismer AC, Arntz HR, Sitter H, Stadbauer KH, Lindner KH. A comparison of vasopressin and epinephrine for out-of-hospital cardiopulmonary resuscitation. N Engl J Med 2004; 350(2):105–113.

37. Lindner KH, Prengel AW, Pfenninger EG, Lindner IM. Angiotensin II augments reflex activity of the sympathetic nervous system during cardiopulmonary resuscitation in pigs. Circulation 1995; 92: 1020–1025.

38. Lindner KH, Prengel AW, Pfenninger EG, Lindner IM. Effect of angiotensin II on myocardial blood flow and acid-base status in a pig model of cardiopulmonary resuscitation. Anesth Analg 1993; 76:485–492.
39. Little CM, Brown CG: Angiotensin II improves myocardial blood flow in cardiac arrest. Resuscitation 1993; 26:203–210.
40. Vaughan Williams EM. Classifying antiarrhythmic actions: by facts or speculation. J Clin Pharmacol 1993; 32:964–977.
41. Balser JR, Nuss HB, Orias DW, et al. Local anesthetics as effectors of allosteric gating. Lidocaine effects on inactivation-deficient rat skeletal muscle Na channels. J Clin Invest 1996; 98:2874–2886.
42. Lie KI, Wellens HJ, van Capelle FJ, Durrer D. Lidocaine in the prevention of primary ventricular fibrillation. A double-blind randomized study of 212 consecutive patients. N Eng J Med 1974; 291:1324–1326.
43. Hine LK, Laird N, Hewitt P, Chalmers TC. Meta-analytic evidence against prophylactic use of lidocaine in acute myocardial infarction. Arch Intern Med 1989; 149:2694–2698.
44. Levine JH, Moore EN, Kadish AH, et al. Mechanisms of depressed conduction from long-term amiodarone therapy in canine myocardium. Circulation 1988; 78:684–691.
45. Kudenchuk PJ, Cobb LA, Copass MK, et al. Amiodarone for resuscitation after out-of-hospital cardiac arrest due to ventricular fibrillation. N Engl J Med 1999; 341:871–878.
46. Dorian P, Cass D, Schwartz B, Cooper R, Gelaznikas R, Barr A. Amiodarone as compared with lidocaine for shock-resistant ventricular fibrillation. N Engl J Med 2002; 346:884–890.
47. Jude JR, Kouwenhoven WB, Knickerbocker GG. Cardiac arrest: report of application of external cardiac massage on 118 patients. JAMA 1961; 178:1063-1070.
48. Von Planta M, Weil MH, Gazmuri RJ, Rackow EC. Myocardial acidosis associated with CO_2 production during cardiac arrest. Circulation 1989; 80:684–692.
49. Kette F, Weil MH, von Planta M, Gazmuri RJ, Rackow EC. Buffer agents do not reverse intramyocardial acidosis during cardiac resuscitation. Circulation 1990; 81:1660–1666.
50. Bleske BE, Warren EW, Rice TL, Gilligan LJ, Tait AR. Effect of high-dose sodium bicarbonate on the vasopressor effects of epinephrine during cardiopulmonary resuscitation. Pharmacotherapy 1995; 15: 660–664.
51. Vukmir RB, Bircher NG, Radovsky A, Safar P. Sodium bicarbonate may improve outcome in dogs with brief or prolonged cardiac arrest. Crit Care Med 1995; 23:515–522.
52. Tang W, Weil MH, Gazmuri RJ. Sun S, Bisera J, Rackow E. Buffer agents ameliorate the myocardial depressant effect of carbon dioxide. Crit Care Med 1990; 18:S182.
53. Sun SJ, Weil MH, Tang W, Fukui M. Effects of buffer agents on post-resuscitation myocardial dysfunction. Crit Care Med 1996; 24:2036–2041.
54. Bjerneroth G. Alkaline buffers for correction of metabolic acidosis during cardiopulmonary resuscitation with focus on Tribonat – a Review. Resuscitation 1998; 37:161–171.
55. Lomasney JW, Cotecchia S, Leftkowitz RJ, Caron MG. Molecular biology of a-adrenergic receptors: implications for receptor classification and for structure-function relationships. Biochim Biophys Acta 1991; 1095:127–139.
56. Link RE, Desai K, Hein L, et al. Cardiovascular regulation in mice lacking a_2-adrenergic receptor subtypes b and c. Science 1996; 273:803.
57. Kable JW, Murrin LC, Bylund DB. In vivo gene modification elucidates subtype-specific function of a_2-adrenergic receptors. J Pharmacol Exper Ther 2000; 293:1.
58. Gavras I, Gavras H. Role of alpha$_2$-adrenergic receptors in hypertension. 1: Am J Hypertens 2001; 14(Pt 2):171S.
59. Ishibashi Y, Duncker DJ, Bache RJ. Endogenous nitric oxide masks alpha$_2$-adrenergic coronary vasoconstriction during exercise in the ischemic heart. Circ Res 1997; 80:196.
60. Klouche K, Weil MH, Tang W, Povoas H, Kamohara T, Bisera J. A selective α-adrenergic agonist for cardiac resuscitation. J Lab Clin Med 2002; 140:27–34.

19

Use of Vasopressor Drugs in Cardiac Arrest

Anette C. Krismer, MD, *Norman A. Paradis,* MD,
Volker Wenzel, MD, *and John Southall,* MD

CONTENTS

INTRODUCTION

The importance of vital organ perfusion in patients suffering cardiac arrest (CA) makes arterial vasomotor tone, and the resultant perfusion pressure, critical in resuscitation from sudden death. After failure of countershock, ventilation, and oxygenation, the target organ for resuscitative pharmacotherapy becomes the arterial vascular smooth muscle cell. Selective stimulation of various vascular smooth muscle cell surface receptors is accomplished through administration of exogenous agents with the intention of altering blood flow away from nonvital organ beds toward the myocardium and brain.

Although there are multiple mechanisms that may affect arterial vascular tone, historically the therapy most commonly used has been catecholamine-induced adrenergic receptor stimulation, with catecholamine epinephrine being the most common drug utilized. However, over the last decade it has become widely known that the utility of epinephrine during cardiopulmonary resuscitation is undefined. There has always been concern that its β-receptor mediated effects, in particular its effects on myocardial oxygen consumption, may actually be deleterious in the setting of ischemia. Of particular note, so-called "high-dose" epinephrine therapy, which had appeared effective with respect to return of spontaneous circulation in laboratory models and uncontrolled clinical trials to, has not been found to improve neurologic outcome in prospective controlled clinical trials. This has led to research into alternative agents, in particular non-adrenergic vasoactive peptides. Other agents, both new and old appear promising. These include α-methyl-norepinephrine and phenylephrine. Recently, vasopressin has been the focus of considerable

From: *Contemporary Cardiology: Cardiopulmonary Resuscitation*
Edited by: J. P. Ornato and M. A. Peberdy © Humana Press Inc., Totowa, NJ

research. In laboratory models of cardiopulmonary arrest (CPA), vasopressin improves vital organ blood flow, cerebral oxygen delivery, rate of return of spontaneous circulation, and neurological recovery compared to epinephrine. In a single study of patients with out-of-hospital ventricular fibrillation (VF), a larger proportion of patients treated with vasopressin survived 24 hours compared with epinephrine. The most recent CPR guidelines of both the American Heart Association (AHA), and European Resuscitation Council recommend 40 units vasopressin or 1 mg epinephrine intravenously in adult patients with VF refractory to electrical countershock.

History

The history of pressor drugs and adrenergic agonists is, to a great extent, synonymous with research on epinephrine and its uses. It was observed in the mid-18th century that extracts of the suprarenal gland raised blood pressure. Starting in 1894, Szymonowicz et al. used adrenal gland extracts to enhance peripheral vasoconstriction and latter to revive asystolic isolated animal hearts *(1)*. In 1896, Gottlieb used adrenal gland extract and thoracic compressions to resuscitate an asystolic rabbit *(2)* and proposed its use to treat CA in humans.

During the first 60 years of the 20th century, epinephrine was used as a vasopressor, with anecdotal use during CA *(3–6)*. Starting in the early 1960s, Redding et al. undertook a series of experiments that are the foundation of modern research on resuscitation. A number of their studies demonstrated the utility of vasoactive amines in the treatment of CA of more than a few minutes duration. Many of their recommendations were incorporated in the AHA guidelines of 1974.

BASIC SCIENCE

The autonomic nervous system is dedicated to maintenance of homeostasis through neuroendocrine changes in visceral function. It is divided into affector and effector limbs, and many autonomic nerves are organized into regional plexuses located outside the central nervous system (CNS). The efferent limb of the autonomic nervous system consists of sympathetic and parasympathetic divisions. Drugs may affect the autonomic nervous system at multiple locations, including the affector limb, the CNS, ganglia, and peripheral innervations of visceral structures.

Preganglionic autonomic fibers, postganglionic parasympathetic fibers, and some postganglionic sympathetic fibers all respond to the neurotransmitter acetylcholine and are termed cholinergic fibers. Most postganglionic sympathetic fibers are termed adrenergic because the neurotransmitter is noradrenaline (norepinephrine). Stimulation of adrenergic or cholinergic tissue receptors, either through autonomic outflow or drug administration, results in typical end-organ responses. Generally, stimulation of one limb of the autonomic nervous system, either the parasympathetic or sympathetic, antagonizes the effects of the other. It is not known, however, if this relationship is significant during CA, which is a state of extreme sympathetic stimulation *(7)*. Modulation of parasympathetic tone, for instance, has not been clearly demonstrated to be important during CA *(8)*, and atropine may have limited utility in treatment of adult VF.

The binding of an adrenergic drug to its receptor causes characteristic changes in the intracellular concentration of second-messenger molecules, which result in the physiologic effects characteristic of the drug. Second messengers include cyclic adenosine monophosphate (cAMP), phosphatidylinositol, and calcium *(9–11)*.

Epinephrine, produced by the chromaffin cells of the adrenal medulla, is stored in chromaffin granules. These cells are innervated by the sympathetic nervous system and release stored epinephrine in response to stimulation. The degree of sympathetic outflow is a function of homeostatic feedback mechanisms and is responsive to various stimuli, such as changes in blood pressure, tissue oxygenation, and environmental stress. The most important endogenous neurohumoral event in CA is the release of adrenomedullary catecholamines as a massive sympathetic response to extreme hypotension *(7)*. It is reasonable to conclude that exogenous epinephrine is not required during early treatment of sudden death as endogenous levels are extraordinarily high.

The first systematic study of adrenergic agonists was performed by Ahlquist *(12)*, who examined the effects of sympathomimetic amines on tissues and delineated two distinct classes of physiologic effect. The first, which he termed α-effects, were excitatory; the second, termed β-effects, were inhibitory. Stimulation of α-receptors typically caused vasoconstriction, and stimulation of β-receptors causes vasodilation. Ahlquist also described an order of potency in each class in descending order for the excitatory α-receptor, were epinephrine, norepinephrine, and isoproterenol; for the inhibitory β-receptor the order was isoproterenol, epinephrine, and norepinephrine.

With apparent contradiction, cardiac stimulation was found to be an "inhibitory" β-receptor stimulation. The α-subtype was later subdivided into smaller classes, α_1 and α_2, with different physiologic effects. Stimulation with α_1-agonists increased cardiac inotropy and chronotropy.

It is important to know that the pathophysiology and pharmacology of the autonomic nervous system during global ischemia and CPR have not been studied beyond simple measurement of levels of circulating hormone. Other than a dramatic increase in circulating catecholamines, it is not known how global ischemia affects autonomic outflow and target organ receptor number and function.

MECHANISM OF ACTION

The treatment of CA with adrenergic agonists predated understanding of their possible mechanisms of action, and our knowledge of these drugs remains incomplete. Although during spontaneous circulation, sympathetic stimulation results in diverse autonomic effects, including changes in inotropy and chronotropy, the importance of the processes during the treatment of CA remains unknown.

CPR is a state of extreme global ischemia, tissue hypoxia, and acidosis. Successful resuscitation depends on reversal of organ hypoxia by improving the supply/demand equilibrium for oxygen. Studies in animal models indicate that the fibrillating myocardium may require blood flow in excess of 40 to 50 mL per minute per 100 g to achieve return of spontaneous circulation *(13)*. Because the oxygen debt increases with the duration of CA, greater blood flows are likely to be required later in resuscitation. Importantly, cellular changes late in resuscitation may interfere with oxygen utilization within the mitochondria and mask the relationship between blood flow and outcome.

Myocardial blood flows during CPR fall rapidly below the needs of the myocardium as the time from loss of circulation increases *(14,15)*. Pressor drugs are administered during CPR to raise arterial pressure and redistribute blood flow to vital organs. Studies in animal models and patients have shown a high correlation between the relaxation phase aortic-to-right-atrial pressure gradient, myocardial blood flow, and return of spontaneous circulation *(15–17)*. It is now widely accepted that this gradient is the *de facto* coronary perfusion pressure during standard external CPR. External chest compression alone is often unable to achieve a perfusion gradient of sufficient magnitude to achieve return of spontaneous circulation after the first few minutes of CA, possibly because vascular smooth muscle cell hypoxia and loss of cellular energy charge cause in a diffuse vasorelaxation. Without exogenous agents, a large fraction of forward flow is directed to organs other than the brain and heart.

Redding and Pearson observed that CPR was only minimally effective without administration of adrenergic agonists *(18)*. In one study, all animals treated with methoxamine or epinephrine had return of spontaneous circulation *(19)*, although the pure β-agonist isoproterenol was less effective than placebo. More recent studies have supported the conclusion that vasoconstriction resulting in increased aortic pressure in the relaxation phase may be the principal mechanism of action by which vasopressor therapy achieves return of spontaneous circulation *(13,17)*.

Redding et al.'s research suggested that α-adrenergic stimulation was of critical importance, although stimulation of β-receptors was not beneficial, possibly even detrimental. In a landmark series of studies, Yakaitis et al. examined the effect of selective combinations of α- and β-receptor stimulation and blockade on resuscitation in an asphyxial-electromechanical dissociation (EMD) model of CA *(20,21)*. Their work supported the hypothesis that peripheral α-receptor stimulation is crucial to the efficacy of adrenergic agents and that epinephrine's β-agonism was of little therapeutic benefit. Recently, Ditchey et al. found that pre-arrest β-receptor blockade resulted in significantly higher aortic and coronary perfusion pressures *(22)*.

Efficacy of Pressors

Although Crile and Dolley had observed that epinephrine improved their ability to restore a heartbeat to dogs in CA around the turn of the century *(23)*, the utility of sympathomimetic amines in the treatment of CA was first systematically studied by Redding and Pearson starting in the 1960s *(19,24–26)*. Research standards at the time, combined with orientation toward treatment of cardiovascular collapse secondary to anesthetic induction, resulted in studies that were limited in size and had a number of methodological limitations. Nonetheless, they convincingly demonstrated the efficacy of adrenergic agents as adjuncts during CPR, a finding that continues to be supported by laboratory research to this day. Redding and Pearson found epinephrine-treated animals were up to nine times more likely to achieve return of spontaneous circulation than those treated with placebo. Indeed, in most laboratory models there is return of spontaneous circulation after the first few minutes of CA by external chest compression alone *(25)*. Addition of pressor drugs extends the window of efficacy for external chest compression to at least 15 minutes *(27)*. Although clinical trials have not clearly demonstrated the efficacy of epinephrine, the preponderance of laboratory studies has confirmed Redding and Pearson's landmark insights.

Brown's research during the 1980s led to a series of studies investigating the efficacy of higher dosages of epinephrine, but there has been no well-controlled clinical trial to investigate the actual utility of epinephrine vs placebo. A small number of studies had purported to demonstrate that use of epinephrine or high-dose epinephrine is correlated with a worse outcome. These studies appear to be fundamentally flawed by the bias that results from total epinephrine dosage being a covariant with total arrest time. Meta-analysis of the controlled high-dose epinephrine clinical trials found little or no decrement in outcome, a finding that, although not supporting use of the drug, militates against there being significant toxicity overall. Nonadrenergic vasoactive peptides, such as vasopressin, hold considerable promise. They may raise perfusion pressure without the increase in oxygen utilization that accompanies administration of drugs such as epinephrine. An intriguing possibility is that they may act synergistically when administered with catecholamines and that concomitant use of adrenergic drugs and vasoactive peptides may allow a lowering of the dosage of each agent.

Individual Adrenergic Agents

A number of sympathomimetic agonists have been considered in therapy for CA. Typically, these drugs have undergone extensive evaluation in animals and humans during spontaneous circulation *(28,29)*, and assessment in CA has been incomplete. The paucity of laboratory studies and direct comparison in controlled clinical trials make choice of a specific drug difficult.

A wide range of adrenergic-receptor agonists is available. Currently, the mixed α- and β-agonist epinephrine is almost universally used. Pure α-agonists such as methoxamine and phenylephrine have been studied and are occasionally used clinically. The α-receptor-agonist isoproterenol was once popular, but is now almost never used in the treatment of CA because of concern that it may decrease perfusion.

There are also a number of vasoactive peptides available. However, at this time, only vasopressin is used clinically *(30)*.

Epinephrine

Epinephrine is the best studied and most widely administered adrenergic agonist used for the treatment of CA. It stimulates α_1- and α_2-receptors almost equally *(31)*, and β_1- and β_2-receptors in a ratio of approx 1:4 *(28,29,32,33)*.

There are no prospective clinical trials that demonstrate the efficacy of epinephrine in improving the outcome of patients suffering CA. Since at least the 1970s, epinephrine has been administered almost universally to patients who have failed basic life support and electrical countershock. This *de facto* "standard" has made performance of placebo-controlled clinical trials extremely difficult. There is, however, a report of a study in which this was done. Woodhouse et al. assigned patients in asystole, or who had failed countershock, to 10-mg epinephrine or placebo *(34)*. Another group was given a standard 1-mg dose of epinephrine. The rates of "immediate survival" and hospital discharge were similar in each group, and these investigators concluded that the use of epinephrine makes "no difference to the outcome of asystole or after two countershocks in those remaining in ventricular fibrillation." They did, however, note that a "change of rhythm to a potentially treatable rhythm occurred more significantly in the 1 mg and 10 mg groups," compared to placebo.

A number of limitations raise doubts about these conclusions. Thirty-eight percent of eligible patients were not randomized because of the concerns of the supervising physicians about entering into the placebo arm of the study *(35)*. Most likely, this study reflects the difficulty of studying therapies that are also predictors of poor prognosis because they are markers of downtime.

There are reasons to be concerned that epinephrine salutary effect on perfusion and the rate of return of spontaneous circulation are counterbalanced by the toxicity of its β-adrenergic effects. Weil and Tang have shown in a series of experiments that use of epinephrine can result in postreperfusion myocardial dysfunction including stone heart.

Berg et al. found a worse 24-hour survival in one animal model. Failure of the randomized clinical trials of high-dose epinephrine to demonstrate an improvement in outcome are also worrisome as effective therapies usually have a detectable dose–response relationship. A reasonable synthesis of the homogenous laboratory data and the heterogenous clinical data is that epinephrine is effective in restoring circulation in patients who have failed CPR and countershock, but that this is at the cost of occasionally significant postreperfusion toxicity.

Epinephrine's Pharmacology in CA

The physiochemistry, bioavailability, volumes of distribution, protein binding, metabolism, elimination, and other standard pharmacological indices have not been delineated for epinephrine during CPR. Almost all that is known about this drug is from laboratory models and humans with spontaneous circulation. It has been so common to extrapolate from the spontaneous circulation to the arrested state that physicians often forget that this has no scientific basis.

The common US formulations of epinephrine as hydrochloride have pH values ranging from 2.5 to 5.0 (36). A potentially important interaction may be that of epinephrine with alkalinizing agents. The AHA guidelines have stated that "epinephrine is inactivated in alkaline solutions and should never be mixed with sodium bicarbonate" (2). Although the use of sodium bicarbonate in CA may be declining, this potential incompatibility remains important, especially for patients with only a single route of intravenous access. In one study, the biological activity of epinephrine decreased 13% after injection through a cannula containing 0.6 mmol/L sodium bicarbonate (42). Although the absolute dictum against mixing of epinephrine and bicarbonate does not appear to be supported by the available data, it seems prudent to avoid the theoretical stoichiometric inactivation if two routes of administration are available. The multidose vial of 30 mL of 1 mg/mL epinephrine commonly used in the United States for high-dose epinephrine therapy contains 0.15% sodium bisulfite. Some decrement in concentration, perhaps 10%, may occur with this particular formulation after storage (37). There are also unpublished reports of up to 30% variability in epinephrine concentrations in the standard 1-mg bolus ampoules, with a tendency toward less than 1 mg. Intravenous administration during CPR is a dynamic and poorly quantified process, in which drugs are injected rapidly, and the admixture space, volume of the intravenous tubing, and admixture site are variable. Whenever possible, it is perhaps best to administer epinephrine to some therapeutic endpoint such as the change in aortic pressure.

Epinephrine and VF

Redding and Pearson noted that dogs in VF were more quickly defibrillated after epinephrine therapy (18), yet Yakaitis found the drug important for achieving return of spontaneous circulation after countershock (38).

"After two minutes of fibrillation epinephrine [becomes] increasingly important for restoration of circulation. The technique of immediate countershock was effective [only] for episodes of fibrillation limited to approximately three minutes."

Niemann and Cairns studied the need for perfusion before defibrillation in a laboratory model with a duration of CA comparable to that seen in human out-of-hospital sudden death (39). Animals were given either immediate countershock or were treated with epinephrine followed by 5 minutes of CPR before countershock. Animals that received epinephrine had a higher rate of return of spontaneous circulation despite longer arrest times. Animals countershocked without adrenergic therapy develop pulseless electrical activity (PEA; *40*).

Epinephrine and Neurological Outcome

Adrenergic agonists improve cerebral blood flow *(15)* in laboratory models. Because the time from onset of arrest to return of spontaneous circulation is the primary determinant of neurological outcome, early use of drugs like epinephrine may shorten arrest time and thus improve outcome. Although preliminary reports from animal models indicate that adrenergic drugs may have a direct neuroprotective effect *(41)*, other studies do not find this effect. Of particular concern, postreperfusion myocardial dysfunction may contribute to a secondary CNS injury. There has been concern that restoration of spontaneous circulation in patients who have suffered irreparable CNS injury may result in a significant burden on families and society *(42)*. In particular, high-dose epinephrine, with its potential to resuscitate patients after prolonged arrest, raises the concern that patients with irreversible brain damage may be revived. Although methodologically limited studies have purported to detect this phenomenon, meta-analysis of the high-dose epinephrine randomized clinical trials has failed to detect this.

Epinephrine's Toxicity

The potential toxicity of epinephrine during and after CA has been of concern since it was advocated as therapy almost 40 years ago, largely as a result of reports of the alarming effects of accidental epinephrine overdoses in patients with intact circulations *(43–46)*. The importance of these effects to patients with arrested circulation is unclear. The severe hypertension that occurs with epinephrine overdose in intact patients is not applicable during CA, and increased oxygen utilization unmatched by increased perfusion would be deleterious. Early concerns that epinephrine might trigger intractable ventricular tachydysrhythmias in CA have not been substantiated. However, this may be because these events are difficult to separate from primary VF.

In some studies, epinephrine increases myocardial oxygen consumption more than supply *(30,47,48)*, and deleterious changes in the ratio of endocardial to epicardial blood flow and in the distribution of pulmonary blood flow have also been reported *(49,50)*. The importance of these effects during resuscitation from CA is unclear because they have been demonstrated in some animal models and patients, but not in others *(42,47, 51)*. The drug's clear ability to improve the rate of return of spontaneous circulation indicates that overall these potential toxicities are more than compensated by improved perfusion *(52)*.

A pattern of myocardial injury, called contraction-band necrosis, has been associated with exposure to high plasma levels of catecholamines *(53,54)*. β-Receptor blockade appears to protect the myocardium from contraction-band necrosis, supporting the hypothesis that pure α-receptor agonists, such as phenylephrine, may be attractive agents. Recently, Weil and Tang have demonstrated that compared to alternative agents, epinephrine is correlated with decrements in myocardial function during the postresuscitation period *(55)*. This has particular import clinically as it may contribute to the refractory shock that often kills patients who have been resuscitated from CA.

During spontaneous circulation, catecholamines may also injure the vascular system *(56,57)* and it is reasonable to conclude that the high doses used in the treatment of CA may injure the vasculature. Although this injury may also contribute to postreperfusion shock, it has not been well studied.

Epinephrine has a well described stimulatory on platelet aggregation. This is particularly worrisome in the treatment of sudden cardiac death as a large fraction of these patients have acute coronary occlusion that results, at least in part, from formation of a coronary thrombus. Platelet aggregation may also play a role in the "no reflow" phenomena, which is felt to contribute to the CNS injury of postanoxic encephalopathy. The effect of epinephrine on platelets is one of the drugs least attractive pharmacologic properties.

The potential of epinephrine to harm pulmonary function has received considerable attention. Pulmonary arteriovenous admixture and alveolar dead space may increase after epinephrine administration (58). In the laboratory, this may cause relative arterial hypoxia and hypercarbia (59). Treatment with the α-agonist methoxamine apparently does not produce similar changes, suggesting that epinephrine may mediate this effect via α-agonism. Clinical experience, however, indicates that such toxicity is hypothetical, as arterial hypocarbia and increased arterial O_2 content are the norm during CPR in humans.

There is longstanding concern that administration of epinephrine during resuscitation might result in untoward effects during the important postresuscitation period (60). Meta-analysis of the high-dose epinephrine randomized clinical trials supports this concern as it indicates that higher dosages of epinephrine may slightly decrease survival. Again, these concerns have focused on β-receptor-mediated injury to the myocardium, vasculature, and some formed elements of blood (61,62). Patients resuscitated after CA of relatively short duration often manifest a brief period of hypertension, most probably from residual epinephrine of adrenal or exogenous origin. In patients who have received large amounts of exogenous epinephrine, hypertension may reach alarming levels and may be associated with tachydysrhythmias. This hypersympathetic state lasts only a few minutes and is usually supplanted by hypotension. Failure to treat this hypotension may result in secondary organ injury.

Epinephrine's Dosage in Cardiac Arrest

Few of the early investigations of epinephrine in CA addressed the issue of dosage, with many studies using a single dose independent of body weight. In 1906, Crile and Dolley gave "one to two cubic centimeters of 1–1000 solution of adrenaline" to dogs (23). This was adrenaline chloride, and the dose has been estimated to have been comparable to approx 0.4 mg/kg. In their early work, Redding and Pearson gave a dose of 1.0 mg and found it to be effective in dogs weighing approx 10 kg, equivalent to 0.1 mg/kg (26). In commenting on epinephrine's use in patients, their 1-mg initial dose was described as "satisfactory," and it was recommended that this be the "standard." Some patients, however, required either a second 1-mg dose or a 2-mg dose (24).

In a 70-kg patient, Redding and Pearson's 1.0-mg dose is equal to 0.014 mg/kg, or approximately an order of magnitude less on a milligram per kilogram basis than in their animal studies. Interestingly, they mention that 1 mg was used "with benefit in children down to 18 months of age" (24). A child of this age would weigh approx 12 kg, and would have received a dose of approx 0.083 mg/kg, almost six times the adult 1-mg dosage. Historically, the 1-mg dose suggested by Redding and Pearson was considered massive, because much smaller doses were known to be dangerous in patients with intact circulation. Indeed, they were "criticized by some for employing such a large dose."

Between the mid-1960s and the 1980s, there were a small number of laboratory studies with alternative dosages of epinephrine. The first, again by Redding and Pearson, used a total dose of 0.2 mg (63). The second, by Jude and coworkers in 1968, used 0.02 and 0.08 mg/kg, and found that the arteriovenous pressure gradient was doubled by the higher dose *(64)*. In the third study, a dose of 0.05 mg/kg produced increased cerebral and myocardial blood flows, but not to levels considered necessary to meet the needs of the myocardium in early fibrillation *(65)*. Other than these studies, the possibility of a dose–response curve for adrenergic agonists during CPR was largely ignored.

In 1985, Kosnik et al. reported the first laboratory study to evaluate the dose–response relationship for epinephrine during CPR *(55)*. They administered 0.015, 0.045, 0.075, and 0.15 mg/kg of epinephrine and measured hemodynamic properties, such as aortic diastolic and coronary perfusion pressures. Although the results were not statistically significant, they did show that only the two higher doses raised and maintained aortic diastolic pressure to approx 30 mmHg for 4 minutes. Shortly thereafter, Ralston et al. demonstrated improved resuscitation rates in animals given progressively higher doses of epinephrine *(66)*. They found that intravenous doses of 0.001, 0.003, 0.01, 0.03, and 0.1 mg/kg produced resuscitation rates of 0, 10, 40, 80, and 90% respectively. Endotracheal epinephrine doses, an order of magnitude higher, produced similar results. These results were important because they clearly demonstrated that dose–response curves could be developed for adrenergic agonists during CPR, and that the optimal dose might be much larger than the standard dose of 1 mg.

Brown and colleagues systematically evaluated the effect of epinephrine and other vasopressors on vital organ blood flow during CPR. These studies combined a radiolabeled-microsphere technique for measurement of myocardial and cerebral blood flows with simultaneous measurement of physiologic variables such as vital organ perfusion pressures, oxygen delivery, and consumption.

These investigators studied the effect of epinephrine, in doses of 0.02, 0.2, and 2.0 mg/kg, on myocardial and cerebral blood flow *(67,68)*. Administration of 0.2 mg/kg was associated with significantly greater organ blood flows than the lowest dose. All agonists tested by Brown et al. improved myocardial O_2 delivery. Only epinephrine 0.2 mg/kg and norepinephrine 0.12 and 0.16 mg/kg, however, increased oxygen delivery to a greater degree than the increase in oxygen consumption. Cerebral blood flow and the rates of return of spontaneous circulation improved with higher dosages for all agonists except methoxamine. Although important, Brown's research was not definitive because long-term neurologic survival was not uniformly evaluated. Nevertheless, they demonstrated that there was a rational pharmacologic basis for use of these drugs during CPR. The dose–response curves and pharmacokinetics may be dramatically different from those during spontaneous circulation, but they are measurable.

Starting in 1987, Lindner et al. evaluated the effects of various epinephrine dosages on hemodynamics and oxygen utilization *(13,69–72)*. The results of these studies generally supported those of Brown et al. in that there was a dose–response relationship between epinephrine and vital organ blood flow and oxygen delivery. Lindner et al. however, found an optimal dosage lower than in the studies by Brown et al.

It seems intuitively reasonable to hypothesize that larger doses of epinephrine may be required as the arrest time increases. Dean and associates addressed this question indirectly when they measured regional blood flow during prolonged resuscitation and found that it declined markedly after 10–20 minutes, despite the continuous infusion of vasopressor *(73)*. Progressively larger infusions of epinephrine were needed to maintain myocardial blood flow late in resuscitation. This suggests that tachyphylaxis to adrenergic agonists occurs or that there is progressive derangement of the CPR circulatory pump mechanism, or both. During the 1980s laboratory studies indicated that higher doses of epinephrine might be effective in improving perfusion during CPR.

The pharmacology of higher epinephrine doses in humans was first studied by Gonzalez et al. *(74)*. They measured changes in radial artery pressure after intravenous administration of 1, 3, and 5 mg of epinephrine in patients who had failed standard therapy and had been transported to the hospital. Only the highest dose significantly raised relaxation-phase pressure. Paradis et al. compared the standard 1-mg dose to 0.2 mg/kg in patients who had failed conventional therapy, including standard dosages of epinephrine *(75)*. Coronary perfusion pressure increased only after administration of high-dose epinephrine. Although these studies were performed late in resuscitation, their applicability to the more important early therapy remains unclear. They do indicate, however, that continued use of 1 mg late in resuscitative efforts is without scientific basis.

Early human studies of high-dose epinephrine, which tended to be performed in patients who had failed conventional doses, reported improvements in variables such as coronary perfusion pressure and the rate of return of spontaneous circulation. In some of these studies, as well as many of the case reports, the patients' return of spontaneous circulation was temporally related to administration of high-dose epinephrine.

In the first well-designed, large clinical trial of high-dose epinephrine, Brown and associates compared 0.02 mg/kg to 0.2 mg/kg epinephrine in 1280 patients suffering out-of-hospital CA *(76)*. This study found no significant difference in clinical outcome between the two groups. In patients with a witnessed arrest, it took approx 17 minutes between the onset of arrest and the first epinephrine administration. Patients with unwitnessed arrest must have received the drug even later. The small number of patients who received their first dose of epinephrine within 10 minutes of CA had a trend toward a higher rate of survival to hospital discharge (23 vs 11%). Patients with electromechanical dissociation had return of spontaneous circulation rates of 47% with high-dose epinephrine vs 33% with standard-dose. These were post hoc subgroups, so the results should not be considered persuasive. There had been concern that administration of high-dose epinephrine might result in an increase in survivors with severe neurologic impairment, but this did not occur. The results in this study did not reach statistical significance, nor do they have statistical power. So we are unable, using this data set, to determine if high-dose epinephrine is better, worse, or the same as standard dose.

Callaham and associates performed a randomized, prospective, double-blind clinical trial comparing standard-dose epinephrine and high-dose epinephrine and norepinephrine in the treatment of prehospital CA *(77)*. They prospectively identified the outcome variables of interest as return of spontaneous circulation in the field, admission to hospital, hospital discharge, and Cerebral Performance Category score. Eight hundred and sixteen patients met inclusion criteria. Thirteen percent of patients receiving high-dose epinephrine regained a pulse in the field vs 8% of those receiving standard dose. Eighteen percent of high-dose epinephrine patients were admitted to the hospital compared to 10% of standard dose. Nevertheless, as in other large studies, there was no statistical difference in hospital discharge. No benefit of norepinephrine compared with high-dose epinephrine was found. High-dose epinephrine did not result in longer hospital or critical care unit stays. These investigators concluded that high-dose epinephrine significantly improves the rate of return of spontaneous circulation and hospital admission without increasing complications.

It is important to note that in the entire study population, 63% of the survivors were among the 11% of patients who were defibrillated by first responders. Therapies that are administered after failure of defibrillation are difficult to study because the sample sizes needed to demonstrate efficacy, or lack of efficacy, are so large.

Table 1
Original Data From the Nine Studies of Interest

Study	No. patients		Dose (mg)		ROSC (%)		Discharge (%)	
	HDE	SDE	HDE	SDE	HDE	SDE	HDE	SDE
Abramson	1456	1459	5,10,15	1	451 (31)	402 (26)	42 (2.9)	46 (3.2)
Brown	648	632	14	1.4	217 (33)	190 (30)	31 (4.8)	26 (4.1)
Callaham	286	260	15	1	37 (13)	22 (8)	5 (1.7)	3 (1.1)
Choux	271	265	5	1	96 (35)	85 (32)	11 (4.1)[a]	5 (1.9)[a]
Gueugniaud	1677	1650	5	1	678 (40)	601 (36)	38 (2.3)	46 (2.8)
Lindner	28	40	5	1	16 (57)	6 (15)	4 (14)	2 (5.0)
Lipman	19	16	10	1	15 (79)	11 (69)	0 (0)	4 (25)
Sherman	78	62	7	0.7	15 (19)	7 (11)	0 (0)	0 (0)
Stiell	317	333	7	1	56 (18)	76 (23)	10 (3.2)	16 (4.8)
Totals	4780	4717			1129 (24)	1003 (21)		

[a] These data are survival at 15 days, because discharge data was not available for this study.
HDE, high-dose epinephrine; SDE, standard-dose epinephrine; ROSC, return of spontaneous circulation.

The Brain Resuscitation Clinical Trial group (BRCT) studied more than 2000 CA patients *(78)*. These patients had either failed electrical countershock or presented with PEA or asystole. Patients were randomly assigned to three doses of either standard- or escalating high-dose epinephrine (5 mg, 10 mg, and 15 mg). Return of spontaneous circulation occurred in 28% of patients receiving standard-dose vs 31% of those receiving escalating high-dose epinephrine. Again, however, high-dose epinephrine resulted in a significant improvement in short-term resuscitation, but did not show a beneficial effect on long-term outcome.

There have now been more than half a dozen randomized clinical trials of high-dose epinephrine. Two recent meta-analyses have attempted to make some sense of this pool of data. Vandycke et al. identified and reviewed five clinical trials with a total of 6339 *(79)*, although Paradis et al. chose broader inclusion criteria and reviewed nine studies for a total of 9497 (Table 1). Paradis notes that there is a small increase in return of spontaneous circulation in the high-dose epinephrine vs standard-dose epinephrine groups, with a number needed to treat of 27, that is, utilization of high-dose epinephrine vs standard-dose epinephrine will cause an additional one return of spontaneous circulation per 27 patients treated. However, neither meta-analysis demonstrated an increase in survival to hospital discharge or improvement in neurological outcome, and Paradis analysis indicated that high-dose epinephrine may slightly decrease the odds of survival.

Alternative Catecholamines: Phenylephrine

As discussed, laboratory studies indicate that it is epinephrine α-adrenergic stimulation that appears to be important in CA. This makes pure α-adrenergic agents, such as phenylephrine or methoxamine, attractive drugs in the treatment of CA. Because of methoxamine's longer half-life, which can result in organ hypoperfusion postresuscitation, we limit our discussion of alternative catecholamines to phenylephrine.

Phenylephrine is a short-acting selective α-adrenergic agonist. It is used as a pressor during anesthesia in patients with spontaneous circulation. Its receptor profile and short half-life make it a theoretically attractive drug for the treatment of CA. The potential of this drug to increase aortic pressure without significant myocardial excitation may be optimal for entities such as VF. Its short half-life provides flexibility in the postresuscitation period during which many patients may not need pressor support.

Animal studies indicate that, compared to placebo, it raises CPR perfusion pressure, the fraction of animals with return of spontaneous circulation, as well as short-term survival. The theoretical benefits of selective α-agonism, as compared to mixed α- and β-agonist such as epinephrine, however, have not been clearly demonstrated. Nevertheless, in situations in which excessive α-receptor stimulation might be contraindicated, such as CA complicating myocardial infarction (MI), phenylephrine is an attractive pressor.

The first studies of phenylephrine were undertaken by Redding and Pearson (25). Their realization that vasoconstriction was important in achieving return of spontaneous circulation led them to study all available pressors, including phenylephrine, metaraminol, and methoxamine. In their asphyxial-electromechanical dissociation model, 10 mg of intracardiac phenylephrine, a dose selected on "theoretical grounds and pilot experiments," resulted in return of spontaneous circulation in 80–90% of animals. In a VF model, they achieved 100% return of spontaneous circulation.

Joyce et al. administered 5 mg of phenylephrine to dogs in an asphyxial-electromechanical dissociation model and found that it raised aortic diastolic pressure and that all animals were resuscitated (80). Holmes, however, found that a dose of 0.05 mg/kg actually lowered cerebral blood flow compared to placebo (65). Brown studied the effect of phenylephrine on myocardial and cerebral blood flows in a porcine VF model (81,82), and found that dosages of 0.1 and 1.0 mg/kg did not significantly improve hemodynamics. A dosage of 10 mg/kg improved aortic diastolic pressure and central blood flow by amounts similar to those with a high dose of epinephrine. Berkowitz found that phenylephrine was able to maintain CPR hemodynamics and oxygen utilization as effectively as epinephrine (42,83). Schleien, using a model with a very short arrest time, had return of spontaneous circulation in 73% of animals, and 100% in a model with 8 minutes of CA (42,84). Brillman had return of spontaneous circulation in 78% of animals using a dose of 10 mg (85). A subsequent study with the same dose had a 75% return of spontaneous circulation and 50% 24-hour survival (27). Ditchey et al. recently observed that the balance between myocardial oxygen supply and demand during CPR could be improved by administering a combination of phenylephrine and propranolol, and that pre-arrest β-blockade improved perfusion pressure (22,86).

Despite the theoretical advantages of phenylephrine, only a single clinical study has been reported (87), the interpretation of which is complicated by a crossover design in which all patients unresponsive to initial therapy received epinephrine. The ultimate rates of return of spontaneous circulation were 31 and 28% for phenylephrine and epinephrine, respectively. The investigators were of the opinion that there were no adverse reactions in patients who had initially received phenylephrine. Unfortunately, this study also used what may have been subtherapeutic and nonequipressor doses of each drug: 1 mg of phenylephrine and 0.5 mg of epinephrine. Significant variability in the effective dose in different laboratories precludes recommendation of a specific dosage. An initial dose of 10 mg appears reasonable. Doses as high as 10 mg/kg, have some basis according to the literature, but until additional clinical trials are performed, the inability to recommend a particular dosage may limit phenylephrine's use. Because this is a generic drug additional research on its efficacy or dosage is unlikely.

Vasopressin: An Endogenous Stress Hormone

A number of fundamental endocrine responses of the human body to CA and CPR have been investigated in the past 10 years *(88–90)*. Circulating endogenous vasopressin concentrations were high in patients undergoing CPR, and levels in successfully resuscitated patients have been shown to be significantly higher than in patients who died *(78)*. This may indicate that the human body discharges vasopressin as an adjunct vasopressor to epinephrine in life-threatening situations such as CA in order to preserve homeostasis. In a clinical study of 60 out-of-hospital CA patients, parallel increases in plasma vasopressin and endothelin during CPR were found only in surviving patients. Both before and after epinephrine administration, plasma epinephrine and norepinephrine concentrations were significantly higher in patients who died when compared with surviving CA victims *(12)*. Thus, plasma concentrations of vasopressin may have a more important effect on CPR outcome than previously thought; and prompted several investigations to assess its role for possible CPR management in order to improve CPR management.

Physiology of Vasopressin

Arginine vasopressin, a hormone that is called antidiuretic hormone as well, has a long evolutionary history. With the emergence of life on land, vasopressin became the mediator of a remarkable reguatory system for the conversation of water. It is an endogenous hormone with osmoregulatory, vasopressor, hemostatic, and central nervous effects. Arginine vasopressin is produced in the magnocellular nuclei of the hypothalamus, and stored in neurosecretory vesicles of the neurohypophysis. The hormone is secreted on osmotic, hemodynamic, and endocrinologic stimuli. Baroreceptor-mediated arginine vasopresin secretion is the primary stimulation release in hypotensive states *(91)*. In plasma, arginine vasopressin is bound to proteins in a concentrations, which ranges from approx 2 to approx 8 pg/mL; serum half-life time varies between approx 8 and approx 15 minutes. Splanchnic and renal enzymatic degradation are primary pathways of inactivation.

Natural vasopressin is a nonapeptide with two cysteine residues forming a bridge between positions 1 and 6. The integrity of this disulfid bond is essential for its biological activity, and amino acid substitutions dictate physiologic actions such as alterations of antidiuretic, or vasopressor function (Table 2). Interestingly, vasopressor effects were observed as early as 1895; it is noteworthy that vasopressin acts directly via V_1-receptors on contractile elements—an effect that can not be reversed by adrenergic blockade or denervation *(92)*. Primary indication of vasopressin and its analogues so far is management of hypothalamic diabetes insipidus, and treating bleeding esophageal varices in some cases.

Vasopressin Receptors

Peripheral effects of arginine vasopressin are mediated by different vasopressin receptors; namely V_1-(V_{1a}), V_2- (V_2), and V_3- (V_{1b}) vasopressin-receptors *(93)*. V_1-receptors have been found in arterial blood vessels, and induce vasoconstriction by an increase in cytoplasmatic ionized calcium via the phosphatidyl–inositol–bisphosphonate cascade *(93)*. In contrast to catecholamine-mediated vasoconstriction, effects of arginine vasopressin are preserved during hypoxia and severe acidosis *(94)*. Physiologically, most arterial beds exhibit vasoconstriction in response to arginine vasopressin *(95,96)*.

Table 2
Vasopressin Analogues With Differences in Their Pharmacologic Profile

Peptide	Simplified amino acid structure	Activity in relation to arginine vasopressin		Comment
		Antidiuretic-effect	Vasopressor-effect	
Arginine vasopressin	Cys-Tyr-Phe-Glu-Asp-Cys-Pro-**L-Arg**-Gly-(NH$_2$)	100	100	ADH/AVP (Pitressin®) (mammals)
Lysine vasopressin	Cys-Tyr-Phe-Glu-Asp-Cys-Pro-**Lys**-Gly-(NH$_2$)	80	60	LVP (Lypressin®) (pigs)
Oxytocin	Cys-Tyr-**Ile**-Glu-Asp-Cys-Pro-**Leu**-Gly-(NH$_2$)	1	1	induces myometrical contractions
Ornithine vasopressin	Cys-Tyr-Phe-Glu-Asp-Cys-Pro-**Orn**-Gly-(NH$_2$)	22	90	POR 8®, esophageal varices
DDAVP	Cys-Tyr-Phe-Glu-Asp-Cys-Pro-**D-Arg**-Gly-(NH$_2$)	1200	0.39	Desmopressin®, increases Factor VIII

Chemical structures and affinity of arginine vasopressin analogues. All peptides shown have disulfid bonds between amino acids on position one and eight. Terlipressin is degraded into lysine vasopressin. ADH, antidiuretic hormone; AVP, arginine vasopressin; LVP, lysine vasopressin; DDAVP, 1-desamino-8-D arginine vasopressin. (Adapted from ref. 91a.)

Similar to oxytocin-mediated paradoxical vasodilatation of vascular smooth muscle, vasodilatation after arginine vasopressin has been described in the pulmonary, coronary, and vertebrobasilar circulation *(97–99)*. The underlying mechanisms seem to be nitric oxide-dependent *(97,100)*. Recently, there is increasing evidence of hemodynamically relevant V_1-receptors on cardiomyocytes. In vitro and animal experiments have demonstrated an increase of intracellular calcium concentration and inotropy after stimulation of myocardial V_1-receptors *(101,102)*.

Hemodynamic Effects of Vasopressin During CPR in Animal Models

During VF, a dose–response investigation of three vasopressin dosages (0.2, 0.4, 0.8 U/kg) compared with the maximum effective dose of 200 µg/kg epinephrine showed that 0.8 U/kg vasopressin was the most effective drug in regards of increasing vital organ blood flow *(103)*. Also, vasopressin significantly improved cerebral oxygen delivery, and VF mean frequency during CPR when compared with a maximum dose of epinephrine *(104)*. Furthermore, effects of vasopressin on vital organ blood flow lasted longer after vasopressin than after epinephrine (approx 4 vs approx 1.5 min); significantly more vasopressin animals could be resuscitated; and vasopressin did not result in bradycardia after return of spontaneous circulation *(105)*. Interestingly, the combination of vasopressin and epinephrine vs vasopressin only resulted in comparable left ventricular (LV) myocardial blood flow, but in significantly decreased cerebral perfusion (Fig.1, *[106]*). The binding of both vasopressin and epinephrine to its receptors causes characteristic changes such as intracellular concentration of phosphatidylinositol and calcium *(107,108)*. In fact, a rodent study evaluating administration of vasopressin, norepinephine, and a combination of vasopressin and norepinephrine showed that V_1- and α-adrenergic receptors saturated the same intracellular transduction pathway *(94)*. Although speculative, this mechanism may have hampered nitric oxide release in the cerebral vasculature induced by vasopressin, and therefore, suppressed cerebral perfusion in our animals receiving a combination of vasopressin and epinephrine. These results are striking because epinephrine selectively spares the cerebral circulation from vasoconstriction when administered during CPR alone.

Drug Delivery Routes of Vasopressin During CPR

Administration of endobronchial drugs during CPR may be a simple and rapid alternative, when intubation is performed before intravenous cannulation *(109)*, and the time interval for intravenous access is prolonged, or when attempts for intravenous access are simply unsuccessful, such as in young children with poor peripheral perfusion. A laboratory model showed that the same dose of intravenous and endobronchial vasopressin resulted into the same coronary perfusion pressure 4 minutes after drug administration (Fig 2.; *110*). This investigation showed that endobronchial vasopressin is absorbed during CPR, increased coronary perfusion pressure significantly within a very short period, and increased the chance of successful resuscitation *(110)*. In contrast, in an animal model the equipotent endobronchial epinephrine dose is approx 10 times higher than the intravenous epinephrine dose during CPR *(66)*. However, endobronchial drug administration may be less appropriate in children, who suffer CA as a result of respiratory disorders. For example, in children suffering CA mostly as a result of severe pneumonia, endobronchial drug delivery is not likely to result in adequate drug absorption, and therefore, may be rather ineffective. In such cases, the endobronchial drug delivery route may render drug absorption erratic as a result of pulmonary oedema and capillary

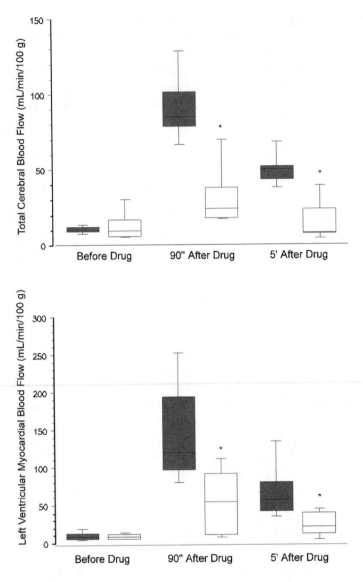

Fig. 1. Combination of vasopressin and epinephrine on left ventricular myocardial blood and cerebral perfusion pressure.

leak, and therefore, may further compromise oxygenation and ventilation in children. Acordingly, the intraosseous route has been recommended for pediatric emergency situations, and is widely taught both in the Americas and internationally by the Paediatric Advanced Life Support and Advanced Trauma Life Support courses (*111*). Additionally, hypovolemia can be rapidly corrected with fluids via an intraosseous catheter, but not via the endobronchial route. Therefore, intraosseous vasopressin may be a valuable alternative for vasopressor administration during CPR, when intravenous access is delayed, or not available. Accordingly, our laboratory studies indicate that the same vasopressin dosage may be administered intravenously, endobronchially, and intraosseously, rendering usage of this vasopressor during CPR simple, rapid, and inexpensive.

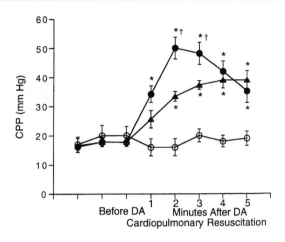

Fig. 2. Intravenous vs endobronchial basopressin.

Repeated Administration of Vasopressin and Epinephrine

Both the AHA and European Resuscitation Council continue to recommend repeated administration of epinephrine during advanced cardiac life support (ACLS; *113,114*), although it is not proven whether repeated epinephrine given during CPR may be effective, or if this strategy may even result in inadvertent catecholamine toxicity. Repeated dosages of vasopressin vs epinephrine were administered, coronary perfusion pressure increased only after the first of three epinephrine injection, but increased after each of three vasopressin injections; accordingly, all vasopressin animals survived, and all pigs resuscitated with epinephrine died *(115)*. Long-term survival after CA may be determined by the ability to ensure adequate organ perfusion during CPR, and in the postresuscitation phase. In the early postresuscitation phase, vasopressin administration resulted in higher arterial blood pressure, but a lower cardiac index; a reversible depressant effect on myocardial function of the vasopressin pigs was observed when compared with epinephrine. However, overall cardiovascular function was not irreversibly or critically impaired after the administration of vasopressin *(116)*. Renal and splanchnic perfusion may be critically impaired during *(117,118)* and after *(119)* successful resuscitation from CA. For example, 30 minutes after return of spontaneous circulation, renal and adrenal blood flow were significantly lower in the vasopressin pigs as compared with the epinephrine group; pancreatic, intestinal, and hepatic blood flow were not significantly different in animals after receiving epinephrine or vasopressin *(120)*.

Renal and Splanchnic Perfusion After Vasopressin

It is unknown whether the vasopressin-mediated pronounced blood shift during CPR from the muscle, skin, and gut toward the myocardium and brain might be deleterious for splanchnic organs, and whether this may contribute to multiorgan failure after return of spontaneous circulation. Furthermore, it is unknown whether a high bolus dose of vasopressin administered during CPR may result in oliguria or anuria as a result of its antidiuretic effects in the postresuscitation phase. In a porcine CPR investigation, vasopressin impaired cephalic mesenteric blood flow during CPR and in the early postresuscitation phase, but did not result in an antidiuretic response. Neither renal blood flow, nor renal function was influenced by vasopressin or epinephrine in this investigation *(121)*.

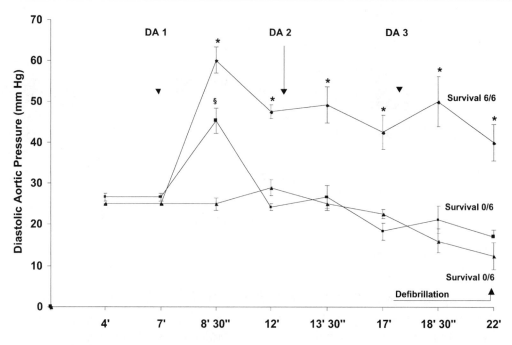

Fig. 3. Vasopressin vs rpinephrine vs saline placebo during prolonged CPR.

Continuous infusion of low-dose dopamine mediated a significant increase in superior mesenteric blood flow after successful CPR with vasopressin by selective vasodilatation of intestinal vessels. Accordingly, administering dopamine may improve gut perfusion, and therefore, may improve gut function in the postresuscitation period *(122)*.

Effects of Vasopressin on Neurological Recovery After CPR

In laboratory investigations of short *(103)* and prolonged *(105)* CA, vasopressin resulted in significantly higher vital organ blood flow and cerebral oxygen delivery than did epinephrine. This implies that vasopressin dilated cerebral arterioles and subsequently, resulted in superior brain perfusion throughout the neuroaxis. In the vasopressin animals, the superior cerebral blood flow lead to a greater cerebral oxygen consumption, but was not the result of an over stimulation of metabolism because cerebral oxygen extraction fell, and oxygen uptake became independent of oxygen delivery *(106)*. The question arises, if increased cerebral blood flow during CPR with vasopressin is beneficial in regards of neurological recovery, or detrimental as a result of fatal complications such as cerebral oedema after return of spontaneous circulation. Although a Glasgow-Coma Score rating was performed after successful CPR with vasopressin vs epinephrine in preliminary clinical studies, the results could unfortunately not be attributed to a single CPR-intervention as a result of many confounding variables. In a porcine model simulating prolonged (22 minutes) of ACLS, all vasopressin animals had return of spontaneous circulation, and all pigs in the epinephrine and saline placebo group died (Fig. 3). After 24 hours of return of spontaneous circulation, the only neurologic deficit of all vasopressin pigs was an unsteady gait, which disappeared within another 3 days *(123)*. This observation confirms that in order to achieve full recovery after CA, both excellent management of basic and ACLS, and careful optimization of organ function in the postresuscitation phase are of fundamental importance *(124)*. Although neurodiag-nostic tests such as evoked potentials, electroencephalogram, or positron emission tomography may not be able to accurately detect pathology *(125)*, we employed cerebral magnetic resonance imaging after successful CPR. Although imaging was performed 4 days after the experiment to ensure that cerebral ischemic regions as a result of extracellular edema would be fully developed, the absence of cerebral cortical and subcortical edema, intraparenchymal hemorrhage, ischemic brain lesions, or cerebral infarction confirmed by T2-weighted magnetic resonance imaging indicates that the vasopressin pigs fully recovered from CA in regards of both anatomical and physiological terms. Thus, laboratory evidence suggests that vasopressin given during CPR may be a superior drug when compared with epinephrine in order to ensure both return of spontaneous circulation and neurological outcome.

Vasopressin as a Continuous Infusion During Vasodilatory Shock

The standard treatment of vasodilatory septic shock includes antibiotics, extracellular volume expansion, vasopressors, and drugs that increase myocardial contractility. Adrenergic catecholamines employed in this setting such as norepinephrine often have a diminished vasopressor action in vasodilatory shock; therefore, alternatives may be very useful. First reports with vasopressin in septic shock described a patient who was successfully resuscitated from CA, but subsequently developed bacterial septicemia, and needed a continuous infusion of both epinephrine and norepinephrine to maintain systolic arterial pressure of approx 90 mmHg. Continuous infusion of vasopressin (0.04 U per minute) then easily improved mean arterial blood pressure, cardiac output remained stable, and urine output increased from approx 6 to more than 50 mL per hour. Stepwise withdrawal of vasopressin subsequently resulted in a decrease in arterial pressure, which again required norepinephrine to maintain systolic arterial pressure at 90–100 mmHg; urine output decreased to 30 mL per hour. Six hours later, systolic arterial pressure was maintained at approx 105 mmHg on vasopressin alone *(126)*. In patients with vasodilatory shock after LV assist device placement or postbypass vasodilatory shock, vasopressin (0.1 U per minute) increased mean arterial pressure, although norepinephrine was decreased *(127,128)*. In the latter study, inappropriately low serum vasopressin concentrations were found before vasopressin administration, indicating endogenous vasopressin deficiency. Thus, it is possible that endogenous vasopressin stores in these patients were simply depleted, or not able to meet the demand to maintain cardiocirculatory homeostasis. Another investigation studying patients on amiodarone and angiotensin-converting enzyme inhibitors with refractory vasodilatation after cardiopulmonary bypass revealed a beneficial potential for continuous vasopressin infusion *(129)*. Similar observations were made in patients with milrinone-induced hypotension, when 0.03 to 0.07 U per minute vasopressin caused an increase in systolic artery pressure from approx 90 to approx 130 mmHg *(130)*. In our experience, 2–4 IU per hour vasopressin as a continuous infusion works best.

These observations may be similar to first experiences in CA patients, when high endogenous vasopressin levels correlated with subsequent survival *(131)*. As such, it is likely that vasopressin as well as the well-established endogenous stress hormone epinephrine plays an important role in regards of arterial blood pressure regulation during shock states such as septicemia, and CPR. Currently, we do not exactly know whether vasopressin acts simply as a backup of the backup vasopressor epinephrine during life-threatening shock states, whether vasopressin or epinephrine alone is better in certain situations, or whether these two hormones have unique adjunct features that we are only starting to understand. A better knowledge of these underlying mechanisms most likely would save many patients—who at this point in time have a relatively small chance to survive.

Clinical Experience With Arginine Vasopressin During Cardiac Arrest

In patients with refractory CA, arginine vasopressin induced an increase in arterial blood pressure, and in some cases, return of spontaneous circulation, in which standard therapy with chest compressions, ventilation, defibrillation, and epinephrine had failed *(132)*. In a small (*N* = 40) prospective, randomized investigation of patients with out-of-hospital VF, a significantly larger proportion of patients treated with arginine vasopressin were successfully resuscitated and survived 24 hours compared with patients treated with epinephrine *(30)*. This was not designed as a mortality study, but even with such small numbers, there was a nonsignificant trend toward an improvement in hospital discharge rate (*p* = 0.16). In a large (*N* = 200) in-hospital CPR trial from Ottawa, Canada, comparable short-term survival was found in both groups treated with either vasopressin or epinephrine, indicating that these drugs may be equipotent when response times of rescuers are short *(133)*. In another clinical evaluation in Detroit, Michigan, 4 of 10 patients responded to arginine vasopressin administration after approx 45 minutes of unsuccessful ACLS, and had a mean increase in coronary perfusion pressure of 28 mmHg *(134)*. This is surprising, because an arterial blood pressure increase with any drug after such a long period of noneffective CPR management would be normally not expeeted. In this study, arginine vasopressin caused an increase in coronary perfusion pressure, and a decrease of epinephrine plasma levels, which is similar to an animal study with increased vital organ blood flow, but decreased catecholamine plasma levels after arginine vasopressin *(135)*. Although speculative, it is possible that baroreceptors in the arterial vasculature registered increased organ perfusion after vasopressin, and subsequently down-regulated endogenous catecholamine secretion—whether this may decrease epinephrine tachyphylaxis and therefore, improve subsequent catecholamine effects, remains under investigation.

A NEW APPROACH: A COMBINATION OF VASOPRESSIN AND EPINEPHRINE

In an experimental model of asphyxia CA in adult, we found that a combination of arginine vasopressin with epinephrine was superior to either arginine vasopressin alone, or epinephrine alone (Fig. 4; *136*). This observation is entirely new and surprising, and may suggest that the usual approach of pharmacological CPR management to administer identical drugs and dosages for patients presenting with CA as a result of dysrhythmia or asphyxia may have to be reconsidered. In fact, it is possible that when the degree of ischemia is fundamental such as during asphyxia, or ACLS is prolonged, a combination of arginine vasopressin with epinephrine could be beneficial. The laboratory experience of this phenomenon may be confirmed by observations from CPR efforts in eight patients who were unsuccessfully resuscitated with epinephrine for approx 10 to 20 minutes, subsequently received 40 units of arginine vasopressin, and subsequently, all patients had return of spontaneous circulation, with three of eight patients being even discharged alive from the hospital *(30)*. This explanation would be in agreement with a Canadian study *(133)*

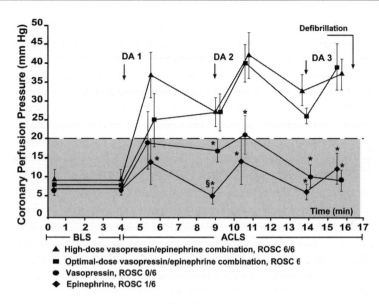

Fig. 4. Asphyxia.

indicating comparable outcome with arginine vasopressin vs epinephrine in in-hospital CA, with a short time of ischemia.

Thus, our usual strategy according to the current CPR guidelines of employing vasopressors during CPR may not sufficiently address the cause of CA, and degree of ischemia. Accordingly, it is possible that the ideal vasopressor and especially, the ideal dosing regimen for CPR is yet to be discovered, rendering a combination of agents possibly necessary; however, development of a CPR "cocktail" may be extremely difficult as a result of multiple potential permutations of different drugs and dosages whenever a combination therapy is employed *(137)*. Laboratory experiments were performed with a combination of arginine vasopressin, epinephrine, and nitroglycerin; however, determining optimal dose–response effects is most likely difficult, and clinical experience is pending *(138)*. Furthermore, vasopressors that improve initial resuscitation may not be the best drugs to improve survival in the postresuscitation phase. The ideal vasopressor for CPR is a drug that significantly increases myocardial and cerebral perfusion during CPR, and yet, if necessary, can be rapidly, but titratibly reversed in the immediate postresuscitation phase *(139)*.

The European Vasopressin Study

From June 1999 to March 2002, we conducted a large multicenter trial in Austria, Germany, and Switzerland, and randomized 1219 out-of-hospital CA patients. Hospital admission and discharge rates were comparable between treatment arms for patients with VF and for PEA, but patients with asystole were more likely to survive when treated with vasopressin. However, if patients could not be successfully resuscitated with the study drugs, additional epinephrine (median dose 5 mg, interquartile range 2–10 mg) significantly ($p = 0.007$) improved hospital admission and discharge in patients who were initially treated with vasopressin first, but not in epinephrine-treated patients. There was no difference in cerebral performance between groups for the entire trial. Our results did not confirm earlier data showing vasopressin to be more effective than epinephrine in the treatment of VF and PEA. Unfortunately, we are unable to state whether this phenomenon may be similar to the observations described with high-dose epinephrine during CPR, when increasing epinephrine dosages were effective in the laboratory, but not in clinical practice. It is clearly a principal problem to extrapolate laboratory CPR to the clinical setting, since species' differences, comparing diseased patients with healthy laboratory animals, or differences in out-of-hospital CPR compared to laboratory conditions are hardly controllable factors of influence.

In contrast to VF and PEA, vasopressin improved the likelihood of asystolic patients reaching the hospital alive in the multicenter study by about 40% over epinephrine. A possible explanation may be the profound ischemia in the asystolic patients. This is in accordance with an in vitro study, where it was demonstrated that vasopressin has vasoconstricting efficacy even in severe acidosis, when catecholamines are less potent. Thus, vasopressin may be more effective than epinephrine in asystolic patients, thereby resulting in better coronary perfusion pressure during cardiac resuscitation. Because improved coronary perfusion pressure during CPR improves survival, vasopressin may be a better option than epinephrine for asystolic patients, who normally have the worst chance of survival. This post hoc observation should be tested in a prospective trial restricted to such patients for whom few treatment options are available. Also, improvement in hospital discharge after treatment with epinephrine following the vasopressin may indicate that the interactions among vasopressin, epinephrine, and the underlying degree of ischemia during CPR may be more complex than was previously thought. When prolonged asphyxia had depleted endogenous epinephrine levels and caused fundamental ischemia in pigs, vasopressin combined with epinephrine tripled coronary perfusion pressure over either epinephrine or vasopressin alone. This suggests that the presence of vasopressin may enhance the effects of epinephrine or vice-versa, especially during prolonged ischemia. These laboratory CPR data are in agreement with the European clinical trial, when about 25 minutes after collapse, at a time that a severe degree of ischemia must be assumed, vasopressin followed by epinephrine was effective, whereas increasing dosages of epinephrine alone were not.

Although half of the survivors with good neurological outcome received the combination of vasopressin and epinephrine, this strategy also resulted in more, albeit not statistically significant, patients in coma than after epinephrine alone. This indicates that the combination of vasopressin and epinephrine effectively resuscitated the heart, but was too late to resuscitate the brain in some patients. When starting CPR, it is difficult to predict postresuscitation brain function. Although our hospital discharge rate (9.7%) compares favorably with that in other reports, 2.2% of our patients had severe neurological impairment. It has to be stated that combining vasopressin and epinephrine improved survival rates, but resulted in unfavorable neurological outcome in some patients. This strategy resulted into unfavorable neurological outcome in 5 of 10 patients who were first found to be in asystole or PEA; in contrast, no asystole or PEA patient receiving 3 mg or more of epinephrine had unfavorable neurological outcome because they simply all died before being discharged. Whether combining vasopressin and epinephrine is beneficial, especially when administered earlier as in our investigation, needs to be confirmed in a prospective study, which is currently on its way in France. Naturally, there is no doubt that we are not doing anybody a favor if we only increase the number of surviving patients with unfavorable neurological outcome. According to the new data from the European vasopressin study, we suggest administering 1 mg epinephrine followed alternately by

1 mg epinephrine and 40 IU vasopressin every 3 minutes in adult cardiac arrest victims, regardless of the initial electrocardiogram rhythm *(147)*.

THE FUTURE OF VASOPRESSORS IN CPR MANAGEMENT

We have shown beneficial effects of arginine vasopressin vs epinephrine in special CPR situations such as epidural anesthesia *(140)*, hypothermia *(141)*, and hypovolemic shock *(143,144)* in the laboratory. In the clinical setting, we observed positive effects of arginine vasopressin in some patients with life-threatening hemorrhagic shock with collapsing arterial blood pressure, who did not respond anymore to adrenergic catecholamines. Although these observations in the laboratory and in individual patients are very promising, they have to be yet confirmed in prospective, randomized clinical trials; however, as a result of the relatively rare occurrence of these special CPR situations, it is unlikely that arginine vasopressin can be studied systematically under these circumstances.

Another area that is extremely complicated to investigate, but definitely needs to be addressed, is the pediatric CA population. As a result of the lack of randomized clinical trials in pediatric emergency cardiac care, some CPR recommendations had to be extrapolated from adult or even laboratory studies. In a porcine preparation, epinephrine was superior to arginine vasopressin in a pediatric CPR model of asphyxia CA *(145)*. We have shown in this pediatric model that a combination of arginine vasopressin and epinephrine was superior to either arginine vasopressin or epinephrine alone; however, this may only apply to pediatric but not adult settings, and definitely warrants especially clinical investigations.

REFERENCES

1. Standards for cardiopulmonary resuscitation (CPR) and emergency cardiac care (ECC). 3. Advanced life support. JAMA 1974; 227(Suppl):852–860.
2. Gottlieb R. Ueber die Wirkung der Nebennierenextrakt auf Herz und Blutdruck. Arch f Exp Path u Pharm Leipzig 1896; 38:99–112.
3. Beck C, Rand HI. Cardiac arrest during anaesthesia and surgery. JAMA 1949; 141:1230–1233.
4. Bodon C. The intracardiac injection of epinephrine. Lancet 1923; 1:586.
5. Gerbode F. The cardiac emergency. Ann.Surg. 1952; 135:431.
6. McCarthy KC. The problem of cardiac arrest. JAMA 1958; 168:2101–2103.
7. Wortsman J, Frank S, Cryer PE. Adrenomedullary response to maximal stress in humans. Am J Med 1984; 77:779–784.
8. Redding JS, Haynes RR, Thomas JD. Drug therapy in resuscitation from electromechanical dissociation. Crit Care Med 1983; 11:681–684.
9. Berridge MJ. Phosphatidylinositol hydrolysis and calcium signaling. Adv Cyclic Nucleotide Res 1981; 14:289–299.
10. Exton JH. Mechanisms involved in alpha-adrenergic phenomena: role of calcium ions in actions of catecholamines in liver and other tissues. Am J Physiol 1980; 238:E3–E12.
11. Gierschig P, Jakops, K,H,. Mechanism for inhibition of adenylate cyclase by alpha-2 adrenergic receptors. In: The alpha-2 adrenergic receptors. Limberd LE, ed. New York: Clifton, 1988, pp. 75–113.
12. Ahlquist. A study of the adrenotropic receptors. Am J Physiol 1948; 153:586–600.
13. Lindner KH, Ahnefeld FW, Bowdler IM. Comparison of different doses of epinephrine on myocardial perfusion and resuscitation success during cardiopulmonary resuscitation in a pig model. Am J Emerg Med 1991; 9:27–31.
14. Ditchey RV, Winkler JV, Rhodes CA. Relative lack of coronary blood flow during closed-chest resuscitation in dogs. Circulation 1982; 66:297–302.
15. Michael JR, Guerci AD, Koehler RC, et al. Mechanisms by which epinephrine augments cerebral and myocardial perfusion during cardiopulmonary resuscitation in dogs. Circulation 1984; 69:822–835.
16. Niemann JT, Rosborough JP, Ung S, Criley JM. Coronary perfusion pressure during experimental cardiopulmonary resuscitation. Ann Emerg Med 1982; 11:127–131.

17. Paradis NA, Martin GB, Rivers EP, et al. Coronary perfusion pressure and the return of spontaneous circulation in human cardiopulmonary resuscitation. JAMA 1990; 263:1106–1113.
18. Redding JS, Pearson JW. Resuscitation from ventricular fibrillation. Drug therapy. JAMA 1968; 203: 255–260.
19. Pearson JW, Redding, J.S. Influence of peripheral vascular tone on cardiac resuscitation. Anesth Analg 1967; 46:746–752.
20. Otto CW, Yakaitis RW, Blitt CD. Mechanism of action of epinephrine in resuscitation from asphyxial arrest. Crit Care Med 1981; 9:321–324.
21. Yakaitis RW, Otto CW, Blitt CD. Relative importance of alpha and beta adrenergic receptors during resuscitation. Crit Care Med 1979; 7:293–296.
22. Ditchey RV, Slinker BK. Phenylephrine plus propranolol improves the balance between myocardial oxygen supply and demand during experimental cardiopulmonary resuscitation. Am Heart J 1994; 127: 324–30.
23. Crile GW, Dolley DH. An experimental research into the resuscitation of dogs killed by anaestheitics and asphyxia. J Exp Med 1906; 8:713–724.
24. Pearson JW, Redding, J.S. The role of epinephrine in cardiac resuscitation. Anesth Analg 1963; 42: 599–606.
25. Pearson JW, Redding JS. Peripheral vascular tone on cardiac resuscitation. Anesth Analg 1965; 44:746–752.
26. Redding JS. Evaluation of drugs for cardiac resuscitation. Anesth 1963; 24:203–207.
27. Brillman J, Sanders A, Otto CW, et al. Comparison of epinephrine and phenylephrine for resuscitation and neurologic outcome of cardiac arrest in dogs. Ann Emerg Med 1987; 16:11–17.
28. Arnold A. Sympathomimetic amine-induced responses of effectors organs subserved by alpha, beta-1, and beta-2 adrenoreceptors. In: Adrenergic Activators and Inhibitors. Handbook of Experimental Pharmacology. Vol. 54/I. Szkekeres, ed. Heidelberg: Springer-Verlag, 1980.
29. Trendelenberg U, Weiner, N. Catecholamines. Handbook of Experimental Pharmacology. Vol. 90/1. Heidelberg: Springer-Verlag, 1988.
30. Lindner KH, Dirks B, Strohmenger HU, et al. Randomised comparison of epinephrine and vasopressin in patients with out-of-hospital ventricular fibrillation. Lancet 1997; 349:535–537.
31. Starke K, Endo T, Taube HD. Relative pre- and postsynaptic potencies of alpha-adrenoceptor agonists in the rabbit pulmonary artery. Naunyn Schmiedebergs Arch Pharmacol 1975; 291:55–78.
32. Szkekeres. Adrenergic activators and inhibitors. Handbook of Experimental Pharmacology. Vol. 54/I. Heidelberg: Springer-Verlag, 1980.
33. Weiner N. Norepinephrine, epinephrine and the sympathomimetic amines. In: Goodman and Gilman's: The Pharmacological Basis of Therapeutics. Gilman AG, Goodman, L.S., eds. New York: MacMillan, 1980, pp. 138–175.
34. Woodhouse SP, Case, C., Cox, S. High and standard dose of adrenaline do not alter survival compared with placebo in cardiac arrest. Resusciation 1995; 30:243–290.
35. Guyatt GH, Sackett DL, Cook DJ. Users' guides to the medical literature. II. How to use an article about therapy or prevention. B. What were the results and will they help me in caring for my patients? Evidence-Based Medicine Working Group. JAMA 1994; 271:59–63.
36. Parker EA, Boomer RJ, Bell SC. Parenteral incompatibilities—past, present and future. Bull Parenter Drug Assoc 1967; 21:197–207.
37. Bonhomme L, Benhamou D, Comoy E, Preaux N. Stability of epinephrine in alkalinized solutions. Ann Emerg Med 1990; 19:1242–1244.
38. Yakaitis RW, Ewy GA, Otto CW, et al. Influence of time and therapy on ventricular defibrillation in dogs. Crit Care Med 1980; 8:157–163.
39. Niemann JT, Cairns CB, Sharma J, Lewis RJ. Treatment of prolonged ventricular fibrillation. Immediate countershock versus high-dose epinephrine and CPR preceding countershock. Circulation 1992; 85:281–287.
40. DeBehnke DJ, Angelos MG, Leasure JE. Use of cardiopulmonary bypass, high-dose epinephrine, and standard-dose epinephrine in resuscitation from post-countershock electromechanical dissociation. Ann Emerg Med 1992; 21:1051–1057.
41. Koide T, Wieloch TW, Siesjo BK. Circulating catecholamines modulate ischemic brain damage. J Cereb Blood Flow Metab 1986; 6:559–565.
42. Gervais HW, Schleien CL, Koehler RC, et al. Effect of adrenergic drugs on cerebral blood flow, metabolism, and evoked potentials after delayed cardiopulmonary resuscitation in dogs. Stroke 1991; 22:1554–1561.

43. Freedman BJ. Accidential adrenaline overdoosage and its treatment with piperoxan. Lancet 1955; 2: 575–578.
44. Hall AH, Kulig KW, Rumack BH. Intravenous epinephrine abuse. Am J Emerg Med 1987; 5:64,65.
45. Levine RD, Orkin LR. Epinephrine overdose; a continuing problem. N Y State J Med 1981; 81:1669,1670.
46. Novey HS, Meleyco LN. Alarming reaction after intravenous administration of 30 mLof epinephrine. Jama 1969; 207:2435,2436.
47. Brown CG, Taylor RB, Werman HA, et al. Myocardial oxygen delivery/consumption during cardiopulmonary resuscitation: a comparison of epinephrine and phenylephrine. Ann Emerg Med 1988; 17: 302–308.
48. Lindner KH, Ahnefeld FW, Pfenninger EG, et al. Effects of epinephrine and norepinephrine on cerebral oxygen delivery and consumption during open-chest CPR. Ann Emerg Med 1990; 19:249–254.
49. Ditchey RV, Lindenfeld J. Failure of epinephrine to improve the balance between myocardial oxygen supply and demand during closed-chest resuscitation in dogs. Circulation 1988; 78:382–389.
50. Livesay JJ, Follette DM, Fey KH, et al. Optimizing myocardial supply/demand balance with alpha-adrenergic drugs during cardiopulmonary resuscitation. J Thorac Cardiovasc Surg 1978; 76:244–251.
51. Brown CG, Katz SE, Werman HA, et al. The effect of epinephrine versus methoxamine on regional myocardial blood flow and defibrillation rates following a prolonged cardiorespiratory arrest in a swine model. Am J Emerg Med 1987; 5:362–369.
52. Paradis NA, Brown CG. High-dose adrenaline and cardiac arrest. Lancet 1988; 2:749.
53. Chappel CI. RG, Bazales T. et al. Comparison of cardiotoxic action of certain sympathomimetic amines. Can J Biochem Physiol 1959; 37:35–42.
54. Todd GL, Baroldi G, Pieper GM, et al. Experimental catecholamine-induced myocardial necrosis. II. Temporal development of isoproterenol-induced contraction band lesions correlated with ECG, hemodynamic and biochemical changes. J Mol Cell Cardiol 1985; 17:647–656.
55. Tang W, Weil MH, Sun S, et al. Epinephrine increases the severity of postresuscitation myocardial dysfunction. Circulation 1995; 92:3089–3093.
56. Haft JI. Cardiovascular injury induced by sympathetic catecholamines. Prog Cardiovasc Dis 1974; 17: 73–86.
57. Waters LL, deSuto-Nagy, G.I. Lesions of the coronary arteries and great vessels of the dog following injection of adrenalin. Their prevention with dibenamine. Science 1950; 111:634–635.
58. Tang W, Weil MH, Gazmuri RJ, et al. Pulmonary ventilation/perfusion defects induced by epinephrine during cardiopulmonary resuscitation. Circulation 1991; 84:2101–2107.
59. Tang W, C. Epinephrine produces both hypoxemia and hypercarbia during CPR. Crit Care Med 1990; 18:276.
60. Berg RA, Otto CW, Kern KB, et al. High-dose epinephrine results in greater early mortality after resuscitation from prolonged cardiac arrest in pigs: a prospective, randomized study. Crit Care Med 1994; 22:282–290.
61. Baroldi G, Silver MD, Lixfeld W, McGregor DC. Irreversible myocardial damage resembling catecholamine necrosis secondary to acute coronary occlusion in dogs: its prevention by propranolol. J Mol Cell Cardiol 1977; 9:687–691.
62. Opie LH, Thandroyen FT, Muller C, Bricknell OL. Adrenaline-induced "oxygen-wastage" and enzyme release from working rat heart. Effects of calcium antagonism, beta-blockade, nicotinic acid and coronary artery ligation. J Mol Cell Cardiol 1979; 11:1073–1094.
63. Redding JS, Pearson JW. Metabolic acidosis: a factor in cardiac resuscitation. South Med J 1967; 60: 926–932.
64. Jude JR, Neumaster T, Kfoury E. Vasopressor-cardiotonic drugs in cardiac resuscitation. Acta Anaesthesiol Scand Suppl 1968; 29:147–163.
65. Holmes HR, Babbs CF, Voorhees WD, et al. Influence of adrenergic drugs upon vital organ perfusion during CPR. Crit Care Med 1980; 8:137–140.
66. Ralston SH, Tacker WA, Showen L, et al. Endotracheal versus intravenous epinephrine during electromechanical dissociation with CPR in dogs. Ann Emerg Med 1985; 14:1044–1048.
67. Brown CG, Werman HA, Davis EA, et al. Comparative effect of graded doses of epinephrine on regional brain blood flow during CPR in a swine model. Ann Emerg Med 1986; 15:1138–1144.
68. Brown CG, Werman HA, Davis EA, et al. The effects of graded doses of epinephrine on regional myocardial blood flow during cardiopulmonary resuscitation in swine. Circulation 1987; 75:491–497.
69. Lindner KH, Ahnefeld FW, Bowdler IM. The effect of epinephrine on hemodynamics, acid-base status and potassium during spontaneous circulation and cardiopulmonary resuscitation. Resuscitation 1988; 16:251–261.

70. Lindner KH, Ahnefeld FW, Bowdler IM. Comparison of epinephrine and dopamine during cardiopulmonary resuscitation. Intensive Care Med 1989; 15:432–438.
71. Lindner KH, Ahnefeld FW, Bowdler IM, Prengel AW. Influence of epinephrine on systemic, myocardial, and cerebral acid-base status during cardiopulmonary resuscitation. Anesthesiology 1991; 74:333–339.
72. Lindner KH, Strohmenger HU, Prengel AW, et al. Hemodynamic and metabolic effects of epinephrine during cardiopulmonary resuscitation in a pig model. Crit Care Med 1992; 20:1020–1026.
73. Dean JM, Koehler RC, Schleien CL, et al. Improved blood flow during prolonged cardiopulmonary resuscitation with 30% duty cycle in infant pigs. Circulation 1991; 84:896–904.
74. Gonzalez ER, Ornato JP, Garnett AR, et al. Dose-dependent vasopressor response to epinephrine during CPR in human beings. Ann Emerg Med 1989; 18:920–926.
75. Paradis NA, Martin GB, Rosenberg J, et al. The effect of standard- and high-dose epinephrine on coronary perfusion pressure during prolonged cardiopulmonary resuscitation. Jama 1991; 265:1139–1144.
76. Brown CG, Martin DR, Pepe PE, et al. A comparison of standard-dose and high-dose epinephrine in cardiac arrest outside the hospital. The Multicenter High-Dose Epinephrine Study Group. N Engl J Med 1992; 327:1051–1055.
77. Callaham M, Madsen CD, Barton CW, et al. A randomized clinical trial of high-dose epinephrine and norepinephrine vs standard-dose epinephrine in prehospital cardiac arrest. Jama 1992; 268:2667–2672.
78. Abramson NS, Safar, P., and Sutton-Tyrrell, K. A randomized clinical trial of escalating doses of high dose epinephrine during cardiac resuscitation. Critical care medicine 1995; 23:A178 (abstract).
79. Vandycke C, Martens P. High dose versus standard dose epinephrine in cardiac arrest - a meta-analysis. Resuscitation 2000; 45:161–166.
80. Joyce SM, Barsan WG, Doan LA. Use of phenylephrine in resuscitation from asphyxial arrest. Ann Emerg Med 1983; 12:418–421.
81. Brown CG, Birinyi F, Werman HA, et al. The comparative effects of epinephrine versus phenylephrine on regional cerebral blood flow during cardiopulmonary resuscitation. Resuscitation 1986; 14:171–183.
82. Brown CG, Werman HA, Davis EA, et al. The effect of high-dose phenylephrine versus epinephrine on regional cerebral blood flow during CPR. Ann Emerg Med 1987; 16:743–748.
83. Berkowitz ID, Gervais H, Schleien CL, et al. Epinephrine dosage effects on cerebral and myocardial blood flow in an infant swine model of cardiopulmonary resuscitation. Anesthesiology 1991; 75:1041–1050.
84. Schleien CL, Koehler RC, Gervais H, et al. Organ blood flow and somatosensory-evoked potentials during and after cardiopulmonary resuscitation with epinephrine or phenylephrine. Circulation 1989; 79:1332–1342.
85. Brillman JA, Sanders AB, Otto CW, et al. Outcome of resuscitation from fibrillatory arrest using epinephrine and phenylephrine in dogs. Crit Care Med 1985; 13:912,913.
86. Ditchey RV, Rubio-Perez A, Slinker BK. Beta-adrenergic blockade reduces myocardial injury during experimental cardiopulmonary resuscitation. J Am Coll Cardiol 1994; 24:804–812.
87. Silfvast T, Saarnivaara L, Kinnunen A, et al. Comparison of adrenaline and phenylephrine in out-of-hospital cardiopulmonary resuscitation. A double-blind study. Acta Anaesthesiol Scand 1985; 29: 610–613.
88. Standards and guidelines for cardiopulmonary resuscitation (CPR) and emergency cardiac care (ECC). JAMA 1986; 255:2841–3044.
89. Guidelines 2000 for cardiopulmonary resuscitation and emergency cardiovascular care. International consensus on science. Resuscitation 2000; 46:1–477 (Generic).
90. Guidelines 2000 for cardiopulmonary resuscitation and emergency cardiovascular care. Part 6: advanced cardiovascular life support: 7C: a guide to the international ACLS algorithms. The American Heart Association in collaboration with the international liaison committee on resuscitation. Circulation 2000; 102:I142–I157.
91. Thrasher TN, Keil LC. Systolic pressure predicts plasma vasopressin responses to hemorrhage and vena caval constriction in dogs. Am J Physiol Regul Integr Comp Physiol 2000; 279:R1035–R1042.
91a. Schmittinger CA, Wenzel V, Stadlbauer KH, et al. Drug therapy during CPR. Anasthesiol Intensivmed Notfallmed Schmerzther 2003; 38:651–672.
92. Hays RM. Agents affecting the renal conservation of water. In: Goodman and Gilman's: The Pharmacological Basis of Therapeutics. Goodman G, Rall, Murad, ed. New York: Macmilian, 1985, pp. 908–919.
93. Birnbaumer M. Vasopressin receptors. Trends Endocrinol Metab 2000; 11:406–410.
94. Fox AW, May RE, Mitch WE. Comparison of peptide and nonpeptide receptor-mediated responses in rat tail artery. J Cardiovasc Pharmacol 1992; 20:282–289.
95. Garcia-Villalon AL, Garcia JL, Fernandez N, et al. Regional differences in the arterial response to vasopressin: role of endothelial nitric oxide. Br J Pharmacol 1996; 118:1848–1854.

96. Moursi MM, van Wylen DG, D'Alecy LG. Regional blood flow changes in response to mildly pressor doses of triglycyl desamino lysine and arginine vasopressin in the conscious dog. J Pharmacol Exp Ther 1985; 232:360–368.

97. Wallace AW, Tunin CM, Shoukas AA. Effects of vasopressin on pulmonary and systemic vascular mechanics. Am J Physiol 1989; 257(Pt 2):H1228–H1234.

98. Okamura T, Ayajiki K, Fujioka H, Toda N. Mechanisms underlying arginine vasopressin-induced relaxation in monkey isolated coronary arteries. J Hypertens 1999; 17:673–678.

99. Suzuki Y, Satoh S, Oyama H, et al. Vasopressin mediated vasodilation of cerebral arteries. J Auton Nerv Syst 1994; 49(Suppl):S129–S132.

100. Russ RD, Walker BR. Role of nitric oxide in vasopressinergic pulmonary vasodilatation. Am J Physiol 1992; 262(Pt 2):H743–H747.

101. Xu YJ, Gopalakrishnan V. Vasopressin increases cytosolic free [Ca2+] in the neonatal rat cardiomyocyte. Evidence for V1 subtype receptors. Circ Res 1991; 69:239–245.

102. Fujisawa S, Iijima T. On the inotropic actions of arginine vasopressin in ventricular muscle of the guinea pig heart. Jpn J Pharmacol 1999; 81:309–312.

103. Lindner KH, Prengel AW, Pfenninger EG, et al. Vasopressin improves vital organ blood flow during closed-chest cardiopulmonary resuscitation in pigs. Circulation 1995; 91:215–221.

104. Prengel AW, Lindner KH, Keller A. Cerebral oxygenation during cardiopulmonary resuscitation with epinephrine and vasopressin in pigs. Stroke 1996; 27:1241–1248.

105. Wenzel V, Lindner KH, Prengel AW, et al. Vasopressin improves vital organ blood flow after prolonged cardiac arrest with postcountershock pulseless electrical activity in pigs. Crit Care Med 1999; 27:486–492.

106. Wenzel V, Linder KH, Augenstein S, et al. Vasopressin combined with epinephrine decreases cerebral perfusion compared with vasopressin alone during cardiopulmonary resuscitation in pigs. Stroke 1998; 29:1462-1467; discussion 1467,1468.

107. Paradis NA, Koscove EM. Epinephrine in cardiac arrest: a critical review. Ann Emerg Med 1990; 19:1288–1301.

108. Lolait SJ, O'Carroll AM, Brownstein MJ. Molecular biology of vasopressin receptors. Ann N Y Acad Sci 1995; 771:273–292.

109. Lindemann R. Endotracheal administration of epinephrine during cardiopulmonary resuscitation. Am J Dis Child 1982; 136:753,754.

110. Wenzel V, Lindner KH, Prengel AW, et al. Endobronchial vasopressin improves survival during cardiopulmonary resuscitation in pigs. Anesthesiology 1997; 86:1375–1381.

111. Kruse JA, Vyskocil JJ, Haupt MT. Intraosseous infusions: a flexible option for the adult or child with delayed, difficult, or impossible conventional vascular access. Crit Care Med 1994; 22:728,729.

112. Voelckel WG, Lindner KH, Wenzel V, et al. Intraosseous blood gases during hypothermia: correlation with arterial, mixed venous, and sagittal sinus blood. Crit Care Med 2000; 28:2915–2920.

113. Anonymous. Guidelines 2000 for cardiopulmonary resuscitation and emergency cardiovascular care. Circulation 2000; 102(Suppl):I1–I384.

114. Anonymous. Guidelines 2000 for cardiopulmonary resuscitation and emergency cardiovascular care. Resuscitation 2000; 46:1–447.

115. Wenzel V, Lindner KH, Krismer AC, et al. Repeated administration of vasopressin but not epinephrine maintains coronary perfusion pressure after early and late administration during prolonged cardiopulmonary resuscitation in pigs. Circulation 1999; 99:1379–1384.

116. Prengel AW, Lindner KH, Keller A, Lurie KG. Cardiovascular function during the postresuscitation phase after cardiac arrest in pigs: a comparison of epinephrine versus vasopressin. Crit Care Med 1996; 24:2014–2019.

117. Lindner KH, Brinkmann A, Pfenninger EG, et al. Effect of vasopressin on hemodynamic variables, organ blood flow, and acid-base status in a pig model of cardiopulmonary resuscitation. Anesth Analg 1993; 77:427–435.

118. Luce JM, Rizk NA, Niskanen RA. Regional blood flow during cardiopulmonary resuscitation in dogs. Crit Care Med 1984; 12:874–878.

119. Strohmenger HU, Lindner KH, Wienen W, Vogt J. Effects of the AT1-selective angiotensin II antagonist, telmisartan, on hemodynamics and ventricular function after cardiopulmonary resuscitation in pigs. Resuscitation 1997; 35:61–68.

120. Prengel AW, Lindner KH, Wenzel V, et al. Splanchnic and renal blood flow after cardiopulmonary resuscitation with epinephrine and vasopressin in pigs. Resuscitation 1998; 38:19–24.

121. Voelckel WG, Lindner KH, Wenzel V, et al. Effects of vasopressin and epinephrine on splanchnic blood flow and renal function during and after cardiopulmonary resuscitation in pigs. Crit Care Med 2000; 28:1083–1088.

122. Voelckel WG, Lindner KH, Wenzel V, et al. Effect of small-dose dopamine on mesenteric blood flow and renal function in a pig model of cardiopulmonary resuscitation with vasopressin. Anesth Analg 1999; 89:1430–1436.

123. Wenzel V, Lindner KH, Krismer AC, et al. Survival with full neurologic recovery and no cerebral pathology after prolonged cardiopulmonary resuscitation with vasopressin in pigs. J Am Coll Cardiol 2000; 35:527–533.

124. Gazmuri RJ, Maldonado FA. Postresuscitation management. In: Weil MH, Tang W, eds. CPR—Resuscitation of the arrested heart. Philadelphia, PA: Saunders, 1999, pp. 179–191.

125. Kampfl A, Schmutzhard E, Franz G, et al. Prediction of recovery from post-traumatic vegetative state with cerebral magnetic-resonance imaging. Lancet 1998; 351:1763–1767.

126. Landry DW, Levin HR, Gallant EM, et al. Vasopressin pressor hypersensitivity in vasodilatory septic shock. Crit Care Med 1997; 25:1279–1282.

127. Argenziano M, Choudhri AF, Oz MC, et al. A prospective randomized trial of arginine vasopressin in the treatment of vasodilatory shock after left ventricular assist device placement. Circulation 1997; 96(Suppl):II-286–II-290.

128. Argenziano M, Chen JM, Choudhri AF, et al. Management of vasodilatory shock after cardiac surgery: identification of predisposing factors and use of a novel pressor agent. J Thorac Cardiovasc Surg 1998; 116:973–980.

129. Mets B, Michler RE, Delphin ED, et al. Refractory vasodilation after cardiopulmonary bypass for heart transplantation in recipients on combined amiodarone and angiotensin-converting enzyme inhibitor therapy: a role for vasopressin administration. J Cardiothorac Vasc Anesth 1998; 12:326–329.

130. Gold JA, Cullinane S, Chen J, et al. Vasopressin as an alternative to norepinephrine in the treatment of milrinone-induced hypotension. Crit Care Med 2000; 28:249–52.

131. Lindner KH, Haak T, Keller A, et al. Release of endogenous vasopressors during and after cardiopulmonary resuscitation. Heart 1996; 75:145–150.

132. Lindner KH, Prengel AW, Brinkmann A, et al. Vasopressin administration in refractory cardiac arrest. Ann Intern Med 1996; 124:1061–1064.

133. Stiell IG, Hebert PC, Wells GA, et al. Vasopressin versus epinephrine for inhospital cardiac arrest: a randomised controlled trial. Lancet 2001; 358(9276):105–109.

134. Morris DC, Dereczyk BE, Grzybowski M, et al. Vasopressin can increase coronary perfusion pressure during human cardiopulmonary resuscitation. Acad Emerg Med 1997; 4:878–883.

135. Wenzel V, Lindner KH, Baubin MA, Voelckel WG. Vasopressin decreases endogenous catecholamine plasma concentrations during cardiopulmonary resuscitation in pigs. Crit Care Med 2000; 28:1096–1100.

136. Mayr VD, Wenzel V, Voelckel WG, et al. Developing a vasopressor combination in a pig model of adult asphyxial cardiac arrest. Circulation 2001; 104:1651–1656.

137. Wenzel V, Lindner KH, Mayer H, et al. Vasopressin combined with nitroglycerin increases endocardial perfusion during cardiopulmonary resuscitation in pigs. Resuscitation 1998; 38:13–17.

138. Lurie KG, Voelckel WG, Iskos DN, et al. Combination drug therapy with vasopressin, adrenaline (epinephrine) and nitroglycerin improves vital organ blood flow in a porcine model of ventricular fibrillation. Resuscitation 2002; 54:187–94.

139. Wenzel V, Ewy GA, Lindner KH. Vasopressin and endothelin during cardiopulmonary resuscitation. Crit Care Med 2000; 28(Suppl):N233–N235.

140. Krismer AC, Hogan QH, Wenzel V, et al. The efficacy of epinephrine or vasopressin for resuscitation during epidural anesthesia. Anesth Analg 2001; 93:734–742.

141. Krismer AC, Lindner KH, Kornberger R, et al. Cardiopulmonary resuscitation during severe hypothermia in pigs: does epinephrine or vasopressin increase coronary perfusion pressure? Anesth Analg 2000; 90:69–73.

142. Kornberger E, Lindner KH, Mayr VD, et al. Effects of epinephrine in a pig model of hypothermic cardiac arrest and closed-chest cardiopulmonary resuscitation combined with active rewarming. Resuscitation 2001; 50:301–308.

143. Voelckel WG, Lurie KG, Lindner KH, et al. Vasopressin improves survival after cardiac arrest in hypovolemic shock. Anesth Analg 2000; 91:627–634.

144. Stadlbauer KH, Wagner-Berger HG, Raedler C, et al. Vasopressin, but not fluid resuscitation ensured survival in a liver trauma model with uncontrolled hemorrhagic shock in pigs. Anesthesiology 2002; 38:693–704.

145. Voelckel WG, Lurie KG, McKnite S, et al. Comparison of epinephrine and vasopressin in a pediatric porcine model of asphyxial cardiac arrest. Crit Care Med 2000; 28:3777–3783.
146. Wenzel V, Lindner KH. Employing vasopressin during cardiopulmonary resuscitation and vasodilatory shock as a lifesaving vasopressor. Cardiovasc Res 2001; 51:529–541.
147. Wenzel V, Krismer AC, Arntz HR, et al. A comparison of vasopressin and epinephrine for out-of-hospital cardiopulmonary resuscitation. N Engl J Med 2004; 350:105–113.

20 Buffer Therapy

Martin von Planta, MD

Contents

INTRODUCTION
PATHOPHYSIOLOGY OF ACID–BASE CHANGES
TREATMENT WITH BUFFER AGENTS
CONCLUSION
REFERENCES

INTRODUCTION

The buffer therapy of acid–base changes during CPR is less controversial than in previous years. Overwhelming experimental and some clinical data failed to demonstrate an improvement in survival after buffer therapy. However, the scant data from randomized controlled trials still impede a clear-cut recommendation on how really to treat cardiopulmonary resuscitation (CPR)-associated acid–base changes.

Conventional closed-chest CPR generates a cardiac output of approx 25% curtailing organ perfusion and oxygen delivery to the tissues. Anaerobiasis with rapid CO_2 generation and slower accumulation of lactic acid results. Continuous CO_2 release from ischemic tissues, decreased CO_2 transport from the underperfused tissues to the lungs decreases alveolar CO_2 elimination accounting for the tissue CO_2 accumulation. Reduced $ETCO_2$ and hypercarbic venous and tissue acidemia and—under conditions of normal ventilation—hypocarbic arterial alkalemia ensue together with arterial and venous lactic acidemia reflecting the "arterio-venous paradox." The accumulation of tissue CO_2 results from local production of CO_2, dissociation of endogenous bicarbonate when anaerobically generated H^+ are buffered and reduced clearance of CO_2 as a result of reduced blood flow. In the heart, intramyocardial PCO_2 drastically increases with low coronary blood flow (Fig. 1).

Varying patterns of acid–base changes are related to the actual flow, the time windows of CPR and the cardiac arrest (CA) location. Arterial pH during well-performed CPR is usually normal, alcalotic (relative hyperventilation) and only late during CPR acidotic. Acid–base changes during out-of-hospital CPR often present a combined metabolic and respiratory acidemia. The triple low-perfusion acid–base abnormality makes the choice of an optimal buffer agent difficult (Table 1). Protection of the airways, adequate ventilation and chest compression to restore oygenated blood flow are the first therapeutic steps before any drug application may be evaluated. If CPR continues, various buffer

From: *Contemporary Cardiology: Cardiopulmonary Resuscitation*
Edited by: J. P. Ornato and M. A. Peberdy © Humana Press Inc., Totowa, NJ

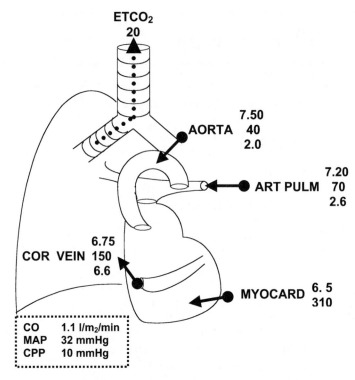

Fig. 1. Low-flow acidemia during CPR. Acid–base changes during CPR with mechanical chest compression and controlled ventilation in pigs. A triple acid–base defect is observed: venous and tissue hypercarbia, arterial hypocarbia, and arterial and venous lactacidemia. pH units; PCO_2 mmHg; lactate mmol/L. Based on refs. *22,24,83*.

Table 1
Potential Buffer Substances for Use During CPR

Anorganic buffers
  Sodium bicarbonate ($NaHCO_3$)
  Sodium carbonate (Na_2CO_3)
Organic buffers
  THAM, tromethamine (CH_2OH_3 C-NH_2)
Buffer mixtures
  Carbicarb (Na_2CO_3 + $NaHCO_3$)
  Tribonate ($NaHCO_3$ + Phosphate + THAM + Acetate)

agents are available of which sodium bicarbonate ($NaHCO_3$) is the most widely used. To date, very few randomized controlled trials are available and neither CO_2-generating ($NaHCO_3$) nor CO_2-consuming buffers (CARBICARB®, TRIBONATE®) were clinically proven to increase return of spontaneous circulation (ROSC) or neurologically intact long-term survival after CPR. In conclusion: the triple acid–base defect associated with CPR is best corrected by restoration of the low-flow state.

PATHOPHYSIOLOGY OF ACID–BASE CHANGES

Reduced Blood Flow and Acid–Base Changes During CPR

During the low-flow state of CPR only limited organ perfusion is maintained by external chest compression with cardiac output around 25% and reduced oxygen delivery to the tissues *(1,2)*. The metabolism shifts from aerobic to anaerobic pathways with production of anaerobic metabolites such as lactic acid and CO_2. Hence, a complex low-perfusion acid–base defect evolves that is only reversed after improvement of blood flow and restoration of adequate tissue oxygenation.

The reduced systemic and pulmonary blood flows curtail alveolar CO_2 elimination. CO_2 release from the tissues after endogenous lactic acid buffering and decreased CO_2 transport from the underperfused tissues to the lungs results in reduced CO_2 elimination accounting for the accumulation of CO_2 in the prepulmonary venous vascular bed and in the tissues (Figs. 2 and 3).

Clinical studies demonstrated $ETCO_2$ decreases with venous and tissue hypercarbic acidosis and time coincident arterial hypocarbic alkalosis *(3–7)*.

Predominantly, hypercarbia and lesser lactacidemia emerged as important acid–base derangements during CPR presenting a therapeutic dilemma. Acid–base changes are an additional epiphenomenon secondary to low flow and not a disease of its own. When cardiac output is reduced, tissue and venous hypercarbia is common. The magnitude of the arterio-venous pH and PCO_2 gradients clinically indicate the severity of the perfusion defect *(8–13)*.

Systemic Acid–Base Changes

The highly diffusable CO_2 molecules rapidly cross the cell membranes into the capillaries increasing venous PCO_2, thereby inducing hypercarbic venous acidemia. Part of this excess CO_2 is then removed during CPR by the small alveolar-capillary gas exchange. The increased ventilation/perfusion ratio during adequate ventilation and decreased cardiac output explains the less acidotic arterial blood than venous blood, i.e., the arterio-venous paradox *(3,14,15)*. Thus, early minor metabolic acidemia may be compensated by concurrent respiratory alkalemia because severe arterial acidemia is usually as a result of inadequate ventilation.

During adequate alveolar ventilation there is increased venous PCO_2, decreased arterial PCO_2, and time coincident decreased $ETCO_2$ *(5,16,17)*. The arterio-venous gradients of pH, PCO_2, and HCO_3^- clinically increased for pH and PCO_2 but not for HCO_3^- *(3,5,9,18,19)*. Differing patterns of arterial acid–base derangements are usually related to the location of CA. Patients resuscitated in wards or in emergency departments had more severe arterial acidemia and hypercarbia than patients resuscitated in intensive care units. Thus, the acid–base changes of prolonged CA, such most out-of-hospital CPR cases, present a combined metabolic and respiratory acidemia *(20)*.

Myocardial Acid–Base Changes and Coronary Perfusion

During myocardial ischemia of CPR anaerobic metabolism generates myocardial H^+, CO_2, and lactate with even greater pH and PCO_2 gradients in the coronary veins *(21–23)*. The intramyocardial CO_2 increases correlated with the coronary perfusion pressure during experimental CPR when coronary blood flow was impaired *(23,24)*.

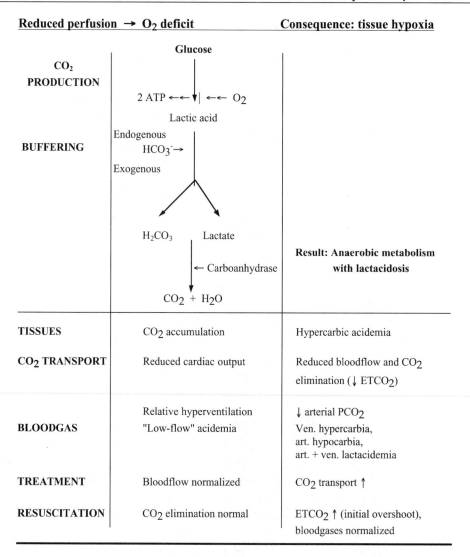

Fig. 2. Pathophysiology of low-perfusion acid–base defect during CPR with restoration of blood flow.

The accumulation of CO_2 within the myocardium reflects the balance of local CO_2 production, dissociation of endogenous myocardial bicarbonate when buffering anaerobically generated H^+ ions and reduced clearance of CO_2 as a result of low blood flow. CO_2 and lactic acid are the predominant determinants of intracellular pH during CPR. Extracellular HCO_3^-, i.e., $NaHCO_3$, exerts its effects on intracellular pH only after a delay as a result of low blood flow and prolonged transfer times from the blood into the intracellular compartment. Bicarbonate buffers anaerobically generated lactic acid increasing intracellular CO_2 and explaining the significant intramyocardial CO_2 increases.

Coronary perfusion pressure is the most important determinant of CPR successes correlating with myocardial blood flow (25–27). Coronary perfusion pressures of 15 mmHg

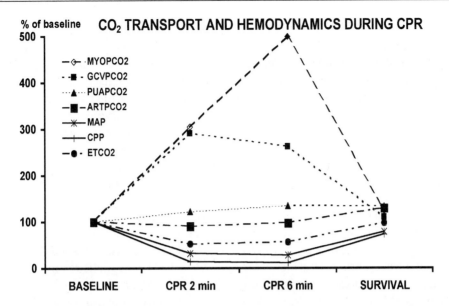

Fig. 3. Normalized carbon dioxide and hemodynamic data during porcine CPR. Normalized PCO_2 changes during CPR and mechanical chest compression and controlled ventilation in pigs. Drastic increases in intramyocardial PCO_2 are associated with lesser in the great cardiac vein and pulmonary artery and aortic PCO_2 decreases. Decreased MAP and CPP are associated with myocardial CO_2 production. $MYOPCO_2$, intramyocardial PCO_2; $GCVPCO_2$, great cardiac vein PCO_2; $PUAPCO_2$, pulmonary artery PCO_2; $ARTPCO_2$, aortic PCO_2; MAP, mean aortic pressure; CPP, coronary perfusion pressure. (Based on refs. *22* and *24*.)

in patients predicted outcome *(28)*. When intramyocardial PCO_2 was above a value of 400 mmHg, coronary perfusion pressure was below 10 mmHg resulting in failure of experimental CPR *(24)*.

Myocardial PCO_2 also correlates with the likelihood of successful recovery of heart function. Critical threshold levels of myocardial PCO_2 above 400 mmHg predicted failure of cardiac recovery after anoxic CA *(23)*. In patients with aortic valve replacement, myocardial PCO_2 predicted the recovery of cardiac function *(29,30)*. Thus, myocardial hypercarbia is a secondary acid–base derangement associated with reduced tissue perfusion.

Intramyocardial Hypercarbia and Its Relationship to Lactate Metabolism

CO_2 is the major determinant of acidosis and decreases in HCO_3^- seem to be of minor importance. In arterial and venous blood, HCO_3^- remains almost unchanged during experimental CPR. In the myocardium, the HCO_3^- was calculated by using the Hendersson-Hasselbach equation assuming the constancy of a pK value of 6.1 *(31)*. Only minor decreases of HCO_3^- were documented, from 21 to 20 mEq/L after a transient increase to 32 mEq/L during the first 5 minutes of CA *(24)*.

Myocardial lactic acidosis is also evident during CPR with increased great cardiac vein lactate indicating either hypoxia or ischemia because lactate increases were consistently identified during myocardial ischemia in experimental animals and in humans *(24,32)*.

Central Nervous System Acid–Base Changes

Brain tissue acid–base changes differ from those in the arterial or venous blood. The rapidly diffusable CO_2 molecules increase cerebrospinal hypercarbia during CPR (33). This central hypercarbia may—when used with $NaHCO_3$—contribute to the prolonged post-CPR cerebral depression observed in resuscitated patients (34). Cerebrospinal CO_2 increases after $NaHCO_3$ induced a "paradoxical" central nervous hypercarbia (35). However, $NaHCO_3$ was not uniformly followed by intrathecal hypercarbia when $NaHCO_3$ was titrated during CPR or with worse outcomes especially when epinephrine was added (36). Continuous infusion of 1 mmol/kg $NaHCO_3$ during canine ventricular fibrillation (VF) and cardiopulmonary bypass was not associated with intracerebral acidosis deterioration (37).

The efficacy of CO_2 consuming buffers was not extensively studied. THAM improved during porcine lactic acidosis cerebrospinal acidemia, but $NaHCO_3$ failed to correct the intrathecal acid–base disturbances (38). CARBICARB® increased and $NaHCO_3$ further decreased intracerebral pH during lactic acidosis (39). 31P magnetic resonance studies demonstrated a paradoxical intracerebral acidosis after $NaHCO_3$ but not after CARBICARB® (40) and low dose CARBICARB® given during asphyxial CA reduced neurologic deficits in rats (41).

Acid–Base Changes, Buffer Agents, and Defibrillation

Conflicting reports resulted when acid–base changes and the effects of buffer agents on defibrillation were investigated. pH ranges from 7.03 to 7.71 were not associated with VF threshold changes or with special defibrillation difficulties during respiratory or metabolic acidosis and alkalosis. VF thresholds remained unchanged during respiratory alkalosis or acidosis (42–46). During metabolic acidosis a reduction in VF thresholds with increased incidence of VF was observed (47). Conversely, protective effects of respiratory alkalosis against VF were demonstrated (48). Only when metabolic acidosis was associated with hypoxia successful defibrillation was prevented (44,45,49). Buffer agents mostly failed to help defibrillation.

Hypercarbia and Survival

Myocardial PCO_2 is a determinant of cardiac resuscitability probably representing an epiphenomenon of reduced blood flow. Thus, intramyocardial hypercarbia is a secondary marker of reduced myocardial blood flow. However, experimental studies suggested that hypercarbia adversely affected outcome even when coronary perfusion pressure was maintained above the critical threshold for survival (50,51). During $FiCO_2$ ventilation concurrent arterial, venous and tissue CO_2 increases as a result of the rapid equilibrium of CO_2 across the membranes were observed. PCO_2 is selectively increased in the venous blood and in the tissues and in the arterial blood only very late in the CPR process. Increased intramyocardial CO_2 levels induced myocardial "carbonarcosis" with decreased contractility accounting for the failure of successful CPR. In this setting, buffer agents may improve postCPR myocardial dysfunction (52).

TREATMENT WITH BUFFER AGENTS

The triple low-perfusion acid–base defect (venous hypercarbia, arterial hypocarbia, and lactic acidemia) make the choice of any buffer agent a therapeutic dilemma. Paramount is the reduction of increased tissue CO_2 and the increase of tissue oxygenation during reduced organ perfusion by adequate ventilation, chest compression, and early defibrillation *(53–55)*. Potentially, anorganic, organic and buffer mixtures are available of which none were clinically proven to increase neurologically intact survival in patients (Tables 1–3).

Sodium Bicarbonate

$NaHCO_3$ dissociates to Na^+ and HCO_3^- converting with H^+ to H_2CO_3 and then to CO_2 and H_2O, which are subsequently excreted by the lungs and kidneys. During normal ventilation and perfusion, the easily excretable CO_2 generated by $NaHCO_3$ is eliminated by the lungs effectively neutralizing excesses of H^+ making $NaHCO_3$ an efficient buffer:

$$H^+ + HCO_3^- \leftrightarrow H_2CO_3 \leftrightarrow H_2O + CO_2$$

Because the pK of the bicarbonate system is 6.1, HCO_3^- should poorly buffer within the clinically relevant pH ranges. However, in 20 patients during CPR, the pK of carbonic acid was equivalent to that of healthy controls *(31)*.

As the transport of CO_2 from the tissues to the lungs and its alveolar removal is impaired during CPR, $NaHCO_3$ may not act as efficient buffer (Figs. 2 and 3). $NaHCO_3$ induced paradoxical tissue and intracellular hypercarbic acidosis *(56–58)* and decreased myocardial contractility *(58,59)*. Significant alkalemia is induced after $NaHCO_3$ *(14,60)* together with increased osmolal and sodium loads *(14,61,62)*, and pediatric intracerebral hemorrhage *(63,64)*. $NaHCO_3$ further induced left shifts of the oxyhemoglobin dissociation curve decreasing P_{50} *(65,66)*. Most importantly is the failure of $NaHCO_3$ to improve defibrillation *(14,25)* or to increase neurologically intact long-term survival *(60,67–72)*. This may be as a result of simultaneous decreases in aortic diastolic pressure and increases in right atrial pressure resulting in decreases in coronary perfusion pressure (Table 4; *73)*.

Nevertheless, these findings are not unequivocal. Laboratory results vary widely as a result of experimental settings, timing and dosages of buffers, timing of blood sampling and perfusion magnitude after epinephrine. Better neurologic outcomes after 24 hours in dogs treated with $NaHCO_3$ and epinephrine were already demonstrated in 1968 *(74)*. Conversely, during porcine CPR the failure of $NaHCO_3$ to improve survival up to 20 minutes of untreated VF was confirmed *(75)*. Recent experimental studies demonstrated after prolonged CAs improved outcomes when $NaHCO_3$ was used in conjunction with epinephrine *(76–78)*. However, a multivariate regression analysis in 773 CA patients documented a significant association between failed CPR and the use of $NaHCO_3$ as well as other ACLS drugs *(79)*. Recently, a retrospective analysis of the timing of $NaHCO_3$ use of a previous randomized clinical trial demonstrated better ROSC in patients when no $NaHCO_3$ was administered during CPR *(80)*. Indeed, the use of $NaHCO_3$ decreased in the 1990s after the publication of the 1986 American Heart Association (AHA) guidelines *(81)*.

The magnitude of acid–base changes followed the dosage of $NaHCO_3$ used during CPR. With doses up to 1.5 mmol/kg, no changes in veno-arterial PCO_2 gradients were observed *(60)*, with doses above of 2 mmol/kg, these gradients transiently increased *(75)*. Tissue pH—approximated by mixed venous pH—increased after $NaHCO_3$ *(9,16,25,70,72)* and paradoxical intracellular pH decreases were observed after high doses of $NaHCO_3$ *(35)*. With less $NaHCO_3$ this effect was not observed *(70,82)* and intramyocardial pH was not reversed but continued to decrease after $NaHCO_3$ as after CARBICARB® and saline placebo *(83)*.

Table 2
Effects of Buffer Agents During Experimental and Human CPR

Author	Year	Main observations
Effects on survival		
Telivuo	1968	No better survival after $NaHCO_3$
Minuck	1977	THAM, $NaHCO_3$ and NaCl are equivalent during CPR
Guerci	1986	$NaHCO_3$ failed to improve survival
von Planta	1988	$NaHCO_3$, THAM and CARBICARB failed to improve survival
Gazmuri	1990	$NaHCO_3$ and CARBICARB failed to improve survival
Roberts	1990	Significantly less surviving patients after $NaHCO_3$
Wiklund	1990	THAM and NaCl improve resuscitability, but not $NaHCO_3$
Levy	1992	$NaHCO_3$ use in human CPR declined without decreases in survival
Dybvik	1995	TRIBONATE® failed to improve survival in humans
Bar-Joseph	1998	$NaHCO_3$ and CARBICARB® promote ROSC
Van Walraven	1998	$NaHCO_3$ in human CPR failed to improve survival
Leong	2001	$NaHCO_3$ may improve survival after prolonged arrest in dogs
Effects on defibrillation		
Turnbull	1966	pH of 7.14–7.60 without influence on fibrillation thresholds
Gerst	1966	During metabolic acidosis more ventricular fibrillation
Dong	1967	Respiratory alkalosis protects against ventricular fibrillation
Yakaitis	1975	pH of 7.03–7.71 without influence on defibrillation
Kerber	1983	Metabolic or respiratory acid–base changes without influence on defibrillation of ventricular fibrillation
Cardiac effects		
Reduction of coronary perfusion pressure (Arterial vasodilatation)		
Huseby	1981	Hyperosmolal solutions are arterial vasodilators
von Planta	1988	THAM reduces coronary perfusion pressure
Kette	1991	Hyperosmolal solutions reduce coronary perfusion pressure
Myocardial acidosis		
Kette	1990	Intramyocardial acidosis not improved after $NaHCO_3$ or CARBICARB®
Myocardial contractility		
Ng	1966	CO_2 and $NaHCO_3$ decrease and THAM increases contractility
Clancy	1967	Na_2CO_3 increases and $NaHCO_3$ decreases contractility
Cingolani	1970	Contractility depends on CO_2, not on pH or HCO_3^-
Poole	1975	CO_2 decreases contractility in isolated rabbit myocardium
Steenbergen	1977	CO_2 decreases contractility in isolated rat myocardium
Graf	1985	Decreases in cardiac output and increases in lactate after $NaHCO_3$
Bersin	1988	$NaHCO_3$ reduces and CARBICARB® increases cardiac output
Sun	1996	Buffers improve post-CPR myocardial dysfunction
Proarrhythmia		
Lawson	1973	Alcalizinization increases ectopic arrhythmias
Douglas	1979	Bolus of $NaHCO_3$ induces ventricular fibrillation in pigs
Effects on the CNS		
CNS acidosis		
Posner	1967	Paradoxical CNS acidosis after $NaHCO_3$ during CPR
Berenyi	1975	Severe hypercarbic acidosis in CNS liquor after $NaHCO_3$
Bureau	1980	$NaHCO_3$ increases CNS liquor lactate

Table 2 *(Continued)*

Author	Year	Main observations
Wiklund	1985	THAM but not $NaHCO_3$ corrects liquor acidosis
Kucera	1989	$NaHCO_3$ reduces intracellular pH, but not CARBICARB
Rosenberg	1989	THAM and $NaHCO_3$ have equivalent effects on brain pH
Katz	2002	CARBICARB® reduces neurologic deficit
CNS damage		
Posner	1967	Prolonged cerebral dysfunction after $NaHCO_3$ during CPR
Thomas	1976	Severe intracranial bleeding after $NaHCO_3$
Huseby	1981	Bolus of $NaHCO_3$ increases intracranial pressure

Metabolic effects

Alkalosis (Reduction of oxygen delivery, reduced P_{50})

Douglas	1979	$NaHCO_3$ reduces arterial and venous oxygen concentration
Bureau	1980	Reduction of oxygen delivery to the CNS after $NaHCO_3$
Bersin	1989	$NaHCO_3$ reduces P_{50} in patients with heart failure
CO_2 production		
Case	1979	Myocardial CO_2 increases during ventricular fibrillation >400 mmHg
Niemann	1984	50 mL 7.5% $NaHCO_3$ liberate 260–280 mmHg CO_2
Kette	1993	High intramyocardial CO_2 is associated with failure of CPR
Hyperosmolality		
Kravath	1970	$NaHCO_3$ induces acute hyperosmolality
Ruiz	1979	Increased osmolality after $NaHCO_3$
Hypernatremia		
Mattar	1974	$NaHCO_3$ induces severe hypernatremia and hyperosmolality
Liver acidosis		
Graf	1985	Reduction of intrahepatic pH and increase of CO_2 after $NaHCO_3$
Bersin	1988	$NaHCO_3$ increases intrahepatic acidosis more than CARBICARB®

The impact of the coronary perfusion pressure on patient survival is well-known *(28)*. Especially after epinephrine, coronary perfusion pressure increased *(84)* and $NaHCO_3$ may be advantageous when combined with epinephrine *(74)*.

Thus, restraint in the initial use of $NaHCO_3$ is advised during CPR (Table 5). $NaHCO_3$ should be abandoned for initial "conventional" CPR, it is not recommended for routine use in CPR! When arrest and CPR times are prolonged, $NaHCO_3$ in reduced dosages (0.5–1.0 mmol/kg iv bolus; half the dose thereafter) guided by actual bicarbonate concentration or base excess may be used. With preexisting metabolic acidemia, hyperkalemia, overdoses, or need to alkalize the urine, NaHCO3 may also be useful *(53–55)*.

Carbicarb® (Na₂CO₃ + NaHCO₃)

CARBICARB® is composed of equimolar amounts of $NaHCO_3$ and Na_2CO_3 consuming CO_2 *(85)*. In dogs with hypoxic lactic acidosis, this buffer mixture normalized arterial pH without increasing arterial CO_2 *(58)*. In a porcine model of CPR, arterial and venous PCO_2 decreased after CARBICARB® *(70)*. Neither mean arterial pressure nor cardiac index decreased after CARBICARB® but significant decreases in the coronary perfusion pressure—attributed to a vasodilator effect of the hyperosmolal buffer mixture with an increase in the right atrial pressure—were observed *(70,73)*. Furthermore, CARBICARB®

Table 3
Composition and Physico-Chemical Properties of Buffer Agents

Substances and properties	Bicarbonate NaHCO₃	Carbicarb® NaHCO₃ + Na₂CO₃	Tribonate® NaHCO₃ + Na₂HPO₄ + THAM + Acetate
Na^+, mmol/L	1000	1000	
HCO_3^-, mmol/L	1000	333	
CO_3 =, mmol/L	0	333	
Osmolality, mOsmoL/L	2000	1667	750
pH of solution	8.0	9.6	8.1
Effect on CO_2	↑	↓	↓
$NaHCO_3$, mmol/L			160
Disodium phosphate, mmol/L			20
THAM, tromethamine, mmol/L			300
Acetate, mmol/L			200

Tris-hydroxy-methyl-amino-methan (THAM):
Buffer capacity: 500 mmol/L

Table 4
Adverse Effects of Sodium Bicarbonate

Alkalemia
Reduced tissue oxygen availability
Increased risk of ventricular arrhythmias
Hyperosmolality
Irreversible cerebral damage
Arterial vasodilation
Decreased coronary perfusion pressure during CPR
CO₂ production
Paradoxical intracellular acidosis
Cerebrospinal fluid acidosis
Decreased myocardial contractility
Survival
Failure to facilitate defibrillation
No improvement of neurologically intact long-term survival

failed to reduce intramyocardial acidosis, myocardial CO_2 production, or to increase ROSC and long-term survival *(83)*. Conversely, CARBICARB® decreased intrahepatic pH *(58)* and did not induce paradoxical intracellular acidosis in the rat brain *(40)*. Hence, these limited data and the lack of controlled human experience do not advise the use of CARBICARB® as a potential buffer substance during CPR.

Tribonate (NaHCO₃ + THAM + Phosphate + Acetate)

The buffer TRIBONATE® (TRIS) is a mixture of $NaHCO_3$, THAM, phosphate and acetate which also consumes CO_2 is predominantly used in Scandinavia. A porcine CPR study demonstrated that TRIBONATE® exerted better intracellular alkalizing effects than $NaHCO_3$, but survival was not better after TRIBONATE® than after NaCl *(72)*. In a prospective clinical trial, 245 TRIBONATE®-treated patients were compared with

Table 5
Recommendations for $NaHCO_3$ Use During CPR

AHA	European Resuscitation Council
Class I: with pre-existing hyperkalemia	Consider $NaHCO_3$ (50 ml of 8.4%) to correct severe metabolic acidosis. When blood gas analysis is not available, consider $NaHCO_3$ after 20–25 minutes of CA.
Class IIa: with diabetic ketoacidosis, overdose (tricyclics, cocaine, diphenhydramine) or need to alkalize the urine.	
Class IIb: with prolonged resuscitation and effective ventilation; after ROSC and long arrest interval.	
Class III: in hypercarbic acidosis (i.e., CPR without intubation).	
Cave: Adequate ventilation and CPR as "major" buffer agent.	
$NaHCO_3$ dose: 0.5–1.0 mmol/kg.	

257 saline placebo controls. Only 10% of the TRIBONATE®-treated patients but 14% of the control patients were discharged alive. A logistic regression demonstrated that TRIBONATE® failed to improve survival *(86)*. Thus, experimental and clinical data do not recommend the use of TRIBONATE® during CPR.

Adverse Effects of Buffers

Table 4 summarizes the adverse effects of $NaHCO_3$. Excesses of buffers may transform acidosis into alkalosis. High pH levels decreased P_{50} reducing tissue O_2 availability because increased hemoglobin affinity impaired tissue oxygen utilization *(87)*. Thus, lactic acidosis may develop as a result of increased anaerobic glycolysis. Alkalemia also has proarrhythmic effects inducing ectopic dysrhythmias potentially triggering fatal ventricular arrhythmias *(88)*.

Increased plasma osmolality above 350 mOsm/kg may induce permanent damage of white matter and intraventricular hemorrhage precluding return of normal brain function *(61,89,90)*. Additionally, rapid osmolality increases are associated with hemodynamically relevant decreases of vascular resistance with transient but marked decreases in coronary perfusion pressures *(73,91)*.

CO_2 stemming from $NaHCO_3$ paradoxically decreases intracellular and spinal fluid pH *(34,35,57,92)*. In vitro myocardial contractility also decreased after $NaHCO_3$ *(93)*. However, these effects were not yet reported in intact animals or patients during CA. Few data documented an improved post-CPR myocardial function after buffer agents *(52)*.

The most important shortcoming of the use of $NaHCO_3$ during CPR is its apparent failure to improve defibrillation success or to increase survival rates after CA. This may mostly be related to decreased oxygen availability, decreases in coronary perfusion pressure, or paradoxical acidosis when $NaHCO_3$ was administered as the only pharmacon. Neither CO_2-generating or CO_2-consuming buffers were extensively tested in patients and their impact on ROSC or long-term survival after CA was yet never conclusively documented.

Post-CPR Phase

During the initial minutes of ROSC, the acid–base abnormalities tend to normalize. Sudden decreases in tissue and venous CO_2 accompany the normalization of tissue and venous pH. During the early phase of ROSC, $ETCO_2$ increases above normal levels. This "overshoot" represents the washout of the retained CO_2 during CPR. Concurrently, arterial blood demonstrates a transient hypercarbia consistent with $ETCO_2$ increases. During continued sufficient ventilation CO_2 normalizes within minutes and arterial pH remains low as a result of the persistence of increased lactate. The slower lactate uptake by the liver, kidney, myocardium, and gut account for the much slower return to normal in contrast to the more rapid decreases of CO_2. Thus, little if at all buffer agents are needed during adequate perfusion and ventilation.

CONCLUSION

Given the fact, that few controlled clinical studies are available at this time, a balanced evaluation of experimental studies with $NaHCO_3$ demonstrated rather detrimental than beneficial effects regarding survival. CARBICARB® failed to mitigate intramyocardial acidosis and its hyperosmolal affected decreased coronary perfusion pressure. With TRIBONATE®, clinical data clearly demonstrated its failure. Thus, alternative buffer agents such as CARBICARB® or TRIBONATE® cannot be recommended for clinical use.

In CPR cases of short duration, adequate ventilation and efficient circulation eliminates generated CO_2. The restoration of sufficient blood flow provides oxygen and counterbalances hypercarbic and metabolic acidemia by concurrent hypocarbic arterial alkalemia obviating the need for a buffer agent. However, during prolonged CPR, or in patients with preexisting hyperkalemia (class I), diabetic ketoacidosis, tricyclic, cocaine or diphenhydramine overdose (class IIa), NaHCO3 together with epinephrine may be indicated (NaHCO3: 0.5–1.0 mmol/kg; Table 5).

Alternative buffer agents such as CARBICARB® or TRIBONATE® cannot be recommend for patient use because there are not enough clinical data available. A randomized controlled trial examining and comparing CO_2 generating or consuming buffer agents during CPR is therefore mandated. Correction of the low-flow state remains the primary therapeutic goal. The correction of the acid–base equilibrium will then follow.

In general, efficient CPR is the best buffer therapy. The acidemia of CPR (arterial hypocarbia, venous and tissue hypercarbia and lactacidemia) is a symptom of low flow. Thus, acid–base changes are a secondary phenomenon of CPR-associated low flow and not a pathophysiologic entity of their own. No randomized clinical trials with buffer agents documented improved ROSC or neurologically intact long-term outcome in patients.

REFERENCES

1. Ditchey RV, Winkler JV, Rhodes CA. Relative lack of coronary blood flow during closed-chest resuscitation in dogs. Circulation 1982; 66:297–302.
2. Weil MH, Bisera J, Trevino RP, Rackow EC. Cardiac output and end-tidal carbon dioxide. Crit Care Med 1985; 13:907–909.
3. Weil MH, Rackow EC, Trevino R, Grundler WG, Falk JL, Griffel MI. Difference in acid-base state between venous and arterial blood during cardiopulmonary resuscitation. N Engl J Med 1986; 315: 153–156.
4. Garnett AR, Ornato JP, Gonzalez ER, et al. End-tidal carbon dioxide monitoring during cardiopulmonary resuscitation. JAMA 1987; 257:512–517.

5. Falk JL, Rackow EC, Weil MH. End-tidal carbon dioxide concentration during cardiopulmonary resuscitation. N Engl J Med 1988; 318:607–611.
6. Sanders AB, Kern KB, Otto CW, et al. End-tidal carbon dioxide during cardiopulmonary resuscitation: a prognostic indicator of survival. JAMA 1989; 262:1347–1352.
7. Callaham M, Barton C. Prediction of outcome of cardiopulmonary resuscitation from end-tidal carbon dioxide concentration. Crit Care Med 1990;18:358–362.
8. Bergman KS, Harris BH. Arteriovenous pH difference - a new index of perfusion. J Ped Surg 1988; 23: 1190–1192.
9. Adrogué HJ, Rashad MN, Gorin AB, Yacoub J, Madias NE. Assessing acid-base status in circulatory failure. Differences between arterial and central venous blood. New Engl J Med 1989; 320:1312–1316.
10. Benjamin E, Paluch TA, Berger SR, Premus G, Wu C, Iberti TJ. Venous hypercarbia in canine hemorrhagic shock. Crit Care Med 1987; 15:516–518.
11. Mecher CE, Rackow EC, Astiz ME, Weil MH. Venous hypercarbia associated with severe sepsis and systemic hypoperfusion. Crit Care Med 1990; 18:585–589.
12. Wendon JA, Harrison PM, Keays R, Gimson AE, Alexander G, Williams R. Arterial-venous pH differences and tissue hypoxia in patients with fulminant hepatic failure. Crit Care Med 1991; 19:1362–1364.
13. Mathias DW, Clifford PS, Klopfenstein HS. Mixed venous blood gases are superior to arterial blood gases in assessing acid-base status and oxygenation during acute cardiac tamponade in dogs. J Clin Invest 1988; 82:833–838.
14. Bishop RL, Weisfeldt ML. Sodium bicarbonate administration during cardiac arrest: Effect on arterial pH, PCO_2, and osmolality. JAMA 1976; 235:506–509.
15. Grundler WG, Weil MH, Rackow EC. Arteriovenous carbon dioxide and pH gradients during cardiac arrest. Circulation 1986; 74:1071–1074.
16. von Planta M, von Planta I, Weil MH, et al. End-tidal carbon dioxide as a hemodynamic determinant of cardiopulmonary resuscitation in the rat. Cardiovasc Res 1989; 23:364-368.
17. Weil MH, Gazmuri RJ, Kette F, et al. End-tidal PCO_2 during cardiopulmonary resuscitation. JAMA 1990; 263:814–816.
18. Ralston SH, Voorhees WD, Showen L, et al. Venous and arterial blood gases during and after cardiopulmonary resuscitation in dogs. Am J Emerg Med 1985; 3:132–138.
19. Chazan JA, McKay DB. Acid-base abnormalities in cardiopulmonary arrest: Varying patterns in different locations in the hospital. N Engl J Med 1989; 320:597–598.
20. Fillmore S, Shapiro JM, Killip T. Serial blood gas studies during cardiopulmonary resuscitation. Ann. Intern. Med. 1970; 72:465–469.
21. Capparelli EV, Chow MSS, Kluger J, Fieldman A. Difference in systemic and myocardial blood acid-base status during cardiopulmonary resuscitation. Crit Care Med 1989; 17:442–446.
22. Gudipati CV, Weil MH, Gazmuri RJ, Deshmukh HG, Bisera J, Rackow EC. Increases in coronary vein CO_2 during cardiac resuscitation. J Appl Physiol 1990; 68:1405–1408.
22. von Planta M, Weil MH, Gazmuri RJ, Bisera J, Rackow EC. Myocardial acidosis associated with CO_2 production during cardiac arrest and resuscitation. Circulation 1989; 80:684–692.
23. MacGregor DC, Wilson GJ, Holness DE, et al. Intramyocardial carbon dioxide tension. A guide to the safe period of anoxic arrest of the heart. J Thor Cardiovasc Surg 1974; 68:101–107.
24. Kette F, Weil MH, Gazmuri RJ, Bisera J, Rackow EC. Intramyocardial hypercarbic acidosis during cardiac arrest and resuscitation. Crit Care Med 1993; 21:901–906.
25. Guerci AD, Chandra N, Johnson E, et al. Failure of sodium bicarbonate to improve resuscitation from ventricular fibrillation in dogs. Circulation 1986; 74 (Suppl 4):75–79.
26. Ralston SH, Voorhees WD, Babbs CF. Intrapulmonary epinephrine during prolonged cardiopulmonary resuscitation: Improved regional blood flow and resuscitation in dogs. Ann Emerg Med 1984; 13:79–86.
27. Sanders AB, Ewy GA, Taft TV. Resuscitation and arterial blood gas abnormalities during prolonged cardiopulmonary resuscitation. Ann Emerg Med 1984; 13:676–679.
28. Paradis NA, Martin GB, Rivers EP, et al. Coronary perfusion pressure and the return of spontaneous circulation in human cardiopulmonary resuscitation. JAMA 1990; 263:1106–1113.
29. Schaff HV, Bixler TJ, Flaherty JT, et al. Identification of persistent myocardial ischemia in patients developing left ventricular dysfunction following aortic valve replacement. Surgery 1979; 86:70–76.
30. Magovern GJJ, Flaherty JT, Kanter KR, Schaff HV, Gott VL, Gardner TJ. Assessment of myocardial protection during global ischemia with myocardial gas tension monitoring. Surgery 1982; 92:373–379.
31. Kruse JA, Hukku P, Carlson RW. Constancy of blood carbonic acid pK' in patients during cardiopulmonary resuscitation. Chest 1988; 93:1221–1224.

32. Opie LH. Effects of regional ischemia on metabolism of glucose and fatty acids. Relative rates of aerobic and anaerobic energy production during myocardial infarction and comparison with effects of anoxia. Circ Res 1976; 38:I52–I74.

33. Javaheri S, Clendending A, Papadakis N, et al. pH changes on the surface of brain and in cisternal fluid in dogs in cardiac arrest. Stroke 1984; 15:553–558.

34. Posner JB, Plum F. Spinal fluid pH and neurologic symptoms in systemic acidosis. N Engl J Med 1967; 277:605–613.

35. Berenyi KJ, Wolk M, Killip T. Cerebrospinal fluid acidosis complicating therapy of experimental cardiopulmonary arrest. Circulation 1975; 52:319–324.

36. Sanders AB, Otto CW, Kern KB, Rogers JN, Perrault P, Ewy GA. Acid-base balance in a canine model of cardiac arrest. Ann Emerg Med 1988; 17:667–671.

37. Rosenberg JM, Martin GB, Paradis NA, et al. The effect of CO_2 and non-CO_2 generating buffers on cerebral acidosis after cardiac arrest: a 31P NMR study. Ann Emerg Med 1989; 18:341–347.

38. Wiklund L, Sahlin K. Induction and treatment of metabolic acidosis: A study of pH changes in porcine skeletal muscle and cerebrospinal fluid. Crit Care Med 1985; 13:109–112.

39. Kucera RR, Shapiro JI, Whalen MA, et al. Brain effects of $NaHCO_3$ and Carbicarb in lactic acidosis. Crit Care Med 1989; 17:1320–1325.

40. Shapiro JI, Whalen M, Kucera R, Kindig N, Filley G, Chan L. Brain pH responses to sodium bicarbonate and Carbicarb during systemic acidosis. Am J Physiol 1989; 256:H1316–H1321.

41. Katz LM, Wang Y, Rockoff S, Bouldin TW. Low-dose carbicarb improves cerebral outcome after asphyxial cardiac arrest in rats. Ann Emerg Med 2002; 39:359–365.

42. Gerst PH, Fleming WH, Malm JR. Relationship between acidosis and ventricular fibrillation. Surg Forum 1964; 15:242–243.

43. Turnbull AD, Dobell ARC. The effect of pH change on the ventricular fibrillation threshold. Surgery 1966; 60:1040–1043.

44. Turnbull AD, MacLean LD, Dobell ARC, et al. The influence of hyperbaric oxygen and of hypoxia on the ventricular fibrillation threshold. J Thorac Cardiovasc Surg 1965; 50:842–848.

45. Yakaitis RW, Thomas JD, Mahaffey JE. Influence of pH and hypoxia on the success of defibrillation. Crit Care Med 1975; 3:139–142.

46. Kerber RE, Pandian NG, Hoyt R et al. Effect of ischemia, hypertrophy, hypoxia, acidosis and alkalosis on canine defibrillation. Am J Physiol 1983; 244:H825–H831.

47. Gerst PH, Fleming WH, Malm JR. Increased susceptibility of the heart to ventricular fibrillation during metabolic acidosis. Circ. Res. 1966; 19:63–70.

48. Dong E, Stinson EB, Shumway NE. The ventricular fibrillation threshold in respiratory acidosis and alkalosis. Surgery 1967; 61:602–607.

49. Kerber RE, Sarnat W. Factors influencing the success of ventricular defibrillation in man. Circulation 1979; 60:226–230.

50. von Planta I, Weil MH, von Planta M, Gazmuri RJ, Duggal C. Hypercarbic acidosis reduces cardiac resuscitability. Crit Care Med 1991; 19:1177–1182.

51. Maldonaldo FA, Weil MH, Tang W, et al. Myocardial hypercarbic acidosis reduces cardiac resuscitability. Anesthesiology 1993; 78:343–352.

52. Sun S, Weil MH, Tang W, Fukui M. Effects of buffer agents on postresuscitation myocardial dysfunction. Crit Care Med 1996; 24:2035–2041.

53. American Heart Association: Guidelines for Cardiopulmonary Resuscitation and Emergency cardiovascular Care. Circulation 2000; 102:I1–I384; Resuscitation 2000; 46; 1–447.

54. American Heart Association: 2000 handbook for emergency cardiovascular care. Resuscitation. Dallas, TX: AHA, 2000.

55. European Resuscitation Council. Summary of guidelines 2000 and sequence of actions for resuscitation. Amsterdam: Elsevier, 2000.

56. Graf H, Leach W, Arieff AI. Evidence for a detrimental effect of sodium bicarbonate therapy in hypoxic lactic acidosis. Science 1985; 227:754–756.

57. Ritter JM, Doktor HS, Benjamin N. Paradoxical effect of bicarbonate on cytoplasmic pH. Lancet 1990; 335:1243–1246.

58. Bersin RM, Arieff AI: Improved hemodynamic function during hypoxia with carbicarb, a new agent for the management of acidosis. Circulation 1988; 77:227–233.

59. Poole-Wilson PA, Langer GA. Effect of pH on ionic exchange and function in rat and rabbit myocardium. Am J Physiol 1975; 229:570–581.

60. von Planta M, Gudipati C, Weil MH, Kraus LJ, Rackow EC. Effects of tromethamine and sodium bicarbonate buffers during cardiac resuscitation. J Clin Pharmacol 1988; 28:594–599.

61. Mattar JA, Weil MH, Shubin H, Stein L. Cardiac arrest in the critically ill: Hyperosmolal states following cardiac arrest. Am J Med 1974; 56:162–168.
62. Lindner KH, Ahnefeld FW, Dick W, Lotz P: Natriumbikarbonatgabe während der kardiopulmonalen Reanimation. Anaesthesist 1985; 34:37–45.
63. Bland RD, Clarke TL, Harden LB. Rapid infusion of sodium bicarbonate and albumin into high-risk premature infants soon after birth: a controlled, prospective trial. Am J Obstet Gynecol 1976; 124:263–267.
64. Thomas DB. Hyperosmolarity and intraventricular hemorrhage in premature babies. Acta Paed Scand 1976; 65:429–432.
65. Douglas ME, Downs JB, Mantini EL, Ruis BC. Alteration of oxygen tension and oxyhemoglobin saturation. Arch Surg 1979; 114:326–329.
66. Bureau MA, Begin R, Berthiaume Y, Shapcott D, Khoury K, Gagnon N. Cerebral hypoxia from bicarbonate infusion in diabetic acidosis. J Pediatrics 1980; 96:968–973.
67. Lee WH, Darby TD, Aldinger EE, Thrower WB. Use of THAM in the management of refractory cardiac arrest. Am Surg 1962; 28:87–89.
68. Telivuo L, Maamies T, Siltanen P, Tala P. Comparison of alkalizing agents in resuscitation of the heart after ventricular fibrillation. Ann Chir Gyn Fenn 1968; 57:221–224.
69. Minuck M, Sharma GP. Comparison of THAM and sodium bicarbonate in resuscitation of the heart after ventricular fibrillation in dogs. Anesth Analg 1977; 56:38–45.
70. Gazmuri RJ, von Planta M, Weil MH, Rackow EC. Cardiac effects of carbon dioxide-consuming and carbon dioxide-generating buffers during cardiopulmonary resuscitation. J Am Coll Cardiol 1990; 15: 482–490.
71. Roberts D, Landolfo K, Light RB, Dobson K. Early predictors of mortality for hospitalized patients suffering cardiopulmonary arrest. Chest 1990; 97:413–419.
72. Wiklund L, Ronquist G, Stjernstrom H, Waldenstrom A. Effects of alkaline buffer administration on survival and myocardial energy metabolism in pigs subjected to ventricular fibrillation and closed chest CPR. Acta Anaesthesiol Scand 1990; 34:430–439.
73. Kette F, Weil MH, Gazmuri RJ. Buffer solutions may compromise cardiac resuscitation by reducing coronary perfusion pressure. JAMA 1991; 266:2121–2130.
74. Redding JS, Pearson JW. Resuscitation from ventricular fibrillation. JAMA 1968; 203:255-260.
75. Federiuk CS, Sanders AB, Kern KB, Nelson J, Ewy G. The effect of bicarbonate on resuscitation from cardiac arrest. Ann Em Med 1991; 20:1173–1177.
76. Vukmir RB, Bircher NG, Radovsky A, Safar P. Sodium bicarbonate may improve outcome in dogs with prolonged cardiac arrest. Crit Care Med 1995; 23:515–522.
77. Bar-Joseph G, Weinberger T, Castel T, et al. Comparison of sodium bicarbonate, Carbicarb, and THAM during cardiopulmonary resuscitation in dogs. Crit Care Med 1998; 26:1397–1408.
78. Leong ECM, Bendall JC, Boyd AC, Einstein R. Sodium bicarbonate improves the chance of resuscitation after 10 minutes of cardiac arrest in dogs. Resuscitation 2001; 51:309–315.
79. van Walraven C, Stiell IG, Wells GA, Hebert PC, Vendemheen K. Do advanced cardiac life support drugs increase resuscitation rates from in-hospital cardiac arrest? Ann Emerg Med 1998; 32:544–553.
80. Bar-Joseph G, Abramson NS, Jansen L, et al. Clinical use of sodium bicarbonate during cardiopulmonary resuscitation – is it used sensibly? Resuscitation 2002; 54:47–55.
81. Levy RD, Rhoden WE, Shearer K, Varley E, Brooks NH. An audit of drug usage for in-hospital cardiopulmonary resuscitation. Eur Heart J 1992; 13:1665–1668.
82. Rothe KF, Diedler J. Comparison of intra- and extracellular buffering of clinically used buffer substances: Tris and bicarbonate. Acta Anaesth Scand 1982; 26:194–198.
83. Kette F, Weil MH, von Planta M, Gazmuri RJ, Rackow EC. Buffer agents do not reverse intramyocardial acidosis during cardiac resuscitation. Circulation 1990; 81:1660–1666.
84. Paradis NA, Martin GB, Rosenberg J, et al. The effect of standard- and high-dose epinephrine on coronary perfusion pressure during prolonged cardiopulmonary resuscitation. JAMA 1991; 265:1139–1144.
85. Filley GF, Kindig NB. Carbicarb. An alkalinizing ion-generating agent of possible clinical usefulness. Trans Am Clin Climat Assoc 1984; 96:141–153.
86. Dybvik T, Strand T, Steen PA. Buffer therapy during out of hospital cardiopulmonary resuscitation. Resuscitation 1995; 29:89–95.
87. Bellingham AJ, Detter JC, Lenfant C. Regulatory mechanism of hemoglobin oxygen affinity in acidosis and alkalosis. J Clin Invest 1971; 50:700–706.
88. Lawson NW, Butler GH, Ray CT. Alkalosis and cardiac arrhythmias. Anest Analg 1973; 52:951–961.
89. Sotos JF, Dodge PR, Meara P, Talbot NB. Studies in experimental hypertonicity. I. Pathogenesis of the clinical syndrome, biochemical abnormalities and cause of death. Pediatrics 1960; 26:925–938.

90. Kravath RE, Aharon AS, Abal G, Finberg L. Clinically significant physiologic changes from rapidly administered hypertonic solutions: Acute osmol poisoning. Pediatrics 1970; 46:267–275.
91. Huseby JS, Gumprecht DG. Hemodynamic effects of rapid bolus hypertonic sodium bicarbonate. Chest 1981; 79:552–554.
92. Arieff AI, Leach W, Park R, Lazarowitz V. Systemic effects of $NaHCO_3$ in experimental lactic acidosis in dogs. Am J Physiol 1982; 242:F586–F591.
93. Ng ML, Levy MN, Zieske HA. Effects of changes of pH and of carbon dioxide tension on left ventricular performance. Am J Physiol 1967; 213:115–120.

21 Anti-Arrhythmic Drugs and Cardiac Resuscitation

Brian Olshansky, MD, Pamela Nerheim, MD, and Richard E. Kerber, MD

CONTENTS

INTRODUCTION

Cardiac arrest (CA) as a result of poorly tolerated ventricular tachycardia (VT) or ventricular fibrillation (VF) is the most common cause of death in many developed countries including the United States. Even with a steady decline in morbidity and mortality from cardiovascular diseases over 30 years *(1)*, approx 60% of the 489,171 deaths attributable to coronary artery disease (CAD) in 1990 were out-of-hospital CA. In 1998, 63% of cardiac deaths were sudden and likely arrhythmic *(2)*. Many of these deaths could have been prevented if the responsible ventricular arrhythmia had been treated with proper resuscitative efforts. Of 350,000 men who died in 1998, 41% had out-of-hospital sudden death, and 22% had a cardiac death in the emergency department (ED) or were dead on arrival. Of 369,000 women who died that year, 52% had out-of-hospital sudden death, and 12% had a cardiac death in the ED or were dead on arrival *(2)*.

Recent data indicate that the rate of VF causing out-of-hospital CA has decreased from 0.85/1000 to 0.38/1000 *(3)* over 20 years with a greater proportion of sudden cardiac deaths as a result of asystole and pulseless electrical activity. Notwithstanding this decline, VF is an enormous problem and a fail safe method to treat and prevent life-threatening arrhythmias remains largely unsolved.

From: *Contemporary Cardiology: Cardiopulmonary Resuscitation*
Edited by: J. P. Ornato and M. A. Peberdy © Humana Press Inc., Totowa, NJ

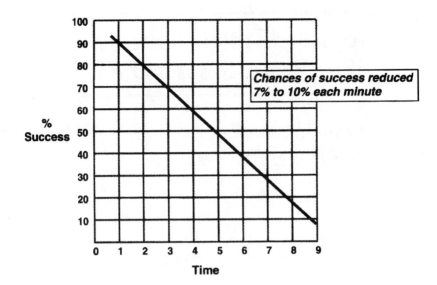

Fig. 1. The chance of successful resuscitation is related to time to defibrillation *(6)*.

A "chain of survival" strategy: early access, early cardiopulmonary resuscitation (CPR), early defibrillation, and early advanced cardiac life support (ACLS), advocated by the American Heart Association (AHA), is crucial for effective resuscitation *(4)*. Unfortunately, survival plummets despite defibrillation and cardiopulmonary resuscitative attempts if "down time" interval exceeds 10 minutes *(5)*. The odds of survival decrease by 7–10% for each additional minute before resuscitation (Fig. 1; *6*). A meta-analysis of 10 studies demonstrated a 9.2% absolute increase in survival with the use of automated external defibrillators (AEDs) by emergency medical technicians simply by providing earlier defibrillation *(7)*.

Resuscitation succeeds only if it is performed early after collapse *(8)*. In Seattle, 27% of patients with witnessed out-of-hospital CA survived to leave the hospital, however, in Chicago, Becker and colleagues reported only a 2% survival rate from out-of-hospital CA *(9)*. Similarly, in New York City, only 1.4% survived to hospital discharge *(10)*. In New York, the mean time to first defibrillation shock was 12.4 minutes whereas in Seattle the first defibrillation shock was delivered within 5.3 minutes after recognition of the CA *(9,11)*. If defibrillation had been provided within 3 to 4 minutes, even in the Seattle experience, survival might have doubled. The chance of survival after an out-of-hospital CA as a result of a ventricular arrhythmia is 40% if one shock is delivered, 30% if two shocks are delivered, 5% if three shocks are delivered and 2% percent after four shocks are delivered *(12)*. Although defibrillation can be effective, the shock must be delivered early, and other initiating conditions must be treatable and treated. Adjunctive therapies may be required.

This chapter will focus on a rational approach to the use of one adjunctive therapy, anti-arrhythmic drug use in the setting of resuscitation and recovery from VF and/or VT CA. The ultimate goal in the use of an anti-arrhythmic drug, as with any resuscitative therapy, is to have a living healthy patient with excellent potential for good quality of life. Other surrogate endpoints such as return of spontaneous circulation or survival to hospitalization alone are not optimal or even acceptable.

Rationale for Using an Anti-Arrhythmic Drug

Early defibrillation, with proper electrode location, shock waveform, and energy delivery, may be successful in terminating VF/VT, but return to a perfusing rhythm is not always possible. Refibrillation is common and occurs in as many as 61% of those who are defibrillated. Up to 35% refibrillate more than once requiring several defibrillation shocks *(13)*. Multiple defibrillation shocks can cause myocardial dysfunction. A drug that would prevent the need for multiple shocks and/or would reduce energy requirements for defibrillation would be desirable *(14)*. Episodes of nonsustained VT can also cause hemodynamic collapse. Anti-arrhythmic drugs, in conjunction with properly performed CPR and effective defibrillation, may facilitate return to a perfusing rhythm and may help maintain it.

Despite the rationale for use of an anti-arrhythmic drug, there are several concerns: (a) time wasted starting intravenous lines to administer the drug, instead of effective CPR and prompt defibrillation, may eliminate any hope of defibrillating the patient *(15)*; (b) lack of uniform guidelines for drug administration can cause confusion and improper management; (c) adverse drug–drug and drug–device interactions are possible; (d) pro-arrhythmia and side effects are frequent; and (e) proof of efficacy is limited.

Pepe *(16)*, in 1993, stated that "while animal data and logical inference support their use, no clinical studies have yet validated advanced life support measures such as intubation, epinephrine, bicarbonate, calcium or anti-arrhythmic drugs in cardiac arrest." In fact, these interventions may actually worsen prognosis in select settings *(17)*. Still, anti-arrhythmic drugs may help in the following specific situations:

- Patients with in- or out-of-hospital, poorly tolerated, VTs that cannot be defibrillated or that recur. Present guidelines suggest use of anti-arrhythmic drugs *after* CPR, defibrillation attempts (at least three) and use of epinephrine or vasopressin *(6,18)*.
- Patients at high risk for having a CA even if one has not yet occurred. Consider the situation of a patient having prolonged episodes of nonsustained, poorly tolerated, VT or sustained monomorphic VT. Such patients may have a life-threatening arrhythmia *prevented* by a stabilizing drug.
- Patients with recurrent ventricular arrhythmias causing repeated implantable cardioverter defibrillator shocks *(19,20)*. The expectation is that the drug will facilitate defibrillation, help decrease VF recurrence rates and ultimately stabilize the patient. In this setting, an anti-arrhythmic drug may also facilitate antitachycardia pacing termination of a VT.
- Patients with CA as a result of a tachyarrhythmia that is not clearly VT. Some patients may have a CA as a result of rapid ventricular rates in response to atrial fibrillation (e.g., the Wolff-Parkinson-White syndrome).

Causes of Ventricular Arrhythmias Causing Cardiac Arrest

The use of anti-arrhythmic drugs, and their benefit, depends on the underlying condition (Table 1). Treating the underlying cause may provide the greatest benefit. Such causes include ischemia, electrolyte abnormalities, metabolic problems, and drug pro-arrhythmia. An anti-arrhythmic drug would not be expected to help in these situations. Polymorphic VT as a result of acute ischemia is best treated with anti-ischemic therapy, not an anti-arrhythmic drug that may simply "fuel the fire." Life-threatening ventricular arrhythmias as a result of metabolic acidosis, drug toxicity, and electrolyte abnormalities

Table 1
Common Causes of Cardiac Arrest as a Result of Ventricular Arrhythmias

Coronary artery disease
  Ischemia
  Infarction
Idiopathic cardiomyopathy
Myocarditis
Drug toxicity
Electrolyte abnormality
Metabolic abnormality
Poisoning
Drug pro-arrhythmia
Infiltrative heart disease (sarcoidosis, amyloidosis)
Idiopathic ventricular fibrillation
Catecholamine-related ventricular fibrillation
Valvular heart disease
Hypertrophic heart disease including hypertrophic cardiomyopathy
Pulmonary embolus
Structural congenital heart disease
Congenital arrhythmic condition (Brugada syndrome, long QT interval syndrome, arrhythmogenic
  RV dysplasia)

may only become worse with anti-arrhythmic drugs. Any drug may be ineffective in the setting of a severe metabolic problem such as acidosis.

Drugs may be responsible for the CA. Digoxin toxicity can cause VT (including bidirectional VT) and VF *(21–23)*. Head injury, *(24)* several types of drugs *(25–33)*, and electrolyte disorders prolong the QT interval (often in a rate-dependent manner) and can cause torsade de pointes. Resolution of this problem requires stopping the offending drug and/or correcting the electrolyte disorder. Anti-arrhythmic drugs generally do not help in this setting, although lidocaine and phenytoin have been used acutely to stabilize some patients with drug-induced torsade de pointes *(34–36)*. Minimizing or eliminating inotropic support may yield dramatic results.

If infarcted, scarred myocardium has created a myocardial substrate for a re-entry, triggered automaticity or an automatic arrhythmia, an anti-arrhythmic drug would be anticipated to have potential benefit. In some instances, the substrate is modified by acute ischemia or sympathetic stimulation. In these cases, an anti-arrhythmic drug may also have benefit. The presence of monomorphic VT suggests that the patient has an underlying substrate for reentry as cause for the problem. It is important to distinguish a monomorphic VT from a supraventricular tachycardia with aberrant conduction so that proper treatment is instituted. It can be difficult to diagnose the etiology of a wide QRS complex tachycardia and even when it appears to have the same morphology as the baseline QRS complex, it can be ventricular in origin *(37–41)*. If the wide QRS tachycardia etiology is not diagnosed, the patient should be treated as if it were VT.

The type of arrhythmia present may indicate the underlying substrate. VF or polymorphic VT may be as a result of ischemia, aortic stenosis, electrolyte abnormality, or drug pro-arrhythmia. The presence of polymorphic VT in select patients such as young individuals who have no obvious underlying structural heart disease suggests the presence of a toxin, an underlying congenital problem such as the long QT interval syndrome, hypertrophic cardiomyopathy or complex congenital heart disease. In the case of the congenital long QT interval syndrome or the Brugada syndrome, anti-arrhythmic drugs should be used sparingly as they may result in death when the patient has otherwise stabilized. Anti-arrhythmic drugs, particularly amiodarone, may have benefit in patients with hypertrophic cardiomyopathy or arrhythmogenic right ventricular dysplasia. Anti-arrhythmic drugs must be considered in relation to the underlying problem responsible for the CA and in light of other drugs being prescribed. There are few data supporting the use of more than one anti-arrhythmic drug during a CA.

The patient and the underlying condition must be considered. Often the arrhythmia is not primary. Aggressive anti-arrhythmic drug treatment of an asymptomatic patient with a well-tolerated arrhythmia may spell disaster.

The Anti-Arrhythmic Drugs (Table 2)

Each anti-arrhythmic drug has specific actions, risks, side effects, and potential for pro-arrhythmia (42,43). They must be considered individually; many have no proven efficacy. Despite extensive basic research regarding anti-arrhythmic drugs as a group, better understanding of mechanistic actions and more accurate classification based on physiologic effects ([44,45] the Sicilian Gambit [46,47] and the Vaughn-Williams-Singh classification [48]), the issue comes down to whether these drugs work in a CA. Intravenous drugs tested include: lidocaine, procainamide, bretylium, amiodarone, and β-blockers.

LIDOCAINE

Lidocaine, as a class IB anti-arrhythmic drug, slows rapid inward sodium current in ventricular myocardium, slows or eliminates conduction in ischemic myocardium and inhibits abnormal automaticity. It does not alter potassium conductance. Lidocaine will not lengthen, and may even shorten, the QT interval. In animal models, lidocaine affects ischemic myocardium preferentially (49–52) but it may block AV conduction and halt escape rhythms, such as idioventricular rhythm and therefore result in death from asystole. Lidocaine may be antifibrillatory but compelling data showing benefit are scant (53).

In a CA, an initial bolus of 1.0 to 1.5 mg/kg IV followed by as second bolus (as there is rapid peripheral distribution) is necessary to rapidly achieve, and then maintain therapeutic but prevent toxic levels. Lidocaine reaches the central circulation after bolus peripheral administration in approx 2 minutes when perfusion is present. The drug can also be given via a tracheal approach at 2–2.5 times the IV dose in 10 mL of saline. Lidocaine may not reach the myocardium effectively in an arrest situation and even if it does, it may not achieve therapeutic levels in the damaged or ischemic myocardium responsible for the arrhythmia as that tissue may be isolated from the circulation by an obstructed coronary artery and/or poor blood flow (this is true for any medications given during an arrest).

Previously, lidocaine has been considered the "first" anti-arrhythmic drug. Its administration is based primarily on established use and historic precedent more than real data. There are few supportive studies. Lidocaine is frequently ineffective and it can be associated with neurological toxicity (Table 3). Patients remain at continued risk for death despite its use. Although lidocaine is well tolerated hemodynamically, patients post-

Table 2
Vaughan-Williams-Singh Anti-Arrhythmic Drug Classification

Class I
   A. Procainamide[a,b], Quinidine[a,b], Disopyramide
   B. Lidocaine[a,b], Phenytoin[a,b], Mexiletine, Tocainide
   C. Flecainide, Propafenone
Class II–β-Adrenergic blockers[a,b]
Class III–Amiodarone[a,b], Sotalol, Dofetilide
Class IV–Verapamil[a]

---

[a] Available intravenously in the United States (intravenous sotalol, not available in the United States).

[b] Possibly useful in cardiac arrest as a result of a life-threatening ventricular arrhythmia.

Table 3
Side Effects of Anti-Arrhythmic Drugs

Class IA: Procainamide–QRS, QT widening, psychosis, hallucinations, anorexia, nausea, hypotension, negative inotropic effect, agranulocytosis, torsades de pointes
Class IB: Lidocaine–neurologic toxicity (at high doses–seizures, confusion, disorientation, fatigue), asystole, hemodynamic impairment (rare), potentiates succinylcholine, metabolism can be impaired by β-blockers
Class II: β-Adrenergic Blockers – (metoprolol, propranolol, esmolol)–hemodynamic collapse, hypotension, bradycardia
Class III: Bretylium–hypotension, hemodynamic collapse, torsade de pointes, increase in QT interval, sinus bradycardia, nausea, vomiting

Amiodarone[a] Event	Total ($N = 1836$)
Hypotension	288 (16%)
Bradycardia	90 (4.9%)
Nausea	72 (3.9%)
Abnormal liver function tests	64 (3.4%)
Heart arrest	55 (2.9%)
Ventricular tachycardia	45 (2.4%)
Congestive heart failure	39 (2.1%)
Fever	37 (2%)

[a] From the Wyeth-Ayerst Database (>2% side effects).

myocardial infarction (MI) given lidocaine prophylactically do not have improved survival and may have worsened outcomes compared to placebo (49,50,52,54–56). There are no randomized controlled trials demonstrating benefit of lidocaine. The lack of efficacy may be as a result of time wasted in administration in lieu of other beneficial therapies (circulation) or that it is given too late. Even considering these possibilities, it is unlikely that lidocaine adds much benefit. Furthermore, lidocaine can increase the energy requirements to defibrillate (57–60).

BRETYLIUM

Bretylium is a class III anti-arrhythmic drug (61) with a long history (62–64). Besides lengthening repolarization (a class III effect) in ventricular myocardium, bretylium releases catecholamines presynaptically on injection followed by a postganglionic adrenergic blocking effect *(65)*. Bretylium has been used for monomorphic and polymorphic VT but there are limited data on efficacy and safety and significant problems with hemodynamic instability and proarrhythmia. The loading dose is 5 mg/kg. Severe hypotension is a common side effect of this drug after the initial release of catecholamines (Table 3; *66*). Since 1999, bretylium has been unavailable from the manufacturer as a result of lack of available raw materials. Although once endorsed as an effective drug *(65)*, it has been removed from the AHA's ACLS treatment algorithms and guidelines. Supportive evidence for its benefit is weak *(67,68)*.

PROCAINAMIDE

Procainamide, as a class IA anti-arrhythmic drug, slows conduction and lengthens repolarization in atrial and ventricular tissue. It can be used for well-tolerated wide-QRS complex tachycardias suspected to be VT or well-tolerated monomorphic VT. It is given at a rate of up to 20 mg per minute until the arrhythmia is suppressed, hypotension ensues, the QRS complex is prolonged by 50% or 17 mg/kg of the drug has been given. Procainamide is potentially effective for monomorphic VT (more so than lidocaine) *(69)* but there are limited data on effectiveness and, serious adverse effects, hemodynamic compromise, negative inotropic effect, long-term and short-term toxicities, torsade de pointes, and other proarrhythmic effects are possible (Table 3; *70*). Like lidocaine, procainamide can increase energy requirements to defibrillate.

Procainamide can lengthen the QT interval and can have a proarrhythmic effect. Procainamide should be avoided in patients with preexisting QT prolongation and in cases of torsade de pointes. It should be avoided in the setting of polymorphic VT if the QT interval is prolonged or is not known. Polymorphic VT not as a result of torsade de pointes, may respond to procainamide (although few data support this use).

AMIODARONE

Amiodarone is a complex drug with class I, II, III, and IV, and other, anti-arrhythmic effects. It has physiologic effects in atrial, AV nodal, and ventricular tissue. The mechanisms by which amiodarone works in a CA are not clear but it is the most effective drug for patients with refractory or recurrent poorly tolerated ventricular tachyarrhythmias. Acute intravenous amiodarone administration may have a different mechanism of action than chronic oral dosing and the actual mechanism(s) of effect is not known. Part of the effect may be a class IA anti-arrhythmic effect, a β-blocking effect and even a class III effect.

There are more controlled data on intravenous amiodarone than any other anti-arrhythmic drug and although many suspect that this is the best anti-arrhythmic drug choice, opinions vary *(71)*. Recent ACLS guidelines incorporate use of intravenous amiodarone in the pulseless VT/VF algorithm *(6)*. Amiodarone can increase the chance to survival to hospitalization but it has not yet been shown to increase survival to hospital discharge *(72,73)*. Amiodarone has potential benefits for control of hemodynamically stable monomorphic VT, polymorphic VT, and wide-complex tachycardia of uncertain origin. Acutely, amiodarone, like bretylium, does not appear to increase the energy requirements to defibrillate although chronically, it does *(59,74,75)*. The drug may have a direct antifibrillatory effect.

The metabolism of amiodarone is complex. When amiodarone is given intravenously, the half-life of amiodarone is relatively short because the volume of distribution is large (70 m/kg) and the dose will be re-distributed into fat, the liver, the heart, and the brain. The half-life of redistribution is a few hours or days with the serum half-life being 12 to

24 hours. There is a close relationship between the serum and the myocardial levels. The presence of amiodarone in the myocardium does not ensure a physiologic effect as the site of action is not well defined (76). Intravenous amiodarone will ultimately become metabolized in the liver to the active metabolite desethylamiodarone, a class III anti-arrhythmic drug. The site of action of intravenous amiodarone and its side effects may in part be related to the metabolite but it is unclear the mechanism by which either works.

Intravenous amiodarone is associated with a 4.9% incidence of bradycardia, 3.9% incidence of nausea, 3.4% incidence of abnormal liver function tests (even fulminant hepatic necrosis and abrupt liver failure; Table 3). Other side effects, including pulmonary toxicity during the acute phase of administration, are relatively rare. Most side effects as a result of intravenous amiodarone are relatively easy to manage. If the patient becomes hypotensive during IV amiodarone infusion, the best approach is to provide intravenous fluid support and to decrease the rate of infusion of the drug. If possible, it is preferential but not mandatory to give intravenous amiodarone via a central line. Amiodarone has been associated with hypotension in up to 16% of patients. This hypotension is usually less severe than that which occurs with procainamide.

Hypotension from intravenous amiodarone appears to be as a result of peripheral vasodilatation but it also can have a negative inotropic influence. Both effects are as a result of the vehicle (Tween-80, polysorbate). Amiodarone is not water soluble but it is possible to make a micellar dispersion (77). However, trials evaluating aqueous intravenous amiodarone have failed to demonstrate clear, convincing, benefit over the standard formulation and there is risk of severe phlebitis. One randomized as yet unpublished trial of aqueous intravenous amiodarone was stopped early as a result of severe adverse side effects (potentially life-threatening phlebitis) and no evidence for additional benefit. The present formulation has side effects that are manageable and acceptable. The drug is available in vials but has a relatively short shelf life.

Amiodarone pro-arrhythmic effects include bradycardia, asystole, and torsade de points but after cardiac arrest, risks appear to be less than for other anti-arrhythmic drugs. Pro-arrhythmia (78) includes polymorphic VT or torsade de pointes. It may be very difficult to distinguish the problem of "amiodarone deficiency" from drug pro-arrhythmia. Assessment of the QT interval may help but if the arrhythmias are worsening despite the amiodarone dose, it may be best to with hold the drug. Some patients require large doses of intravenous amiodarone to stabilize. If, after intravenous amiodarone is given, the patient has recurrent episodes of polymorphic VT or VF and does not seem to be stabilizing, the physician should consider the possibility that amiodarone might be pro-arrhythmic and consider stopping the drug early. The issue is confusing because amiodarone commonly increases the QT interval without inducing torsade de pointes (79) and yet it can also cause polymorphic VT without even lengthening the QT interval.

In an arrest situation, a bolus of 300 mg intravenously is appropriate but if the patient is in sinus rhythm and is between episodes of recurrent CA, a dose of 150 mg is appropriate. Repeat boluses may be needed to stabilize a patient. Although a total of six 150-mg boluses are recommended additionally to intravenous infusion, some patient may require more than nine boluses in a 24-hour period to achieve stability.

Most patients who survive a CA do not require an anti-arrhythmic drug but if amiodarone was required to achieve initial stability, then continuation of amiodarone is appropriate until other therapies can be implemented. Several algorithms have been developed and recommended to transition from intravenous to oral amiodarone dosing.

In the process of transition, the total intravenous dose given, the severity and recurrence of the arrhythmia, the capability of the gastrointestinal tract to absorb the drug must be considered. In general, if a patient was loaded well on intravenous amiodarone and has continued on an infusion, there should be an overlap between the intravenous and the oral doses. The oral dose given after 1 to 2 days of intravenous bolus and infusion should generally begin at 800 to 1200 mg per day before the intravenous drug is stopped. Then, after several days, if the patients remain stable, the dose can be decreased to 600 to 800 mg a day in divided dosages. The rest of the load depends on all other clinical variables; total loading may take up to 1 month.

The cost of amiodarone was once a concern but intravenous amiodarone has come down substantially in price recently as it is now nonproprietary. The current cost is less than $7 for a 150-mg vial.

INTRAVENOUS β-BLOCKERS

β-Blockers can prevent ischemia and reinitiation of VT and VF by several mechanisms *(80–82)*. Unfortunately, β-blockers may impair hemodynamics and worsen heart failure (Table 3). The drugs most commonly given in this setting are metoprolol and esmolol. There are data describing the decreased mortality in patients with CAD in individual trials *(83–85)* and in a meta-analysis *(86)*. Data supporting β-adrenergic blocker use for acute treatment of ventricular arrhythmias are limited, but encouraging.

Case reports and patients with "electrical storm" (*see* section on Electrical Storm) may benefit. β-Blockers with concomitant atrial pacing may suppress exercise-induced repetitive polymorphic ventricular ectopy, paroxysms of bidirectional VT, and bursts of slow idiopathic polymorphic and monomorphic VT *(87,88)*. High-dose propranolol was used in conjunction with extra-corporeal life support and an intra-aortic balloon pump to treat refractory VT *(89)*. β-Blockers may augment the efficacy of amiodarone as was shown in a randomized crossover study of 20 patients with ejection fraction of 0.28 ± 0.8 and recurrent or incessant VT *(90)*. Other data suggest this drug class may be antifibrillatory and have additive effects to amiodarone *(91)*.

It does not make sense to use a β-adrenergic blocker with a β-adrenergic stimulant. Before starting a β-blocker, dobutamine, isoproterenol or epinephrine should be withdrawn. The side effects of β-blockers—hypotension, bradycardia, and cardiovascular collapse—may limit their use in the setting of a resuscitative effort.

DO ANTI-ARRHYTHMIC DRUGS HELP IN CARDIAC RESUSCITATION? THE CLINICAL TRIAL DATA

The early data on anti-arrhythmic drug effects collected on resuscitated patients were case reports or nonrandomized and retrospective trials. This, in part, is a result of the difficulty in obtaining data and performing studies in such patients. Not surprisingly, by the time the anti-arrhythmic is given, the chance of survival is vanishingly small. The patient population and the resuscitation methods differ from the modern era of resuscitation. Also, the approach to resuscitation may have been overly aggressive; patients received the "kitchen sink" so that it was difficult to determine the benefit, or lack thereof, for any specific intervention.

Initial studies used bretylium and lidocaine *(54,59,62–64,67,69)*. Lidocaine and bretylium were ineffective in experimental cardiac arrest and in clinical resuscitation *(61)*. Lidocaine was "not useful for improving outcome in patients who persist in VF" *(15)*. It increased the chance for asystole and delayed the use of needed shocks. In 1989,

Armengol studied 20 patients with 31 episodes of wide complex tachycardia treated with lidocaine. Nineteen percent (six episodes in five patients) had successful termination of tachycardia. However, in three of these five patients, lidocaine was ineffective against a recurrence of tachycardia (92). Other studies evaluating lidocaine in monomorphic VT show that it is relatively ineffective (69,93,94).

In 1994, Nasir evaluated the use of lidocaine in patients with spontaneous or induced monomorphic VT but *without MI*. Of 128 patients, only 10 (8%) had successful termination with lidocaine. None of these drugs was remarkably beneficial (93).

In 1994, Ho compared the efficacy of lidocaine and sotalol in 33 patients with spontaneous sustained VT. The investigator crossed over the patients to the other drug if the initial drug was ineffective after 15 minutes. VT was terminated by lidocaine in 18 % and by sotalol in 69% (94).

Gorgels studied 29 patients comparing procainamide to lidocaine in 1996. Nineteen percent of the lidocaine patients and 79% of the procainamide patients had successful termination of VT (69). Procainamide is a difficult drug to use in a resuscitative effort because it needs to be given relatively slowly. This is as a result of its negative inotropic effect and its vasodilatory effect. The infusion can take more than 30 minutes. This drug is best used for well-tolerated VT or for those patients who have intermittent episodes of tachycardia.

One large trial evaluated 773 in-hospital CA patients, 245 of whom (32%) had VT or VF (17). Of these, 585 could be resuscitated with return of spontaneous circulation. A multivariate analysis of outcome vs anti-arrhythmic drug treatment in these 245 patients controlling for age, gender, rhythm, cause of arrest, and chronic cardiorespiratory disease indicated risk reduction with lidocaine ($N = 42$) OR 0.53 (95% CI = 0.31–0.90) and possibly with bretylium ($N = 36$) OR = O.56 (0.26–1.23). These data, although relatively scant, provide evidence for a positive benefit from these anti-arrhythmic drugs.

Initial reports focused on intravenous amiodarone after other drugs had failed. These small trials showed that intravenous amiodarone had promise. Mostow (95) evaluated intravenous amiodarone in the early 1980s, in 36 patients. In an uncontrolled trial, he showed that intravenous amiodarone markedly reduced recurrent episodes of poorly tolerated VT. In patients unresponsive, or resistant, to other anti-arrhythmic therapies, Morady ($N = 15$; 96) showed an 80% response for VT, Helmy ($N = 46$; 97) showed a 59% response for VT and VF, Klein ($N = 13$; 98) showed a 54% response for VT, Ochi ($N = 22$; 99) showed a 64% response for VT and VF, Schutzenberger ($N = 15$; 100) showed a 60% response for VT and VF and Mooss ($N = 350$; 101) showed a 63% response for VT. These small but compelling trials opened the way to controlled clinical trials of intravenous amiodarone.

RANDOMIZED TRIALS EVALUATING ANTI-ARRHYTHMIC DRUG EFFICACY IN CA: THE VALUE OF INTRAVENOUS AMIODARONE

Controlled trials assessed the potential benefit of intravenous amiodarone during resuscitation. These trials have included in- and out-of-hospital episodes of VT and VF and have included patients with various clinical presentations. The first controlled studies involved patients with recurrent VT and VF refractory to all other medical therapy. These patients had exposure to many anti-arrhythmic drugs. The combination of these drugs may have been synergistic or antagonistic. There are no randomized clinical trials

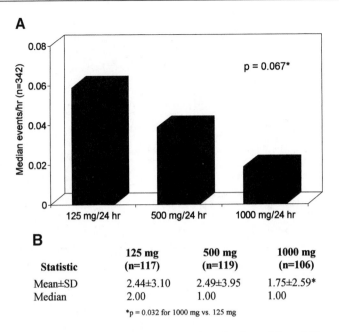

Fig. 2. (A) IV amiodarone dose-ranging study *(102)*. *Cochran-Mantel-Haenszel procedure.
(B) Total supplemental boluses of IV amiodarone.

assessing the survival benefit of a combination of anti-arrhythmic drugs or a β-blocker plus amiodarone (compared to no combination) in patients having out-of-hospital CA. Later trials evaluated the use of intravenous amiodarone as the sole anti-arrhythmic drug.

Dose-Ranging Studies

Two multicenter trials were dose ranging, evaluating patients randomized to different doses of intravenous amiodarone. The first trial, reported by Scheinman (Fig. 2; *102)* used intravenous amiodarone at 125 mg per 24 hours, 500 mg per 24 hours, and 100 mg per 24 hours but patients could get additional boluses. To be enrolled in this trial, patients had to experience two episodes of VT and/or VF over 24 hours. Most of these patients were in-patients. The doses of IV amiodarone prescribed were: 125 mg ($N = 117$), 500 mg ($N = 119$), and 1000 mg ($N = 106$) over 24 hours. All patients were given lidocaine, procainamide and often bretylium before amiodarone and all patients were refractory to these drugs. This study did not achieve statistical significance in the mean number of VT events per hour (total events = 342, $p = 0.067$ between groups, intention to treat) and there was no survival difference. There was a trend to an improved outcome at the highest dose of compared to the lowest dose of intravenous amiodarone (0.02 events per hour at the highest dose compared to 0.06 events per hour at the lowest). Those taking the higher dose needed fewer boluses of intravenous amiodarone and therefore considering the extra boluses, many patients in all three arms received similar total doses of amiodarone *(102)*. The mean additional 150 mg boluses for those with the lowest starting dose was 2.44 (median = 2) doses compared to 1.75 (median = 1) doses for the highest dose ($p = 0.032$). Patients in this trial were critically ill and refractory to all other treatment. Many responded extraordinarily well to amiodarone and survived when they

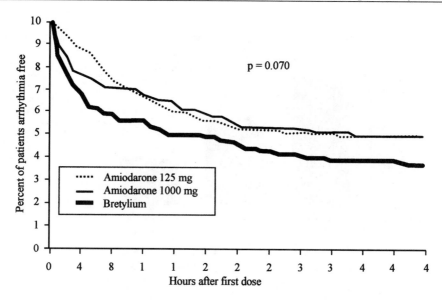

Fig. 3. IV amiodarone vs IV bretylium *(104).*

had no chance otherwise. The investigators who participated in the trial were often pleased and surprised with patient outcomes.

A second dose ranging trial by the Intravenous Amiodarone Multicenter Trial Group included 273 patients refractory to IV lidocaine, bretylium, and procainamide *(103)*. This study evaluated the response rate and safety of intravenous amiodarone in 273 patients with recurrent, hypotensive VT (blood pressure <80 mmHg systolic) or fibrillation refractory to lidocaine, procainamide, and bretylium. Patients were randomized to receive 500 mg, 1000 mg, or 2000 mg over 24 hours by a 150 mg bolus followed by an infusion. One hundred and ten of 237 patients (40%) who completed the 6-hour load survived the 6- to 24-hour maintenance period without recurrent hypotensive ventricular tachyarrhythmias when intravenous amiodarone was used as a single anti-arrhythmic drug. Twenty-nine of 237 patients (12%) responded to amiodarone in combination with another drug. Thirty-six patients (15%) were withdrawn from the study during the first 6 hours, 17 (7%) died, 14 (6%) were withdrawn as a result of adverse effects, and 5 (2%) were withdrawn as a result of intractable arrhythmias. There were no significant dif-ferences between groups in the percentage in 24 hours with a successful response but there was a trend to improved success in the higher dose group. Of patients whose arrhythmias were not controlled during the 6- to 24-hour period, 14 (5%) died and 7 (3%) were withdrawn because of adverse effects. There was no clear dose–response relationship in this trial with respect to success rates (primary end-point), time to first tachycardia recurrence (post hoc analysis), or mortality (secondary end-point) over 24 hours.

Amiodarone vs Bretylium

In another multicenter trial (Fig. 3; *104*), intravenous amiodarone was compared to bretylium in patients who were refractory to procainamide (as possible to give) and lidocaine (all patients). The study entry criteria included patients refractory to defibril-

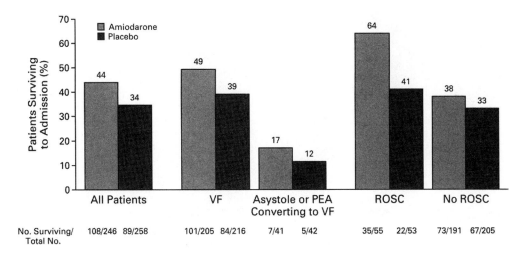

Fig. 4. The ARREST trial *(72)*.

lation (at that time monophasic shocks) or with recurrent episodes of VT or VF. Patients did not need to be refractory to procainamide and did not receive bretylium before study. Doses of intravenous amiodarone (125 and 1000 mg over 24 hours) were compared to bretylium 5 mg/kg. Three hundred and two patients were enrolled in this double-blind, randomized trial. Recurrent ventricular arrhythmias were less for patients receiving the higher dose of amiodarone compared to the lower dose but there were no differences between the bretylium group and the group taking higher doses of amiodarone ($p = 0.07$). In a post hoc analysis of this intention to treat study, patients placed on bretylium had more frequent recurrences of VT. Nearly 50% were crossed over to amiodarone. Based on these mainly in-patient studies without placebo control, it appears that intravenous amiodarone is somewhat superior to bretylium. The intravenous amiodarone boluses given in these trials were not necessarily given during a CA but were often given between recurrent episodes of CA.

THE ARREST TRIAL

Data regarding resuscitation in the field came from the Amiodarone after Resuscitation of Out-of-Hospital CA as a result of VF (ARREST) trial (Figs. 4,5; *72*). This single-center randomized placebo-controlled trial performed in Seattle involved patients who experienced out-of-hospital CA and had persistent or recurrent episodes of VT or ventricular and thus failed standard resuscitation measures including intubation, epinephrine, and defibrillation. Subjects were randomized blindly to a 300-mg intravenous amiodarone bolus or a placebo bolus. The primary endpoint was the survival rate to admission to the hospital as the study was not powered to assess mortality (Fig. 4). Secondary endpoints included adverse drug effects, time to return of spontaneous circulation, survival to hospital discharge, and neurological status at hospital discharge.

Of 504 patients enrolled, predictors of hospital admission included: initial rhythm of VF ($p < 0.001$), dispatch to advanced life support unit ($p < 0.001$), transient return of

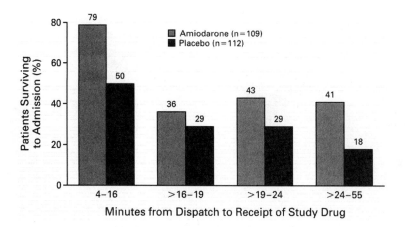

Fig. 5. The ARREST trial *(72).*

spontaneous circulation before therapy ($p < 0.001$), arrest at home or at a nursing home ($p < 0.003$), anti-arrhythmic drug before treatment ($p < 0.04$), and amiodarone ($p < 0.02$). Amiodarone was associated with better survival to hospital admission whether the drug was administered early or late (Fig. 5) (OR = 1.6, 95% CI, 1.1 to 2.4; $p = 0.02$).

Amiodarone was associated with more hypotension and bradycardia and there was no survival benefit to hospital discharge. This raises the concern that amiodarone might simply extend hospital stay and increase hospital cost with no palpable benefit.

In the ARREST trial, another concern was that the time the anti-arrhythmic drug was given in the "field" was quite late, even in the circumstances of a planned trial. The drug was given 15 to 25 minutes after the arrest. By that time, it would not be unexpected for a patient to die from a CA despite administration of an effective drug. Even if amiodarone were given centrally, it may have no effect as it might not ultimately reach the myocardium.

Several issues became apparent: (a) an anti-arrhythmic drug may be beneficial but for it to be effective, it must be given early; (b) the best method to give an anti-arrhythmic drug remains uncertain; (c) even in the best of circumstances, the anti-arrhythmic drug may not help improve survival; and (d) the best initial dose of amiodarone is not known but 300 mg was associated with few side effects and this dose, larger than Food and Drug Administration recommendations, may have additional benefits over 150 mg intravenously (which may be better in less urgent situations).

In the ARREST Trial, intravenous amiodarone appears capable of facilitating return of a perfused rhythm compared to placebo but lidocaine was not tested in a head-to-head comparison.

THE ALIVE TRIAL

The Amiodarone vs Lidocaine In Pre-Hospital Refractory VF Evaluation (ALIVE) trial *(105)* was also a single-center trial (Figs. 6,7). Patients experiencing out-of-hospital CA, refractory to standard resuscitative maneuvers, were recruited similar to those in the ARREST trial. Patients were given intravenous lidocaine 1.5 mg/kg and intravenous amiodarone placebo (vehicle) or intravenous lidocaine placebo and intravenous amiodarone 2.5 mg/kg (blinded double dummy as a result of differences in preparation

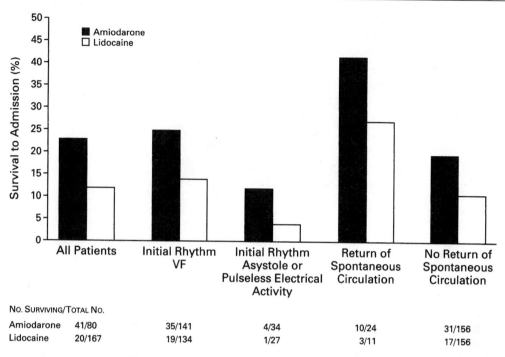

No. Surviving/Total No.				
Amiodarone 41/80	35/141	4/34	10/24	31/156
Lidocaine 20/167	19/134	1/27	3/11	17/156

Fig. 6. The ALIVE trial *(105)* subgroup survival.

of the two drugs). As in the ARREST trial, patients were required to fail three defibrillation shocks, intubation, and epinephrine and had to have persistent or recurrent hemodynamically intolerable VT or VF to be enrolled.

The primary endpoint was survival to hospital admission (Fig. 6). The study was powered to assess the primary endpoint to increase hospital admission from 25 to 40% ($\alpha = 0.05$; $\beta = 0.2$). The amiodarone group ($N = 179$) was compared to the lidocaine group ($N = 165$). There were no differences in age, sex, weight, history of heart disease (present in more than 60%), witnessed arrest (more than 75%) or bystander CPR (more than 25%). The last recorded rhythm before drug administration was VF in more than 90%. On average, five shocks were given before drug administration. The time to first defibrillation shock was 11 minutes, the time to the intravenous administration was 13, minutes and the time to study drug was 25.2 ± 8.0 minutes in the amiodarone arm and 24.1 ± 7.0 minutes in the lidocaine arm.

In the ALIVE trial, the number surviving to hospital admission was greater in the amiodarone arm with a risk ratio of 2.17 (1.21, 3.23). The survival to hospitalization for amiodarone patients was 25.2%, whereas with lidocaine it was 13.3 ($p = 0.02$) when the rhythm was VF. When it was not, 13.5% of those given amiodarone survived compared to 0% given lidocaine ($p = 0.06$). Those given amiodarone whether given early or late (Fig. 7) were more likely to survive to hospitalization than those given lidocaine. The rate of survival to hospital admission depended on the time between dispatch of the emergency medical service and time of administration of the study drug. Those receiving amiodarone fared better when the drug was given early. The treatment and the time effects of amiodarone were both significant (treatment effect $p = 0.005$, time effect

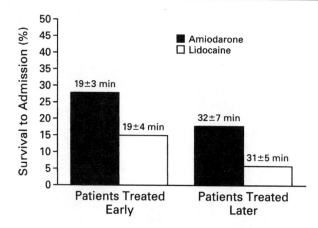

Fig. 7. Survival rate to hospital admission by time of dispatch of EMS crew to administration of drug *(105)*.

$p < 0.001$, interaction between time/treatment $p = 0.26$, multiple logistic-regression analysis).

Survival and better outcomes were associated with earlier administration of an anti-arrhythmic drug and amiodarone was better than lidocaine. The data were further strengthened by the fact that the use of an anti-arrhythmic drug is dependent on the time course for administration. There was no mortality benefit from either anti-arrhythmic drug but the study was not powered to assess this survival to hospital discharge.

WHEN SHOULD ANTI-ARRHYTHMIC DRUGS BE USED IN CARDIAC ARREST?

Based on ACLS guidelines *(6)*, anti-arrhythmic drug therapy is not high on the list of first-line approaches to treat life-threatening ventricular arrhythmias (Table 4). There are no class I indications for the use of anti-arrhythmic drugs. Based on the present data it is reasonable to consider an anti-arrhythmic drug *after defibrillation attempts and CPR* have been undertaken appropriately for those with CA as a result of a ventricular arrhythmia. The rhythm causing the arrest must be scrutinized, as it may be a bradyarrhythmia unresponsive to an anti-arrhythmic drug. It may be sinus tachycardia or a supraventricular tachycardia that will not respond to an anti-arrhythmic drug as expected. The rhythm could be a wide QRS but "perfusing" rhythm that should not be suppressed. It is also important to recognize that an anti-arrhythmic drug will not work effectively if it is given too late in the course of the resuscitation effort as severely damaged cardiac muscle will not respond to anti-arrhythmic drug.

A team effort in a resuscitation attempt should include proper defibrillation, proper CPR, and simultaneous preparation for more advanced therapies such as anti-arrhythmic drugs utilization, preferably via a central line.

Summary of Anti-Arrhythmic Drug Data (Table 4)

The greatest amount data available concerning the benefit of an anti-arrhythmic drug in the face of resuscitation from ventricular tachyarrhythmia favors use of intravenous

Table 4

ACLS Guideline Recommendations

Wide complex tachycardia, type unknown, stable

Attempt diagnosis: 12 lead ECG (*adenosine de-emphasized*)

If unable to make a diagnosis:

   EF normal: cardioversion, procainamide or *amiodarone*

   EF <40%, heart failure or unknown: cardioversion or *amiodarone*

Stable VT Monomorphic/Polymorphic

Monomorphic VT: cardioversion or

   EF normal: procainamide (IIa), sotalol (IIa), amiodarone (IIb), lidocaine (IIb)

   EF poor: amiodarone 150 mg IV/10 minute or lidocaine 0.5–0.75 mg/kg IV push

   If ineffective, synchronized cardioversion

Polymorphic VT: cardioversion or

   Normal QT (consider: ischemia, electrolyte or metabolic problem and treat).

      EF normal: β-Blocker or lidocaine or amiodarone or procainamide

      EF impaired: amiodarone 150 mg/10 minute or lidocaine 0.5–0.75 mg/kg IV push

      Then, cardioversion, as needed

   Prolonged QT baseline (Torsade de Pointes)

      Correct electrolytes, stop offending agent

      Magnesium sulfate, overdrive pacing, isoproterenol, phenytoin (?), lidocaine (?)

      If ineffective, cardioversion

VF/Pulseless VT

   CPR, defibrillation three times (200 J, 200 J–300 J, 360 J) or equivalent biphasic shocks (150 J–200 J). If unsuccessful: vasopressin 40 U IV (class IIb) or epinephrine 1 mg q3–5 minute (class indeterminate) and then defibrillate at maximum output. If ineffective:

Anti-Arrhythmic drug

   First: Amiodarone 300 mg IV push, can repeat 150 mg IV once (class IIb)

   Second: Lidocaine 1.0–1.5mg/kg IV push q3–5 minutes up to 3 mg/kg (class indeterminate)

      $Mg^{+2}SO_4$ 1–2 g IV if polymorphic VT/hypomagnesaemia (class IIb)

      Procainamide 30 mg per minute up to 17mg/kg (class IIb)

   Bicarbonate prolonged arrest (class IIb), hyperkalemia (class I), bicarbonate responsive acidosis (class IIa), tricyclic overdose (class IIa), or to alkalinize urine for aspirin overdose (classIIa); not for hypercarbia

   Defibrillate at maximal output

Summary of ACLS Guidelines – Use of Anti-Arrhythmic Drugs

   Amiodarone (class IIb) and procainamide (class IIb) before lidocaine and adenosine for hemodynamically stable wide-complex tachycardia, and unstable VT/VF.

   Amiodarone for *stable* monomorphic and polymorphic VT (class IIa).

   Amiodarone – more evidence-based support than any other anti-arrhythmic drug.

   Lidocaine – acceptable for shock-refractory and/or pulseless VT (evidence is poor, studies are weak). ("Indeterminate" recommendation). Not for routine prophylaxis.

   Magnesium sulfate – hypomagnesemia and Torsade de Pointes (class IIb)

ACLS, advanced cardia life support; EF, ejection fraction; VT, ventricular tachycardia; IV, intravenous; VF, ventricular fibrillation. (From ref. *6*.)

amiodarone. The AHA ACLS guidelines give intravenous amiodarone a class "IIb" indication. Lidocaine has an "indeterminate" indication but it is not contraindicated (6).

This recommendation is based on data from randomized controlled clinical trials in various settings. No trial has yet demonstrated survival benefit of amiodarone or any other anti-arrhythmic drug in CA. Clearly, the benefit of resuscitation comes from aggressive cardiopulmonary resuscitation and appropriate and rapid defibrillation. This must be the first-line approach.

On the other hand, if this approach is ineffective despite appropriate delivery of defibrillation shocks and appropriate CPR, it is possible that an anti-arrhythmic drug will improve the outcome. If it is to help, the anti-arrhythmic drug must be given early and must be given so that the drug can reach the myocardium at risk. No study has yet demonstrated that an alternative delivery approach would be beneficial (such as injection directly into the left ventricle).

Thus anti-arrhythmic drugs are second line therapies: intravenous procainamide in relatively well-tolerated sustained monomorphic VT, IV lidocaine when there is a prolongation in the QT interval, and IV amiodarone as for patients with recurrent or refractory VT or fibrillation despite appropriate defibrillation attempts.

Is Intravenous Magnesium Sulfate Effective?

Magnesium use is controversial but most data do not support its use in CA (106–111). One report was a randomized placebo-controlled trial of patients without clinical need for magnesium (including Torsade de Pointes) who had in-hospital CA (112). Fifty-six patients were treated with either 2 g of magnesium sulfate followed by an infusion of 8 g over 24 hours or placebo. The primary endpoint was return of spontaneous circulation least 1 hour after CA. The secondary endpoints were survival to 24 hours, survival to hospital discharge, and neurological outcome. Magnesium showed no significant benefit.

In an open label prospective study, Miller et al. (106) assessed patients at a single center who had in-hospital CA as a result of a ventricular tachyarrhythmia refractory to three defibrillation shocks and intravenous epinephrine dose (three defibrillation attempts). Twenty-nine patients received magnesium sulfate and defibrillation shocks; 33 received shocks alone. The groups were similar although those randomized to magnesium sulfate had a 5-minute longer code (14.2 vs 19.8 minutes). There was only a trend toward benefit with magnesium resuscitation in 21% (7/33) vs 35% (10/29) ($p = 0.21$).

Other studies have evaluated intravenous magnesium with discrepant results (107,110). The body of evidence does not support intravenous magnesium in resuscitation unless the patient has torsade de pointes (113) or is magnesium deficient.

What to Do If Intravenous Anti-Arrhythmic Drugs
Do Not Stabilize the Patient in the Face of Resuscitation

Recurrent or refractory episodes of VT or VF may occur despite aggressive defibrillation attempts and the use of intravenous anti-arrhythmic drugs. Evaluation should include consideration of the potential mechanisms involved. Treatment should address influences of ischemia, drug pro-arrhythmia, inotropic drug effects and other initiators. Some patients have a ventricular ectopic beat on a T wave responsible for triggering recurrent VF. This may be in part as a result of bradycardia. Backup pacing may help these patients. Methods to decrease sympathetic tone may also be beneficial but β-blockers may be too risky. Sympathetic tone can be decreased by ventricular assist devices such as an intra aortic balloon pump or a left ventricular assist device *(114)*. They also decrease ischemia and myocardial stretch both of which may be responsible for recurrent episodes of CA *(115)*.

Specific Situations

IMPLANTABLE CARDIOVERTER DEFIBRILLATORS AND ANTI-ARRHYTHMIC DRUGS

Amiodarone or procainamide may slow the VT and make it more resistant to an implantable cardioverter defibrillator (ICD) shock *(116)*. If the VT slows, it may be below the programmed detection limit of the implantable defibrillator and the device will not deliver a shock for VT. Procainamide can increase defibrillation thresholds *(117)*. Lidocaine also will increase defibrillation thresholds sometimes dramatically (bretylium does not *[60,118]*). Intravenous amiodarone does not seem to increase defibrillation thresholds as much. Anti-arrhythmic drugs may also make the rhythm more amenable to pacing termination through the ICD.

The Brugada Syndrome

This congenital syndrome is as a result of a "channelopathy" in which there is a defect in the I_{to} (transient outward current *[119,120]*) and/or the inward Na^+ current. When inward Ca^{+2} currents (ICa) are overwhelmed by I_{to}, the action potential duration may shorten leading to re-entry as a result of heterogeneous repolarization. Class I anti-arrhythmic drugs can make this problem worse *(119,121–123)*. If this problem is diag-nosed, anti-arrhythmic drugs should be avoided as none are shown to be safe in this condition even though quinidine may have unique effects.

Catecholaminergic Polymorphic Ventricular Tachycardia

This syndrome has been associated with abnormality in the protein hRyR2, the ryanodine receptor, found inside the cell. This regulates release of calcium ions in the cell *(124)*. There are abnormalities in this receptor in arrhythmogenic right ventricular dyspla-sia as well *(125)*. Patients with this congenital syndrome can respond well to β-adrenergic blockade.

Congenital Long QT Interval Syndrome

This is a congenital condition in which CA is triggered by the long QT interval allow-ing polymorphic VT or VF to occur *(119,126)*. There are several genetic abnormalities in repolarization causing this life-threatening problem. Acutely, no anti-arrhythmic drug, except for perhaps lidocaine, is appropriate in this setting as procainamide and amiodarone may make the problem of recurrent ventricular tachyarrhythmias even worse by length-ening repolarization. There is often a family history of CA in these individuals. Suspect this problem in a young patient at low risk for cardiac conditions.

Acquired Long QT Interval Syndrome

Torsade de Pointes is a polymorphic VT in association with a prolonged QT interval. (QTc >0.45 seconds). In a retrospective review of 190 patients with out-of-hospital CA, 117 patients (62%) had monomorphic VT and 73 (38%) had polymorphic VT. Of the 73 patients with polymorphic VT, 49% had a prolonged QTc. In this review, patients with a prolonged QTc who were treated with ACLS had an equal rate of out-of-hospital return of spontaneous circulation to those with a normal QTc interval *(127)*. This problem is common and must be considered before giving a drug that lengthens the QT interval even more (such as procainamide, bretylium, or amiodarone). The treatment is well-reviewed elsewhere *(125)*.

HYPOTHERMIA

Hypothermia can lengthen the QT interval and cause severe bradycardia *(129–132)*. When the body warms up too fast especially as the temperature reaches 90° F (although the data differ), VF is common *(133–137)*. The goal is to repeatedly defibrillate and warm slowly. Anti-arrhythmic drugs are not shown to be effective and may be harmful in this instance.

Cocaine-Induced Cardiac Arrest

Cocaine use can be associated with VF or unstable VT by several mechanisms *(138,139)*. β-Blockers in such patients may cause coronary vasoconstriction and should be avoided (class III indication, i.e., not indicated). There are no clear data supporting the use of an anti-arrhythmic drug in this setting. Cocaine can also influence, and lengthen, the QT interval so that intravenous amiodarone may be dangerous. Cocaine can also have class I anti-arrhythmic drug properties. In patients with cocaine-induced VF, when recurrent, treat for MI first. No specific data support the use of an anti-arrhythmic drug.

ELECTRICAL STORM

Electrical storm consists of multiple recurrences of VF or poorly tolerated VT requiring defibrillation. It is seen in the setting of acute ischemia, acute infarction, decompensated heart failure and drug toxicity. The cause should be determined if possible. The mortality is high. Intravenous amiodarone given aggressively and at high doses can help stabilize the patients. Other therapies to consider include: elimination of inotropic agents, an intra-aortic balloon pump, a ventricular assist device, β-adrenergic blockade or even stellate ganglionic blockade *(114,140)*.

Credner et al. studied 136 patients who received ICDs for sustained VT or CA as a result of VF. Fourteen (10%) had subsequent electrical storms. These patients were treated with intravenous β-blockers and the class I anti-arrhythmic drug ajmaline. If the electrical storm did not abate, they were then treated with intravenous amiodarone. Three patients had termination of ventricular arrhythmia with β-blockers and ajmaline, and the rest had suppression with amiodarone *(139)*.

Evaluating treatment efficacy of electrical storm related to an acute MI, Nademanee *(138)* compared sympathetic blockade to an ACLS. Forty-nine patients were randomized to receive after initial ACLS followed by lidocaine, procainamide and if needed, bretylium. The sympathetic blockade group received β-blockers or a left stellate ganglionic blockade. Forty-one patients received general anesthesia. Mortality at one week was 82% in the anti-arrhythmic drug group (all died of refractory VF) vs 22% in the sympathetic blockage group *(138)*. This study may support the use of sympathetic blockade but there are several caveats: (a) amiodarone was not tested; (b) not all electrical storms may respond to this treatment as there may be multiple mechanisms involved; and (c) sympathetic blockade may be associated with adverse effects.

Data from prior studies using intravenous amiodarone have included patients with electrical storm. Such patients may respond well to intravenous amiodarone and this should be considered a first-line anti-arrhythmic drug approach to these patients in lieu of other concomitant therapies (including β-blockade *[102,104]*) but amiodarone may make the problem worse by inducing refractory VF. Assessment of the QT interval may be helpful as well as observation of the trigger for recurrent arrhythmias. If the QT has substantially prolonged, if the patient is markedly bradycardic between episodes or if there are paroxysms of polymorphic nonsustained VT, consider stopping the intravenous amiodarone, as it may be pro-arrhythmic.

What If a Patient is Already Taking an Anti-Arrhythmic Drug?

Before giving an anti-arrhythmic rule out pro-arrhythmia. If the patient is fully loaded on amiodarone, there is no use in giving more. If the patient is not fully loaded with amiodarone, give more. Combinations of lidocaine and amiodarone are not proven to be effective but they may be worth a try.

Long-Term Treatment

The long-term management of a patient who has suffered a CA requires careful assessment of available therapies. Patients who arrest after cardiac surgery, even with stabilization and intravenous amiodarone, generally require an ICD *(140)*. This is true for most patients who have a CA as a result of VT or VF. An ICD should be implanted after acute stabilization unless the patient has suffered an acute MI and has intact left ventricular function, that is, has an explainable cause for arrest that can be treated effectively and completely. Long-term drug therapy in lieu of ICD for select patients depends on clinical status. Treat underlying problems as best possible. β-Blockers should be used liberally if not contraindicated. The ACC/AHA guidelines for ICD implantation have been revised recently *(141)*.

CONCLUSION

Anti-arrhythmic drugs may improve outcomes in select patients requiring resuscitation from a potentially fatal ventricular arrhythmia but use of such drugs is presently a second-line approach after other methods have failed. Substantial benefit is unlikely when the "down-time" interval is prolonged. Anti-arrhythmic drugs can facilitate recovery in select cases of CA, but the present data do not mandate earlier use of an anti-arrhythmic drug in lieu of other lifesaving therapies. For a drug to be beneficial, although it must be considered early in the arrest and may be a useful adjunct as part of a team effort in a multimodality approach to patient resuscitation.

REFERENCES

1. Statistics, N.C.f.H., Advance report of final mortality statistics, 1990. Monthly Vital Statistics Report 1993; 41.
2. Zheng ZJ, et al. Sudden cardiac death in the United States, 1989 to 1998. Circulation 2001; 104:2158–2163.
3. Cobb LA. Changing incidence of out of hospital ventricular fibrillation. JAMA 2002; 288: 3008–3013.
4. Cummins RO, et al. Improving survival from sudden cardiac arrest: the "chain of survival" concept. A statement for health professionals from the Advanced Cardiac Life Support Subcommittee and the Emergency Cardiac Care Committee, American Heart Association. Circulation, 1991; 83:1832–1847.
5. Cummins RO, et al. Survival of out-of-hospital cardiac arrest with early initiation of cardiopulmonary resuscitation. Am J Emerg Med 1985; 3:114–119.
6. Guidelines 2000 for Cardiopulmonary Resuscitation and Emergency Cardiovascular Care. Circulation 2000; 102(8 Suppl)11:1–291.
7. Watts DD. Defibrillation by basic emergency medical technicians: effect on survival. Ann Emerg Med 1995; 26:635–639.

8. White RD, Hankins DG, Bugliosi TF. Seven years' experience with early defibrillation by police and paramedics in an emergency medical services system. Resuscitation 1998; 39:145–151.

9. Becker, LB, et al. Outcome of CPR in a large metropolitan area—where are the survivors? Ann Emerg Med 1991; 20:355–361.

10. Lombardi G, Gallagher J, Gennis P. Outcome of out-of-hospital cardiac arrest in New York City. The Pre-Hospital Arrest Survival Evaluation (PHASE) Study. JAMA 1994; 271:678–683.

11. Mayfield T. 200 city survey. EMS in the nation's most-populous cities. JEMS 1998; 23:50–69.

12. Herlitz J, et al. Rhythm changes during resuscitation from ventricular fibrillation in relation to delay until defibrillation, number of shocks delivered and survival. Resuscitation 1997; 34:17–22.

13. White RD, Russell JK. Refibrillation, resuscitation and survival in out-of-hospital sudden cardiac arrest victims treated with biphasic automated external defibrillators. Resuscitation 2002; 55:17–23.

14. Gazmuri, RJ. Effects of repetitive electrical shocks on postresuscitation myocardial function. Crit Care Med, 2000 28(Suppl):N228–232.

15. Weaver WD, et al. Effect of epinephrine and lidocaine therapy on outcome after cardiac arrest due to ventricular fibrillation. Circulation 1990; 82:2027–2034.

16. Pepe PE, et al. Cardiac arrest presenting with rhythms other than ventricular fibrillation: contribution of resuscitative efforts toward total survivorship. Crit Care Med 1993; 21:1838–1843.

17. van Walraven C, et al. Do advanced cardiac life support drugs increase resuscitation rates from in-hospital cardiac arrest? The OTAC Study Group. Ann Emerg Med 1998; 32:544–553.

18. Guidelines 2000 for Cardiopulmonary Resuscitation and Emergency Cardiovascular Care. Part 6: advanced cardiovascular life support: section 5: pharmacology I: agents for arrhythmias. The American Heart Association in Collaboration with the International Liaison Committee on Resuscitation. Circulation 2000; 102(8 Suppl):I112–I128.

19. Santini M, Pandozi C, Ricci R. Combining antiarrhythmic drugs and implantable devices therapy: benefits and outcome. J Interv Card Electrophysiol 2000; 4(Suppl):65–68.

20. Manolis AG, et al. Electrical storms in an ICD-recipient with 429 delivered appropriate shocks: therapeutic management with antiarrhythmic drug combination. J Interv Card Electrophysiol 2002; 6:91–94.

21. Curione M, et al. An electrocardiographic criterion to detect AV dissociation in wide QRS tachyarrhythmias. Clin Cardiol 1988; 11:250–252.

22. Bigger JT, Jr. Digitalis toxicity. J Clin Pharmacology 1985; 25:514–521.

23. Hauptman PJ, Kelly RA. Digitalis. Circulation 1999; 99:1265–1270.

24. Rotem M, et al. Life-threatening Torsade de Pointes arrhythmia associated with head injury. Neurosurgery 1988; 23:89–92.

25. Roden DM. Torsade de pointes. Clin Cardiol 1993; 16:683–686.

26. Glassman AH, Bigger JT, Jr. Antipsychotic drugs: prolonged QTc interval, Torsade de pointes, and sudden death. Am J Psychiatry 2001; 158:1774–1782.

27. Pathak A, et al. Celecoxib-associated Torsade de pointes. Ann Pharmacother 2002; 36:1290, 1291.

28. Cantani A, Mocini V. Antihistamines and the Torsade de point in children with allergic rhinitis. Eur Rev Med Pharmacol Sci 2001; 5:139–142.

29. Krantz MJ, et al. Torsade de pointes associated with very-high-dose methadone. Ann Intern Med, 2002; 137:501–504.

30. Kakar A, Byotra SP. Torsade de pointes probably induced by sparfloxacin. J Assoc Physicians India, 2002; 50:1077–1078.

31. Milberg P, et al. Divergent proarrhythmic potential of macrolide antibiotics despite similar QT prolongation: fast phase 3 repolarization prevents early after depolarizations and Torsade de pointes. J Pharmacol Exp Ther 2002; 303:218–225.

32. Farkas A, Lepran I, Papp JG. Proarrhythmic effects of intravenous quinidine, amiodarone, D-sotalol, and almokalant in the anesthetized rabbit model of Torsade de pointes. J Cardiovasc Pharmacol 2002; 39:287–297.

33. Alter P, Tontsch D, Grimm W. Doxepin-induced Torsade de pointes tachycardia. Ann Intern Med 2001; 135:384–385.

34. Raehl CL, Patel AK, LeRoy M. Drug-induced torsade de pointes. Clin Pharm 1985; 4:675–690.

35. Kay GN, et al. Torsade de pointes: the long-short initiating sequence and other clinical features: observations in 32 patients. J Am Coll Cardiol 1983; 2:806–817.

36. Bansal AM, et al. Torsade de pointes: successful acute control by lidocaine and chronic control by tocainide in two patients—one each with acquired long QT and the congenital long QT syndrome. Am Heart J 1986; 112:618–621.

37. Wellens HJ, Brugada P. Diagnosis of ventricular tachycardia from the 12-lead electrocardiogram. Cardiol Clin 1987; 5:511–525.

38. Brugada P, et al. A new approach to the differential diagnosis of a regular tachycardia with a wide QRS complex. Circulation 1991; 83:1649–1659.
39. Rinkenberger RL, Naccarelli GV. Evaluation and acute treatment of wide complex tachycardias. Crit Care Clin 1989; 5:599–641.
40. Sager PT, Bhandari AK. Wide complex tachycardias. Differential diagnosis and management. Cardiol Clin 1991; 9:595–618.
41. Olshansky B. Ventricular tachycardia masquerading as supraventricular tachycardia: a wolf in sheep's clothing. J Electrocardiol 1988; 21:377–384.
42. Naccarelli GV, Wolbrette DL, Luck JC. Proarrhythmia. Med Clin North Am 2001; 85:503–526.
43. Nestico PF, Morganroth J, Horowitz LN. New antiarrhythmic drugs. Drugs 1988; 35:286–319.
44. Whalley DW, Wendt DJ, Grant AO. Basic concepts in cellular cardiac electrophysiology: Part I: Ion channels, membrane currents, and the action potential. Pacing Clin Electrophysiol 1995; 18:1556–1574.
45. Whalley DW, Wendt DJ, Grant AO. Basic concepts in cellular cardiac electrophysiology: Part II: Block of ion channels by antiarrhythmic drugs. Pacing Clin Electrophysiol 1995; 18(Pt 1):1686–1704.
46. Rosen MR. Consequences of the Sicilian Gambit. Eur Heart J 1995; 16(Suppl):32–36.
47. The 'Sicilian Gambit'. A new approach to the classification of antiarrhythmic drugs based on their actions on arrhythmogenic mechanisms. The Task Force of the Working Group on Arrhythmias of the European Society of Cardiology. Euro Heart J 1991; 12:1112–1131.
48. Chaudhry GM, Haffajee CI. Antiarrhythmic agents and proarrhythmia. Crit Care Med 2000; 28(Suppl): N158–N164.
49. Hondeghem LM. Selective depression of the ischemic and hypoxic myocardium by lidocaine. Proc West Pharmacol Soc 1975; 18:27–30.
50. Borer JS, et al. Beneficial effect of lidocaine on ventricular electrical stability and spontaneous ventricular fibrillation during experimental myocardial infarction. Am J Cardiol 1976; 37:860–863.
51. Spear JF, Moore EN, Gerstenblith G. Effect of lidocaine on the ventricular fibrillation threshold in the dog during acute ischemia and premature ventricular contractions. Circulation 1972; 46:65–73.
52. Lazzara R, et al. Effects of lidocaine on hypoxic and ischemic cardiac cells. Am J Cardiol 1978; 41: 872–879.
53. Herlitz J, et al. Lidocaine in out-of-hospital ventricular fibrillation. Does it improve survival? Resuscitation 1997; 33:199–205.
54. Lie KI, et al. Efficacy of lidocaine in preventing primary ventricular fibrillation within 1 hour after a 300 mg intramuscular injection. A double-blind, randomized study of 300 hospitalized patients with acute myocardial infarction. Am J Cardiol 1978; 42:486–488.
55. MacMahon S, et al. Effects of prophylactic lidocaine in suspected acute myocardial infarction. An overview of results from the randomized, controlled trials. JAMA 1988; 260:1910–1916.
56. Hine LK, et al. Meta-analytic evidence against prophylactic use of lidocaine in acute myocardial infarction. Arch Intern Med 1989; 149:2694–2698.
57. Dorian P, et al. Lidocaine causes a reversible, concentration-dependent increase in defibrillation energy requirements. J Am Coll Cardiol 1986; 8:327–332.
58. Echt DS, et al. Evaluation of antiarrhythmic drugs on defibrillation energy requirements in dogs. Sodium channel block and action potential prolongation. Circulation 1989; 79:1106–1117.
59. Kerber RE, et al. Effect of lidocaine and bretylium on energy requirements for transthoracic defibrillation: experimental studies. J Am Coll Cardiol 1986; 7:397–405.
60. Peters RW, et al. Lidocaine-related increase in defibrillation threshold. Anesth Analg 1997; 85:299–300.
61. Vachiery JL, et al. Bretylium tosylate versus lidocaine in experimental cardiac arrest. Am J Emerg Med 1990; 8:492–495.
62. Leveque PE. Anti-arrhythmic action of bretylium. Nature 1965; 207:203–204.
63. Bacaner MB. Quantitiative comparison of bretylium with other antifibrillatory drugs. Am J Cardiol 1968; 21:504–512.
64. Bacaner M. Bretylium tosylate for suppression of induced ventricular fibrillation. Am J Cardiol 1966; 17:528–534.
65. Rapeport WG. Clinical pharmacokinetics of bretylium. Clin Pharmacokinet 1985; 10:248–256.
66. Euler DE, et al. Deleterious effects of bretylium on hemodynamic recovery from ventricular fibrillation. Am Heart J 1986; 112:25–31.
67. Chandrasekaran S, Steinberg JS. Efficacy of bretylium tosylate for ventricular tachycardia. Am J Cardiol 1999; 83:115–117.

68. Ornato JP, et al. Future directions for resuscitation research. III. External cardiopulmonary resuscitation advanced life support. Resuscitation 1996; 32:139–158.
69. Gorgels AP, et al. Comparison of procainamide and lidocaine in terminating sustained monomorphic ventricular tachycardia. Am J Cardiol 1996; 78:43–46.
70. Lazzara R. Antiarrhythmic drugs and Torsade de pointes. Eur Heart J 1993; 14 (Suppl):88–92.
71. Stewart CE. Amiodarone for ACLS: a critical evaluation. Emerg Med Serv 2001; 30:61–67.
72. Kudenchuk PJ, et al. Amiodarone for resuscitation after out-of-hospital cardiac arrest due to ventricular fibrillation. NEJM 1999; 341:871–878.
73. Dorian P, Philippon F. The management of acute ventricular tachycardia or fibrillation. Can J Cardiol 2000; 16(Suppl C):16C–19C.
74. Boriani G, et al. High defibrillation threshold at cardioverter defibrillator implantation under amiodarone treatment: favorable effects of D,L-sotalol. Heart & Lung 2000; 29:412–416.
75. Kuhlkamp V, et al. Effect of amiodarone and sotalol on the defibrillation threshold in comparison to patients without antiarrhythmic drug treatment. Int J Cardiol 1999; 69: 271–279.
76. Anastasiou-Nana MI, et al. Amiodarone concentration in human myocardium after rapid intravenous administration. Cardiovasc Drugs Ther 1999; 13:265–270.
77. Somberg JC, et al. Intravenous lidocaine versus intravenous amiodarone (in a new aqueous formulation) for incessant ventricular tachycardia. Am J Cardiol 2002; 90:853–859.
78. Tomcsanyi J, et al. Early proarrhythmia during intravenous amiodarone treatment. Pacing Clin Electrophysiol 1999; 22(Pt 1):968–970.
79. van Opstal JM, et al. Chronic amiodarone evokes no Torsade de pointes arrhythmias despite QT length-ening in an animal model of acquired long-QT syndrome. Circulation 2001; 104:2722–2727.
80. Wiesfeld AC, et al. Beta adrenergic blockade in the treatment of sustained ventricular tachycardia or ventricular fibrillation. Pacing Clin Electrophysiol 1996; 19:1026–1035.
81. Andresen D, et al. Beta blockers: evidence versus wishful thinking. Am J Cardiol 1999; 83:64D–67D.
82. Reiter MJ, Reiffel JA. Importance of beta blockade in the therapy of serious ventricular arrhythmias. Am J Cardiol 1998; 82:9I–19I.
83. Anonymous. Timolol-induced reduction in mortality and reinfarction in patients surviving acute myocar-dial infarction. NEJM 1981; 304:801–807.
84. Hjalmarson A, et al. Effect on mortality of metoprolol in acute myocardial infarction. A double-blind randomised trial. Lancet 1981; 2:823–827.
85. Gottlieb SS, McCarter RJ, Vogel RA. Effect of beta-blockade on mortality among high-risk and low-risk patients after myocardial infarction NEJM 1998; 339: 489–497.
86. Perez-Castellano N, et al. Benefit of pacing and beta-blockers in idiopathic repetitive polymorphic ven-tricular tachycardia. J Cardiovasc Electrophysiol 2001; 12:1304–1307.
87. Fisher JD. A patient with polymorphic ventricular tachycardia controlled by beta-blockers and atrial pacing. J Cardiovasc Electrophysiol 2002; 13:202.
88. Kurose M, et al. Successful treatment of life-threatening ventricular tachycardia with high-dose propra-nolol under extracorporeal life support and intraaortic balloon pumping. Jpn Circ J 1993; 57:1106–1110.
89. Bashir Y, et al. A prospective study of the efficacy and safety of adjuvant metoprolol and xamoterol in combination with amiodarone for resistant ventricular tachycardia associated with impaired left ventricular function. Am Heart J 1992; 124:1233–1240.
90. Ogunyankin KO, Singh BN. Mortality reduction by antiadrenergic modulation of arrhythmogenic sub-strate: significance of combining beta blockers and amiodarone. Am J Cardiol 1999; 84:76R–82R.
91. Olson DW, et al. A randomized comparison study of bretylium tosylate and lidocaine in resuscitation of patients from out-of-hospital ventricular fibrillation in a paramedic system. Ann Emerg Med 1984; 13 (Pt 2):807–810.
92. Armengol RE, et al. Lack of effectiveness of lidocaine for sustained, wide QRS complex tachycardia. Ann Emerg Med 1989; 18:254–257.
93. Nasir N Jr., et al. Evaluation of intravenous lidocaine for the termination of sustained monomorphic ventricular tachycardia in patients with coronary artery disease with or without healed myocardial infarction. Am J Cardiol 1994; 74:1183–1186.
94. Ho DS, et al. Double-blind trial of lignocaine versus sotalol for acute termination of spontaneous sustained ventricular tachycardia. Lancet 1994; 344:18–23.
95. Mostow ND, et al. Amiodarone: intravenous loading for rapid suppression of complex ventricular arrhythmias. J Am Coll Cardiol 1984; 4:97–104.
96. Morady F, et al. Intravenous amiodarone in the acute treatment of recurrent symptomatic ventricular tachycardia. Am J Cardiol 1983; 51:156–159.

97. Helmy I, et al. Use of intravenous amiodarone for emergency treatment of life-threatening ventricular arrhythmias. J Am Coll Cardiol 1988; 12:1015–1022.

98. Klein RC, et al. Efficacy of intravenous amiodarone as short-term treatment for refractory ventricular tachycardia. Am Heart J 1988; 115(Pt 1):96–101.

99. Ochi RP, et al. Intravenous amiodarone for the rapid treatment of life-threatening ventricular arrhythmias in critically ill patients with coronary artery disease. Am J Cardiol 1989; 64:599–603.

100. Schutzenberger W, et al. Clinical efficacy of intravenous amiodarone in the short term treatment of recurrent sustained ventricular tachycardia and ventricular fibrillation. Br Heart J 1989; 62:367–371.

101. Mooss AN, et al. Efficacy and tolerance of high-dose intravenous amiodarone for recurrent, refractory ventricular tachycardia. Am J Cardiol 1990; 65:609–614.

102. Scheinman MM, et al. Dose-ranging study of intravenous amiodarone in patients with life-threatening ventricular tachyarrhythmias. The Intravenous Amiodarone Multicenter Investigators Group. Circulation 1995; 92:3264–3272.

103. Levine JH, et al. Intravenous amiodarone for recurrent sustained hypotensive ventricular tachyarrhythmias. Intravenous Amiodarone Multicenter Trial Group. J Am Coll Cardiol 1996; 27:67–75.

104. Kowey PR, et al. Randomized, double-blind comparison of intravenous amiodarone and bretylium in the treatment of patients with recurrent, hemodynamically destabilizing ventricular tachycardia or fibrillation. The Intravenous Amiodarone Multicenter Investigators Group. Circulation 1995; 92:3255–3263.

105. Dorian P, et al. Amiodarone as compared with lidocaine for shock-resistant ventricular fibrillation. NEJM 2002; 346:884–890.

106. Miller B, et al. Pilot study of intravenous magnesium sulfate in refractory cardiac arrest: safety data and recommendations for future studies. Resuscitation 1995; 30:3–14.

107. Roffe C, Fletcher S, Woods KL. Investigation of the effects of intravenous magnesium sulphate on cardiac rhythm in acute myocardial infarction. Br Heart J 1994; 71:141–145.

108. Allegra J, et al. Magnesium sulfate in the treatment of refractory ventricular fibrillation in the prehospital setting. Resuscitation 2001; 49:245–249.

109. Hassan TB, Jagger C, Barnett DB. A randomised trial to investigate the efficacy of magnesium sulphate for refractory ventricular fibrillation. Emerg Med J 2002; 19:57–62.

110. Woods KL, Fletcher S. Long-term outcome after intravenous magnesium sulphate in suspected acute myocardial infarction: the second Leicester Intravenous Magnesium Intervention Trial (LIMIT-2). Lancet 1994; 343:816–819.

111. Iseri LT, Allen BJ, Brodsky MA. Magnesium therapy of cardiac arrhythmias in critical-care medicine. Magnesium 1989; 8:299–306.

112. Thel MC, et al. Randomised trial of magnesium in in-hospital cardiac arrest. Duke Internal Medicine Housestaff. Lancet 1997; 350:1272–1276.

113. Tzivoni D, et al. Treatment of Torsade de pointes with magnesium sulfate. Circulation 1988; 77: 392–297.

114. Geannopoulos CJ, Wilber DJ, Olshansky B. Control of refractory ventricular tachycardia with biventricular assist devices. Pacing Clin Electrophysiol 1991; 14:1432–1434.

115. Kiseleva I, et al. Mechanoelectric feedback after left ventricular infarction in rats. Cardiovasc Res 2000; 45:370–378.

116. Movsowitz C, Marchlinski FE. Interactions between implantable cardioverter-defibrillators and class III agents. Am J Cardiol 1998; 82:41I–48I.

117. Babbs CF, et al. Elevation of ventricular defibrillation threshold in dogs by antiarrhythmic drugs. Am Heart J 1979; 98:345–350.

118. Chow MS, et al. The effect of lidocaine and bretylium on the defibrillation threshold during cardiac arrest and cardiopulmonary resuscitation. Proc Soc Exp Biol Med 1986; 182:63–67.

119. Nemec J, Shen WK. Congenital long QT syndromes and Brugada syndrome: the arrhythmogenic ion channel disorders. Expert Opin Pharmacother 2001; 2:773–797.

120. Naccarelli GV, Antzelevitch C. The Brugada syndrome: clinical, genetic, cellular, and molecular abnormalities. Am J Med 2001; 110:573–581.

121. Brugada J, Brugada P, Brugada R. The syndrome of right bundle branch block ST segment elevation in V1 to V3 and sudden death—the Brugada syndrome. Europace 1999; 1:156–166.

122. Chen SM, et al. Brugada syndrome without mutation of the cardiac sodium channel gene in a Taiwanese patient. J Formos Med Asso 2000; 99:860–862.

123. Priori SG, et al. Task force on sudden cardiac death of the European Society of Cardiology. Eur Heart J 2001; 22:1374–1450.

124. Priori SG, et al. Mutations in the Cardiac Ryanodine Receptor Gene (hRyR2) Underlie Catecholaminergic Polymorphic Ventricular Tachycardia. Circulation 2001; 103:196–-200.

125. George CH, et al. In situ modulation of the human cardiac ryanodine receptor (hRyR2) by FKBP12.6. Biochem J 2003; 370(Pt. 2):579–589.
126. Witchel HJ, Hancox JC. Familial and acquired long QT syndrome and the cardiac rapid delayed rectifier potassium current. Clin Exp Pharmacol Physiol 2000; 27:753–766.
127. Brady WJ, DeBehnke DJ, Laundrie D. Prevalence, therapeutic response, and outcome of ventricular tachycardia in the out-of-hospital setting: a comparison of monomorphic ventricular tachycardia, polymorphic ventricular tachycardia, and Torsades de pointes. Acad Emerg Med 1999; 6:609–617.
128. Roden DM. A practical approach to Torsade de pointes. Clin Cardiol 1997; 20:131.
129. Kuo CS, et al. Mechanism of ventricular arrhythmias caused by increased dispersion of repolarization. Eur Heart J 1985:6(Suppl):63–70.
130. Bjornstad H, Tande PM, Refsum H. Cardiac electrophysiology during hypothermia. Implications for medical treatment. Arctic Med Res 1991; 50(Suppl):71–75.
131. Kalla H, Yan GX, Marinchak R. Ventricular fibrillation in a patient with prominent J (Osborn) waves and ST segment elevation in the inferior electrocardiographic leads: a Brugada syndrome variant? J Cardiovasc Electrophysiol 2000; 11:95–98.
132. Farstad M. et al. Rewarming from accidental hypothermia by extracorporeal circulation. A retrospective study. Eur J Cardiothorac Surg 2001; 20:58–64.
133. Antunes E, et al. The differential diagnosis of a regular tachycardia with a wide QRS complex on the 12-lead ECG: ventricular tachycardia, supraventricular tachycardia with aberrant intraventricular conduction, and supraventricular tachycardia with anterograde conduction over an accessory pathway. Pacing Clin Electrophysiol 1994; 17:1515–1524.
134. Elrifai AM, et al. Rewarming, ultraprofound hypothermia and cardiopulmonary bypass. J Extra Corpor Technol 1993; 24:107–112.
135. Gregory JS, et al. Comparison of three methods of rewarming from hypothermia: advantages of extracorporeal blood warming. J Trauma 1991; 31:1247–1251; discussion 1251, 1252.
136. Brunette DD, McVaney K. Hypothermic cardiac arrest: an 11 year review of ED management and outcome. Am J Emerg Med 2000; 18:418–422.
137. Karch SB. Cardiac arrest in cocaine users. Am J Emerg Med 1996; 14:79–81.
138. Nademanee K, et al. Treating electrical storm : sympathetic blockade versus advanced cardiac life support-guided therapy. Circulation 2000; 102:742–747.
139. Credner SC, et al. Electrical storm in patients with transvenous implantable cardioverter-defibrillators: incidence, management and prognostic implications. J Am Coll Cardiol 1998; 32:1909–1915.
140. Telfer EA, et al. Implantable defibrillator use for de novo ventricular tachyarrhythmias encountered after cardiac surgery. Pacing Clin Electrophysiol 2002; 25:951–956.
141. Gregoratos G, et al. ACC/AHA/NASPE 2002 guideline update for implantation of cardiac pacemakers and antiarrhythmia devices: summary article. A report of the American College of Cardiology/American Heart Association Task Force on Practice Guidelines (ACC/AHA/NASPE Committee to Update the 1998 Pacemaker Guidelines). J Cardiovasc Electrophysiol 2002; 13: 1183–1199.

22 Electrolyte Disturbances and Cardiopulmonary Resuscitation

Domenic A. Sica, MD

INTRODUCTION

Sudden cardiac death (SCD) annually affects 400 to 460,000 individuals in the United States, accounting for half the mortality rate as a result of coronary heart disease. SCD remains a major unresolved public health problem. Pathophysiologically, SCD arises from a harmful interplay of myocardial structure, and function. Structural abnormalities furnish the anatomic substrate for SCD and include the myocardial repercussions of coronary artery disease (CAD), left ventricular hypertrophy (LVH) and/or dilation, and specific electrophysiological anatomic abnormalities. The functional issues capable of destabilizing a chronic electrophysiological abnormality include transient ischemia and reperfusion, systemic issues (e.g., electrolyte disturbances, pH changes, and hemodynamic dysfunction), autonomic fluctuations (both at a systemic and a tissue level), and proarrhythmic effects of various drugs. We center the discussion in this chapter on two aspects of electrolyte abnormalities; first, the role they play in the origin of SCD and second how the therapies employed during cardiopulmonary resuscitation (CPR) can result in specific electrolyte abnormalities. Cardiopulmonary arrest (CPA) can occur in a wide spectrum of patient types, some with underlying cardiac abnormalities receiving active treatment others without any obvious cardiovascular (CVR) malady. It is in the instance of the former that electrolyte disturbances can precede and on occasion incite a CPA *(1)*. Such electrolyte abnormalities can have multiple origins, relating to either intercurrent illnesses or administered medications. In most cases those circumstances impacting potassium (K^+) and magnesium (Mg^{++}) homeostasis are of most importance. The electrophysiologic basis of CPA can be quite complex and a detailed discussion of the electrophysiologic effects of electrolyte abnormalities extends beyond the scope of this chapter. The reader is directed to several excellent discussions on this topic *(1–4)*.

From: *Contemporary Cardiology: Cardiopulmonary Resuscitation*
Edited by: J. P. Ornato and M. A. Peberdy © Humana Press Inc., Totowa, NJ

BLOOD SAMPLING

Diagnosing an electrolyte abnormality in the time period surrounding CPR can prove challenging. A number of issues must be considered before a blood chemistry value is accepted as accurate. First, the urgency of the situation at the time of CPA may supercede the "correct" tube being used for a biochemical analyte; thus, rather than a "red-top" tube, a "purple-top" or "green-top" tube may be inadvertently chosen. Non-red-top tubes—such as these—can contain K^+-EDTA or K^+-heparin, respectively, which can confuse the interpretation of the reported K^+ value. Second, the sampling location is an important consideration in the interpretation of reported values for acid–base parameters and serum K^+. Ineffective compressions can result in a low-flow state; thus, venous blood obtained from the lower extremity may reveal a serum K^+ value (usually elevated) more so reflecting localized conditions of K^+ release rather than the prevailing systemic concentration of K^+. This sampling misrepresentation can be minimized by measurement of serum K^+ from an arterial sample. Finally, blood gases obtained during cardiac arrest (CA) are sample site-dependent relative to oxygenation (thoracic sampling with a higher PO_2 than femoral sampling [5]) and/or underestimate the drop in arterial pH and rise in pCO_2 otherwise evident from inspection of mixed venous blood (6,7).

FREQUENCY OF ELECTROLYTE DISTURBANCES

In the Anti-Arrhythmics Vs Implantable Defibrillators (AVID) trial, patients resuscitated from ventricular tachycardia (VT) or ventricular fibrillation (VF) were randomized to anti-arrhythmic drug therapy vs an implantable cardioverter defibrillator if they did not have a potentially treatable or correctable cause of VT/VF. A registry was maintained of all patients screened for the AVID trial irrespective of VT/VF etiology. The AVID registry included 2013 patients of which 278 had a presenting ventricular arrhythmias considered to be as a result of a transient or potentially correctable cause. Of the 278 patients with a presumed transient cause for their arrhythmias 9.7% (27/278) had a basis for their event, which was attributed to an electrolyte abnormality (8). However, these data require careful interpretation because the physicians in this study had considerable discretion in the definition of an index arrhythmia as being "caused by hypokalemia." In fact, in clinical practice it is quite difficult to conclusively identify cases in which hypokalemia is the sole cause of VT/VF because mild hypokalemia can be the result, as well as the cause of VT/VF (9,10). Typically, for hypokalemia to cause VT/VF there must exist an underlying milieu of vulnerability, such as that seen in the peri-infarct period or following administration of proarrhythmic medications (11).

Sodium Disturbances

ETIOLOGIES: HYPONATREMIA

Clinically relevant hyponatremia is uncommon in the general outpatient population in that the kidney is remarkably efficient in maintaining sodium (Na^+) and water (H_2O) balance. The kidney synchronizes several physiologic processes including: glomerular filtration, proximal tubular and thick ascending limb solute/solvent handling and collecting tubule H_2O permeability to effectively excrete a H_2O load. When this circuit is intact it is difficult to exceed the diluting capacity (ability to excrete a H_2O load) of the kidney; thus, in normal individuals consciously ingesting large volumes of dilute fluids intake in the order of 30-L per day is required before hyponatremia occurs. Intake of this order before hyponatremia develops presupposes an adequate dietary solute load (Na^+ and protein) to support excretion of the ingested H_2O. The presence of an adequate dietary solute load is not a priori a safe assumption. Restrictions on dietary Na^+ and protein intake are common, either prescribed or self-imposed, and can seriously limit the solute load available for excretion and thereby allow dilutional hyponatremia to occur at a much reduced level of intake (12).

If hyponatremia occurs in normal individuals it is generally as a consequence of Na^+ and H_2O losses with replacement of such losses with H_2O based solutions alone. This form of hyponatremia is typically self-limited and responds rapidly to isotonic fluid replacement. Of those diseases associated with both hyponatremia and an inherent increased risk of CPA congestive heart failure (CHF) and/or CAD are probably the lead conditions. Hyponatremia frequently complicates the clinical course of the patient with CHF, especially in its later stages (13). The hyponatremia of CHF is characterized by an excess of total body Na^+ and H_2O with the latter predominating; thus, the characteristic dilutional hyponatremia of the CHF patient.

Na^+ retention is a primary process in CHF and stems from combined renal and cardiac functional abnormalities supported by the neurohumoral abnormalities that predominate in CHF (14). The decline in renal blood flow (RBF) and reduced glomerular filtration rate (GFR) in the CHF patient will further the likelihood of developing and/or progressing hyponatremia in the CHF patient. CHF may compromise any or all of the requirements for excretion of dilute urine, a problem only further exacerbated by the frequent presence of an excessive thirst drive (15). The low-end serum Na^+ values in advanced CHF are typically around 125 mEq/L. This level of plasma hypoosmolality is generally associated with few symptoms above and beyond those dictated by the severity of the CHF syndrome (16). CHF patients with serum Na^+ values less than 135 mEq/L have more profound neurohumoral activation and a greater reduction in hepatosplachnic and RBF. Hyponatremia is a fairly ominous prognostic factor in CHF patients (17,18). Hyponatremia patients are relatively unstable hemodynamically and are prone to hypotension and excessive falls in GFR when given angiotensin-converting enzyme (ACE) inhibitors; accordingly, their existence is more tenuous (19,20).

Relationship to CPA and Treatment Considerations

One difficulty in linking serum Na^+ disturbances to CPA has been the virtual absence of descriptive information surrounding the event (21,22). However, it can be presumed that the average serum Na^+ values will tend to be lower in CPA patients because a significant number of subjects at risk for CPA have either abnormal cardiac and/or renal function (conditions frequently associated with hyponatremia). Moreover, events surrounding CPA may increase the likelihood of hyponatremia. For example, if volume resuscitation occurs with hypotonic fluids, the chances of developing dilutional hyponatremia increase at least, in part, because transient renal dysfunction can occur in the post-CPR state (23,24). As an aftereffect of this change in renal function volume loads will be less efficiently eliminated. However, severe progressive acute renal failure (ARF) after CPR is rare. Pre-CPA hemodynamics, if abnormal, seems to be more so associated with the onset of ARF than is the degree of hypoperfusion, which occurs during resuscitation (23,24).

Finally, the American Heart Association (AHA) Guidelines consider vasopressin to be an effective vasopressor and recommend it as an alternative to epinephrine for the treatment of adult shock refractory VF CPA *(25)*. The recommended dosage is 40 units intravenously in place of the first dose of epinephrine in the pulseless VT/VF algorithm. The vasopressin dose recommended—to augment vital organ perfusion during CPR—is considerably in excess of that required for an antidiuretic effect. It has been hypothesized that vasopressin administered during CPR can result in oliguria or anuria because of its antidiuretic effect and thereby increases the risk of hyponatremia in the postresuscitation period. When studied, this has not been observed suggesting that the level of urine output following CPR and vasopressin administration is an amalgam of several concurrent processes including: vasopressin effects on RBF, GFR, and tubular function as well as the state of systemic hemodynamics and cardiac function *(26)*.

Etiologies: Hypernatremia

Hypernatremia develops whenever water intake falls below the sum of renal and extrarenal water losses. All hypernatremic states are hypertonic. The most common causes of clinically significant hypernatremia derive from three pathogenic mechanisms: impaired thirst, solute or osmotic diuresis, excessive losses of water, either through the kidneys or extrarenally, and combinations of these individual derangements.

An inadequate intake of water occurs in patients who are comatose or who are otherwise unable to communicate thirst. Rarely, patients will have a primary thirst deficiency. Partial thirst defects, however, are not uncommon. Such defects are most commonly seen in older patients *(27)*. Osmotic diuresis occurs in the setting of uncontrolled glycosuria or when mannitol is given. In the instance of a prolonged osmotic diuresis, net H_2O losses may be of a sufficient magnitude that hypernatremia develops., A very high Na^+ intake and/or the administration of normal saline or hypertonic Na^+ containing substances increases the likelihood of hypernatremia in patients with partial impairment of urinary concentrating ability *(28)*. Extrarenal losses of free H_2O can be striking in the case of profound sweating. Excess renal losses of free H_2O typically relate to some impairment in antidiuretic hormone (ADH) production. The complete absence of ADH is marked by urine outputs in the range of 1 L per hour and can result in the rapid development of severe hypernatremia. Combinations of these individual derangements—as is occasionally seen in CHF—can result in hypernatremia *(29,30)*.

Relationship to CPA and Treatment Considerations

Hypernatremia, like the illnesses it is associated with, is not inherently coupled to a specific risk for CPA. If hypernatremia is observed it most typically occurs in the time period following successful resuscitation. Several pathogenic variations of hypernatremia, linked to hypoxemic encephalopathy, have been described following CPR. These include transient diabetes insipidus *(31)*, a more complete form of diabetes insipidus *(32)*, and a variant of nephrogenic diabetes insipidus *(33)*. The development of diabetes insipidus following CPR augurs a poor prognosis in that it suggests significant anoxic brain injury. In the time period following CPR hypernatremia may also develop in concert with the administration of hypertonic sodium bicarbonate ($NaHCO_3$ *[34]*). The AHA no longer recommends the routine use of $NaHCO_3$ in CAs; accordingly $NaHCO_3$-related hypernatremia is now much less common. However, when hypertonic Na^+-containing solutions are administered their use does not appreciably affect defibrillation efficacy of electrical treatment of VF *(35)*.

Calcium Disturbances

ETIOLOGIES: HYPOCALCEMIA

True hypocalcemia is generally the result of two processes: decreased gut calcium (Ca^{++}) absorption or decreased Ca^{++} resorption from bone. Because 98% of total body Ca^{++} is located within the skeleton, sustained hypocalcemia rarely occurs independent of abnormalities of either parathyroid hormone (PTH) or vitamin D (calcitriol), hormones which acutely mobilize Ca^{++} from bone. Total circulating plasma calcium is comprised of three components: ionized calcium (50%), protein-bound calcium (40%), and calcium complexed with small organic anions (10%). A low *total* calcium value alone may not represent *true* or "physiologically relevant" hypocalcemia because this value drops as the serum albumin concentration falls (for each 1-g/dL decrease in serum albumin concentration from its normal value of 4-g/dL, a 0.8-mg/dL fall in total serum calcium concentration occurs). Physiologically relevant hypocalcemia exists only when the *ionized* Ca^{++} concentration drops below the reference range of 4.2 to 5.0 mg/dL (1.05 to 1.25 mmol/L). Ca^{++} binding to albumin is also influenced by the systemic pH (for each 0.1 decrease in pH, Ca^{++} increases approx 0.2-mg/dL). Such correction issues should be used only in lieu of direct measurement of ionized serum calcium.

The causes of hypocalcemia are too numerous to mention. Of these causes however, hypomagnesemia—typically in relationship to loop diuretic therapy—is the one most relevant to patients susceptible to CPA (see section on Magnesium Disturbances). Loop diuretic therapy typically increases Ca^{++} excretion. In order to maintain a "normal" Ca^{++} concentration in this setting it must be mobilized from bone—a process controlled by PTH. When magnesium (Mg^{++}) deficiency exists this will not occur because both PTH secretion and its end-organ effect at the bone level are arrested. This sequence of events then leads to hypocalcemia, which can be significant and refractory to therapy until the Mg^{++} deficit is corrected.

Relationship to CPA and Treatment Considerations

Ionized calcium values tend to fall during CPA, which may relate to dysfunctional transcellular ionic transport mechanisms *(36–38)*. The level of ionized hypocalcemia appears similar between arterial and mixed-venous blood samples *(38)*. Because Ca^{++} plays an essential role in excitation-contraction coupling its use then seemed logical in the setting of CPR; accordingly, intravenous calcium chloride was used in cardiac resuscitation efforts in patients with bradyasystolic arrest (irrespective of the plasma Ca^{++} concentration [39]). It is no longer used for this indication because survival benefits have not been observed with its use *(40)* and there is evidence that the high blood levels induced by Ca^{++} may induce cerebral vasospasm *(41–43)* and impact the extent of reperfusion injury in the heart and brain *(43,44)*. Intravenous Ca^{++} is of benefit however for hyperkalemia, hypermagnesemia, or calcium-channel blocker toxicity-related CPA. Intravenous Ca^{++} is also indicated when hypocalcemia is known to exist during CPR; however, it is not known whether administration of intravenous Ca^{++} under these circumstances provides direct cardiopulmonary benefits or merely normalizes the serum Ca^{++} value. When necessary, a 10% solution of calcium chloride can be given in a dose of 2–4-mg/kg and repeated as necessary at 10-minute intervals.

ETIOLOGIES: HYPERCALCEMIA

Pathologically, three general mechanisms may lead to the development of hypercalcemia: (a) increased mobilization of calcium from bone, by far the most common and important mechanism; (b) increased absorption of calcium from the gastrointestinal (GI) tract; and (c) decreased urinary excretion of calcium. Increased bone resorption of Ca^{++} is typically a silent process because it seldom causes hypercalcemia unless significant dehydration (and a drop in GFR) has occurred. Patients taking thiazide diuretics may also develop moderate hypercalcemia. Although the mechanisms for the hypercalcemia with thiazide diuretics are not fully understood; issues such as a reduction in urinary Ca^{++} excretion and extracellular fluid (ECF) volume contraction are likely involved. Hyper-calcemia is an uncommon occurrence in coronary heart disease- and CPA-prone patients.

Relationship to CPA and Treatment Considerations

Hypercalcemia has a positive inotropic effect on the cardiovascular system. Ca^{++} also increases peripheral resistance with hypertension occurring in 20 to 30% of patients with chronic hypercalcemia. The most significant change in the electrocardiogram of the hypercalcemic patient is a shortening of the QT interval, which seems not to specifically increase the risk of CPA. The QT interval change with hypercalcemia is neither linear nor curvilinear in nature; accordingly, the magnitude of change can be quite unpredictable. The EKG changes of hypercalcemia disappear with normalization of serum Ca^{++} levels. Because the positive inotropic effect of digitalis is enhanced by Ca^{++}, digitalis toxicity may be induced or aggravated by hypercalcemia. This interaction occurs much less frequently because digoxin and intravenous calcium chloride (during CPR) are clinically used more sparingly.

Acid–Base Abnormalities/Relationship to CPA

A full discussion on the various acid–base disturbances in clinical medicine is beyond the scope of this chapter. Only select aspects of acid–base abnormalities are commented on in this section. Acid–base abnormalities are typically divided into two categories: respiratory and metabolic and in either instance case can be either the cause or a consequence of CPA. The acid–base changes exhibited by the CPA patient are sequential and predictable. In the pre-CPA stage any of a variety of acid–base abnormalities may exist. Individual disorders, such as metabolic and/or respiratory acidosis, are the ones most commonly associated with CPA. Metabolic and/or respiratory acidosis may not increase the likelihood of a CPA per se unless significant hypoxia and/or a fall in systemic pH (<7.20) are accompanying features. During CPR both respiratory and metabolic acidosis can independently develop in a time-wise fashion, linked respectively to the level of effective alveolar ventilation and tissue perfusion. During closed-chest compression mixed venous blood is generally acidotic (pH ~7.15) and hypercarbic ($PaCO_2$ ~74 mmHg) (6). Many of the specific risks, which accompany CPA, relate to the level to which pH drops, which is most importantly an issue of time. Brief and extended CAs generally lead to different patient outcomes at least, in part, as a result of the progressive nature of metabolic and respiratory acidosis (45,46). During CPR, tissue hypoxia and cellular anaerobic metabolism are common, occurring in tandem with the marked fall in cardiac output during closed chest compression (47). When combined with an increase in lactate production, coincident to a shift to anaerobic glycolysis, acidosis (systemic and cellular) can be significant. Under these conditions intracellular myocardial PCO_2 can rapidly increase reaching concentrations considerably in excess of 90 mmHg (48). Acidemia affects several aspects of cellular electrophysiology including resting membrane potential, threshold potential and conduction velocities, which establishes it as a pro-arrhythmic state *(49)*. Additionally, hypoxia and acidosis reversibly depress myocardial function *(50)*. Moreover, the systemic response to vasopressors may be diminished in the presence of acidosis, which may also influence the success rate of CPR *(51)*. Well-performed CPR can stabilize and ultimately improve the respiratory and metabolic acidosis of CPA. Arterial blood pH during well-performed closed-chest compression typically falls within the normal range *(6,52–53)*; however, venous blood pH persists in the acidemic range *(6)*. The manner in which CPR is conducted is important. For example, severe arterial acidosis during closed-chest compression is usually as a result of inadequate ventilation *(54)*. Therein, the proficiency with which external chest compression occurs and/or the correct placement of an endotracheal tube become relevant considerations. Alternatively, if a patient is overventilated or excess base is given, pH values can quickly reverse and alkalemia emerge.

Use of Buffers During CPA

In the past, administration of $NaHCO_3$ was recommended during closed-chest compression in the belief that the H^+ ion produced during anaerobic metabolism would be buffered. However, $NaHCO_3$ itself contains a high concentration of carbon dioxide (CO_2; 260–280-mmHg *[55]*). In plasma, the CO_2 is released; because gases (CO_2) gain entry into cells more rapidly than do charged molecules (HCO_3^-)—the result therein is a paradoxical rise in intracellular PCO_2 and a substantial drop in intracellular pH. A rise in intracellular PCO_2 can be problematic in several ways. For example, within heart muscle cells as intracellular PCO_2 increases there follows a fall in cardiac contractility and potentially a drop in blood pressure *(56)*. A paradoxical acidosis can also develop in cerebrospinal fluid following $NaHCO_3$ administration and may contribute to the prolonged confusion occasionally seen after CPR *(57)*.

The recent AHA recommendations de-emphasize the role of $NaHCO_3$ and suggest that acid–base control during CA requires much less $NaHCO_3$ than had previously been advocated *(25)* because there are no convincing data proving treatment with $NaHCO_3$ is of benefit during closed chest compression *(58,59)*. As is the case with any form of metabolic acidosis, if alveolar ventilation is adequate, the acidemia is partially, if not completely corrected *(60)*. $NaHCO_3$ administration is not without adverse consequences because several deleterious effects including respiratory acidosis, hypernatremia, and hyperosmolality have been described *(61)*. Ideally, $NaHCO_3$ should be administered when a calculated base deficit exists, which requires the determination of arterial blood pH and PCO_2.

$NaHCO_3$ administration should rarely precede more established interventions, such as defibrillation, ventilation with endotracheal intubation, and pharmacologic therapies. If needed, 1 mEq/kg of $NaHCO_3$ should be administered; subsequent doses should be administered only if the state of acidemia is not adequately resolved with the original dose. Ready-to-use, prefilled injection syringes containing 8.4% $NaHCO_3$ (50-mEq/ 50-mL) are available for use during CPR. Repeat dosing of $NaHCO_3$ is oftentimes empiric because in the course of CPR the serum HCO_3 value can prove difficult to interpret (and likewise the pH) relating to the non-steady-state nature of the measurement. It takes some time (hours) for HCO_3 to equilibrate in cellular compartments, a process which will automatically reduce the serum HCO_3 value. $NaHCO_3$ may be most useful during the immediate postresuscitation period, when a profound metabolic acidosis can occur; particularly, in those patients who remain hemodynamically compromised. In such situations a sustaining infusion of $NaHCO_3$ may be preferable.

Magnesium Disturbances

ETIOLOGIES: HYPOMAGNESEMIA AND HYPERMAGNESEMIA

Mg $^{++}$ is the second most common intracellular cation in the human body with a free cytosolic concentration around 0.5-mmol/L *(62)*. Mg^{++} is distributed in three major compartments in the body: approx 65% in the mineral phase of bone, about 34% in muscle and 1% in plasma and interstitial fluid. Unlike, plasma Ca^{++}, which is 40% protein-bound, only approx 20% of plasma Mg^{++} is protein-bound. Consequently, changes in plasma protein concentrations have less effect on total plasma Mg^{++} concentration than on total plasma Ca^{++} concentrations. Mg^{++} is important in many cell membrane functions, including the gating of Ca^{++} channels, thereby mimicking many of the effects of calcium-channel blockade. Mg^{++} is a necessary cofactor for any biochemical reaction involving adenosine triphosphate (ATP), and is essential for the proper functioning of the Na$^+$-K$^+$ and calcium ATPase pumps, which are critical to the maintenance of a normal resting membrane potential. Intracellular Mg^{++} deficiency can lead to abnormalities in myocardial membrane potential, which then serves as a trigger for cardiac arrhythmias *(63,64)*. Deficiency states or abnormalities in Mg^{++} metabolism also play important roles in ischemic heart disease, CHF, sudden cardiac death, diabetes mellitus, and/or hypertension *(65)*. However, Mg^{++} deficiency has yet to be established as an independent CVR mortality risk factor in such conditions *(66)*.

Mg^{++} deficiency occurs in association with various medical disorders, but is particularly common in diabetes mellitus *(67)*, CHF *(68–70)*, and following diuretic use *(71)*. Recognition of K$^+$ deficiency and/or its correction follows fairly standard guidelines; alternatively, the circumstances are much different for Mg^{++} deficiency because serum values poorly reflect total body Mg^{++} stores *(62)*. K$^+$ repletion in a hypokalemic patient can prove difficult unless underlying Mg^{++} deficiency is first corrected *(67)*. Hypomagnesemia is also a cause of hypocalcemia as the result of its decreasing parathyroid hormone release and/or action *(72)*. This form of hypocalcemia responds to small amounts of supplemental Mg^{++} but can redevelop unless the Mg^{++} deficit is fully replaced *(73)*. The occurrence of diuretic-related hypokalemia and/or hypomagnesemia, in either CHF and/or hypertension, can be considerably lessened by K$^+$-sparing diuretics.

Hypermagnesemia generally results from an excessive intake of Mg^{++} or overzealous replacement of presumed losses in the presence of advanced functional renal failure, as may be seen in the later stages of CHF. Excessive oral intake is generally a consequence of the inappropriate use of Mg^{++} supplements, Mg^{++}-containing antacids or cathartic agents. The diagnosis of hypermagnesemia should be considered in patients who present with symptoms of hyporeflexia, lethargy, refractory hypotension, shock, prolonged QT interval, respiratory depression, or CA *(74)*.

Relationship to CPA and Treatment Considerations

Mg^{++} deficiency impairs the function of the Na-K-ATPase enzyme, which, in turn, lowers intracellular K$^+$. As a result, the resting membrane potential becomes less negative, thereby lowering the threshold for arrhythmias *(75,76)*. In addition to its effect on the Na-K-ATPase pump, Mg^{++} deficiency has potential arrhythmogenic effects through an interaction with several different types of K$^+$ channels localized to cardiac cells *(77)*.

The arrythmogenic effect of Mg^{++} deficiency is further supported by the observation that there is an inverse correlation between myocardial irritability and serum Mg^{++} concentrations; a finding that is particularly evident in CHF *(78,79)*. Moreover, considerable evidence exists linking Mg^{++} deficiency with an increased incidence of both supraventricular and ventricular arrhythmias *(80,81)*.

Studies in animals appear to support the theory that Mg^{++} administration increases cell resistance to the development of arrhythmias, a phenomenon that may be independent of the serum Mg^{++} concentration. For example, Mg^{++} infusions have been shown to raise the threshold for both ventricular premature contractions and VF induction in normal denervated (heart–lung preparations) and whole-animal digitalis-treated hearts *(78)*. Evidence of the salutary effects of intravenous Mg^{++} in treating both ventricular premature contractions and supraventricular and ventricular tachyarrhythmias has also been available for many years *(82)*. For example, 0.2 mEq/kg of $MgSO_4$ given over 1-hour to CHF patients reduces the frequency of ectopic beats in a 6-hour postdosing monitoring period *(83)* and MgCl given as a 10-minute bolus (0.3-mEq/kg) followed by a 24-hour maintenance infusion (0.08 mEq/kg/hr) also reduces the hourly frequency of ectopic beats *(84)*. Oral Mg^{++} replacement (15.8 mmol MgCl/day for 6 weeks) has been shown to reduce ventricular irritability during chronic CHF treatment despite the fact that serum Mg^{++} insignificantly changes (0.87 ± 0.07 to 0.92 ± 0.05 mmol/L *[85]*). The risk of arrhythmia development is particularly high in hypomagnesemic individuals concurrently receiving digitalis *(86)*.

Finally, numerous anecdotal reports have been published attesting to the utility of Mg^{++} in cases of refractory ventricular arrhythmias, although most of these cases were probably associated with Mg^{++} deficiency. Interestingly, K^+-sparing diuretics, compounds that also exhibit Mg^{++}-sparing effects, do not carry the same increased risk for SCD observed with non-K^+-sparing diuretics *(87)*. Despite these observations and the theoretical benefits of Mg^{++} with regards to the development of arrhythmias, there have been few controlled studies evaluating the specific efficacy of Mg^{++} as an antiarrhythmic agent in the treatment of ventricular arrhythmias. Furthermore, it is unclear whether the potential effectiveness of Mg^{++} in these situations represents a pharmacological effect of Mg^{++} or whether it merely reflects correction of an underlying deficiency state. Whatever its potential role in the management of VF *(88–90)* supraventricular arrhythmias *(91)*, and "run-of-the-mill" ventricular arrhythmias *(82,92)*, Mg^{++} clearly does have a time-honored and proven place in the treatment of ventricular arrhythmias associated with either digoxin toxicity or drug-induced torsade de pointes *(77,93,94)*.

Difficulty in establishing the diagnosis of Mg^{++} deficiency is as a result of the lack of reliable laboratory tests and the non-specific nature of the symptoms accompanying Mg^{++} deficiency *(62)*. Mg^{++} deficiency should be suspected when other electrolyte abnormalities are present because it tends to coexist with abnormalities such as hypocalcemia and hypokalemia *(95,96)*.

Electrocardiographic changes such as prolongation of the Q-T and P-R intervals, widening of the QRS complex, ST segment depression, and low T waves, as well as supraventricular and ventricular tachyarrhythmias should also raise the index of suspicion for Mg^{++} deficiency *(97,98)*.

Parenteral Mg^{++} administration is the most effective way to correct a hypomagnesemic state and should be the route used when replacement is necessary during medical emergencies. A variety of Mg^{++} treatment regimens have been tried in the setting of CPA, being given not to replace a physiologic deficit but rather to take advantage of its pharmacologic properties. These pharmacologic regimens have utilized $MgSO_4$ doses ranging from 2 to 5 g *(88,90)*. Total body deficits of Mg^{++} present a different circumstance in the patient prone to CPA; therein, preemptive treatment is warranted. For acute administration during VT or VF with known or suspected hypomagnesemia or for torsade de pointes, 1 or 2 g of $MgSO_4$ can be administered over 5 to 10 minutes. Caution should be used when Mg^{++} is administered intravenously to safeguard against hypotension, bradycardia, or asystole. When present, Mg^{++} deficits are typically in the order of magnitude of 1–2 mEq/kg/b.w. To this end, rapid correction of an Mg^{++} deficit can be accomplished with between 32 and 64-mEq per day of $MgSO_4$ intravenously infused. Alternatively, oral Mg^{++} replacement can occur with any of a wide range of Mg^{++} salts and/or Mg^{++} containing antacids. Ongoing Mg^{++} losses, as occur in patients subject to long-term diuretic therapy, oftentimes are best treated by use of an Mg^{++} sparing diuretic, such as spironolactone.

Potassium Disturbances

ETIOLOGIES: HYPOKALEMIA AND HYPERKALEMIA

The economy of K^+ in the body is typically separated into elements of both external and internal balance. The GI and renal systems both influence external K^+ balance, with a normally functioning gut typically conserving or eliminating K^+ based on total body stores. The GI abnormalities most relevant to external K^+ balance include diarrhea and vomiting. Diarrheal states are characterized by significant K^+ (and Mg^{++}) losses with stool K^+ content reaching values as high as 90 mmol/L. Vomiting is another GI disturbance commonly accompanied by hypokalemia, although its origin is not as a consequence of GI losses—gastric fluid typically contains no more than 10-mmol of K^+/L—but rather as the result of increased renal K^+ losses in association with metabolic alkalosis. GI issues do not often result in hyperkalemia except when such issues produce a level of volume contraction sufficient to reduce GFR in the setting of a high K^+ intake and/or the ingestion of potassium-sparing medications *(99)*.

Renal issues influencing external K^+ balance include urinary flow rate, ECF volume, diuretic use, Na^+ intake, acid–base balance, mineralocorticoid excess, renal tubular diseases and/or renal failure, and Mg^{++} depletion *(100)*. Diuretic therapy is the leading drug-related cause of hypokalemia and relates to both the dose and type of diuretic used as well as the level of dietary Na^+ intake.

Renal failure is among the lead causes of hyperkalemia. K^+ homeostasis is typically well-maintained until a GFR of 30-mL per minute except in the instance of diabetes in which a tendency to develop hyperkalemia emerges at higher GFR levels (typically at 60-mL per minute). Hyperkalemia of a renal origin also occurs in the context of medication administration, particularly when the GFR is reduced. A number of CVR medications have been implicated in this regard including aldosterone-receptor antagonists—such as spironolactone, ACE inhibitors, angiotensin-receptor blockers, and heparin *(101–103)*.

An average 70-kg adult maintains a total body K^+ content of approx 3500 mmol, the majority of which (98%) resides intracellularly; accordingly, less than 2% of total body K^+ is located within the ECF space. The persistence of this relationship results in a very high intracellular-to-extracellular ratio (10:1) for K^+, a cellular gradient that is maintained routinely by the Na^+/K^+ ATPase pump. Internal K^+ balance is modulated further by a range of other issues, including hydrogen (H^+) ion concentration, plasma tonicity, catecholamine concentrations, plasma insulin, and possibly plasma aldosterone *(104)*. The impact of many of these issues on serum K^+ is variable. For example, the influence of H^+ concentration on transcellular shifts of K^+ has proven to be much less than first thought *(105)* and is most prominent in the presence of inorganic acidoses *(106)*.

Plasma tonicity remains a critical factor in transcellular K^+ fluxes and is a probable explanation for the rise in K^+ that commonly follows mannitol administration or that which occurs in the setting of hyperglycemia (107). Both insulin and β-adrenergic active catecholamines encourage intracellular migration of K^+ by stimulating cell membrane Na^+/K^+ ATPase (108). It remains unclear whether aldosterone affects transcellular K^+ distribution; alternatively, aldosterone remains an important determinant of renal K^+ handling (109).

Correctly establishing that transcellular shifts of K^+ are affecting a serum K^+ concentration is an important clinical exercise. Hypokalemia is not always associated with true depletion of body K^+ stores. K^+ redistribution is a frequently observed phenomenon, most often seen in stressful situations, such as at the time of an AMI, when endogenous catecholamine release exerts a $β_2$-adrenergic-mediated effect to force intracellular migration of K^+. Other clinical situations in which intracellular K^+ movement may be observed to a sufficient degree so to be clinically relevant include insulin administration (e.g., in the treatment of hyperglycemia) or during $β_2$ agonist use (i.e., during CA, in the course of postoperative blood pressure support in the cardiothoracic surgery patient, and/or in the course of symptomatic management of acute or chronic asthma).

Redistributional hypokalemia occurs independent of the underlying state of total body K^+ balance. Therefore, laboratory values obtained during such situations cannot be used to accurately predict whether a true total body deficit of K^+ exists or, in the instance of a mixed picture—a patient with a known basis for a K^+ deficit and the presence of issues associated with redistribution—to establish the true level of the deficit. When redistributional hypokalemia is treated, it should be treated cautiously, with an understanding that when the precipitating factor is removed—which can occur rapidly—continued administration of K^+ in the absence of a stimulus for transcellular K^+ shifts can lead to development of hyperkalemia. Thus, estimation of total body K^+ status in the presence of hypokalemia is, at best, a cautious clinical guess.

Relationship to CPA and Treatment Considerations

Because K^+ serves as the primary ion mediating cardiac repolarization, the hypokalemic state is highly arrhythmogenic, particularly in the presence of digoxin or anti-arrhythmic drug therapy. Falling extracellular K^+ levels alter repolarizing electrical currents across the cardiac cell membrane such that during phases 2 and 3 of repolarization, the cell reinitiates isolated or repeated action potentials (early afterdepolarizations). Thus, hypokalemic states produce complex effects on myocardial refractory periods and the potential for triggered arrhythmias. In contrast, hyperkalemia causes slowed conduction and conduction block, which if sufficiently progressive, can result in asystole. Hyperkalemia may also attenuate the effects of antiarrhythmic agents and repolarizing K^+ currents (110).

Electrocardiographically, hypokalemia produces a flattening or inversion of the T wave with concomitant prominence of the U wave, usually with prolongation of the QT interval. The ECG pattern of hypokalemia is not specific and is similar to that seen following administration of antiarrhythmic agents, or phenothiazines, or in left ventricular hypertrophy or marked bradycardia (111). Clinically, arrhythmias associated with hypokalemia include atrial fibrillation and multifocal atrial tachycardias. The most concerning and life-threatening arrhythmias associated with K^+ deficiency states are ventricular tachyarrhythmias, which range from an increase in the frequency of premature ventricular contractions, linearly related to the fall in serum K^+ concentrations, to nonsustained VT and triggering of monomorphic and polymorphic VT, including torsade de pointes and VF. Low K^+ levels can also prolong repolarization and QT intervals.

Data gathered from relatively small studies show a striking relationship between serum K^+ levels and the development of ventricular arrhythmias in patients admitted with acute myocardial infarction (MI) *(112,113)*. The catecholamine surge that occurs during an acute MI causes a rapid, transient cellular shift of K^+, resulting in a short-lived but dramatic fall in serum K^+ of approx 0.5–0.6 mmol/L, which in certain instances may be more extreme *(114)*. Accordingly, in an autopsy study, myocardial K^+ content was significantly lower in subjects who died of CA (0.063 mmol/g wet weight) than in those who died from trauma (0.074 mmol/g wet weight; $p < 0.025$). Myocardial Mg^{++} concentrations also were significantly lower *(115)*. This latter observation is of some relevance to the arrhythmogenic potential of transcellular K^+ shifts. It should be appreciated, however, that the association of low K^+ levels with an increased risk of primary VF in acute MI patients is confounded by the size of the infarct. Larger infarctions are typically accompanied by a greater increase in plasma catecholamines and therefore a greater intracellular flux of K^+; thus, the lower K^+ values may not directly relate to arrhythmia risk but rather reflect a larger infarct size with its attendant risk. As shown in the β-Blocker Heart Attack Trial (BHAT) and the Norwegian Timolol Studies, β-blocker therapy lessens the catecholamine surge, independently reduces transcellular K^+ shifts, and thereby maintains a normokalemic state *(116–118)*. Additionally, hypokalemia is often found in patients during and following resuscitation from a CA, which is a secondary phenomenon as a result of catecholamine-induced K^+ shift into the cells. In this regard, hypokalemia is found in up to 50% of survivors of out-of-hospital VF *(119,120)*.

Transcellular K^+ shifts in the setting of acute MI must always be viewed in the context of the underlying state of K^+ balance and/or the prevailing serum K^+ value in the affected patient. Thus, a patient who had normal or high-normal serum K^+ values before the acute MI would likely experience a drop in serum K^+ into a range that would modestly increase their risk for subsequent ventricular arrhythmias. In contrast, a hypertensive patient taking a K^+-wasting diuretic could be subject to a much greater arrhythmogenic risk because they would experience transcellular shifts of K^+ in the presence of varying degrees of total body K^+ depletion.

Hypokalemia contributes to arrhythmic deaths in cardiac patients, but it is not the only cause. Additionally, resuscitation from refractory VF is less likely to be successful if hypokalemia and/or hypomagnesemia are present. The question has also been raised to the appropriateness of cardioverter defibrillator placement in patients having an electrolyte abnormality (a correctable cause of a life-threatening ventricular arrhythmia according to AHA/American College of Cardiology Practice Guidelines) and VT or VF. The available information would suggest that patients with structural heart disease and an abnormal serum K^+ concentration at the time of an initial episode of sustained VT or VF are at high risk for a recurrent ventricular arrhythmia; therefore, implantable defibrillator therapy may be a reasonable option *(8,9,121)*.

Potassium-wasting diuretics, although shown to reduce mortality and the incidence of strokes, abdominal aortic aneurysms, and hypertensive deaths, are associated with an increased incidence of SCD *(122)*. Diuretic-related hypokalemia is particularly prominent in patients receiving loop and thiazide diuretics in combination. Findings from older trials and more recent studies demonstrate the importance of K^+ and diuretics on SCD *(123,124)*. A multivariate retrospective analysis of diuretic use in the Studies of Left Ventricular Dysfunction (SOLVD) trial showed that patients taking any diuretic had significantly greater increased relative risk of SCD (1.37 vs 1.00; $p = 0.009$ *[125]*). When analyzed by diuretic type, patients taking K^+-wasting diuretics had a significantly higher risk of fatal arrhythmias (1.33; $p = 0.02$), although use of K^+-sparing diuretics either as monotherapy or in combination with other diuretics was not independently associated with an increased risk of arrhythmic death (0.90; $p = 0.6$). Similarly, data from the prospective United Kingdom Heart Failure Evaluation and Assessment of Risk Trial (UK-Heart) show serum K^+ to be one of four independent predictors of SCD *(126)*.

Hypokalemia in the patient with CA and refractory VF must be treated aggressively. K^+ should be administered intravenously under such circumstances. Guidelines for K^+ replacement that are acceptable in the less emergent clinical circumstance may be inadequate to correct hypokalemia in a timely enough fashion during CPA. There has been no regimen for K^+ replacement formally tested during CPA. Because of the urgency of the situation during CPA it is not unreasonable to give 10–20 mEq of potassium chloride as a "run" over 10–15 minutes. K^+ should initially be given in glucose-free solutions as glucose may further lower K^+. This dose can be repeated as necessary during the rechecking of serum levels; however, treatment provided for a serum K^+ value obtained during or immediately after CPR must occur in the context of the significant transcellular K^+ shifts having occurred.

Hyperkalemia as a cause of CPA is a very specific circumstance that can prove quite responsive to treatment. Urgent treatment of hyperkalemia is typically based on electrocardiogram changes (and/or CPA), immediate intervention is critical. Following the intravenous administration of a calcium salt (calcium chloride is preferred), the initiation of short-term measures can be launched by either a single or combined regimen of the three agents that effect a transcellular shift of K^+ - insulin with glucose, β_2-agonism (albuterol), and $NaHCO_3$. *(127)*. Serum K^+ can drop as much as 1–2 mEq with therapy designed at effecting transcellular shifts. A change in serum K^+ of this order of magnitude is typically sufficient to reestablish an effective cardiac rhythm in a patient otherwise having sustained CPA from hyperkalemia. However, the transcellular shifting of K^+ is a temporary phenomenon and steps should be taken to effect bulk removal of K^+; from the body by either gastrointestinal or renal routes (inclusive of hemodialysis in which so indicated).

SUMMARY

A number of electrolyte abnormalities can trigger CPA and, in turn, can be caused by events surrounding successful resuscitation. Potassium and magnesium abnormalities remain most important in this regard. Maintaining potassium and magnesium balance in patients prone to CPA can prove to be a difficult task but not one that cannot be accomplished if careful attention is paid to supplement therapy and the use of potassium/magnesium sparing diuretics.

REFERENCES

1. Part 8: advanced challenges in resuscitation. Section 1: Life-threatening electrolyte abnormalities. European Resuscitation Council. Resuscitation 2000; 46:253–259.

2. Ramaswamy K, Hamdan MH. Ischemia, metabolic disturbances, and arrhythmogenesis: mechanisms and management. Crit Care Med 2000; 28(Suppl):N151–157.
3. Delva P. Magnesium and cardiac arrhythmias. Mol Aspects Med. 2003; 24:53-62.
4. Kleeman K, Singh BN. Serum electrolytes and the heart. In: Clinical Disorders of Fluid and Electrolyte Metabolism, 3rd edition. Maxwell MH, Kleeman CR, eds. New York: McGraw-Hill, 1980, pp. 145–180.
5. Sanders AB, Ewy GA, Taft TV. Reliability of femoral artery sampling during cardiopulmonary resuscitation. Ann Emerg Med 1984; 13:680–683.
6. Weil MH, Rackow EC, Trevino R, et al. Difference in acid-base state between venous and arterial blood during cardiopulmonary resuscitation. N Engl J Med 1986; 315:153–156.
7. Steedman DJ, Robertson CE. Acid base changes in arterial and central venous blood during cardiopulmonary resuscitation. Arch Emerg Med 1992; 9:169–176.
8. Wyse DG, Friedman PL, Brodsky MA, et al. Life-threatening ventricular arrhythmias due to transient or correctable causes: high risk for death in follow-up. J Am Coll Cardiol 2001; 38:1718–1724.
9. Salerno DM, Murakami MM, Winston MD, Elsperger KJ. Postresuscitation electrolyte changes: role of arrhythmia and resuscitation efforts in their genesis. Crit Care Med 1989; 17:1181–1186.
10. Isner JM, Harten JT. Factitious lowering of the serum potassium level after cardiopulmonary resuscitation. Implications for evaluating the arrhythmogenicity of hypokalemia in acute myocardial infarction. Arch Intern Med 1985; 145:161–162
11. Viskin S, Halkin A, Olgin JE. Treatable causes of sudden death: not really "treatable" or not really the cause? J Am Coll Cardiol 2001; 38:1725–1727.
12. Sica DA, Gehr T: Diuretic use in congestive heart failure. Cardiol Clin 1989; 7:87–97.
13. Lee WH, Packer M. Prognostic importance of serum sodium concentration and its modification by converting-enzyme inhibition in patients with severe chronic heart failure. Circulation 1986; 73:257–267.
14. Schrier RW, Ecder T. Gibbs memorial lecture. Unifying hypothesis of body fluid volume regulation: implications for cardiac failure and cirrhosis. Mt Sinai J Med 2001; 68:350–361.
15. Sica DA. Pharmacotherapy in congestive heart failure: angiotensin II and thirst: therapeutic considerations. Congest Heart Fail 2001; 7:325–328.
16. Dargie HJ, Cleland JG, Leckie BJ, et al. Relation of arrhythmias and electrolyte abnormalities to survival in patients with severe chronic heart failure. Circulation 1987; 75:IV98–IV107.
17. Panciroli C, Galloni G, Oddone A, et al. Prognostic value of hyponatremia in patients with severe chronic heart failure. Angiology 1990; 41:631–638.
18. Lee WH, Packer M. Prognostic importance of serum sodium concentration and its modification by converting-enzyme inhibition in patients with severe chronic heart failure. Circulation 1986; 73:257–267.
19. Packer M, Lee WH, Kessler PD, et al. Identification of hyponatremia as a risk factor for the development of functional renal insufficiency during converting enzyme inhibition in severe chronic heart failure. J Am Coll Cardiol 1987; 10:837–844.
20. Oster JR, Materson BJ. Renal and electrolyte complications of congestive heart failure and effects of therapy with angiotensin-converting enzyme inhibitors. Arch Intern Med 1992; 152:704–710.
21. Buylaert WA, Calle PA, Houbrechts HN. Serum electrolyte disturbances in the post-resuscitation period. The Cerebral Resuscitation Study Group. Resuscitation 1989; 17 (Suppl):S189–S196
22. Eisenberg IJ. Electrolyte measurements during in-hospital cardiopulmonary resuscitation. Crit Care Med 1990; 18:25–28.
23. Domanovits H, Schillinger M, Mullner M, et al. Acute renal failure after successful cardiopulmonary resuscitation. Intensive Care Med 2001; 27:1194–1199.
24. Domanovits H, Mullner M, Sterz F, et al. Impairment of renal function in patients resuscitated from cardiac arrest: frequency, determinants and impact on outcome. Wien Klin Wochenschr 2000; 112:157–161.
25. AHA Scientific Statement: International Guidelines 2000 for Cardiopulmonary Resuscitation and Emergency Cardiovascular Care. Circulation 2000; 102(Suppl I):I-1–I-384.
26. Voelckel WG, Lindner KH, Wenzel V, et al. Effects of vasopressin and epinephrine on splanchnic blood flow and renal function during and after cardiopulmonary resuscitation in pigs. Crit Care Med 2000; 28:1083–1088.
27. Rolls BJ, Phillips PA. Aging and disturbances of thirst and fluid balance. Nutr Rev 1990; 48:137–144.
28. Ujhelyi MR, Winecoff AP, Schur M, et al. Influence of hypertonic saline solution infusion on defibrillation efficacy. Chest 1996; 110:784–790.
29. Kaufman AM, Kahn T. Congestive heart failure with hypernatremia. Arch Intern Med 1986; 146:402, 403.
30. Kahn T. Hypernatremia with edema. Arch Intern Med 1999; 159:93–98.
31. Kordas J, Kotulski J, Zolnierczyk J. Transient diabetes insipidus following cardiologic resuscitation in a patient with myocardial infarct. Wiad Lek 1975; 28:1701–1708.

32. Rothschild M, Shenkman L. Diabetes insipidus following cardiorespiratory arrest. JAMA 1977; 238: 620–621.
33. Beasley EW 3rd, Phillips LS. Polyuria and refractory hypernatremia after cardiopulmonary arrest. Am J Med 1987; 82:347–349.
34. Aufderheide TP, Martin DR, Olson DW, et al. Prehospital bicarbonate use in cardiac arrest: a 3-year experience. Am J Emer Med 1992; 10:4–7.
35. Ujhelyi MR, Winecoff AP, Schur M, et al. Influence of hypertonic saline solution infusion on defibrillation efficacy. Chest 1996; 110:784–790.
36. Gando S, Igarashi M, Kameue T, Nanzaki S. Ionized hypocalcemia during out-of-hospital cardiac arrest and cardiopulmonary resuscitation is not due to binding by lactate. Intensive Care Med 1997; 23: 1245–1250.
37. Niemann JT, Cairns CB. Hyperkalemia and ionized hypocalcemia during cardiac arrest and resuscitation: possible culprits for postcountershock arrhythmias? Ann Emerg Med 1999; 34:1–7.
38. Gando S, Tedo I, Kubota M. A comparison of serum ionized calcium in arterial and mixed venous blood during CPR. Ann Emerg Med 1990; 19:850–856.
39. Ornato JP, Gonzalez ER, Morkunas AR, et al: Treatment of presumed asystole during pre-hospital cardiac arrest: superiority of electrical countershock Am J Emer Med 1985; 3:395–399.
40. Stempien A, Katz AM, Messineo FC. Calcium and cardiac arrest. Ann Intern Med 1986; 105:603–606.
41. Kirsch JR, Dean JM, Rogers MC: Current concepts in brain resuscitation. Arch Intern Med 1986; 146:1413–1419.
42. Dembo DH: Calcium in advanced life support. Crit Care Med 1981; 9:358–359.
43. Follette DM, Fey K, Buckberg GD, et al. Reducing postischemic damage by temporary modification of reperfusate calcium, potassium, pH, and osmolarity. J Thorac Cardiovasc Surg 1981; 82:221–238.
44. Zimmerman AN, Hulsmann WC: Paradoxical influence of calcium ions on the permeability of the cell membrane of the isolated rat heart. Nature 1966; 211:646, 647.
45. Vukmir RB, Bircher NG, Radovsky A, Safar P. Sodium bicarbonate may improve outcome in dogs with prolonged cardiac arrest. Crit Care Med 1995; 23:515–522.
46. Levy MM. An evidence-based evaluation of the use of sodium bicarbonate during cardiopulmonary resuscitation. Crit Care Clin 1988; 14: 457–483.
47. Weil MH, Ruiz CE, Michaels S, Rackow EC. Acid-base determinants of survival after cardiopulmonary resuscitation. Crit Care Med 1985; 13: 888–892.
48. MacGregor DC, Wilson GJ, Holmes DE, et al. Intramyocardial carbon dioxide tension: a guide to the safe period of anoxic arrest of the heart. J Thorac Cardiovasc Surg 1974; 68:101–107.
49. Orchard CH, Cingolani HE. Acidosis and arrhythmias in cardiac muscle. Cardiovasc Res 1994; 28: 1312–1319.
50. Teplinsky K, O'Toole M, Olman M, et al. Effect of lactic acidosis on canine haemodynamics and left ventricular function. Am J Physiol 1990; 258:1193–1199.
51. Wenzel V, Linder KH, Krismer AC, et al. Repeated administration of vasopressin but not epinephrine maintains coronary perfusion pressure after early and late administration during prolonged cardiopulmonary resuscitation in pigs. Circulation 1999; 99:1379–1384.
52. Jaffe AS. New and old paradoxes. Acidosis and cardiopulmonary resuscitation. Circulation 1989; 80:1079–1083.
53. Grundler W, Weil MH, Yamaguchi M, et al. The paradox of venous acidosis and arterial alkalosis during CPR. Chest 1984; 86:282.
54. Ornato JP, Gonzalez ER, Coyne MR, et al. Arterial pH in out-of-hospital cardiac arrest: response time as a determinant of acidosis. Am J Emerg Med 1985; 3:498–502.
55. Niemann JT, Rosborough JP. Effects of acidemia and sodium bicarbonate therapy in advanced cardiac life support. Ann Emerg Med 1984; 13:781–784.
56. Clancy RL, Cingolani HE, Taylor RR, et al. Influence of sodium bicarbonate on myocardial performance. Am J Physiol 1967; 212:917–923.
57. Berenyi KJ, Wolk M, Killip T. Cerebrospinal fluid acidosis complicating therapy of experimental cardiopulmonary arrest. Circulation 1975; 52:319–324.
58. Guerci AD, Chandra N, Johnson E, et al. Failure of sodium bicarbonate to improve resuscitation from ventricular fibrillation in dogs. Circulation 1986; 74(Pt 2):IV75–IV79.
59. Dybvik T, Strand T, Steen PA. Buffer therapy during out of-hospital cardiopulmonary resuscitation. Resuscitation 1995; 29:89–95.
60. Bishop RL, Weisfeldt ML. Sodium bicarbonate administration during cardiac arrest: Effect of arterial pH, P_{CO2} and osmolality. JAMA 1976; 235:506–509.

61. Imai T, Kon N, Kunimoto F, et al. Exacerbation of hypercapnia and acidosis of central venous blood and tissue following administration of sodium bicarbonate during cardiopulmonary resuscitation. Jpn Circ J 1989; 53:298–306.
62. Saris NE, Mervaala E, Karppanen H, et al. Magnesium: an update on physiological, clinical, and analytical aspects. Clin Chim Acta 2000; 294:1–26.
63. Reinhart RA. Clinical correlates of the molecular and cellular actions of magnesium on the cardiovascular system. Am Heart J 1991; 121:1513–1521.
64. Chakraborti S, Chakraborti T, Mandal M, et al. Protective role of magnesium in cardiovascular diseases: a review. Mol Cell Biochem 2002; 238:163–179.
65. Fox C, Ramsoomair D, Carter C. Magnesium: its proven and potential clinical significance. South Med J 2001; 94:1195–1201.
66. Eichhorn EJ, Tandon PK, DiBianco R, et al. Clinical and prognostic significance of serum magnesium concentration in patients with severe chronic congestive heart failure: the PROMISE Study. J Amer Coll Cardiol 1993; 21:634–640.
67. Agus ZS: Hypomagnesemia. J Am Soc Nephrol 1999; 10:1616–1622.
68. Cohen N, Alon I, Almoznino-Sarafian D, et al. Metabolic and clinical effects of oral magnesium supplementation in furosemide-treated patients with severe congestive heart failure. Clin Cardiol 2000; 23:433–436.
69. Leier CV, Dei Cas L, Metra M. Clinical relevance and management of the major electrolyte abnormalities in congestive heart failure: hyponatremia, hypokalemia, and hypomagnesemia. Am Heart J 1994; 128:564–74.
70. Cermuzynski L, Gebalska J, Wolk R, Makowska E. Hypomagnesemia in heart failure with ventricular arrhythmias. Beneficial effects of magnesium supplementation. J Intern Med 2000; 247:78–86.
71. Wester PO, Dyckner T. Diuretic treatment and magnesium losses. Acta Med Scand 1981; 647(Suppl): 145–152.
72. Chase LR, Slatopolsky E. Secretion and metabolic efficiency of parathyroid hormone in patients with severe hypomagnesemia. J Clin Endocrinol Metab 1974; 38:363–371.
73. Leicht E, Schmidt-Gayk H, Langer HJ, et al. Hypomagnesaemia-induced hypocalcaemia: concentrations of parathyroid hormone, prolactin and 1,25-dihydroxyvitamin D during magnesium replenishment. Magnes Res 1992; 5:33–36.
74. Mordes JP, Swartz R, Arky RA. Extreme hypermagnesemia as a cause of refractory hypotension. Ann Intern Med 1975; 83:657, 658.
75. Dyckner T, Wester PO. Ventricular extrasystoles and intracellular electrolytes before and after potassium and magnesium infusions in patients on diuretic treatment. Am Heart J 1979; 97:12–18.
76. McLean RM. Magnesium and its therapeutic uses: a review. Is J Med 1994; 96:63–76.
77. Delva P. Magnesium and cardiac arrhythmias. Mol Aspects of Med 2003; 24:53–62.
78. Ghani MF, Rabah M. Effect of magnesium chloride on electrical stability of the heart. Is Heart J 1977; 94:600–602.
79. Gottlieb SS, Fisher ML, Pressel MD, et al. Effects of intravenous magnesium sulfate on arrhythmias in patients with congestive heart failure. Amer Heart J 1993; 125:1645–1650.
80. Iseri LT. Magnesium and cardiac arrhythmias. Magnesium 1986; 5:111–126.
81. Tsuji H, Venditti FJ Jr., Evans JC, et al. The association of levels of serum K and magnesium with ventricular premature complexes (the Framingham Heart Study). Am J Cardiol 1994; 74:232–235.
82. Arsenian MA. Magnesium and cardiovascular disease. Prog Cardiovasc Dis 1993; 35:271–310.
83. Sueta CA, Clarke SW, Dunlap SH, et al. Effect of acute magnesium administration on the frequency of ventricular arrhythmia in patients with heart failure. Circulation 1994; 89:660–666.
84. Gottlieb SS, Fisher ML, Pressel MD, et al. Effects of intravenous magnesium sulfate on arrhythmias in patients with congestive heart failure. Amer Heart J 1993; 125:1645–1650.
85. Bashir Y, Sneddon JF, Staunton HA, et al. Effects of long‑term oral magnesium chloride replacement in congestive heart failure secondary to coronary artery disease. Am J Cardiol 1993; 72:1156–1162.
86. Crippa G, Sverzellati E, Giorgi-Pierfranceschi M, Carrara GC. Magnesium and cardiovascular drugs: interactions and therapeutic role. Ann Ital Med Int 1999; 14:40–45.
87. Hoes AW, Grobbee DE, Lubsen J, et al. Diuretics, β-blockers, and the risk for sudden cardiac death in hypertensive patients. Ann Intern Med 1995; 123:481–487.
88. Allegra J, Lavery R, Cody R, et al. Magnesium sulfate in the treatment of refractory ventricular fibrillation in the prehospital setting. Resuscitation 2001; 49:245–249.
89. Allen BJ, Brodsky MA, Capparelli EV, et al. Magnesium sulfate therapy for sustained monomorphic ventricular tachycardia. Am J Cardiol 1989; 64:1202–1204.

90. Fatovich DM, Prentice DA, Dobb GJ. Magnesium in cardiac arrest (the magic trial). Resuscitation 1997; 35:237–241.
91. Toraman F, Karabulut EH, Alhan HC, et al. Magnesium infusion dramatically decreases the incidence of atrial fibrillation after coronary artery bypass grafting. Ann Thorac Surg 2001; 72:1256–1261.
92. Zehender M, Meinertz T, Faber T, et al. Antiarrhythmic effects of increasing the daily intake of magnesium and potassium in patients with frequent ventricular arrhythmias. Magnesium in Cardiac Arrhythmias (MAGICA) Investigators. J Am Coll Cardiol 1997; 29:1028–1034.
93. Perticone F, Adinolfi L, Bonaduce D. Efficacy of magnesium sulfate in the treatment of torsade de pointes. Am Heart J 1986; 112: 847–849.
94. Tzivoni D, Banai S, Schuger C, et al. Treatment of torsade de pointes with magnesium sulfate. Circulation 1988; 77:392–397.
95. Whang R, Oei TO, Aikawa JK, et al Predictors of clinical hypomagnesemia. Hypokalemia, hypophosphatemia, hyponatremia and hypocalcemia. Arch Intern Med 1984; 144:1794–1796.
96. Gettes LS. Electrolyte abnormalities underlying lethal and ventricular arrhythmias. Circulation 1992; 85(Suppl):I70–I76.
97. Chen WC, Fu XX, Pan ZJ, Qian SZ. ECG changes in early stage of magnesium deficiency. Am Heart J 1982; 104:1115–1116.
98. Iseri LT, Freed J, Bures AR. Magnesium deficiency and cardiac disorders. Am J Med 1975; 58:837–846.
99. Schepkens H, Vanholder R, Billiouw JM, Lameire N. Life-threatening hyperkalemia during combined therapy with angiotensin-converting enzyme inhibitors and spironolactone: an analysis of 25 cases. Am J Med 2001; 110:438–441.
100. Halperin ML, Kamel KS. Potassium. Lancet. 1998; 352:135–140.
101. Bozkurt B, Agoston I, Knowlton AA. Complications of inappropriate use of spironolactone in heart failure: when an old medicine spirals out of new guidelines. J Am Coll Cardiol 2003; 41:211–214.
102. Obialo CI, Ofili EO, Mirza T. Hyperkalemia in congestive heart failure patients aged 63 to 85 years with subclinical renal disease. Am J Cardiol 2002; 90:663–665.
103. Perazella MA. Drug-induced hyperkalemia: old culprits and new offenders. Am J Med 2000; 109: 307–314.
104. Madias JE, Shah B, Chintalapally G, et al. Admission serum potassium in patients with acute myocardial infarction: its correlates and value as a determinant of in-hospital outcome. Chest 2000; 118:904–913.
105. Adrogue HJ, Madias NE. Changes in plasma potassium concentration during acute acid-base disturbances. Am J Med. 1981; 71:456–467.
106. Ponce SP, Jennings AE, Madias NE, Harrington JT. Drug-induced hyperkalemia. Medicine (Baltimore) 1985; 64:357–370.
107. Makoff DL, da Silva JA, Rosenbaum BJ, et al. Hypertonic expansion: acid-base and electrolyte changes. Am J Physiol. 1970; 218:1201–1207.
108. Clausen T, Everts ME. Regulation of the Na, K-pump in skeletal muscle. Kidney Int 1989; 35; 1–13.
109. Field MJ, Giebisch GJ. Hormonal control of renal potassium excretion. Kidney Int 1985; 27:379–387.
110. Yang T, Roden DM. Extracellular potassium modulation of drug block of I_{Kr}. Implications for torsade de pointes and reverse-use dependence. Circulation. 1996; 93:407–411.
111. Fletcher GF, Hurst JW, Schlant RC. Electrocardiographic changes in severe hypokalemia. A reappraisal. Am J Cardiol 1967; 20:628–631.
112. Salerno DM, Asinger RW, Elsperger J, et al. Frequency of hypokalemia after successfully resuscitated out-of-hospital cardiac arrest compared with that in transmural acute myocardial infarction. Am J Cardiol 1987; 59:84–88.
113. Nordrehaug JE, Johannessen K-A, von der Lippe G. Serum potassium concentration as a risk factor of ventricular arrhythmias early in acute myocardial infarction. Circulation 1985; 71:645–649.
114. Struthers AD, Whitesmith R, Reid JL. Prior thiazide diuretic treatment increases adrenaline-induced hypokalemia. Lancet 1983; 1:1358–1361.
115. Johnson CJ, Peterson DR, Smith EK. Myocardial tissue concentrations of magnesium and potassium in men dying suddenly from ischemic heart disease. Am J Clin Nutr 1979; 32:967–970.
116. Nordrehaug JE, Johannessen K-A, von der Lippe G, et al. Effect of timolol on changes in serum potassium concentration during acute myocardial infarction. Br Heart J. 1985; 53:388–393.
117. Valladares BK, Lemberg L. Catecholamines, potassium, and beta-blockade. Heart Lung 1986; 15: 105–107.
118. Salerno DM, Murakami M, Elsperger KJ. Effects of pretreatment with propranolol on potassium, calcium, and magnesium shifts after ventricular fibrillation in dogs. J Lab Clin Med 1989; 114:595–603.

119. Thompson RG, Cobb LA. Hypokalemia after resuscitation from out-of-hospital ventricular fibrillation. JAMA 1982; 248:2860–2863.
120. Ornato JP, Gonzalez ER, Starke H, et al. Incidence and causes of hypokalemia associated with cardiac resuscitation. Am J Emerg Med 1985; 3:503–506.
121. Michaud GF, Strickberger SA. Should an abnormal serum potassium concentration be considered a correctable cause of cardiac arrest? J Am Coll Cardiol 2001; 38:1224, 1225.
122. Psaty BM, Smith NL, Siscovick DS, et al. Health outcomes associated with antihypertensive therapies used as first-line agents. A systematic review and meta-analysis. JAMA 1997; 277:739–745.
123. Medical Research Council Working Party on Mild to Moderate Hypertension. Ventricular extrasystole during thiazides treatment: substudy of MRC mild hypertension trial. BMJ 1983; 287:1249–1253.
124. Cohen JD, Neaton JD, Prineas RJ, Daniels KA, for the Multiple Risk Factor Intervention Trial Research Group. Diuretics, serum potassium, and ventricular arrhythmias in the Multiple Risk Factor Intervention Trial. Am J Cardiol 1987; 60:548–554.
125. Cooper HA, Dries DL, Davis CE, et al. Diuretics and risk of arrhythmic death in patient with left ventricular dysfunction. Circulation. 1999; 100:1311–1315.
126. Nolan J, Batin PD, Andrews R, et al. Prospective study of heart rate variability and mortality in chronic heart failure. Results of the United Kingdom Heart Failure Evaluation and Assessment of Risk Trial (UK-Heart). Circulation. 1998; 98:1510–1516.
127. Kim HJ, Han SW. Therapeutic approach to hyperkalemia. Nephron 2002; 92(Suppl):33–40.

23 Cardiac Arrest in Pregnancy

Alison A. Rodriguez, MD
and Gary A. Dildy, III, MD

CONTENTS

INTRODUCTION

Cardiac arrest (CA) in pregnancy is an uncommon occurrence with an incidence of about 1 in every 30,000 deliveries *(1)*. The causes are quite numerous, but the management is essentially the same with the exception of a few modifications regarding the fetus. In this chapter, causes of maternal mortality are reviewed along with potential interventions to decrease its incidence. A general overview of maternal and fetal physiology and how it pertains to the resuscitation of the mother will also be provided. Pharmacological agents used in the resuscitative protocol and their effects on the fetus are discussed. Finally, the issue of perimortem cesarean delivery is addressed, along with the difficult questions that must be answered within minutes of deciding who should and should not be considered for this drastic, potentially lifesaving procedure.

MATERNAL MORTALITY

For the purpose of this discussion, maternal mortality will be expressed in terms of the maternal mortality ratio (MMR), which is defined as the number of maternal deaths per 100,000 live births *(2)*. By definition, maternal death is a death that occurs during pregnancy or within 1 year of pregnancy termination *(3)*. Certain criteria must be met in order for a death to be classified as pregnancy-related. Specifically, death must be caused by pregnancy complications, a sequence of events initiated by pregnancy, or exacerbation of an unrelated event by the changes associated with pregnancy *(3)*. Not included in the MMR are the deaths occurring in women with fetal demises, elective or spontaneous

From: *Contemporary Cardiology: Cardiopulmonary Resuscitation*
Edited by: J. P. Ornato and M. A. Peberdy © Humana Press Inc., Totowa, NJ

abortions, ectopic pregnancies, and molar pregnancies. These also contribute significantly to overall maternal mortality, especially in the first trimester *(3)*.

Both maternal and infant mortality provide important insight into the general state of health of the country in question *(4)*. In the United States, the MMR has declined significantly from the 1930s to 2004 from 670 to 7.5 maternal deaths per 100,000 live births *(4)*. Although this is a significant achievement, it still does not meet the *Healthy People 2000: National Health Promotion and Disease Prevention Objective* of no more than 3.3 maternal deaths per 100,000 live births overall and no more than 5 maternal deaths per 100,000 live births for black women *(5)*. Black women are about four times more likely than white women to die from causes related to pregnancy *(5)*. From 1960 to 1990, the MMR for black women was considerably higher than for white women in every age group and for each major cause of death *(2)* with no significant improvement noted from 1987 to 1996 *(6)*. From 1987 to 1990, the leading causes of maternal death in the United States were hemorrhage (29%), pulmonary embolism (20%), and pregnancy-induced hypertension (18%); the remainder resulted from amniotic fluid embolism, infection, anesthesia-related complications, cardiomyopathy, and cerebrovascular accidents *(5,7)*. Causes of maternal death changed very little from 1974 to 1985, with the exception of a relative reduction in deaths related to anesthesia and a relative increase in deaths as a result of cardiomyopathy and infection *(3)*. Intentional and unintentional injuries are common causes of nonmaternal or nonpregnancy-related deaths, with homicide and suicide accounting for 48% of such causes *(8)*. Motor vehicle accidents were the most common cause of unintentional injury accounting for nonmaternal death *(8)*, and in one series, trauma was the most common nonobstetric cause of death *(9)*. It should be noted that the number of pregnancy-related deaths is probably underestimated as a result of both underreporting and misclassification *(10)*.

In developing countries, maternal mortality is much higher with some of the highest rates seen in parts of Africa and South Asia *(11)*. The estimated global maternal mortality, according to the World Health Organization, in 1996 was 585,000 per year with 99% occurring in developing countries and 1% occurring in developed counties *(11)*. The etiologies in these regions are different and more commonly as a result of hemorrhage, poor nutrition, anemia, malaria, unsafe abortion, and obstructed labor *(12)*.

Many measures must be taken to decrease maternal mortality worldwide. These include, in part, preconceptional counseling, family planning, improved nutrition, avoidance of illicit substances, better access to quality obstetric care, vaccinations, blood transfusion, operative vaginal delivery, and cesarean section *(12,13)*.

MATERNAL PHYSIOLOGY

There are numerous maternal physiological adaptations induced by pregnancy (Table 1); the most relevant changes occur in the cardiovascular, pulmonary, gastrointestinal, and uteroplacental systems. Each of these are discussed separately.

Cardiovascular

Beginning in the first trimester, blood volume begins to rise, increasing by about 30 to 50% and plateauing after the 30th week of gestation *(14)*. Both plasma volume and red cell mass increase, but the former does so to a greater extent, producing a "dilutional anemia" *(15)*. This hypervolemia of pregnancy serves as a protective mechanism against hemorrhage during delivery and also compensates for the decreased venous return and

Table 1
Summary of Maternal Physiological Changes in Pregnancy

System	Increase	Decrease
Cardiovascular	Cardiac output Blood volume	Blood pressure COP/CPWP
Respiratory	Minute ventilation Tidal volume O_2 consumption	Functional residual capacity
Gastrointestinal	Risk of regurgitation	pH of gastric contents Esophageal sphincter pressure Gastric motility
Uteroplacental	Blood flow	Reduced if uterine compression of great vessels

Modified from ref. *45*.

cardiac output when in the supine and erect positions *(16)*. Similar to blood volume, cardiac output also increases by 30 to 50%, reaching its peak at about 28 to 32 weeks of gestation *(17)*. Both an increase in heart rate and stroke volume contribute to this rise in cardiac output *(18)*. Both blood volume and cardiac output increase to a greater extent in twin gestations *(19)*. The changes in blood pressure are as a result of a fall in peripheral vascular resistance, which accounts for the drop of about 10 mmHg in mean blood pressure at 30 weeks of gestation *(15)*. Both systemic vascular resistance and pulmonary vascular resistance fall because of the hormonal changes of pregnancy and the low resistance of the placental vasculature. Finally, the colloid oncotic pressure–pulmonary capillary wedge pressure gradient decreases, possibly predisposing the gravid woman to an increased risk of pulmonary edema with increased pulmonary capillary permeability or cardiac preload *(20)*.

Pulmonary

There are significant anatomic as well as functional changes in the pulmonary system of the pregnant female. The gravid uterus, especially in the third trimester, may decrease the vertical diameter of the chest by as much as 4 cm *(15)*. In order to compensate for this, the ribs tend to flare and the anterior–posterior and transverse diameters of the chest increase by 2 cm *(15)*. The functional residual capacity is decreased as a result of these anatomic changes *(21)*. The vital capacity is unchanged, but there is a significant increase in both the tidal volume and minute ventilation as a result of the stimulatory effect of progesterone on the respiratory centers in the brain *(21)*. This "hyperventilation of pregnancy" accounts for the compensated respiratory alkalosis apparent on blood gas measurements performed on pregnant women. It is important to note that moderate hypoxemia occurs in about one-quarter of healthy term patients as they are in the supine position, as well as a widened alveolar-arterial oxygen gradient *(22)*. Maternal positioning affects arterial oxygenation and thus it makes sense that arterial blood gas samples should be drawn in the sitting position, if possible *(22)*. The final and most important point to emphasize is that the oxygen consumption is greater than 30% above normal in the term pregnant patient *(15)*. This increased oxygen consumption causes a more profound and more rapid decrease in oxygen tension during periods of apnea (i.e., cardiopulmonary collapse, intubation) and necessitates the need for prompt reoxygenation in these situations *(23)*.

GASTROINTESTINAL

The two major adaptations observed in the gastrointestinal tract during pregnancy are decreased motility and decreased pressure of the lower esophageal sphincter *(24)*. It is thought that the high levels of progesterone cause relaxation of smooth muscle leading to the above changes, with a resultant delay in gastric emptying and increased risk of regurgitation *(25)*. As pregnancy progresses and the uterus enlarges, mechanical compression also plays a role in the obstruction of gastric emptying *(15)*. The hormone gastrin is also increased during pregnancy. Gastrin lowers the pH of stomach contents to an even greater degree *(26)*. The combination of all of these factors predisposes the pregnant patient to aspiration of gastric contents, especially during times of sedation and unconsciousness *(27)*. Aspiration of gastric contents is the most common cause of anesthesia-related maternal mortality *(15)*. Prophylaxis with antacids and manual cricoid pressure in preparation for endotracheal intubation are of paramount importance *(28)*.

UTEROPLACENTAL

As gestation progresses, the uterus increases in size and weight from 30 to 1000 g, more than 10 times its nonpregnant state *(15)*. This requires augmentation of blood flow. By 37 weeks gestation, the uterine blood flow is 500 mL per minute, which translates into about 10% of the total cardiac output *(29)*. The uteroplacental blood flow is greatly influenced by maternal body position. When a woman at term is supine, the stroke volume is only 30% of the nonpregnant value *(17)*. In the supine position, complete obstruction of the inferior vena cava by the gravid uterus has been reported to occur in the majority of patients *(30)*. This obstruction causes a significant decrease in both cardiac output and venous return *(30)*, which can be partially relieved by changing from the supine to the left lateral decubitus position. Most of the decrease in blood flow is to the placenta and intervillous space, with no significant change in myometrial flow *(31)*.

FETAL PHYSIOLOGY

Oxygenation of the fetus is highly dependent on adequate cardiac output and blood flow to the placenta. The placenta ultimately functions as the fetal lungs and is the organ of fetal gas exchange *(32)*. There are several mechanisms unique to the fetus that ensure adequate oxygenation. The fetal circulation is a highly specialized system designed specifically for this *(33)*. Fetal hemoglobin has an increased oxygen carrying capacity and a higher affinity for oxygen, which shifts the fetal oxygen dissociation curve to the left of the maternal curve *(34)*. In other words, for a given partial pressure of oxygen, a greater percentage of oxygen saturation will be observed in the fetus compared to the mother. Fetal arterial chemoreceptors detect hypoxia and mediate the fetal response through parasympathetic pathways *(35)*. Profound fetal bradycardia is the usual response to severe hypoxia, as seen in CA *(36)*.

ETIOLOGIES OF CARDIAC ARREST IN PREGNANCY

As stated before, CA in pregnancy is rare and usually occurs in young, otherwise healthy women. Therefore, it becomes important to be aware of causes more likely to be encountered in this unique situation (Table 2). These causes vary in severity and reversibility, with some having a high-associated mortality and others not. Amniotic fluid embolism (also known as anaphylactoid syndrome of pregnancy) carries a high mortality despite aggressive management *(37)*. Others, like pulmonary embolism, eclampsia,

Table 2
Common Causes of CA in Pregnancy

Amniotic fluid embolism
Pulmonary embolus
Hemorrhage
Magnesium sulfate toxicity
Anesthesia complications
Cardiomyopathy
Trauma

magnesium sulfate overdose, anesthesia complications, cardiomyopathy, and acute hemorrhage, have more variable outcomes *(38)*. There are numerous case reports in the literature describing CA in pregnancy from less common causes including myocardial infarction (MI) as a result of administration of intravenous ergonovine *(39)*, severe vagotonia secondary to spinal anesthesia *(40)*, acute MI *(41)*, and penetrating trauma *(42)*. Regardless of the etiology, the basic life support (BLS) and advanced cardiac life support (ACLS) principles still apply with some modifications for treating the pregnant female.

PREGNANCY AND CARDIOPULMONARY RESUSCITATION: SPECIAL CONSIDERATIONS

The main principles of BLS during pregnancy remain the same. For one rescuer, two breaths should be given for every 15 chest compressions. For two rescuers, one breath for every 5 chest compressions *(43)*. Chest compressions should be performed on a hard surface with the heels of the hands placed on the lower one-third of the sternum in order to depress it 3.5 to 5 cm *(43)*. This may be difficult to accomplish in pregnancy secondary to the gravid uterus and enlarged breasts *(44)*. The effectiveness of chest compressions is hindered greatly by the obstructive effect of the enlarged uterus on the great vessels. In the most ideal situation, chest compressions produce a cardiac output that is 30% of normal. It then stands to reason that this obstruction must be relieved. This can be done in several ways. Manual displacement of the uterus, tilting the operating room table to the left, placing a wedge under the right hip, and using the Cardiff resuscitation wedge are all acceptable methods to accomplish this *(45)*.

Because of the increased oxygen consumption in pregnancy, hypoxemia occurs much more rapidly and the threshold for anoxic brain injury is lowered *(46)*. The heart is even more sensitive than the brain to anoxia *(47)*, making early intubation and 100% oxygen delivery imperative *(1)*. In ventricular fibrillation (VF) and pulseless ventricular tachycardia (VT), early and rapid defibrillation is the key to optimizing survival *(48)*. The fetal heart rate is not affected by defibrillating current *(41)*.

The primary and secondary surveys of the ACLS protocol along with some additions for pregnancy are shown in Table 3. None of the drugs used in the management of VF, VT, pulseless electrical activity, asystole, or any of the arrhythmias are contraindicated absolutely in pregnancy *(45)*. Some of these drugs do have potential fetal effects, but it is important to remember that if cardiac output to the mother is not restored, the fetal mortality will invariably be 100%. There is some controversy surrounding the use of sodium bicarbonate in pregnancy because it can cross the placenta, increase fetal pCO_2, and potentially worsen fetal acidemia *(49)*. If perimortem cesarean section is performed,

Table 3
ACLS Protocol: Primary and Secondary Surveys With Pregnancy Modifications

Primary survey	Secondary survey
Airway—is it open? (No change)	**A**—Intubate (Intubate sooner because of more rapid onset of anoxia and risk of aspiration)
Breathing—Is the patient moving air? (Remember the increased O_2 consumption)	**B**—Check ET tube placement and oxygenation (No change)
Circulation—Check pulse (Place patient on her left side to decrease aortocaval compression)	**C**—Obtain IV access, administer medications as indicated (No absolute contraindications to resuscitation medications in pregnancy)
Defibrillation if no pulse present (No effect on fetal heart rate change)	**D**—Differential diagnosis (Causes may be different in pregnancy)
	Expedite delivery of the fetus (Perimortem C-section within 4 minutes of arrest)

Modified from ref. *51*.

many of the drugs will not reach adequate concentrations in the fetal circulation to be of any consequence. If a code has been running for 4 to 5 minutes and there has been no stabilization in maternal condition, perimortem cesarean section is the next step to be considered in the resuscitation protocol.

PERIMORTEM CESAREAN SECTION

Cesarean sections have been performed for nearly 3000 years. A common misconception is that the word "caesarean" comes from the birth of Julius Caesar, however, it actually comes from a ruling made by the king of Rome in the eighth century BC called the *Lex Regis de Inferendo*. This law stated that if a pregnant woman was to die, the fetus must be removed from her abdomen as soon as possible, in order to provide the child with a separate burial. Under the ruling of Emperor Julius Caesar, this law became known as the *Lex Caesare (50)*.

The decision to perform a perimortem cesarean section is a difficult one and must be made within minutes of initiating maternal resuscitation. Several factors must be considered when making this decision *(51)*:

* How much time has elapsed since the onset of CA?
* Have adequate cardiopulmonary resuscitation (CPR) and appropriate drug therapy been administered?
* What is the gestational age of the fetus?
* Does the fetus have a chance to survive neurologically intact?
* Will the mother benefit from the removal of a previable fetus?
* Is the mother's injury fatal or reversible?
* Is there adequate support (obstetrics, pediatrics, anesthesia) and equipment available?

Table 4
The Decision Tree to Perimortem Cesarean Section

Question	Comment
How much time has elapsed since the onset of CA?	Best outcome is <4 minutes for both mother and fetus
Have adequate CPR and appropriate drug therapy been administered?	Cannot declare CPR unsuccessful unless all interventions have been carried out correctly.
What is the gestational age of the fetus?	If unknown, ultrasound may be helpful if available.
Does the fetus have a chance to survive neurologically intact?	If <24 weeks, very poor chance for survival with normal neurological function
Will the mother benefit from removal of the previable fetus?	Possible, especially if >20 weeks.
Is the mother's injury fatal or reversible?	If fatal, reasonable to proceed directly to cesarean section
Is there adequate support available?	Involve pediatrics, obstetrics, and anesthesia as soon as possible

Modified from ref. *52*. CA, cardiac arrest; CPR, cardiopulmonary resuscitation.

The answers to these questions will determine both maternal and fetal outcome under most circumstances (Table 4).

Over the last century, causes of maternal mortality have shifted from chronic, slowly progressive diseases (cholera, tuberculosis, dysentery) to more acute causes (anesthesia, embolism, cerebrovascular *[46]*). This is relevant in that babies born via postmortem cesarean section from mothers with chronic diseases have a decreased chance for survival than those born from previously healthy mothers who died acutely *(46)*. In situations in which a woman is believed to be at risk for sudden CA, provisions should be made to have a cesarean section tray at the bedside *(45)*. Informed consent should be obtained beforehand, if possible. If informed consent is not feasible, a cesarean section should still be performed if indicated to provide the best possible outcome for both the mother and fetus *(45,46,52,53)*.

The American College of Obstetricians and Gynecologists has published guidelines for managing pregnancies at the threshold of fetal viability. The neonatal survival rate is 0% at 21 weeks and 75% at 25 weeks (Table 5; *54*). Emphasis is placed on the reality that infants born prior to 24 weeks are not likely to survive and that of those surviving, the likelihood of normal neurological function is extremely low *(55)*. If gestational age is unknown and ultrasound is available, it may be reasonable to perform a quick measurement of the fetal head using the biparietal diameter (BPD) as a rough estimate of gestational age. The accuracy of dating pregnancies with ultrasound decreases with increasing gestational age, especially if only one parameter is used in the determination. A BPD on an 18-week fetus may be off by plus or minus 8 days (95% CI) as opposed to a discrepancy of 3 weeks in the third trimester *(56)*. BPD measurements of 58, 59, and 60 mm correspond to an average estimated gestational age of 23.9, 24.2, and 24.6 weeks, respectively *(57)*.

Table 5
Percent Neonatal Survival by Gestational Age

Completed weeks of gestation	Percentage of survival
21	0
22	21
23	30
24	50
25	75
26	80
27	90

Modified from ref. *56*; data from ref. *55*.

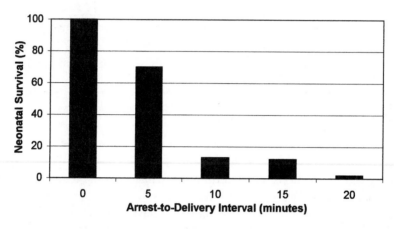

Fig. 1. Percent of infants surviving postmortem cesarean section as a function of time. (Modified from ref. *46*.)

As discussed previously, CPR in the pregnant female is relatively inefficient as a result of the compression of the great vessels by the gravid uterus and the resultant decrease in cardiac output and venous return. It is therefore imperative to relieve this compression by either manually displacing the uterus or placing the patient in a left lateral position. If this is not successful, preparations should be made to perform a perimortem cesarean section *(58)*.

Cesarean delivery should be initiated within 4 minutes of CA and the infant should be delivered by the fifth minute for an optimal outcome *(46)*. With removal of the fetus and placenta, the contraction of the uterus will "autotransfuse" blood into the systemic circulation and may help restore perfusion and enhance the effectiveness of chest compressions *(59)*. Timing of perimortem cesarean section is critical for neonatal outcome. Fetal survival is highest (70%) within the first 5 minutes and drastically declines after this interval along with the chance of normal neurological function (Fig. 1; *46*). Even if more than 15 minutes has elapsed, it is still reasonable to perform a cesarean section because there is 100% fetal mortality if no action is taken *(60)*. In one reported case, the emergency team did not arrive until 25 minutes after a maternal shooting with thoracic aorta injury.

Table 6
The Technical Points of Perimortem Cesarean Section

Vertical skin incision
Classical uterine incision may be quicker
One minute from incision to delivery
Usually bloodless
Avoid injury to bowel and bladder
Notify pediatrics, obstetrics, and anesthesia
Continue CPR throughout procedure

The pulse and blood pressure were unobtainable at that time and another 20 minutes elapsed before arrival to the hospital. Cesarean delivery was performed 2 minutes later with neonatal survival and only minimal neurological dysfunction noted at 18 months of age (42). Inability to auscultate fetal heart tones does not exclude the possibility of a neonatal survival (58).

Prior to performing a perimortem cesarean section, several technical points should be considered (Table 6). A vertical skin incision is recommended because it is the fastest way to enter the abdomen (50). Some authors advocate classical hysterotomy for prompt delivery, however, we do not necessarily recommend this approach if the lower uterine segment is adequately developed. In the third trimester of pregnancy with a thin lower uterine segment, a low transverse uterine incision is likely to be more expeditious and associated with less morbidity than a classical uterine incision. The only instrument in these circumstances needed to perform the surgery is a scalpel (61). Care should be taken to avoid injury to the surrounding organs and good hemostasis should be obtained in the event of maternal survival (46). The bloodless nature of this procedure and the relaxed muscles of the abdomen make this an easier procedure to perform (58). Finally, it is essential that CPR be continued throughout the procedure and that the maternal pulse is checked immediately after completion of the surgery (62).

Prior to Katz's article in 1986, there were no reports of any physician being found liable for performing a perimortem cesarean section (46), but this is a legitimate concern in today's litigious society. As stated previously, informed consent is desirable if it can be obtained. Inability to obtain signed informed consent should not delay an indicated, potentially lifesaving procedure. Meticulous documentation in the medical record is also critical and must reflect both the basis on which the decision to perform a perimortem cesarean section was made and all procedures implemented leading up to that point.

In summary, CA in pregnancy, although rarely encountered, offers the resuscitation team the opportunity to intervene on behalf of two patients, the mother and her fetus. The etiologies of CA during pregnancy may differ somewhat from those in the general population, and some are unique to pregnancy. Both maternal and fetal well-being must be considered under these circumstances, and a basic understanding of the physiological changes of pregnancy is important when managing these patients. None of the drugs used in the BLS and ACLS protocols are contraindicated absolutely in pregnancy and should be used when indicated. Perimortem cesarean section can be a lifesaving procedure for both the mother and the fetus and should be initiated if hemodynamic stability is not restored within 4 minutes of the onset of CA.

REFERENCES

1. Takouri MSM, Seraj MA, Channa AB. Advisory Statement of the International Liaison Committee on Resuscitation (ILCOR). CPR in pregnancy. Middle East J of Anesth 1998;14:399–405.

2. Differences in maternal mortality among black and white women—United States, 1990. MMWR 1995;44:6,7,13,14.

3. Berg CJ, Atrash HK, Koonin LM, Tucker M. Pregnancy-related mortality in the United States, 1987-1990. Ob Gyn 1996;88:162–167.

4. Maternal mortality—United Stated, 1982–1996. MMWR 1998;47:705–707.

5. Koonin LM, MacKay AP, Berg CJ, Atrash HK, Smith JC. Pregnancy-related mortality surveillance-United States, 1987-1990. MMWR 1997;46:17–36.

6. State-specific maternal mortality among black and white women—United States, 1987-1996. MMWR 1999;48:492–496.

7. Kaunitz AM, Hughes JM, Grimes DA, et al. Causes of maternal mortality in the United States. Ob Gyn 1985;65:605–612.

8. Rochat RW, Koonin LM, Atrash HK, Jewett JF. Maternal mortality in the United States: Report from the Maternal Mortality Collaborative. Ob Gyn 1988;72:91–97.

9. Jacob S, Bloebaum L, Shah G, Varner MW. Maternal mortality in Utah. Ob Gyn 1998;91:187–191.

10. Atrash HK, Alexander S, Berg CJ. Maternal mortality in developed countries: Not just a concern of the past. Ob Gyn 1995;86:700–705.

11. Ghosh MK. Maternal mortality: A global perspective. J Reprod Med 2001;46:427–433.

12. Goodburn E, Campbell O. Reducing maternal mortality in the developing world: Sector-wide approaches may be the key. Br Med J 2001;322:917–920.

13. Opportunities to reduce maternal and infant mortality. MMWR 1999;48:856.

14. Ueland K. Maternal cardiovascular dynamics. VII. Intrapartum blood volume changes. Am J Ob Gyn 1976;126:671–677.

15. Gibbs CP. Maternal physiology. Clin Ob Gyn 1981;24:525–543.

16. Pritchard JA. Changes in blood volume during pregnancy and delivery. Anesthesiology 1965;26:393–399.

17. Ueland K, Novy MJ, Peterson EN, Metcalfe J. Maternal cardiovascular dynamics. IV. The influence of gestational age on the maternal cardiovascular response to posture and exercise. Am J Ob Gyn 1969;104:856–864.

18. Ueland K, Metcalfe J. Circulatory changes in pregnancy. Clin Ob Gyn 1975;18:41–50.

19. Veille JC, Morton MJ, Burry KJ. Maternal cardiovascular adaptations to twin pregnancy. Am J Ob Gyn 1985;153:261–263.

20. Clark SL, Cotton DB, Lee W, Bishop C, et al. Central hemodynamic assessment of normal term pregnancy. Am J Ob Gyn 1989;161:1439–1442.

21. Cugell DW, Frank NR, Gaensler ED, et al. Pulmonary function in pregnancy: I. Serial observations in normal women. Am Rev Tuberc 1953;67:568–597.

22. Awe RJ, Nicotra MB, Newson TD, Viles R. Arterial oxygenation and alveolar-arterial gradients in term pregnancy. Ob Gyn 1979;53:182–186.

23. Archer GW, Marx GF. Arterial oxygen tension during apnea in parturient women. Br J Anesth 1974;46:358–360.

24. Dinnick OP. Hiatus hernia: An anesthetic hazard. Lancet 1961;1:400–473.

25. Macfie AG, Magides AD, Richmond MN, Reilly CS. Gastric emptying in pregnancy. Br J Anesth 1991;67:54–57.

26. Attia RR, Ebeid AM, Fischer JE. Gastrin: Placental, maternal, and plasma cord levels: Its possible role in maternal residual gastric acidity (abstract). American Society of Anesthesiologists Annual Meeting. 1976:547.

27. Roberts RB, Shirly MA. Reducing the risks of acid aspiration during cesarean section. Anesth Analg 1974;53:859–868.

28. Sellick BA. Cricoid pressure to control regurgitation of stomach contents during induction of anesthesia. Lancet 1961;2:404–406.

29. Metcalfe J, Romney SL, Ramsey LH, et al. Estimation of uterine blood flow in normal human pregnancy at term. J Clin Invest 1955;34:1632–1643.

30. Kerr MG. The mechanical effects of the gravid uterus in late pregnancy. J Ob Gyn Br Commonw 1965:513.

31. Kauppila A, Koskiner M, Puolakka J, et al. Decreased intervillous and unchanged myometrial flow in supine recumbency. Ob Gyn 1980;55:203–205.

32. Koffler H. Fetal and neonatal physiology. Clin Ob Gyn 1981;24:545–553.

33. Rudolph AM, Heymann MA. The fetal circulation. Ann Rev of Med 1968;19:195–206.

34. Bunn HF, Jandl JH. Control of fetal hemoglobin function within the red cell. NEJM 1970;282:1414–1420.

35. Rulolph AM. The fetal circulation and its response to stress. J Dev Physiol 1984;6:11–19.

36. Gimovsky ML. Fetal heart rate monitoring. Casebook: Fetal heart rate monitoring during respiratory and cardiac arrest. J Perinat 1997;17:495–499.

37. Clark SL, Hankins GD, Dudley DA, et al. Amniotic fluid embolism: Analysis of the national registry. Am J Ob Gyn 1995;172:1158–1169.

38. Kloeck W, Cummings RD, Chamberlain D, et al. Special resuscitative situations: An advisory statement from the International Liaison Committee on Resuscitation. Circul 1997;95:2196–2210.

39. Tsui BC, Stewart B, Fitzmaurice A, Williams R. Cardiac arrest and myocardial infarction induced by postpartum intravenous ergonovine administration. Anesthesiology 2001;94:363–364.

40. Thrush DN, Downs JB. Vagotonia and cardiac arrest during spinal anesthesia. Anesthesiology 1999;91:1171–1173.

41. Curry JL, Quintana FJ. Myocardial infarction with ventricular fibrillation during pregnancy treated by direct current with fetal survival. Chest 1970;58:82–84.

42. Lopez-Zeno JA, Carlo WA, O'Grady JP, Fanaroff AA. Infant survival following delayed postmortem cesarean delivery. Ob Gyn 1990;76:991–992.

43. Datta S, Nasr NF, Khorasani A, Datta R. Current concepts in cardiopulmonary resuscitation in adults. J Indian Med Assoc 1999;97:259–264.

44. Lee RV, Rodgers BD, White LM, Harvey RC. Cardiopulmonary resuscitation of pregnant women. Am J Med 1986;81:311–318.

45. Dildy GA, Clark SL. Cardiac arrest during pregnancy. Ob Gyn Clin N Amer 1995;22:303–314.

46. Katz VL, Dotters DJ, Droegemueller W. Perimortem cesarean delivery. Ob Gyn 1986;68:571–576.

47. Plum F. Vulnerability of the brain and heart after cardiac arrest. NEJM 1991;324:1278–1280.

48. Cummings RO (ed.): Advanced Cardiac Life Support Provider Manual, 5th ed. Dallas: American Heart Association, 2001.

49. Satin AJ, Hankins GDV. Cardiopulmonary resuscitation in pregnancy. In: Critical Care Obstetrics, 2nd ed. Clark SL, Cotton DB, Hankins GDV, et al, eds. Boston: Blackwell Scientific, 1991:579–598.

50. Whitten M, Irvine LM. Postmortem and perimortem cesarean section: what are the indications? J Royal Soc of Med 2000;93:6–9.

51. Anonymous. Part 8: Advanced challenges in resuscitation. Section 3: Special challenges in ECC. 3F: Cardiac arrest associated with pregnancy. Resuscitation 2000;46:293–295.

52. Behmey CA. Cesarean section delivery after death of the mother. JAMA 1961;176:617–619.

53. Weber CE. Postmortem cesarean section: Review of the literature and case reports. Am J Ob Gyn 1971;110:158–163.

54. Lemons JA, Korones SB, Papile LA, Stoll BJ, et al. Very low birth weight outcomes of the National Institute of Child Health and Human Development Neonatal Research Network, January 1995 through December 1996. NICHD Research Network. Pediatrics 2001;107:E1.

55. Depp R, Lemons JA. Perinatal care at the threshold of viability. American College of Obstetricians and Gynecologists Practice Bulletin 2002;100:617–624.

56. Hadlock FP. Sonographic estimation of fetal age and weight. Radiologic Clin of N Amer 1990;28:39–50.

57. Weber CE. Postmortem cesarean section: Review of the literature and case reports. Am J Ob Gyn 1971;110:158–163

58. Hadlock FP, Deter RL, Harrist RB, et al. Fetal biparietal diameter: A critical reevaluation of the relation to menstrual age by means of real time ultrasound. J Ultrasound Med 1982;1:97–104.

59. Kam CW. Perimortem cesarean sections. J Accident Emerg Med 1994;11:57–58.

60. Chen HF, Chien NL, Huang GD, et al. Delayed maternal death after perimortem cesarean section. Acta Ob Gyn Scand 1994;73:839–841.

61. Cardosi RJ, Porter KB. Cesarean delivery of twins during maternal cardiopulmonary arrest. Ob Gyn 1998;92:695–697.

62. Parker J, Balis N, Chester S., et al. Cardiopulmonary arrest in pregnancy: Successful resuscitation of mother and infant following immediate cesarean section in labour ward. Aust NZ J Ob Gyn 1996; 36:207–210.

63. DePace NL, Betesh JS, Kotler MN. Postmortem cesarean section with recovery of both mother and offspring. JAMA 1982;248:971–973.

24 Cardiopulmonary Resuscitation Following Drowning

Jerome H. Modell, MD
and Andrea Gabrielli, MD

CONTENTS

DEFINITIONS AND DESCRIPTIONS

Several definitions and multiple terminology have appeared since the 1950s regarding the description of victims who suffer a fatal or near-fatal event from being submerged in water and other liquids. Some of the descriptors have had modifications placed on them and, furthermore, their meaning was somewhat lost when translated into some languages other then English. Because drowning is a global problem, at the World Congress on Drowning in Amsterdam, The Netherlands, in 2002, a group was convened from multiple countries to develop a definition of "drowning" that would be applicable in multiple languages worldwide *(1)*. Although unanimity may not have been present on every term discussed, there clearly was a consensus to simplify the terminology for international application. What follows is the consensus of that group with comment and, in some cases, slight modification representing the bias of the authors of this chapter.

Drowning is the process resulting from primary respiratory impairment from submersion or immersion in a liquid medium. Implicit in this definition is that a liquid-to-air interface must be present at the entrance to the individual's airway, thus, precluding the possibility of the individual to breathe air. Although it is possible to suffer a drowning episode in multiple types of liquid, this chapter is confined to the most common use of the terminology, namely, drowning in water.

The drowning process is a continuum beginning when the individual's airway is initially below the surface of the liquid. At this time, the individual first will voluntarily hold his or her breath. Some victims will swallow significant quantities of water during this time. This period of voluntary breath-holding, which has been found in human volunteers to last an average of 87 seconds at rest and shorter with exercise *(2)*, is followed by an involuntary period of laryngospasm secondary to water in the oropharynx or at the level of the larynx acting as a foreign body *(3)*. During this period of breath-

From: *Contemporary Cardiology: Cardiopulmonary Resuscitation*
Edited by: J. P. Ornato and M. A. Peberdy © Humana Press Inc., Totowa, NJ

holding and laryngospasm, the patient cannot breathe gas, therefore, oxygen is depleted and carbon dioxide is not eliminated. This results in the patient becoming hypercarbic, hypoxic, and acidotic (4).

As blood levels of carbon dioxide increase and levels of oxygen decrease, respiratory efforts become very active but no exchange of air occurs because of the obstruction at the larynx. Victims who subsequently recover and recall this period, frequently describe it as being quite terrifying and painful as they struggle to create intense negative intrapleural pressure breathing against a closed glottis (5). As the patient's arterial oxygen tension drops further, laryngospasm abates, and the patient then actively breathes water. Further evidence of the magnitude of negative pressure created during laryngospasm is the fact that the lungs of drowning victims frequently demonstrate significant hyperinflation at autopsy (6).

The amount of liquid a drowning victim breathes varies considerably between victims (4). Studies comparing the biochemical changes occurring in humans after a drowning episode with those in experimental animals, suggest that, although the volume of liquid actually inhaled varies considerably from one victim to another, only 15% of persons who die in the water aspirate in excess of 22 mL per kg of water (7), and the percentage is considerably less in those who survive (4). Changes occur in the lung, body fluids, and electrolyte concentrations, which are dependent on both the composition and volume of the liquid aspirated (8–10).

A victim can be rescued at any time during the drowning process and given appropriate resuscitation measures in which case, the process is interrupted. The individual may recover with the initial resuscitation efforts or with subsequent therapy aimed at eliminating hypoxia, hypercarbia, and acidosis, and restoring normal organ function. If the patient is not removed from the water, then circulatory arrest will occur, and, in the absence of effective resuscitative efforts, multiple organ dysfunction and death will result, primarily from tissue hypoxia.

Although the tolerance to hypoxia of various tissues is different, it should be noted that the brain is the organ most at risk for permanent detrimental changes from relative brief periods of hypoxia. The following question is frequently asked: "How long can one be submerged and still be rescued and resuscitated back to a normal life?" Although, obviously, there are no controlled human studies, nor should there be on this subject, the limiting time factor is likely the duration that cerebral hypoxia can be tolerated before irreversible changes occur. Irreversible damage to brain tissue is reported to begin approx 3 minutes after the PaO$_2$ falls below 30 mmHg under normothermic conditions in otherwise normal people (11). Such data suggests that if the individual is rescued and effective resuscitation efforts are applied within 3 minutes of the cessation of respiration, i.e., submersion in water, that the vast majority of such victims should be able to be resuscitated and suffer no permanent brain damage. Furthermore, because the period of voluntary breath-holding and laryngospasm is thought to last for approx 1.5 to 2 minutes (2,12), persons who are retrieved within that time frame will likely not suffer lung damage secondary to the aspiration of liquid. Once the 3-minute time frame has been exceeded, although some normal survivors are reported, it becomes less likely that normal survival will result from resuscitation efforts. This time frame may be prolonged if hypothermia occurs rapidly because it decreases the cerebral requirement for oxygen.

Trained divers have been shown to be able to voluntarily hold their breath for much longer periods of time, approaching 4 to 5 minutes without complication (13). Persons who become hypothermic as a result of immersion or submersion in extremely cold water will rapidly develop hypothermia, which protects the brain by decreasing its oxygen requirement and prolongs survival (14). In the latter case, seemingly miraculous recoveries of patients who have been submerged for more than 20 minutes have been reported (15). It should be noted, however, that hypothermia is a two-edged sword; although it can protect the brain from oxygen deprivation, it also can cause death in the water secondary to its effect on the conduction system of the heart, resulting in circulatory arrest either by asystole or ventricular fibrillation (VF [16]).

The drowning process can be altered by the initiating event. For example, if the individual suffers trauma, develops syncope or unconsciousness, has a circulatory arrest either by asystole or VF as the precipitating event, hyperventilates prior to breath-holding underwater, has a convulsive disorder that leads them to become incapacitated thereby becoming submerged, the individual's judgment and/or motor function is impaired by significant parenteral levels of depressant drugs including alcohol, each of these events will have an effect on the drowning process per se. For example, in the individual who suffers a concussion from a blow to the head, subsequent recollection of the events is unlikely. If trauma results in a cervical fracture, disastrous damage to the spinal cord may occur acutely and, thus, motor function may be lost below that level. If the individual has a circulatory arrest either by asystole or VF as a precipitating event, respiration will cease, and it is highly unlikely that significant amounts of water will be breathed into the lung because active respiration is necessary for this to occur (17). If the individual hyperventilates prior to breath-holding underwater, it has been shown that the breath-holding breaking point can be extended until the level of hypoxia is so severe that consciousness is lost and the individual then actively breathes water (2,12). The effect of drug usage is variable depending on the level of depression and the patient's response. There is considerable variation in tolerance to depressant drugs and alcohol and their effects on performance and orientation. To better understand what to expect in each victim, the initiating event should be reported in, every case if it is known.

When one experiences a drowning episode, the result can be death or survival. Furthermore, survival can be without residual damage or with residual damage to varying degrees; e.g., from minor neurologic difficulty to one that has no normal function other then continuation of an effective heartbeat with or without spontaneous respiration.

The terms "drown" and "near-drown" have been used for decades in an attempt to separate these outcomes (18). At the World Congress on Drowning, however, it became apparent that their meaning was not felt to be clear when translated into some languages (1). Furthermore, one could have no signs of spontaneous physiologic function and, therefore, be "drowned" but once resuscitative efforts were applied, they would respond positively and survive to varying degrees and, thus, the term applied to them would have to be changed to "near-drown" (19). Then there are those who do not die acutely but die later of complications from their drowning episode. In this case, the question is were they "near-drowned" or were they "drowned?"

The definition of "drowned" we believe to be fairly clear, namely, death secondary to undergoing the drowning episode. "Near-drowned" presents a significantly greater problem of understanding. We believe that the term "drowned" should be retained for both those who die acutely in the water and those who die later of consequences directly resultant from the submersion episode. However, we agree with the consensus of the World Congress members that "near-drowned" may lead to unnecessary confusion and, therefore, should be replaced by terminology such as "the individual survived the drowning episode" and then describe the ultimate condition of the individual.

Other terms that have appeared in the literature over the past few decades that we believe are confusing and should be abandoned discussed here.

Dry vs Wet Drowning

Because all drowning occurs in liquid, by definition, they are all wet. This terminology has been used by some to categorize drowning victims into those who aspirate liquid into the lungs and those who do not. Frequently, it is not possible to determine at the scene of the accident whether the individual actually did aspirate water. This is particularly true when the quantity of water aspirated is small. Furthermore, if evidence of fluid aspiration is not detected in the individual who dies or is discovered dead in the water, the diagnosis may be suspect (20). In these cases, one should look for other explanations such as acute mechanical standstill of the heart, from asystole or VF or, for that matter, whether the individual actually was alive when they first became submerged.

Active vs Passive vs Silent Drowning

This terminology has been used by some to separate those victims who are observed to be struggling at the surface of the water from those who are first discovered when they are actually submerged and motionless. It has been shown with underwater cameras that even in victims who were not seen to be in difficulty on the surface of the water by observers, they may have had unrecognized active motion although submerged. We believe, therefore, that these terms should be abandoned in favor of the terms "witnessed" when the episode is witnessed from the onset of submersion/immersion to the time of rescue or "unwitnessed" when a body is found in the water without anybody seeing how it got there.

Secondary Drowning

This terminology has been used by some to describe a situation when a precipitating event from another origin, for example, syncope, causes a victim to be below the surface of the water and then they drown. On the other hand, some use this terminology to describe a victim who appears to be recovering from a drowning episode in the hospital and then develops adult respiratory distress syndrome. Not only is this terminology confusing but, also, in the latter instance, a patient does not experience a second submersion or drowning episode, therefore, this terminology should be abandoned.

PATHOPHYSIOLOGY

There have been extensive studies both in animals (7–9,14,18,21–34) and in humans (4,6,20,35–40) over the past century in an attempt to quantitate the changes that occur as a result of a drowning episode. What has consistently been shown over and over again is that acutely, drowning produces asphyxia (i.e., hypoxia, hypercarbia, and acidosis). The hypercarbia is the result of absent or ineffective ventilation and is readily correctable when aggressive mechanical ventilation is instituted. The hypoxia that occurs initially is not as readily correctable and may be persistent for long periods of time (8–10). This hypoxia is first as a result of apnea and, then, primarily of intrapulmonary shunting from alveoli that are perfused but not being ventilated or not being ventilated adequately (32). The acidosis is mixed, and the respiratory component rapidly disappears with effective ventilation. One is, however, frequently left with significant metabolic acidosis as a result of anaerobic metabolism during the period of time that profound tissue hypoxia secondary to absent or ineffective respiration and cardiac output was present. The hallmark of this high anion gap metabolic acidosis is an increased level of serum lactic acid.

Although intrapulmonary shunting occurs after both freshwater and seawater aspiration, the etiology is different *(33)*. In the case of freshwater, the aspirated water alters the surface tension properties of pulmonary surfactant. Thus, the alveoli become unstable and do not maintain their normal shape or patency, resulting in an increase in both absolute and relative intrapulmonary shunt *(32,33)*. Seawater does not change the surface tension properties of pulmonary surfactant, but, because it is hypertonic, it pulls fluid from the circulation into the alveoli, thus, producing obstruction to gas exchange at the alveolar level. Bronchoconstriction also has been reported after aspiration of even small quantities of water *(28)*.

Freshwater, being hypotonic, is absorbed very rapidly into the circulation and because of the transient hypervolemia that occurs and the change in the surface tension properties of pulmonary surfactant, pulmonary edema results. The pulmonary edema is most commonly described as frothy or foamy and blood-tinged. This coloring is secondary to the presence of free plasma hemoglobin from the rupture of some red blood cells as a result of the absorption of hypotonic fluid into the circulation in the face of hypoxia *(41)*. Pulmonary edema also occurs when seawater is aspirated, secondary to a semipermeable membrane effect because the seawater is hypertonic compared to plasma. Even though the etiology of the hypoxia is different between freshwater and seawater aspiration, the result of both is to increase intrapulmonary shunt, which requires aggressive therapy *(32,42,43)*.

Extensive studies of serum electrolyte concentrations after drowning have shown that only 15% of individuals who die in the water, aspirate more than 22 mL per kg of water. In patients who survive, the percentage is much less and, thus, significant changes in serum electrolyte concentrations that require treatment, are rarely observed *(7)*. The only exception, possibly being persons who drowned in the Dead Sea *(44)*.

The treatment of the respiratory lesion requires providing mechanical ventilatory support in a fashion that will restore an adequate functional residual capacity and keep the alveoli open during all phases of the respiratory cycle, thus, decreasing the intrapulmonary shunt. Obviously, if foreign material such as sand, silt or plant life is aspirated into the lung, it may produce obstruction and it should be removed via bronchoscopy.

The cardiovascular changes that occur during a drowning episode can best be ascribed to inadequate oxygenation. Although fatal arrhythmia such as VF is rarely documented in human drowning victims, VF can occur with profound hypoxia, especially if very significant changes in serum potassium and serum sodium result from the movement of fluid and rupture of red blood cells. Although a wide variety of cardiac arrhythmias have been reported *(45)*, particularly in animal models, rarely do they require specific therapy other than improving oxygenation and correcting severe metabolic acidosis. More common problems are profound hypoxia and the leak of fluid into the lung as pulmonary edema resulting in a relative hypovolemia in the patient. It has been shown by multiple investigators that to treat this hypovolemia it may be necessary to infuse significant amounts of intravenous fluid to maintain an adequate effective circulating blood volume, even in the face of pulmonary edema *(26,43)*. Without such therapy, even though the arterial oxygen tension might have improved with mechanical ventilatory support, the delivery of oxygen to the tissues remains compromised and incompatible with supplying adequate tissue oxygenation *(43)*. Use of vasopressors and other pharmacologic agents may be indicated as a temporary crutch, so to speak, in these patients, however, they are not a substitute for providing adequate oxygenation and adequate intravascular fluid volume. If the latter are established, it is highly unlikely that pharmacologic support of the heart will be necessary.

Detrimental changes in renal function are rarely seen in persons recovering from near-drowning. However, when present, they likely are the result of inadequate perfusion and oxygenation rather than anything specific in regard to the drowning episode per se. Some have emphasized the need for the kidneys to clear free plasma hemoglobin after fresh-water drowning, however, significant levels of free plasma hemoglobin have rarely been reported in such patients. This, likely, is as a result of the fact that for red blood cells to rupture and release enough hemoglobin into the plasma during a drowning episode to require specific therapy for its clearance, it requires transfer of substantial volumes of free water into the circulation in the face of hypoxia *(41)*. As stated above, this rarely occurs.

RESCUE AND RESUSCITATION

To ensure survival after a drowning episode, it is imperative that one never lose sight of the fact that time is of the essence. The longer one is without the ability to breathe air, the more profound is the hypoxia and the risk of permanent damage to vital tissues. Thus, those who are entrusted with guarding swimming facilities must never lose sight of the fact that continual vigilance is required to recognize a victim in distress, and to remove them from the water and begin resuscitative measures in timely fashion. Frequently, bodies are discovered motionless in a pool without anyone in attendance being able to pinpoint the length of time that the individual was submerged. In many cases, lifeguards report that they thought the individual was "fooling around" and, therefore, they did not affect a timely rescue. Also, lifeguards may be assigned other duties such as pool maintenance and tending to concession stands, thus, precluding them from timely recognition of a victim in trouble and prompt rescue.

Frequently, bathers are permitted to deliberately hyperventilate on the side of the pool before becoming submerged to see "how long they can hold their breath" or "how far they can swim underwater." These practices are to be condemned. If an individual is not noted to be making purposeful movements for more then 10 seconds, rescue attempts should be initiated *(46)*. The individual responsible for safety at the pool should always be in proper attire and in position to affect such a rescue and complete it within 20 seconds of the recognition of the problem.

When removing the victim from the water, care should be taken to avoid complicating neck injuries when they are suspected. In such cases, the patient should be floated onto a long back-board. Gentle immobilization of the head should be accomplished, securing it in a neutral position. However, if the neck appears to be obviously deformed and the patient has pain with neck movement, the neck should be immobilized in the existing position.

If the individual is apneic, the airway should rapidly be cleared of foreign material, a patent airway secured, and mouth-to-mouth resuscitation should be started immediately. It is preferable to begin artificial ventilation in the water if it can be accomplished without jeopardizing the safety of the rescuer. It should be remembered that not all victims are in a state of CA when the rescue attempt begins. They may be in a state of vasoconstriction or have a significant bradycardia, in which case, if effective ventilation is started, the myocardium will be reoxygenated and increased cardiac activity will result in improved tissue perfusion.

On removing the individual from the water, he or she should rapidly be assessed for the presence of both spontaneous respiration and cardiac activity. In the absence of these, the airway should be inspected rapidly to ensure that there is no mechanical obstruction, and artificial respiration and cardiac compression should be instituted without delay. Recently, some have proposed that chest compression alone and without artificial respiration should be attempted in victims of dysrhythmic CA *(47)*. It must be emphasized that these recommendations do not apply to the drowning victim because the pathophysiologic lesion in the lungs requires active attempts at re-inflation and stabilization of the alveoli. Therefore, CA following drowning is more likely as a result of asphyxia.

If equipment is available at the site for administering supplemental oxygen, it should be delivered in the highest concentration possible under existing conditions. Electrical activity of the heart should quickly be evaluated and an automatic defibrillator applied if indicated. A pulse oximeter will frequently be of assistance in determining the effectiveness of oxygenation. However, many pulse oximeters do not work well if the individual is cold and vasoconstricted or if there is excessive movement.

Although one should rapidly inspect the airway for the presence of obstructing material, the abdominal thrust maneuver, which had been advocated by some in the past, has been thoroughly debated and found not to be of value in treating a drowning victim unless solid material is actually blocking the conducting airway *(48)*.

Patient Transport and Emergency Medical Services

Neither equipment nor properly trained personnel are usually available at the site to provide advanced cardiac life support (ACLS) including endotracheal intubation, intravenous access, drug therapy, and electrical defibrillation. However, these measures should be instituted when indicated and when the proper equipment and properly trained personnel are available. It is crucial that someone other than the individual rescuing and resuscitating the patient, contact emergency medical services (EMS) as rapidly as possible so that they can respond in a timely fashion and make ACLS treatment available to the victim.

A word of caution to EMS personnel. If one is not familiar with a technique, treatment of the acute drowning victim is not the appropriate place to experiment with something for the first time. This caution is especially pertinent when talking about delaying or abandoning mechanical ventilation with a bag and mask in favor of attempting to place an endotracheal tube and the endotracheal tube then ending up in the esophagus rather than in the trachea. People die from lack of ventilation and oxygen, not from lack of an endotracheal tube or other similar type of appliance.

Whenever a drowning victim has to be transported to a location or facility such as a hospital emergency room, it is important that a call be made promptly to inform the emergency room personnel of the exact circumstances, type of treatment instituted and condition of the patient en route so that they will be prepared to accept the patient and to render appropriate therapy as soon as the patient arrives.

When moving a critically ill drowning victim it is imperative to remember the fragility of such patients because they can decompensate in a matter of a few seconds or minutes if appropriate therapy is withdrawn. Examples of such situations are movement from the scene to the EMS vehicle, from the EMS vehicle to the hospital emergency department (ED) or from the hospital ED to other hospital locations for testing, such as radiology, or for treatment, such as the intensive care unit. Thus, every attempt should be made to continue essential therapy at all times.

Treatment in the Emergency Department

In the ED, a thorough evaluation of the patient should be performed, keeping in mind that the most serious problems that require immediate therapy are pulmonary insufficiency and cardiovascular instability resulting in inadequate delivery of oxygen to vital tissues. If the individual is responding fully, does not require respiratory or cardiovascular support, and has a normal oxyhemoglobin saturation while breathing room air, it is unlikely that the individual has aspirated a significant amount of water, and observation may be all that is necessary.

At the other extreme is the patient who is still unconscious and requires extensive pulmonary and cardiovascular support in an attempt to normalize vital signs and produce adequate cardiac output and tissue oxygenation. Thus, one cannot prescribe cookbook treatment that would apply to every victim. However, the treating physician should keep in mind that increased intrapulmonary shunt and poorly matched ventilation-to-perfusion ratios are the rule rather than the exception for one who has aspirated a significant quantity of water.

Therapy must be aimed at improving ventilation-to-perfusion ratios and restoring adequate residual lung volume to optimally oxygenate the blood. A relative hypovolemia frequently is present as a result of fluid shifts between the lung and the circulation. These can be accentuated by the increase in mean intrathoracic pressure that occurs with mechanical ventilatory support. Thus, evaluation of effective circulating blood volume and replenishment of intravascular fluid volume to physiologic levels is important as a primary concern.

Although currently some controversy exists regarding when to treat metabolic acidosis in persons who have suffered a CA, we believe that the adverse effect of acidosis on the pulmonary vasculature and cardiac function is sufficient so that metabolic acidosis producing a pH of less than 7.2 should be treated with intravenous sodium bicarbonate. If the patient is a victim of seawater drowning and has aspirated sufficient water to produce a hypernatremia, one might be better advised to use an agent such as THAM to avoid compounding the hypernatremia. However, once again, it should be noted that the quantity of water aspirated is seldom sufficient to produce such significant changes in serum electrolyte concentrations; except perhaps when the drowning occurs in water of extreme hypersalinity such as the Dead Sea *(44)*.

Changes in serum electrolyte concentrations and hemoglobin and hematocrit of sufficient magnitude to justify specific therapy are rare, as are alterations in renal function other then those that might be expected in the hypovolemic, hypoxic, or markedly acidotic patient.

The patient's level of consciousness on admission to the emergency room has been shown to markedly influence outcome *(49,50)*. The most important consideration here is to provide for adequate oxygenation and perfusion and to avoid producing increased intracranial pressure, if possible. Treatments aimed specifically at preservation of cerebral function have not been shown to be particularly beneficial to date *(50,51)*.

If the patient requires diagnostic testing in a distant location such as the radiology department, it is imperative that adequate personnel and equipment accompany the patient to ensure that optimum therapy is not interrupted at any time during transport or when performing the procedure. Likewise, transportation to the intensive care unit should be done with a "full team approach." Should optimum therapy be interrupted during any of these time periods, adverse consequences should be anticipated.

Drowning episodes in cold water may produce significant hypothermia. There are several methods of rewarming that have been recommended including, but not necessarily limited to, heating blankets, warmed intravenous fluids, warmed humidification of breathing circuits, gastric lavage, and cardiopulmonary bypass. The method used should be tailored to the resources available and the condition of the patient. It must be remembered, however, that rewarming peripheral tissues before the patient's circulation is capable of supplying adequate amounts of oxygenated blood can compound the situation and increase the degree of metabolic acidosis.

In-Hospital Therapy

Expert intensive care is vital to survival, once optimal prehospital and ED management has been performed. Hemodynamic instability after CA, respiratory insufficiency, and severe neurologic impairment, are all criteria for admission to the intensive care unit (ICU). The administrative structure of the hospital's critical care service dictates the setting to which the patient is admitted. A recent attempt to classify survivors of drowning based on the severity of symptoms on a scale of 1 to 6 recommends ICU admission for all pediatric patients requiring high concentrations of oxygen, with or without the need for invasive ventilation *(52)*.

Respiratory Support

Although the degree of intrapulmonary shunting after drowning is variable from one patient to the next, if the patient is breathing adequately to clear carbon dioxide, the single most important method of treatment in reversing hypoxemia is the application of continuous positive airway pressure (CPAP). The amount of CPAP applied must be individualized because the degree of atelectasis, the amount of pulmonary edema and the magnitude of the intrapulmonary shunt varies between patients. In great measure this will depend on the type and quantity of the water aspirated. Although the mechanism for producing the intrapulmonary shunt is different between freshwater and seawater *(33)*, Lee found no statistically significant difference between the PaO_2/FiO_2 ratio in patients after the two kinds of aspiration *(53)*.

The pathophysiologic mechanism involved in freshwater drowning is lowering of the sodium concentration in the alveolus, thus changing the surface tension characteristics of pulmonary surfactant *(33,54)*. The alteration in the surface tension properties of pulmonary surfactant increases alveolar surface tension on compression of the surfactant layer and results in alveolar volume loss. Also, pulmonary capillaries become more permeable, resulting in an increase in interstitial lung water that eventually compresses alveoli and promotes volume loss and causes pulmonary edema. Based on the severity of the acute respiratory derangement this "abnormal surfactant state" has been termed acute lung injury (ALI) or acute respiratory distress syndrome (ARDS *[55]*).

ALI and ARDS represent a final common pathway that accompanies a number of physiologic insults that may occur after drowning including respiratory obstruction, aspiration of water or gastric contents, and global hypoxemia from cardiovascular insufficiency or CA. Unfortunately, ALI and ARDS often can be clinically and radiologically confused with acute pulmonary edema from left ventricular (LV) dysfunction or fluid overload of different etiologies.

Both CPAP and positive end-expiratory pressure (PEEP) have the capability to restore lung volume and improve oxygenation in many patients with decreased lung volume and especially functional residual capacity. However, there are some differences in their function. By definition, CPAP means that airway pressure remains positive during all phases of the respiratory cycle. With PEEP, during the inspiratory phase of a spontaneous breath, circuit pressures drop to 0 or become negative as a result of a vigorous inspiratory effort by the patient. Because PEEP with spontaneous ventilation increases the work of breathing it may increase pressure gradients between the pulmonary vasculature and the alveoli, thereby leading to more pulmonary edema. Also, it does not forcibly inflate alveoli with abnormal surfactant after freshwater drowning (32). Thus, CPAP is more beneficial than PEEP for spontaneously breathing drowning victims (42,56).

Both CPAP and PEEP increase expiratory pressure, thus air is trapped within the lungs during the expiratory phase of respiration. This results in an increase in residual lung volume in many patients with ARDS. As alveolar units re-expand, intrapulmonary shunt decreases and improvement is seen in oxygenation and compliance. The increase in compliance decreases the work of breathing (57). The degree of lung volume restoration roughly correlates with the improvement in oxygenation. As lung volume increases toward normal, gas exchange continues to improve. It has been shown however, that although the above beneficial effect is found with CPAP in many victims of both fresh and seawater drowning (56,58), unless mechanical breaths are added, PEEP may not improve the ventilation-to-perfusion ratio after freshwater drowning (32,42,56). Also, in some freshwater drowning victims CPAP alone does not produce an adequate response and mechanical breaths should be added (42).

When ARDS develops and oxygen desaturation occurs, an FiO_2 of 1.0 is recommended to attempt to restore adequate oxygenation. Increased work of breathing, severe hypoxemia and hypercarbia are all indications for instituting mechanical ventilation. Ordinarily, CPAP is titrated to achieve an oxygen saturation greater than 95% with the lowest possible inspired oxygen (FiO_2) levels down to an FiO_2 of 0.5 or less. We routinely increase CPAP at the bedside in increments of 3–5 cm H_2O in an attempt to achieve an oxygen saturation of 95%. Then, the FiO_2 is gradually decreased to reach a PaO_2/FiO_2 of greater than 300 mmHg. Increased dead space ventilation and decreased preload are the two most important adverse effects that can limit the use of CPAP. Once adequate PaO_2/FiO_2 has been achieved, CPAP can slowly be weaned based on improvement of patient lung compliance and general clinical conditions.

MECHANICAL VENTILATION

CPAP therapy alone is not sufficient in the case of the patient who is apneic, hypoventilating, hypercarbic, or shows little to no improvement in ventilation-to-perfusion matching although breathing spontaneously. In these patients, mechanical ventilatory breaths must also be provided. In general, mechanical ventilation in patients with ALI or ARDS can be applied either noninvasively or invasively, i.e., face mask vs endotracheal tube, respectively. Noninvasive ventilation is reserved for milder cases of ARDS or pulmonary edema, when the patient is awake, cooperative, triggering spontaneous ventilation, and have their swallowing and protective laryngeal reflexes intact. Although successful experience with noninvasive positive pressure ventilation (NPPV) for patients with respiratory failure other than from COPD is growing (59), potential complications include gastric distention, nasal congestion, regurgitation and aspiration of stomach contents, nasal bridge ulceration, and eye irritation (60). Several modes of mechanical ventilation and adjunct therapies are available; although not specifically used in drowning, their use has proven valuable in the ventilatory support of any patient with ALI or ARDS. A list of the most commonly used forms in drowning victims follows.

CONTROLLED MECHANICAL VENTILATION

Controlled mechanical ventilation (CMV) provides total ventilation and it does not permit spontaneous breathing. It usually is indicated only in patients who are apneic, deeply comatose, deeply sedated, or paralyzed. All breaths delivered with CMV are positive pressure breaths, therefore, mean intrathoracic pressure is increased with potential deleterious hemodynamic effects. Most notable of these is the impedance of venous return, thus effectively causing a relative hypovolemia and decreased cardiac output *(43)*.

INTERMITTENT MANDATORY VENTILATION

Intermittent mandatory ventilation (IMV) combines mechanical ventilatory breaths with spontaneous breathing and is better tolerated than CMV by most patients *(61)*. Allowing some spontaneous breathing reduces mean intrathoracic pressure, which increases venous return and maintains better cardiac output. It also may reduce the incidence of barotrauma. The number of mechanical breaths used are those necessary to supplement the patient's own spontaneous ability to maintain adequate minute ventilation. As the patient is recovering, the ventilator rate is gradually reduced by one to two breaths per minute down to a minimum of two breaths per minute . IMV remains the mainstay of all our ventilator support. It may be coupled with other modes such as pressure support ventilation (PSV).

PRESSURE SUPPORT VENTILATION

The primary benefit of this ventilatory mode is to reduce the inspiratory work of breathing. The patient maintains control of the inspiratory-to-expiratory ratio, inspiratory time, and frequency during the spontaneous efforts. The mechanical breath delivered during PSV usually discontinues once flow decreases to 25% of peak inspiratory flow. Adjustable pressure support parameters include the time necessary to reach maximal flow or rate of rise of PSV. A shorter pressure rise time is generally used to reduce work of breathing in patients with the highest inspiratory flow demand.

PSV has the capability to reduce or eliminate both imposed (apparatus and airway resistance) and physiologic (lung and chest wall static compliance) work of breathing. Therefore, the clinician may reduce or eliminate the extra-imposed work of breathing and keep the physiologic work of breathing within tolerable limits, by choosing the appropriate level of PSV.

Despite a careful, stepwise approach to mechanical ventilation in ALI and ARDS, iatrogenic complications are frequent. Several potentially protective measures have been evaluated to reduce the incidence of barotrauma from increased peak airway pressure in patients with severely reduced total lung compliance. However, strong evidence-based medicine in favor of their use is still lacking.

NITRIC OXIDE

Inhaled nitric oxide (NO) appears to act selectively on the pulmonary vascular bed and only in those areas associated with adequate ventilation, locally reversing hypoxic pulmonary vasoconstriction and increasing oxygenation. However, outcome in terms of mortality or number of days alive and off of mechanical ventilation between patients treated with NO and those not treated has not changed when the effect of NO is studied in a prospective randomized fashion *(62)*. Nevertheless, reducing the level of mechanical ventilatory support or FiO_2 needed to achieve adequate oxygenation is a potential benefit that could reduce barotrauma and the side effects of treatment.

PRONE POSITIONING

Rotation of patients from supine to prone may cause rapid improvement in oxygenation that may last for up to 12 hours *(63)*. With this maneuver, there is a relatively high risk of inadvertent extubation and removal of invasive monitors; nevertheless, oxygenation improves mainly because the nondependent dorsal portion of the lung has a higher air-to-tissue ratio *(64)*. Obviously, the risks and benefits need to be considered before using this technique in any specific patient.

BRONCHODILATOR THERAPY

Small airway closure has been shown to occur even with aspiration of relatively small amounts of water *(25)*. Thus, bronchodilator therapy should be considered in patients when bronchospasm is thought to be present.

CORTICOSTEROIDS

The rationale for use of corticosteroids in ARDS seems to be limited to the fibroproliferative phase, to reduce the incidence of pulmonary fibrosis *(65)*. However, its efficacy for use in drowning victims has not been shown either in large retrospective clinical studies *(4)* or in prospective animal studies *(66)*. Corticosteroids can interfere with normal pulmonary healing and increase the rate of sepsis. Corticosteroids have been associated with higher mortality in one study, probably as a result of the immunosuppressant effect in patients with sepsis *(67)*. In another, their use has shown, after aspiration of gastric contents, to increase pulmonary granuloma formation *(68,69)*.

SURFACTANT

ARDS from drowning involves both quantitative (seawater) and qualitative (freshwater) alterations in lung surfactant *(33,70)*. Although the use of exogenous surfactant has been shown to lower mortality in neonates with respiratory distress syndrome *(71)*, this effect in adults has been disappointing, and its prohibitive cost makes its use infrequent *(72)*.

PROPHYLACTIC ANTIBIOTICS

The use of broad-spectrum antibiotics may enhance the emergence of resistant organisms. An exception represents survival from drowning in heavily contaminated water such as stagnant ponds or public spas, where pseudomonas species are endemic. Our initial choice in this situation is usually a fourth-generation cephalosporin with broad Gram-negative coverage. In other patients, antibiotics are not recommended unless the patient develops evidence of infection, in which case cultures and sensitivities will guide the choice of antibiotics to be given.

Cardiovascular Support

By the time a drowning victim reaches the ICU, cardiac arrhythmias are rarely a problem. If witnessed in the ED or the ICU, the most common cause of arrhythmias is severe hypoxia and providing adequate ventilation and oxygenation will usually restore a normal rhythm. If not, then drug therapy or, in the case of severe ventricular arrhythmias, electrical intervention is appropriate.

Hypotension may require initial pharmacologic support but it should be remembered that the hypotension seen in drowning victims is predominantly as a result of fluid shifts resulting in hypovolemia *(26,43)*. This hypovolemia may be accentuated when mechanical ventilatory techniques that increase mean intrathoracic pressure are used *(43)*.

Experimental studies have shown that whereas mechanical ventilation and CPAP will decrease intrapulmonary shunt and increase PaO_2, because of the detrimental effect on cardiac output, tissue perfusion is compromised. Attempting to increase oxygen delivery by use of vasopressors and inotropes was not productive, but fluid administration to increase blood volume resulted in an increased cardiac output and oxygen delivery (43).

Precise fluid replacement is dependent on an accurate assessment of effective circulating blood volume. To this end, monitoring the patient with a pulmonary artery catheter or transesophageal echocardiography is extremely helpful.

Central Nervous System Support

The two most important issues influencing morbidity and mortality in victims surviving drowning are severe respiratory insufficiency and permanent neurologic impairment secondary to cerebral hypoxia. Despite improvement in emergency and intensive pulmonary and cardiovascular care, neurological outcome in drowning patients is directly related to the initial duration of hypoxia from the onset of submersion until effective CPR is provided. The Glasgow Coma Scale (GCS) score mirrors this during the first few hours after submersion.

The most common cerebral lesion results from cytotoxic injury as a result of global central nervous system hypoxemia. Cerebral edema, which usually is not clinically evident or is mild on presentation, reaches its peak by day two to three after the submersion event. One would think that successful intensive care management of these patients would reflect the ability to control the intracranial pressure (ICP) and limit secondary brain injury from inadequate cerebral perfusion and hypoxia through standard protocols. Therefore, monitoring of the intracranial pressure is often recommended in patients with a GCS score compatible with severe central nervous system injury (eight and below), in conjunction with what is described in detail in the neurosurgical guidelines for traumatic brain injury (73). Unfortunately, monitoring of ICP has not been shown to increase normal survival after drowning.

Seizure prophylaxis is immediately initiated in patients with CNS compromise, and ventilatory rate is titrated to achieve a $PaCO_2$ of 35 to 40 mmHg. However, a lower level of $PaCO_2$ has been recommended in the past to decrease intracranial pressure in some of these patients. Unfortunately, the decrease in ICP is accompanied by a reduction in cerebral blood flow (74), which can result in cerebral ischemia (75). There are no data to support the use of barbiturates or steroids to lower refractory ICP (51). Despite adequate control of the intracranial pressure, and maintenance of the cerebral perfusion pressure with aggressive brain resuscitation modalities, the majority of patients who were severely comatose on arrival to the ICU, die or leave the ICU in a persistent vegetative state, because the damage from the initial event was so severe it is irreversible (49,50).

Miscellaneous Considerations

Control of Blood Glucose Levels

Aggressive blood glucose control (<110 mg/dL) with insulin infusion recently has been associated with a reduced mortality, from 8 to 4.3%, when compared with intermittent doses of subcutaneous regular insulin in an heterogeneous large group of critically ill patients that were prospectively randomized (76). Although this study included a variety of patients admitted to the ICU with hypoxic or hypercapnic respiratory failure, the reduction in mortality from multiple-organ failure suggests a possible benefit in patients surviving episodes of drowning who require prolonged ICU hospitalization. Interestingly, critical-illness polyneuropathy was reduced 44% in the insulin infusion group. It is our practice to control the patient's blood sugar level with an insulin infusion in any critically ill patient with a level above normal. A glucose-based crystalloid infusion is used when blood sugar is below 200 mg/dL, to limit the risk of hypoglycemia. Blood glucose level is usually checked every 1 or 2 hours.

RENAL SUPPORT

Albuminuria, hemoglobinuria, oliguria, and anuria, although rare, have all been described in drowning victims secondary to acute tubular necrosis from hypoxemia, rhabdomyolysis or both. Hypothermia leads to reduced blood flow to the skin and muscle, preserving core temperature and central organ perfusion. The acute pathophysiology of acute rhabdomyolysis is probably secondary to tissue hypoxia from acute vessel constriction as a result of the competitive need for heat conservation. Skeletal myolysis and increased circulating myoglobin will result. Acute renal failure may be aggravated by acute tubular necrosis secondary to hemodynamic instability.

Acute tubular necrosis and rhabdomyolysis require early and vigorous treatment directed at correcting hypovolemia, improving oxygenation and enhancing heme protein elimination. Volume replacement therapy aims to restore normal blood flow and enhance renal oxygen supply. The medullary-ascending limb of Henle's loop is most vulnerable to hypoxic injury. Invasive monitoring may be necessary to provide adequate intravascular volume. A central venous pressure or pulmonary wedge pressure around 15 mmHg is a reasonable hemodynamic goal if ventricular function is normal. Higher pressures may be necessary in patients with a significant increase in mean intrathoracic pressure. Right ventricular ejection fraction, a pulmonary artery catheter, or transthoracic or transesophageal echocardiography can be used if the interpretation of preload by invasive monitoring is difficult, as it often is in patients requiring major ventilator support. The window of opportunity for restoration of intravascular volume and volume expansion is likely within 6 hours or less of the acute event.

If rhabdomyolysis is present, enhancing heme protein elimination helps to limit tubular damage. Systemic alkalinization of the urine with sodium bicarbonate increases the solubility and, therefore, the elimination of heme protein (77). A urine pH of between 7.0 and 8.0 produces a myoglobin solubility of around 80% and is a reasonable goal. However, in a patient with low urine output, massive doses of sodium bicarbonate may be associated with volume overload secondary to an acute increase in intravascular osmolarity (78). In these cases, when the hemodynamic goal is mild hypervolemia, the weak diuretic, acetazolamide, may be a valid alternative. Acetazolamide increases the excretion of bicarbonate in urine as a result of the inhibition of the carbonic anhydrase enzyme. However, diuretics, particularly in patients on significant ventilatory support, may adversely affect venous filling and cardiac output. Three other therapeutic agents have been used successfully to preserve renal function in patients with acute rhabdomyolysis: dopamine, loop diuretics, and mannitol. All three drugs enhance recovery of renal function by optimizing the relationship between renal oxygen supply and demand after a hypoxic insult (79).

Manipulating the renal output by means of significantly altering the effective circulating blood volume in drowning victims frequently has a detrimental effect on pulmonary and cardiovascular function. Therefore, a fine-tuned balancing act is frequently required to not adversely affect one organ system while treating another.

OTHER CONCERNS

Severe metabolic acidosis from low systemic oxygen delivery and resulting anaerobic metabolism should be corrected. We recommend correction of the base deficit with bicarbonate or acetate solutions to maintain a pH no lower than 7.2. Mechanical ventilation is adjusted frequently with the help of arterial blood gas determinations to maintain $PaCO_2$ between 35 and 40 mmHg. Lactic acid levels are checked frequently for a few hours after resuscitation. In fact, although base deficit and single absolute levels of lactic acidosis do not necessarily correlate with the development of multiple organ failure and survival, the rate of lactic acid clearance does (80). Because significant electrolyte abnormalities requiring specific therapy rarely are observed in the drowning victim, normal saline is given as replacement fluid in drowning victims. Isotonic solution also provides less chance of aggravating cerebral edema.

PREVENTION

An awareness of the hidden dangers of recreational activities in and around water, and close supervision of infants, children, and adolescents is the secret to preventing a significant number of drowning incidents. Swimming pools should be enclosed by security fences to prevent small children from entering the water inadvertently or unsupervised. By identifying age-related drowning risks, communities can reduce drowning rates. Effective CPR and water safety skills should be encouraged in the community, particularly for parents with small children who own home pools. Furthermore, children who can swim should never do so alone or without adult supervision. Everyone participating in water sports should wear an approved personal flotation device. Adolescents need to be taught to swim and informed about the dangers of alcohol and other drug consumption during water sport activities. Between 13 and 19 years of age, risk-taking behavior increases significantly in boys therefore extra counseling is warranted. Alcohol should never be consumed, regardless of age, while swimming or engaging in water sports. Swimming with a partner is particularly important for individuals with medical conditions that may abruptly alter their level of consciousness, such as seizure disorders, cardiac disease, and several metabolic diseases. Emergency gear for rescuing and resuscitating drowning victims should be readily available at pool-side. The specific gear required may vary with the size, access, and ownership of the facility.

The community expects the government to enforce safety rules, to promote health education through medical and nonmedical personnel, and to punish individuals who transgress basic safety rules and regulations. Despite recent advances in CPR and more sophisticated intensive care medicine, drowning victims with poor GCS scores have a high likelihood of living in a vegetative state as a result of the initial injury. When this occurs, making life or death decisions regarding withdrawal of life support by relatives and health professionals represents a significant stressful problem. At the time of this writing, prevention is still the most fundamental way to limit neurologic disasters from drowning.

ACKNOWLEDGMENTS

The authors thank Anita Yeager and DeNae Flentje for their editorial and secretarial assistance, respectively.

REFERENCES

1. Idris AH, Berg R, Bierens J, et al. Recommended guidelines for uniform reporting of data from drowning: the "Utstein Style". Circulation 2003; 108:2565–2574.
2. Craig AB, Jr. Causes of loss of consciousness during underwater swimming. J Appl Physiol 1961; 16: 583–586.
3. Swann HG. Resuscitation in semi-drowning. In: Whittenberg JF, ed. Artificial Respiration: Theory and Application. New York: Harper and Roe, 1962, pp. 202–224.
4. Modell JH, Graves SA, Ketover A. Clinical course of 91 consecutive near-drowning victims. Chest 1976; 70:231–238.
5. Lowson JA. Sensations in drowning. Edinburgh Med J 1903; 13:41–45.
6. Fuller RH. The 1962 Wellcome prize essay. Drowning and the post-immersion syndrome. A clinico-pathologic study. Milit Med 1963; 129:22–36.
7. Modell JH, Davis JH. Electrolyte changes in human drowning victims. Anesthesiology 1969; 30: 414–420.
8. Modell JH, Moya F, Newby EJ, et al. The effects of fluid volume and seawater drowning. Ann Intem Med 1967; 67:68–80.
9. Modell JH, Moya F. Effects of volume of aspirated fluid during chlorinated fresh water drowning. Anesthesiology 1966; 27:662–672.
10. Modell JH, Gaub M, Moya F, Vestal B, Swarz H. Physiologic effects of near-drowning with chlorinated fresh water, distilled water and isotonic saline. Anesthesiology 1966; 27:33–41.
11. Leach RM, Treacher DS. A13C of oxygen: oxygen transport–2. Tissue hypoxia. Br Med J 1998; 317: 1370–1373.
12. Craig Jr AB. Underwater swimming and loss of consciousness. JAMA 1961; 176:255–258.
13. Ferrett G, Costa M, Ferrigno M, et al. Alveolar gas composition exchange during deep breath-hold diving and dry breath holds in elite divers. J Appl Physiol 1991; 70:794–802.
14. Gray SW. Respiratory movement of rat during drowning and influence of water temperature upon survival after submersion. Am J Physiol 1951; 167:95–102.
15. Kvittingen TD, Naess A. Recovery from drowning in fresh water. Br Med J 1963; 1:1315–1317.
16. Movritzen CV, Andersen MN. Myocardial temperature gradients and ventricular fibrillation during hypothermia. J Thorac Cardiovasc Surg 1965; 49:937–944.
17. Cot C. Les asphyxies accidentecelles (submersion, electrocution, intoxication, oxycarbonique) etude clinique, therapeutique et preventive. Paris: Editions Medicales N. Maloine 1931.
18. Modell JH. The Pathophysiology and Treatment of Drowning and Near-drowning. Springfield, IL: Charles C. Thomas, 1971, p. 9.
19. Modell JH. Drown vs. near-drown: a discussion of definitions, editorial. Crit Care Med 1981; 9:341–352.
20. Modell JH, Bellefleur M, Davis JH. Drowning without aspiration: is this an appropriate diagnosis? J Forensic Sci 1999; 44:119–123.
21. Loughead DW, Janes JM, Hall GE. Physiological studies in experimental asphyxia and drowning. Can Med Assoc J 1939; 40:423–428.
22. Swann HG, Spafford NR. Body salt and water changes during fresh and sea water drowning. Texas Rep Biol Med 1951; 9:356–382.
23. Swann HG, Brucer M, Moore C, et al. Fresh water and sea water drowning. A study of the terminal cardiac and biochemical events. Texas Rep Biol Med 1947; 5:423–437.
24. Halmagyi DFJ, Colebatch HJH. Ventilation and circulation after fluid aspiration. J Appl Physiol 1961; 16:35–40.
25. Colebatch HJH, Halmagyi DFJ. Lung mechanics and resuscitation after fluid resuscitation. J Appl Physiol 1961; 16:684–696.
26. Redding JS, Voight GC, Safer P: Treatment of sea water aspiration. J Appl Physiol 1960; 15:1113–1116.
27. Colebatch HJH, Halmagyi DFJ. Reflex pulmonary hypertension of fresh water aspiration. J Appl Physiol 1963; 18:179–185.
28. Colebatch HJH, Hahnagyi DFJ. Reflex airway reaction to fluid aspiration. J Appl Physiol 1962; 17: 787–794.
29. Fainer DC, Martin CG, Ivy AC. Resuscitation of dogs from fresh water drowning. J Appl Physiol 1951; 3:417–426.
30. Redding JS, Cozine RA. Restoration of circulation after fresh water drowning. J Appl Physiol 1961; 16:1071–1074.

31. Redding JS, Voight GC, Safer P. Drowning treated with intermittent positive pressure breathing. J Appl Physiol 1960; 15:849–854.
32. Modell JH, Moya F, Williams HD, et al. Changes in blood gases and AaD02 during near-drowning. Anesthesiology 1968; 29:456–465.
33. Giamniona ST, Modell JH. Drowning by total immersion. Effects on pulmonary surfactant of distilled water, isotonic saline and sea water. Am J Dis Child 1967; 114:612–616.
34. Spitz WV, Blanke RV. Mechanism of death in fresh-water drowning. I. An experimental approach to the problem. Arch Path (Chicago) 1961; 71:661–668.
35. Modell JH, Davis JH, Giammona ST, et al. Blood gas and electrolyte changes in human near-drowning victims. JAMA 1968; 203:337–343.
36. Fainer DC. Near-drowning in sea water and fresh water. Ann Intern Med 1963; 59:537–541.
37. Hasan S, Avery WE, Fabian C, et al. Near-drowning in humans. A report of 36 cases. Chest 1971; 59: 191–197.
38. Fuller RH. The clinical pathology of human near-drowning. Proc Roy Soc Med 1963; 56:33–38.
39. Moritz AR. Chemical methods for the determination of death by drowning. Physiol Rev 1944; 24: 70–88.
40. Butt MP, Jalowayski A, Modell JH, et al. Pulmonary function after resuscitation from near-drowning. Anesthesiology 1970; 32:275–277.
41. Modell JH, Kuck EJ, Ruiz BC, et al. Effect of intravenous vs. aspirated distilled water on serum electrolytes and blood gas tensions. J Appl Physiol 1972; 32:579–584.
42. Bergquist RE, Vogelhut MM, Modell JH, et al. Comparison of ventilatory patterns in the treatment of fresh water near-drowning in dogs. Anesthesiology 1980; 52:142–148.
43. Tabeling BB, Modell JH. Fluid administration increases oxygen delivery during continuous positive pressure ventilation after freshwater near-drowning. Crit Care Med 1983; 11:693–696.
44. Yag IR, Stalnikowicz R, Michaeli J. Near-drowning in the Dead Sea-electrolyte imbalances and therapeutic implications. Arch Intern Med 1985; 145:50–53.
45. Modell JH: The Pathophysiology and Treatment of Drowning and Near-drowning. Springfield, IL: Charles C. Thomas, 1971, pp. 61–66.
46. Ellis J. National Pool and Water Park Lifeguard Training Manual. Boston: Jones & Bartlet, 2000.
47. The American Heart Association in collaboration with the International Liaison Committee on Resuscitation. Guidelines 2000 for Cardiopulmonary Resuscitation and Emergency Cardiovascular Care, Circulation 2000; 102(Suppl):233–235.
48. Rosen P, Stoto M, Harley J, et al (eds). The use of the Heimlich Maneuver in near-drowning. Committee on the treatment of near-drowning victims. Washington DC: Institute of Medicine, 1994.
49. Conn A, Montes J, Barker G. Cerebral salvage in near-drowning following neurologic classification by triage. Can J Anaesth 1980; 27:201–210.
50. Modell JH, Graves SA, Kuck EJ. Near-drowning: correlation of level of consciousness and survival. Can Anaesth Soc J 1980; 27:211–215.
51. Bohn DJ, Biggart WD, Smith CR, et al. Influence of hypothermia, barbiturate therapy and intracranial pressure monitoring on morbidity and mortality after near-drowning. Crit Care Med 1986; 14:529–534.
52. Orlowski JP, Szpilman D. Pediatric critical care: Drowning. Rescue, resuscitation and reanimation. A new Millenium. Pediatr Clin North Am 2001; 48:627–646.
53. Lee KH. A retrospective study of near drowned victims admitted to the intensive care unit. Ann Acad Med Singapore 1998; 27:344–346.
54. Goodwin SR. Aspiration syndromes. In: Civetta JM, Taylor RW, Kirby RR (eds). Critical Care. Philadelphia, PA: Lippincott-Raven, 1997, pp. 1861–1875.
55. Bachofen M, Weibel ER. Alterations of the gas exchange apparatus in adult respiratory insufficiency associated with septicemia. Am Rev Respir Dis 1977; 116:589–615.
56. Ruiz BC, Calderwood HW, Modell JH. Effect of ventilatory patterns on arterial oxygenation after near-drowning with fresh water. A comparative study in dogs. Anesth Analg 1973; 52:570–576.
57. Suter PS, Fairley HB, Isenberg MD. Optimum end-expiratory airway pressure in patients with acute pulmonary failure. N Engl J Med 1975; 292:284–289.
58. Modell JH, Calderwood HW, Ruiz BC, et al. Effects of ventilatory patterns on arterial oxygenation after near-drowning in sea water. Anesthesiology 1974; 40:376–384.
59. Antonelli M, Conti G, Rocco M, et al. A comparison of noninvasive positive-pressure ventilation and conventional mechanical ventilation in patient with acute respiratory failure. N Eng J Med 1998; 339: 429–435.
60. Rabatin JT, Gay PC: Noninvasive ventilation. Mayo Clin Proc 1999; 74:817–820.

61. Downs JB, Klein EF Jr, Desautels D, et al. Intermittent manditory ventilation: a new approach to weaning patients from mechanical ventilators. Chest 1973; 64:331–335.
62. Dellinger RP, Zimmennan JL, Taylor RW et al. Effects of inhaled nitric oxide in patients with acute respiratory distress syndrome: Results of a randomized phase II trial. Crit Care Med 1998; 26:15–23.
63. Jolliet P, Bulpa P, Chevrolet J. Effects of the prone position on gas exchange and hemodynamics in severe acute respiratory distress syndrome. Crit Care Med 1998; 26:1977–1985.
64. Pelosi P, Tubiolo D, Mascheroni D et al. Effects of the prone position on respiratory mechanics and gas exchange during acute lung injury. Am J Respir Crit Care Med 1998; 157:387–393.
65. Meduri GU, Headley AS, Golden E et al. Effect of prolonged methylprednisolone therapy in unresolving acute respiratory distress syndrome: A randomized controlled trial. JAMA 1998; 280:159–165.
66. Calderwood HW, Modell JH, Ruiz BC. The ineffectiveness of steroid therapy for treatment of freshwater near-drowning. Anesthesiology 1975; 43:642–650.
67. Bone RC, Fisher Jr. CJ, Clemmer TP et al. Early methylprednisolone treatment for septic syndrome and the adult respiratory distress syndrome. Chest 1987; 92:1032–1036.
68. Wynne JW, Modell JH. Respiratory aspiration of stomach contents. Ann Intern Med 1977; 87:66–474.
69. Wynne JW, Reynolds JC, Hood Cl, et al. Steroid therapy for pneurnonitis induced in rabbits by aspiration of food stuff. Anesthesiology 1979; 51:11–19.
70. Petty TL, Reiss OK, Paul GW et al. Characteristics of pulmonary surfactant in adult respiratory distress syndrome associated with trauma and shock. Am Rev Respir Dis 1977; 115:531–536.
71. Corbet A, Bucciarelli R, Goldman S et al. Decreased mortality among small premature infants treated at birth with a single dose of synthetic surfactant: A multicenter controlled trial. J Pediatr 1991; 118:227–234.
72. Anzueto A, Baughman RP, Guntupalli KK et al. Aerosolized surfactant in adults with sepsis-induced acute respiratory distress syndrome. N Engl J Med 1996; 334:1417–1421.
73. Bullock RM, Chestnut RM, Clifton GL, et al. Guidelines for the management of severe traumatic brain injury. J Neurotrauma 2000; 17:451–627.
74. Fortune JB, Feustel PJ, deLuna C, et al. Cerebral blood flow and blood volume in response to O_2 and CO_2 changes in normal humans. J Trauma 1995; 39:463–471.
75. Weckesser M, Posse S. Oltholf U, et al. Functional imaging of the visual cortex with bold contrast MRI: hyperventilation decreases signal response. Magn Reson Med 1999; 41:213–216.
76. Van den Berghe G, Wouters P, Weekers F, et al. Intensive insulin therapy in critically ill patients. N Engl J Med 2001; 345:1359–1367.
77. Better OS, Stein JH. Early management of shock and prophylaxis of acute renal failure in traumatic rhabdomyolysis. N Engl J Med 1990; 322:825–829.
78. Eneas JF, Schoenfeld PY, Humphreys MH. The Effect of infusion of mannitol-sodium bicarbonate on the clinical course of myoglobinuria. Arch Intem Med 1979; 139:801–805.
79. Gelman S. Preserving renal function during surgery. In: International Anesthesia Research Society Review Course Lectures. Baltimore, MD: Williams and Wilkins, 1992, pp. 88–92.
80. Bakker J, Gris P, Coffemils M, et al. Serial blood lactate levels can predict the development of multiple organ failure following septic shock. Am J Surg 1996; 171:221–226.

25 Cardiopulmonary Resuscitation and Early Management of the Lightning Strike Victim

Mary Ann Cooper, MD
and Sara Ashley Johnson, MD

CONTENTS

INTRODUCTION

In the past 40 years, lightning has killed more people than any other storm-related phenomena except floods *(1)*. On average, lightning causes 75 to 100 deaths per year *(1)*. The number of nonfatal injuries is estimated to be 10 times the number of deaths, but the exact number is not precisely known because of incomplete reporting *(2)*. A risk table for lightning injury is available at www.lightningsafety.noaa.gov and is excerpted as Table 1.

Contrary to popular belief, death caused by lightning is not as a result of burns. Severe burns are uncommon because the majority of lightning energy flashes around the outside of the individual and is simply not around long enough to burn through the skin in most cases, although secondary steam, hot metal, and other incidental superficial burns may be observed *(3,4)*. Lightning is a nervous system injury. Of the 90% who survive lightning strike injury, a significant number have disability from brain injury, neurocognitive deficits, or chronic pain syndromes *(4–6)*. A lightning strike victim is highly unlikely ($p < 0.0001$) to die unless he or she has suffered cardiopulmonary arrest (CPA) immediately at the time of the strike *(5)*. Although complications of postarrest anoxia or depression and suicide may lead to death after the acute event, the only immediate cause of death is cardiac arrest (CA) at the time of the strike *(5)*. Although autonomic injury is known to occur and many patients report arrhythmias and chest pain, the etiology and occurrence of long-term cardiac sequelae is unclear and poorly documented *(4)*.

From: *Contemporary Cardiology: Cardiopulmonary Resuscitation*
Edited by: J. P. Ornato and M. A. Peberdy © Humana Press Inc., Totowa, NJ

Table 1
Odds of Becoming a Lightning Victim

US 2000 Census population	280,000,000
Reported deaths 85, injuries 315	1/700,000
Actual deaths 120, injuries 1050	1/230,000
Life expectancy of 80 years	1/3000
Ten people affected for every one hit	1/300

Unlike triage in common multicasualty situations, with lightning, anyone who shows signs of life such as moaning or groaning will survive, albeit perhaps with sequelae, and may be attended to later (4). Because the only cause of immediate death is CPA, the goal of treating lightning strike victims is to resuscitate and stabilize those in arrest. Besides prevention, probably the best way to minimize acute lightning-related death is to optimize cardiopulmonary resuscitation (CPR) and postresuscitation care. This chapter provides the background information necessary to understand the pathophysiology of lightning strikes and the injury patterns they produce, describe the initial management of all lightning strike victims, and detail the specific management of victims based on clinical presentation and electrocardiogram (EKG) findings.

MECHANISM OF LIGHTNING STRIKES

Although lightning may occur in many forms, the most common discharge is the negative cloud to ground (CG) stroke. Lightning occurs when sufficient charge differential is built up in a cloud to cause electrical discharges. Discharges begin as horizontal intercloud lightning that jumps in spurts 30 to 50 meters long. It branches, then retreats to the source only to refill the main established streamer channel and branch again at the endpoint of each of the 30- to 50-meter lengths, repeating this cycle over and over again in a matter of milliseconds.

This alternating retreat and branching is what causes the sawtooth appearance of lightning. Some spurts never progress past their first or second generation and in most storms the majority of the streamers remain in the cloud unseen or perhaps causing only a brightening of the cloud. In the average storm, about 10% will approach the ground at some stage as downward leaders. Downward leaders continue branching in 30- to 50-meter segments until they get close to the ground. This branching and retreating mechanism in part explains why lightning does not "always hit the tallest object." The downward leader only "sees" a 30- to 50-meter radius from the tip of its last division so that when lightning does not hit the obvious "tallest" structure in an area it is usually because that structure is outside this 30- to 50-meter radius. Thus, the goal posts on a football field are unlikely to protect someone standing in the middle of the field (4).

As the storm cloud moves across the land, an opposite, usually positive charge is induced in the ground. Surges of charge move through any upward projecting object, whether it is a tree, a TV tower, a person, or a blade of grass and produce upward streamers. Occasionally, these may be seen as St Elmo's Fire. More often, the upward streamers are invisible and not appreciated except perhaps as static electricity causing one's hair to stand on end (4).

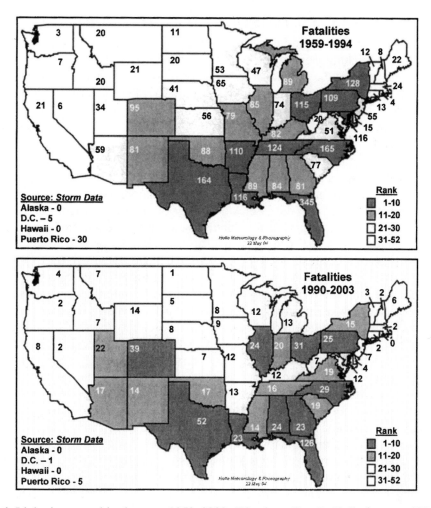

Fig. 1. Lightning casualties by state 1959–2003. (Thanks to Ron L. Holle for use of Fig. 1.)

One or more of these upward streamers may connect with a downward streamer to complete the cloud to ground channel in a process called attachment. There are often multiple upward streamers that do not form a connection but are of a magnitude sufficient to cause injury *(7,8)*. After attachment occurs, several spaced strong surges of energy rush upward as return strokes and down again as dart leaders, causing the flickering and brightening that we see in the main lightning pathway.

In the United States, there are approx 20 million CG flashes detected each year, most frequently in the summer months *(9)*. More than half of lightning strikes have two ground contact sites or more. CG lightning is most common in the southeastern United States, but deaths and injuries are most common along the Gulf and Atlantic coasts, the major US river valleys and over the Rocky Mountains (Fig. 1). Injuries peak in July and in the mid-afternoon hours on Saturdays and Sundays. One-third of lightning injuries are work-related *(1,4)*.

MECHANISMS OF LIGHTNING INJURY

In attempting to define the injury mechanism for a particular person, the question arises: "Does the lightning energy go down through or around the person from the cloud to the ground, up from the ground to the cloud or by some other mechanism?"

At least five mechanisms of lightning strike injury have been identified: direct hit, side splash to a person from another object, contact when the person is holding onto an object such as a fence that is struck, ground current/ground arcing and uncompleted upward streamer, hypothesized by engineers for years but only recently documented in the medical literature (4,10). Further complicating the issue is the fact that the majority of the energy probably flashes around ("flashover") rather than through the person (4).

Although it is reasonable to infer that a direct strike is more likely to cause death, there is no hard evidence that this is the case. Although theoretically knowledge of the mechanism of injury should be helpful in anticipating the level of care required, pragmatically it is nearly impossible to tell which mechanism has injured a particular victim. When there are witnesses, they are often too upset or injured themselves to give a good account. Lightning strike is so instantaneous that even the most focused and expectant observer has difficulty telling where the energy traveled. Further complicating the history is that victims often have few or no burns. Even in those that do, the burns cannot be used to tell where the energy has traveled as the burns are often secondary to sweat or rainwater that has heated up and caused steam burns, from hot metal burns from necklaces, belts, pocket coins, or other secondary burns. The terms "entry" and "exit" have no meaning with lightning injuries (3). The first organized study of lightning injuries in 1980 gives some clues of prognosis (5). Those with burns about the head are more likely to have CA and die as are those with burns to both legs. However, burns from one arm to a leg or between arms were not associated with a higher incidence of death or CA.

Many survivors have amnesia for the event (5). However, they will almost always and quite innocently reconstruct a composite mechanism of injury consistent with what they have heard from the paramedics who transported them, from their physicians, their relatives, from what they read and from any burns that they may have received. This reconstruction may or may not have any relationship to what actually happened (4). However, the story is usually harmless and attempting to dissuade the survivor or their family from their believed mechanism is a waste of time, does not improve outcome and generally leads to dissatisfaction on all sides.

The lightning literature is clouded with assumptions to the mechanisms of injury and their outcomes. Unfortunately, most of the lightning cardiac literature consists of case reports with almost no organized studies relating mechanism of injury, EKG findings, outcome, or other cardiac questions.

Direct Hit

Perhaps the most dramatic strike is a "direct hit." Classically, this occurs in unsheltered, open areas such as sporting or farm fields, golf courses, or mountains. Although specific data has not been reported, direct hits are assumed to be the mechanism most likely to cause CA or severe cardiac damage because the force of the strike is transmitted directly to the individual and not decreased by the interposition of trees or other objects.

In a 1993 study of cardiovascular effects of lightning strikes, Robert Lichtenberg described four patients reportedly with direct strikes by lightning, three of whom had myocardial injury. One victim suffered CPA in the field, arrived in the emergency department (ED) in asystole. Despite aggressive resuscitation and a return to sinus tachycardia, this patient was pronounced dead 36 hours later. The remaining two victims had ST segment elevation on their EKGs, elevated cardiac enzymes, and echocardiographic evidence of global ventricular dysfunction *(11)*. In 1981, B.L. Chia described a 23-year-old woman reportedly directly hit by lightning, who arrived in the hospital in pulmonary edema, which was successfully treated with diuretics and digoxin *(12)*.

CONTACT AND SIDE-SPLASH INJURIES

Contact and side-splash injuries are probably much more common than direct hits. In "contact" injuries, lightning strikes an object such as a tree or fence and a portion of the strike's energy travels to anyone touching the object. A side-splash injury occurs when lightning strikes an object but some of the energy splashes through the air to a nearby person. People who gather under trees during thunderstorms are often injured in this way and sometimes lightning may be witnessed to travel sequentially from one victim to another.

Numerous reports of cardiac sequelae following contact and side-splash injuries exist *(11,13–16)*, ranging in severity from Lichtenberg's three patients, all of whom had nonspecific ST-T wave changes but no echocardiographic abnormality *(11)*, to J. P. Kleiner's report of a man whose tent was struck by lightning who developed ventricular failure requiring diuretics and a 3-week hospital stay *(13)*. Although the vast majority of side-splash injuries occur outdoors, a not insignificant number occur inside buildings, often via telephone wires or from plumbing or electrical fixtures *(4,17)*.

GROUND CURRENT

When lightning strikes the earth, the energy spreads radially, and may pass up through people or animals near the lightning contact point. Sports teams, soldiers on maneuvers, and other groups of people have been injured in this way with mortality ranging from 0 to 23% *(18–23)*. Kitigawa has recently further divided the ground current effect: one where current flows through the ground with little energy flow to those standing on it and therefore minor injury, and ground arcing where energy arcs above the surface of the ground, through or around the person as part of its pathway, similar to side splash. The second type of injury, although it may occur on flat surfaces, is more likely to be seen on uneven terrain and mountains and is more likely to cause severe injuries because of the greater energy exposure of the person *(24)*.

Lichtenberg described 12 patients affected by ground current strikes: although three had nonspecific ST-T wave changes on electrocardiogram, only one had CK-MB release, and none had an abnormal echocardiogram *(11)*.

UPWARD STREAMERS

A fifth mechanism for injury by lightning has been hypothesized by lightning and electrical researchers for many years but only recently have cases been specifically studied for this mechanism *(7,8,10,23,25)*. Upward streamers are surges of charge that begin at the ground, rush up through or around the person but do not connect with the downward leader from a cloud to complete the lightning channel *(10)*. Upward streamers may occur a kilometer or more from the charged cloud. Cooper described a case in which an upward streamer passed through a member of an electrical crew. Paramedics arrived to find the patient in ventricular fibrillation (VF). Despite defibrillation and intubation, the patient never regained a perfusing rhythm and was pronounced at the ED *(10)*. Because this mechanism is newly documented, no cases of hospital management for surviving patients are available for review.

MANAGEMENT OF LIGHTNING VICTIMS
Diagnosis

When witnesses are available or when the individual is alert enough to provide his or her own history, making the diagnosis of lightning strike is not difficult. However, when found confused and alone outdoors, a lightning strike victim may be initially thought to have had an intracranial hemorrhage, a seizure, or suffered an assault *(4)*. Because lightning can injure victims indoors, the diagnosis should be considered in anyone found confused and unconscious during or shortly after a thunderstorm, particularly when no other mechanism of illness is evident *(4,17)*.

Physical clues that a patient has been struck by lightning include clothing partially or completely exploded off, linear or punctate burns, missing shoes, ruptured tympanic membranes, and the rare but pathognomonic keraunographic markings or Lichtenberg figure (it is not known if this is any relation to R. Lichtenberg *[4]*). These are an evanescent feather or fern-like pattern that usually disappears within a few hours and are not true burns. Historically, they were attributed to the imprint of plants the individual had been near when struck but more recently thought to represent a fractile pattern from electrons tracking over the skin during lightning strike *(4,26)*.

Causes of Cardiac Arrest From Lightning

It has been hypothesized that a primary arrest occurs from the strike energy itself similar to the short asystole that occurs after defibrillation but that a healthy heart resumes cardiac activity after the lightning insult. The respiratory arrest lasts much longer causing a secondary CA that may be irrecoverable *(4,5)*. It was further hypothesized that early and adequate ventilatory support could make a difference in the outcome of the individual.

Simulated lightning strike to animals in the laboratory has confirmed this sequence of primary arrest and pause, often with recovery, but prolonged respiratory arrest and secondary CA with higher shock doses *(26,27)*. Even the animals that survived had arrythmias for a short period of time. However, in the fatally injured, ventricular tachycardia (VT), bradycardia, intermittent and variable blocks, sometimes fibrillation, and eventually (secondary) asystolic CA developed *(26,27)*. Recent unreported animal studies have also confirmed a significant effect on heart rate variability from autonomic nervous system injury at the time of the strike *(27)*.

Some early references recommended very prolonged resuscitation for lightning victims based on a mechanism of "suspended animation" for lightning survivors in which the brain and other organs are protected by some unknown mechanism so that resuscitation might be successful and without deficits if it were carried for a much longer time than would be considered useful by most clinicians. A more recent case series of survivors with QT prolongation after the strike hypothesized that this may contribute to a torsade mechanism that has been confused with "suspended animation" perhaps with some perfusion, no palpable pulses but yet some recovery *(28)*. There is no reason to believe that CA from lightning is more brain "protective" than other forms of CA to young healthy individuals.

Studies have not been done to determine the relative contributions of autonomic nervous system injury, direct damage to conducting and pacing pathways or to the heart itself, injury to respiratory and cardiac control centers in the brain, timing of the lightning strike during the cardiac cycles, or other as yet unknown mechanisms to the CA or how these affect recovery or long-term cardiac effects.

INITIAL RESUSCITATION AND STABILIZATION OF LIGHTNING STRIKE VICTIMS

In treating the lightning strike victim, the first step is to establish airway, breathing, and circulation, as well as assure the safety of the individual and the rescue crew who are often responding during an active thunderstorm. It may be necessary to move the victim to a safer area before adequate resuscitation attempts can begin

Unfortunately, not enough research has been done with lightning victims or animal models to allow tailored recommendations for cardiac resuscitation of lightning victims. Established ACLS protocols should be followed with victims of lightning strike who are unresponsive and without spontaneous respirations in the field: an airway should be established, and CPR performed until a cardiac rhythm can be determined. More directed treatment with cardioversion, defibrillation and/or epinephrine, atropine, and other standard ACLS medications should proceed according to the most recent guidelines. The resuscitation of lightning victims may be complicated by hypothermia from wet clothing or cold conditions on mountains and other high-risk lightning areas.

It is also too early to tell if the growing availability of automatic external defibrillators (AEDs) to first responders or in sports venues, schools, and other areas will produce better outcomes for lightning victims, although this author is aware of three separate recent unpublished cases in which the use of an AED resulted in successful resuscitation. An AED trial application can cause no harm provided other resuscitation and rescue protocols continue as well.

There is no reason to believe that CA from lightning is more brain "protective" than other forms of cardiac arrest to young healthy individuals. Old anecdotal reports of "suspended animation" and miraculous cures after very prolonged resuscitation have not been substantiated in more recent literature and should be probably included among the large number of other lightning myths that abound (3). However, consistent with historical evidence in the literature, ventilatory assistance may need to be prolonged after a successful cardiac resuscitation.

CESSATION OF RESUSCITATION

The decision to abandon resuscitation efforts should be guided by the clinical scenario including how long the person has been without adequate resuscitation and their response after standard ACLS measures have been started. What constitutes a reasonable period will depend on the most recent ACLS guidelines and the judgment and experience of the clinicians involved in the lightning strike victim's care but certainly if there is no response within thirty minutes, termination of resuscitation should be considered as it is unlikely that the individual will survive with useful brain function after this length of time. When arrest occurs in a wilderness setting far from the benefits of electrical intervention, drugs, and medical care, rescuers should be absolved of any guilt in terminating resuscitation efforts if there is no response within twenty or thirty minutes or when rescuers become exhausted, whichever occurs first (4,29).

EVALUATION AND TREATMENT OF MORE STABLE LIGHTNING STRIKE VICTIMS

In lightning strike victims with stable airway and a cardiac rhythm, adequate ventilation should be assured and a secondary survey performed. Although this chapter focuses on the cardiopulmonary manifestations of lightning strike, it should be noted that lightning victims may suffer a number blunt injuries including pulmonary contusions, back and brain injuries and occasionally fractures from both the explosive nature of the strike around them or from being thrown by the intense muscle contractions induced by the electrical energy *(4,30,31)*. All trauma victims should be undressed in order to identify other injuries as well as to remove wet clothes that may be contributing to hypothermia.

Carotid and femoral pulses are usually palpable in lightning strike victims who are not in CA. If the patient is hypotensive without palpable distal pulses, cardiogenic, hypovolemic, and spinal shock should be ruled out. However, in many cases of lightning strike, distal pulses may be affected even in the presence of normal blood pressure and cardiovascular stability. A significant number of lightning victims may exhibit keraunoparalysis with cool, mottled, pulseless extremities, which is thought to be the result of sympathetic instability and intense vasospasm *(4,31)*. In Cooper's study of severely injured lightning strike victims, a full two-thirds had some degree of lower extremity paralysis, in which the affected extremities were cool, mottled, insensate, and pulseless *(5)*.

The vast majority of lightning strike victims not in arrest or congestive heart failure on arrival to the hospital will have normal cardiovascular exams and electrocardiograms. These patients are unlikely to deteriorate *(4,5,11)*. Asymptomatic patients with normal electrocardiograms and no other injuries requiring admission do not need cardiac enzymes measured and may be safely discharged from the ED with instructions to follow up with their primary-care physician.

EKG CHANGES

Several types of EKG abnormalities in lightning strike victims have been described.

QT PROLONGATION

In 1987, A.B.D. Palmer described a case of lightning induced q-t segment prolongation *(15)*. The patient had a modestly prolonged QTc (0.36 seconds) on admission. Thirty-eight hours later, the QTc was an impressive 0.68 seconds, and by day 3, the QTc had shortened to 0.5 seconds. Fortunately, this patient's rhythm never degenerated into torsades de pointe or VF.

In 1993, Andrews reviewed literature involving lightning strike victims and their electrocardiograms, and found that what Palmer had published as an isolated case report was far from uncommon. When a precise QTc could be calculated from available data, 63% were prolonged *(28)*. Additionally, the overall trend mirrored that described by Palmer: QTc intervals became increasingly prolonged in the first few days of recovery and slowly returned to normal.

Although the mechanism by which a lightning strike delays ventricular repolarization prolonging the QTc interval is not well understood, the implications are clear. The increased risk of developing torsade de pointes VT must be considered so that monitored admission of lightning strike victims with this abnormality is probably prudent. In many cases, the QTc will normalize over a few days. If this fails to occur, Holter monitoring and electrophysiological studies may be considered *(15)*.

NONSPECIFIC T-WAVE AND ST-T CHANGES

T-wave inversion and ST-T changes that do not fit typical coronary ischemia patterns are often observed in lightning strike victims. Most of these patients are asymptomatic and the vast majority of the ECG changes resolve spontaneously over a period of days to weeks *(4,11–14)*. It may be that these usually self-limited changes are as a result of direct myocardial damage caused by the lightning rather than vascular ischemia. Of the six patients Lichtenberg studied with nonspecific ST-T wave changes, all had normal echo cardiograms and uneventful recoveries *(11)*.

ANATOMICAL ST-ELEVATION AND T-WAVE INVERSION

There are several documented cases of ST segment elevation after lightning strike *(11,15,32)*. Lichtenberg described a patient, reportedly directly struck, who presented with ST elevation in the anterior and precordial leads and anterior wall motion abnormalities on echocardiogram *(11)*. The patient never developed heart failure and wall motion returned to normal in a few days. Jackson and Palmer described patients with elevated ST segments in the inferior leads who remained asymptomatic, and whose electrocardiogram changes resolved within several days *(15,32)*. T-Wave inversion consistent with vascular ischemic patterns has been reported *(12,13)* in both anterior and inferior patterns. Electrocardiograms normalized in a few weeks in all of these cases

ECG changes such may be caused by injury to the coronary arteries or by spasm resulting from high levels of catecholamines after lightning strike *(4,10)*. When the damage to underlying muscle is extensive enough, congestive heart failure and pulmonary edema can develop *(11–13)*. Kleiner described an 18-year-old who developed severe shortness of breath three hours after being struck *(13)*. The patient's chest x-ray showed severe pulmonary edema and Swan-Ganz catheterization measured his pulmonary capillary pressure at 25 mmHg. The patient improved with diuretic therapy and did not require inotropic support.

Patients with changes on EKG should be evaluated for signs of congestive heart failure. If significant comorbidities such as age or underlying heart disease exist, they may warrant echocardiogram, telemetry admission, or other interventions.

LONG-TERM PROBLEMS

There are several common complaints of lightning survivors that may be cardiac in origin: palpitations, chest pain, hypertension, dizziness, and near syncope *(4)*.

Many survivors complain of palpitations for a considerable period of time after lightning injury. They may also complain of shortness of breath, dizziness, and other symptoms so that from the history alone it is difficult to tell whether the palpitations are as a result of panic attacks or are true arrhythmias. No malignant arrhythmias have been reported as sequelae of lightning injury but there are also no reports in the literature of investigations of these complaints.

Some survivors experience frequent chest pain. Although a cardiac work up is usually indicated, it is often negative so that the etiology for the chest pain in these cases remains unclear. Some may be as a result of musculoskeletal injury from blunt injury caused by the strike *(4)*. Other reasons have not been investigated in relationship to lightning.

There have been a number of cases of worsened hypertension or new hypertension documented after a lightning strike. Although lightning is well known to cause autonomic damage, it has not been studied as an independent cause of hypertension.

Dizziness and tinnitus, frequent complaints of lightning survivors, is most often from damage to the eighth cranial nerve. Near syncope may be confused with new onset temporal lobe, partial complex seizure or hypothalamic seizures, which may have an onset as late as 2 years after the injury. Unfortunately, routine electroencephalograms measure only surface seizure activity and miss 50–100% of seizures that occur in deeper structures, further burdening many of these patients with the diagnosis of "pseudoseizure."

Table 2
Lightning Safety Guidelines

Know the weather forecast before starting an outdoor activity.
Have a Lightning Safety Plan that includes safer places to go as well as
    the time to get there.
Know your local weather patterns and keep an eye on the sky.
At the first sight of lightning or sound of thunder, begin implementation of
    your Lightning Safety Plan.
Safer areas include substantial buildings and fully enclosed metal vehicles
    with the windows rolled up.
Avoid tall structures such as towers, mountains, and trees.
Avoid open fields, open vehicles, and being near or in water.
Avoid contact with metal conductors or using small "shelters."
Do not resume outside activity until 30 minutes after the last lightning and
    last thunder.

Prevention

Although no place can be guaranteed to be totally safe from lightning strike, certain precautions can be taken to minimize the risks of lightning injury. Lightning warnings by the National Weather Service is uncommon, unlike many other disasters for which the government issues warnings hours to days in advance, so the individual must be responsible for making the best choices for their own personal safety as well as others for whom they may be responsible. Lightning Safety Guidelines for individuals, small groups and very large groups such as sports stadia audiences are outlined in Table 2 and are available in greater detail from other sources *(29,33–35)*. These guidelines, adopted by the National College Athletic Association in 1987, the National Athletic Trainers Association in 2000, and the entire Dallas Public School system in 2000 are becoming more widespread in both sporting, occupational and public venues.

CONCLUSIONS AND PREVENTION

Although lightning is the second largest storm killer annually in the United States, exceeded only by floods, it is still reasonably uncommon to suffer any lasting cardiac damage as a result. For those patients who arrest from lighting strike, recent advances in the acute care of CAs—improvements in the emegency medical services system, increased availability of AEDs and decreased time to resuscitation, and optimized intensive care for those who survive the initial insult—are likely to increase survival. Additionally, knowledge culled from the dozens of case reports of cardiac effects of lightning strike makes it easier for emergency physicians and cardiologists to predict which patients are likely to recover and which require monitoring.

Even as the treatment of lightning strike victims improves, we should not forget that injury from lightning strikes is, more often than not, preventable. Lightning Safety Guidelines, now published in many venues, can help individuals and organizations to develop lightning safety action plans that can prevent injury Table 3 *(29,33–35)*.

Table 3
Components of a Lightning Action Plan

Develop a Lightning Safety Plan
Train personnel to be familiar with the plan
Access up-to-date weather information
If detection or warning systems are used, train personnel in their use.
Designate safer areas
Plan for routing and evacuating people
Display appropriate signage
Educate of the event's participants about the Plan
Use a Warning Signal—different from All Clear Signal
Carry out regular plan drills
Review and modify plan as needed

REFERENCES

1. Curran EB, Rolle RL, Lopez RE. Lightning casualties and damages in the United States from 1959–1993. J Clim 2000; 13:3338–3363.
2. Cherington M, Walker J, Boyson M, et al. Closing the gap on the actual numbers of lighting casualties and death. In: Proceedings of the 11th Conference on Applied Climatology. January 10–15, 1999. Dallas, TX: American Meteorological Society 1999, pp. 379,380.
3. Cooper MA. Myths, miracles, and mirages. Semin Neurol 1995;15:358–361.
4. Cooper MA, Andrews CJ, Holle RL et al. Lightning Injuries. In: Auerbach PS, ed. Wilderness Medicine: Management of Wilderness and Environmental Emergencies, 3th ed. St. Louis, MO: Mosby, 2001, pp. 72–110.
5. Cooper MA. Lightning injuries: prognostic signs for death. Ann Emerg Med 1980; 9:133–138.
6. Cooper MA. Disability, Not Death is the Main Problem. National Weather Digest 2001; 25:43–47.
7. Mackeras D. Protection from Lightning. In: Lightning Injuries: Electrical, Medical, and Legal Aspects. Andrews CJ, Cooper MA, Darveniza M, Mackerras D, ed. Boca Raton: CRC Press 1992, pp. 145–156.
8. Uman MA. Physics of Lightning Phenomena. In: Andrews CJ, Cooper MA, Darveniza M, Mackerras D, eds. Lightning Injuries: Electrical, Medical, and Legal Aspects. Boca Raton: CRC Press 1992, pp. 6–22.
9. Huffines GR, Orville RE. Lighting ground flash density and thunderstorm duration in the contiguous United States: 1989–1996. J Appl Meterorol 1999; 38:1013.
10. Cooper MA. A fifth mechanism of lightning injury. Acad Emerg Med 2002; 9:172–173.
11. Lichtenberg R, Dries D, Ward K, Marshall W, Scanlon P. Cardiovascular effects of lightning strikes. J Am Coll Cardiol 1993; 21:531–536.
12. Chia BL. Electrocardiographic abnormalities of congestive cardiac failure due to lightning stroke. Cardiology 1981; 68:39–53.
13. Kleiner JP, Wilkin JH. Cardiac effects of lightning stroke. JAMA 1978; 230:2757–2759.
14. Kleinot S, Klachko DM, Keeley KJ. The cardiac effects of lightning injury. S Afr Med J 1966; 30:1131–1133.
15. Palmer AB. Lightning injury causing prolongation of the Q-T interval. Postgrad Med J 1987; 63:891–893.
16. Subramanian N, Somasundaram B, Periasamy JK. Cardiac injury due to lightning—report of a survivor. Indian Heart J 1985; 37:72–73.
17. Andrews CJ, Darveniza M. Telephone-mediated lightning injury: an Australian survey. J Trauma 1989; 29:665–671.
18. Epperly TD, Stewart JR. The physical effects of lightning injury. J Fam Pract 1989; 29:267–272.
19. Dollinger SJ. Lightning-strike disaster among children. Br J Med Psychol 1985; 58:375–383.
20. Arden GP, Harrison SH, Lister J, et al. Lightning accident at Ascot. Br Med J 1956; 1:1350–1353.
21. Buechner HA, Rothbaum JC. Lightning stroke injury: a report of multiple casualties resulting from a single lightning bolt. Mil Med 1961; 153:755–762.

22. Carte AE, Anderson RB, Cooper MA. A large group of children struck by lightning Ann Emerg Med 2002; 39:665–670.
23. Anderson R, Jandrell IR, Nematswerani HE. The Upward Streamer Mechanism Versus Step Potentials as a Cause of Injuries from Close Lightning Discharges. Transaction of the South African Institute of Electrical Engineers. March 2002, pp. 33–43.
24. Kitigawa N, Ohashi M, Ishikawa T. The Substantial Mechanisms of Step Voltage Effects. J Atmospheric Electricity 2001; 21:87–94.
25. Krider, EP, Ladd CG. Upward streamers in lightning discharges to mountainous terrain. Weather 1975; 30:77–81.
26. Andrews CJ. Studies in aspects of lightning injury, doctoral dissertation, Brisbane, Austrailia: University of Queensland, 1993.
27. Kotsos T, Gandhi MV, Neideen T, Cooper MA. Acute Cardiac Effects of Simulated Lightning in Rodents. , Chicago, IL: Bioengineering World Conference, July 27, 2000.
28. Andrews CJ, Colquhoun DM, Darveniza M. The QT interval in lightning injury with implications for the "cessation of metabolism" hypothesis. J Wilderness Med 1993; 3:155–166.
29. Zimmerman C, Cooper MA, Holle RL. Lightning safety guidelines. Ann Emerg Med 2002; 29:660–663.
30. Ohashi M, Hosoda Y, Fujishiro Y, et al. Lightning Injury as a Blast injury of Skull, Brain, and Visceral Lesions: Clinical and Experimental Evidences. The Keio Journal of Medicine 2001; 50:257–262.
31. ten Duis HJ, Klasen HJ, Reenalda PE. Keraunoparalysis, a 'specific' lightning injury. Burns Incl Therm Inj 1985; 12:53–57.
32. Jackson SH, Parry DJ. Lightning and the heart. Br Heart J 1980; 33:353–357.
33. Holle RL, Lopez RE, Zimmermann C. Updated Recommendations for Lightning Safety—1998. Bull of the Amer Met Soc 1999; 80:2035–2040.
34. Lightning Safety, 1998–99 NCAA Sports Medicine Handbook, 11th Edition, Ed. Michael V. Earle, August 1998, pp. 12–14.
35. Walsh K, Bennett B, Cooper MA, Holle R, Kithil R, Lopez R. National Athletic Trainers' Association Position Statement: Lightning Safety for Athletics and Recreation, Journal of Athletic Training 2000; 35:471–477.

26 Hypothermic Cardiac Arrest

Daniel F. Danzl, MD

CONTENTS

INTRODUCTION
TEMPERATURE REGULATION
PATHOPHYSIOLOGY
SUMMARY
REFERENCES

INTRODUCTION

The contemporary allure of hypothermia is regularly sparked by the apparent "reanimations" of profoundly cold patients in prolonged cardiac arrest (CA). Recently, a physician who was resuscitated from 13.7°C presented her own case report at an international conference *(1)*. There are also promising ongoing investigations of mild therapeutic hypothermia for traumatic intracranial hypertension and stroke *(2–4)*. Nevertheless, hypothermia remains more of a geographically and seasonally pervasive physiological threat than a therapy *(5–8)*.

Pathophysiological changes occur during hypothermia, which is defined as a core temperature less than 35°C. With primary hypothermia, the healthy individual's compensatory responses to heat loss through conduction, convection, radiation, and evaporation are simply overwhelmed. On the other hand, secondary hypothermia caused by many cardiopulmonary and other systemic diseases is consistently underreported *(9)*.

Therapeutic interventions including active rewarming become essential below 32°C. Interpretation of the literature is complicated by the fact that selection bias in this very heterogenous patient population affects the interpretation of the therapeutic response attributed to a specific rewarming modality. There is no single best approach to rewarming. Prognostic indicators that negatively impact outcome in hypothermia most commonly include not only the duration of CA, but also coexistent infection, toxin ingestion, and various medical illnesses and trauma *(10)*.

In addition to severe hypothermia, active rewarming is also indicated for cardiovascular instability, an inadequate rate or failure to rewarm, endocrinologic insufficiency, traumatic or toxicologic peripheral vasodilatation, or secondary hypothermia that impairs thermoregulation. The usual options for active core rewarming include: heated inhalation, heated infusion and irrigation of various sites, diathermy, and a variety of extracorporeal rewarming modalities. There are also a variety of methods to provide active external rewarming, including heated forced air blankets.

From: *Contemporary Cardiology: Cardiopulmonary Resuscitation*
Edited by: J. P. Ornato and M. A. Peberdy © Humana Press Inc., Totowa, NJ

TEMPERATURE REGULATION

Normal heat loss occurs through five mechanisms. Assuming an average basal metabolic rate, 55–65% of this loss is through radiation. Conduction normally accounts for only approx 2–3% of the heat loss, but this may increase up to five times in the presence of wet clothing and up to 25 times in cold water. Convection, evaporation, and respiration account for the remainder of the heat loss.

Shivering thermogenesis markedly increases the basal metabolic rate and oxygen consumption. Shivering is modulated by the posterior hypothalamus and the spinal cord *(11)*. The preoptic anterior hypothalamus orchestrates nonshivering heat conservation and dissipation. Serotonergic and dopaminergic neurons exert immediate control through the autonomic nervous system and delayed control through the endocrine system. Thermal suppression or activation of the sympathetic nervous system with cold-induced release of norepinephrine also occurs. Cold stimulates the hypothalamus to release thyrotropin-releasing hormone, which activates the anterior pituitary gland. Thyroid-stimulating hormone causes the release of thyroxine *(12)*.

As the temperature drops, vasoconstriction, shivering, and nonshivering basal and endocrinologic thermogenesis also conserve and generate heat. From 32° to 24°C, a progressive depression of the basal metabolic rate occurs without shivering thermogenesis. At temperatures less than 24°C, autonomic and endocrinologic mechanisms for heat conservation are gradually inactivated *(13)*.

PATHOPHYSIOLOGY

There are consistent physiologic characteristics for the three significant levels of hypothermia (Table 1). The cardiovascular system is depressed. Because the bradycardia of hypothermia results from decreased spontaneous depolarization of the pacemaker cells, bradydysrhythmias are refractory to atropine. Hypothermia also decreases the mean arterial pressure and the cardiac index.

The J (Osborn) wave is seen at the junction of the QRS complex and ST segment (Fig. 1; *14*). This deflection appears to result from hypothermic ion flux alterations, with delayed depolarization or early repolarization of the left ventricular wall. It can also be seen during local cardiac ischemia, with sepsis or central nervous system (CNS) lesions, and on occasion in young normothermic patients. Some J waveform abnormalities can simulate a myocardial injury current. Of note, because hypothermic electrocardiogram (EKG) changes are not easily computer programmable, inadvertent thrombolytic therapy has occurred in unrecognized and potentially coagulopathic hypothermic patients *(15)*.

Virtually all atrial and ventricular dysrhythmias commonly develop in moderate to severe hypothermia. Re-entrant dysrhythmias result from decreased conduction velocity coupled with an increased myocardial conduction time and a decreased absolute refractory period. Independent electrical foci also precipitate dysrhythmias. Because the conduction system is more sensitive to the cold than the myocardium, cardiac cycle prolongation occurs. Atrial fibrillation, without a rapid ventricular response, commonly develops when the core temperature is less than 32°C. This rhythm usually converts spontaneously during rewarming, although mesenteric embolization is a hazard in chronic cases.

Hypothermia also causes a decrease in transmembrane resting potential, which, in turn, decreases the threshold for ventricular dysrhythmias. Ventricular fibrillation (VF)

Table 1
Physiologic Characteristics of Significant Hypothermia

State	Core temperature		Characteristics
	°C	°F	
Moderate	33	91.4	Amnesia, dysarthria, ataxia, and apathy develop; maximum respiratory stimulation; tachycardia and tachypnea then progressive bradycardia and hypoventilation; cold diuresis
	32	89.6	EEG abnormalities; J waves
	31	87.8	Extinguished shivering thermogenesis
	30	86	Atrial fibrillation and other dysrhythmias; poikilothermia; pulse and cardiac output two-thirds normal; insulin ineffective
	29	85.2	Progressive decrease in level of consciousness, pulse, and respiration; pupils dilated.
Severe	28	82.4	VF susceptibility; 50% decrease in oxygen consumption and pulse
	27	80.6	Hyporeflexia and no motion
	26	78.8	Major acid–base disturbances; no reflexes or response to pain
	25	77	Loss of cerebral autoregulation; cardiac output 45% normal; pulmonary edema may develop
	24	75.2	Significant hypotension
	23	73.4	No corneal or oculocephalic reflexes
	22	71.6	Maximum risk of VF; 75% decrease in oxygen consumption
Profound	20	68	Lowest resumption of cardiac electromechanical activity; pulse 20% of normal
	19	66.2	Flat EEG
	18	64.4	Asystole commonly occurs
	14.2	57.6	Lowest accidental hypothermia survival in an infant (76)
	13.7	56.7	Lowest accidental hypothermia survival in an adult (1)
	9	48.2	Lowest therapeutic hypothermia survival (75)

EEG, electroencephalogram; VF, ventricular fibrillation.

can result from an independent focus or by a re-entrant phenomenon. When the heart is cold, there is a large dispersion of repolarization that facilitates the development of a conduction delay. The action potential is also prolonged, and this increases the temporal dispersion of the recovery of excitability. Asystole and VF may occur spontaneously when the core temperature falls below 25°C. Putative ancillary causes include tissue hypoxia, physical jostling, electrophysiologic or acid–base disturbances, and autonomic dysfunction.

The term *core temperature afterdrop* refers to a further decline in an individual's core temperature after removal from the cold. The two major processes that contribute to core temperature afterdrop are simple temperature equilibration across a gradient and circulatory changes. Countercurrent cooling of the blood, which is perfusing cold tissues, results in a temperature decline until the gradient is eliminated (16,17).

Hypothermia initially stimulates respiration. This is followed by a progressive decrease in the respiratory minute volume (RMV), which is proportional to the decreasing metabolism. As a result, carbon dioxide production decreases 50% with an 8°C fall in temperature. The normal stimuli for respiratory control are altered in severe hypothermia, and carbon dioxide retention with respiratory acidosis can occur. Numerous other pathophysiologic issues adversely affect the respiratory system. These include cold-induced viscous bronchorrhea, decreased ciliary motility, and pulmonary edema (Table 2).

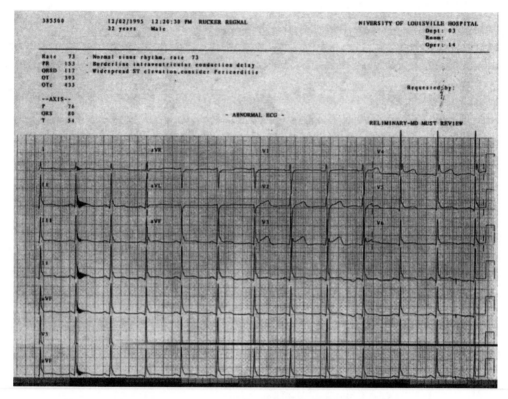

Fig. 1. Prominent J waves are commonly not computer interpretable.

Table 2
Hypothermia Oxygenation Issues

Beneficial	Detrimental
Linear disease in oxygen consumption	Shivering and rewarming will acutely increase consumption
Increased oxygen solubility in plasma	Tissue perfusion impaired by hyperviscosity and vasoconstriction
Acidosis and hypercapnia shift the oxyhemoglobin dissociation curve to the right	Temperature depression shifts the oxyhemo-globin dissociation curve to the left
	Pulmonic dysfunction—V/Q mismatch, atelectasis, bronchorrhea

The CNS is also progressively depressed, and cerebral metabolism decreases 6–7% for each 1°C decline in temperature. Significant alteration of the brain's electrical activity is noted below 33.5°C, and the electroencephalogram begins to silence around 19–20°C. Cerebral autoregulation is maintained via an increase in vascular resistance until 25°C. In severe hypothermia there is a disproportionately higher redistribution of blood flow to the brain.

Simple exposure to cold induces a diuresis regardless of an individual's state of hydration. Severe hypothermia causes an initial relative central hypervolemia as a consequence of peripheral vasoconstriction. Cold diuresis may act as a volume regulator to diminish the vasoconstriction-induced capacitance vessel overload. Hypothermia depresses renal blood flow, reducing it by 50% at 27–30°C. The kidneys then excrete a large amount of dilute urine, termed "the cold diuresis." Cold diuresis is essentially glomerular filtrate, which does not efficiently clear nitrogenous waste products (18).

As a result of the hypothermic pathophysiology, the physical examination and "vital signs" are often misleading. A relative tachycardia disproportionate to the temperature may reflect secondary issues such as hypovolemia, hypoglycemia, or an overdose. Relative hyperventilation implies an underlying metabolic acidosis or CNS dysfunction. Although the Glasgow Coma Scale is not prognostic during hypothermia, the level of consciousness should be consistent with the temperature unless there is additional anoxic, toxic, traumatic, or infectious impairment.

Management

Hypothermia should be preferably monitored at two sites with continuous core temperature evaluation (19). Readings are least accurate during the transition between cooling, core temperature afterdrop, and rewarming. The rectal temperature can lag behind the brain, and cardiac rewarming and is influenced by lower extremity temperatures and probe placement. The probe should be inserted to 15 cm and not placed in cold feces.

On the other hand, the tympanic temperature equilibrates most rapidly with the core temperature and is closest to the hypothalamic temperature. The reliability of infrared thermography, however, remains uncertain. If the patient is tracheally intubated, an esophageal probe will record falsely elevated with heated inhalation. Nevertheless, the trend line comparing the esophageal and rectal temperature is often helpful.

Pulse oximetry during conditions of poor perfusion, vasoconstriction, and hypothermia may not be accurate (20,21). Similarly, end-tidal carbon dioxide measurements only reliably assess tissue perfusion and tracheal tube placement at normal temperatures. Most of the commercially available devices will not function because airway rewarming requires complete humidification.

Gentle endotracheal intubation is safe during hypothermia (9). Issues that could precipitate dysrhythmias include failure to preoxygenate, mechanical jostling, acid–base changes, or electrolyte fluctuations. Decreased gastric motility and gastric dilatation also occur commonly. The abdominal examination is unreliable because the cold can induce rectus muscle rigidity. A large percentage of moderate and severely hypothermic patients have diminished or absent bowel sounds.

During resuscitation and rewarming, monitor the patient's volume status. Fluids administered intravenously should be heated to 40–42°C (22). Counter-current heat exchangers, and a variety of other blood-warming devices, efficiently heat crystalloids and blood (23). In select cases, central venous pressure measurements may be useful. The clinician should avoid insertion of the central venous catheter into a potentially irritable right atrium. An arterial catheter for continuous monitoring of intra-arterial blood pressure may also facilitate treatment of selected profoundly hypothermic patients. The risk–benefit ratio for pulmonary wedge pressure measurements is an even larger concern than in normothermia. The placement of pulmonary artery catheters theoretically risks perforation of a cold stiff pulmonary artery (24).

Laboratory Evaluations

The ideal acid–base strategy causes the fewest cardiac and CNS complications during rewarming *(25)*. Blood gas analyzers routinely warm blood to 37°C, which increases the partial pressure of dissolved gases. This results in an arterial blood gas (ABG) showing higher oxygen and carbon dioxide levels and a lower pH than the patient's actual in vivo values. The correction of ABGs for temperature is unnecessary as a guide to therapy *(26,27)*. In fact, attempting to maintain a corrected pH at 7.4 and pCO_2 at 40 mmHg during hypothermia depresses cerebral and coronary blood flow, cardiac output, and increases the incidence of VF *(28)*. To accurately interpret uncorrected ABGs, the values should simply be compared with the normal values at 37°C *(29)*.

The buffering capacity of blood is markedly impaired by the cold. In normothermia, when the pCO_2 increases 10 mmHg, the pH decreases 0.08 units. At 28°C, this decrease in pH doubles. Because the neutral pH point of water at 37°C is pH of 6.8, the normal 0.6 unit pH offset between blood and intracellular water should be maintained at all temperatures. Just as the neutral pH rises with cooling, so should actual blood pH.

Intracellular electrochemical neutrality ensures optimal enzymatic function at all temperatures *(26)*. Relative alkalinity affords myocardial protection and improves electrical stability of the heart *(28)*. When the uncorrected pH and pCO_2 are 7.42 and 40 mmHg, respectively, there is acid–base balance at any core temperature. This approach to guide resuscitation is termed the α stat or ectothermic strategy. In induced hypothermia, low concentrations of carbogen (1–5% CO_2 with oxygen) can facilitate acid–base management. Carbogen may eventually prove valuable in the treatment of hypothermia because it flattens and shifts the oxyhemoglobin dissociation curve to the right during conditions with minimal CO_2 production, and helps maintain the uncorrected pCO_2 around 40 mmHg.

A patient's hematocrit (Hct) may be deceptively high as the result of a decreased plasma volume. The Hct level increases 2%/1°C fall in temperature. Therefore, a normal Hct level in a moderate to severely hypothermic patient suggests a pre-existing anemia or acute blood loss.

Frequent evaluation of serum electrolytes is essential, because there are no safe predictors of their values. Changes continuously occur in both membrane permeability and in the efficiency of the sodium-potassium pump. The patient's pre-existing physiologic status, the severity and chronicity of hypothermia, and the method of rewarming will alter the serum electrolyte values.

Hypothermia usually induces an increased natriuresis. Preexisting gastrointestinal losses or previous diuretic treatment may also contribute to sodium loss. Patients with normal sodium and osmolality values may have preexisting sodium overload as a result of cirrhosis, nephrosis, or congestive heart failure. Most patients with chronic hypothermia will be free-water depleted, which will elevate their sodium and osmolality values.

The plasma potassium level reflects the underlying pathophysiology. The most clinically relevant abnormality is hyperkalemia, which is often associated with metabolic acidosis, rhabdomyolysis, or renal failure. An important caveat is that hypothermia enhances the cardiac toxicity and obscures the premonitory EKG changes associated with hyperkalemia. Conditions associated with hypokalemia include preexisting diabetic ketoacidosis, hypopituitarism, inappropriate secretion of antidiuretic hormone, previous diuretic therapy, and alcoholism *(30)*.

The blood urea nitrogen (BUN) and creatinine levels will often be elevated as a result of impaired glomerular filtration or with pre-existing renal disease. With dynamic hypothermic fluid shifts, the hematocrit and the BUN levels are inadequate indicators of a patient's actual fluid status.

An acute cold exposure initially causes hyperglycemia through catecholamine-induced glycogenolysis, diminished insulin release, and inhibition of cellular membrane glucose carrier systems. Chronic hypothermia with antecedent shivering produces glycogen depletion that predisposes to hypoglycemia. The symptoms of hypoglycemia may be masked by hypothermia, and a cold-induced renal glycosuria may be observed in hypoglycemic patients.

When hyperglycemia persists during rewarming, the cause may be hemorrhagic pancreatitis or diabetic ketoacidosis. Because insulin is progressively ineffective below 32°C, active rewarming is essential.

A physiologic increase in coagulation occurs with hypothermia, and a disseminated intravascular coagulation type of syndrome occurs. The causes are multifactorial, including catecholamine or steroid release, simple circulatory collapse and release of tissue thromboplastin from cold, ischemic tissue (31).

In hypothermic patients, the activated clotting factor enzymes are depressed by the cold (32). The clotting prolongation is proportional to the number of steps in the cascade. Because the kinetic tests of coagulation are always performed in the laboratory at 37°C, there will be a disparity between the clinically evident in vivo coagulopathy and the deceptively "normal" prothrombin time or partial thromboplastin time or international normalized ratio reported by the laboratory (33). The only effective treatment is rewarming, not administration of clotting factors. Additionally, cold-induced thrombocytopenia may result from either direct bone marrow suppression or hepatosplenic sequestration. Platelet dysfunction is also caused by decreased thromboxane B_2 production (34,35).

Hypothermia compromises host defenses. Many of the usual signs of infection, complicating cardiopulmonary and other diseases, will not be present. In addition to the absence of fever, the absence of leukocytosis does not exclude infection. Splenic, hepatic, and splanchnic sequestration in hypothermia decreases leukocyte counts.

Shaking, rigors, and chills during sepsis mimic shivering. Diminished bone marrow release and circulation of neutrophils, along with impaired neutrophil migration and bacterial phagocytosis, predispose to infection. Routine antibiotic prophylaxis is only warranted, especially at the age extremes, if the clinical picture is consistent with sepsis or if there is failure to rewarm.

Cold exposure normally induces adrenal unresponsiveness to adrenocorticotrophic hormone (ACTH). As a result, decreased adrenal reserve can be misdiagnosed in hypothermia. An acute cold stress initially stimulates cortisol secretion that may already be elevated as a result of an underlying stress. The percentage of cortisol bound to protein is increased with hypothermia, and therefore the active free fraction is decreased. If a patient fails to rewarm, consider the possibility of adrenocortical insufficiency or steroid dependence.

Empiric treatment with thyroxine should be reserved for patients thought to be myxedematous. Thyroid hormone replacement is recommended if a history of hypothyroidism is present, a suggestive neck scar is present, or the patient's rate of rewarming is too slow. Administration of intravenous levothyroxine results in a smooth effect after the onset of action at 6–12 hours. This is evidenced by improvement in the vital signs and the rewarming rate. If there is no improvement, L-triiodothyronine should also be given every 6 hours through a nasogastric tube (30).

Cardiac Pharmacology

The efficacy of most cardiac and other medications is temperature dependent, because protein binding increases during hypothermia and liver metabolism is decreased. Predictably, the effects of hypothermia on the autonomic nervous system vary. In primate studies, the sympathetic nervous system responds rapidly to cooling from 37 to 31°C *(36)*. It then switches off around 29°C, which suggests that some catecholamine support is useful in that temperature range *(37)*. Low-dosage catecholamine infusions should be considered in euvolemic patients who do not respond to rewarming and remain disproportionately hypotensive.

Atrial Arrhythmias

All atrial arrhythmias, including atrial fibrillation (AF), should normally have a slow ventricular response during hypothermia. If a rapid ventricular response is observed, common causes include hypovolemia, hypoglycemia or a cyclic antidepressant overdose. AF is commonly found below 32°C and usually converts spontaneously during rewarming. Digitalis, like insulin, is ineffective and not indicated. Hypothermia renders the negative inotropic effects of calcium channel blockers redundant.

The electrophysiologic AH interval prolongation is unresponsive to atropine. Mesenteric embolization is a potential hazard when the rhythm spontaneously converts to sinus rhythm during rewarming, although with chronic hypothermia, there is usually a coagulopathy.

In essence, all new atrial arrhythmias will usually convert spontaneously during rewarming, and should be considered innocent. Efforts should be directed toward correcting any acid–base, fluid, and electrolyte imbalances, although avoiding administration of atrial anti-arrhythmics.

Ventricular Arrhythmias

The prophylaxis and treatment of ventricular arrhythmias is more problematic. The past cardiac history from the hypothermia patient is often unavailable. Pre-existing chronic premature ventricular contractions may be suppressed during hypothermia and recur during rewarming. Most hypothermia-induced ventricular dysrrhythmias convert spontaneously during rewarming. As a result, ventricular arrhythmias should generally be treated expectantly. The terminal cardiac arrest rhythm in monitored hypothermic patients is commonly not VF, but asystole *(38)*. In hypothermia, asystole that develops during rewarming is not a more ominous rhythm than VF.

Temperature depression progressively decreases the conduction velocity and increases the action potential duration (APD). As a result, the ideal ventricular anti-arrhythmic would not further decrease conduction through the His-Purkinje system but would shorten the APD. Lengthening the APD only in warmer regions would reduce dispersion and stabilize the rhythm.

In normothermia, the class IA ventricular antidysrhythmics have numerous unfavorable characteristics including negative inotropic and indirect anticholinergic effects. These agents moderately decrease conduction velocity and depolarization, although prolonging the APD and repolarization. One agent in this group, procainamide, increases the incidence of VF during hypothermia. Another drug in this group, quinidine, surprisingly has prevented VF during induced profound hypothermia. The cardiac effects of disopyramide are unclear.

Class 1B ventricular antidysrhythmics, in contrast, minimally slow conduction and depolarization although shortening the APD and repolarization. Clinically, lidocaine appears to have minimal effects. Class 1C agents such as encainide and flecainide, although unstudied in this setting, would appear pharmacologically hazardous. Conduction and depolarization are markedly slowed, and the APD and repolarization are prolonged.

Although class III agents prolong the APD, they possess variable direct antifibrillatory action. Bretylium tosylate produces a chemical sympathectomy and is both an anti-arrhythmic and an antifibrillatory agent. Bretylium increases the VF threshold, the APD and the effective refractory period (EFP). Interestingly, at least at normal temperatures, the antifibrillatory effects occur more acutely than the anti-arrhythmic effects.

The effect of bretylium on plasma catecholamines and electrically induced arrhythmias is reported in hypothermia. Because catecholamine levels increase during cooling, the demonstrated protection appears to be as a result of an alteration of the electrophysiologic properties of the cardiac tissues (39).

Bretylium tosylate has been very effective in several animal studies. Unlike under normothermic conditions, bretylium increases the VF threshold prior to increasing the APD and the ERP when cold (40). Clinical chemical defibrillations with bretylium in severely hypothermic humans are reported (41,42). The optimal dosage and ideal infusion rates are unknown but normothermic guidelines are commonly observed. The commercial availability of bretylium varies internationally.

The safety of amiodarone, another class III agent that possesses antifibrillatory activity, is unknown during hypothermic conditions. Magnesium sulfate at an intravenous dose of 100 mg/kg has spontaneously defibrillated many CPB patients with induced hypothermia.

Cardiac pacing for hypothermia-induced bradydysrhythmias is rarely indicated during rewarming. External noninvasive pacing by means of large low-resistance electrodes would appear to be a preferable alternative to potentially hazardous transvenous pacing (43). New bradydysrhythmias that develop after rewarming rarely require pacing.

Blood flow during CPR also differs in hypothermia (44). The consensus guideline is that CPR should be initiated unless do-not-resuscitate status is documented and verified, obvious lethal injuries are present, any signs of life are present, rescuers are endangered by evacuation delays or overriding triage considerations, or chest wall compression is impossible (9). The role of a "thoracic pump" with the heart as a passive conduit during closed chest compressions is an attractive hypothesis to explain clinical observations. The "thoracic pump" model suggests that phasic alterations in the intrathoracic pressure generated by compressions are applied equally to all thoracic vessels and cardiac chambers. Competent venous valves are located at the thoracic outlet. These valves prevent retrograde transmission of increased intrathoracic pressure into the venous circulation. The resultant arteriovenous pressure gradients generate supradiaphragmatic antegrade flow.

During compression systole, blood circulates through the left side of the heart, which is functionally a passive conduit. During compression, blood moves through the mitral valve into the systemic circulation. The mitral valve remains patent during systole and blood continues to circulate through the left side of the heart.

Mechanical cardiac "massage" requires some degree of pliancy and may be a misnomer during hypothermic conditions. Consider the description of one survivor following 120 minutes of closed-chest compression: "At thoracotomy, the refrigerated . . . heart was found to be hard as stone and it is hardly conceivable how effective external cardiac massage could have been *(45)* . . . ."

Clearly, closed-chest compressions are effective under hypothermic conditions in humans. In the multicenter survey of 428 hypothermic cases, 9 of 27 patients receiving field-initiated CPR survived, as did 6 of 14 who had CPR initiated in the emergency department *(9)*. Regional blood flow during hypothermic cardiac arrest in swine is reported *(44)*. The cardiac output, cerebral and myocardial blood flows averaged 50, 55, and 31% of those achieved during normothermic conditions with closed-chest compressions. Unlike normothermic conditions, blood flow did *not* decrease over time.

Rewarming Options

The indications for using active rewarming techniques include: cardiovascular instability, poikilothermia (below 32.2°C), inadequate rate or failure to rewarm, endocrinologic insufficiency, traumatic or toxicologic induced peripheral vasodilation, or secondary hypothermia (Table 3; *46–48*). Heat can be provided externally or internally *(49)*. Forced-air warming systems will efficiently transfer heat directly to the skin *(50–52)*. The air exits apertures on the patient side of the cover, which allows a convective transfer of heat. Forced-air rewarming can decrease shivering and the attendant metabolic stress, without inducing rewarming shock and core temperature afterdrop *(53)*.

In contrast, immersion in a bath of 40°C complicates monitoring or resuscitation. Other rewarming options include plumbed garments that recirculate warm fluids, hot water bottles, heating pad and radiant sources. Thermal injury to vasoconstricted hypoperfused skin is a common hazard with local heat application.

Arteriovenous anastomoses rewarming is another non-invasive AER technique *(54–56)*. Exogenous heat is provided by immersion of the lower parts of the extremities (hands, forearms, feet, calves) in 44–45° C water. Heat opens the arteriovenous anastomoses (AVA) that are 1 mm below the epidermal surface in the digits *(57)*. A permutation of AVA rewarming is negative pressure rewarming, which is intended to open the AVAs. To initiate negative pressure rewarming, the forearm is inserted through an acrylic tubing sleeve device fitted with a neoprene collar. After a –40 mmHg vacuum pressure is created, heat is applied over the dilated AVA *(58)*. The clinical utility of this technique, if any, remains to be determined.

Active Core Rewarming

Airway rewarming, as an adjunct to the other active core rewarming (ACR) techniques, is noninvasive, assures adequate oxygenation, and will decrease respiratory heat loss. The respiratory tract is a very limited site for heat exchange. A sufficient respiratory minute volume (RMV) and complete humidification are necessary for maximal heat delivery *(59)*. The efficiency of heated mask ventilation is also being explored. Another option is heated inhalation through face mask continuous positive airway pressure (CPAP *[60]*). A thermal countercurrent heat exchanger, known as the rete mirabile, is present in the cerebrovascular bed of humans. In theory, preferentially rewarming the brainstem could facilitate earlier resumption of central thermoregulatory control. Additional benefits of airway rewarming include the stimulation of pulmonary cilia, a decrease in pulmonary secretion viscosity, and a reduction of cold-induced bronchorrhea. Pulmonic absorption occurs without adverse affects on surfactant or increased pulmonary congestion.

Table 3
Indications for Active Rewarming

1. Poikilothermia
2. Cardiovascular instability/collapse
3. Vasodilation—toxicologic or traumatic
4. Secondary hypothermia—endocrine, predisposing issues
5. Inadequate passive rate of rewarming

Maintenance of sufficient oxygenation is critical in moderate and severe hypothermia. The effects of hypothermia, pH, $PaCO_2$, and the level of 2,3-diphosphoglycerate on the shift of the oxyhemoglobin dissociation curve decrease the capacity of hemoglobin to unload oxygen to the tissues (61). Despite lower metabolic requirements, this decrease in "functional" hemoglobin, combined with a depressed RMV, results in minimum oxygen reserves (Table 2).

Most humidifiers are manufactured in accordance with the International Standards regulations. The humidifier will not exceed 41°C close to the patient outlet with a 6-foot tubing length. Strategies to circumvent the 41°C ceiling include reduction of tubing length, adding additional heat sources, disabling the humidifier safety system, and placing the temperature probe outside the patient circuit (62). All modified equipment should be labeled to avoid routine use. A volume ventilator with a heated cascade humidifier can also deliver CPAP or positive end-expiratory pressure (PEEP) if needed during rewarming.

Heated Irrigation

Heat transfer from irrigation fluids depends on the surface area available for heat exchange. Gastric or colonic irrigation can cause fluid and electrolyte fluxes, and is rarely worth the effort. On the other hand, closed thoracic lavage rewarming in accidental hypothermia is more efficient (63). Two large-bore thoracostomy tubes are inserted into one or both hemithoraces. One is placed anteriorly in the second or third intercostal space at the midclavicular line. The other is placed in the posterior axillary line at the fifth to sixth intercostal space. Sterile normal saline ideally in 3-L bags is heated to 40° to 42°C and infused and drained in a nonrecycled sterile system (64).

The efficiency of heat transfer varies with the flow rate and dwell times. Pleural adhesions can prevent adequate drainage, which must be ensured to prevent intrathoracic hypertension. Unless there are other indications for a thoracostomy tube, thoracic lavage should be reserved for severely hypothermic patients who do not respond to standard techniques (65,66). Left-sided thoracostomy tube insertion into perfusing patients could easily induce VF.

The option of closed sterile thoracic lavage seems a natural selection during CA resuscitations. In perfusing patients, this technique should clearly be considered potentially hazardous unless extra-corporeal rewarming capability is immediately available. The clinically reported infusion rates range from 180–550 mL per minute. The overall rate of rewarming should easily equal or exceed that achievable with peritoneal lavage, with the added benefit of preferential mediastinal rewarming. Additionally, closed-chest compressions during CA can maintain perfusion. Open cardiac massage of a rigid contracted heart may not be possible in severe cases prior to bypass. Thus, mediastinal irrigation should be avoided when bypass is impossible (45).

Mediastinal irrigation and direct myocardial lavage should only be considered in patients without spontaneous perfusion. After a standard left lateral thoracotomy incision, leave the pericardium intact unless an effusion or tamponade is present. The heart is bathed in 1–2 L of an isotonic solution heated to 40°C for several minutes. The fluid is suctioned and the lavage repeated. Internal defibrillation is attempted at 1–2°C intervals after the myocardial temperature exceeds 26–28°C. When a perfusing rhythm is achieved, lavage is continued until the myocardial temperature exceeds 32°C. A median sternotomy approach allows ventricular decompression in addition to direct defibrillation.

Peritoneal lavage should not be routinely used in treating stable mildly hypothermic patients. In severe cases, the transfer of heat is lower than that achieved with cardiac bypass or hemodialysis. The most common irrigant is normal saline or lactated Ringers, but standard 1.5% dextrose dialysate solution with optional potassium supplementation is another option. The isotonic dialysate is heated to 40–45°C. Up to 2 L are then infused (10–20 cc/kg), retained for 15–20 minutes, and subsequently aspirated. The usual clinical exchange rate is 6 L per hour, which yields rewarming rates of 1–3°C per hour. An alternative to consider in severe cases is a larger catheter placed with the Seldinger technique. The higher drainage capability will markedly increase the exchange rates and minimize dwell times necessary for maximal thermal transfer. The flow rate via gravity through regular tubing is approx 500 cc per minute, which can be tripled under infusion pressure (67).

A unique advantage of peritoneal dialysis when hemodialysis in unavailable is overdose and rhabdomyolysis detoxification. Additionally, direct hepatic rewarming reactivates detoxification and conversion enzymes. Peritoneal dialysis will worsen preexistent hypokalemia. Vigilant electrolyte monitoring is essential prior to empiric modification of the dialysate. The presence of adhesions from previous abdominal surgery will increase the complication rate and minimize heat exchange. This technique can be used in combination with all available rewarming techniques in CA patients.

EXTRACORPOREAL REWARMING

The four common techniques to directly rewarm blood are hemodialysis, venovenous rewarming, arteriovenous rewarming, and cardiopulmonary bypass (CPB; Table 4).

Standard *hemodialysis* is portable, efficient, and should be considered in perfusing patients with electrolyte abnormalities, renal failure, or intoxication with a dialyzable substance. Two-way flow catheters allow cannulation of a single vessel. A Drake-Willock single-needle dialysis catheter can be used with a portable hemodialysis machine and external warmer. After central venous cannulation, exchange cycle volumes of 200–250 mL per minute are possible.

Although heat exchange is less than with standard two-vessel hemodialysis, the ease of percutaneous subclavian vein placement is a major advantage. Hemodialysis via two separate single-lumen catheters placed in the femoral vein can achieve continuous blood flow at 450–500 mL per minute. Hemodialysis can be performed heparin-free and can transfer more heat than peritoneal lavage.

Extracorporeal *venovenous rewarming* is another option for warming and recirculating blood. With this technique, blood is removed, usually from a central venous catheter, heated to 40°C, and returned via a second central or large peripheral venous catheter. Flow rates of 150–400 mL per minute are achievable (68). The circuit is not complex and is more efficient than many other nonbypass modalities. There is no oxygenator and

Table 4
ECR Considerations

HD	Widely available
	Adjust electrolyte/toxicologic derangements
	Exchange cycle volumes 200–500 mL per minute
	ROR 2–3°C per hour
VV	Circuit nonbypass modality
	Volume infusion to augment cardiac output
	Flow rates of 150–400 mLl per minute
	ROR 2–3°C per hour
AVR	Percutaneous Seldinger technique
	Requires arterial cannulation and BP >60 mmHg
	No need for perfusionist/pump/anticoagulation
	Average flow rates 225–375 mL per minute
	ROR 3–4°C per hour
CPB	Perfusate core temperature gradient—consider 5–10°C
	Flow rates 3–7 L per minute (average 3–4 L per minute)
	ROR 5–9.5°C per hour
	Full circulatory support

HD, hemodialysis; VV, venovenous; AVR, arteriovenous; CPB, cardiopulmonary bypass; ECR, extracorporeal rewarming; ROR rate of rewarming.

because the method does not provide full circulatory support, volume infusion is the only option to augment inadequate cardiac output.

Continuous arteriovenous rewarming (CAVR) is another option when the systolic blood pressure is at least 60 mmHg. CAVR involves the use of percutaneously inserted femoral arterial and contralateral femoral venous catheters *(69)*. The Seldinger technique is used to insert the 8.5 Fr catheters. Because the catheters are 8.5 Fr, the patient must weigh at least 40 kg. Heparin-bonded tubing circuits obviate the need for systemic anticoagulation. CAVR has principally been performed on hypothermic traumatized patients.

The blood pressure of spontaneously perfusing hypothermic patients creates a functional arteriovenous fistula by diverting part of the cardiac output out the femoral artery through a counter-current heat exchanger. The heated blood is then returned with admixed heated crystalloids via the femoral vein. Additional fluids are infused for hypotension, and the rate of rewarming exceeds hemodialysis. CAVR does not require the specialized equipment and perfusionist necessary for cardiopulmonary bypass. The average flow rates are 225–375 ml per minute, resulting in a rate of rewarming of 3–4°C per hour.

For CPB, the standard femoral–femoral circuit includes arterial and venous catheters, a mechanical pump, a membrane or bubble oxygenator, and a heat exchanger *(70)*. A 16–30-Fr venous cannula is inserted via the femoral vein to the junction of the right atrium and inferior vena cava. The tip of the shorter 16–20-Fr arterial cannula is inserted 5 cm or just proximal to the aortic bifurcation. Supplemental transesophageal echocardiography may be required to evaluate the ventricular load and valvular function.

Systemic anticoagulation, which previously limited clinical applicability, can be selectively avoided. Heparin-coated perfusion equipment, and the use of nonthrombogenic pumps, are options. Another favorable hemodynamic factor is the enhanced physiologic fibrinolysis seen in the first hour of CPB.

Heated, oxygenated blood is returned via the femoral artery. Femoral flow rates of 2–3 L per minute can elevate the core temperature 1–2°C every 3–5 minutes. Most pumps are capable of generating full flow up to 7 L per minute. In one review the mean CPB temperature increase was 9.5°C per hour *(71)*. The optimal temperature gradient and bypass rewarming rates are unclear. An excessive temperature gradient between brain tissue and circulant may adversely affect electroencephalogram regeneration. Another concern is the possibility of increased bubbling if high perfusate temperature gradients are used. Most current investigators use 5°C or 10°C gradients *(72)*.

The major advantage of CPB in perfusing patients is the preservation of flow if mechanical cardiac activity is lost during rewarming *(73)*. Potential candidates for CPB are patients who do not respond to less invasive rewarming techniques, those with completely frozen extremities, and those with rhabdomyolysis that is accompanied by major electrolyte disturbances *(74)*.

With any of these four techniques, rapid acceleration of the rate of rewarming per se does not necessarily improve survival rates. Complications of rapid rewarming in severe hypothermia include disseminated intravascular coagulation, pulmonary edema, hemolysis, and acute tubular necrosis.

Extracorporeal blood rewarming should be attempted in hypothermic cardiac arrest patients when no contraindications to CPR exist. Patients with secondary hypothermia are often not appropriate candidates. Extracorporeal blood rewarming is unlikely to succeed below 10–12°C *(25)*. Resuscitation should be terminated if frozen or clotted intravascular contents are identified. The most vexing decision often centers on the issue of potential survivability. There may never be a validated neurologically predictive instrument in hypothermia. Cardiopulmonary arrest (CPA) is more favorable when it is a direct result of hypothermia, in contrast to asphyxia, acidosis, or cardiac arrest and the subsequent postmortem decline in core temperature. Because outcome is difficult to predict, the type and severity of the underlying or precipitating disease process is the major determinant *(1,75,76)*. Patient age is not an independent predictor of mortality *(77)*.

Trauma, infection, and toxin ingestions also affect survival unpredictably *(78)*. The search for a valid triage marker of death continues *(79,80)*. Grave prognostic indicators include evidence of intravascular thrombosis (fibrinogen less than 50 mg/dL), cell lysis (hyperkalemia more than 10 mEq/L), and ammonia levels greater than 250 μmol/L, and anoxia with severe acidosis *(81)*.

SUMMARY

Because hypoxemia is the rule following hypothermic CA, the goal with supplemental oxygen should be normoxia. The prolonged use of 100% oxygen after the return of spontaneous circulation may increase oxidative brain injury by generating reactive oxygen species including superoxide and hydrogen peroxide. The clinician should minimize positive end-expiratory pressure unless it is essential to maintain normoxia, because it decreases cerebral venous outflow.

As in normothermia, cerebral vasculature autoregulation may be lost after global brain ischemia, and yet hypocarbia-induced vasoconstrictive mechanisms remain intact. Therefore, avoid protracted hyperventilation without carbogen because hypothermic CO_2 production may be minimal.

Posthypothermic hyperglycemia is also potentially detrimental, because glucose levels over 250 mg/dL are associated with lactate generation and exacerbation of metabolic acidosis. During resuscitation, avoid dextrose containing solutions without evidence of hypoglycemia. Global brain ischemia can also induce seizures. The role of seizure prophylaxis during hypothermia is unclear, as is the role of continuous electroencephalogram monitoring in select cases. Diphenylhydantoin or fosphenytoin, which do not mask the evolving neurological examination during rewarming, would seem to be the agents of choice. If seizures are clinically evident, aggressive treatment is indicated, because seizures dramatically increase the brain's metabolic demands at any temperature.

When reperfusion is re-established, the initial transient hyperemic period is characterized by increased CBF with low oxygen consumption. This lasts for minutes, and is followed by the "no reflow" phase, which lasts for hours. Some of this delayed hypoperfusion is as a result of a secondary vasospasm. Reperfusion after rewarming is also characterized by both cytotoxic edema during ischemia, and vasogenic edema as a result of blood–brain barrier injury.

In summary, the final common pathway for the demise of many hypothermic patients is a very dynamic neuronal injury. During rewarming, avoid issues known to exacerbate the adverse neuronal responses to cerebral ischemia: hypoperfusion, hypoxia, hyperglycemia, hyperoxia, and seizures. The initial ideal target temperature during rewarming may well be less than 37°C.

REFERENCES

1. Gilbert M, Busund R, Skagseth A, Nilsen PA, Solbo JP. Resuscitation from accidental hypothermia of 13.7 degrees C with circulatory arrest [letter]. Lancet 2000; 355:375,376.
2. Kammersgaard LP, Rasmussen BH, Jorgensen HS. Feasibility and safety of inducing modest hypothermia in awake patients with acute stroke through surface cooling: A case-control study: the Copenhagen Stroke Study. Stroke 2000; 31:2251–2256.
3. Jiang J, Yu M, Zhu C. Effect of long-term mild hypothermia therapy in patients with severe traumatic brain injury: 1-year follow-up review of 87 cases [see comments]. J Neurosurg 2000; 93:546–549.
4. Marion DW, Penrod LE, Kelsey SF, et al. Treatment of traumatic brain injury with moderate hypothermia. N Engl J Med 1997; 336:540–546.
5. Mills WJ, Jr. Field care of the hypothermic patient. Int J Sports Med 1992; Suppl:S199–S202.
6. Miller JW, Danzl DF, and Thomas DM. Urban accidental hypothermia: 135 cases. Ann E Emerg Med 1980; 9:456–461.
7. Marsigny B. Medical mountain rescue in the Mont-Blanc massif. Wilderness Environ Med 1999; 10: 152–156.
8. Hypothermia-related deaths—Alaska, October 1998–April 1999, and trends in the United States, 1979–1996. MMWR 2000; 1949:11–14.
9. Danzl DF, Pozos RS, Auerbach PS, et al. Multicenter hypothermia survey. Ann of Emerg Med 1987; 16:1042–1055.
10. Irwin BR. A case report of hypothermia in the wilderness. Wild Environ Med 2002; 13:125–128.
11. Pozos RS, Israel D, McCutcheon R, Wittmers LE, Jr, Sessler D. Human studies concerning thermal-induced shivering, postoperative "shivering," and cold-induced vasodilation. Ann Emerg Med 1987; 16:1037–1041.
12. Giesbrecht GG. Cold stress, near drowning and accidental hypothermia: a review. Aviat Space Environ Med 2000; 71:733–752.
13. Sessler DI. Perioperative heat balance. Anesthesiology. 2000; 92:578–596.
14. Vassallo SU, Delaney KA, Hoffman RS, Slater W, Goldfrank LR. A prospective evaluation of the electrocardiographic manifestations of hypothermia. Acad Emerg Med 1999; 6:1121–1126.
15. Danzl DF, O'Brien DJ. The ECG computer program: mort de froid. J Wilderness Med 1992; 3:328,329.
16. Giesbrecht GG, Johnston CE, Bristow GK. The convective afterdrop component during hypothermic exercise decreased with delayed exercise onset. Aviat Space Environ Med 1998; 69:17–22.
17. Hayward JS, Eckerson JD, Kemna D. Thermal and cardiovascular changes during three methods of resuscitation from mild hypothermia. Resuscitation 1984; 11:21–33.
18. Lloyd EL. Accidental hypothermia. Resuscitation 1996; 32:111–124.

19. Nicholson RW, Iserson KV. Core temperature measurement in hypovolemic resuscitation. Ann Emerg Med 1991; 20:62–65.

20. Clayton DG, Webb RK, Ralston AC, Duthie D, Runciman WB. A comparison of the performance of 20 pulse oximeters under conditions of poor perfusion [see comments]. Anaesthesia 1991; 46:3–10.

21. Kober A, Scheck T, Lieba F, et al. The influence of active warming on signal quality of pulse oximetry in prehospital trauma care. Anes Anal 2002; 95:961–966.

22. Silbergleit R, Satz W, Lee DC, McNamara RM. Hypothermia from realistic fluid resuscitation in a model of hemorrhagic shock. Ann Emerg Med 1998; 31:339–343.

23. Handrigan MT, Wright RO, Becker BM, Linakis JG, Jay GD. Factors and methodology in achieving ideal delivery temperatures for intravenous and lavage fluid in hypothermia. Am J Emerg Med 1997; 15:350–353.

24. Cohen JA, Blackshear RH, Gravenstein N, Woeste J. Increased pulmonary artery perforating potential of pulmonary artery catheters during hypothermia. J Cardiothoracic Vas Anest 1991; 5:234–236.

25. Danzl DF, Pozos RS. Accidental hypothermia. N Engl J Med 1994; 331:1756–1760.

26. Baraka AS, Baroody MA, Haroun ST, et al. Effect of alpha-stat versus pH-stat strategy on oxyhemoglobin dissociation and whole-body oxygen consumption during hypothermic cardiopulmonary bypass. Anest Anal 1992; 74:32–37.

27. Delaney KA, Howland MA, Vassallo S, Goldfrank, LR. Assessment of acid-base disturbances in hypothermia and their physiologic consequences [review]. Ann Emerg Med 1989; 18:72–82.

28. Kroncke GM, Nichols RD, Mendenhall JT, Myerowitz PD, Starling JR. Ectothermic philosophy of acid-base balance to prevent fibrillation during hypothermia. Arch Surg 1986; 121:303,304.

29. McInerney JJ, Breakell A, Madira W, Davies TG, Evans PA. Accidental hypothermia and active rewarming: the metabolic and inflammatory changes observed above and below 32 degrees C. Emerg Med J 2002; 19:219–223.

30. Danzl DF, Lloyd E. Treatment of Accidental Hypothermia. In: Pandolf KB, Burr RE, Wenger CB, Pozos, RS, eds. Medical Aspects of Harsh Environments, vol.1. In Zajtchuk R, Bellamy RF, eds. Textbook of Military Medicine. Washington, DC: Department of the Army, Office of the Surgeon General, and Borden Institute, 2001:491-529.

31. Cosgriff N, Moore EE, Sauaia A, et al. Predicting life-threatening coagulopathy in the massively transfused trauma patient: hypothermia and acidoses revisited. J Trauma 1997; 42:857–861.

32. Eddy VA, Morris JA, Jr, Cullinane DC. Hypothermia, coagulopathy, and acidosis. Surg Clin North Am 2000; 80:845–854.

33. Rohrer MJ and Natale AM. Effect of hypothermia on the coagulation cascade. Crit Care Med 1992; 20: 1402–1405.

34. Watts, DD, Trask A, Soeken K, et al. Hypothermic coagulopathy in trauma: effect of varying levels of hypothermia on enzyme speed, platelet function, and fibrinolytic activity. J Trauma 1998; 44:846–854.

35. Reed RL, Bracey AW, Jr, Hudson JD, Miller TA, Fischer RP. Hypothermia and blood coagulation: dissociation between enzyme activity and clotting factor levels. Circ Shock 1990; 32:141–152.

36. Chernow B, Lake CR, Zaritsky A, et al. Sympathetic nervous system "switch off" with severe hypothermia. Crit Care Med 1983; 11:677–680.

37. Weiss SJ, Muniz A, Ernst AA, Lippton HL. The physiological response to norepinephrine during hypothermia and rewarming. Resuscitation 1998; 39:189–195.

38. Rankin AC, Rae AP. Cardiac arrhythmias during rewarming of patients with accidental hypothermia. Br Med J 1984; 289:874–877.

39. Orts A, Alcaraz C, Delaney KA, Goldfrank LR, Turndorf H, Puig MM. Bretylium tosylate and electrically induced cardiac arrhythmias during hypothermia in dogs. Am J Emerg Med 1992; 10:311–316.

40. Murphy K, Nowak RM, Tomlanovich MC. Use of bretylium tosylate as prophylaxis and treatment in hypothermic ventricular fibrillation in the canine model. Ann Emerg Med 1986; 15:1160–1166.

41. Kochar G, Kahn SE, Kotler MN. Bretylium tosylate and ventricular fibrillation in hypothermia [letter]. Ann Int Med 1986; 105:624.

42. Danzl DF, Sowers MB, Vicario SJ, Thomas DM, Miller JW. Chemical ventricular defibrillation in severe accidental hypothermia. Ann Emerg Med 1982; 11:698,699.

43. Dixon RG, Dougherty JM, White LJ, Lombino D, Rusnak RR. Transcutaneous pacing in a hypothermic-dog model. Ann Emerg Med 1997; 29:602–606.

44. Maningas PA, DeGuzman LR, Hollenbach SJ, Volk KA, Bellamy RF. Regional blood flow during hypothermic arrest. Ann Emerg Med 1986; 15:390–396.

45. Althaus U, Aeberhard P, Schupbach P. Management of profound accidental hypothermia with cardiorespiratory arrest. Ann Surg 1982; 195:492–495.

46. Danzl DF. Hypothermia. Seminars in Respiratory and Critical Care Medicine 2002; 23:57–68.
47. Lazar HL. The treatment of hypothermia. New Engl J Med 1997; 337:1545–1547.
48. Rogers I. Which rewarming therapy in hypothermia? A review of the randomized trials. Emerg Med 1997; 9:213–220.
49. Grief R, Rajek A, Laciny S, Bastanmehr H, Sessler DI. Resistive heating is more effective than metallic-foil insulation in an experimental model of accidental hypothermia: a randomized controlled trial. Ann Emerg Med 2000; 35:337–345.
50. Kornberger E. Forced air surface rewarming in patients with severe accidental hypothermia. Resuscitation 1999; 41:105–111.
51. Giesbrecht GG, Bristow GK. Recent advances in hypothermia research. Ann NY Acad Sci 1997; 813: 676–681.
52. Goheen MS, Ducharme MB, Kenny GP, et al. Efficacy of forced-air and inhalation rewarming by using a human model for severe hypothermia. J Appl Physiol 1997; 83:1635–1640.
53. Steele MT, Nelson MJ, Sessler DI, et al. Forced air speeds rewarming in accidental hypothermia. Ann Emerg Med 1996; 27:479–484.
54. Vangaard L, et al. Arteriovenous anastomoses (AVA) rewarming in 45°C water is effective in moderately hypothermic subjects. FASEB J 1998; 12:A90.
55. Grahn D, Brock-Utne JG, Watenpaugh DE, Heller HC. Recovery from mild hypothermia can be accelerated by mechanically distending blood vessels in the hand [see comments]. J Appl Physiol 1998; 85:1643–1648.
56. Taguchi A. Negative pressure rewarming vs. Forced air warming in hypothermic postanesthetic volunteers. Anesth Analg 2001; 92:261–266.
57. Ducharme MB, Giesbrecht GG, Frim J, et al. Forced-air rewarming in –20 degrees C simulated field conditions. Ann NY Acad Sci 1997; 813:676–681.
58. Soreide E, Grahn DA, Brock-Utne JG, Rosen L. A non-invasive means to effectively restore normothermia in cold stressed individuals: a preliminary report. J Emerg Med 1999; 17:725–730.
59. Weinberg AD. The role of inhalation rewarming in the early management of hypothermia. Resuscitation 1998; 36:101–104.
60. Canivet JL, Larbuisson R, Lamy M. Interest of face mask-CPAP in one case of severe accidental hypothermia. Acta Anaesthesiol Belg 1989; 40:281–283.
61. Fisher A, Foex P, Emerson PM, Darley JH, Rauscher LA. Oxygen availability during hypothermic cardiopulmonary bypass. Crit Care Med 1977; 5:154–158.
62. Wallace W. Does it make sense to heat gases higher than body temperature for the treatment of cold water near-drowning or hypothermia? A point of view paper. Alaska Med 1997; 39:75–77.
63. Winegard C. Successful treatment of severe hypothermia and prolonged cardiac arrest with closed thoracic cavity lavage. J Emerg Med 1997; 15:629–632.
64. Hall KN and Syverud SA. Closed thoracic cavity lavage in the treatment of severe hypothermia in human beings. Ann Emerg Med 1990; 19:204–206.
65. Iversen RJ, Atkin SH, Jaker MA, Quadrel MA, Tortella BJ, Odom JW. Successful CPR in a severely hypothermic patient using continuous thoracostomy lavage. Ann Emerg Med 1990; 19:1335–1337.
66. Brunette DD, Biros M, Mlinek EJ, Erlandson C, Ruiz E. Internal cardiac massage and mediastinal irrigation in hypothermic cardiac arrest. Am J Emerg Med 1992; 10:32–34.
67. Levitt MA, Kane V, Henderson J, Dryjski M. A comparative rewarming trial of gastric versus peritoneal lavage in a hypothermic model. Am J Emerg Med 1990; 8:285–288.
68. Heise D, Rathgeber J, Burchardi H. Severe, accidental hypothermia: active rewarming with a simple extracorporeal veno-venous warming-circuit. Anaesthesist 1996; 45:1093–1096.
69. Gentilello LM, Jurkovich GJ, et al. Is hypothermia in the victim of major trauma protective or harmful? A randomized, prospective study. Ann Surg 1997; 226:439–447.
70. Walpoth BH, Locher T, Leupi F, Schupbach P, Muhlemann W, Althaus U. Accidental deep hypothermia with cardiopulmonary arrest: extracorporeal blood rewarming in 11 patients. European J Cardio Thoracic Surg 1990; 4:390–393.
71. Splittgerber FH, Talbert JG, Sweezer WP, Wilson RF. Partial cardiopulmonary bypass for core rewarming in profound accidental hypothermia. Am Surgeon 1986; 52:407–412.
72. Bolgiano E, Sykes L, and Barish RA. Accidental hypothermia with cardiac arrest: recovery following rewarming by cardiopulmonary bypass. J Emerg Med 1992; 10:427–433.
73. Brunette DD. and McVaney K. Hypothermic cardiac arrest: an 11 year review of ED management and outcome. Am J Emerg Med 2000; 18:418–422.

74. Roggla M, Frossard M, Wagner A, Holzer M, Bur A, Roggla G. Severe accidental hypothermia with or without hemodynamic instability: rewarming without the use of extracorporeal circulation. Wiener Klinische Wochenschrift 2002; 114:315–20.

75. Niazi SA and Lewis FJ. Profound hypothermia in man: report of a case. Ann Surg 1958; 147:264–266.

76. Dobson JAR, Burgess JJ. Resuscitation of severe hypothermia by extracorporeal rewarming in a child. J Trauma 1996; 40:483–485.

77. Danzl DF, Hedges JR, and Pozos RS. Hypothermia outcome score: development and implications. Crit Care Med 1989; 17:227–231.

78. Walpoth BH, Walpoth-Aslan BN, Mattle HP, et al. Outcome of survivors of accidental deep hypothermia and circulatory arrest treated with extracorporeal blood warming. N Engl J Med 1997; 337:1500–1505.

79. Pillgram-Larsen J, Svennevig JL, et al. Accidental hypothermia. Risk factors in 29 patients with body temperature of 30 degrees C and below [Norwegian]. Tidsskrift for Den Norske Laegeforening 1991; 111:180–183.

80. Schaller MD, Fischer AP, Perret CH. Hyperkalemia: a prognostic factor during acute severe hypothermia. JAMA 1990; 264:1842–1845.

81. Hauty MG, Esrig BC, Hill JG, Long WB. Prognostic factors in severe accidental hypothermia: experience from the Mt. Hood tragedy. J Trauma 1987; 27:1107–1112.

27 Cardiopulmonary Resuscitation in Trauma

Rao R. Ivatury, MD and Kevin R. Ward, MD

INTRODUCTION

Cardiopulmonary resuscitation (CPR) in a patient with multiple injuries involves a different approach than in a nontrauma patient. Although the basic principles are the same as dealt with in other chapters of this book, CPR in the trauma victim has to address prevention of cardiopulmonary failure from problems exclusive to the injured patient. This chapter concentrates on these issues and highlights some of the recent developments in the field.

CARDIOPULMONARY SUPPORT IN THE EMERGENCY DEPARTMENT

Prompt resuscitation of the trauma patient in the emergency department (ED) includes control and/or maintenance of the airway, reversal of life-threatening events (e.g., tension pneumothorax, cardiac tamponade), maintenance of cellular aerobic metabolism by supplemental oxygenation and assisted ventilation, and restoration of normovolemia. One important caveat has developed in volume replacement in recent years: in a bleeding trauma patient, especially after penetrating trauma, aggressive attempts at stabilization of the cardiovascular state by fluid infusion *before* definitive control of bleeding is achieved may lead to a higher morbidity and mortality. This is not a new concept but a resurrection of Cannon's observations after World War I. He pointed out that "hemorrhage in the case of shock may not have occurred to a marked degree because blood pressure has been too low and flow too scant to overcome the obstacle offered by a clot. If the pressure is raised before the surgeon is ready to check any bleeding that may take place, blood that is sorely needed may be lost" *(1)*. The effect of massive, early fluid resuscitation was recently examined critically in hypotensive prehospital trauma patients. Kaweski et al. *(2)* reviewed the records of 6855 hypotensive trauma patients. Fifty-six

From: *Contemporary Cardiology: Cardiopulmonary Resuscitation*
Edited by: J. P. Ornato and M. A. Peberdy © Humana Press Inc., Totowa, NJ

percent of these patients received prehospital fluid resuscitation. Fluid challenge in this group of patients did not improve survival. Bickell et al. *(3)* conducted a prospective trial comparing immediate and delayed fluid resuscitation in 598 adults with penetrating torso injuries who presented with a prehospital systolic blood pressure of less than 90 mmHg. Patients assigned randomly to the immediate-resuscitation group received standard fluid resuscitation before and after they reached the hospital. Those assigned to the delayed-resuscitation group received intravenous cannulation but no fluid resuscitation until they reached the operating room (OR). When fluid resuscitation was delayed, 203 (70%) survived and were discharged from the hospital, as compared with 193 of the 309 patients (62%) surviving when immediate fluid resuscitation was provided ($p = 0.04$). In delayed-resuscitation patients who survived to the postoperative period, 55 (23%) had one or more complications (adult respiratory distress syndrome, sepsis syndrome, acute renal failure, coagulopathy, wound infection, or pneumonia), as compared with 69 of the 227 patients (30%) in the immediate-resuscitation group, a difference that approached statistical significance. The duration of hospitalization was shorter in the delayed-resuscitation group. The authors concluded that delay of aggressive fluid resuscitation until operative control of bleeding is accomplished improves the outcome of hypotensive patients with penetrating torso injuries. These clinical data are supported by animal models of uncontrolled hemorrhagic shock, induced either by intra-abdominal large-vessel injury to the ileocolic artery, or by tail resection. In these models, infusion of hypertonic saline (HTS) or large volumes of normal saline increases rebleeding, hemodynamic collapse, and increased short-term mortality *(4–11)*. The concept appears to be applicable even in blunt trauma animal models *(12,13)*. Vigorous boluses of crystalloid infusion after "massive" or "moderate" splenic injury in rats also increases bleeding and shortens survival time *(14–17)*. Thus, excessive early crystalloid infusion only increases bleeding and shortens survival time in the early critical "golden hour" after injury. These data support the concept that avoiding fluid resuscitation until definitive control of bleeding is achieved or deliberate "hypotensive resuscitation" with a limited volume of crystalloid or colloid solutions until bleeding can be controlled surgically results in better survival *(18)*.

EMERGENCY DEPARTMENT THORACOTOMY AND OPEN-CHEST CARDIAC COMPRESSION

It is crucial to provide the most efficient adequate cardiac and cerebral perfusion in a hypovolemic patient with traumatic hemorrhagic shock. Multiple rib fractures and flail chest can interfere with effective external chest compression. The past decade has seen an ever-increasing enthusiasm for ED thoracotomy (EDT) in trauma centers because it can optimize blood flow using direct cardiac massage, relieve traumatic pericardial tamponade, and allow control of intrathoracic hemorrhage. Closed-chest compression often results in poor cardiac index and other hemodynamic parameters even in nontraumatic arrest patients. Babbs *(19)* developed an electrical model of the human circulatory system with heart and blood vessels modeled as resistive-capacitive networks, pressures in the chest, abdomen, and vascular compartments as voltages, blood flow as electric current, blood inertia as inductance, and the cardiac and venous valves as diodes. Simulations included two modes: the cardiac pump mechanism, in which the atria and ventricles of the model were pressurized simultaneously, as occurs during open chest cardiac massage; and the thoracic pump mechanism, in which all intrathoracic elements of the model were pressurized simultaneously, as is likely to occur in closed chest compression. The two mechanisms were compared for the same peak applied pressure (80 mmHg). Pure cardiac pump CPR generated near normal systemic perfusion pressures throughout the compression cycle. Pure thoracic pump CPR generated much lower systemic perfusion pressure, only during the diastolic phase of the compression cycle. Cardiac pump CPR produced total flows of 2500–3300, myocardial flows of 150–250 and cranial flows of 600–800 mL per minute, depending on the compression rate. In contrast, thoracic pump CPR produced a total flow of approx 1200-myocardial flow of 70, and cranial flow of 450 mL per minute, independently of the compression rate. The author concluded that direct cardiac compression is an inherently superior hemodynamic mechanism because it can generate greater perfusion pressure throughout the compression cycle. Similar results were reported by Sanders et al. *(20)*. Reider et al. *(21)* compared the hemodynamic effectiveness of closed-chest cardiac massage (CCCM) with closed subdiaphragmatic massage (CSDM) and four open transdiaphragmatic cardiac massage techniques during cardiac arrest (CA) with an open abdomen in dogs. CCCM resulted in the lowest cardiac index (CI), mean arterial pressure (MBP), and carotid blood flow (CBF) of all cardiac massage techniques tested. CSDM was not statistically superior to CCCM but did result in a 23% increase in CI and a 54% increase in CBF. Transdiaphragmatic retrocardiac massage through an incision in the diaphragm resulted in the highest hemodynamic parameters of the four open transdiaphragmatic techniques and had significantly higher values than those for CCCM. Open-chest manual compression was also found to be as effective as open-chest compression-active-decompression (CAD). Therefore, open-chest compression is vital in the trauma patient who is in extremis and is the rationale for EDT in urban centers. The objectives of EDT for the "agonal" trauma patient are as follow: (a) maintenance of coronary and cerebral perfusion by relief of cardiac tamponade and/or restoration of efficient cardiac contractility; and (b) control of hemorrhage by cardiorrhaphy, compression of bleeding intrathoracic vessels, and/or reduction of intra-abdominal blood loss by temporary occlusion of the thoracic aorta. The ultimate objective is to improve survival in these desperate patients, a goal that has been achieved with variable success in different series *(22)*.

EDT has not improved survival in the majority of patients, even though it appears to have value in important subgroups (e.g., patients with penetrating cardiac injuries). There are additional concerns with EDT: the cost of indiscriminate, futile resuscitative attempts in patients already dead and the risk for disease transmission to the surgical team. These issues demand a critical analysis of patient selection for the procedure *(23)*.

In a recent collective review of 111 stab wound (SW) and 239 gunshot wound (GSW) patients who had EDT, Boyd and associates *(24)* noted a survival of 18% for SW and 2% for GSW of chest. The survival was 10% for abdominal SW and 6% for abdominal GSW. When multiple sites were injured, survival was 5–6%. Rhee et al. *(25)* reviewed 24 studies that included 4620 cases of EDT for both blunt and penetrating trauma over the past 25 years. The overall survival rate was 7.4%. Normal neurological outcomes were noted in 92.4% of surviving patients. Survival rates were 8.8% for penetrating injuries (6.8% for SW and 4.3% for GSW) and 1.4% for blunt injuries. Survival rates were 10.7% for thoracic injuries, 4.5% for abdominal injuries, and 0.7% for multiple injuries. Cardiac injuries had the highest survival rate (19.4%). If signs of life were present on arrival at the hospital, survival rate was 11.5% in contrast to 2.6% if none were present. Absence of signs of life in the field yielded a survival rate of 1.2%. Similar data were provided by a recent series *(26)*. EDT, therefore, plays an important in the CPR of selected patients with trauma, particularly in penetrating wounds of the chest. The technical details and potential pitfalls of the procedure have been described in detail elsewhere *(23)*.

Hypertonic Saline for Resuscitating Trauma Patients

Hypertonic solutions are the new, potentially beneficial tools for shock/trauma resuscitation. Compared with isotonic fluids, the lesser volumes of hypertonic solutions are associated with equivalent or improved systemic blood pressure, cardiac output, and survival in experimental animals. A positive cardiac inotropic effect is documented, as is a decrease in systemic vascular resistance. Restoration of normal cellular transmembrane potential is enhanced, indicating a reversal of the cellular abnormalities induced by hemorrhagic shock. As long as 24 hours after the shock episode, blood pressure is maintained more effectively than with conventional crystalloid solutions. A solution of 7.5% saline has been shown to be more effective with respect to survival than 0.9, 5, or 10% saline solutions. Improved tissue perfusion occurs as indicated by reduced lactate values. An early increase in urine output, decreased fluid retention, and improved late pulmonary function are also seen *(27–33)*. Possible mechanisms by which hypertonic saline-dextran (HSD) maintains circulation in hemorrhagic shock include rapid shift of fluid from intracellular to extracellular space, improved peripheral perfusion, and increased cardiac contractility.

Despite the abundance of animal studies in support of HTS resuscitation, only a few clinical trials are available to establish its role. Bunn et al. *(34)* from the Cochrane group reviewed the available literature data on all randomized trials comparing hypertonic to isotonic crystalloid in patients with trauma, burns, or undergoing surgery. Seventeen trials were identified with 869 participants. The pooled relative risk for death in trauma patients was 0.84 (95% CI 0.61–1.16), in patients with burns 1.49 (95% CI 0.56–3.95), and in patients undergoing surgery 0.62 (95% CI 0.08–4.57). The authors concluded that there are not enough data to argue for the superiority of hypertonic crystalloid over isotonic crystalloid for the resuscitation of patients with trauma, burns, or those undergoing surgery. The final recommendations must await further trials, large enough to detect a clinical difference.

HTS is on a firmer ground in the resuscitation and maintenance in head-injured patients *(35)*. Two recent reviews summarize the current status *(36,37)*. Although the exact mechanisms by which HTS acts on the injured brain remain unclear, animal human studies suggest that HTS possesses osmotic, vasoregulatory, hemodynamic, neurochemical, and immunologic properties. HTS improves and maintains mean arterial pressure (MAP) better than the high volumes required of isotonic resuscitation and the consequent increase in intracranial pressure (ICP). Cerebral perfusion pressure (CPP) may be improved with HTS resuscitation, leading to better perfusion of injured areas of brain. Unfortunately, these increases in CPP and cerebral oxygen delivery (CDO_2) are transient, with a rebound rise in ICP or fall in CPP to pre-infusion levels *(38–41)*. HTS also appears to counteract hypoperfusion and vasospasm via an increase in vessel diameter and through plasma volume expansion. Additionally, HTS can attenuate the rise in ICP experienced with hyperemia. The endothelial cell edema that is well documented after trauma may be reversed by HTS, improving perfusion to multiple organs including the brain *(37,42)*.

Animal models of brain injury suggest that HTS decreases leukocyte adherence and migration and may alter production of certain prostaglandins. It has been demonstrated to increase circulating levels of cortisol and adrenocorticotropic hormone *(44,45)*. Neutrophil margination and trafficking are also decreased with HTS, possibly via alterations in chemo-attractant production *(46–50)*. As a result, HTS appears to afford some degree of protection against serious bacterial illness *(51,52)*.

Numerous animal models demonstrate the efficacy of HTS in reducing ICP. There are few human trials, generally limited to patients who have failed conventional management. Worthley et al. *(53)* and Einhaus and associates *(54)* documented small case series of patients with intractable intracranial hypertension who were treated successfully with HTS. Suarez et al. *(41)* described eight patients (one with brain injury, one with brain tumor, and others with subarachnoid hemorrhage) in whom HTS was used for ICP control after failure of mannitol. Schatzmann et al. *(55)* observed similar effects of a single 100-mL bolus of 10% HTS to treat 42 separate episodes of intracranial hypertension refractory to standard therapy in six patients with severe brain injury. Simma et al. *(56)* were the first to perform a prospective, randomized trial in severely head-injured pediatric patients to receive either 1.7% HTS or Ringer's Lactate (LR) as maintenance fluid for the first 72 hours after admission. They observed that patients receiving HTS had lower ICP values and required fewer interventions to manage ICP elevations. These patients also required less fluid to maintain blood pressure and had a decreased incidence of respiratory distress syndrome. Survival was improved for patients receiving HTS. Similar results were reported by Horn et al. *(57)* in a prospective study of patients with traumatic subarachnoid .

The role of HTS as a resuscitation fluid was studied by Vassar and associates in a series of studies *(29,58,59)*. Dextran was added to HTS on the basis of its potential to augment the favorable hemodynamic effects of HTS. They observed higher systolic blood pressure with smaller fluid volumes of HTS in their prospective study involving 166 trauma patients. The improvement in survival to discharge in patients treated with HTS vs controls did not reach statistical significance for the entire population but was statistically significant for the subgroup of patients with severe head injury. The same group of investigators performed a multicenter trial to compare 7.5% HTS, 7.5% HTS/6% dextran, 7.5% HTS/12% dextran, and LR (250 mL of each) in hypotensive trauma patients, and again observed improvements in systolic blood pressure with HTS *(29)*. There was no difference in overall survival. Survival was significantly higher than predicted in patients receiving HTS but not LR. Subgroup analysis of patients with an initial Glasgow Coma Score of 8 or less revealed significant improvements in survival to hospital discharge with use of HTS. Dextran appeared to confer no additional benefit over HTS alone.

The side effects of hypertonic saline therapy are more theoretical than real. Osmotic demyelination syndrome (ODS), acute renal insufficiency, and hematologic abnormalities including increased hemorrhage, coagulopathy, and red cell lysis have been described but have not been linked directly to HTS treatment *(36)*. In summary, hypertonic saline resuscitation of trauma victims is a concept with considerable promise but larger studies are needed to establish its ultimate role.

Cardiopulmonary Support in the OR: The Concept of "Damage Control"

The trauma patient with massive injuries faces many potential landmines in the OR. In addition to the ongoing bleeding from injuries, the patient rapidly faces the "triad of death": acidosis, hypothermia, and coagulopathy, all intertwined and contributing to one another. The concept of abbreviating operations, also termed "damage-control" surgery has evolved in recent times *(60–68)* in an effort to break this vicious cycle of complications.

"Damage control" was a term originally coined by the US Navy in reference to "the capacity of a ship to absorb damage and maintain mission integrity." First discussed by Stone in 1983 *(60)*, the technique involved "saving the day for another day in battle" by truncation of laparotomy, intra-abdominal packing for tamponade of nonsurgical bleeding from coagulopathy, and subsequent completion of definitive surgical repair when the patient is in a better physiological state. Damage control consists of three separate phases:

- Rapid control of hemorrhage and contamination; intra-abdominal packing and temporary abdominal closure (phase I)
- Correction of hypothermia by rewarming; correction of coagulopathy; fluid resuscitation and optimization of tissue perfusion (phase II)
- When normal physiology has been restored, re-exploration for definitive management of injuries and abdominal closure (phase III).

Phase I

The indication for damage control is, in general, a severity of anatomic and physiological injury that is beyond the ability of the patient or the surgeon to handle in a time frame that would likely result in patient survival. The triggers for abbreviating the laparotomy are *(67,68)*:

- Massive blood loss (10–15 units of packed red blood cells),
- Injury Severity Score greater than 35, hypotension, hypothermia (temperature <34°C), clinical coagulopathy, and acidosis (pH <7.2)
- Inadequate resources in terms of personnel, equipment, and specialty backup.

Occasionally, with injury to the liver, pelvis, or large muscle beds, packing must be done and prompt angiography performed to embolize and control bleeding from intraparenchymal or intramuscular vessels. In the case of major vascular injuries, the patient may need resection of the injured vessel and/or temporary intraluminal shunting to accomplish distal perfusion; definitive vascular reconstruction is performed at a later stage. Closure of the packed abdomen is best accomplished by temporary measures; leaving the fascia open to prevent abdominal compartment syndrome (discussed in greater length below).

Phase II

The second phase of damage control consists of resuscitation in the intensive care unit (ICU) to optimize tissue perfusion, correct hypothermia, and correct coagulopathy. Acidosis associated with hypovolemic shock contributes to coagulopathic bleeding, worsening the shock state. The goal is complete restoration of aerobic metabolism, as indicated by normalization of serum lactate levels, base deficit, mixed venous oxygen saturation, and in some patients, tissue end-points such as gastric mucosal pH (as discussed elsewhere in this volume).

Correction of hypothermia is crucial to break the vicious cycle of triad of death *(61,67,68)*. Passive external rewarming techniques include simple covering of the patient to minimize convective heat loss. Active external rewarming techniques include fluid-circulating heating blankets, convective warm air blankets, and radiant warmers. Active core rewarming techniques include warmed airway gases, heated peritoneal or pleural lavage, warmed intravenous fluid infusion, and extracorporeal rewarming. Countercurrent heat exchange mechanisms are excellent for rapid infusion of warmed banked blood products. Continuous arteriovenous rewarming is an excellent technique that is driven by the patient's blood pressure and is currently the procedure of choice in massively injured patients.

Dilution of coagulation issues and platelets by fluid resuscitation, decreased total and ionized calcium concentration, hypothermia, severity of injury, shock, and metabolic acidosis may all contribute to coagulopathy. Replacement of clotting issues and platelets based on clinical coagulopathy rather than laboratory values are the accepted approach in these desperate circumstances.

PHASE III

This consists of a return to the OR for definitive organ repair, and fascial closure if possible. The operation should be undertaken when the patient is on his or her way to correction of hypothermia, acidosis, and coagulopathy. A complete correction is not always necessary. However, continuing transfusion needs, uncorrectable acidosis, or increasing bladder pressures suggest ongoing bleeding and the need for reexploration. If the patient is on the way to correct the acidosis and is, at least, improving the coagulopathy, he or she is ready for phase III of the damage control. At reoperation, hemostasis is secured, the peritoneal cavity is irrigated thoroughly, and the bowel anastomoses or repair are completed. Definitive vascular repair, if needed, is accomplished. Persistent visceral edema may limit abdominal closure in many patients. Usually it is necessary to continue with prosthetic (plastic material) closure until favorable circumstances permit skin or fascial closure at a subsequent stage. Some access to providing enteral feeding is desirable and must be weighed against the dangers of opening a thick, edematous bowel. The patient is returned to the ICU for continued resuscitation, gradual ventilator weaning, aggressive nutritional support, and antibiotic therapy, as indicated.

The open abdomen management has undergone significant refinements recently with the advent of a "vacuum-pack" technique as described by Barker and associates (69). After the completion of abdominal exploration, a polyethylene sheet is placed over the peritoneal viscera and beneath the peritoneum of the abdominal wall to prevent adhesions between the bowel and the fascial edges. Next, a moist sterile surgical towel(s) is folded to fit the abdominal wall defect and is placed over the polyethylene sheet. The edges of the towel are positioned below the skin edges. Two large drains are placed on top of the towel. The wound is then covered with a plastic drape backed with iodophor-impregnated adhesive. Each drain tube is connected to bulb suction. Each bulb suction is connected to a limb of a Y-adapter. The Y-adapter is connected to a suction source at 100–150 mmHg continuous negative pressure. Suction to the drains is maintained until reexploration is required. At reexploration, the wound will be considerably smaller and the fascial edges may be approximated in a significant number of patients. If there is still tension between the fascial edges, the process is repeated and multiple explorations may be necessary to close the fascia. An example of vacuum pack is shown in Fig. 1.

Barker and associates (69) reported on 216 vacuum packs performed in 112 trauma patients. Sixty-two patients (55.4%) went on to primary closure and 25 patients (22.3%) underwent polyglactin mesh repair of the defect followed by wound granulation and eventual skin grafting. Similar excellent results with some variant of vacuum-pack technique were reported by other authors (70–72). Damage control has become an important tool in the management of the severely injured patient. The concept is being extended to other phases of trauma care (prehospital), other injuries (orthopedic and vascular), and other populations (pediatric). A recent cumulative analysis has collected about 1000 patients with a 50% survival (64). Rotondo et al. (61) found a remarkable salvage rate of more than 70% in a subset of major vascular injuries. The challenges for the future are to define the indications better, to reduce the morbidity of repeated operations and advance the management of open abdomen.

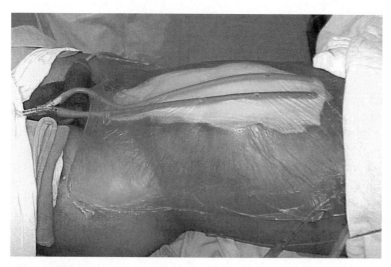

Fig. 1. Illustration of a method of "vacuum-pack" technique of open abdomen management.

Cardiopulmonary Support in the ICU:
The Increasing Problem of "Abdominal Compartment Syndrome"

Increased intra-abdominal pressure (IAP) occurs in a variety of clinical situations such as accumulation of ascites, bowel distension from ileus or mechanical obstruction, following the reduction into the peritoneal cavity of large, chronic hernia contents that have "lost their domain" and excessive crystalloid resuscitation of patients with burns, multiple trauma, abdominal catastrophes. Intra-abdominal hypertension (IAH), or markedly increased IAP, is common after extensive abdominal trauma from accumulation of blood and clot, bowel edema or congestion from injury to mesenteric vessels, excessive crystalloid resuscitation and perihepatic or retroperitoneal packing after "damage-control" laparotomy. IAH can lead to the classic abdominal compartment syndrome (ACS), characterized by a tensely distended abdomen, elevated intra-abdominal and peak airway pressures, inadequate ventilation with hypoxia and hypercarbia, disturbed renal function, and an improvement of these features after abdominal decompression. The adverse physiological sequelae of increased abdominal pressure are becoming increasingly common in ICU patients. It is imperative to monitor IAP in severely ill patients who are at the brink of physiological exhaustion *(73–80)*.

IAP can be monitored indirectly by using bladder pressure, either continuously or intermittently. A simple technique consists of instilling 50 mL of saline into the urinary bladder through the Foley catheter. The tubing of the collecting bag is clamped and a needle is inserted into the specimen-collecting port of the tubing proximal to the clamp and is attached to a manometer. Bladder pressure measured in cm H_2O is the height at which the level of the saline column stabilizes with the symphysis pubis as the 0 point. The IAP can be measured either in mmHg or cm of H_2O (1 mmHg = 1.36 cm of H_2O). The exact level at which IAP should be called IAH that requires treatment has not been defined. Burch and associates *(77)* described a grading system of elevated IAP: grade I (10–15 cm of H_2O), grade II (15–25 cm of H_2O), grade III (25–35 cm of H_2O), and grade IV (>35 cm of H_2O). They suggested that most of the patients with grade III and all of the

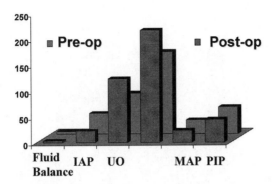

Fig. 2. Effects of abdominal decompression on intra-abdominal pressure (IAP), urine output (UO), mean arterial pressure (MAP), and peak inspiratory pressure (PIP). (Data from ref. *88a*.)

patients with grade IV elevations in IAP should have abdominal decompression. As is discussed in greater detail below, splanchnic hypoperfusion is noted at an IAP level of 15 mmHg (20.4 cm of H_2O). Therefore, our practice is to consider a persistent elevation of IAP beyond 20 to 25 cm H_2O as IAH and institute therapy.

Hemodynamic and Respiratory Consequences of IAH

Venous return and cardiac output fall despite a normal arterial pressure as the IAP rises above 10 mmHg. Beyond an IAP of 25 mmHg, a marked increase in end-inspiratory pressures is noted *(73–80)*. Barnes et al. *(81)* showed that the compliance of the peritoneal cavity fell as IAP increased from 0 to 40 mmHg. Intrathoracic pressures increased. Cardiac output and stroke volume were reduced by 36% after an IAP elevation to 40 mmHg. Flow in the celiac, superior mesenteric, and renal arteries fell by 42, 61, and 70%, respectively, possibly related to neural, hormonal or intrinsic influences. Whole-body O_2 consumption, pH, and arterial pO_2 decreased. Since these reports, multiple reports recorded the changes in hemodynamic parameters with increased IAP and the dramatic benefits of decompression on the cardiovascular status (Fig. 2).

Renal Effects of IAH

Anuria can be produced in animal models by increasing the IAP above 30 mmHg without a significant drop in systemic blood pressure. This is a reversible phenomenon and the urine output increases with a drop in IAP. Other observed effects are a decrease in renal plasma flow, glomerular filtration rate, and glucose reabsorption, independent of the effect on cardiac output. In a prospective study of postoperative patients, Sugrue et al. *(82)* noted renal impairment (defined as a serum creatinine >1.3 mg/L or an increase in serum creatinine of >1mg/L within 72 hours of surgery) was observed in 33% of the patients, of whom 20 of 29 or 69% had raised IAP.

IAH and Splanchnic Flow

Caldwell and Ricotta *(83)* documented a reduction in blood flow to all abdominal viscera except the adrenal glands using radio-labeled microspheres in an animal model.

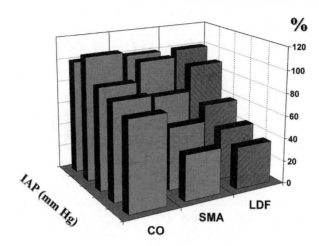

Fig. 3. Effect of increasing intra-abdominal pressure (IAP) on cardiac output (CO), Superior mesenteric artery flow (SMA) and laser Doppler flow (LDF) in intestinal mucosa. (Modified from ref. *88a*.)

As noted above, Barnes et al. *(81)* observed a marked decrease in the blood flow through renal, celiac, and superior mesenteric vessels at an IAP of 40 mmHg. Diebel and associates showed that the mesenteric and mucosal blood flow in anesthetized pigs declined progressively to 61% of the base line with an IAP above 20 mmHg and 28% of the baseline at an IAP of 40 mmHg (Fig. 3). Corresponding to these changes, the intestinal mucosa (as studied by the tonometer) developed severe acidosis (Fig. 3). Similar reductions were observed in hepatic arterial, portal and hepatic microcirculatory blood flow *(84,85)*. Using fluorescence quenching optodes in the submucosa of the ileum in ventilated swine to measure mucosal partial pressure of oxygen, Bongard et al. *(86)* demonstrated a progressive fall in bowel tissue oxygen partial pressure (TPO_2) as the IAP was increased although the subcutaneous TPO_2 remained unchanged. Abdominal decompression in patients with IAH reduced the IAP and reversed these changes *(87)*.

A severe systemic inflammatory response corresponds with this splanchnic hypoperfusion. Rezende-Neto and associates induced IAH in Sprague-Dawley rats. As compared with controls, IAH caused a significant decrease in mean arterial pressure. After abdominal decompression the pressure returned to baseline levels. A significant decrease in arterial pH was also noted. Increase in the levels of tumor necrosis factor-α and interleukin (IL)-6 was noted 30 minutes after abdominal decompression. Plasma concentration of IL-1b was elevated after 60 minutes of IAH. Lung neutrophil accumulation was significantly elevated only after abdominal decompression. Histopathological findings showed intense pulmonary inflammatory infiltration including atelectasis and alveolar edema. Doty and colleagues *(89)* observed in an experimental study that hemorrhage followed by reperfusion and a subsequent insult of IAH caused significant gastrointestinal mucosal acidosis, hypoperfusion, as well as systemic acidosis. These changes, however, were not associated with a significant bacterial translocation as judged by polymerase chain reaction measurements, tissue, or blood cultures.

Oda et al. *(90)* hypothesized that sequential hemorrhagic shock (HS) and ACS would result in a greater cytokine activation and polymorphonuclear neutrophil (PMN)-mediated lung injury than with either insult alone. Twenty Yorkshire swine (20–30 kg) were studied. Group 1 ($n = 5$) was hemorrhaged to a mean arterial pressure of 25–30 mmHg for 60 minutes and resuscitated to baseline mean arterial pressure. Intra-abdominal pressure was then increased to 30 mmHg above baseline and maintained for 60 minutes. Group 2 ($n = 5$) was subjected to hemorrhagic shock alone and group 3 ($n = 5$) to abdominal compartment syndrome alone. Group 4 ($n = 5$) had sham experiment without either of these insults. Portal and central vein cytokine levels were equivalent but were significantly higher in group 1 (hemorrhagic shock + abdominal compartment syndrome) than in other groups. baseline lung lavage (BAL) PMNs were higher ($p < 0.05$) in group 1 ($4.1 \pm 2.0 \times 10^6$) than in the other groups (0.6 ± 0.5, 1.4 ± 1.3, and 0.1 ± 0.0 times 10^6, respectively) and lung myeloperoxidase activity was higher ($p < 0.05$) in group 1 ($134.6 \pm 57.6 \times 10^6/g$) than in the other groups (40.3 ± 14.7, 46.1 ± 22.4, and $7.73 \pm 4.4 \times 10^6/g$, respectively). BAL protein was higher ($p < 0.01$) in group 1 (0.92 ± 0.32 mg/mL) compared with the other groups (0.22 ± 0.08, 0.29 ± 0.11, and 0.08 ± 0.06 mg/mL, respectively). The authors concluded that, in this clinically relevant model, sequential insults of ischemia-reperfusion (hemorrhagic shock and resuscitation) and ACS were associated with significantly increased portal and central venous cytokine levels and more severe lung injury than caused by either insult alone.

These experimental reports and the clinical series, described below establish unrecognized, untreated IAH as a major contributor to the classic and complete ACS and contribute to systemic inflammatory syndrome and multiorgan failure.

IAH and Intracranial Pressure

Josephs and associates *(91)* noted that elevated IAP during laparoscopy caused a significant elevation in ICP. Bloomfield and coworkers *(92–94)* confirmed the effect of elevated IAP on ICP in animals without head injury as well as in a patient with head injury. The precise mechanism of the effects of increased IAP on ICP and CPP are not yet elucidated. Bloomfield and colleagues suggest *(94)*, based on their porcine model, that elevated central venous pressure as a result of elevated IAP may interfere with venous drainage from cerebral venous outflow, increase the size of the intracranial vascular bed and raise the ICP.

Frequency of IAH and ACS

Ertel and associates *(95)* presented a combined prospective and retrospective study of 311 patients who had severe abdominal and pelvic trauma and had "damage-control" laparotomy. They defined ACS as significant respiratory compromise, renal dysfunction or hemodynamic instability, and in a small number of patients, bladder pressures more than 25 mmHg. The syndrome developed in 5.5% of patients from intra-abdominal bleeding or visceral edema. In a series of penetrating trauma patients undergoing "damage-control" laparotomy, Ivatury and associates *(74)* noted that 33% of the patients developed IAH (IAP >20 cms of H_2O). Meldrum and associates *(96)* noted a 14% prevalence in 145 patients with abdominal injuries. ACS was defined as IAP greater than 20 mmHg with dysfunction of cardiovascular, respiratory, or renal systems. It is, therefore, evident that the frequency of the complication varies with the definition. In a prospective study from Miami, Florida *(97)*, 15 (2%) of 706 patients had intra-abdominal hypertension. Six of the 15 patients with intra-abdominal hypertension had abdominal compartment syndrome. Half of the patients with abdominal compartment syndrome died, as did two of the remaining nine patients with intra-abdominal hypertension.

Secondary Abdominal Compartment Syndrome

ACS can occur in the absence of abdominal injury. Maxwell and associates *(98)* reported on six patients with secondary "hemorrhagic shock" in the absence of abdominal injuries in 46 patients who had visceral edema. Bladder pressures in this group averaged 33 ± 3 mmHg. The syndrome is probably related to excessive resuscitation volumes (average 19 liters of crystalloid and 29 units of packed cells). We have noted this phenomenon in patients with blunt nonabdominal injuries as well as in burn patients. The term secondary ACS has been applied to describe patients who develop ACS but do not have abdominal injuries. Secondary ACS appears to be a highly lethal event, as substantiated by the series from Denver *(99)*. Fourteen patients (13 male, aged 45 ± 5 years) developed ACS 11.6 ± 2.2 hours following resuscitation from shock. Eleven (79%) required vasopressors. The worst base deficit was 14.1 ± 1.9. Resuscitation included 16.7 ± 3.0 L crystalloid and 13.3 ± 2.9 red blood cell units. Decompressive laparotomy improved intra-abdominal, systolic, and peak airway pressures, as well as urine output. Mortality was 38% among trauma, and 100% among nontrauma, patients. In another recent study *(100)*, 11 (9%) of 128 standardized shock resuscitation patients developed secondary ACS. All presented in severe shock (systolic blood pressure 85 ± 5 mmHg, base deficit 8.6 ± 1.6 mEq/L), with severe injuries (injury severity score 28 ± 3) and required aggressive shock resuscitation (26 ± 2 units of blood, 38 ± 3 L crystalloid within 24 hours). The mortality rate was 54%. These data reinforce the notion that secondary ACS is an early but, if appropriately monitored, recognizable complication in patients with major nonabdominal trauma who require aggressive resuscitation.

Abdominal Compartment Syndrome and IAH

This substantial volume of experimental and clinical data supports the hypothesis that IAH is associated with a significant adverse effect on splanchnic perfusion that is further aggravated by the unfavorable systemic cardiorespiratory consequences of IAH. Current studies suggest that IAH (defined as IAP >20–25 cm of H_2O) and ACS may not be synonymous, as was suggested in the past *(73,74)*. IAH may be an earlier phenomenon that, when uncorrected, leads to the full manifestations of ACS. Splanchnic hypoperfusion and gut mucosal acidosis commence at much lower abdominal pressures, long before the manifestations of ACS become clinically evident. For example, Ivatury et al. *(74)* analyzed 70 patients who had catastrophic penetrating abdominal trauma. Of these, 42 patients had their gut mucosal pH monitored and 11 of them developed IAH; 7 of the 11(64%) had acidotic pHi (7.15 ± 0.2) with IAH, despite having a high CI (3.8 ± 1.2), DO_2I (646 ± 250) and VO_2I (174 ± 44) and normal PaO_2/FiO_2 (289 ± 98) and $PaCO_2$ (40 ± 9). The pHi improved after abdominal decompression in five and none developed ACS. Only two patients with IAH and low pHi had established ACS. Diebel and associates *(85)* noted a similar phenomenon of IAH and gastric mucosal acidosis without the other manifestations of ACS. Sugrue et al. *(101)* evaluated postoperative patients prospectively with IAP and pHi monitoring. Patients with a pHi less than 7.32 were 11.3 times more likely to have an IAP greater than 20 mmHg compared to patients with normal pHi. Abnormal pHi was also associated with a poor outcome.

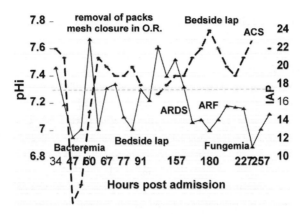

Fig. 4. Intensive care unit course of a patient with extensive abdominal injuries from a gunshot wound of the abdomen. Note the inverse relationship between intra-abdominal pressure (IAP) and gastric mucosal pH (pHi). Note the persistent elevation of IAP and decrease in pHi at the onset of multiorgan failure (157 hours). These parameters could not be corrected before the patient's death a few days later. ARF, acute renal failure; ARDS, acute respiratory distress syndrome; Lap, laparotomy.

The complications of IAH and ACS appear to be particularly serious after prior insults of traumatic shock and resuscitation. With a few exceptions mentioned in the prior section on IAH and splanchnic flow, many of the earlier studies only addressed the adverse effects of IAH alone. Both experimental and clinical data now support the concept that these sequential insults predispose the patient to multiorgan failure and death. In a series of experiments, Friedlander and Simon *(102,103)* substantiated the amplifying effect of IAH on top of ischemia-reperfusion on superior mesenteric arterial flow as well as pulmonary dysfunction. In a clinical study, Raeburn and associates *(104)* analyzed patients requiring postinjury damage-control surgery. The patients were divided into groups depending on whether or not they developed ACS. ACS was defined as an IAP greater than 20 mmHg in association with increased airway pressure or impaired renal function. ACS developed in 36% of the 77 patients with a mean IAP prior to decompression of 26 ± 1 mmHg. The ACS group was not significantly different from the non-ACS group in patient demographics, Injury Severity Score, ED vital signs, or ICU admission indices (blood pressure, temperature, base deficit, CI, lactate, international normalized ratio, partial thromboplastin time, and 24-hour fluid). The initial peak airway pressure after surgery was higher in patients who went on to develop ACS. The development of ACS was associated with increased ICU stays, days of ventilation, complications, multiorgan failure, and mortality (Fig. 4).

Management of IAH

IDENTIFICATION OF PATIENTS "AT RISK" AND PREVENTION OF IAH

Patients who are at increased risk for IAH include those with the following:

1. *Pre-operative hypovolemic shock and massive fluid resuscitation*: burns, peritonitis, pancreatitis, ruptured abdominal aortic aneurysm (AAA), gastrointestinal hemorrhage, multiple or multisystem injuries.
2. *Increased intra-abdominal fluid accumulation*: Ascites, excessive resuscitation fluids, coagulopathy and abnormal bleeding, acute abdominal pathology, ruptured AAA, pelvic

and retroperitoneal hematomas, intestinal obstruction and hemoperitoneum from nonoperative management of solid organ injury.

3. *Mechanical increase in pressure:* Pelvic and retroperitoneal hematoma, "damage-control" surgery with intra-abdominal packing, sudden intra-abdominal reduction of long-standing hernial contents, tension pneumothorax, massive hemothorax, "chronic" abdominal compartment syndrome from morbid obesity, intestinal obstruction.

It is important to anticipate IAH and attempt prophylaxis by "open abdomen" in these patients. The "open abdomen" approach offers several advantages. It provides a rapid method of abbreviating the laparotomy and transporting the patient to the ICU for resuscitation. In a significant number of patients, it may actually prevent IAH. In recent reports, Mayberry and associates *(105,106)* analyzed 73 consecutive patients who had an absorbable mesh closure of the abdomen, 47 at the initial celiotomy (group 1) and 26 at a subsequent celiotomy (group 2). The two groups had similar injury severity but group 2 had a higher incidence of postoperative ACS (35 vs 0%). A similar statistically significant reduction in IAH was also noted by Ivatury and colleagues *(74)*.

It is also important to keep in mind that prophylactic open abdomen and nonclosure of fascia does not always prevent IAH and ACS, as has been observed by several investigators *(74,97, 99,104,107)*. These patients, therefore, should have close IAP monitoring in the postoperative period.

Treatment of IAH and ACS

We suggest that a critical level of 25 cm of H_2O (18.3 mmHg) should trigger careful monitoring of IAP and prompt treatment if it continues to increase. The first step in the evaluation of an increased IAP, especially in the presence of agitation and restlessness, is to sedate and, if necessary, chemically paralyze the patient. If the bladder pressures are still high and/or systemic manifestations of IAH (as described above) are evident, the appropriate treatment, in most instances, is abdominal decompression by laparotomy.

Recently, two studies emphasized the nonoperative approach to ACS in burn patients *(108,109)*. The first study *(108)* evaluated the utility of percutaneous drainage (PD) of peritoneal fluid compared with decompressive laparotomy in burn patients. Nine of 13 (69%) study patients developed IAH that progressed to abdominal compartment syndrome in five (31%). All were treated with PD using a diagnostic peritoneal lavage catheter. Five patients underwent PD successfully, and their IAH did not progress to ACS. Four patients with greater than 80% total body surface area burns and severe inhalation injury did not respond to PD and required decompressive laparotomy. There was no evidence of bowel edema, ischemia, or necrosis. All patients requiring decompressive laparotomies died either from sepsis or respiratory failure. The second study *(109)* reported similar success with percutaneous drainage in ACS in three burn victims. Similar paracentesis treatment of IAH was described in patients with liver injury being treated nonoperatively by Yang et al. *(110)*.

In summary, the current evidence suggests that routine use of IAP monitoring is indicated in all patients "at risk" (includes most of the massively injured patients or critically ill patients in the ICU). The critical level of IAP that becomes IAH is around 20–25 cm of H_2O. IAH may be an earlier phenomenon that, when persistent or neglected, may lead to the complete manifestations of ACS. ACS may become manifest at much lower pressures than recognized previously. Prophylaxis and aggressive and prompt treatment of IAH is recommended to prevent ACS from becoming an irreversible syndrome and culminate in cardiopulmonary arrest in the severely ill or the multiply injured patient.

REFERENCES

1. Cannon WB, Faser J, Cowell EM. The preventive treatment of wound shock. JAMA 1918; 47:618.
2. Kaweski SM, Sise MJ, Virgilio RW. The effect of prehospital fluids on survival in trauma patients. J Trauma 1990; 30:1215–1219.
3. Bickell WH, Wall MJ Jr, Pepe PE, et al. Immediate versus delayed fluid resuscitation for hypotensive patients with penetrating torso injuries. N Engl J Med 1994; 331:1105–1109.
4. Gross D, Landau EH, Assalia A, Krausz MM. Is hypertonic saline resuscitation safe in "uncontrolled" hemorrhagic shock? J Trauma 1988; 28:751–756.
5. Bickell WH, Bruttig SP, Wade CE. Hemodynamic response to abdominal aortotomy in the anesthetized swine. Circ Shock 1989; 28:321–332.
6. Krausz MM, Horn Y, Gross D. The combined effect of small volume hypertonic saline and normal saline solutions in uncontrolled hemorrhagic shock. Surg Gynecol Obstet. 1992; 174:363–368.
7. Kowalenko T, Stern SA, Dronen SC, Wang X. Improved outcome with hypotensive resuscitation of uncontrolled hemorrhagic shock in a swine model. J Trauma 1992; 33:349–353.
8. Gross D, Landau EH, Klin B, Krausz MM. Treatment of uncontrolled hemorrhagic shock with hypertonic saline solution. Surg Gynecol Obstet 1990; 170:106–112.
9. Bickell WH, Bruttig SP, Millnamow GA, O'Benar J, Wade CE. The detrimental effects of intravenous crystalloid after aortotomy in swine. Surgery 1991; 110:529–536.
10. Krausz MM, Bar-Ziv M, Rabinovici R, Gross D. "Scoop and run" or stabilize hemorrhagic shock with normal saline or small-volume hypertonic saline? J Trauma 1992; 33:6–10.
11. Stern SA, Dronen SC, Birrer P, Wang X. The effect of blood pressure on hemorrhage volume and survival in a near-fatal hemorrhage model incorporating a vascular injury. Ann Emerg Med 1993; 22:155–163.
12. Matsuoka T, Hildreth J, Wisner DH. Liver injury as a model of uncontrolled hemorrhagic shock: resuscitation with different hypertonic regimens. J Trauma 1995; 39:674–680.
13. Matsuoka T, Hildreth J, Wisner DH. Uncontrolled hemorrhage from parenchymal injury: is resuscitation helpful? J Trauma 1996; 40:915–922.
14. Solomonov E, Hirsh M, Yahiya A, Krausz MM. The effect of vigorous fluid resuscitation in uncontrolled hemorrhagic shock following massive splenic injury. Crit Care Med 2000; 28:749–754.
15. Krausz MM, Bashenko Y, Hirsh M. Crystalloid or colloid resuscitation of uncontrolled hemorrhagic shock after moderate splenic injury. Shock 2000; 13:230–235.
16. Krausz MM, Bashenko Y, Hirsh M. Crystalloid and colloid resuscitation of uncontrolled hemorrhagic shock following massive splenic injury. Shock 2001; 16:383–388.
17. Abu-Hatoum O, Bashenko Y, Hirsh M, Krausz MM. Continuous fluid resuscitation and splenectomy for treatment of uncontrolled hemorrhagic shock after massive splenic injury. J Trauma 2002; 52:253–258.
18. Kaweski SM, Sise MJ, Virgilio RW. The effect of prehospital fluids on survival in trauma patients. J Trauma 1990; 30:1215–1219.
19. Babbs CF, Thelander K, Engoren M, Severyn F, Fenn-Buderer N, DeFrank M. Theoretically optimal duty cycles for chest and abdominal compression during external cardiopulmonary resuscitation: Cardiac output, coronary blood flow, and blood gases during open-chest standard and compression-active-decompression cardiopulmonary resuscitation. Resuscitation 2002; 55:309–316.
20. Sanders AB, Kern KB, Ewy GA, Atlas M, Bailey L. Improved resuscitation from cardiac arrest with open-chest massage. Ann Emerg Med 1984; 13(Pt 1):672–675.
21. Rieder CF, Crawford BG, Iliopoulos JI, Thomas JH, Pierce GE, Hermreck AS. A study of the techniques of cardiac massage with the abdomen open. Surgery 1985; 98:824–830.
22. Ivatury RR. Emergency Room Thoracotomy. In: Ivatury RR, Cayten CG, eds. The Textbook of Penetrating Trauma. Baltimore: Williams & Wilkins, 1996.
23. Ivatury RR, Rohman M. Emergency department throacotomy for trauma: a collective review. Resuscitation 1987; 15:23.
24. Boyd M, Vaneck VW, Bourguet CC. Emergency room thoracotomy: when is it indicated? J Trauma 1992; 33:714-721.
25. Rhee PM, Jordan MR, Rich N. Survival after emergency department thoracotomy: review of published data from the past 25 years. J Am Coll Surg 2000; 190:288–298.
26. Ladd AP, Gomez GA, Jacobson LE, Broadie TA, Scherer LR III, Solotkin KC. Emergency room thoracotomy: updated guidelines for a level I trauma center. Am Surg 2002; 68:421–424.
27. Wade CEJ, Grady JJ, Fabian T, Younas RN, Kramer GC. Efficacy of hypertonic 7.5% saline and 6% dextran-70 in treating trauma: a meta-analysis of controlled clinical studies. Surgery 1997; 122:609–616.

28. Holcroft JW, Vassar MJ, Turner JE, Derlet RW, Kramer GC. 3% NaCl and 7.5% NaCl/dextran 70 in the resuscitation of severely injured patients. Ann Surg 1987; 206:279–288.

29. Vassar MJ, Fischer RP, O'Brien PE, et al. A multicenter trial for resuscitation of injured patients with 7.5% sodium chloride. Arch Surg 1993; 128:1003–1013.

30. Krausz MM. Controversies in shock research: hypertonic resuscitation pros and cons. Shock 1995; 3:69–72.

31. Dronen SC, Stern SA, Wang X, Stanley M. A comparison of the response of near-fatal acute hemorrhage models with and without a vascular injury to rapid volume expansion. Am J Emerg Med 1993; 11:331–335.

32. Sindlinger JF, Soucy DM, Greene SP, Barber AE, Illner H, Shires T. The effects of isotonic saline volume resuscitation in uncontrolled hemorrhage. Surg Gynecol Obstet 1993; 177:545–550.

33. Krausz MM, David M, Amstislavsky T. Hypertonic saline treatment of uncontrolled hemorrhagic shock in awake rats. Shock 1994; 2:267–270.

34. Bunn F, Roberts I, Tasker R, Akpa E. Hypertonic versus isotonic crystalloid for fluid resuscitation in critically ill patients. Cochrane Database Syst Rev 2002; (1):CD002045.

35. Novak L, Shackford SR, Bourguignon P, et al. Comparison of standard and alternative prehospital resuscitation in pressure driven hemorrhagic shock and head injury. J Trauma. 1999; 47:834–844.

36. Doyle JA, Davis DP, Hoyt DB. The use of hypertonic saline in the treatment of traumatic brain injury. J Trauma 2001; 50:367–83.

37. Shackford S. Effect of small-volume resuscitation on intracranial pressure and related cerebral variables. J Trauma 1997; 42(Suppl):S48–S53.

38. Ducey J, Lamiell J, Gueller G. Cerebral electrophysiologic effects of resuscitation with hypertonic saline-dextran after hemorrhage. Crit Care Med 1990; 18:744–749.

39. Gemma M, Cozzi S, Piccoli S, Magrin S, De Vitis A, Cenzato M. Hypertonic saline fluid therapy following brain stem trauma. J Neurosurg Anesthesiol 1996; 8:137–141.

40. Qureshi A, Wilson D, Traystman R. Treatment of elevated intracranial pressure in experimental intracerebral hemorrhage: comparison between mannitol and hypertonic saline. Neurosurgery 1999; 44:1055–1063.

41. Suarez J, Qureshi A, Bhardwaj A, et al. Treatment of refractory intracranial hypertension with 23.4% saline. Crit Care Med 1998; 26:1118–1122.

42. Corso CO, Okamoto S, Leiderer R, Messmer K. Resuscitation with hypertonic saline dextran reduces endothelial cell swelling and improves hepatic microvascular perfusion and function after hemorrhagic shock. J Surg Res 998; 80:210–220.

43. Cudd TA, Purinton S, Patel NC, Wood CE. Cardiovascular, adrenocorticotropin, and cortisol responses to hypertonic saline in euvolemic sheep are altered by prostaglandin synthase inhibition. Shock 1998; 10:32–36.

43. Corso CO, Okamoto S, Reuttinger D, Messmer K. Hypertonic saline dextran attenuates leukocyte accumulation in the liver after hemorrhagic shock and resuscitation. J Trauma 1999; 46:417–423.

44. Angle N, Hoyt DB, Cabello-Passini R, Herdon-Remelius C, Loomis W, Junger WG. Hypertonic saline resuscitation reduces neutrophil margination by suppressing neutrophil L selectin expression. J Trauma 1998; 45:7–13.

45. Angle N, Hoyt DB, Coimbra R, et al. Hypertonic saline resuscitation diminishes lung injury by suppressing neutrophil activation after hemorrhagic shock. Shock 1998; 9:164–170.

46. Junger WG, Hoyt DB, Davis RE, et al. Hypertonicity regulates the function of human neutrophils by modulating chemoattractant receptor signaling and activating mitogen-activated protein kinase p38. J Clin Invest 1998; 101:2768–2779.

47. Patrick DA, Moore EE, Offner PJ, Johnson JL, Tamura DY, Silliman CC. Hypertonic saline activates lipid-primed human neutrophils for enhanced elastase release. J Trauma 1998; 44:592–598.

48. Coimbra R, Junger WG, Hoyt DB, Liu FC, Loomis WH, Evers MF. Hypertonic saline resuscitation restores hemorrhage-induced immunosuppression by decreasing prostaglandin E2 and interleukin-4 production. J Surg Res 1996; 64:203–209.

49. Tokyay R, Zeigler ST, Kramer GC, et al. Effects of hypertonic saline dextran resuscitation on oxygen delivery, oxygen consumption, and lipid peroxidation after burn injury. J Trauma 1992; 32:704–713.

50. Coimbra R, Hoyt DB, Junger WG, et al. Hypertonic saline resuscitation decreases susceptibility to sepsis after hemorrhagic shock. J Trauma 1997; 42:602–607.

51. Worthley LI, Cooper DJ, Jones N. Treatment of resistant intracranial hypertension with hypertonic saline. Report of two cases. J Neurosurg 1988; 68:478–481.

52. Einhaus S, Croce M, Watridge C, Lowery R, Fabian T. The use of hypertonic saline for the treatment of increased intracranial pressure. J Tenn Med Assoc 1996; 89:81–82.
53. Schatzmann C, Heissler H, Kˆnig K, et al. Treatment of elevated intracranial pressure by infusions of 10% saline in severely head injured patients. Acta Neurochir Suppl (Wien) 1998; 71:31–33.
54. Simma B, Burger R, Falk M, Sacher P, Fanconi S. A prospective, randomized, and controlled study of fluid management in children with severe head injury: lactated Ringer's solution versus hypertonic saline. Crit Care Med 1998; 26:1270.
55. Horn P, Meunch E, Vajkoczy P, et al. Hypertonic saline solution for control of elevated intracranial pressure in patients with exhausted response to mannitol and barbiturates. Neurol Res 1999; 21:758–764.
56. Vassar MJ, Perry CA, Gannaway WL, Holcroft JW. 7.5% sodium chloride/dextran for resuscitation of trauma patients undergoing helicopter transport. Arch Surg 1991; 126:1065–1072.
57. Vassar M, Perry C, Holcroft J. Prehospital resuscitation of hypotensive trauma patients with 7.5% NaCl versus 7.5% NaCl with added dextran: a controlled trial. J Trauma 1993; 34:622–632.
58. Stone HH, Strom PR, Mullins RJ. Management of the major coagulopathy with onset during laparotomy. Ann Surg 1983; 197:532–535.
59. Rotondo MF, Schwab CW, McGonigal MD, et al. Damage control: an approach for improved survival in exsanguinating penetrating abdominal injury. J Trauma 1993; 35:375–383.
60. Burch JM, Ortiz VB, Richardson RJ, et al. Abbreviated laparotomy and planned re-operation for critically injured patients. Ann Surg 1992; 215:476–484.
61. Moore EE. Staged laparotomy for the hypothermia, acidosis and coagulopathy syndrome. Am J Surg 1996; 172:405–410.
62. Shapiro MB, Jenkins DH, Schwab CW, Rotondo MF. Damage control: collective review. J Trauma 2000; 49:969–978.
63. Vargo DJ, Battistella FD. Abbreviated thoracotomy and temporary chest closure: an application of damage control after thoracic trauma. ArchSurg 2001; 136:21–24.
64. Johnon JW, Gracias VH, Schwab CW, et al. Evolution in damage control for exsanguinating penetrating abdominal injury. J Trauma 2001; 51:261–269.
65. Asensio JA, McDuffie L, Petrone P, et al. Reliable variables in the exsanguinated patient which indicate damage control and predict outcome. Am J Surg 2001; 182:743–751.
66. Hoey BA, Schwab CW. Damage control surgery. Scand J Surg 2002; 91:92–103.
67. Barker DE, Kaufman HJ, Smith LA, Ciraulo DL, Richart CL, Burns RP. Vacuum pack technique of temporary abdominal closure: a 7-year experience with 112 patients. J Trauma 2000; 48:201–206.
68. Miller PR, Thompson JT, Faler BJ, Meredith JW, Chang MC. Late fascial closure in lieu of ventral hernia: the next step in open abdomen management. J Trauma 2002; 53:843–849.
69. Garner GB, Ware DN, Cocanour CS, et al. Vacuum-assisted wound closure provides early fascial reapproximation in trauma patients with open abdomens. Am J Surg 2001; 182:630–638.
70. Markley MA, Mantor PC, Letton RW, Tuggle DW. Pediatric vacuum packing wound closure for damage-control laparotomy. J Pediatr Surg 2002; 37:512–514.
71. Ivatury RR, Diebel L, Porter JM et al. Intra-abdominal hypertension and the abdominal compartment syndrome. Surg Clin North Am 1997; 77:783–800.
72. Ivatury RR, Porter JM, Simon RJ et al. Intra-abdominal hypertension after life threatening abdominal trauma: incidence, prophylaxis and clinical relevance to gastric mucosal pH and abdominal compartment syndrome. J Trauma 1998; 44:1016–1021.
73. Saggi BH, Sugerman HJ, Ivatury RR et al. Abdominal compartment syndrome. J Trauma 1998; 45: 597–609.
74. Schein M, Wittmann DH, Aprahamian CC et al. The abdominal compartment syndrome: the physiological and clinical consequences of elevated intra-abdominal pressure. J Amer Coll Surg 1995; 180:747–753.
75. Burch JM, Moore EE, Moore FA et al. The abdominal compartment syndrome. Surg Clin North Amer 1996; 76:833–842.
76. Sugerman HJ, Windsor A, Bessos M et al. Intra-abdominal pressure, sagittal abdominal diameter, and obesity comorbidity. J Intern Med 1997; 241:71–79.
77. Morris JA Jr, Eddy VA, Blinman TA et al. The staged celiotomy for trauma. Issues in unpacking and reconstruction. Ann Surg 1993; 217:576–586.
78. Loi P, De Backer D, Vincent JL. Abdominal compartment syndrome. Acta Chir Belg 2001; 101:59–64.
79. Barnes GE, Laine GA, Gaim PY, et al. Cardiovascular responses to elevation of intra-abdominal hydrostatic pressure. Am J Physiol 1985; 248:R208–R213.
80. Sugrue M, Jones F, Janjua KJ, Deane SA, Bristow P, Hillman K. Temporary abdominal closure: a prospective evaluation of its effects on renal and respiratory physiology. J Trauma 1998; 45; 914–921.

81. Caldwell CB, Ricotta JJ. Changes in visceral blood flow with elevated intra-abdominal pressure. J Surg Res 1987; 43:14–20.

82. Diebel LN, Wilson RF, Dulchavshy SA. Effect on increased intra-abdominal pressure on hepatic arterial, portal venous, and hepatic microcirculatory blood flow. J Trauma 1992; 33:279–283.

83. Diebel LN, Dulchavshy SA, Wilson RF. Effect on increased intra-abdominal pressure on mesenteric arterial and intestinal mucosal blood flow. J Trauma 1992; 33:45–49.

84. Bongard F, Pianim N, Dubecz S, Klein S. Adverse consequences of increased intra-abdominal pressure on bowel tissue oxygenation. J Trauma 1995; 39:519–525.

85. Chang MC, Miller PR, D'Agostino R Jr, Meredith JW. Effects of abdominal decompression on cardiopulmonary function and visceral perfusion in patients with intra-abdominal hypertension. J of Trauma 1998; 44:440–445.

86. Rezende-Neto JB, Moore EE, Melo De Andrade MV, et al. Systemic inflammatory response secondary to abdominal compartment syndrome: stage for multiple organ failure. J. Trauma 2002; 53:1121–1128.

87. Doty JM, Oda J, Ivatury RR, et al. The effects of hemodynamic shock and increased intra-abdominal pressure on bacterial translocation. J Trauma 2002; 52:13–17.

88. Oda J, Ivatury RR, Blocher CR, Malhotra AJ, Sugerman HJ. Amplified cytokine response and lung injury by sequential hemorrhagic shock and abdominal compartment syndrome in a laboratory model of ischemia-reperfusion. J Trauma 2002; 52:625–631.

88a. Ivatury RR, Cayten CG. (eds.) The Textbook of Penetrating Trauma. Baltimore, MD: Williams & Wilkens, 1996.

89. Josephs LG, Este-McDonald JR, Birkett DH et al. Diagnostic laparoscopy increases intracranial pressure. J Trauma 1994; 36:815–819.

90. Bloomfield GL, Ridings PC, Blocher CR, Marmarou A, Sugerman HJ. Effects of increased intra-abdominal pressure upon intracranial and cerebral perfusion pressure before and after volume expansion. J Trauma 1996; 40:936–943.

91. Bloomfield GL, Ridings PC, Blocher CR, Marmarou A, Sugerman HJ. A proposed relationship between increased intra-abdominal, intra-thoracic, and intracranial pressure. Crit Care Med 1997; 25:496–503.

92. Ertel W, Oberholzer A, Platz A, et al. Incidence of Abdominal compartment syndrome after "damage-control" laparotomy in 311 patients with severe abdominal and/or pelvic trauma. Crit Care Med 2000; 28:1747–1753.

93. Meldrum DR, Moore FA, Moore EE, Franciose RJ, Sauaia A, Burch JM. Prospective characterization and selective management of the abdominal compartment syndrome. Am J Surg 1997; 174:667–672.

94. Hong JJ, Cohn SM, Perez JM, Dolich MO, Brown M, McKenney MG. Prospective study of the incidence and outcome of intra-abdominal hypertension and the abdominal compartment syndrome. Br J Surg 2002; 89:591–596.

95. Maxwell RA, Fabian TC, Croce MA et al. Secondary abdominal compartment syndrome: an underappreciated manifestation of severe hemorrhagic shock. J Trauma 1999; 47:995–999.

96. Biffl WL, Moore EE, Burch JM, Offner PJ, Franciose RJ, Johnson JL. Secondary abdominal compartment syndrome is a highly lethal event. Am J Surg 2001; 182:645–648.

97. Balogh Z, McKinley BA, Cocanour CS, Kozar RA, Holcomb JB, Ware DN, Moore FA. Secondary abdominal compartment syndrome is an elusive early complication of traumatic shock resuscitation. Am J Surg 2002; 184:538–543.

98. Sugrue M, Jones F, Lee A, Buist MD, Deane S, Bauman A, Hillman K, Intraabdominal pressure and gastric intramucosal pH: is there an association? World J Surg 1996; 20:988–991.

99. Friedlander MH, Simon RJ, Ivatury R, DiRaimo R, Machiedo GW. Effect of hemorrhage on superior mesenteric artery flow during increased intra-abdominal pressures. J Trauma 1998; 45:433–439.

100. Simon RJ, Friedlander MH, Ivatury RR, DiRaimo R, Machiedo GW. Haemorrhage lowers the threshold for intra-abdominal hypertension-induced pulmonary dysfunction. J Trauma 1997; 42:398–403.

101. Raeburn CD, Moore EE, Biffl WL, et al. The abdominal compartment syndrome is a morbid complication of postinjury damage control surgery. Am J Surg 2001; 182:542–546.

102. Mayberry JC, Mullins RJ, Crass RA et al. Prevention of abdominal compartment syndrome by absorbable mesh prosthesis closure. Arch Surg 1997; 132:957–961.

103. Mayberry JC. Prevention of the abdominal compartment syndrome. Lancet 1999; 354:1749–1750.

104. Offner PJ, de Souza AL, Moore EE, et al. Avoidance of abdominal compartment syndrome in damage-control laparotomy after trauma. Arch Surg 2001; 136:676–681.

105. Latenser BA, Kowal-Vern A, Kimball D, Chakrin A, Dujovny N. A pilot study comparing percutaneous decompression with decompressive laparotomy for acute abdominal compartment syndrome in thermal injury. J Burn Care Rehabil. 2002; 23:190–195.

106. Corcos AC, Sherman HF. Percutaneous treatment of secondary abdominal compartment syndrome. J Trauma 2001; 51:1062–1064.
107. Yang EY, Marder SR, Hastings G, Knudson MM. The abdominal compartment syndrome complicating nonoperative management of major blunt liver injuries: recognition and treatment using multimodality therapy. J Trauma 2002; 52:982–986.

28 Monitoring Techniques During Resuscitation

Kevin R. Ward, MD, R. Wayne Barbee, PhD, and Rao R. Ivatury, MD

INTRODUCTION

Shock is a complex entity defined traditionally as a state in which the oxygen utilization or consumption needs of tissues are not matched by sufficient delivery of oxygen. This mismatch commonly results from states of altered tissue perfusion. From this perspective, cardiopulmonary arrest represents the most extreme of shock states.

Figure 1 represents the basic relationship between oxygen consumption (VO_2) and oxygen delivery (DO_2) that is pertinent to individual organs as well as to the whole body *(1–3)*. As noted, VO_2 can remain constant over a wide range of DO_2. This is possible because most tissue beds are capable of efficiently increasing the extraction of oxygen. This will be reflected by decreasing venous oxygen saturation from each organ. However, when DO_2 reaches a critical threshold, tissue extraction of oxygen cannot be further increased to meet tissue demands. It is at this point that VO_2 becomes directly dependent on DO_2 (DO_2crit) and cells begin to convert to anaerobic metabolism as manifested by increases in certain metabolic products such as lactate, nicotinamide adenine dinucleotide (NADH), and reduced cytochrome oxidase. The point of DO_2crit is the point of dysoxia or ischemia in which tissue DO_2 cannot meet tissue oxygen demand *(2)*. Oxygen debt can be defined as the amount of cumulative difference of VO_2 between baseline and that spent below DO_2crit. As will be discussed latter, the level of accumulated oxygen debt in shock states is linked critically with survival *(4,5)*.

Several unique physiological aspects and principles of cardiac arrest (CA) and cardiopulmonary resuscitation (CPR) exists that will limit the usefulness of many monitoring modalities, some of which will be more useful in the postresuscitation period. These include the following:

1. CA produces a global state of ischemia wherein all organ systems especially those most metabolically active (heart and brain) experience severe ischemia within minutes. DO_2crit

From: *Contemporary Cardiology: Cardiopulmonary Resuscitation*
Edited by: J. P. Ornato and M. A. Peberdy © Humana Press Inc., Totowa, NJ

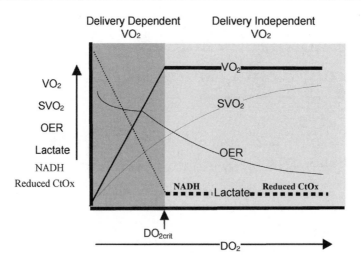

Fig. 1. Biphasic relationship between oxygen delivery (DO_2) and oxygen consumption (VO_2). Oxygen extraction ratio (OER) increases and mixed venous oxygen saturation (SvO_2) decreases in response to decreased DO_2. Below a critical DO_2 (DO_2crit), VO_2 becomes delivery dependent. DO_2 below DO_2crit results in the beginning of anaerobic metabolism as noted by an increase in a variety of cellular products including lactate, NADH, and reduced cytochrome oxidase (CtOx). The DO_2crit of various organ systems can occur at points either above or below whole body DO_2crit depending on the metabolic and blood flow regulatory characteristics of the organ system and the rapidity of the reductions in DO_2. $DO_2 = CO \times CaO_2$ (normal range: 460–650 mL/min/m²); $VO_2 = CO \times (CaO_2 - CvO_2)$ (normal range: 96–170 mL/min/m²); CaO_2 (arterial oxygen content) $= (Hb \times 1.39 \times SaO_2) + (0.003 \times PaO_2)$; $CvO_2 = (Hb \times 1.39 \times SvO_2) + (0.0003 \times PvO_2)$. CO, Cardiac output; PaO_2, arterial oxygen tension; Hb, hemoglobin, SvO_2 normal range 70–80%.

is surpassed immediately. As opposed to other shock states such as those produced by hemorrhage or sepsis, there is no compensatory state prior to sudden death CA. Thus every minute of CA results in a greater temporal-based oxygen debt than other etiologies of shock. This state of profound whole-body ischemia is further complicated by the fact that the brain and heart, which are usually spared globally from dysoxia until the late stages of other forms of shock, almost immediately (within minutes) reach dysoxia in CA. Additionally, depending on the cause of the arrest, individual organ regions may have undergone significant ischemia (such as the case of acute myocardial infarction) prior to arrest or globally, in the case of asphyxial arrest and thus accumulated a signifi-cant degree of regional or whole-body oxygen debt prior to the actual arrest.

2. Traditional CPR is incapable of restoring DO_2 to the point of VO_2 independence. This is especially true of the brain in which high-energy phosphate depletion occurs within minutes and cannot be restored with CPR. Only return of spontaneous circulation or alternative methods of CPR such as open-chest cardiac massage or cardiopulmonary bypass (CPB) can produce this.

3. Optimal outcomes from CA are, for the most part linked, directly to pre-arrest events and the duration of arrest. Thus, the goal of CPR is to achieve hemodynamic changes capable of producing ROSC within seconds to minutes as opposed to the minutes to hours time frame that can be used to affect favorable hemodynamic changes during the postresuscitation period. To date, the major hemodynamic factor determining the ability to produce ROSC is coronary perfusion pressure (CPP).

With these issues in mind, it is apparent that the immediate goal of CPR is to restart the heart as soon as possible to limit the total time of ischemia especially to the brain, and the heart itself. Because of this compressed timeframe, selected monitoring end-points must have the ability to detect targeted processes or parameters, which are linked with ROSC and which are capable of changing within seconds of interventions (i.e., CPP). Monitors must have corresponding response times and be capable of being applied to the patient and reporting data within seconds.

MONITORING DURING CPR

Traditional Monitoring

Monitoring during CPR has traditionally consisted of carotid or femoral pulse palpation along with electrocardiogram (EKG) evaluation in one or more leads. Although the lack of a palpable pulse during CPR may indicate inadequate forward flow, quantification of forward flow cannot be estimated in the presence of a palpable CPR generated pulse because pressures generated by chest compressions may be transmitted equally to both the major arterial and venous vessels *(6)*. Additionally, inability to palpate a pulse has not been demonstrated to conclusively rule out spontaneous forward flow in certain rhythms such as pulseless electrical activity (PEA) *(7)*. Additionally, myocardial blood flow is not dependent on palpated arterial systolic pressure but instead on CPP, which is defined as the difference between aortic diastolic and coronary sinus (or right atrial) diastolic pressure *(8)*. EKG monitoring during CPR will indicate the electrical status of the heart but not mechanical activity. Although perhaps the best attainable in certain circumstances, these two monitoring modalities do not provide reliable information regarding the effectiveness of CPR (both mechanical and pharmacologic interventions) or prognosis given current treatment recommendations.

Central Hemodynamic or Global Monitoring

CORONARY PERFUSION PRESSURE

Laboratory data has clearly demonstrated the relationship between CPP and myocardial blood during CPR and the need to reach a certain threshold of CPP in order to achieve ROSC *(8–10)*. Clinical studies have confirmed the link between CPP and ROSC and have clearly demonstrated that using current treatment resuscitative treatment modalities as recommended by the American Heart Association (AHA), a minimum CPP of 15 mmHg is necessary to achieve ROSC if initial defibrillation attempts fail *(11,12)*. This is necessary although not always sufficient to achieve ROSC and issues such as significant coronary artery lesions, down-time and others will mean that despite reaching a CPP of 15 mmHg, ROSC is not possible. For example, not only are myocardial oxygen requirements of ventricular fibrillation (VF) higher than for example the asystolic heart, fibrillation has been demonstrated to cause mechanical compression of subendocardial vessels *(13,14)*. Higher opening pressures and flow may be required to achieve ROSC in these circumstances *(15,16)*. Additionally, vasopressors such as epinephrine have been demonstrated in some instances to further increase the imbalance between myocardial oxygen demand and delivery despite increasing myocardial blood flow *(9)*.

Clinical studies have demonstrated that CPP can be positive or negative during CPR and cannot be distinguished by palpation of a pulse alone (Fig. 2; *17*). Although monitoring of CPP is the most reliable direct indicator of the adequacy of chest compression

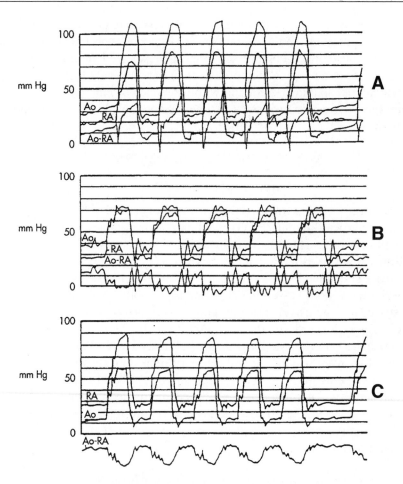

Fig. 2. Aortic (Ao), right atrial (RA), and coronary perfusion (Ao-RA) pressure tracings during human cardiopulmonary resuscitation: (a) positive coronary perfusion pressure (CPP) generated during both compression and relaxation phases of chest compressions; (b) positive CPP generated only during relaxation phase of chest compressions; and (c) negative CPP throughout compression cycle. The degree of CPP cannot be predicted by palpation of CPR produced peripheral pulses. (From ref. *17*.)

and pharmacological interventions, its major drawbacks is that it requires time and resources (equipment and human) because access to both the arterial and central venous vasculature is required to determine arterial diastolic and central venous diastolic pressure. Additionally, pressure transduction supplies and equipment are required to verify pressure tracings and calculate CPP because most pressure monitors, although capable of reporting systolic and diastolic arterial pressure, will report central venous pressure (CVP) as a mean value.

Animal data indicates that the ability to achieve a diastolic arterial pressure of at least 40 mmHg is predictive of ROSC and is likely related to achieving a threshold CPP, however clinical CPP data to substantiate this is lacking and critical CPPs can be achieved in humans without achieving a diastolic arterial blood pressure of 40 mmHg *(18)*. Furthermore, it may be impossible to achieve a diastolic arterial pressure of 40 mmHg in some individuals using traditional closed-chest compressions.

Measurement of CPP in the manner described above is possible in an in-hospital setting especially in intensive care units in which patients may be instrumented already. Unfortunately, this important variable is often ignored. The measurement is also possible in most emergency departments (EDs) with proper staffing and preparation and should be taken advantage of especially in circumstances in which central vascular access is obtained for the purposes of drug administration. Unfortunately, it does not appear that simply monitoring diastolic CVP alone can predict CPP. In reality, because it is becoming increasingly popular to carry out CA resuscitations in their entirety in the prehospital setting, it is unlikely that real-time direct CPP monitoring will ever become a standard in EDs or other settings. Its application in the prehospital setting is simply not feasible from a technical and time standpoint.

ARTERIAL BLOOD PRESSURE MONITORING

Use of oscillometric or other noninvasive blood pressure monitoring techniques will be unreliable in their ability to measure arterial blood pressure during CPR. These methods require detection of pulsations in the cuff or other detector transmitted by the artery. Although these techniques provide acceptable levels of variance from intra-arterial measures in stable patients, levels of variance are increased greatly in states of critical illness. Motion produced during CPR as well as the low pressure produced will require a sensitivity not required of standard applications of the technology (19). If knowledge of systolic pressure is desired, use of a manually inflated pressure cuff along with a Doppler device is recommended remembering that diastolic pressure cannot be determined in this manner. It must be emphasized, however, that achieving a target systolic pressure alone during CPR has never been associated with ROSC, thus use of noninvasive blood pressure monitoring will be of little value during CPR. Because of the physiology of CA and CPR-induced perfusion pressures, significant changes in systolic blood pressure may occur without favorable changes in CPP. Direct arterial blood pressure monitoring will be useful in distinguishing true electromechanical dissociation (EMD) from pseudo-EMD in which patient body habitus or significantly low pulse pressure prevents detection of pulsatile flow by pulse detection or end-tidal CO2 monitoring (discussed later [7]).

During the postresuscitation phase, invasive arterial blood pressure monitoring is recommended because of the noted unreliability of noninvasive measures during labile states (19). Because a minimal perfusion pressure of 70 mmHg is suggested to stay in the autoregulatory range of the brain and to maintain CPP, invasive arterial pressure will be helpful in ensuring this. Invasive monitoring will also make acquisition of arterial blood gases easier.

LABORATORY TESTING

Intermittent venous and arterial blood sampling for gas or chemistry analysis is of limited utility during CPR and basically will have no application in the out-of-hospital setting. Use of whole blood gas and electrolyte measurements (now available at many institutions and in point-of-care testing kits) can provide hemoglobin levels in addition to potassium levels within minutes. These may, of course, be helpful in excluding hyperkalemia and severe anemia as a cause or arrest or inhibitor of attempts at resuscitation. Co-oximetry measurement of hemoglobin for evidence of carbon monoxide poisoning would be helpful in the right circumstances. Severely elevated carboxyhemoglobin levels are likely to preclude successful resuscitation using standard resuscitation techniques

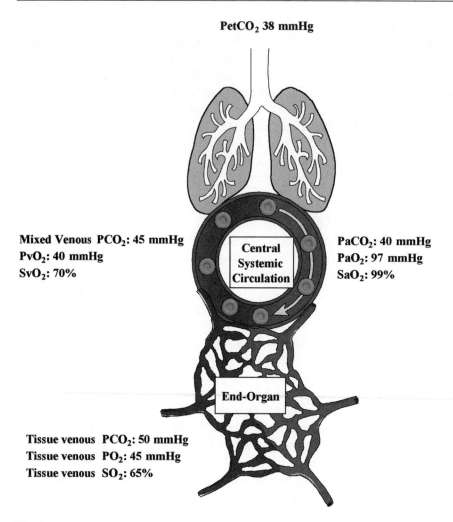

PetCO$_2$ 38 mmHg

Mixed Venous PCO$_2$: 45 mmHg
PvO$_2$: 40 mmHg
SvO$_2$: 70%

Central Systemic Circulation

PaCO$_2$: 40 mmHg
PaO$_2$: 97 mmHg
SaO$_2$: 99%

End-Organ

Tissue venous PCO$_2$: 50 mmHg
Tissue venous PO$_2$: 45 mmHg
Tissue venous SO$_2$: 65%

Fig. 3. Representative blood and tissue gas levels of the normal circulation. Mixed venous values represent aggregate values from all organ systems. Thus, tissue venous values are not necessarily identical to mixed venous values but can be higher or lower depending on the individual organ system's level of metabolic activity. The majority of blood volume at the level of the tissue is contained in the venous compartment.

given the fact that a state of functional anemia will exists in combination with the poor perfusion produced by CPR thus further reducing DO$_2$. Typical blood gas findings during CPR include severe venous respiratory acidosis and arterial respiratory alkalosis that are reflective of the large dead space created in the lungs by CA and the poor forward blood flow produced by chest compressions as compared to the normal circulation (Figs. 3,4; [2–23]). SaO$_2$ is usually 99% with PO$_2$ levels well above 100 mmHg.

Lactate monitoring during CPR itself has been examined as a means to determine down and to titrate therapy (24–26). Normal lactate levels (in the absence of liver failure) are less than 2 mmol/L. Lactic acidosis existing during CPR and the initial postresuscitation period is as a result of inadequate DO$_2$ (type A lactic acidosis). However, single measures will have limited value. Changes in lactate will not occur rapidly enough during

PetCO$_2$ 15 mmHg

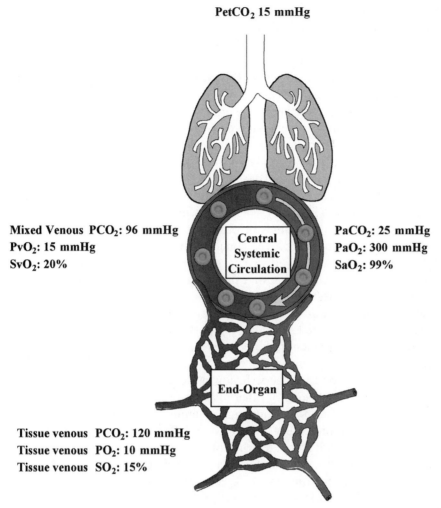

Mixed Venous PCO$_2$: 96 mmHg
PvO$_2$: 15 mmHg
SvO$_2$: 20%

Central Systemic Circulation

PaCO$_2$: 25 mmHg
PaO$_2$: 300 mmHg
SaO$_2$: 99%

End-Organ

Tissue venous PCO$_2$: 120 mmHg
Tissue venous PO$_2$: 10 mmHg
Tissue venous SO$_2$: 15%

Fig. 4. Representative blood and tissue gas levels of the circulation produced during CA and CPR. As a result of the tremendous reductions in blood flow produced by CPR a dead space in the lungs is created thus producing gaps between mixed venous PCO$_2$, PetCO$_2$, and PaCO$_2$. The severe reductions in DO$_2$ to each organ system results in very high oxygen extraction at the level of the tissue, which produces very low tissue venous PO$_2$ and thus SO$_2$ levels. The very high venous PCO$_2$ levels are as a result of both decreased removal of aerobically and anaerobically produced CO$_2$ (*see* Fig. 5). As with Fig. 3, the mixed venous values represent aggregate values of all organ systems.

CPR to allow changes in therapy. In fact, it can be argued that better CPR may result in increasing lactate levels because of wash out phenomena (removal of lactate sequestered in tissue beds into the central circulation) and/or because of enhanced delivery of substrate to cells, which are still below the point of DO$_2$crit thus resulting in additional lactate production. Additionally, lactate levels at the beginning of CPR may differ among individuals based in the etiology of arrest. For example, a person with asthma who experienced significant hypoxemia prior to arrest will have higher levels of lactate and a higher oxygen debt compared to the victim of sudden death. Lactate levels during CPR have not been demonstrated in humans to correlate with neurologic outcome (*27*).

The major utility of lactate monitoring will be in the postresuscitation setting as a useful endpoint to guide postresuscitation hemodynamic management. Lactate levels will be universally elevated immediately after ROSC, therefore use of lactate as a postresuscitation endpoint to the adequacy of DO_2 will require serial measurement. It is thus not the absolute level of lactate that is prognostic in shock as much as it is the ability to halt dysoxic lactate production and clear it (28–31). Lactate clearance of at least 5–10% an hour should be a goal. Rising lactate levels or the inability to clear lactate indicates continuing accumulation of oxygen debt and thus DO_2 levels below DO_2crit or significant regional dysoxia (3,29). Therapies aimed at increasing DO_2 or reducing VO_2 should be instituted.

It is not uncommon to observe elevated or rising lactate levels in the postresuscitation period despite normal or elevated systemic blood pressures. This should be interpreted as an indication of severe microcirculatory shunting, which may be secondary to excessive circulating levels of catecholamines or other vasocative mediators (32). In this setting, the presence of elevated lactate levels concomitant with elevated central or mixed venous hemoglobin oxygen saturation again indicates severe microcirculatory injury and portends a poor outcome (32,33). Nonintuitive therapies such as vasodilator therapy may be required to reverse this state.

Although lactic acid and base deficit are highly correlated, hyperlactatemia (levels 2–5 mmol/L) may be observed in the latter phases of postresuscitation care in the absence of metabolic acidosis as a consequence of processes that increases the glycolytic flux of glucose to lactate such as catecholamine administration (34). Despite this, clinicians should aggressively rule out occult hypoperfusion as a cause of elevated lactate levels.

Postresuscitation laboratory testing of other markers or compounds as indicators of myocardial function, neuronal injury, immune and inflammatory function, and so on, will inevitably come into being as our ability to treat CA and the postresuscitation syndrome evolves. Much of this will result from advances in our understanding of the molecular basis and complex interplay between systems in the pathology and treatment of the disease. One could envision performing bedside genomic and proteomic profiling in the postresuscitation period to understand prognosis better or to develop individual pharmacogenomics approaches to therapy for the patient.

PULSE OXIMETRY

The technique of pulse oximetry utilizes two wavelengths of light (red and infra-red) to determine the percentages of oxy and deoxy hemoglobin. This is determined by isolating the small increase in blood volume occurring at the site of measurements in response to systole and comparing it to background absorption, which includes blood, bone, skin, and other tissue components. The technique thus requires pulsatile flow in order to make the measurement. There has been confusion to the role of pulse oximetry during CPR. Because of the physiology of CPR that produces low systemic blood flows and significant increases in physiologic dead space along with ventilation that uses high flow oxygen, arterial blood gases reveal hemoglobin oxygen saturations of 99% as PaO_2 levels are uniformly above 100 mmHg (20,35). Thus in the absence of significant anemia, obtaining maximum arterial oxygen content during CPR is rarely a problem. In terms of its use to monitor the effectiveness of chest compressions, use of SpO_2 monitoring to observe the produced plethysmograph is unreliable as a result of various issues including such things as nail polish, temperature induced vasoconstriction of digits, shunting as a result of reductions in CPR blood flow, and others. Additionally to this, studies have demonstrated very low pulsatile blood flow is capable of producing a plethysmograph *(36,37)*. Various manufacturers have developed very bright light emitting diodes and sensitive detectors, which can pick up very weak signals. They have even developed sensitive motion artifact rejection software. Most manufacturers "auto scale" the detected plethysmograph for the user thus information on signal intensity is not available. Thus, the ability to detect a peripheral SpO_2 produced plethysmograph is not indicative of adequate CPR.

Examination of the characteristics of the plethysmograph determined by pulse oximetry has not been examined for its ability to correlate with central hemodynamics produced by closed-chest compressions and pharmacologic interventions although it may warrant study. It is likely, however, that interpatient variations produced by arterial vascular disease and other issues will preclude its use as a sensitive guide to resuscitation.

END-TIDAL CO$_2$ MONITORING

Capnometry is the measurement of the concentration of CO_2 in the airway during inspiration and expiration. Capnography refers to the graphic display of this measurement over time. The measurement of CO_2 concentrations at the very end of expiration is termed end-tidal CO_2 ($PetCO_2$). Measurement of CO_2 in respiratory gases can be performed by several methods with infrared spectroscopy being the most common. $PetCO_2$ can also be measured qualitatively and semi-quantitatively using pH-sensitive filter papers containing metacresol purple, which changes color in response to varying concentrations of CO_2 as a result of the formation of hydrogen ions *(38,39)*.

Beginning with the work of Kalenda and Smallhout, the value of $PetCO_2$ monitoring for the resuscitation of victims of CA has been demonstrated repeatedly *(40)*. The value of $PetCO_2$ monitoring lies in its ability to closely reflect alveolar CO_2. Alveolar CO_2 is determined by the combination of CO_2 production (VCO_2), pulmonary capillary blood flow (i.e., cardiac output), and alveolar ventilation. As such, alveolar CO_2 and $PetCO_2$ are linearly related to VCO_2. VCO_2 depends on two different issues: pulmonary excretion and metabolic production of CO_2. In low-flow states with steady-state ventilation, VCO_2 declines secondary to decreased delivery of CO_2 to the lungs and to ventilation/perfusion mismatches in the lung resulting in an enormous increases in dead space (up to 0.7 in the setting of CPR *[41]*). This results in a widening of the arterial PCO_2 to $PetCO_2$ gradient and is further reflected by mixed venous hypercarbia. Although difficult to measure, VCO_2 also declines secondary to reductions in actual CO_2 production from decreases in DO_2 *(21,42,43)*. Although sometimes described as logarithmic, VCO_2 and thus $PetCO_2$ basically have almost the same biphasic relationship with DO_2 as does VO_2 (Fig. 5). As such, DO_2crit as been determined by following changes in VCO_2 and $PetCO_2$ and does not significantly differ compared to determination using changes in VO_2 or lactate production *(42,44)*. Concomitant with reductions in DO_2 will be increases in tissue CO_2 as decreases in blood flow will reduce the amount of aerobically produced CO_2 that is removed from tissue, creating a tissue respiratory acidosis *(45–47)*. Additional tissue CO_2 will be produced after DO_2crit is reached as metabolic acids such a lactic acid is buffered by tissue bicarbonate although tissue CO_2 production as a whole will be decreased in accordance with decreases in VO_2 *(48)*.

VCO_2 and thus $PetCO_2$ are linearly related to DO_2 during states of oxygen supply dependent metabolism. Because during CPR, oxygen content does not significantly change, then the major component of DO_2 tracked by VCO_2 or $PetCO_2$ is cardiac output. This is, of course, advantageous during CPR because as discussed earlier, CPR is a state in which VO_2 is directly dependent on DO_2.

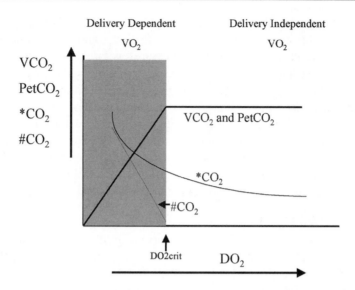

Fig. 5. Biphasic relationship between DO_2 and VCO_2. Note the similarities between the relationships as compared to Fig. 1. When minute ventilation is held constant, DO_2crit can be determined by reductions in VCO_2 and thus $PetCO_2$. This corresponds to the point of delivery dependent VO_2. *CO_2 represents CO_2 that accumulates as a result of decreased removal of aerobically produced CO_2 secondary to decreases in flow (respiratory acidosis). #CO_2 represents additional tissue CO_2 production and accumulation as a result of buffering of metabolic acids produced by anaerobic metabolism after DO_2crit is reached. Overall VCO_2 is decreased as a result of drops in VO_2. Quantities of CO_2 as depicted on the y-axis are not drawn to scale but instead are depicted to demonstrate their temporal relationship to each other in reference to changes in DO_2.

Again, in order for this to be valid, both alveolar ventilation (minute ventilation) and VCO_2 must be assumed to be relatively constant. If this is assumed, then changes in $PetCO_2$ will reflect changes in the pulmonary capillary blood flow or cardiac output. In this setting, although $PetCO_2$ correlates with cardiac output, it does not correlate with actual $PaCO_2$ during CPR in humans because of the large increase in pulmonary dead space produced.

Although VCO_2 production during CPR is difficult to measure, there are not likely to be wide swings. Additionally, the extremely high concentrations of CO_2 in the mixed venous blood pool (>60 mmHg) and large pulmonary dead space ensure that small changes in VCO_2 do not cause appreciable changes in $PetCO_2$ *(21)*. Only ROSC or improved artificial circulation (e.g., with open-chest massage) will result in a dramatic and sustained increase in $PetCO_2$. Minute ventilation should be held relatively constant if one is to use $PetCO_2$ as an indicator of cardiac output.

Both animal and human data have demonstrated that PetCO2 correlates with CPP and cerebral perfusion pressure (CePP) during CPR *(49–51)*. The correlation between $PetCO_2$ and CPP and CePP is as a result of its relationship with cardiac output in the low-flow setting of CPR. This can be predicted based on the known relationship between mean arterial pressure and cardiac output when peripheral vascular resistance (PVR) is constant. Thus, when PVR is not significantly changing, increases in cardiac output will result in increases in organ blood flow with the increase in cardiac output being noted by an increase in PetCO2 if minute ventilation and VCO_2 are constant.

These correlations between $PetCO_2$, CPP, CePP, and cardiac output may be uncoupled by epinephrine and other vasopressors administered during CPR. Animal and human studies have demonstrated that $PetCO_2$ decreases when large doses of epinephrine are used during CA despite significant increases in CPP and myocardial and cerebral blood flow (10,52). Initially thought to be as a result of increases in shunt fraction, it has been found that this effect is as a result of actual decreases in CPR produced cardiac output as a result of increases in afterload (10). Thus, although cardiac output is decreased, DO_2 to the myocardium and cerebrum are increased as a result of the redistribution of blood volume, much of which lies in the aorta. Although consistently shown in animals, the effect of epinephrine administration during CPR on reducing $PetCO_2$ in humans has been variable (53,54). When decreases in $PetCO_2$ occur after epinephrine administration, they correlate with the timing of increases in central arterial levels of epinephrine and the concomitant vasopressor effect. The length of time these changes last, if they occur clinically has not been well quantified. Interestingly, such changes in $PetCO_2$ may be potentially useful for timing subsequent epinephrine or other vasopressor dosing or in understanding if CPR is producing enough forward flow to distribute intravenously administered vasopressors to the systemic circulation.

Because sodium bicarbonate contains and produces CO_2, its bolus administration during CPR will cause a variable but significant transient rise in $PetCO_2$. The timing of this increase is within 1 minute of administration, last usually less than 2 minutes depending on whether minute ventilation changes (55).

End-tidal CO_2 can be used as a feedback to optimize chest compressions during CPR. Monitoring $PetCO_2$ during CA may detect unrecognized CPR provider fatigue (49,56). Because an effective threshold for chest compressions has been demonstrated, $PetCO_2$ may be of value in detecting compression thresholds whether manual or mechanical chest compressions are used (57,58). Changes in pulse pressure as detected by palpation of CPR-produced peripheral pulses do not necessarily correlate with flow (6). $PetCO_2$ on the other hand, provides evidence of improvements or deterioration in real-time forward flow given that one recognizes the possible effects of bicarbonate and vasopressor agents on $PetCO_2$. One effective strategy might be to perform CPR at a rate and compression depth to produce the maximum $PetCO_2$ values. Chest compressions need not be halted during CPR to palpate pulses if $PetCO_2$ monitoring is performed.

In cases of mechanical causes of PEA, $PetCO_2$ monitoring should be valuable in indicating the immediate success of such therapeutic maneuvers as needle decompression of tension pneumothorax, pericardiocentesis for relief of cardiac tamponade, or fluid resuscitation for hypovolemia. $PetCO_2$ monitoring might also be deemed to be helpful in determining which patients with PEA have true electromechanical dissociation vs those with significant cardiac contractions but in whom a pulse cannot be palpated as a result of obesity, vasoconstriction, or hypothermia. Paradis et al. found a significant number of patients with PEA to have arterial pulse pressures when invasively monitored, with several patients having systolic blood pressures of 90 mmHg (7). $PetCO_2$ monitoring would have demonstrated values significantly greater than 0 mmHg in these patients when no chest compressions are performed.

Several investigators have reported $PetCO_2$ values during CPR that may offer prognostic information concerning chances of obtaining ROSC. These include averaging $PetCO_2$ values over 20 minutes of resuscitation, taking initial and maximal $PetCO_2$ values, measuring $PetCO_2$ changes after epinephrine administration and measuring $PetCO_2$ values during resuscitation of various presenting rhythms such as asystole or

PEA *(59–64)*. Levine and colleagues have demonstrated that a $PetCO_2$ value of less than 10 mmHg after 20 minutes of resuscitation in out-of-hospital CA with PEA has a 100% predictive value of no ROSC *(63)*. Similar results have been observed in other out-of-hospital studies as well as in the in-hospital setting *(53,54,60,61)*. Others have demonstrated that an initial PetCO2 value of less than 15 mmHg has a 91% predictive value for no ROSC. The use of high-dose epinephrine (>10 mg) changes but does not eliminate the ability of $PetCO_2$ to predict ROSC. Two studies have demonstrated that reductions in $PetCO_2$ after epinephrine administration result in positive predictive values for ROSC ranging from 29 to 53% and negative predictive value ranging from 92 to 100% *(53,54)*. Nonetheless, it should be remembered that epinephrine doses of greater than 1 mg may decrease or have no effect on $PetCO_2$ *(54)*.

Although no formal guidelines or recommendations have been made by any organization concerning the use of $PetCO_2$ to guide CPR efforts, the following is suggested. For $PetCO_2$ less than 10 mmHg, the clinician should modify the ongoing resuscitation. Better standard CPR (e.g., increased rate or depth of compression) should be performed. If despite optimal performance of CPR, $PetCO_2$ values remain less than 10 mmHg and the clinical scenario warrants aggressive intervention, the clinician should consider an alternative method of CPR such as open-chest cardiac massage. If despite optimal resuscitative efforts, the $PetCO_2$ cannot be raised to greater than 10 mmHg and the patient's dysrhythmia is not amenable to electrical therapy, ceasing resuscitation efforts in a normothermic arrest patient should be considered *(55)*.

Because values are low during CPR and mixed venous PCO_2 is so high, ROSC should be immediately detected by significant increases in $PetCO_2$. $PetCO_2$ values have been shown to be the first changes noted after ROSC *(55,65,66)*. On ROSC, there is a rapid rise in $PetCO_2$ that will generally overshoot values of 40 mmHg. This overshoot stems from the large tissue and venous respiratory acidosis that has existed because the onset of arrest. Elevated $PetCO_2$ may persist for some time as CO_2 is washed out of various tissue beds. $PetCO_2$ monitoring can be helpful at this time in adjusting minute ventilation as a guide to bringing $PaCO_2$ back to baseline because ROSC will reduce dead space back to levels in which $PetCO_2$ can be used to estimate $PaCO_2$. This will assist in using ventilation to control systemic pH. Similarly, $PetCO_2$ monitoring can help detect deterioration in perfusion after resuscitation. Sudden drops in $PetCO_2$ after ROSC when no changes in ventilation have been made can be interpreted as significant deterioration in cardiac output consistent returning to a state below DO_2crit *(42,44)*. In these instances, re-arrest is likely to be imminent if not action is taken.

In summary, $PetCO_2$ monitoring is an ideal monitoring tool for use during CPR and in the postresuscitation period as a result of its linear relationship with cardiac output in low-flow states and the relationship between cardiac output and critical perfusion pressures such as CPP and CePP. Its link with these central hemodynamic events during CPR allows real-time changes to be detected within seconds of interventions given current CA treatment protocols. For purposes of diagnostic and treatment decisions, $PetCO_2$ monitoring during CPR should be carried out with devices using infrared technology so that quantitative values can be obtained and inspection of the capnogram can take place.

Cardiac Output and Oxygen Consumption Monitoring

There are now numerous invasive and noninvasive means to monitor cardiac output. These range from traditional thermodilution methods using the pulmonary artery catheter to less invasive methods, which utilize impedance cardiography, esophageal Doppler technology, rebreathing of CO_2 (CO_2 Fick method) and others *(67–70)*. Although the use of noninvasive methods to measure cardiac output during CPR is tempting, the efficacy of such an approach is questionable especially in light of the proven utility of $PetCO_2$ monitoring described previously. If the goal of CPR is to produce the highest cardiac output and CPP to achieve ROSC in the shortest period of time, it would be difficult to justify actual cardiac output monitoring during CPR. Furthermore, given the low cardiac outputs and motion that CPR produces, it is doubtful that any cardiac output readings obtained with these techniques would have the required accuracy and precision to be useful.

Cardiac output monitoring may be more useful in the postresuscitation setting as a means to recognize cardiac dysfunction and to optimize global DO_2. Use of cardiac output as an end-point unto itself is ill advised because significant end-organ hypoperfusion can exist despite normal and even supernormal cardiac output *(71–77)*. Instead, a more appropriate use of cardiac output monitoring may be as a guide to volume resuscitation in determining optimal preload (volume challenges provided until no further increase in cardiac output obtained). Additionally, its use in conjunction with markers of end-organ perfusion (discussed below) may assist in identifying the points in which pharmacologic therapy to increase cardiac output has been maximized and in turn the need to institute additional circulatory adjuncts such as intra-aortic balloon pumping. The method of cardiac output monitoring used is not as important as how and when it is used.

Measurement of VO_2 in states of critical illness is very underutilized. Although its use during CPR will be uninformative because a state of severe DO_2-dependent VO_2 is present, it use during the postresuscitation phase of care has shown promise in being predictive of survival. There are two major methods of measuring VO_2 *(1)*. These include the use of the indirect or reverse Fick method, which requires insertion of a pulmonary artery catheter for determination of cardiac output and the arterial to mixed venous difference in oxygen content and the use of indirect calorimetry. The latter is believed to be more accurate because it eliminates the potential for mathematical coupling of VO_2 with cardiac output that is believed to occur *(1)*. Additionally, it takes into account actual oxygen utilization of the lung itself, which can be substantial in some situations *(78)*.

Rivers et al. reported the use of VO_2 monitoring after CA and found that failure to achieve of VO_2 greater than 90 mL per minute per m^2 within the first 6 hours of arrest was associated with a 100% mortality at 24 hours after ROSC *(32)*. The reasons for this appear to be twofold. First there is as expected a component of cardiogenic shock in which DO_2 is impaired from a cardiac output perspective. However, importantly but under-recognized is that the oxygen extraction ratio in these individuals is lower than expected and is accompanied by the presence of venous hyperoxia *(32,33)*. This indicates the likely presence of an impairment in microcirculatory DO_2 as a result of microcirculatory occlusion or shunting, which contributes to the accumulation of a fatal level of oxygen debt.

A very valuable surrogate of VO_2 monitoring is mixed venous (SvO_2) or central venous ($ScvO_2$) hemoglobin oxygen saturation monitoring. The use of mixed venous hemoglobin oxygen saturation (SvO_2) has long been advocated as a means to detect tissue hypoxia in the critically ill or injured patient because it is a reflection of oxygen extraction that in turn is a reflection of the adequacy of DO_2 *(72)*. Normal values average 75%. SvO_2 reflects the aggregate balance between tissue oxygen delivery and consumption or the extraction ratio of all tissues and is thus a reflection of global DO_2 (Fig. 1). It is not difficult to understand the potential value of such a measure as an early warning system in identifying reductions in DO_2 prior to DO_2crit as well as the need for increasing DO_2

even after reaching a state of VO_2 independent DO_2. However, placement of a pulmonary artery catheter is difficult in the immediate postresuscitation period (and in fact may not be needed) and impossible during CPR. Although not truly mixed, a suitable surrogate of SvO_2 may be $ScvO_2$ monitoring *(79–82)*. $ScvO_2$ has been advocated for use during CPR (79). Similar to tissue CO_2 measurements, $ScvO_2$ values will be significantly below baseline demonstrating maximum oxygen extraction. Rivers and colleagues have found that similar to CPP thresholds, there appears to be a $ScvO_2$ threshold below which patients undergoing CPR cannot be resuscitated. In there studies, no patient with an $ScvO_2$ of less than 30% could be resuscitated. All but one patient who achieved ROSC obtained an $ScvO_2$ during CPR of at least 40%. These findings should be reflective of the adequacy of DO_2 based on the cardiac output produced during CPR. Unfortunately, the study by Rivers did not simultaneously report $PetCO_2$ levels and thus it is unclear if $ScvO_2$ monitoring would have any significant advantage over $PetCO_2$ monitoring during CA that would justify it use.

Similar, however, to some of the tissue specific methods of monitoring discussed below, the real value of $ScvO_2$ or SvO_2 monitoring will likely be in the postresuscitation setting as a means to exclude occult tissue hypoxia and to determine the adequacy DO_2. Of special note is the ability of the technique to detect venous hyperoxia as a manifestation of severe microcirculatory injury especially after high dose vasopressor use *(32)*. In this setting $ScvO_2$ levels are noted to be significantly elevated in the presence of elevated lactate levels indicating the likely presence of significant shunting *(32,38)*. In this setting, the body is not consuming oxygen (again likely as a result of problems with microcirculatory DO_2) and measures that increase microcirculatory DO_2 must be considered quickly before fatal levels of oxygen debt are reached. Such measures might include intra-aortic balloon pumping, use of vasodilators, or use of extracorpreal circulation techniques. Although studies examining the use of both SvO_2 and tissue specific indicators of oxygenation such as gastric tonometry in other shock states such as trauma and sepsis (discussed below) have demonstrated the superiority of tissue-specific measures over SvO_2, these studies have not applied the techniques ultra early. It is therefore unclear if there would be cases in the immediate postarrest period in which $ScvO_2$ would be normal but tissue-specific measures would be abnormal. The transition from perfusion limited shock states (hemorrhage, cardiogenic) to those associated with significant inflammation (sepsis) make the interpretation of both SvO_2, $ScvO_2$ and tissue-specific measures such as gastric tonometry more difficult *(71,72,84)*. However, recent evidence suggest that early use of $ScvO_2$ will be capable of identifying significant tissue hypoxia (much of it occult) and will be useful as an end-point to guide treatment and in identifying states of venous hyperoxia after CA *(32,82,85)*. The technique has the added advantage of allowing the user to monitor CVP and thus assist in optimizing preload.

ULTRASOUND

Rapid access and use of ultrasound in the emergent setting is becoming a more common reality given advances in the quality and portability of devices. In the setting of CA, ultrasound can rapidly assist the clinician in distinguishing between true EMD and pseudo-EMD during treatment of PEA. It will also assist the clinician in diagnosing other causes of PEA or arrest such as pericardial tamponade (in addition to guiding pericardiocentesis) and in diagnosing exsanguinating intra-abdominal or intrathoracic hemorrhage. The use of special ultrasound variations such as transesophageal echocardiography that provide higher resolution visualization of the heart and mediastinal structures, may be useful in identifying other causes of CA such as pulmonary embolism or aortic dissection and in detecting severe valvular abnormalities *(86)*. Finally, the use of ultrasound for echocardiography in the postresuscitation period could be extremely useful in judging the degree of postarrest myocardial dysfunction and in making decisions on how to assist the failing heart. Ultrasound may also be used to assist in vascular cannulation of central vessels when blind cannulation using anatomical landmarks is unsuccessful *(87,88)*. The major limitations to the use of ultrasound in the settings above are the experience and skills of the operator. Making the diagnosis of pericardial tamponade or intra-abdominal hemorrhage will require less skill than determining the degree of myocardial dysfunction in the postresuscitation setting.

Tissue-Specific Monitoring

Figure. 1 demonstrates the biphasic relationship between VO_2 and VCO_2 with DO_2 existing not only for the whole body but also for individual organ systems that may have DO_2 crit values, which differ from whole-body DO_2 crit. Studies have demonstrated, for example in hemorrhagic shock that the DO_2 crit of the splanchnic bed occurs at a higher global DO_2 than the DO_2crit of the whole body *(48,89,90)*. However, as noted earlier, CA immediately results in a state of profound delivery-dependent VO_2 so that all organ systems are immediately past their DO_2crit values. As such, each would demonstrate evidence of profound tissue hypoxia and flow stagnation as represented by very low venous hemoglobin oxygen saturations and elevated venous or tissue CO_2 levels. The advantage of monitoring one tissue over another in this setting is difficult to defend. However, tissue-specific monitoring in the postresuscitation setting may make sense based in the characteristics of the tissue and the goals to be achieved.

Tissue CO_2 Monitoring

Several monitoring options are available to monitor tissue CO_2 and have been studied in various shock states. These include transcutaneous CO_2 ($PtcCO_2$) skin monitoring, interstitial fiberoptic PCO_2, gastric mucosal CO_2 via gastric tonometry ($PgCO_2$), and most recently, sublingual tonometry ($PslCO_2$ *[72,91–99]*). $PtcCO_2$, $PgCO_2$, and $PslCO_2$ are noninvasive, whereas interstitial PCO_2 monitoring requires probe insertion into tissue parenchyma. The details regarding how CO_2 is actually measured by these techniques has been well described *(72)*. All of these methods are based on the diffusion of CO_2 from tissue. Each of these techniques will reflect the balance between supply of CO_2 to the tissue, CO_2 production by the tissue, and CO_2 removal of the tissue. This balance does not mean all tissue compartments contribute equally. Values will be a composite of vascular and interstitial levels in the immediate environment of the sensor. Because the majority of blood volume in tissues in venous (approx 70%), the tissue CO_2 concentrations will mainly reflect venous PCO_2 concentrations *(100,101)*. The ability of these measures, however, to reflect the balance between DO_2 and VO_2 or to reflect perfusion pressures or other real-time hemodynamic changes during CPR has not been studied. It is unknown how high CO_2 concentrations can reach in each tissue after CA in humans. However, in animal models, some tissue beds reach levels well over 100 mmHg *(102)*. The majority of CO_2 accumulation in each tissue will be secondary to inability to remove aerobically produced CO_2 that was being produced prior to ischemia. As mentioned previously, additional CO_2 will be produced in response to metabolic acids (mainly lactate) produced after the onset of ischemia by the cells as they are buffered by endogenous bicarbonate stores. Interpretation of real-time changes in tissue PCO_2 in response to interventions will be challenging compared to use in other shock settings in which there is significantly more flow and more time for trending. If improvements in forward flow are not accompanied by an increase in minute ventilation, arterial PCO_2 will be increased thus more CO_2 will be delivered to the tissue (22). Use of vasopressors to improve CPP and CePP will most likely result in decreases in peripheral tissue flow, thus potentially further reducing removal of CO_2 during CPR. It is doubtful that tracking tissue CO_2 changes will be meaningful during the short duration of CA, especially given the redistribution of blood flow, which occurs during CPR and in response to vasopressor administration. Response times are unlikely to be rapid enough to guide the resuscitation effort. Although this seems counterintuitive based on the previous discussion of $PetCO_2$ monitoring, it must be remembered that $PetCO_2$ is reflecting CO_2 at the end of its journey from the tissue beds. Its rapid breath-by-breath analysis makes its response time to interventions difficult to improve on. The only thing that can be said with certainty is that on ROSC, tissue PCO_2 should rapidly decline as CO_2 is removed from previously stagnant tissue beds and aerobic metabolism is re-established.

The real value of tissue CO_2 monitoring will be in the postresuscitation phase of care in which it can be used to assist in assuring resolution of end-organ perfusion abnormalities. $PgCO_2$ and perhaps $PslCO_2$ may be particularly helpful. The splanchnic bed is particularly sensitive to reductions in systemic blood flow in part because the responsiveness of its vasculature to the myriad of vasoactive mediators associated with shock (103,104). Of special concern in the victim of CA are the mediators angiotensin II, vasopressin, endothelin, and epinephrine. Endogenous levels of these agents are significantly elevated during shock and of course will be even higher in the postresuscitation phase if vasopressin and epinephrine are administered during the arrest to achieve ROSC or in the postresuscitation period to maintain blood pressure (105,106). These and other vasopressor agents provided for blood pressure support in shock states have been demonstrated to contribute to intestinal mucosal ischemia (103,107). This in turn has been hypothesized to lead a breach of the intestinal mucosal barrier, allowing bacteria and other toxic mediators into the systemic circulation, which leads to sepsis and multisystem organ failure (108–112). This paradigm, which is generally accepted in other shock states has not been well studied in the setting of CA (104). The postresuscitation experience of patients who received vasopressin during CPR has not been well described and no clinical studies regardless of vasopressin use have been reported that have examined the incidence of splanchnic hypoperfusion or ischemia as determined by $PgCO_2$ monitoring. Regardless, the need for vasopressor support in the postresuscitation phase is high and will be complicated by a large component of cardiogenic shock. Monitoring of splanchnic blood flow by either $PgCO_2$ or $PslCO_2$ as performed in other shock states makes sense especially in the very early stages of postresuscitation care because, as with other shock states, there is clear evidence that occult splanchnic ischemia can exists in the presence of normal systemic variable such as blood pressure, heart rate, cardiac output, and mixed venous hemoglobin oxygen saturation (71,113,114).

$PgCO_2$ monitoring has been used successfully to guide the resuscitation of trauma patients and those with septic and cardiogenic shock (74,94,115). This technique essentially monitors intraluminal CO_2 in the stomach, which has diffused from the stomach mucosa. A modified nasogastric tube containing a CO_2 permeable balloon is placed in the stomach. Air is circulated intermittently through the balloon. CO_2 diffuses from the mucosa into the balloon in which it is circulated proximally and measured via an infrared detector in the same manner as PetCO$_2$. This CO$_2$ value has been used previously to estimate the intramucosal pH (pHi) by substituting it for arterial CO$_2$ in the Henderson-Hasselbach equation. Use of this formula assumes that arterial HCO$_3$—and mucosal HCO$_3$—are equivalent. pHi values of less than 7.32 are considered abnormal. The technique also assumes constant minute ventilation. A more robust use of the technology uses PgCO$_2$–PaCO$_2$ or PgCO$_2$–PetCO$_2$ gap to detect abnormalities in perfusion because this does not require the previous assumptions regarding HCO$_3$—and in addition does not require strict maintenance of normocapnia because hypo- or hyperventilation, although effecting PgCO$_2$ will not effect the gap. Given the arterial to alveolar pCO$_2$ gap is approx 4 mmHg, it is felt that a PgCO$_2$–PaCO$_2$ or PgCO$_2$–PetCO$_2$ gap greater than 11–14 mmHg is abnormal and reflective of perfusion abnormalities *(95)*. Although the response time of current PgCO$_2$ methodologies will not lend themselves to using during CPR, they should prove to be quite valuable during the postresuscitation period. As with other shock state, normalization of the PgCO$_2$–PaCO$_2$ or PgCO$_2$–PetCO$_2$ gap will help ensure that occult tissue hypoxia is not present, thus helping to avoid further accumulation of oxygen debt and its associated complications.

The development of PslCO$_2$ monitoring as a substitute for PgCO$_2$ monitoring to detect shock and guide its treatment is a recent development. Several studies appear to support the premise that the sublingual surface of the tongue may be as sensitive to disturbances in perfusion as the rest of the gastrointestinal (GI) tract perhaps owing that its shares the same embryonic origin as the rest of the gut *(45,46,96,97,116–119)*. This technique uses fiberoptic determination of CO$_2$ within a disposable cover (similar to oral electronic thermometer), which allows diffusion of CO$_2$ from the sublingual surface into the space between the cover and sensor. The advantage of this technique is that the response time is faster because the sensor is more or less in direct contact with tissue surface as opposed to PgCO$_2$ balloon, which is in the middle of a large lumen (the stomach). The disadvantage is that it is still as of yet difficult to perform continuous monitoring. As with PgCO$_2$, or any other tissue CO$_2$ monitoring technique, the gap of the measure using either PaCO$_2$ or PetCO$_2$ should be utilized in order to avoid misinterpretation of PslCO$_2$ in the setting of hyper or hypocarbia. Definitive values of this gap or of absolute PslCO$_2$ levels have not been determined, but it is likely that they will not differ from those of the PgCO$_2$–PaCO$_2$ or PgCO$_2$–PetCO$_2$ gap. Although use of the PslCO$_2$–PetCO$_2$ gap may have potential value in monitoring during actual CPR, it is likely that it will have no advantage over simple PetCO$_2$ monitoring. As suggested above, it is plausible that the use of vasopressors would actually increase PslCO$_2$ despite increasing CPP above a critical threshold for ROSC.

Similarly, PtcCO$_2$ monitoring of the skin and/or interstitial tissue PCO$_2$ monitoring of tissues such as skeletal muscle may be useful in the postresuscitation setting in assuring resolution of end-organ tissue perfusion abnormalities. Both should be used similar that described for PgCO$_2$ and PslCO$_2$. Continued elevation of CO$_2$ as measured by these methods in the presence of normocapnia have been associated with an increased mortality *(91,98,99,120,121)*. Of note is that the technology used to measure interstitial PCO$_2$ is the same used in the development of continuous arterial blood gas monitoring and is thus also capable of simultaneous measurement of PO$_2$ and pH. The disadvantage of the technique is that it is slightly invasive, and can only sense the environment several micrometers from the sensor. It also requires a considerable calibration time (on the order of 30 minutes).

Tissue Oxygen Monitoring

Similar to tissue CO_2 monitoring, several options exist to monitor tissue oxygenation, which provides information regarding the balance between DO_2 and VO_2 of the tissue. These include transcutaneous PO_2 ($PtcO_2$) monitoring from the skin, interstitial PO_2 monitoring from tissue parenchyma, and tissue hemoglobin oxygen saturation (StO_2) using near infrared absorption spectroscopy (NIRS). The general principles making tissue oxygenation monitoring potentially helpful are the same as those discussed above concerning tissue PCO_2.

Of special interest is the use of StO_2 monitoring using NIRS. Visible light (450–700 nm) penetrates tissue only short distances because it is usually strongly attenuated by various tissue components, which absorb and scatter at these wavelengths. In the NIR spectrum (700–1100 nm), however, photons are capable of deeper penetration (several centimeters or more) even through bone. It is also within this spectral region that oxygen-dependent electronic transitions of the metalloproteins hemoglobin and cytochrome oxidase (the terminal electron acceptor in the mitochondrial electron transport chain) absorb light. These chromophores absorb NIR radiation differentially based on their concentration and interaction with oxygen. These changes in absorption can be measured using NIRS technology. The Beer-Lambert law provides the physical and mathematical basis for NIRS although it is modified to account for the inhomogeneous media that the NIR light traverses. The depth of penetration and volume of tissue begin interrogated by NIRS is dependent on the distance between optodes. The technique of NIRS differs from that of pulse oximetry because pulse oximetry targets only the arterial component of blood flow.

The basis for using NIRS to monitor the state of tissue oxygenation is similar to that of tissue PCO_2 monitoring in that it relies on the compartmentalization of blood volume, which in most systems is believed to be proportioned among the arteriolar, capillary and venular compartments in a ratio of 10:20:70%, respectively (100,101). Thus, the values obtained by NIRS closely parallel those of venous hemoglobin leaving the tissue. This essentially allows it to be used in the same manner as SvO_2 and $ScvO_2$, except that instead of representing an aggregate reflection of the balance between DO_2 and VO_2 for the entire body, it becomes the reflection of such in an individual organ (skeletal muscle, brain, and so on). In addition to being noninvasive, the use of StO_2 monitoring may prove more sensitive over $ScvO_2$ or SvO_2 if the organ being interrogated is sensitive to changes in DO_2.

The vast majority of NIRS technology has been used to monitor the oxygenation status of the brain in neonates and in adults undergoing operative procedures that may effect the brain such as carotid endarterectomy, or cardiopulmonary bypass (122,123). It is also being aggressively studied in the setting of trauma by using skeletal muscle or GI tract as the end-organ of interest (124–127). Normal NIRS derived StO_2 values for brain and skeletal muscle range from 60 to 80%. The use of NIRS during both CA and in the postresuscitation phase has been reported only for the brain (128–131). For use in the brain, special bilateral probes are placed on the forehead. This is necessary because it reduces the amount of skeletal muscle that the NIR light must traverse. The NIRS spectra between hemoglobin and myoglobin cannot be distinguished from each other. This is important because myoglobin exist in almost equal proportions to hemoglobin in skeletal muscle with the P50 for myoglobin being only 5 mmHg (132,133). There is some evidence that when used as an indicator of skeletal muscle oxygenation, the NIRS signal is derived mainly from myoglobin and not hemoglobin within the tissue (134). This would limit its use during CPR and potentially the postresuscitation period if skeletal muscle was chosen and the end-organ to guide resuscitation efforts. Based on these issues, when used for brain oxygenation monitoring, the NIRS signal is reported then to derive from the frontal lobes. The bilateral probes have their origin in allowing comparison between the cerebral circulations of both hemispheres during surgical procedures in which the circulation to one hemisphere may be compromised. As expected, StO_2 values are so low during CPR they cannot be registered in many instances. There is some evidence, however, that during CPR, higher cerebral StO_2 values are associated with ROSC [128]. This is not surprising given the redistribution of blood flow during CA and the relationship between myocardial and cerebral blood flow with CPR-produced cardiac output described earlier. Similar to $PetCO_2$ monitoring, StO_2 values should immediately increase on ROSC. Additional studies will need to be performed to include a larger number of patients to understand if, as with $PetCO_2$ monitoring, there is a threshold cerebral StO_2 values below which victims cannot achieve ROSC. Unfortunately, no studies to date have measured cerebral StO_2 values concomitantly with $PetCO_2$ monitoring to understand if StO_2 values are simply a reflection of cardiac output and therefore CPP and CePP similar to $PetCO_2$. If it is, it may be hard to justify StO_2 monitoring during CPR over the technology of $PetCO_2$ monitoring that also is capable of providing information concerning proper airway management and sudden hemodynamic collapse after ROSC.

It is tempting to suggest the use of cerebral StO_2 monitoring in the postresuscitation phase to guide therapy. Although it may be a valid assumption that the circulation to the frontal lobes during CA is indicative of blood flow to the rest of the brain (because the cerebral circulation is maximally dilated), use of cerebral StO_2 monitoring during the postresuscitation phase may be more complicated. It is well known that the brain undergoes a complicated pattern of heterogeneous blood flow and oxygen extraction in the postresuscitation period along with the potential for decreased global cerebral DO_2 [135–139]. Although there is potential for use of cerebral oximetry in this setting, it has met with mixed results [128,131]. When compared to jugular venous bulb oximetry (a measure of global cerebral oxygen utilization), NIR cerebral oximetry values are higher, indicating that they may not be reflective of global cerebral blood flow and oxygenation, especially given that the majority of blood flow heterogeneity and damage will occur in the regions of the hippocampus and basal ganglia, which are supplied by different circulation than the frontal lobes. Because of blood flow heterogeneity and differences in regional cerebral metabolic activity, it may be difficult to understand changes in cerebral StO_2 values as being secondary to changes in blood flow vs extraction as a result of increased metabolism. Infarction of a region of brain tissue being interrogated may result in increases in StO_2 [129]. It is unclear how the use of therapeutic hypothermia will effect the potential for NIRS use in the brain in the postresuscitation period.

As mentioned earlier, NIR StO_2 monitoring of skeletal muscle as an end-organ during CPR or in the postresuscitation period will require further study. Use of NIR StO_2 monitoring of the GI tract is still in the experimental stages of development.

Although the potential exists to use NIRS to determine the redox status of the cytochrome oxidase (the terminal electron acceptor in the mitochondrial transport chain) and thus the point of DO_2crit for the organ being monitored, this has proven to be extraordinarily challenging in part because the reduced form of cytochrome oxidase does not have an absorption spectrum and because the amount of cytochrome oxidase is so much smaller compared to hemoglobin. Thus, in order to use NIRS to monitor the redox state of the mitochondria, monitoring must take place prior to changes in the redox state. This obviously limits value for monitoring during CA or the postresuscitation state.

Ventricular Waveform Analysis

It has long been held that VF represented a simple chaotic dysrhythmia with little structure. It had been observed that the initial VF rhythm appeared "coarse" and later became "fine" in appearance as the arrest continued and that course VF seemed to be more amendable to treatment than fine VF. Often, defibrillation of fine VF resulted in postcountershock asystole or PEA, which was difficult to resuscitate. Several studies seem to clearly indicate that deterioration of the VF waveform occurs in response to depletion of intramyocardial high-energy phosphates, which may make it more prone to injury from the countershock itself. In fact, several studies have demonstrated that treatment of VF with chest compressions and epinephrine prior to countershock appears to increase the chances of successful defibrillation into a perfusing rhythm *(140–142)*. Before the last decade, little had been done to objectively analyze the rhythm for patterns, which could predict response to treatment.

Various aspects of the VF waveform have been analyzed in various models of CA. These include amplitude, median frequency, dominant frequency, edge frequency, centroid frequency, and peak power frequency *(143–149)*. Of these, the parameter of median frequency appears to hold the most promise in predicting successful defibrillation. The median frequency correlates directly with myocardial blood flow in animal models of CPR. Digital filtering is effective at removing CPR-induced artifact such that spectral analysis of the VF waveform may proceed without the need to interrupt chest compressions. Although median frequency has shown promise in predicting down time, the animal and human models studied were those in which the initial rhythm was VF and there was no intervening therapy prior to spectral analysis.

The attractiveness of using spectral analysis of the VF waveform is its apparent direct link to myocardial blood flow (demonstrated in animal models). This will be particularly important in humans in whom significant coronary artery occlusions may exist, which impede myocardial blood flow despite what appears to be good CPR-produced cardiac output and CPP based on $PetCO_2$ analysis.

Use of VF analysis tools is of course limited to VF and will thus not be helpful in gauging the response of asystole, PEA or pulseless ventricular tachycardia (VT) to treatment nor predict outcome. An important aspect of VF waveform analysis technology that will require study is its performance in settings in which VF is not the initial rhythm encountered or in which patients have repetitive episodes of VF with intervening rhythms including ROSC followed by re-fibrillation. Despite this, incorporation of this type of technology in defibrillators including automated external defibrillators holds great potential to improve outcomes from VF. Although the data is compelling, this technology awaits a definitive prospective trial. The major impediment to use of such technology will be the mammoth re-education of health care providers who have been taught for decades to defibrillate first and then provide adjunctive treatments.

Postresuscitation Monitoring

Resuscitation of the CA victim does not end with ROSC. The immediate post-ROSC period represents a complex shock state with components of both traditional cardiogenic shock from ischemia, and microvascular shunting as a result of vasopressor use and occurrence of microthrombi. It is during this time that rapid institution of both global and tissue-specific goal-directed measures of oxygen transport should take place to optimize the potential for both satisfactory cardiovascular and neurologic outcomes (*see* Fig. 1).

Table 1

Monitoring End-Points During CPR

CPP	>15 mmHg
PetCO$_2$	>10 mmHg (prior to vasopressor administration)
ScvO$_2$	>40%

Postresuscitation Monitoring Goals

Global End-Points

Mean Arterial Pressure	70–90 mmHg
CVP/PCWP	10–15/15–18 mmHg (or pressure, which results in no further improvement in CO)
Hemoglobin	>10 g/dL
Lactate	<2.0 mM
SaO$_2$	94–99%
ScvO$_2$/SvO$_2$	70–80%
VO$_2$	> 90 mL/min/m^2

Tissue-Specific End-Points

pHi	>7.32
PgCO$_2$–PaCO$_2$ gap	<15 mmHg
PgCO$_2$–PetCO$_2$ gap	<15 mmHg
PslCO$_2$–PaCO$_2$ gap	<15 mmHg
PslCO$_2$-PetCO$_2$ gap	<15 mmHg
StO$_2$	>65% (skeletal muscle, brain, or gastrointestinal tract)

The time of ROSC does not ensure that a state of VO$_2$-independent DO$_2$ exists. It is thus incumbent on the clinician to institute such monitoring techniques that can assist in assuring that both overt and occult tissue hypoxia is being resolved. The importance of this cannot be overemphasized. Both animal and clinical studies have demonstrated the effect of cumulative oxygen debt on mortality or in developing significant morbidity such as multisystem organ failure. Studies in critically ill surgery patients demonstrate little or no mortality when oxygen debt is less than 4100 mL/m^2. Mortality increases to 50% and 95% when cumulative oxygen debt is 4900 mL/m^2 and 5800 mL/m^2, respectively *(4,5)*. In contrast for a 70-kg individual with a baseline VO$_2$ of 120 mL/min/m^2, a 30-minute CA would create an oxygen debt of only 3600 mL/m^2. Rivers demonstrated that significant additional oxygen debt can accumulate after ROSC that cannot be quantified by blood pressure and other conventional means *(32,33)*. It is thus apparent that significant ongoing accumulation of oxygen debt is possible during the postresuscitation period. Deferring aggressive postresuscitation care until for example, the patient is moved from the ED into the intensive care unit is ill conceived and runs the risk of allowing patients to develop cumulative oxygen debts, which are not consistent with prolonged survival.

Although there are many end-points to choose from, those that can be instituted rapidly within the first minutes of ROSC are preferred and may be able to guide the clinical team to determine whether additional monitoring and therapy is warranted. Our preference is to use a combination of global and tissue-specific techniques in a goal-directed fashion. The techniques and principles discussed are applicable to all forms of initial resuscitation including trauma. Table 1 lists those end-points that should be considered during CPR to gauge the effectiveness of the resuscitation as well as end-points that might be considered to optimize the postresuscitation effort. Although many may consider these experimental, they are far and beyond more objective and sensitive than the use of traditional heart rate and blood pressure monitoring.

REFERENCES

1. Chittock DR, Ronco JJ, Russell JA. Monitoring of oxygen transport and oxygen consumption. In: Principles and Practice of Intensive Care Monitoring. Tobin MJ, ed. New York: McGraw-Hill, 1998, pp. 317–343.
2. Schumacker PT, Cain SM. The concept of a critical oxygen delivery. Intensive Care Med 1987; 13: 223–229.
3. Vincent JL. Lactate and biochemical indexes of oxygenation. In: Tobin MJ, ed. Principles and Practice of Intensive Care Monitoring. New York: McGraw-Hill, 1998, pp. 369–376.
4. Shoemaker WC, Appel PL, Kram HB. Tissue oxygen debt as a determinant of lethal and nonlethal postoperative organ failure. Crit Care Med 1988; 16:1117–1120.
5. Shoemaker WC, Appel PL, Kram HB. Role of oxygen debt in the development of organ failure sepsis, and death in high-risk surgical patients. Chest 1992; 102:208–215.
6. McDonald JL. Systolic and mean arterial pressures during manual and mechanical CPR in humans. Ann Emerg Med 1982; 11:292–295.
7. Paradis NA, Martin GB, Goetting MG, Rivers EP, Feingold M, Nowak RM. Aortic pressure during human cardiac arrest. Identification of pseudo- electromechanical dissociation. Chest 1992; 101: 123–128.
8. Kern K, Niemann J. Coronary perfusion pressure during cardiopulmonary resuscitation. In: Paradis N, Halperin H, Nowak R, eds. Cardiac Arrest: The science and practice of resuscitation medicine. Baltimore, MD: Williams and Wilkins, 1996, pp. 270–284.
9. Ditchey RV, Lindenfeld J. Failure of epinephrine to improve the balance between myocardial oxygen supply and demand during closed-chest resuscitation in dogs. Circulation 1988; 78:382–389.
10. Chase PB, Kern KB, Sanders AB, Otto CW, Ewy GA. Effects of graded doses of epinephrine on both noninvasive and invasive measures of myocardial perfusion and blood flow during cardiopulmonary resuscitation. Crit Care Med 1993; 21:413–419.
11. Paradis NA, Martin GB, Rivers EP, et al. Coronary perfusion pressure and the return of spontaneous circulation in human cardiopulmonary resuscitation [see comments]. JAMA 1990; 263:1106–1113.
12. Paradis NA, Martin GB, Rosenberg J, et al. The effect of standard- and high-dose epinephrine on coronary perfusion pressure during prolonged cardiopulmonary resuscitation. Jama 1991; 265: 1139–1144.
13. Downey J. Compression of the coronary arteries by the fibrillating canine heart. Circ Res 1976; 39:53–57.
14. Downey JM, Chagrasulis RW, Hemphill V. Quantitative study of intramyocardial compression in the fibrillating heart. Am J Physiol 1979; 237:H191–H196.
15. Kern KB, Lancaster L, Goldman S, Ewy GA. The effect of coronary artery lesions on the relationship between coronary perfusion pressure and myocardial blood flow during cardiopulmonary resuscitation in pigs. Am Heart J 1990; 120:324–333.
16. Kern KB, de la Guardia B, Ewy GA. Myocardial perfusion during cardiopulmonary resuscitation (CPR): effects of 10, 25 and 50% coronary stenoses. Resuscitation 1998; 38:107–111.
17. Martin GB, Carden DL, Nowak RM, Lewinter JR, Johnston W, Tomlanovich MC. Aortic and right atrial pressures during standard and simultaneous compression and ventilation CPR in human beings. Ann Emerg Med 1986; 15:125–130.
18. Niemann JT, Criley JM, Rosborough JP, Niskanen RA, Alferness C. Predictive indices of successful cardiac resuscitation after prolonged arrest and experimental cardiopulmonary resuscitation. Ann Emerg Med 1985; 14:521–528.
19. Lodato RF. Arterial pressure monitoring. In: Tobin MJ, ed. Principles and practice of intensive care monitoring. New York: McGraw-Hill, 1998. pp. 733–749.
20. Angelos MG, DeBehnke DJ, Leasure JE. Arterial blood gases during cardiac arrest: markers of blood flow in a canine model. Resuscitation 1992; 23:101,111.
21. Weil MH, Rackow EC, Trevino R, Grundler W, Falk JL, Griffel MI. Difference in acid-base state between venous and arterial blood during cardiopulmonary resuscitation. N Engl J Med 1986; 315: 153–156.
22. Gazmuri RJ, von Planta M, Weil MH, Rackow EC. Arterial PCO2 as an indicator of systemic perfusion during cardiopulmonary resuscitation. Crit Care Med 1989; 17:237–240.
23. von Planta M. Acid-base and electrolyte management. In: Weil MH, Tang W, eds. CPR: Resuscitation of the arrested Heart. Philadelphia, PA: W.B. Saunders, 1999, pp. 37–52.
24. Carden DL, Martin GB, Nowak RM, Foreback CC, Tomlanovich MC. Lactic acidosis as a predictor of downtime during cardiopulmonary arrest in dogs. Am J Emerg Med 1985; 3:120–124.

25. Carden DL, Martin GB, Nowak RM, Foreback CC, Tomlanovich MC. Lactic acidosis during closed-chest CPR in dogs. Ann Emerg Med 1987; 16:1317–1320.
26. Prause G, Ratzenhofer-Comenda B, Smolle-Juttner F, et al. Comparison of lactate or BE during out-of-hospital cardiac arrest to determine metabolic acidosis. Resuscitation 2001; 51:297–300.
27. Mullner M, Sterz F, Domanovits H, Behringer W, Binder M, Laggner AN. The association between blood lactate concentration on admission, duration of cardiac arrest, and functional neurological recovery in patients resuscitated from ventricular fibrillation. Intensive Care Med 1997; 23:1138–1143.
28. Tuchschmidt JA, Mecher CE. Predictors of outcome from critical illness. Shock and cardiopulmonary resuscitation. Crit Care Clin 1994; 10:179–195.
29. Vincent JL, Dufaye P, Berre J, Leeman M, Degaute JP, Kahn RJ. Serial lactate determinations during circulatory shock. Crit Care Med 1983; 11:449–451.
30. Bakker J, Coffernils M, Leon M, Gris P, Vincent JL. Blood lactate levels are superior to oxygen-derived variables in predicting outcome in human septic shock. Chest 1991; 99:956–962.
31. Bakker J, Gris P, Coffernils M, Kahn RJ, Vincent JL. Serial blood lactate levels can predict the development of multiple organ failure following septic shock. Am J Surg 1996; 171:221–226.
32. Rivers EP, Rady MY, Martin GB, et al. Venous hyperoxia after cardiac arrest. Characterization of a defect in systemic oxygen utilization. Chest 1992; 102:1787–1793.
33. Rivers EP, Wortsman J, Rady MY, Blake HC, McGeorge FT, Buderer NM. The effect of the total cumulative epinephrine dose administered during human CPR on hemodynamic, oxygen transport, and utilization variables in the postresuscitation period. Chest 1994; 106:1499–1507.
34. Luchette FA, Robinson BR, Friend LA, McCarter F, Frame SB, James JH. Adrenergic antagonists reduce lactic acidosis in response to hemorrhagic shock. J Trauma 1999; 46:873–880.
35. Tucker KJ, Idris AH, Wenzel V, Orban DJ. Changes in arterial and mixed venous blood gases during untreated ventricular fibrillation and cardiopulmonary resuscitation. Resuscitation 1994; 28:137–141.
36. Jay GD, Hughes L, Renzi FP. Pulse oximetry is accurate in acute anemia from hemorrhage. Ann Emerg Med 1994; 24:32–35.
37. Severinghaus JW, Spellman MJ, Jr. Pulse oximeter failure thresholds in hypotension and vasoconstriction. Anesthesiology 1990; 73:532–537.
38. Hess DR. Capnometry. In: Tobin MJ, ed. Principals and Practice of Intensive Care Monitoring. New York: McGraw-Hill, 1998, pp. 377–400.
39. Ward KR, Yealy DM. End-tidal carbon dioxide monitoring in emergency medicine, Part 1: Basic principles. Acad Emerg Med 1998; 5:628–636.
40. Kalenda Z. The capnogram as a guide to the efficacy of cardiac massage. Resuscitation 1978; 6:259–263.
41. Hindman BJ. Sodium bicarbonate in the treatment of subtypes of acute lactic acidosis: physiologic considerations. Anesthesiology 1990; 72:1064–1076.
42. Dubin A, Murias G, Estenssoro E, et al. End-tidal CO_2 pressure determinants during hemorrhagic shock. Intensive Care Med 2000; 26:1619–1623.
43. Relman AS. Letter. N Engl J Med 1986; 315:1618.
44. Guzman JA, Lacoma FJ, Najar A, Kruse JA. End-tidal partial pressure of carbon dioxide as a noninvasive indicator of systemic oxygen supply dependency during hemorrhagic shock and resuscitation. Shock 1997; 8:427–431.
45. Sato Y, Weil MH, Tang W. Tissue hypercarbic acidosis as a marker of acute circulatory failure (shock). Chest 1998; 114:263–274.
46. Jin X, Weil MH, Sun S, Tang W, Bisera J, Mason EJ. Decreases in organ blood flows associated with increases in sublingual PCO_2 during hemorrhagic shock. J Appl Physiol 1998; 85:2360–2364.
47. Schlichtig R, Mehta N, Gayowski TJ. Tissue-arterial PCO_2 difference is a better marker of ischemia than intramural pH (pHi) or arterial pH-pHi difference. J Crit Care 1996; 11:51–56.
48. Schlichtig R, Bowles SA. Distinguishing between aerobic and anaerobic appearance of dissolved CO_2 in intestine during low flow. J Appl Physiol 1994; 76:2443–2451.
49. Sanders AB, Atlas M, Ewy GA, Kern KB, Bragg S. Expired PCO_2 as an index of coronary perfusion pressure. Am J Emerg Med 1985; 3:147–149.
50. Kern KB, Sanders AB, Voorhees WD, Babbs CF, Tacker WA, Ewy GA. Changes in expired end-tidal carbon dioxide during cardiopulmonary resuscitation in dogs: a prognostic guide for resuscitation efforts. J Am Coll Cardiol 1989; 13:1184–1189.
51. Lewis LM, Stothert J, Standeven J, Chandel B, Kurtz M, Fortney J. Correlation of end-tidal CO_2 to cerebral perfusion during CPR. Ann Emerg Med 1992; 21:1131–1134.
52. Martin GB, Gentile NT, Paradis NA, Moeggenberg J, Appleton TJ, Nowak RM. Effect of epinephrine on end-tidal carbon dioxide monitoring during CPR. Ann Emerg Med 1990; 19:396–398.

53. Cantineau JP, Merckx P, Lambert Y, Sorkine M, Bertrand C, Duvaldestin P. Effect of epinephrine on end-tidal carbon dioxide pressure during prehospital cardiopulmonary resuscitation. Am J Emerg Med 1994; 12:267–270.

54. Callaham M, Barton C, Matthay M. Effect of epinephrine on the ability of end-tidal carbon dioxide readings to predict initial resuscitation from cardiac arrest. Crit Care Med 1992; 20:337–343.

55. Ward KR, Yealy DM. End-tidal carbon dioxide monitoring in emergency medicine, Part 2: Clinical applications. Acad Emerg Med 1998; 5:637–646.

56. Ward KR, Menegazzi JJ, Zelenak RR, Sullivan RJ, McSwain NE, Jr. A comparison of chest compressions between mechanical and manual CPR by monitoring end-tidal PCO2 during human cardiac arrest. Ann Emerg Med 1993; 22:669–674.

57. Babbs CF, Voorhees WD, Fitzgerald KR, et al. Relationship of blood pressure and flow during CPR to chest compression amplitude. Ann Emerg Med 1983; 12:527–532.

58. Ornato JP, Gonzalez ER, Garnett AR, Levine RL, McClung BK. Effect of cardiopulmonary resuscitation compression rate on end-tidal carbon dioxide concentration and arterial pressure in man. Crit Care Med 1988; 16:241–245.

59. Callaham M, Barton C. Prediction of outcome of cardiopulmonary resuscitation from end-tidal carbon dioxide concentration. Crit Care Med 1990; 18:358–362.

60. Sanders AB, Kern KB, Otto CW, Milander MM, Ewy GA. End-tidal carbon dioxide monitoring during cardiopulmonary resuscitation. A prognostic indicator for survival. JAMA 1989; 262:1347–1351.

61. Cantineau JP, Lambert Y, Merckx P, et al. End-tidal carbon dioxide during cardiopulmonary resuscitation in humans presenting mostly with asystole: a predictor of outcome. Crit Care Med 1996; 24: 791–796.

62. Asplin BR, White RD. Prognostic value of end-tidal carbon dioxide pressures during out-of-hospital cardiac arrest. Ann Emerg Med 1995; 25:756–761.

63. Levine RL, Wayne MA, Miller CC. End-tidal carbon dioxide and outcome of out-of-hospital cardiac arrest. N Engl J Med 1997; 337:301–306.

64. Wayne MA, Levine RL, Miller CC. Use of end-tidal carbon dioxide to predict outcome in prehospital cardiac arrest. Ann Emerg Med 1995; 25:762–767.

65. Sanders AB, Ewy GA, Bragg S, Atlas M, Kern KB. Expired PCO2 as a prognostic indicator of successful resuscitation from cardiac arrest. Ann Emerg Med 1985; 14:948–952.

66. Garnett AR, Ornato JP, Gonzalez ER, Johnson EB. End-tidal carbon dioxide monitoring during cardiopulmonary resuscitation. Jama 1987; 257:512–515.

67. De Maria AN, Raisinghani A. Comparative overview of cardiac output measurement methods: has impedance cardiography come of age? Congest Heart Fail 2000; 6:60–73.

68. Valtier B, Cholley BP, Belot JP, de la Coussaye JE, Mateo J, Payen DM. Noninvasive monitoring of cardiac output in critically ill patients using transesophageal Doppler. Am J Respir Crit Care Med 1998; 158:77–83.

69. Botero M, Lobato EB. Advances in noninvasive cardiac output monitoring: an update. J Cardiothorac Vasc Anesth 2001; 15:631–640.

70. Murias GE, Villagra A, Vatua S, et al. Evaluation of a noninvasive method for cardiac output measurement in critical care patients. Intensive Care Med 2002; 28:1470–1474.

71. Ivatury RR, Simon RJ, Havriliak D, Garcia C, Greenbarg J, Stahl WM. Gastric mucosal pH and oxygen delivery and oxygen consumption indices in the assessment of adequacy of resuscitation after trauma: a prospective, randomized study. J Trauma 1995; 39:128–134; discussion 34–36.

72. Ward KR, Ivatury RR, Barbee RW. Endpoints of resuscitation for the victim of trauma. J Intensive Care Med 2001; 16:55–75.

73. Porter JM, Ivatury RR. In search of the optimal end points of resuscitation in trauma patients: a review. J Trauma 1998; 44:908–914.

74. Maynard N, Bihari D, Beale R, et al. Assessment of splanchnic oxygenation by gastric tonometry in patients with acute circulatory failure [see comments]. JAMA 1993; 270:1203–1210.

75. Gutierrez G, Bismar H, Dantzker DR, Silva N. Comparison of gastric intramucosal pH with measures of oxygen transport and consumption in critically ill patients. Crit Care Med 1992; 20:451–457.

76. Gutierrez G, Palizas F, Doglio G, et al. Gastric intramucosal pH as a therapeutic index of tissue oxygenation in critically ill patients [see comments]. Lancet 1992; 339:195–199.

77. Marik PE. Gastric intramucosal pH. A better predictor of multiorgan dysfunction syndrome and death than oxygen-derived variables in patients with sepsis. Chest 1993; 104:225–229.

78. Light RB. Intrapulmonary oxygen consumption in experimental pneumococcal pneumonia. J Appl Physiol 1988; 64:2490–2495.

79. Rivers EP, Martin GB, Smithline H, et al. The clinical implications of continuous central venous oxygen saturation during human CPR. Ann Emerg Med 1992; 21:1094–1101.

80. Rady MY, Rivers EP, Martin GB, Smithline H, Appelton T, Nowak RM. Continuous central venous oximetry and shock index in the emergency department: use in the evaluation of clinical shock. Am J Emerg Med 1992; 10:538–541.

81. Scalea TM, Hartnett RW, Duncan AO, et al. Central venous oxygen saturation: a useful clinical tool in trauma patients. J Trauma 1990; 30:1539–1543.

82. Ander DS, Jaggi M, Rivers E, et al. Undetected cardiogenic shock in patients with congestive heart failure presenting to the emergency department. Am J Cardiol 1998; 82(7):888-91.

83. Nguyen HB, Rivers EP, Muzzin A, Knoblich B, Havstad S, Tomlanovich M. Central venous oxygen saturation/lactic acid index as an early indicator of survival of patients in shock (abstract). Acad Emerg Med 2000; 7:586,587.

84. Gomersall CD, Joynt GM, Freebairn RC, Hung V, Buckley TA, Oh TE. Resuscitation of critically ill patients based on the results of gastric tonometry: a prospective, randomized, controlled trial. Crit Care Med 2000; 28:607–614.

85. Rivers EP, Nguyen HB, Havstad S, et al. Early goal-directed therapy in the treatment of the systemic inflammatory response syndrome (SIRS): An outcome evaluation of emergency department intervention (abstract). Acad Emerg Med 2000; 5:427.

86. Ma MH, Huang GT, Wang SM, et al. Aortic valve disruption and regurgitation complicating CPR detected by transesophageal echocardiography. Am J Emerg Med 1994; 12:601,602.

87. Hilty WM, Hudson PA, Levitt MA, Hall JB. Real-time ultrasound-guided femoral vein catheterization during cardiopulmonary resuscitation. Ann Emerg Med 1997; 29:331–336; discussion 37.

88. Hrics P, Wilber S, Blanda MP, Gallo U. Ultrasound-assisted internal jugular vein catheterization in the ED. Am J Emerg Med 1998; 16:401–403.

89. Schlichtig R, Kramer DJ, Pinsky MR. Flow redistribution during progressive hemorrhage is a determinant of critical O2 delivery. J Appl Physiol 1991; 70:169–178.

90. Bowles SA, Schlichtig R, Kramer DJ, Klions HA. Arteriovenous pH and partial pressure of carbon dioxide detect critical oxygen delivery during progressive hemorrhage in dogs. J Crit Care 1992; 7: 95–105.

91. Tremper KK, Mentelos RA, Shoemaker WC. Effect of hypercarbia and shock on transcutaneous carbon dioxide at different electrode temperatures. Crit Care Med 1980; 8:608–612.

92. Tremper KK, Shoemaker WC, Shippy CR, Nolan LS. Transcutaneous PCO2 monitoring on adult patients in the ICU and the operating room. Crit Care Med 1981; 9:752–755.

93. Shoemaker WC, Thangathurai D, Wo CC, et al. Intraoperative evaluation of tissue perfusion in high-risk patients by invasive and noninvasive hemodynamic monitoring. Crit Care Med 1999; 27:2147–2152.

94. Ivatury RR, Simon RJ, Islam S, Fueg A, Rohman M, Stahl WM. A prospective randomized study of end points of resuscitation after major trauma: global oxygen transport indices versus organ-specific gastric mucosal pH. J Am Coll Surg 1996; 183:145–154.

95. Hurley R, Chapman MV, Mythen MG. Current status of gastrointestinal tonometry. Current Opin Crit Care 2000; 6:130–135.

96. Weil MH, Nakagawa Y, Tang W, et al. Sublingual capnometry: a new noninvasive measurement for diagnosis and quantitation of severity of circulatory shock [see comments]. Crit Care Med 1999; 27:1225–1229.

97. Nakagawa Y, Weil MH, Tang W, et al. Sublingual capnometry for diagnosis and quantitation of circulatory shock. Am J Respir Crit Care Med 1998; 157(Pt 1):1838–1843.

98. McKinley BA, Parmley CL, Butler BD. Skeletal muscle PO2, PCO2, and pH in hemorrhage, shock, and resuscitation in dogs. J Trauma 1998; 44:119–127.

99. McKinley BA, Ware DN, Marvin RG, Moore FA. Skeletal muscle pH, P(CO2), and P(O2) during resuscitation of severe hemorrhagic shock. J Trauma 1998; 45:633–636.

100. Guyton AC. The systemic circulation. In: Guyton AC, ed. Textbook of Medical Physiology. 6th ed. Philadelphia, PA: W.B. Saunders, 1981, p. 219.

101. Shepherd JT. Circulation to skeletal muscle. In: Shepherd JT, Abboud FM, Geiger SR, eds. Handbook of Physiology. Bethesda, MD: American Physiology Society, 1983, pp. 319–370.

102. von Planta M, Weil MH, Gazmuri RJ, Bisera J, Rackow EC. Myocardial acidosis associated with CO2 production during cardiac arrest and resuscitation. Circulation 1989; 80:684–692.

103. Reilly PM, Bulkley GB. Vasoactive mediators and splanchnic perfusion. Crit Care Med 1993; 21:S55–S68.

104. Ward KR. Visceral organ ischemia and reperfusion in cardiac arrest. In: Paradis N, Halperin H, Nowak R, eds. Cardiac Arrest: The science and practice of resuscitation medicine. Baltimore, MD: Williams and Wilkins, 1996, pp. 160–184.

105. Morris DC, Dereczyk BE, Grzybowski M, et al. Vasopressin can increase coronary perfusion pressure during human cardiopulmonary resuscitation. Acad Emerg Med 1997; 4:878–883.

106. Wortsman J, Paradis NA, Martin GB, et al. Functional responses to extremely high plasma epinephrine concentrations in cardiac arrest. Crit Care Med 1993; 21:692–697.

107. Toung T, Reilly PM, Fuh KC, Ferris R, Bulkley GB. Mesenteric vasoconstriction in response to hemorrhagic shock. Shock 2000; 13:267–273.

108. Abello PA, Buchman TG, Bulkley GB. Shock and multiple organ failure. Adv Exp Med Biol 1994; 366:253–268.

109. Baron P, Traber LD, Traber DL, et al. Gut failure and translocation following burn and sepsis. J Surg Res 1994; 57:197–204.

110. Deitch EA, Bridges W, Berg R, Specian RD, Granger DN. Hemorrhagic shock-induced bacterial translocation: the role of neutrophils and hydroxyl radicals. J Trauma 1990; 30:942–951; discussion 51–52.

111. Deitch EA. The role of intestinal barrier failure and bacterial translocation in the development of systemic infection and multiple organ failure. Arch Surg 1990; 125:403,404.

112. Deitch EA. Multiple organ failure. Pathophysiology and potential future therapy. Ann Surg 1992; 216:117–134.

113. Guzman JA, Kruse JA. Splanchnic hemodynamics and gut mucosal-arterial PCO_2 gradient during systemic hypocapnia. J Appl Physiol 1999; 87:1102–1106.

114. Guzman JA, Lacoma FJ, Kruse JA. Relationship between systemic oxygen supply dependency and gastric intramucosal PCO_2 during progressive hemorrhage. J Trauma 1998; 44:696–700.

115. Janssens U, Graf J, Koch KC, vom Dahl J, Hanrath P. Gastric tonometry in patients with cardiogenic shock and intra-aortic balloon counterpulsation [In Process Citation]. Crit Care Med 2000; 28:3449–3455.

116. Sato Y, Weil MH, Tang W, Sun S, Xie J, Bisera J, et al. Esophageal PCO_2 as a monitor of perfusion failure during hemorrhagic shock. J Appl Physiol 1997; 82:558–562.

117. Povoas HP, Weil MH, Tang W, Moran B, Kamohara T, Bisera J. Comparisons between sublingual and gastric tonometry during hemorrhagic shock. Chest 2000; 118:1127–1132.

118. Povoas HP, Weil MH, Tang W, Sun S, Kamohara T, Bisera J. Decreases in mesenteric blood flow associated with increases in sublingual PCO_2 during hemorrhagic shock. Shock 2001; 15:398–402.

119. Marik PE. Sublingual capnography: a clinical validation study. Chest 2001; 120:923–927.

120. Tatevossian RG, Wo CC, Velmahos GC, Demetriades D, Shoemaker WC. Transcutaneous oxygen and CO_2 as early warning of tissue hypoxia and hemodynamic shock in critically ill emergency patients. Crit Care Med 2000; 28:2248–53.

121. McKinley BA, Butler BD. Comparison of skeletal muscle PO_2, PCO_2, and pH with gastric tonometric $P(CO_2)$ and pH in hemorrhagic shock [see comments]. Crit Care Med 1999; 27:1869–1877.

122. Owen-Reece H, Smith M, Elwell CE, Goldstone JC. Near infrared spectroscopy. Br J Anaesth 1999; 82:418–426.

123. Reich D. Near-infrared spectroscopy: theory and applications. J Cardiothorac Vasc Anesth 1996; 10:406–418.

124. Cairns CB, Moore FA, Haenel JB, et al. Evidence for early supply independent mitochondrial dysfunction in patients developing multiple organ failure after trauma. J Trauma 1997; 42:532–536.

125. McKinley BA, Marvin RG, Cocanour CS, Moore FA. Tissue hemoglobin O2 saturation during resuscitation of traumatic shock monitored using near infrared spectrometry. J Trauma 2000; 48:637–642.

126. Cohn SM, Varela JE, Giannotti G, et al. Splanchnic perfusion evaluation during hemorrhage and resuscitation with gastric near-infrared spectroscopy. J Trauma 2001; 50:629–634.

127. Varela JE, Cohn SM, Giannotti GD, et al. Near-infrared spectroscopy reflects changes in mesenteric and systemic perfusion during abdominal compartment syndrome. Surgery 2001; 129:363–370.

128. Mullner M, Sterz F, Binder M, Hirschl MM, Janata K, Laggner AN. Near infrared spectroscopy during and after cardiac arrest—preliminary results. Clin Intensive Care 1995; 6:107–111.

129. Nemoto EM, Yonas H, Kassam A. Clinical experience with cerebral oximetry in stroke and cardiac arrest. Crit Care Med 2000; 28:1052–1054.

130. Newman DH, Freed J, Callaway CW. Cerebral oximetry and ventilation rate changes in out-of-hospital cardiac arrest. Ann Emerg Med 2002; 40:77.

131. Buunk G, van der Hoeven JG, Meinders AE. A comparison of near-infrared spectroscopy and jugular bulb oximetry in comatose patients resuscitated from a cardiac arrest. Anaesthesia 1998; 53:13–19.

132. Moller P, Sylven C. Myoglobin in human skeletal muscle. Scand J Clin Lab Invest 1981; 41:479–482.
133. Nemeth PM, Lowry OH. Myoglobin levels in individual human skeletal muscle fibers of different types. J Histochem Cytochem 1984; 32:1211–1216.
134. Tran TK, Sailasuta N, Kreutzer U, et al. Comparative analysis of NMR and NIRS measurements of intracellular PO2 in human skeletal muscle. Am J Physiol 1999; 276(Pt 2):R1682–R1690.
135. Sterz F, Leonov Y, Safar P, et al. Multifocal cerebral blood flow by Xe-CT and global cerebral metabolism after prolonged cardiac arrest in dogs. Reperfusion with open-chest CPR or cardiopulmonary bypass. Resuscitation 1992; 24:27–47.
136. Wolfson SK, Jr., Safar P, Reich H, et al. Dynamic heterogeneity of cerebral hypoperfusion after prolonged cardiac arrest in dogs measured by the stable xenon/CT technique: a preliminary study. Resuscitation 1992; 23:1–20.
137. Leonov Y, Sterz F, Safar P, Johnson DW, Tisherman SA, Oku K. Hypertension with hemodilution prevents multifocal cerebral hypoperfusion after cardiac arrest in dogs. Stroke 1992; 23:45–53.
138. Oku K, Kuboyama K, Safar P, et al. Cerebral and systemic arteriovenous oxygen monitoring after cardiac arrest. Inadequate cerebral oxygen delivery. Resuscitation 1994; 27:141–152.
139. Mullner M, Sterz F, Domanovits H, Zeiner A, Laggner AN. Systemic and cerebral oxygen extraction after human cardiac arrest. Eur J Emerg Med 1996; 3:19–24.
140. Niemann JT, Cairns CB, Sharma J, Lewis RJ. Treatment of prolonged ventricular fibrillation. Immediate countershock versus high-dose epinephrine and CPR preceding countershock. Circulation 1992; 85:281–287.
141. Niemann JT, Cruz B, Garner D, Lewis RJ. Immediate countershock versus cardiopulmonary resuscitation before countershock in a 5-minute swine model of ventricular fibrillation arrest. Ann Emerg Med 2000; 36:543–546.
142. Cobb LA, Fahrenbruch CE, Walsh TR, et al. Influence of cardiopulmonary resuscitation prior to defibrillation in patients with out-of-hospital ventricular fibrillation. JAMA 1999; 281:1182–1188.
143. Brown CG, Griffith RF, Van Ligten P, et al. Median frequency—a new parameter for predicting defibrillation success rate. Ann Emerg Med 1991; 20:787–789.
144. Brown CG, Dzwonczyk R, Martin DR. Physiologic measurement of the ventricular fibrillation ECG signal: estimating the duration of ventricular fibrillation. Ann Emerg Med 1993; 22:70–74.
145. Dzwonczyk R, Brown CG, Werman HA. The median frequency of the ECG during ventricular fibrillation: its use in an algorithm for estimating the duration of cardiac arrest. IEEE Trans Biomed Eng 1990; 37:640–646.
146. Strohmenger HU, Lindner KH, Keller A, Lindner IM, Pfenninger E, Bothner U. Effects of graded doses of vasopressin on median fibrillation frequency in a porcine model of cardiopulmonary resuscitation: results of a prospective, randomized, controlled trial. Crit Care Med 1996; 24:1360–1365.
147. Strohmenger HU, Lindner KH, Keller A, Lindner IM, Pfenninger EG. Spectral analysis of ventricular fibrillation and closed-chest cardiopulmonary resuscitation. Resuscitation 1996; 33:155–161.
148. Noc M, Weil MH, Tang W, Sun S, Pernat A, Bisera J. Electrocardiographic prediction of the success of cardiac resuscitation. Crit Care Med 1999; 27:708–714.
149. Weaver WD, Cobb LA, Dennis D, Ray R, Hallstrom AP, Copass MK. Amplitude of ventricular fibrillation waveform and outcome after cardiac arrest. Ann Intern Med 1985; 102:53–55.

29 Myocardial Dysfunction Postresuscitation

Alejandro Vasquez, MD and Karl B. Kern, MD

CONTENTS

RESUSCITATION TODAY

Real strides have been made in the last decade in the treatment of sudden cardiac death. Survival rates from out-of-hospital cardiac arrest (CA) have been reported as low as 1 and 2% in large cities *(1,2)*. Communities with rapid emergency response teams have reported better results with survival rates from 15 to 30% *(3)*. Within the last few years providing early defibrillation by equipping nonmedical first responders with automated external defibrillators (AEDs) has been a crucial step in improving survival from out-of-hospital CA. Recent reports from Rochester, Minnesota, where police are now providing early defibrillation, have shown a community-wide survival rate of 40% for patients whose initial rhythm is ventricular fibrillation (VF *[4]*). Casinos in which security personnel were trained to use AEDs have reported overall survival rates from VF of 59% for victims of sudden CA on property *(5)*. Similarly, the Chicago Airport Authority experience has been impressive *(6,7)*. After placing AEDs in the terminals of both O'Hare and Midway airports, they found a 56% neurologically normal survival rate for VF CA within the first 24 months of starting this public access defibrillation program.

Another important recent advance in improving survival from sudden cardiac death has been the success of intravenous amiodarone administered in the field for refractory VF CA. Two clinical trials (Amiodarone in Out-of-Hospital Resuscitation of Refractory Sustained Ventricular Tachyarrythmias [ARREST] and Amiodarone vs Lidocaine in Pre-Hospital Refractory Ventricular Fibrillation Evaluation [ALIVE]) have now shown improved survival to hospital admission in patients treated with amiodarone vs placebo (ARREST *[8]*) or lidocaine (ALIVE *[8,9]*).

In the United States alone, an estimated 400,000 individuals will suffer CA this year *(10)*. An initial resuscitation rate of 15–25% of this group would produce about 100,000

From: *Contemporary Cardiology: Cardiopulmonary Resuscitation*
Edited by: J. P. Ornato and M. A. Peberdy © Humana Press Inc., Totowa, NJ

early survivors. If recently reported advances can be achieved in general communities across the United States, then initial resuscitation rates could be as good as 40–50%, translating into as many as 200,000 individuals resuscitated initially.

Such improvements in the treatment of sudden death are impressive and encouraging. However, many initially resuscitated individuals do not survival to leave the hospital. Current estimates of survival to hospital discharge are only 25–35% of those initially resuscitated *(11,12)*. This late loss of those resuscitated initially is a large and yet often ignored problem. Such devastating losses can literally wipe out all the recent gains by early defibrillation and effective advanced cardiac life support drug therapy leaving only 10–15% of all CA victims. We must improve the postresuscitation long-term survival rate to realize a true advance in the survival of cardiac arrest victims.

POSTRESUSCITATION DEATHS

Why do those who are originally resuscitated die before leaving the hospital? The vast majority of such deaths occur from either central nervous system (CNS) damage or myocardial failure, manifested as cardiogenic shock or recurrent CA. In reporting a series of out-of-hospital CAs, Schoenenberger et al. found that approximately one-third of such postresuscitation deaths were from brain damage, one-third from myocardial failure, and one-third from a variety of causes including infection *(13)*. The need to better understand and treat such postresuscitation deaths has recently highlighted at the recent American College of Cardiology 31st Bethesda Conference on Emergency Cardiac Care *(14)* and at the National Institutes of Health's 2000 "PULSE" Conference on scientific priorities and strategic planning for resuscitation research and lifesaving therapies *(15)*.

What is Postresuscitation Myocardial Dysfunction?

The first detailed description of cardiac dysfunction following CA and successful resuscitation came from the Safar Center for Resuscitation Research at the University of Pittsburgh *(16)*. Using their canine VF CA model, these investigators studied myocardial filling pressures and cardiac output before and after resuscitation following normothermic CA periods of 7.5, 10, and 12.5 minutes of "no flow." Central venous pressures were elevated initially post resuscitation after all three periods of CA, but returned to pre-arrest baseline levels by 1 hour. Pulmonary capillary "wedge" pressure rose by about 40% in all three groups immediately after resuscitation, but remained elevated at 6 hours only in the group receiving 12.5 minutes of untreated CA. Cardiac index (CI) decreased by an average of 25% in all animals by 4 hours postresuscitation, but remained depressed only in the 12.5-minute group by 6 hours postresuscitation. Left ventricular (LV) stroke work index was also depressed about 25–30% at 2–6 hours postresuscitation. Interpretation of the data is confused by the postresuscitation care, which allowed the use of norepinephrine for hypotension within the first 2 hours, then dopamine, fentanyl, and pancuronium between the hours 2 and 24.

Researchers at the Institute for Critical Care Medicine in Palm Springs, California measured dP/dt and pressure volume relationships in isolated perfused hearts from Sprague-Dawley rats, which had been resuscitated following VF CA *(17)*. Fifteen rats underwent 4 minutes of untreated VF followed by 5 minutes of cardiopulmonary resuscitation (CPR) before defibrillation. Hearts were harvested at 2 minutes and 20 minutes postresuscitation, isolated, and then perfused using a modified Langendorff preparation. Serial measurements of LV-developed pressure, dP/dt, and pressure-volume relation-

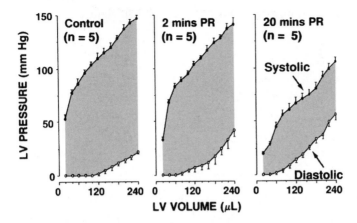

Fig. 1. Left ventricular pressure-volume curves. Left ventricular dysfunction after resuscitation. Pressure-volume relationships after progressive increase in left ventricular balloon volumes. Effects on the generated ventricular systolic and diastolic pressures are shown in hearts harvested at 2 min after resuscitation (2 min PR) and 20 min after resuscitation (20 min PR). LV, left ventricular; PR, postresuscitation. Values are mean ± SD. Adapted from ref. *17*, with permission.

ships showed a progressive deterioration in LV function in the first 20 minutes postresuscitation. Both systolic and diastolic function declined, with a decrease in contractility and a decrease in ventricular compliance (Fig. 1.)

This same group of investigators also performed a study of LV function using a conductance catheter in an in vivo porcine model of CA and resuscitation *(18)*. Thirteen animals underwent 4 minutes of untreated VF then 8 minutes of CPR before electrical defibrillation was attempted. Seven animals were successfully resuscitated. An additional seven animals were utilized as "sham" controls, in which CA was never induced. LV pressure-volume relationships and hemodynamics were measured pre-arrest and at 30, 60, 240, and 360 minutes postresuscitation. Progressive increases in both diastolic and systolic volumes were noted. Ventricular dilatation was associated with a reduction in stroke volume (although cardiac output remained constant via compensatory increases in heart rate) and ventricular work. A dramatic rightward shift in the pressure-volume relationship occurred characteristic of impairment in LV contractile function. The rate of LV pressure decrease did not change, suggesting no alteration in lusitropic properties. Figure 2 illustrates these pressure-volume relationships. These results differ from their previous report in which diastolic function was noted to be abnormal postresuscitation *(17)*.

At the same time, we at the University of Arizona Sarver Heart Center, also studied postresuscitation myocardial dysfunction in a swine model of prolonged VF CA *(19)*. Twenty-eight domestic swine (26 ± 1 kg) underwent both invasive and noninvasive measurements of ventricular function before and after 10 or 15 minutes of untreated CA. Contrast left ventriculograms, ventricular pressures, cardiac output, isovolumetric relaxation time (tau), and transthoracic Doppler-echocardiographic studies were performed. The aim of this study was to define the nature, extent, and duration of postresuscitation myocardial dysfunction in an in vivo porcine model of prolonged VF CA. Twenty-three of 28 animals were successfully resuscitated and postresuscitation data obtained. LV ejection fraction (EF) showed a significant reduction 30 minutes after resuscitation,

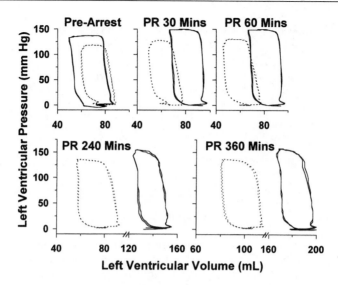

Fig. 2. Left ventricular pressure-volume loops. Rightward shift of pressure-volume loops in a successfully resuscitated animal (solid line) compared with changes in an animal subjected to "sham cardiac arrest" (dashed line). PR, postresuscitation. (Adapted from ref. *18*, with permission.)

Table 1
Left Ventricular Angiographic Data

	Pre-arrest	30-minute PR	2-hour PR	5-hour PR	24-hour PR	48-hour PR
EF (%)	54 ± 2	26 ± 3[a,b]	27 ± 3[a,b]	30 ± 4[a,b]	42 ± 2[a]	54 ± 3
EDV	31 ± 5	32 ± 5	29 ± 2	32 ± 5	35 ± 4	31 ± 6
ESV	15 ± 2	24 ± 4[a,b]	22 ± 2[a,b]	22 ± 3[a,b]	19 ± 2	13 ± 3
SV	17 ± 3	9 ± 2[a,b]	7 ± 1[a,b]	10 ± 2[a,b]	16 ± 2	18 ± 4
PSP/ESV	7 ± 1		5 ± 1[a,b]	5 ± 0[a,b]	5 ± 1[a,b]	5 ± 1[a] 10 ± 1[a]

Note: All volumes are in milliliters.

[a] *p* < 0.05 vs pre-arrest baseline.

[b] *p* < 0.005 vs 48-hour postresuscitation.

PR, postresuscitation; EF, ejection fraction; EDV, end-diastolic volume; ESV, end-systolic volume; SV, stroke volume; PSP/ESV peak systolic pressure to end-systolic volume ratio. (Adapted from ref. *19,* with permission.)

which progressively worsened through the first 5 hours postresuscitation. Partial recovery was seen by 24 hours, and full recovery was seen by 48 hours (Table 1). The systolic LV dysfunction was a diffuse, global process with wall motion abnormalities seen in all ventricular walls (Fig. 3). End-systolic and end-diastolic LV volumes were calculated from the contrast ventriculograms. No change in end-diastolic volume was seen after resuscitation, but end-systolic volume increased consistently when measured at 30 minutes, 2 hours, and 5 hours after resuscitation (Table 1). Similarly, stroke volume was also compromised in all groups during the first 5 hours postresuscitation. Peak LV systolic pressure divided by end-systolic volume, a commonly calculated ratio for measurement of load-independent global myocardial contraction, decreased significantly in all groups over the same follow-up period (Table 1).

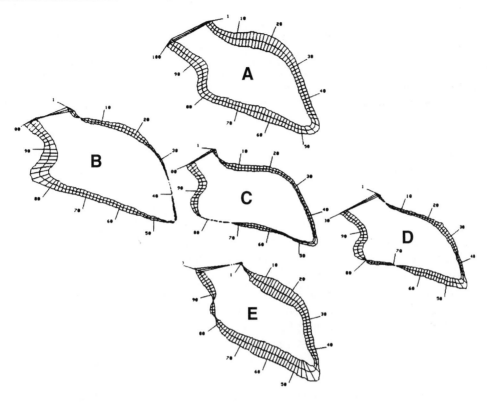

Fig. 3. Contrast left ventriculograms after resuscitation. Contrast left ventriculograms from one animal (swine) illustrating the progressive global hypokinesis seen after successful resuscitation from prolonged cardiac arrest. Baseline (**A**); 30 minutes PR (**B**) 2 hours PR (**C**); 5 hours PR (**D**); 48 hours PR (**E**). From ref. *19,* wth permission.

Table 2
Left Ventricular Hemodynamic Data

	Pre-arrest	30-minute PR	2-hour PR	5-hour	24-hour	48-hour
LVEDP	11 ± 1^{b}	18 ± 2^{a}	$22 \pm 3^{a,b}$	$21 \pm 3^{a,b}$	14 ± 2	7 ± 1
CO	18 ± 1	16 ± 1	13 ± 1^{a}	13 ± 0^{a}	14 ± 1^{a}	19 ± 1
"Tau"	29 ± 1	38 ± 4	46 ± 3^{a}	41 ± 3	34 ± 2	26 ± 1

[a] $p < 0.05$ vs pre-arrest baseline.
[b] $p < 0.005$ vs 48-hour postresuscitation
CO, cardiac output (mL per minute); LVEDP, left ventricular end-diastolic pressure; PR, postresuscitation; "Tau," isovolumetric relaxation time (ms). (Adapted from ref. *19,* with permission.)

Hemodynamic changes seen after resuscitation included a dramatic rise in LV end-diastolic pressure (LVEDP), a fall in cardiac output measured by thermodilution technique, and an increase in isovolumic relaxation time or "tau" (Table 2). These changes demonstrate significant diastolic LV dysfunction as well as the systolic dysfunction seen by the angiographic measurements.

Table 3
Left Ventricular Echocardiographic Data

	Pre-arrest	5-hour PR	24- to 48–hour PR
Fractional shortening (%)	29 ± 1	23 ± 1[a,b]	28 ± 2
Mitral deceleration time (ms)	98 ± 5	61 ± 3[a,b]	88 ± 4[a]
LV isovolumic relax time (ms)	72 ± 3	91 ± 3[a,b]	73 ± 4

[a]$p < 0.05$ vs pre-arrest baseline.
[b]$p < 0.005$ vs 48-hour postresuscitation.
PR, postreuscitation; LV, left ventricular. (Adapted from ref. 19, with permission.)

Transthoracic echocardiographic studies collaborate these findings, showing diminished systolic ventricular function as a decreased fractional shortening and diminished diastolic ventricular function by a decreased mitral valve deceleration time as well as an increased isovolumetric relaxation time at 5 hours postresuscitation (Table 3).

This was the first report in an in vivo model of CA to elucidate the time course and transient quality of both LV systolic and diastolic dysfunction after successful CPR. Maximal dysfunction was seen at 6 hours with partial resolution by 24 hours and full recovery by 48 hours, indicating a true "stunning" phenomenon. After 15 minutes of VF, no data could be obtained at 24 hours because all such subjects died overnight. Such data suggest that transient LV failure postresuscitation can be life threatening. Only after the CA interval was shortened to 10 minutes was 24-hour survival accomplished and follow-up data on LV function obtained.

In some respects, these two porcine studies (18,19) complemented each other, but also disagreed in particular whether diastolic function was abnormal after resuscitation from prolonged CA. Other studies of ischemic injury to the myocardium have suggested that lusitropic properties are not spared, but are, in fact, the most sensitive to such injury (20,21).

RIGHT VENTRICULAR FUNCTION POSTRESUSCITATION

That LV function is impaired transiently following resuscitation from prolonged CA seems clear from the experimental data. Is right ventricular (RV) function also compromised? Does the right ventricle also recover? What is the time course before its function returns to normal? These questions were addressed in a recent experimental study at the University of Arizona (22). RV function was studied before and after 15 minutes of VF CA in 28 swine, 16 of which received no treatment to define the natural history of RV dysfunction postresuscitation. RVEF decreased, although end-diastolic pressure increased (Table 4). RV systolic and diastolic properties were both affected. In comparison to the left ventricle (19), RV dysfunction following resuscitation appears to occur earlier and resolve more rapidly. RV dysfunction peaked at 30 minutes and showed improvement by 2 hours, whereas LV dysfunction peaked about 6 hours and showed improvement at 24 hours. The global ischemic insult of prolonged CA presumably has different effects on the two ventricles. The thin-walled right ventricle has less myocardial mass and appears to be more resilient to the ischemia of CA. Clinical experience with RV infarction suggests the same. Right ventricles almost always make a full functional recovery even after extensive ischemic insults and injuries (23).

Table 4
Right Ventricular Dysfunction Postresuscitation

	Baseline	30 minutes	2 hours	5 hours
RVEF	50 ± 2	34 ± 2[a]	40 ± 28[a,b]	41 ± 2[a,b]
RVEDP	5 ± 1	8 ± 1[a]	4 ± 1[b]	5 ± 1[b]
Heart rate	122 ± 24	160 ± 14[a]	136 ± 21	127 ± 20

[a] $p < 0.05$ vs baseline.

[b] $p < 0.05$ vs 30 minute postresusciation.

RVEF, right ventricular ejection fraction; RVEDP, right ventricular end-diastolic pressure. (Adapted from ref. *22*, with permission.)

VF vs Non-VF CA: Effect on Postresuscitation Myocardial Dysfunction

Does the type of CA affect the development of postresuscitation myocardial dysfunction? The data show that resuscitation following prolonged VF CA can result in substantial impairment of both systolic and diastolic function of both the left and right ventricles. VF is known to be an energy-consuming dysrhythmia. High-energy phosphates are depleted quickly during VF *(24)*. Would non-VF causes of CA produce less myocardial stunning if successfully treated and resuscitation achieved? Weil et al. attempted to answer these questions by studying asphyxial CA (mean aortic pressure less than 30 mmHg) vs VF CA in their murine model of postresuscitation myocardial dysfunction *(25)*. Postresuscitation myocardial function was compared between two groups of animals, one undergoing asphyxial and the other VF CA. The two groups were standardized in the duration of CA and in the number of defibrillation shocks (including shocks given to the asphyxial group to make them comparable to the VF group). Greater impairment of CI, dP/dt_{40}, $-dP/dt_{40,}$ and LVEDP was seen in those with VF CA compared to those with asphyxial CA. Further studies to include EF, pressure-volume relationships, and tau would be helpful.

Clinical Evidence for Postresuscitation Myocardial Dysfunction

Postresuscitation myocardial dysfunction has also been described clinically. Numerous case reports have suggested that transient LV failure can occur after successful resuscitation *(26,27)*. We recently published such a case involving a previously healthy young woman with no known cardiac disease who required both fluid resuscitation and subsequently CPR for 5 minutes for postdelivery bleeding and CA. Echocardiography 6 hours postresuscitation showed generalized LV hypokinesis with an EF of 35%. Over the subsequent 3 days, full recovery of LV function occurred with a final echocardiogram showing a LVEF of greater than 55% *(28)*.

Several clinical resuscitation trials have noted the occurrence of myocardial dysfunction postresuscitation. Of the 778 patients enrolled in the two international "Brain Resuscitation Clinical Trials" (I and II), 65% of those initially resuscitated died within 1 week *(11,12)*. More than half of those who expired manifested evidence of significant postresuscitation myocardial dysfunction either as hypotension/shock or malignant ventricular arrhythmias with recurrent sudden death.

Table 5
Hemodynamic and Angiographic Data

	Myocardial dysfunction	No myocardial dysfunction	p
N	73	75	0.92
Heart rate (bpm)	105 (75–143)	85 (48–118)	< 0.05
LVEDP (mmHG)	19 (10–32)	12 (5–25)	<0.01
LVEF (%)	32 (25–40)	43 (35–50)	<0.01
Coronary occlusion	51%	37%	0.06
Two- or three-vessel CAD	52%	51%	0.99
Significant CAD	74%	71%	0.98

bpm, beats per minute; LVEDP, left ventricular end-diastolic pressure; LVEF, left ventricular ejection fraction. (Adapted from Laurnet I, et al., poster presentation, American College of Cardiology 49th annual Scientific Sessions, Anaheim, CA and ref. *29*, with permission.)

Table 6
Resuscitation Data

	Myocardial dysfunction	No myocardial dysfunction	p
N	73	75	0.92
Collapse to CPR (minutes)	5 (1–5)	5 (2–9)	0.59
CPR to ROSC (minutes)	25 (14–38)	15 (7–30)	< 0.01
VF as initial rhythm	70%	66%	0.75
Number of defibrillation shocks	3 (1–6)	2 (1–3)	< 0.01
Epinephrine dose (mg)	10 (3–15)	2 (0–10)	< 0.01

CPR, cardiopulmonary resuscitation; ROSC, return to spontaneous circulation; VF, ventricular fibrillation. (Adapted from Laurnet I, et al., poster presentation at the American College of Cardiology 49th annual Scientific Sessions, Anaheim, CA and ref. *29*, with permission.)

Laurent and coworkers in France reported a series of 148 patients admitted to the hospital after successful resuscitation following out-of-hospital CA *(29)*. All patients underwent acute cardiac catheterization and coronary angiography. Seventy-three patients (49%) developed myocardial dysfunction manifested early by tachycardia and an elevated LVEDP, then later at 6–8 hours postresuscitation developing hypotension (mean arterial pressure <75 mmHg) and low cardiac output (CI <2.2 L/min/m^2). Table 5 summarizes the hemodynamic and angiographic differences between those patients who developed the postresuscitation myocardial dysfunction syndrome and those that did not.

Significant differences in the resuscitation efforts between the two groups were noted. The time from CA to restoration of circulation was longer, the amount of epinephrine received higher, and the number of defibrillation shocks greater in those who developed the myocardial dysfunction (Table 6). These differences in resuscitation characteristics suggest a longer and more difficult effort is more likely to produce myocardial dysfunction postresuscitation.

Table 7
Recovery of Cardiac Index Postresuscitation

	Survivors	Nonsurvivors
N	59	14
8 hours PR	2.1 (1.4–2.9)	2.4 (1.3–3.8)
12 hours PR	2.6 (1.9–3.5)	2.4 (1.9–2.8)
24 hours PR	3.2 (2.7–4.2)	2.6 (2.3–3.0)
72 hours PR	3.7 (2.9–4.5)	2.9 (2.2–3.6)

Note: Cardiac index (l per minute/m^2). PR, postresusci-tation. (Adapted from Laurnet I, et al., poster presentation at the American College of Cardiology 49th Annual Scientific Sessions, Anaheim, CA and ref. *29*, with permission.)

Table 8
Issues Influencing Postresuscitation Myocardial Dysfunction

Duration of untreated cardiac arrest
Duration of resuscitation effort
Use of vasoconstrictive medications
Use of buffer agents
Use of high-dose defibrillation
Type of waveform used for defibrillation (monophasic vs biphasic)

In accordance with the previously outlined experimental data showing that such postresuscitation myocardial dysfunction is generally transient, the patients who developed such typically showed improvement in LV function by 24 hours. Cardiac index showed a nadir at 8 hours postresuscitation, then partially improving by 24 hours, with further improvement noted by 72 hours (Table 7). If such improvement did not occur by 24 hours, the myocardial pump failure generally led to refractory shock and death. Of those patients with postresuscitation myocardial dysfunction, 14 (19%) expired in this fashion.

A second series of patients evaluated for postresuscitation myocardial dysfunction was reported by investigators in Austria *(30)*. Twenty patients resuscitated from out-of-hospital (as well as four control patients) had transesophageal echoes at and 24 hours postresuscitation. LV contractility was calculated using the load-independent parameter of mean velocity of circumferential fiber shortening (Vcf$_c$) and the meridional wall stress. Patients resuscitated had a mean z score of –7.0 at 4 hours and –3.7 at 24 hours indicating significant LV systolic dysfunction, compared to controls (0.0 and 0.7). The authors concluded that severe LV systolic dysfunction is present after resuscitation from CA although the cause remains speculative.

Factors Effecting Postresuscitation Myocardial Dysfunction

A number of factors have been shown to impact the degree of myocardial dysfunction seen after resuscitation (Table 8). Perhaps most important is the underlying state of the myocardium prior to CA. Experimental models to date have employed healthy rats or swine, without precedent myocardial or coronary disease. The degree of postresuscitation myocardial dysfunction in such cases is clearly the result of the insults of CA and subsequent resuscitation. On the other hand, the two reported clinical series *(29,30)* found a majority of the resuscitated CA victims had evidence of at least peri-arrest myocardial infarction that can also influence ultimately the postresuscitation myocardial function.

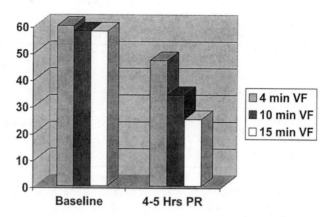

Fig. 4. Ejection fractions postresuscitation: effect of ventricular fibrillation duration. (Adapted from ref. *31*, with permission.)

Unfortunately, no clinical series to date has been able to collect known LV function data prior to the CA. Hence, the pre-arrest state of LV function in these clinical series is not known.

Duration of CA

The duration of CA should affect the degree of subsequent myocardial dysfunction if such dysfunction reflects (in part) the injury from global ischemia during the "no-flow" period. Experimental and clinical data suggests that this is the case. We found that swine undergoing 15 minutes of untreated VF had worse LV function than did swine undergoing only 10 minutes of untreated VF *(19)*. Tang and coworkers found that swine undergoing 10 minutes of untreated VF had worse EFs postresuscitation than those undergoing only 4 minutes of untreated VF *(31)*. Figure 4 illustrates these composite data and the relationship between duration of untreated VF and resultant postresuscitation LVEF.

Laurent et al., in their clinical series, found a similar relationship between the length of resuscitation effort and subsequent postresuscitation myocardial dysfunction *(29)*. They found no difference in time from collapse to CPR between those who developed postresuscitation myocardial dysfunction and those who did not, but did find a significant difference in the duration of resuscitation effort until the return of spontaneous circulation (Table 6). Other statistical differences were found in the amount of epinephrine utilized and the number of shocks delivered (Table 6). Both these parameters speak to a more difficult resuscitation in those who develop postresuscitation myocardial dysfunction.

Pressors

Epinephrine has been the α-adrenergic vasopressor of choice for cardiac resuscitation for more than 40 years. Epinephrine probably adversely affects postresuscitation myocardial dysfunction through disproportionate increases in myocardial oxygen consumption via a β-adrenergic-mediated mechanism and by persistent increases in systemic vascular resistance postresuscitation. Tang et al. demonstrated this concept using an established rodent model of cardiac resuscitation *(32)*. Forty rats divided in two groups were assigned to undergo VF-induced CA for 4 and 8 minutes, respectively. Four therapeutic subsets were established within each group to receive epinephrine alone, epinephrine with esmolol, phenylephrine or placebo, within 4 minutes of CPR initiation. All animals were defibrillated at 8 minutes of CPR. LV pressure, dP/dt_{40}, and negative dP/dt were measured continuously for an interval of 240 minutes after successful cardiac resuscitation. The duration of survival after successful resuscitation was decreased and the total energy required for successful defibrillation was significantly increased in epinephrine-treated and placebo-treated animals when compared with phenylephrine and epinephrine–esmolol-treated animals after 4 or 8 minutes of untreated VF. Myocardial contractility, as measured by dP/dt_{40}, was significantly decreased in all animals after successful resuscitation but the change was more dramatic when the duration of untreated CA increased from 4 to 8 minutes. Impairment of myocardial contractility was greater in animals treated with epinephrine or placebo compared to those receiving epinephrine and esmolol or phenylephrine. The lack of difference in postresuscitation LV function between animals receiving epinephrine and those receiving saline placebo was unexplained by the authors. The severity of postresuscitation myocardial dysfunction was reduced significantly when epinephrine was administered in combination with esmolol, supporting the proposed β-agonist-mediated detrimental effect of epinephrine on postresuscitation myocardial dysfunction. This study also demonstrated again the existence of postresuscitation diastolic dysfunction, which was increased in the placebo- and epinephrine-treated groups.

β-Agonist and to some extent α-1 agonist stimulation may result in increased myocardial oxygen consumption through its inotropic and chronotropic effects, even with fibrillating ventricles. Based on the results from the previous study and considering that no α-2 agonist receptors have been found in the myocardium, Sun et al. conducted a study to assess the effects of the selective α-2 agonist α-methylnorepinephrine (α-MNE [33]). Using the same rodent model described above, 20 rats were studied to measure LV pressure, dP/dt_{40}, negative dP/dt and cardiac index for an interval of 240 minutes after resuscitation. CPR was initiated after 8 minutes of untreated VF. Either α-MNE, epinephrine, or saline placebo was injected 2 minutes after the start of precordial compression. As an additional control, one group of animals was pretreated with the α_2-receptor blocker, yohimbine, before injection of α-MNE. Defibrillation was attempted 4 minutes later. Coronary perfusion increased equally on both the epinephrine and α-MNE treated groups. Systolic and diastolic dysfunction occurred expectedly in all groups, but those receiving α-MNE had significantly less dysfunction. This contrasted with animals treated with epinephrine or with saline placebo in which there was greater impairment of myocardial contractility and relaxation. The beneficial effects of α-MNE were completely blocked by pretreatment with yohimbine.

α-Blockers have been avoided traditionally in resuscitation as a result of the ease with which these drugs cross the blood–brain barrier. In the CNS, α_2-adrenergic agonists exert a negative inotropic and chronotropic action with a subsequent there decline in myocardial contractility and arterial blood pressure. Investigators did not note this effect with α-methylnorepinephrine in this study. More recent data from the same laboratory document the effects of α-methylnorepinephrine in a swine model of CA (34). Fourteen male domestic pigs underwent 7 minutes of untreated VF, followed by CPR and either α-MNE (100 μg/kg) or epinephrine (20 μg/kg) after 2 minutes of precordial compression. Following an additional 4 minutes of precordial compression, defibrillation was attempted. LV systolic and diastolic function was quantitated with the use of transesophageal echo-Doppler imaging. Coronary perfusion increased equally with both epinephrine and α-MNE, and all animals were successfully resuscitated. α-MNE was as effective as epinephrine in restoring spontaneous circulation, but resulted in less postresuscitation myo-cardial dysfunction. EF in the postresuscitation follow-up period of 4 hours was $52 \pm 7\%$ in the α-MNE treated group and $36 \pm 8\%$ in the epinephrine treated group ($p < 0.01$).

Besides the concern about excessive stimulation of β-receptors, the beneficial aspect of vasoconstrictors during CPR (to improve coronary perfusion pressure [CPP] by vasoconstricting the peripheral circulation), may become a problem in the postresus-citation phase. Our group studied endothelin, a potent vasoconstrictor without β-adren-ergic effects, during swine CPR (35). The purpose of this study was to compare the effectiveness of standard-dose epinephrine vs standard-dose epinephrine plus endothelin in improving successful resuscitation and survival outcomes. Animals underwent 2 min-utes of unassisted CPR followed by 6 minutes of ventilation and chest compressions after which they were assigned to receive 1 mg epinephrine or 1 mg epinephrine plus 0.1 mg endodthelin-1 randomly. CPR was provided for 10 minutes after initial drug administra-tion before defibrillation was attempted. The addition of endothelin-1 to standard-dose epinephrine improved CPP and the initial rates of ROSC significantly, but the intense vasoconstriction in the postresuscitation period resulted in very narrow pulse pressures, then progressive hypotension, resulting in significantly higher mortality rates. This sug-gested that excessive vasoconstriction postresuscitation produces significant myocardial dysfunction resulting in detrimental effects on post-CA survival.

BUFFERS

Controversy exists about the use of buffers during CPR. Initial data demonstrated that buffers were ineffective when used during the initial phases of cardiac resuscitation, as they were unable to modify myocardial pH and had no beneficial effect on the rate of successful resuscitation (36,37). This was attributed to systemic vasodilatation that pre-sumably impacted CPP adversely during resuscitation. Recently, other studies have examined the effect of buffer solutions on post resuscitation myocardial dysfunction.

Sun et al., using their well-described rodent model, studied the effect of both carbon dioxide (CO_2)-generating and CO_2-consuming buffers on postresuscitation myocardial dysfunction (38). They studied 40 rats divided in two groups undergoing 4 and 8 minutes of unassisted VF, respectively. Four different subsets were established within each group and were assigned to receive sodium bicarbonate (CO_2 generating buffer, Carbicarb®), tromethamine (CO_2-consuming buffer), hypertonic saline, or placebo. There was less depression in dP/dt_{40} and less increase in LV diastolic pressure, as well as greater duration of survival (hours) was in the Carbicarb® and tromethamine-treated animals when com-pared with hypertonic saline-treated animals after 4 minutes of untreated VF. However, the administration of each buffer agent, including sodium bicarbonate, resulted in less myocardial dysfunction and increased duration of survival when compared with hyper-tonic saline placebo after 8 minutes of untreated VF. These findings suggest that hypercarbia can contribute to postresuscitation myocardial dysfunction, and that CO_2-consuming buffers may alleviate some of that dysfunction.

A second study from the same investigator using their rodent model evaluated if the combination of buffers and adrenergic agents was useful in preventing or improving postresuscitation myocardial dysfunction (39). The first group was assigned to receive sodium bicarbonate, tromethamine, or 0.9% sodium chloride in a blinded fashion, before the administration of epinephrine and the β-blocker esmolol. The second group received the same treatment in reverse order. Sixteen rats underwent 8 minutes of untreated VF-induced CA, followed by CPR as previously described. Buffers and adrenergic agents were given at 2 and 4 minutes of CPR. Resuscitation was attempted with up to three 2-J countershocks after 16 minutes of CA and 8 minutes after the start of precordial compression. Myocardial function was assessed from measurements of LV pressure, cardiac output, isovolumic contractility (dP/dt$_{40}$), and myocardial relaxation (–dP/dt). In each instance, as opposed to their previous report, a greater impairment of postresuscitation myocardial function and decreased postresuscitation survival was observed after the use of buffer agents. The authors speculated that the mechanism for this adverse effect of buffers is through arterial pH-mediated increases in myocardial oxygen requirements and intensified myocardial ischemia. Given these results, they recommend caution in using buffer agents during CPR or postresuscitation.

DEFIBRILLATION: ENERGY

The amount of energy delivered during defibrillation has also been studied as a potential cause in the degree of resulting myocardial dysfunction after resuscitation. The magnitude and duration of the transthoracic electrical shock has always been suspected as being responsible for myocardial injury. Several initial studies in intact animals under physiologic conditions (not in CA) demonstrated that the magnitude and duration of a transthoracic shock was not detrimental to the overall myocardial function postresuscitation. Work performed by our group supported this notion by failing to demonstrate a relationship between the amount of energy (Joules) delivered during normal sinus rhythm and any subsequent post shock myocardial dysfunction (19). Xie et al. however, using a rodent VF CA model demonstrated that high-energy defibrillation (during VF) can be an important contributor to postresuscitation myocardial dysfunction and ultimately can impact postresuscitation survival (40). Using their group's standard measurements, including LV diastolic pressure, dP/dt$_{40}$, and -dP/dt, they found a correlation between defibrillation energy and subsequent degree of postresuscitation myocardial dysfunction. Unfortunately, the maximal dose per kilogram employed (20 J/kg) was well above that recommended clinically (5 J/kg). Hence, any conclusions about the effects of clinically relevant doses are difficult to ascertain.

Other investigators searching for a mechanism by which defibrillation could contribute to postresuscitation LV dysfunction have shown that free radicals are generated after defibrillation when electrodes are applied directly to the endocardium (41). Generation of free radicals could be explained by damaged sarcolemma and mitochondria, calcium overload, impaired mitochondrial function, and impaired oxidative metabolism.

DEFIBRILLATION: WAVEFORM

Tang et al. reported that the type of waveform used in defibrillation can influence the degree of myocardial dysfunction that ensues following resuscitation (42). In a study of 20 swine undergoing 4 or 7 minutes of untreated VF, they compared the effects of biphasic vs conventional monophasic defibrillation on the degree of postresuscitation myocardial dysfunction. After 4 minutes of untreated VF, the LV stroke volume, EF, fractional area change, and LV-end diastolic volume were significantly greater in the group defibrillated with biphasic waves. The same findings were noted when the VF duration was increased to 7 minutes. Furthermore, successful resuscitation and survival was greater in the biphasic group, although those differences were not significant. Niemann et al., however, found no relationship between defibrillation waveform and post-resuscitation myocardial function (43). Studying 38 swine (26–36 kg) submitted to 5 minutes of untreated VF then defibrillated with either monophasic (200 J, 300 J,

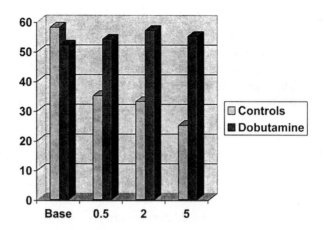

Fig. 5. Postresuscitation ejection fraction and dobutamine. (Adapted from ref. *47*, with permission.)

360 J) or biphasic (150 J, 150 J, 150 J), they could not demonstrate any differences in postresuscitation cardiac output, dP/dt, or peak LV pressure. The sensitivity of these LV function measurements has been questioned *(44)*, nonetheless the issue of whether the type of defibrillation waveform contributes to postresuscitation ventricular dysfunction appears not yet resolved.

Current Treatment Options for Postresuscitation Myocardial Dysfunction

Several treatments for postresuscitation myocardial dysfunction have been proposed and studied. Recognizing the similarities of postresuscitation myocardial "stunning" with the global stunning seen after some cardiac surgery particularly postcardiac transplantation, we explored the use of a β-adrenergic agonist (dobutamine), which is commonly used in the immediate postcardiac surgery period *(45)*. Previous work has shown this agent to be a significant inotrope capable of enhancing LV function including stunned myocardium *(46)*.

Using our previously published porcine model of postresuscitation systolic and diastolic LV dysfunction *(19)*, we studied the effect of dobutamine infusions (10 μg/kg per minute in 14 animals and 5 μg/kg per minute in 5 animals) begun 15 minutes after resuscitation and compared to no treatment in 8 control animals *(47)*. The marked deterioration in systolic and diastolic LV function postresuscitation seen in the control animals was ameliorated in the dobutamine-treated animals (Fig. 5). Measurement of isovolumic relaxation of the left ventricle (tau) demonstrated a similar benefit of the dobutamine infusion for overcoming postresuscitation diastolic dysfunction. Tau rose, indicating decreased LV compliance in control animals whereas it remained constant in the dobutamine-treated animals (Fig. 6). LVEDP rose significantly in the control group but not in the dobutamine group when comparing pre-arrest and 5-hour data (Fig. 7). Of particular concern was the increased heart rate seen in the dobutamine-treated group. Average heart rate at 30 minutes postresuscitation in animals treated with 10 μg/kg per minute of dobutamine was 190 ± 12 beats per minute (bpm) as opposed to only 134 ± 8 bpm in the control group ($p < 0.05$). As a result of the excessive heart rate increase seen in the animals receiving 10 μg/kg per minute of dobutamine, additional animals were

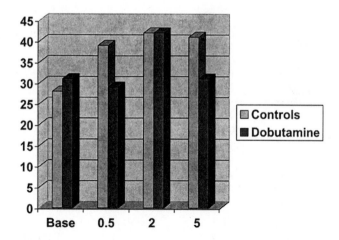

Fig. 6. Postresuscitation tau and dobutamine. (Adapted from ref. *47*, with permission.)

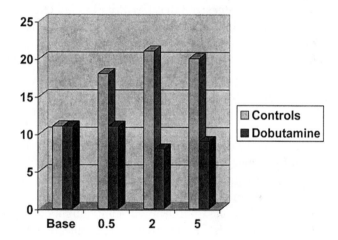

Fig. 7. Postresuscitation left ventricular end-diastolic pressure and dobutamine. (Adapted from ref. *47*, with permission.)

studied post hoc using the same protocol except for a lower dose of dobutamine (5 μg/ kg per minute). Heart rate response was significantly less with 5 μg/kg per minute, however LVEF did not improve as much as with the 10 μg/kg per minute dose.

Concern about raising heart rate (thereby increasing myocardial oxygen consumption in a "sick" heart postresuscitation) stimulated a search for alternative treatments. Intra-aortic balloon counterpulsation (IABP) seemed like a good choice. A commonly employed therapy for severe but reversible heart failure (particularly with acute ischemic disease), aortic counterpulsation has no intrinsic chronotropic effects, but has been shown to decrease LV work while still maintaining adequate peripheral perfusion. IABP aids cardiac performance primarily through reduction in afterload. This is reflected typically in a reduced systolic arterial pressure (generally decreased by 10–20%). Rather than increase myocardial oxygen demand it improves myocardial oxygen delivery by increasing coronary perfusion secondary to an increase in diastolic aortic pressure.

Table 9
Optimal Dobutamine Dosing Postresuscitation: EF (%)

Time PR dose (µg/kg per minute)	Pre-arrest	25-minute PR	30-minute PR	2-hour PR	4-hour PR	6-hour PR
0	49	35	35	34	28	33
2.5	49	33	34	43	37	41
5	47	29	38	45	46	48
7.5	42	27	43	44	45	46

EF, ejection fraction; PR, postresuscitation.

We therefore designed a preliminary study to examine the efficacy of the IABP vs dobutamine in the treatment of postresuscitative dysfunction in an established preclinical CA model (48). We hypothesized that IABP will be a better therapy than dobutamine because of its ability to improve acute myocardial dysfunction without increasing the subsequent heart rate.

Ten domestic swine (49 ± 3 kg) underwent 15 minutes of untreated VF before being successfully resuscitated. LV systolic and diastolic function was measured at pre-arrest baseline, at 30 minutes and at 6 hours postresuscitation. Five animals were treated immediately after resuscitation with IABP and five were given dobutamine (5 µg/kg per minute).

At 30 minutes postresuscitation, pulmonary capillary wedge pressure and LVEDP were significantly higher (16 vs 7mmHg and 20 vs 11 mmHg), whereas LV isovolumic relaxation (tau) was significantly longer (34 vs 20 ms) in the IABP treated vs the dobutamine treated animals. Likewise, at 6 hours postresuscitation LV EF was significantly less (20% vs 38%), and LVEDP significantly higher (18 vs 10 mmHg) in the IABP group. Heart rate was not different between the groups at any time postresuscitation.

Dobutamine was superior to IABP for treatment of postresuscitation LV systolic and diastolic dysfunction, at least in our experimental model without antecedent coronary artery disease (CAD). The hypothesized advantage of IABP for treatment of postresuscitation myocardial stunning without excessively raising the heart rate like dobutamine was not realized. The role for IABP in the clinical arena in which the typical victim of sudden cardiac death has substantial coronary disease remains undefined.

What's the best dose of dobutamine in the setting of postresuscitation care? We recently explored the optimal dose of dobutamine for postresuscitation myocardial dysfunction in our swine model (49). Twenty animals were studied for 6hours after successful resuscitation, with five each receiving 0, 2, 5, or 7.5 µg/kg per minute of dobutamine. Drug infusions were begun at 30 minutes postresuscitation. We found that both the 5 and 7.5 µg/kg per minute doses completely reversed the decline in EF. Both doses were significantly better than either 2 µg/kg per minute or controls for improving systolic LV function (Table 9). However, both also raised the heart rate at 6 hours postresuscitation above that seen with either 2 µg/kg per minute or placebo controls. Only the higher dose of 7.5 µg/kg per minute had an adverse effect on myocardial oxygen consumption.

In exploring other avenues of treatment, Weil, Tang, and coworkers examined the possibility that ischemic preconditioning could ameliorate postresuscitation myocardial dysfunction *(50)*. Using a rodent CA model, five different strategies were tested including: (a) ischemic preconditioning by repetitive episodes of short duration VF; (b) administration of a potassium adenosine triphosphate (ATP) channel activator (cromakalim); (c) administration of a potassium ATP channel blocker (glibenclamide) 1 minute after VF; (d) administration of a potassium ATP channel blocker (glibenclamide) 45 minutes before ischemic preconditioning; and (e) administration of placebo. The potassium ATP channel activator lowered CPP during CPR significantly, but produced a reduction of postresuscitation myocardial dysfunction and an increase in postresuscitation survival. Ischemic preconditioning by repetitive VF episodes also reduced postresuscitation myocardial dysfunction significantly. LV dP/dt_{40}, CI, and negative dP/dt_{40} were all improved in rats undergoing preconditioning (whether by potassium ATP channel activation or by repetitive VF episodes) when compared to placebo controls at 1, 2, 3, and 4 hours postresuscitation. Forty-eight-hour survival was better in preconditioned animals than either those receiving placebo or the potassium ATP channel blocker. Of note, providing preconditioning through the pharmacological activation and opening of the potassium ATP channel during cardiac resuscitation provided similar protective effects for postresuscitation myocardial function as did ischemic preconditioning.

These same investigators reported preliminary data on the use of 21-aminosteroids for the treatment of postresuscitation myocardial dysfunction at the American Heart Association's (AHA) Scientific Sessions 2000 *(51)*. Such compounds have been shown to minimize reperfusion injury mediated by liberation of free radicals. Weil, Tang, and associates tested their administration for improved postresuscitation function and better neurologically normal survival. VF was induced in 10 rats, left untreated for 8 minutes, and then CPR was performed for an additional 6 minutes prior to defibrillation. A 21-aminosteroid (U-74389G-Upjohn) was injected into the right atrium 1 minute prior to starting CPR in five animals with placebo injected into the others. CI, dP/dt_{40}, negative dP/dt_{40}, LVEDP were all better postresuscitation in the group treated with the 21-aminosteroid. Neurological deficit scores were less in the active treatment group (33 ± 66 vs 151 ± 63; $p < 0.05$), and duration of postresuscitation survival was also greater (57 ± 22 vs 29 ± 16 hours; $p < 0.05$). These investigators concluded that 21-aminosteroids administered during CPR improve post resuscitation myocardial function, neurological outcome, and postresuscitation survival. Whether similar results can be achieved by their administration after resuscitation is unknown.

FUTURE DIRECTIONS IN STUDYING POSTRESUSCITATION MYOCARDIAL DYSFUNCTION

The possibility of improving long-term outcome following CA by better understanding, preventing, or treating postresuscitation myocardial dysfunction is exciting and promising. Several intriguing pathways have been suggested recently for future study in this regard *(15)*.

The possibility of preventing much of the myocardial dysfunction following resuscitation from prolonged CA by inducing a state of suspended animation or hibernation during CA is appealing. Hibernating animals tolerate ischemic and reperfusion conditions as they enter and emerge from hibernation without apparent injury. Remarkably, such animals regulate their local and systemic oxygen needs, reducing them to levels in which ischemic injury does not occur, even when oxygen delivery is substantially compromised. Heart rate may decline to 5% of normal levels during hibernation, yet no ischemia seems to occur nor does the rhythm degenerate into VF or complete asystole. After arousal and with restoration of normal heart rates and oxygen delivery, no reperfusion injury is evident. Molecular signaling mechanisms and intracellular cascades are just now being defined and discovered. Application of such discoveries in the field of resuscitation science hold great hope for extending the time limits for successful resuscitation with reduced postresuscitation injuries.

Hypothermia is another recognized therapeutic modality with promise in the field of resuscitation. Two recent clinical reports *(52,53)* have shown improved CNS outcome in CA survivors treated with mild hypothermia postresuscitation. Very little has yet been done examining the effects of hypothermia on myocardial function postresuscitation. One report calls for caution however, after showing increased histological damage to the myocardium after induction of postresuscitation moderate (28–32°C) hypothermia *(54)*. No functional assessment of LV or RV function was performed in this study however.

SUMMARY

Myocardial dysfunction postresuscitation is now well described and characterized in both experimental models and in clinical studies. Both systolic and diastolic functions are affected. Both the left and right ventricles can be involved. Global decreases in systolic and diastolic function are temporary, and full recovery is possible. Large animal models used in translational experiments suggest that 48 hours is required for full recovery. Clinically, this period may be longer depending on the precedent ventricular function and underlying CAD. Severe compromise of myocardial function can occur and lead to death from acute pump failure, shock. and recurrent CA if therapy is not undertaken. Successful reversal of both LV and RV dysfunction postresuscitation has been achieved with dobutamine in experimental models. Preconditioning with potassium ATP channel activation may also improve both postresuscitation myocardial dysfunction and outcome.

REFERENCES

1. Lombardi G, Gallagher J, P. G. Outcome of out-of-hospital cardiac arrest in New York City: the Pre-Hospital Arrest Survival Evaluation (PHASE) study. JAMA 1994; 271:678–683.
2. Becker L, Ostrander M, Barrett J, Kondos G. CPR Chicago: outcome of cardiopulmonary resuscitation in a large metropolitan area-where are the survivors? Ann Emerg Med 1991; 20:355–361.
3. Cummins R, Ornato J, Theis W, Pepe P. Improving Survival From Sudden Cardiac Arrest: The "Chain of Survival" Concept. Circulation 1991; 83:1832–1847.
4. White R, Hankins D, Bugliosi T. Seven years' experience with early defibrillation by police and paramedics in an emergency medical services system. Resuscitation 1998; 39:145–151.
5. Valenzuela TD, Roe DJ, Nichol G, Clark LL, Spaite DW, Hardman RG. Outcomes of rapid defibrillation by security officers after cardiac arrest in casinos. [see comments.]. N Engl J Med 2000; 343: 1206–1209.
6. Willoughby P, Caffrey S. Improved survival with an airport-based PAD program. Circulation 2000; 102:II–828.
7. Caffrey S, Willoughby P, Pepe P, Becker L. Public use of automated external defibrillators. N Engl J Med 2002; 347:1242–1247.
8. Kudenchuk PJ, Cobb LA, Copass MK, et al. Amiodarone for resuscitation after out-of-hospital cardiac arrest due to ventricular fibrillation. [see comments.]. N Engl J Med 1999; 341:871–878.
9. Dorian P, Cass D, Schwartz B, Cooper R, Gelaznikas R, Barr A. Amiodarone as compared with lidocaine for shock-resistant ventricular fibrillation. N Engl J Med 2002; 346:884–890.
10. Centers for Disease Control and Prevention (CDC). State-Specific Mortality From Sudden Cardiac Death—United States, 1999. MMWR 2002; 51; 123–126.
11. Group BRCTIS. Brain Resuscitation Clinical Trial I Study Group: A randomized clinical study of thiopental loading in comatose survivors of cardiac arrest. N Engl J Med 1986; 314:397–403.

12. Group BRCTIS. Brain Resuscitation Clinical Trial II Study Group: A randomized clinical study of a calcium-entry blocker (lidoflazine) in the treatment of comatose survivors of cardiac arrest. N Engl J Med 1991; 324:1125–1131.

13. Schoenenberger RA, von Planta M, von Planta I. Survival after failed out-of-hospital resuscitation. Are further therapeutic efforts in the emergency department futile? Arch Int Med 1994; 154:2433–2437.

14. Ewy GA, Ornato JP. 31st Bethesda Conference: Emergency Cardiac Care (1999), Bethesda Conference Report, Bethesda, Maryland. 1999; Vol. 35. J Am Coll Cardiol.

15. Becker LB, Weisfeldt ML, Weil MH, et al. The PULSE initiative: scientific priorities and strategic planning for resuscitation research and life saving therapies. Circulation 2002; 105:2562–2570.

16. Cerchiari EL, Safar P, Klein E, Cantadore R, Pinsky M. Cardiovascular function and neurologic outcome after cardiac arrest in dogs. The cardiovascular post-resuscitation syndrome. Resuscitation 1993; 25:9–33.

17. Tang W, Weil MH, Sun S, Gazmuri RJ, Bisera J. Progressive myocardial dysfunction after cardiac resuscitation. Crit Care Med 1993; 21:1046–1050.

18. Gazmuri RJ, Weil MH, Bisera J, Tang W, Fukui M, McKee D. Myocardial dysfunction after successful resuscitation from cardiac arrest. Crit Care Med 1996; 24:992–1000.

19. Kern KB, Hilwig RW, Rhee KH, Berg RA. Myocardial dysfunction after resuscitation from cardiac arrest: an example of global myocardial stunning. J Am Coll Cardiol 1996; 28:232–240.

20. Patel B, Kloner RA, Przyklenk K, Braunwald E. Postischemic myocardial "stunning": A clinically relevant phenomenon. Ann Intern Med 1988; 108:626–628.

21. Wijns W, Serruys P, Slager C, et al. Effect of coronary occlusion during percutaneous transluminal angioplasty in humans on left ventricular chamber stiffness and regional diastolic pressure-radius relations. J Am Coll Cardiol 1986; 7:455–463.

22. Meyer RJ, Kern KB, Berg RA, Hilwig RTW, Ewy GA. Post-resuscitation right ventricular dysfunction: delineation and treatment with dobutamine. Resuscitation. 2002; 55:187–191.

23. Bowers TR, O'Neill WW, Grines C, Pica MC, Safian RD, Goldstein JA. Effect of Reperfusion on Biventricular Function and Survival after Right Ventricular Infarction. N Engl J Med 1998; 338:933–940.

24. Kern KB, Garewal HS, Sanders AB, et al. Depletion of myocardial adenosine triphosphate during prolonged untreated ventricular fibrillation: effect on defibrillation success. Resuscitation 1990; 20:221–229.

25. Kamohara T, Weil MH, Tang W, et al. A comparison of myocardial function after primary cardiac and primary asphyxial cardiac arrest. Am J Respir Crit Care Med 2001; 164:1221–1224.

26. Deantonio HJ, Kaul S, Lerman BB. Reversible myocardial depression in survivors of cardiac arrest. Pacing Clin Electrophysiol 1990; 13:982–985.

27. Bashir R, Padder FA, Khan FA. Myocardial stunning following respiratory arrest. Chest 1995; 108: 1459–1460.

28. Kern KB. Post resuscitation left ventricular dysfunction: acute reversible heart failure. Cardinale (French) 1998; 10:16–18.

29. Laurent I, Spaulding C, Monchi M, et al. Transient shock after successful resuscitation: clinical evidence for post-cardiac arrest myocardial stunning. J Am Coll Cardiol 2000; 35:399A.

30. Mullner M, Domanovits H, Sterz F, et al. Measurement of myocardial contractility following successful resuscitation: quantitated left ventricular systolic function utilizing non-invasive wall stress analysis. Resuscitation 1998; 39:51–59.

31. Tang W, Weil MH, Sun S. Low-energy biphasic waveform defibrillation reduces the severity of postresuscitation myocardial dysfunction. Crit Care Med 2000; 28:N222–N224.

32. Tang W, Weil MH, Sun S, Noc M, Yang L, Gazmuri RJ. Epinephrine increases the severity of postresuscitation myocardial dysfunction. Circulation 1995; 92:3089–3093.

33. Sun S, Weil MH, Tang W, Kamohara T, Klouche K. Alpha-Methylnorepinephrine, a selective alpha2-adrenergic agonist for cardiac resuscitation. J Am Coll Cardiol 2001; 37:951–956.

34. Klouche K, Weil MH, Tang W, Povoas H, Kamohara T, Bisera J. A selective alpha(2)-adrenergic agonist for cardiac resuscitation. J Lab Clin Med 2002; 140:27–34.

35. Hilwig RW, Berg RA, Kern KB, Ewy GA. Endothelin-1 vasoconstriction during swine cardiopulmonary resuscitation improves coronary perfusion pressures but worsens postresuscitation outcome. Circulation 2000; 101:2097–2102.

36. Kette F, Weil MH, von Planta M, Gazmuri RJ, Rackow EC. Buffer agents do not reverse intramyocardial acidosis during cardiac resuscitation. Circulation 1990; 81:1660–1666.

37. Kette F, Weil MH, Gazmuri RJ. Buffer solutions may compromise cardiac resuscitation by reducing coronary perfusion pressure. [see comments.] [erratum appears in JAMA 1991 Dec 18; 266(23):3286.]. JAMA 1991; 266:2121–2126.

38. Sun S, Weil MH, Tang W, Fukui M. Effects of buffer agents on postresuscitation myocardial dysfunction. Crit Care Med 1996; 24:2035–2041.
39. Sun S, Weil MH, Tang W, Povoas HP, Mason E. Combined effects of buffer and adrenergic agents on postresuscitation myocardial function. J Pharm Exp Ther 1999; 291:773–777.
40. Xie J, Weil MH, Sun S, et al. High-energy defibrillation increases the severity of postresuscitation myocardial dysfunction. Circulation 1997; 96:683–688.
41. Caterine MR, Spencer KT, Pagan-Carlo LA, Smith RS, Buettner GR, Kerber RE. Direct current shocks to the heart generate free radicals: an electron paramagnetic resonance study. J Am Coll Cardiol 1996; 28:1598–1609.
42. Tang W, Weil MH, Sun S, et al. The effects of biphasic and conventional monophasic defibrillation on postresuscitation myocardial function. [see comments.]. J Am Coll Cardiol 1999; 34:815–822.
43. Niemann JT, Burian D, Garner D, Lewis RJ. Monophasic versus biphasic transthoracic countershock after prolonged ventricular fibrillation in a swine model. [see comments.]. J Am Coll Cardiol 2000; 36:932–938.
44. Sun S, Klouche K, Tang W, Weil MH. The effects of biphasic and conventional monophasic defibrillation on postresuscitation myocardial function. [letter; comment.]. J Am Coll Cardiol 2001; 37:1753,1754.
45. Cohn LH. Dobutamine in the postcardiac surgery patient. In: Chatterjee K, ed. Dobutamine: A Ten-Year Review. Indianapolis, IN: Eli Lilly, 1989, pp. 123–128.
46. Berrizbeitia LD, Piccione W, Austin JC, et al. Inotropic response of the salvaged myocardium after acute coronary occlusion. Ann Thorac Surg 1986; 41:58–64.
47. Kern KB, Hilwig RW, Berg RA, et al. Postresuscitation left ventricular systolic and diastolic dysfunction. Treatment with dobutamine. Circulation 1997; 95:2610–2613.
48. Tennyson H, Kern KB, Hilwig RW, Berg RA, Ewy GA. Treatment of post resuscitation myocardial dysfunction: aortic counterpulsation versus dobutamine. Resuscitation 2002; 54:69–75.
49. Vasquez A, Kern K, Hilwig R, Heidenreich JW, Berg RA, Ewy GA. Dobutamine for post-resuscitation left ventricular dysfunction: an assessment of optimal dosing. Resuscitation 2004; 61:199–207.
50. Tang W, Weil MH, Sun S, Pernat A, Mason E. K(ATP) channel activation reduces the severity of postresuscitation myocardial dysfunction. Am J Physiol Heart Circ Physiol 2000; 279:H1609–H1615.
51. Kamohara T, Weil MH, Tang W, Sun S, Klouche K, Zhao D. Improved function and survival after administration of 21-aminosteriods during CPR. Circulation 2000; 102:II–571.
52. The Hypothermia after Cardiac Arrest Study G. Mild therapeutic hypothermia to improve the neurologic outcome after cardiac arrest. [see comments.] [erratum appears in N Engl J Med 2002 May 30; 346(22):1756.]. N Engl J Med 2002; 346:549–556.
53. Bernard SA, Gray TW, Buist MD, et al. Treatment of comatose survivors of out-of-hospital cardiac arrest with induced hypothermia. [see comments.]. N Engl J Med 2002; 346:557–563.
54. Leonov Y, Sterz F, Safar P, Radovsky A. Moderate hypothermia after cardiac arrest of 17 minutes in dogs. Effect on cerebral and cardiac outcome. Stroke 1990; 21:1600–1606.

30 Postresuscitation Cerebral Dysfunction

Prevention and Treatment

Antonio E. Muñiz, MD, FACEP, FAAP, FAAEM

INTRODUCTION

Permanent brain damage caused by ischemia and reperfusion that results from disease processes such as stroke and cardiac arrest (CA) with resuscitation has been estimated to affect approx 200,000 patients in the United States annually *(1)*. Neuronal damage from stroke and CA occur by different mechanistic models of injury. In ischemic stroke, only a portion of the brain is at risk, and the ischemia is only complete in the center of the vulnerable area. This central area of dense ischemia is surrounded by a penumbral zone in which blood flow is diminished but not completely lost. As opposed to CA with resuscitation, flow ceases altogether and the entire brain is at risk for a transient period of complete ischemia followed by reperfusion *(2)*.

Neuronal impairment after ischemia and reperfusion from CA is determined by many elements, including arrest (no-flow) time, resuscitation (low-flow) time, reperfusion (no-flow, hyperemic phase, and global and multifocal hypoperfusion) severity, and temperature. The enormous significance of the postresuscitation phase for long-term outcome is often underestimated. Nevertheless, the time from onset of cardiopulmonary arrest (CPA) until restoration of an effective spontaneous circulation is, probably the single most vital determinant of long-term, neurologically intact survival from CPA. The majority of neuronal-injuring processes occur not during the actual CA or resuscitation but throughout reperfusion.

The idea of cerebral resuscitation was first introduced by Peter Safar in the 1970s and started with the concept of "brains too good to die" after cardiac standstill *(3)*. Despite

From: *Contemporary Cardiology: Cardiopulmonary Resuscitation*
Edited by: J. P. Ornato and M. A. Peberdy © Humana Press Inc., Totowa, NJ

all the marvelous and exciting improvement in resuscitation techniques in the last few decades, neurological recovery continues to be the major limiting factor in acquiring a meaningful quality of life postresuscitation. Cerebral injury occurring after CA and resuscitation becomes a primary focus in the management priorities in the postresuscitation phase of care. Unfortunately, recent estimates show that only 3–10% of cardiopulmonary resuscitation (CPR) attempts outside of the hospital setting result in survival without brain damage *(4,5)*. The poor tolerance of neurons to global ischemia accounts for much of the morbidity and mortality associated with CA. Additionally, in the last two decades, research focused on amelioration of neuronal injury has been extensive but at best frustrating, principally because the mechanisms responsible for the injury caused by cerebral ischemia and reperfusion are extremely complicated and multifactorial in nature and not yet entirely understood.

In addition to cerebral dysfunction following global ischemia, other factors contribute to the morbidity and mortality after CA, which may hinder recuperation from neuronal injury. These include cardiovascular and hemodynamic derangements, respiratory insufficiency, and hyperthermia, all of which are common after the return of spontaneous circulation (ROSC *[6,7]*). Although the multiorgan dysfunction syndrome from other causes such as hemorrhagic or septic shock has been linked by an intermediary state termed systemic inflammatory response syndrome (SIRS), there is limited evidence for a clear relationship between that syndrome and the postresuscitation syndrome *(8,9)*. Instead, it appears more likely that protracted derangements of hemodynamic and respiratory function, many of which may be iatrogenic in nature, in the postresuscitation period are fundamentally responsible. The postresuscitation syndrome proved to affect primarily the brain, but also to some extent the extracerebral organs, even when systemic blood pressure, arterial blood gases, and blood volume were normalized. This syndrome is identified by protracted tissue acidosis and reduced cardiac output and tissue perfusion.

Shortly after resuscitation, patients may display a wide range of physiological conditions. Patients may regain normal hemodynamic and cerebral function. On the other hand, many remain comatose with cardiopulmonary insufficiency. All patients require meticulous, repeated assessments to establish the status of their neurologic and cardiopulmonary systems. Postresuscitation goals include preservation of brain function and optimization of respiratory, cardiovascular, metabolic, renal, and hepatic function in order to arrest secondary organ injury. Additionally, it includes an assessment and treatment for the cause of the CA.

To improve on the survival after ROSC, one fundamental objective is the complete reestablishment of regional cerebral perfusion. In normal circumstances, cerebral blood flow is autoregulated such that it is independent of perfusion pressure over a wide range of blood pressures, usually between a mean arterial blood pressure (MABP) of 50 to 150 torr *(10)*. After global brain ischemia, however, autoregulation is lost, and perfusion becomes contingent on arterial pressure primarily. Consequently, the occurrence of postresuscitation hypotension, a common phenomenon, can reduce cerebral blood flow severely and result in further brain damage *(11)*. Therefore, after restoration of spontaneous circulation, MABP should be at least normalized, and attaining a blood pressure higher than pre-arrest values by administration of fluids or vasopressors may be even more beneficial *(2)*.

A consistent problem in the postresuscitation phase is counting on simple vital signs to indicate adequate resuscitation. Simple restoration of blood pressure, even in the presence of excellent coronary perfusion alone and improvement in tissue gas exchange do not necessarily correlate with better survival *(12)*. However, if spontaneous ventilation and circulation do not occur early, then successful cerebral resuscitation usually does not happen. These commonly used endpoints fail to indicate appropriate resuscitation of end-organs and restoration of their blood supply which contribute to continued organ dysfunction after an ischemic and reperfusion injury (13,14).

Particularly vulnerable neurons die, in part, because of a complex cascade of events during reperfusion. Reverting the patient to the level of pre-arrest neurological function is the ultimate goal of resuscitation. This objective has been termed cardiopulmonary–cerebral resuscitation (CPCR) by Dr. Safar (15). Cerebral dysfunction occurring after flow is reestablished is contingent on the severity and duration of the ischemic insult (16). The shorter the interval between onset of CA and restoration of systemic and cerebral blood flow, the greater the success of resuscitation and likelihood of hospital discharge (17). Prevention of postresuscitation cerebral dysfunction is dependent on decreasing the downtime interval and increasing perfusion to the brain and heart during CPR. The best method for decreasing the downtime interval and reducing the severity of the postresuscitation syndrome is summarized in the American Heart Association's (AHA) "chain of survival," which calls for early activation of the emergency medical services, early CPR, early defibrillation, and early advanced life support (18). Cerebral viability appears to require at least 20% of normal cerebral blood flow, which standard external CPR cannot reliably generate (19). Occasionally, optimal standard CPR may produce a sufficiently high cerebral blood flow, but cannot sustain electroencephalogram (EEG) activity or cerebral oxygenation (20).

Numerous techniques have been designed to improve blood flow during cardiac standstill. Several new experimental CPR methods have been shown to augment cerebral blood flow and outcomes in animal models and some have been shown to improve outcome in limited human trails. Recently, mild induced hypothermia has been the only clinically effective therapeutic protocol for amelioration of brain damage caused by ischemia and reperfusion. Clinical trials of therapies directed at reducing the extent of ultimate neuronal damage by use of either barbiturate, calcium antagonist, excitatory amino acid blockers, oxygen-free radical inhibitors, and protein synthesis modulators have been at best disappointing. The limitation of most therapies currently being developed to attenuate neuronal damage after CA is that they affect a single pathway implicated in the ischemic and reperfusion syndrome. Neuronal injury as a result of ischemia and reperfusion is a complex and multifactorial disease. Thus, it is unlikely that a single therapeutic option is going to be effective (15,21,22). Recently, the 5-minute limit for neuronal survival from normothermic arrest has recently been extended to 11 minutes with the use of a combination treatment regime (23). The complex pathogenesis of neuronal damage from ischemia and reperfusion is more likely to be amenable to a combination of therapies directed at specific mechanisms for injury (15,24).

The ultimate goal of CPR research is to find methods that can improve survival and postresuscitation quality of life in patients with CA. To accomplish this, an understanding of the pathways implicated in neuronal death and neuronal repair during ischemia and reperfusion and the issues that modulate these processes are critical. Experimental studies performed at the cellular level have begun to define vital determinants in the process of cerebral dysfunction and have shown promise toward improving neurological outcome. Further understanding of the elemental pathways involved in the pathophysiology of neuronal injury and repair may allow for a paradigm shift in therapeutic approaches. Because the mechanism for neuronal injury is multifactorial, therapy directed at the most prominent mechanisms that lead to brain damage must be developed. This chapter provides an overview of the present knowledge about the mechanisms underlying cerebral dysfunction from ischemia and reperfusion. Additionally, it describes treatment modalities, some speculative, for the amelioration of cerebral dysfunction associated with CA.

CEREBRAL DYSFUNCTION: PATHOPHYSIOLOGY

Standard CPR often allows ROSC, but cannot be relied on to protect the brain from injury during resuscitation. Disruption of blood flow to the brain for even a few minutes with restoration of perfusion sets in motion a cascade of cellular derangements resulting in continued neuronal damage. These cascades appear to be triggered in part by cellular energy depletion during ischemia from CA and circulation of oxygenated, acidotic blood during reperfusion. After global ischemia from CA, reperfusion and reoxygenation of tissues is necessary to restore energy metabolism and cell viability and remove toxic metabolites. Reperfusion, although essential for reestablishing energy metabolism and cell viability, results in generation of oxygen-free radicals, release of excitatory amino acids, nitric oxide and inflammatory mediators, increase in intracellular calcium and many additional derangements at the cellular level. All of these processes create a tissue milieu responsible for the postresuscitation syndrome. Following a CA with no flow of greater than 10 minutes with subsequent reperfusion generates the cerebral postresuscitation syndrome or postischemic-anoxic encephalopathy. This syndrome consists of a series of multiple organ system derangements, which may hinder recovery from CA even when systemic arterial pressure, arterial blood gases, and blood volume are maintained at normal levels.

The precise mechanisms by which ischemia and reperfusion causes neuronal injury and produces cerebral postresuscitation syndrome has not been established firmly and is generally assumed to be multifactorial (15,22,25–27). Many of these processes are still speculative and are being studied actively. Some of the mechanisms for neuronal injury include the following:

1. Depletion of adenosine triphosphate (ATP).
2. Derangements in neuronal ion membrane.
3. Perfusion abnormalities.
4. Brain tissue acidosis.
5. Reoxygenation chemical cascades leading to generation of oxygen-free radicals and release of excitatory amino acids resulting in cellular death.
6. Influx of calcium flux and sodium with cell swelling
7. Nitric oxide release.
8. Post-arrest activation of the inflammatory mediators.
9. Loss of protein translation competence.
10. Calpain-mediated proteolysis.
11. Derangements as a result of blood stasis.
12. Inhibition of growth-factor signal transduction.
13. Induction of apoptosis.
14. Extracellular organ and tissue derangements (see Fig. 1).

Based on conventional staining, morphological evidence shows that most structural cellular damage in vulnerable neurons occurs during reperfusion in two phases (28,29). Cytosolic microvacuolization is noted within the first 15 minutes of reperfusion, although a substantial degree of normalization occurs over the next hour. Further morphological evidence of progressive damage to these neurons is then seen throughout the following

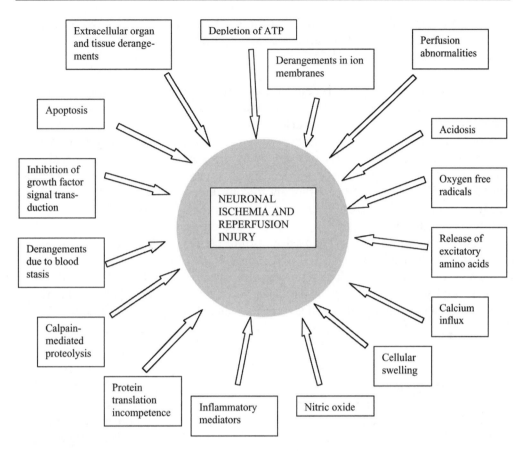

Fig. 1. A schematic representation of the mechanism involved in ischemia and reperfusion neuronal injury.

6 hours. At about 24 hours post-arrest and notably by 48 to 72 hours post-arrest the irreversible morphologic changes can be seen scattered on light microscopy in some neurons (30,31). The histological features of necrotic cell death include mitochondrial and nuclear swelling, dissolution of organelles, and condensation of chromatin around the nucleus. These events are followed subsequently by the rupture of nuclear and cytoplasmic membranes and the degradation of DNA by random enzymatic cleavage (31). The ongoing neuronal damage occurring 48 to 72 hours after reperfusion from CA raises hope that new promising resuscitative therapies may be effective in ameliorating neuronal damage (32).

Ischemic brain edema results from both cell swelling (cytotoxic edema) and increased blood vessel permeability (vasogenic edema). Although intracranial pressure remains normal after survivable CA, extracellular-to-intracellular fluid and electrolytes shifts occur early during ischemia leading to cytotoxic edema (30,33). Vasogenic edema may occur later during reperfusion following severe insults and is made worse by hypoxia or hypercapnia (30,34). Reperfusion restores blood flow, bringing oxygen, glucose, and leukocytes to the injured neurons. Several tissue and leukocyte-derived mediators, (e.g., oxygen-free radicals, nitric oxide [NO]), and proteases) are released. These mediators promote microvascular permeability, damage the blood–brain barrier (BBB) and are responsible for the generation of vasogenic edema *(35)*. Vasogenic edema plays a critical role because of the increased risk for hemorrhage from damaged blood vessels and excess fluid *(36)*.

Other mechanisms of cerebral edema formation have been described in focal ischemic models, but have yet to be proven in global ischemia from CA. An abnormality in a brain water transport protein, called aquaporin 4 (AQP4) can contribute to brain edema *(37)*. Another pathway thought to contribute to ischemia and reperfusion injury is through the formation and release of matrix metalloproteinases (MMPs *[38]*). They constitute a family of at least 20 zinc-containing serine proteases. After a focal ischemic and reperfusion injury, the MMPs are thought to contribute to the breakdown of the BBB integrity and have been involved in several phases of inflammation *(39)*.

If the brain edema is untreated, it will lead to an increase in intracranial pressure (ICP) as a result of the brain being enclosed in a rigid cranial vault with limited room for expansion. Further increases in ICP will eventually lead to compression of cerebral tissue, decreased cerebral perfusion pressure, impaired cerebral blood flow, and further neuronal injury. Characterizing the pathogenesis of cerebral edema formation may one day lead to therapeutic agents that may attenuate neurological damage after a CA.

CEREBRAL BLOOD FLOW

Normal Brain

Under normal circumstances, autoregulation preserves global cerebral blood flow (gCBF) constant at about 50 ml/100g brain tissue per minute, within a broad range of mean arterial pressure. CBF is maintained despite varying cerebral perfusion pressure (CPP). CPP is represented by the equation of MABP minus ICP and is maintained generally between 50 and 150 mmHg.

Brain cells require a continuous supply of oxygen and glucose, two primary substrates for brain metabolism. High-energy phosphates are produced primarily from oxidative metabolism of glucose. A significant amount of the ATP is used to maintain ionic equilibrium across neural membranes by the Na^+-K^+ ATPase, Ca^{2+} ATPase, and pathways involved in the synthesis, reuptake, and metabolism of neurotransmitters *(40)*.

Ischemic Brain

When CPP is below 50 mmHg, CBF starts to decrease. When CPP is reduced below 40 to 50 mmHg, autoregulatory reserve is exhausted, CBF decreases, and oxygen extraction increases. When CPP is reduced below about 30 mmHg, oxygen extraction is at maximal, although cerebral oxygen consumption decreases *(41)*. During incomplete ischemia, as seen with standard CPR, the viability of normal neurons becomes threatened by CPP less than 30 mmHg, gCBF less than 15 mL/100 g of brain tissue per minute or cerebral venous oxygen partial pressure (PO_2) of less than 20 torr *(42,43)*. The brain tolerates low flow (CBF 10% of normal) better than no flow or trickle flow (<5 mL/100 g of brain tissue per minute *[44]*). Trickle flow is usually meant to imply very low blood flow that is adequate to provide sufficient glucose delivery for anaerobic glycolysis but only able to support very limited oxidative phosphorylation.

During a CA there is either loss or rightward shift of autoregulation *(45)*. With loss of autoregulation, CBF becomes contingent on CPP. One must keep MABP at a higher level than expected to maintain cerebral perfusion adequate during a resuscitation. This has been confirmed in an animal model, in which a higher CPP was required to restore CBF and ATP when CPR was delayed for 6 minutes than if CPR was initiated immediately following induction of ventricular fibrillation (VF [46]).

Perfusion Failure

No cell depends more on oxygen and glucose than a neuron. The vulnerability to oxygen deprivation derives from the brain's predominantly aerobic metabolism, lack of energy reserves, and significant activity of ion-transporting pathways. With sudden CA at normothermia, loss of oxygen delivery to the brain and loss of consciousness occur within 10 seconds, although EEG activity becomes isoelectric within 20 seconds (43,47). Following sudden CA, high-energy phosphates are depleted more rapidly in the brain than in most other organs and because of limited reserves results in energy failure. Reduced oxygen delivery causes cells to revert to anaerobic metabolism. Anaerobic metabolism of tissue stores of glucose and glycogen produces small amounts of ATP for several minutes. During anaerobic metabolism, consumption of a unit of glucose results in the formation of lactic acid and 2 ATP molecules as compared to 32 ATP molecules generated via aerobic pathways (48). The currently accepted maximal period of time of normothermic no flow that is consistently reversible to complete recovery of neuronal function is less than 5 minutes (49). Evidence for this 5-minute limit includes maximal depletion of brain glucose and ATP stores with no activity of the membrane Na^+-K^+ ATPase pump (50). This 5-minute limit is being challenged by the observation that occasional animals or humans recover after 10 minutes of arrest time (51). However, even though there is complete gross neurological recovery after normothermic VF of 5 minutes in a dog model, there is some evidence of early damage to vulnerable neurons on histological examinations of the brain (52).

During cerebral ischemia, intracellular calcium loading, increased extracellular concentration of excitatory amino acids, and brain tissue lactic acidosis set the stage for reoxygenation injury (43,53–55). These mechanisms seem to be in part responsible for the phenomenon of "selective vulnerability" of neurons from an ischemic and reperfusion injury. These neurons include specifically the cornu ammonis-1 (CA-1) and CA4 sector of hippocampus, thalamic reticular nucleus, cortical layers III, V, and VI, and cerebellar Purkinje cells (1,56).

Cerebral perfusion abnormalities occur both during CA and after return of spontaneous circulation. Reperfusion, but not autoregulation, is recovered with the initiation of CPR. When a patient is resuscitated successfully and there is ROSC, the brain appears to pass through four stages of abnormal perfusion and substrate delivery, which leads to further injury, especially to vulnerable neurons.

These stages are as follows:

- Immediate multifocal absence of reperfusion ("no-reflow phenomenon"). This has been readily prevented by maintaining normal postresuscitation blood pressures or with slightly elevated blood pressures (24,57). Early postresuscitation hypotension can be detrimental by not overcoming the absent reperfusion in vulnerable neurons.
- Transient global hyperemia lasting between 5 and 40 minutes (33,58). Increasing the duration of ischemia usually increases the duration of hyperemia, except after extremely long ischemic times when severe brain edema may restrict reperfusion altogether (59). The mechanism of vasodilation is multifactorial and includes elevated extracellular concentrations of potassium and adenosine and decreases in extracellular pH and calcium (60). Using xenon studies in dogs, this hyperemia is relatively heterogeneous among

brain regions and areas with diminished perfusion are likely as a result of swollen astrocytes that impede blood flow (61). The uneven distribution may account for why some neurons are not vulnerable to ischemic injury.

• Delayed, prolonged global and multifocal hypoperfusion throughout the brain and is evident 2 to 12 hours postarrest (33,58,62). gCBF is reduced to 50% of pre-arrest values, however global oxygen uptake returns to normal or above pre-arrest values (53,60). Cerebral venous PO_2 may show a critically low level (<20 mmHg), reflecting mismatching of oxygen delivery and uptake (63). The etiology is most likely multifactorial and includes vasospasm, edema formation, blood cell aggregates, and excessive release of endothelins (64).

• This stage is characterized by either: (a) resolution, when normal CBF and oxygen uptake return to normal and consciousness occurs; (b) persistent coma, when both CBF and oxygen uptake remains low; or (c) secondary hyperemia with associated decrease oxygen uptake and eventual neuronal death (2,22,58,63). This reduction occurs even if cerebral perfusion is normal. Any elevation of ICP or reduction in systemic MABP may reduce CPP and further compromise CBF and ultimately leads to more neuronal injury. Physiological mechanisms responsible for persistent hypoperfusion may involve impairment of endothelial-dependent vasodilation in arterioles or CBF responses to CO_2; hypoxia or blood pressure; decreased red blood cell deformability; increased platelet aggregation; pericapillary cellular edema; and abnormal calcium fluxes (43,65,66).

Reoxygenation Chemical Cascades

Reoxygentation (Fig. 2), although effective and a prerequisite for restoring energy charge, also has been implicated in the chemical cascades that ultimately result in lipid peroxidation with destruction of plasma membranes and neuronal DNA (67). These cascades include intracellular calcium loading, release of excitatory amino acids, generation of oxygen-free radicals, free iron mobilization, and intracellular acidosis. These cascades have been demonstrated in vitro and in extracerebral organs. However, only partial evidence of their presence have been recognized in the brain (68). Excitatory amino acids and lactic acid are removed quickly during reperfusion, although ionic balance takes longer time to be restored to normal (69). Although there may be transient elevation of intracellular calcium after an arrest, treatable surges in brain intracellular calcium after arrest remain yet to be demonstrated (1). Some of these molecular changes could merely be an epiphenomena of permanent brain injury, whereas other chemical events might explain why dying neurons can be found side by side with surviving cells.

The pathogenesis of postresuscitation cerebral dysfunction is complex. Cell injury develops not only as a direct result of oxygen deprivation and ATP depletion during the interval of CA but also as a result of cellular events that develop only after reperfusion with oxygenated blood has been established. There are two main theories explaining the injury caused to selectively vulnerable neurons. The excitotoxic amino acid neurotransmitter theory focuses largely on events during ischemia, although the oxygen-free radical theory focuses primarily on events during reperfusion. These theories are not mutually exclusive, and considerable evidence supports each of them independently. There is evidence that calcium entry into a cell is mediated by both energy depletion and glutamate receptor activation during ischemia. Furthermore, substantial evidence exists for membrane damage caused by both calcium activation of lipases and oxygen-free radical generation during reperfusion. Unfortunately, treatments directed at only one of the mechanisms have not yet been shown to be beneficial.

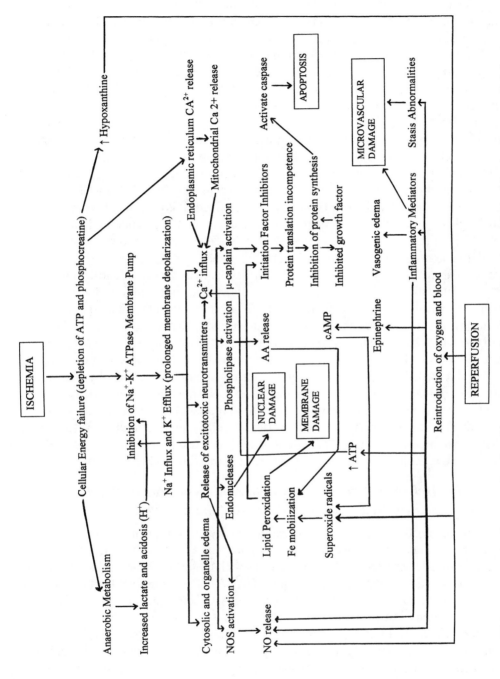

Fig. 2. Schematic diagram of molecular processes during ischemia and reperfusion that lead to neuronal death.

Normal Neuronal Cell Membrane Function

To understand the initial neurological derangement that accompanies global cerebral ischemia, one must first understand the normal physiologic conditions that occur in the neuron. Because of the marked permeability of cellular membranes to potassium, the distribution of potassium largely determines the cellular membrane potential. ATP is used primarily to maintain an elevated intracellular potassium by exchanging 3 Na^+ for 2 K^+. These changes result in an intracellular concentration of potassium 40 times that of the extracellular concentration (70). Extracellular calcium is increased by 1 Ca^{2+} in exchange for 2 Na^+. The net result of these active processes is that extracellular sodium concentration are 10 times greater than intracellular concentration and extracellular calcium is 10,000 times greater than intracellular concentration (71).

When an influx of calcium occurs, most of it is buffered rapidly or sequestered intracellularly, resulting in only small, brief increases in cytosolic Ca^{2+} (72). Such bufferering may become saturated if a large influx of Ca^{2+} is sustained, as is postulated to occur during global ischemia. The regulation of $[Ca^{2+}]_i$ is achieved by the plasma membrane Ca^{2+}/ Mg^{2+}-ATPase (Ca^{2+} gate), the ATP-dependent uptake of Ca^{2+} into the endoplasmic reticulum and mitochondria, and by the arachidonic acid (AA) cascade. The Na^+/Ca^{2+} exchanger normally represents the principal efflux pathway for Ca^{2+}. It utilizes the usual Na^+ gradient to allow Ca^{2+} efflux but is capable of reversal under circumstances in which $[Na+]_i$ is elevated, such as with depletion of ATP during ischemia and membrane depolarization (73). The release of bound Ca^{2+} from the endoplasmic reticulum is believed to occur from stimulation of specific membrane receptors that causes activation of phospholipase C enzyme. This enzyme hydrolyzes the membrane lipid phosphatidyllinositol, yielding the second messengers inositol-1,4,5 triphosphate (IP3) and/or by free arachidonic acid. IP3 mobilizes Ca^{2+} stores from the endoplasmic reticulum. Release of Ca^{2+} bound in mitochondria is not thought to occur until the endoplasmic reticulum stores are depleted. The initial response of many different cell types to stimulation, such as in ischemia and reperfusion, is an increase in $[Ca^{2+}]_i$ as a result of release of intracellular endoplasmic reticulum-bound Ca^{2+}, an influx of extracellular Ca^{2+}, or both.

During Ischemia: Excitotoxic Amino Acid Neurotransmitter Theory of Neuronal Death and Calcium Overload

This theory is often referred to as the excitotoxicity theory of neuronal death because damage is prominent in neurons with excitatory neurotransmitter receptors, such as those for glutamate and aspartate, and not in neurons with inhibitory neurotransmitter receptors, such as those for γ-aminobutyric acid (GABA). The amino acids glutamate and aspartate are ubiquitous excitatory amino acid (EAA) neurotransmitters, eliciting fast excitatory responses at postsynaptic receptor sites, primarily of dendritic origin (74). There are two classes of glutamate receptors, the ionotropic receptor, which are ligand-gated ion channels, and the metabotropic glutamate receptors, which are coupled to cellular effectors via guanosine triphosphate (GTP)-binding proteins. The types of receptors on selectively vulnerable neurons include: two subtypes of glutamate ionotropic receptors that are activated by either N-methyl-D-aspartate (NMDA), or α-amino-3-hydroxyl-5-methyl-4-isoxazole proprionic acid (AMPA); and the metabotropic receptors, activated selectively by quisqualate (Q).

Signal transmission between neurons is mediated by release from presynaptic neurons of chemical neurotransmitters that bind to postsynaptic membrane surface receptors and activate them. One of the first events during ischemia is the net loss of intracellular potassium *(75)*. This intracellular potassium loss occurs when there is approx 50% reduction in CBF *(71)*. The mechanism of this efflux is not understood well, because this K^+ efflux during early ischemia is not associated with an equal gain in intracellular sodium *(76)*. The K^+ efflux occurs well before the cells are energy depleted.

With advance global ischemia, cellular energy stores are exhausted and approaches 0 within about 4 minutes *(77)*. The EAA neurotransmitter theory states that the rapid depletion in cerebral phosphocreatine (PCr) and ATP during ischemia induces an inhibition of the Na^+-K^+ ATPase membrane pump. The effect is a net efflux of $K^+$and a net influx of Na^+ *(27,68)*. Increased tissue acidosis causes H^+ accumulation with further influx of Na^+ via the Na^+/H^+ exchanger *(78)*. The rise in intracellular Na^+ also leads to an osmotically driven net influx of water, which is responsible for causing cytosolic edema. A net influx of Ca^{2+} occurs when intracellular sodium is exchanged with extracellular calcium by way of the Na^+/Ca^{2+} exchanger *(79)*. The increase in intracellular Ca^{2+} mobilizes a set of events, including lipolysis during ischemia followed by free fatty acid metabolism and generation of superoxide radical (O_2^-) during reperfusion.

These electrolyte derangements create a prolonged depolarization of the plasma membrane that leads to a release into the extracellular fluid of an immense amount of the neurotransmitters glutamate and aspartate *(80)*. Excitotoxic neurotransmitters bind to two inotropic receptors that are distinctively activated by NMDA or AMPA on the selectively vulnerable neurons. The rise in extracellular glutamate causes an extended and excessive activation of these receptors. The result is opening of channels that indirectly or directly cause an increase in the influx of calcium into the cytosol of the cell *(15,53,81)*. Increased intracellular calcium itself activates glutamate release from presynaptic vesicles containing the neurotransmitter *(77)*. Re-uptake of glutamate is inhibited by AA or products of lipid peroxidation and results in further activation of inotropic receptors *(82)*. AMPA receptor activation specifically opens a Na^+ channel. Na^+ influx occurs along a steep electrochemical gradient, which also allows Cl^- to enter via normal or activated anion channels. A secondary effect of the Na^+ influx is the translocation of osmotically obliged water into the cell leading to cytosolic edema. The increased intracellular Na^+ is speculated to induce reversal of the normal Ca^{2+} extrusion through the Na^+/Ca^{2+} antiporter, thereby resulting in a further increase in intracellular Ca^{2+}. Activation of the NMDA receptor opens a Ca^{2+} channel, allowing Ca^{2+} influx. The Ca^{2+} conductance is strongly antagonized by Mg^{2+}, which blocks the channel in a voltage-dependent manner *(83)*.

The metabotropic glutamate receptor subtypes do not control ion channels directly but are linked by GTP-binding proteins to second messenger systems, involving phospholipase C and phopholipase D enzymes. Activation can lead to a rise in inositol-1,4,5 triphophate (IP3) which act to release Ca^{2+} from intracellular stores *(84)*.

Excessive intracellular calcium ions leads to activation of calcium-dependent enzymes, including phopholipases, protease μ-calpain, and endonucleases, which degrade membrane lipids and specific proteins, respectively *(85,86)*. The phospholipases are a ubiquitous family of enzymes, found both in the cytosol, plasmalemma, and mitochondrial membrane, that hydrolyze functional groups from phospholipids *(87)*. Increases in $[Ca^{2+}]_i$ specifically activates phopholipase A2, which cleaves fatty acyl chains from the position of phopholipids (PL) into free fatty acids, particularly AA. The degree of lipolysis during ischemia in the selectively vulnerable neurons is significantly greater than in other areas of the brain *(88)*. AA causes increased activity of the cyclooxygenase pathway to produce

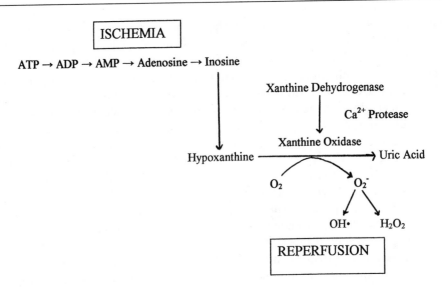

Fig. 3. Schematic diagram of superoxide generation by the xanthine/xanthine oxidase system after ischemia and reperfusion.

prostaglandins, including thromboxane A2, and the lipoxygenase pathway to produce leukotrienes. These products operate as neurotransmitters and signal transducers in neurons and glial cells and activate thrombotic and inflammatory pathways in the microcirculation.

During no flow, the hydrolysis of ATP to AMP leads to an accumulation of adenosine, inosine, and hypoxanthine (Fig. 3). Increased intracellular calcium causes Ca^{2+}-activated proteases, such as μ-calpein, which augment the conversion of the enzyme xanthine dehydrogenase to xanthine oxidase (XO), priming the neuron for the production of oxygen-free radical superoxide (O_2^-) during reperfusion when oxygen is reintroduced (89). XO catalyzes the oxidation of hypoxanthine to xanthine and uric acid by O_2, with the formation of O_2^-. This results from the creation during reperfusion of incompletely reduced O_2 species that occur from electrophilic attack of cellular molecules and a deficiency in enzymes that detoxify these potent oxidizers and their precursors (90). This ultimately results in destruction of cytoskeleton proteins and nuclear DNA.

Identification of this massive early shift of calcium was subsequently followed by interest in the hypothesis that neuronal calcium overloading was the fundamental process initiating chemical cascades resulting in neuronal death (53,91). The hypothesis predicts that some cells have a higher density of calcium channels in their plasma membranes, thereby making these neurons more vulnerable during ischemia to injury (92). Additionally, sections of the brain that were most vulnerable to ischemic cell death showed the greatest changes in Ca^{2+} (93). Accumulating evidence supports the concept that Ca^{2+} overload and ischemic neuronal injury may be linked to cellular Na^+ overload (94). Studies that have employed voltage-gated Ca^{2+} channel blockers have mostly been ineffective in reducing neuronal injury partly as a result of the Na^+/Ca^{2+} exchanger as the mediator of the injury (95). However, evidence for implicating Na^+ loading is lacking and further research is required to define its role with more precision.

The calcium hypothesis has been recently been challenged on grounds that it is not known whether a rise in free cytosolic calcium concentration precedes or merely is a consequence of neuronal death. Proponents against this theory have shown that EAAs are not required for the occurrence of intracellular calcium overload. Energy depletion and persistent depolarization result in calcium influx *(43)*. Although it has been shown that an ischemia-induced increase in extracellular glutamate is restored quickly to basal levels following reperfusion, a secondary elevation of glutamate has been observed in vivo *(96)*. Furthermore, microscopic studies have documented that neuronal calcium overloading is corrected rapidly within 15 minutes of reperfusion. Therefore, persistent calcium overloading is not a problem during early reperfusion, when progressive ultrastructural damage is seen. Additionally, breakdown of cytoskeletal components and loss of ordered membrane function can occur without an increase in intracellular Ca^{2+} and that depletion of ATP is the main detrimental factor to the survival of the cell *(97)*. It has been theorized that lipolysis during ischemia may occur from agonist-dependent activation of phospholipase C instead of from Ca^{2+} activation of phospholiase A2 *(98)*. These results do not eliminate the possibility that calcium influx is a significant mediator of early ischemic neuronal damage, and in fact it is well known that a marked increase in intracellular Ca^{2+} accelerates other reactions that are harmful to the survival of the cell *(92)*.

During Reperfusion and Reoxygenation: Oxygen-Derived Free Radicals Theory

Respiring cells are able to reduce molecular oxygen (dioxygen, O_2) by four electrons to water (H_2O) via cytochrome c oxidase, without creating any free intermediary species of reduced O_2. Most cells have added mechanisms, enzymatic or nonenzymatic, by which O_2 can be reduced by only, one, two, or three electrons giving rise to superoxide radical (O_2^-), hydrogen peroxide (H_2O_2) and the highly reactive hydroxyl radical (OH•), respectively (89). The term oxygen-derived free radicals is applied to compounds derived from molecular oxygen that have acquired fewer than four electrons. The sites for production of free radicals include the mitochondrial respiratory chain, sequences catalyzed by cyclooxygenase and lipooxygenase, autoxidation of certain compounds, and the XO reaction.

In the oxygen-free radical theory, selective neuron vulnerability occurs primarily during reperfusion. There are two principal theories for the generation of free radicals, which include XO and iron. Forms of oxygen-free radicals implicated in reperfusion injury include the superoxide anion, hydrogen peroxide, and the highly reactive hydroxyl ion *(89)*. The oxygen-derived free radicals species can hinder various cell functions *(99)*. There is increasing evidence that these species may be the causative agents in a number of pathologic conditions, including cerebral ischemia-reoxygenation injury *(100)*. Selectively vulnerable neurons are particularly prone to oxygen free radical-induced damage, specifically lipid peroxidation. These neurons are deficient in glutathione peroxidase and are surrounded by iron-laden supporting cells that release this iron during ischemia and reperfusion *(101)*.

It now appears likely oxygen-free radical species, notably OH•, are formed by iron catalysis of the reaction between O_2^- and H_2O_2 *(102)*. Glial cells have abundant stores of oxidized (ferric) iron, mostly in ferritin and transferrin, in which the iron is unable to function as a catalyst for oxygen-free radical reactions *(103)*. Production of the hydroxyl radical (OH•) in biological systems may happen nonenzymatically through a three-electron reduction of molecular oxygen. Stoichiometry of the reaction between O_2^- and H_2O_2 to form OH• is illustrated by the Haber-Weiss reaction *(15,89,99,104)*:

$$O_2^- + H_2O_2 \Leftrightarrow OH^- + OH• + O_2$$

The same net result may be catalyzed with a transition metal ion complex as described by the Fenton reaction. Increased O_2^- further leads to a rise in OH•, as a result of the Fenton reaction with iron liberated from ferritin in the mitochondria:

$$Fe^{2+} + H_2O_2 \Leftrightarrow Fe^{3+} + OH^- + OH•,$$

The excess O_2^- formed from these reactions can serve as an electron donor and reduces insoluble irons (Fe^{3+}), stored in glia to soluble iron (Fe^{2+} *[99,105]*). These soluble ferrous ions participate in the production of other partially reduced oxygen species that are very powerful oxidizers, such as hydroxyl radical (OH•) or peroxynitrite ($ONOO^-$). Peroxynitrite, produced by the reaction of O_2^- with NO has been implicated as the lipid peroxidation-initiating radical species during reperfusion *(106)*.

These resistant oxidizers overwhelm the cells antioxidant system and injure the plasma membrane of neurons by peroxidation of unsaturated fatty acids *(107)*. The resultant abnormal configuration of the fatty acids would then alter the permeability and fluidity of the membrane. Peroxidation of membrane phospholipids may result in severe neuronal injury owing to lysis of intracellular organelles and of the cell as a whole. Additionally, and probably more significant, membranes contain receptors, ion channels, and other proteins with functions that are likely to be impaired by alterations in the phospholipids. Lipid peroxidation also appears to be implicated in the genesis of the postischemic hypoperfusion phenomenon, which has been prevented by the administration of super-oxide dismutase, deferoxamine or U74006F, a lipid peroxidation chain terminator *(44,108)*.

The hydroxyl radical is a potent oxidant of some amino acids residues, purine, and pyrimidine bases in proteins and nucleic acids, respectively. These result in enzyme inactivation and splitting of DNA strands *(73,109)*. Oxygen-derived free radicals may also be generated by activated neutrophils, but their role in neuronal injury is less apparent *(110)*. The plasma membrane of activated neutrophils harbors the nicotinamide adenine dinucleoide phosphate (NADPH) oxidase system, which enables the neutrophil to produce reactive oxidizing agents. This enzyme participates in the production of superoxide anion and hydrogen peroxide both of which injure host tissue but are short-lived and are rapidly used up in other reactions. The combination of NADPH oxidase-derived H_2O_2 with myeloperoxidase, a constituent of the neutrophils' intracellular granule system, how-ever, generates an oxidizing agent of great destructive potential.

The most significant source of incompletely reduced O_2 species is metabolism during reperfusion of the free fatty acids accumulated during ischemia. During reperfusion, oxidative metabolism of the AA released from lipids during ischemia results in reduction of O_2 by one electron, thereby creating O_2^- *(43)*. Cyclooxygenase catalyzes the addition of two molecules of O_2 to an unsaturated fatty acid, such as AA to form prostaglandin G2, which is peroxidized quickly to prostaglandin H2 with simultaneous release of O_2^- *(77)*. The rise in O_2^- leads to an increase H_2O_2 production as a result of the intracellular action of the enzyme superoxide dismutase (SOD). H_2O_2 generated through SOD is removed by either intracellular catalase or through various peroxidases.

Confirmation of injury mediated by oxygen radicals during reperfusion includes identification of spin-trapped radicals and lipid peroxidation products, and fluorescence microscopic demonstration that lipid peroxidation products are concentrated in the selectively vulnerable neurons during the first 90 minutes of reperfusion *(86)*. Exogenous administration of toxic oxygen metabolites creates structural and functional alterations reminiscent of those seen after ischemia.

Enzymatic lipolysis and lipid peroxidation may function synergistically in plasma membrane destruction during reperfusion. Peroxidized fatty acids are superior substrates for phospholipases. Additionally, some of the products of lipid peroxidation stimulate the activity of phospholipase, whereas others inhibit the activity of the lipid repair enzymes lysophosphatidylcholine acyltransferese and fattyacyl-CoA synthetase during reperfusion *(111,112)*.

Reoxygenation restores ATP through oxidative phosphorylation, which may lead to massive uptake of calcium into the mitochondria, which are already swollen from an increased osmolality *(80)*. Thus, mitochondria loaded with bound calcium may become dysfunctional by rupturing and releasing free radicals. Increased calcium intracellularly by itself and by triggering free-radical reactions may result in lipid peroxidation, membrane destruction, and ultimately neuronal death.

During ischemia and reperfusion, loading of the neuron with calcium is believed to be the key ingredient that drives its death. This event, as described above, leads to a wide variety of pathological processes. Proteases, lipases, and nucleases are released, which may contribute to activation of genes or gene products critical to the progression of programmed cell death or inactivation of genes or gene products normally inhibiting this process. Activation of NO synthase by calcium can generate NO, which can combine with superoxide produce peroxynitrite *(113)*. This and OH• can both lead to DNA injury and programmed cell death or protein and membrane peroxidation, respectively. Nerve growth factor (NGF), nuclear immediate early response genes, heat shock protein, free radical scavengers, adenosine, and other endogenous defenses attempt to counteract the neuronal injury.

Protein Synthesis Impairment

After successful ROSC, the reperfusion phase is characterized by significant changes in protein-synthesis machinery. New protein synthesis is a prerequisite for long-term survival after damage incurred from cerebral ischemia and reperfusion *(114)*. Recovery of neurons is almost entirely dependent on active transcription and repair of DNA injury. The derangement in protein synthesis in response to ischemia and reperfusion is not regionally homogenous. The selectively vulnerable neurons display a generalized and prolong diminished capacity for new protein synthesis following ischemia and reperfusion *(115)*. As little as 3 minutes of ischemia triggers inhibition of protein synthesis during reperfusion *(116)*. Ischemic times greater than 5 minutes result in delayed protein translation recovery in surviving neurons *(117)*.

The severity and duration of the ischemia, as well as the intraischemic temperature are the main factors influencing the reversibility of the initiation block for protein synthesis. The significance of renewing protein synthesis for the complete functional and metabolic recovery of neurons during the reperfusion period is evident from the finding that necrosis is preceded by persistently suppressed protein synthesis in selectively vulnerable regions of the brain *(115)*. The functional recovery of neuronal activity has only been seen in cases in which protein synthesis was restored *(118)*.

Protein synthesis is a complex process requiring: (a) high-energy phosphates, (b) intact DNA, (c) intact transcription machinery, (d) posttranscriptional processing and nucleo-cytoplasmic transport of mRNA from the site of transcription to the site of translation, and (e) intact translation machinery. Each of these steps in the process plays a role in the normal regulation of gene expression and are potential sites of disruption following ischemia and reperfusion. Translation of mRNA into proteins requires the presence of active ribosomal subunits, translation issues, aminoacyl-tRNAs, amino acids, an energy supply, and an appropriate ionic environment. Ischemia and reperfusion appears to alter some, but not all of these processes. For example, ischemia does not change the intracellular levels of amino acids and ribosomes can tolerate extended periods of ischemia without significant injury *(119)*. However, it seems that the key alteration is that newly formed mRNA is not effectively reaching the cytoplasm following ischemia and reperfusion, suggesting a disorder of the nucleocytoplasmic transport *(120)*.

Initiation of protein synthesis is a highly regulated process that requires multiple translation initiation issues. Persistent suppression of eukaryotic initiation factor (eIF), which is needed for continuous protein synthesis is responsible for overall depression of protein synthesis. Because protein synthesis is a very endergonic process, depletion of ATP and GTP stores during ischemia is responsible for the termination of protein synthesis *(120)*. However, energy failure cannot account fully for the extended suppression of protein synthesis seen during ischemia, because these high-energy phosphates are restored shortly after reperfusion *(120)*.

There is additional evidence that protein synthesis may be suppressed irreversibly by an initiation inhibitor during early reperfusion, thereby inhibiting the nucleocytoplasmic transport of mRNA *(121)*. Assembly of the initiation complex is a complex process involving more than 140 proteins and requiring at least nine initiation issues in the eukaryotic cell *(122)*. The eukaryotic translation initiation factor 2 (eIF2) plays a key role in the initiation of translation. eIF2 is a heterotrimeric protein consisting of three subunits α, β, γ. The inhibition of protein synthesis involves specifically the phosphorylation of serine-51 on the α-subunit (elF-2 α *[123,124]*). Phosphorylation of as little as little as 25% of eIF2 α can be sufficient to suppress protein translation completely *(123)*. Additionally serine-51 phophorylation of elf-2 α is known to be activated by iron and lipid peroxidation, suggesting that free radical generation during reperfusion are an important step in the inhibition of protein synthesis *(125)*.

During early reperfusion, several lines of evidence suggest that protein synthesis is suppressed by inhibition of translation. Ribosomal sedimentation profiles obtained from brain tissue during reperfusion demonstrates polysome disaggregation into monomeric ribosomal subunits, suggesting that polypeptide chain initiation of translation is blocked *(126)*. Ultrastructural evaluation of these neurons shows that most of the structural injury actually occurs with reperfusion *(1)*. The vulnerable neurons demonstrate peroxidative damage to unsaturated fatty acids in the plasma membrane, chromatin clumping, and prominent alterations in the structure of the Golgi apparatus that is responsible for assembling the plasma membrane *(127)*. This leads to the inability of the ribosomes to maintain its normal function of protein synthesis.

Translational competence in the brain after ischemia and reperfusion is not homogeneous with areas of the cortex, hippocampus, and caudate showing severe and extended inhibition of protein synthesis, although the brain stem and midbrain are relatively unaffected *(128)*. In general, neurons destined to die do not recuperate the ability to synthesize proteins *(128,129)*. After reperfusion, immunohistochemical staining of several brain proteins, including tubulin, neuron-specific enolase, and brain-specific creatine kinase, demonstrate a gradual loss of protein synthesis in the selectively vulnerable neurons over several days after reperfusion *(130)*.

Growth Factors' Signal Transduction

Cell growth, proliferation, and differentiation are regulated in part by growth factors *(131)*. The brain has receptors for several growth factors, including insulin, fibroblast growth factor (FGF), and NGF*(132–134)*. Additionally, key aspects of the protein-translation system, in particular phosphorylation of the eIF-2 α, are controlled in part through the signal-transduction system that is activated by growth factor receptors. All of these growth factors have been located in the selectively vulnerable neurons of the hippocampus and neocortex. Similarly, transforming growth factor (TGF)-β insulin-like growth factor (IGF)-1, and epidermal growth factor (EGF) have been isolated in brain *(135,136)*. Insulin is a member of a growth factor known as IGF-1, and NGF. IGF-1 has 90% peptide sequence homology with insulin and NGF has 60% homology with insulin.

Growth factors are important in neurite sprouting and synapse formation during development and in maintaining synapses in mature brain. The mechanisms by which these growth factors determine cellular growth and differentiation are not understood completely. These growth factors bind to protein receptors in the plasma membrane and possess a tyrosine kinase activity at the cytosolic face of the plasmalemma *(137)*. Activation of the receptor enables the tyrosine kinase to add phosphate groups to specific tyrosinases in neurons. This leads to transcription of the so-called immediate early genes, which comprise the proto-oncogenes *c-fos* and *c-jun*. These act as third messengers in the stimulus–genomic response to growth factors and cell stress. Proteins of the *c-fos* family form heterodimers with proteins of the *c-jun* family and interact with the activator protein (AP)-1 complex to facilitate initiation and regulate transcription in the nucleus. AP-1-responsive genes are speculated to have vital roles in the mechanisms of cellular proliferation and differentiation and may play a role in the repair of the plasma membrane *(138)*.

c-fos mRNA and *c-jun* mRNA are expressed during early reperfusion, and synthesis of their gene products also occur early in reperfusion. Synthesis of these gene products occurs primarily in neurons resistant to ischemia. Synthesis of early gene products is poor in vulnerable neurons destined to ischemic injury, presumably because of the generalized inhibition of protein synthesis at the translational step *(138)*. In the brain, however, the selectively vulnerable neurons have increased concentrations of receptors for growth factors of the insulin family and increased concentrations of tyrosine-phosphorylated proteins in their nuclei.

There are important interrelations between induction of *c-fos* and *c-jun* and the translation of other stress proteins *(139)*. Another family of proteins expressed after ischemia are the heat shock proteins, named because of their discovery in cells exposed to heat stress. Cerebral ischemia and reperfusion elicit the production of both growth factors and proto-oncogene products in certain neurons. Heat shock proteins appear to be involved in facilitating folding of proteins, aid in membrane synthesis and can be induced by growth factors *(140)*. Heat shock mRNAs and proteins are expressed in the brain during reperfusion *(141)*. Heat shock genes begin transcriptional activation of new mRNA coding for a set of proteins that provide a mechanism for repair, salvage, and intracellular disposition of damaged macromolecules. After global ischemia, the selectively vulnerable neurons transcribe large amounts of a 70 kDa heat shock protein (*hsp-70*), but translation is diminished when compared to surviving neurons in other areas of the brain *(141)*. It is unclear whether synthesis of heat shock proteins actually confers neuroprotection or whether lack of translation that ordinarily occurs in postischemic vulnerable neurons is simply an epiphenomenon associated with overall depression of protein synthesis. These results convey the important association of early transcription and translation of *c-fos*, *c-jun*, and *hsp-70* with neuronal survival.

Apoptosis

Neuronal cell death may occur by two separate processes, necrosis or apoptosis *(142,143)*. Necrotic cell death in the brain is a passive form of cell death and is preceded by acute ischemia or traumatic injury. It occurs in the selectively vulnerable neurons by the processes discussed above, which lead to the generation of free radicals and EAAs. Necrosis usually affects large numbers of contiguous cells and leads to swelling of the cytoplasm and of the mitochondria and other organelles within it. The ultimate result is rupture of plasma membranes with lysis of the cell, which leads to an intense inflammatory reaction to occur. It is characterized histologically by nuclear and cytoplasmic disintegration with the loss of membrane integrity and loss of lysosomal contents.

Apoptotic cell death, also known as programmed cell death, is an active process of self-destructive cell death. It is initiated by the cell on the basis of information from its developmental history, from the environment or from activation of mechanisms encoded in the genomes of all higher eukaryotic cells *(144)*. It is a process that requires protein synthesis. Appreciation of the significance of apoptosis in cell death has only developed during the last decade, and some of the mechanisms still remain poorly understood. Nevertheless, it can be a feature of both acute and chronic neurological diseases and has been implicated in the pathogenesis of both focal and global ischemia *(31,145–147)*.

In apoptosis, a biochemical cascade activates proteases that destroy molecules that are necessary for cell survival and others that institute a program of cell suicide. There are distinctive morphological changes during apoptosis that include shrinkage of the cell, marked condensation of chromatin (heterochromatin), extensive alterations in the microtubular array, fragmentation of the nucleus, and formation of broad cytoplasmic protuberances at the surface of the cell. After cellular death, there is fragmentation of the cell by separation of the protuberances to form multiple small membrane-bound bodies ("apoptotic bodies") that contain intact morphological intact organelles and/or dense clumps of condensed chromatin *(148)*. The later stages are characterized by internucleosomal cleavage of DNA into fragments of about 180 base pairs *(149)*. Unlike necrotic cell death, the structural integrity of the plasma membrane remains intact, as does that of organelles. Other features of apoptosis are a reduction in the membrane potential for the mitochondria, intracellular acidification, generation of free radicals, and externalization of phosphotidylserine residues *(150)*. In apoptosis, cells do not release their contents into the interstitial fluid and death occurs without an inflammatory reaction through early activation of endogenous nuclear endonucleases. Once nuclear DNA is cut and cellular death ensured, macrophages are recruited for phagocytosis. After an ischemic insult, apoptosis occurs in areas that are not affected severely by the ischemia. For example, after ischemia, necrotic cell death occurs in the center of the lesion, in which hypoxia is most severe, and apoptosis occurs in the penumbra, in which collateral blood flow attenuates the degree of hypoxia *(151)*.

There is growing evidence that some neuronal death after ischemia is mediated by the activity of cysteine-requiring aspartate-directed proteases (caspases), the protease responsible for apoptosis in mammals *(152)*. The interleukin-1-converting enzyme (ICE) family of cysteine proteases, now also known as caspases, is another group of apoptosis-regulating genes that may play a role in ischemic brain injury *(153)*. The ICE family consists of 11 members (caspases-1 to 11). When overexpressed, these caspases cause apoptosis in cultured cells *(154)*. Caspase-3 has been shown to induce apoptosis after glutamate excitototxicity following transient global ischemia *(155)*.

Caspases are members of a distinct family of cysteine proteases that share the ability to cleave substrates on the carboxyl side of aspartate residues *(156)*. The caspases are synthesized as inactive proenzymes (procaspases) that contain an N-terminal prodomain, a large subunit, and a small subunit. Activation results from proteolytic cleavage of the procaspases into its three components, ordinarily via the action of other, activated caspases. Binding to plasma membrane receptors, such as, FAS (Apo-1), tumor necrosis factor receptor, and tumor necrosis factor-related apoptosis-inducing ligand receptor, leads to several signaling proteins to the cytoplasmic domains of the receptors. This will eventually result in apoptosis by activation of caspase proteases *(157)*. These receptors contain a cytoplasmic motif composed of 68 amino acids, termed the "death domain," which is a protein–protein interaction zone evident in many of the proteins in this system *(158)*. Ligand binding to these receptors leads to recruitment of upstream caspases *(158)*. Caspase-mediated neuronal death is more extensive after transient than permanent focal brain ischemia and may contribute to delayed loss of neurons from the penumbral region of infarcts.

After brain ischemia, activation of caspases is largely dependent on the translocation from the cytoplasm to mitochondria of Bax, Bak, and other BH3-only members of the *bcl-2* family. Once in the mitochondria they oligomerize and insert into the outer mitochondrial membrane. This contributes to the formation of pores that causes release of cytochrome *c*, procaspase-9, and apoptosis activating factor-1 (Apaf-1) from the mitochondrial intermembrane space *(159)*. *Bcl-2* family members are the main regulators that control cytochrome *c* and other apoptosis-promoting factors from mitochondria. The mechanism, however, by which ischemia induces this translocation is still poorly understood.

Release of cytochrome *c* into the cytoplasm has been associated with activation of caspase-3 by operating in conjunction with two other cytosolic protein factors, procaspase-9 and Apaf-1 *(160)*. Caspase-3 mRNA and protein have been shown to be increased for a more prolonged period of time in the hippocampus cells, which are selectively vulnerable to ischemic injury, than in other sections of the brain *(155)*. Furthermore, inhibition of ICE- or caspase-3 protease affords protection in rodent brains exposed to ischemia *(161)*. Thus, caspase-3 and other related caspases could be important mediator of neuronal death under ischemic conditions.

Caspase-3 may mediate ischemic cell death through several mechanisms. Mature caspase-3 can cleave specific cellular proteins. The best described is poly(ADP-ribose) polymerase (PARP), an enzyme involved in DNA repair and maintenance of genomic integrity, including proliferation, differentiation, and transformation *(162)*. PARP catalyzes the covalent binding of ADP-ribose subunits from its substrate, nicotinamide adenine dinucleotide (NAD), to numerous nuclear proteins, including PARP itself. Formation of poly (ADP-ribose) is a unique posttranslational modification that can be induced by DNA strand breaks following oxygen-free radical damage or exposure to NO *(163)*. Under many apoptotic conditions, PARP is cleaved by caspase-3 to generate both 85 and 24 kDa fragments *(164)*. Once cleaved, PARP appears to facilitate apoptosis by interrupting DNA binding and repair *(165)*. It is unknown if the cleavage of PARP is the cause of neuronal death or if is just a product of overall cellular destruction in the final stages of the apoptotic cascade. However, under focal ischemia, inhibition of PARP has been shown to improve neuronal survival *(166)*. Additionally, rats deficient in PARP were resistant to brain injury after transient focal ischemia *(167)*.

Other mechanisms by which caspase-3 might produce neuronal death following ischemia is by activating other caspases or activation of caspase-activated deoxyribonuclease (CAD), a key DNA-cleavage enzyme responsible for DNA fragmentation during apoptosis *(168)*. Further research into identifying specific cellular substrates for caspase-3 at initial stages of neuronal death would aid in the defining the role of this protease in ischemic brain injury and potentially contrive new therapeutic agents for the prevention of neuronal cell death.

Although programmed cell death is mediated largely by caspases, apoptosis can occur in the absence of caspase activity. Mediators implicated include apoptosis-inducing factor (AIF), endonuclease G and DNase II *(169,170)*. Caspase-independent neuronal apoptosis has been demonstrated following ischemia and excitotoxic stimulation with NMDA receptors *(171)*. The exact mechanism has not yet been elucidated but it is noteworthy that these insults are associated with depletion of ATP and intracellular acidosis.

Acidosis

Normal intracellular pH in the brain is approx 7.1 and normal extracellular pH is about 7.3 *(172)*. This trancellular pH gradient is the net result of intracellular production of acids, proton, and bicarbonate antiporters, and membrane voltage *(172)*. During global cerebral ischemia, intracellular pH falls to 6.2 within 6 minutes *(173)*. CA and the consequent interruption of blood flow to metabolically active tissues leads to intense hypercarbia and metabolic acidosis at the tissue level *(174)*. These derangements are the result of a shift from aerobic to anaerobic metabolism and the accumulation of end products such as CO_2, lactate, and hydrogen ions. When conventional closed-chest resuscitation is performed, the systemic and regional blood flow generated rarely surpasses 25% of normal, thus failing to meet the necessary tissue metabolic demands *(175)*. As a result, tissue acidosis persists during conventional resuscitation efforts and resolves only after restoration of spontaneous cardiac activity with the reestablishment of normal perfusion *(176)*.

A chief source of protons during complete ischemia is the hydrolysis of ATP and other nucleoside triphosphates *(177)*. Another source of protons is anaerobic glycolysis whereby 1 mole of glucose forms 2 moles of ATP and 2 moles of lactate anions. Glycolysis during hypoxia results in anaerobic metabolism and buildup of lactic acid, until all glucose is depleted. When these two moles of ATP are eventually hydrolyzed, approx 2 moles of protons are produced, although the exact proportion depend on the pH and Mg^{2+} concentration *(40)*. During ischemia the amount of total protons generated depend on the glucose and glycogen stores in tissue before the onset of the ischemia *(178)*. Additionally, proton production is also contingent on the continued delivery of glucose to the brain and therefore the arterial glucose concentration *(178)*.

Under general conditions, changes in the intracellular pH are buffered passively by proteins, inorganic phosphates, and bicarbonate ions. Active control of intracellular pH associated with changes in acid loads is mediated by transporters, including Na^+/H^+ exchanger, the Cl^-/HCO_3^- exchanger, and Na^+/HCO_3^- cotransporter *(172)*. During complete ischemia CO_2 is not removed and bicarbonate ions are an ineffective buffer. Noticeable changes in Na^+ and Cl^- gradients during ischemia render extrusion of acid equivalents by antiporters unfavorable. With reperfusion, CO_2 is cleared within a few minutes and tissue pH increases by about 0.3–0.4 *(179)*. However, full recovery of tissue pH requires approx 15 minutes and is highly dependent on the duration of ischemia *(180)*.

Evidence that acidosis contributes to ischemic injury is largely based on studies in which tissue pH have been manipulated by changing the serum glucose levels and thereby influencing the magnitude of anaerobic glycolysis during ischemia *(181)*. Conditions promoting the anaerobic metabolism of glucose to lactate in the ischemic brain dramatically enhance ischemic brain damage *(43)*. Induction of hyperglycemia prior to ischemia augments neuronal damage *(182,183)*. Additionally, the severity of neuronal damage depends on the magnitude and duration of hyperglycemia *(183)*. Postischemic hyperglycemia may enhance anaerobic glycolysis and delay pH recovery when intraischemic acidosis is severe *(184)*.

The mechanism by which acidosis increases ischemic injury remains speculative. It is predominantly thought that by changing protein charge, acidosis affects functions of a wide array of enzymes, receptors, ion channels, and intracellular messenger systems. Acidosis might augment ischemic injury by allowing further increases in intracellular Ca^{2+} through NMDA-mediated mechanisms *(185)*. Acidosis may promote damage from oxygen-free radicals during reoxygenation and allow lipid peroxidation by mobilizing iron *(186)*. Lactic acidosis destabilizes iron bound to protein via carbonate bridges. On reoxygenation, superoxide anion is produced, which in the presence of iron, enhances formation of hydroxyl radicals involved in lipid peroxidation via Fenton reaction *(187)*. Additionally, lipid peroxidation is optimal in an acidic environment *(188)*.

Blood Derangement

Coagulation disturbances after CA have been characterized by hypocoagulability *(189)*. It occurs approx 30 minutes after resuscitation and consists of prolonged clotting times, decreased platelets and fibrinogen. Generally, it normalizes approx 24 hours later.

On the other hand, some animal models of CA have documented increased blood coagulability accompanied by microvascular thrombosis and small emboli *(190)*. Microthrombi have been found in cerebral microvessels 5 to10 minutes following the onset of CA *(190,191)*. Experimental and clinical studies have shown that CA and resuscitation are associated with a striking activation of blood coagulation, without adequate activation of endogenous fibrinolysis *(192)*. The d-dimer and plasminogen activator inhibitor type 1 are not increased or only slightly elevated, suggesting that hypercoagulability was not sufficiently balanced by activation of the endogenous fibrinolytic system *(192)*. Hence, the disseminated formation of microvascular fibrin and microthrombosis throughout the entire microcirculation that follows the activation of blood coagulation without appropriate concomitant endogenous fibrinolysis may result in generalized impairment of the microcirculatory blood flow during reperfusion *(192)*. Hypercoagulability and microvascular thrombosis have been implicated to cause the noreflow phenomenon *(191,193)*. These changes are usually reversed by 1 week. Additionally, administration of heparin or thrombolytic agents to animals before CA leads to a significant increase in survival rate and neurological outcome *(194)*.

Inflammatory Reaction

The normal brain is considered an immune-privileged organ in which the BBB subdues the inflammatory response and hinders infiltration of inflammatory cells although the ischemic brain is unable to perform these functions. There is growing evidence that acute inflammation contributes to neuronal damage after ischemia and reperfusion *(195)*. Inflammatory reactions after ischemia and reperfusion have been demonstrated to occur in extracerebral organs, focal or global brain ischemia and brain trauma *(196)*. The mechanism for inflammatory injury can de divided into three broad categories: (a) adverse effects on blood rheology during reperfusion; (b) vasculature injury; and (c) cytotoxic injury to neurons.

Leukocytes are much less deformable than red blood cells and therefore require greater pressure to go through narrow capillaries. During reperfusion, capillaries have reduced diameter, which are as a result of swelling of perivascular astrocytes. It is thought that the mechanism causing the delayed hypoperfusion seen following global ischemia may represent the lingering effects of leukocyte-induced perfusion defects. Despite this belief, during CA, depletion of neutrophils with antineutrophil serum-ameliorated delayed hypoperfusion but failed to improve neurological outcome over a 24-hour period *(197)*.

Leukocytes are likely candidates to cause reperfusion injury because they are important sources for generating oxyradicals and hydrolytic enzymes and in addition produce both leukotrienes and platelet-activating factor (PAF), which are known to damage endothelium *(303)*. Until recently, leukocytes were thought to be implicated only in the very late phases of cerebral reperfusion, days after the CA. However, leukocytes aggregate in areas of poor blood flow in the brain during the first few hours of postischemic reperfusion *(199)*. In fact, leukocyte depletion prior to global ischemia has been demonstrated to ameliorate early recovery of somatosensory-evoked response amplitude *(200)*. Despite that, attempts to attenuate postischemic leukocyte aggregation using therapy to inhibit neutrophil chemotaxis and adhesion have not been as effective in the brain as in the heart *(201)*. Therefore, the role of leukocytes in ischemia and reperfusion injury still requires clarification.

Complement activation may lead to increased vascular permeability, activation of blood coagulation, platelet aggregation, and decreased regional blood flow *(202)*. Activation of the complement cascade produces an elevated serum concentration of anaphylatoxins C3a and C5a and generation of C5b-9 and are increased dramatically following CA *(203)*. C3a, C5a, and C5b-9 leads to rapid expression of adhesion molecules on both endothelium and leukocytes *(204)*. A leukocyte activated by complement can release elastase, secondary mediators, and oxygen-free radicals *(205)*. Additionally, the terminal complement complex C5b-9 directly induces endothelial and tissue cell swelling, which leads to narrowing and blocking of small vessels *(202)*. Therapy directed at depleting or inhibiting complement have been shown in animal models to reduce tissue injury after cerebral ischemia and reperfusion *(206)*.

Tissue and/or endothelial injury can result in production of adhesion molecules, cytokines, chemokines, and other mediators, triggering local involvement of systemic inflammatory cells in an interaction between blood and damaged tissue. Cells secrete a diverse amount of proteins called cytokines that control cell–cell interactions and leukocyte–endothelial cell interactions. Cytokines are soluble, cell-secreted, nonimmunoglobulin proteins that include entities such as interleukins (ILs), interferon, growth factors, and colony-stimulating factors *(207)*. Following ischemia and reperfusion there is synthesis and local release of several proinflammatory cytokines by macrophages, leukocytes, and endothelial cells. Cytokines play a pivitol role in generation of the inflammatory response after global ischemia and reperfusion and therefore may represent a novel method at which therapeutic modalities for ameliorating neuronal injury can be targetted.

One critically important effect of these inflammatory cytokines is to induce the expression of cell surface adhesion receptors on a variety of cell types, which may serve to localize phagocytic cells to areas of inflammation. Adhesion molecules expressed on the surface of the microvascular endothelium play a vital role in modulating the leukocyte–endothelial cell interaction associated with the acute inflammation following ischemia and reperfusion. Three of the best characterized endothelial cell adhesion molecules are P-selectin, E-selectin, and intracellular adhesion molecule-1 (ICAM-1 [208]). These adhesion molecules bind to circulating leukocytes and facilitate their migration into the brain. Once in the brain, the macrophage and microglial response to injury may either be beneficial by scavenging necrotic debris or detrimental by facilitating cell death in neurons that would otherwise recover.

P-selectin is normally found in the α-granulaes of platelets and in Weibel-Palade secretory bodies within endothelial cells. Following stimulation with complement, thrombin, or histamine, P-selectin is mobilized to the endothelial cell surface within minutes, remains there transiently, is associated with reversible leukocyte rolling, and is rapidly removed by endocytosis (209). Leukocyte rolling is an obligatory initial step leading to subsequent leukocytes adhesion to the endothelium (210). Recent studies demonstrate that IL-1 and tumor necrosis factor (TNF-α) enhance biosynthesis of endothelial P-selectin (211). Hypoxia induces the synthesis of IL-1 and TNF-α by mononuclear cells (212). In comparison, activation of endothelial cells by oxyradicals results in a sustained expression of P-selectin leading to leukocyte rolling and adhesion (213). Therefore, failure to reinternalize P-selectin may be caused by impaired regulatory mechanism when microvascular endothelium is overwhelmed by oxygen-free radicals generated during reperfusion.

E-selectin is not constitutively present on endothelium, but its expression, which requires new protein synthesis and is maximal by 4 hours, is induced by cytokines and lipopolysaccharide (209). The absence of E-selectin on unstimulated endothelium coupled with its inducible expression on activated endothelium suggests that this adhesion molecule may lead circulating leukocytes to sites of ischemia and reperfusion-induced inflammatory injury (208).

ICAM-1 is an inducible cell surface glycoprotein that is expressed constitutively on endothelium (214). Exposure of endothelial cells to cytokines leads to maximal expression of ICAM-1 within 4 to 8 hours, which persists for 24 hours (214). It plays a role in leukocyte adherence but not in leukocyte rolling (214,215). Upregulation of ICAM-1 expression during reperfusion is mediated by proxidant-reactive transcription factor nuclear factor κB (NF-κB [216]).

Leukocytes can be targeted to the site of inflammation by a highly coordinated and dynamic sequence of events in which each of the known adhesion molecules has a distinct role. The initial adhesive interaction between leukocytes and the endothelium involves upregulation of adhesion molecules (P-selectin, E-selectin, and ICAM-1) on the surface of the endothelium, abutting the site of inflammatory injury. The endothelium releases PAF and IL-8. PAF, a potent mediator of increased vascular permeability, granulocyte chemotaxis, and arachidonate-independent platelet aggregation, has been demonstrated to cause cerebral hypoperfusion and hypermetabolism (217). PAF and other pro-inflammatory substances may then interact with CD11/CD18 while simultaneously inducing the shedding of L-selectin *(218,219)*. This strengthens the leukocyte–endothelial cell adhesive interaction, which then is followed by extravasation of leukocyte into the tissue. After extravasation, synthesis of oxidant and degranulation occur, leading to tissue injury. Degranulation of neutrophils and release of several enzymes, such as elastase and myeloperoxidase cause further endothelial injury *(220)*.

Substantial experimental evidence supports the concept that inhibition of leukocyte–endothelial cell interactions during ischemia and reperfusion by blocking intracellular adhesion molecules ameliorates leukocyte activation and adherence to endothelium, and affords protection of the microcirculation *(221)*. Most chemotactic agents, cytokines, and oxidants that have been implicated in the pathogenesis of ischemia and reperfusion are known to induce neutrophil adherence by β2-integrins (CD11/CD18)-dependent mechanisms *(218,219)*. Additionally, antibodies against the CD18 component of the CD11/CD18 complex lessen ischemic-reperfusion-induced leukocyte sequestration, adherence, and extravasation, as well as tissue injury and dysfunction *(219,222)*.

Microglia may also play a role in ischemic damage. These cells are activated within a few minutes following global ischemia and proliferate and transform into ameboid shape and express many of the same mediators as activated macrophages. Microglia engulf cellular debris from dead neurons, express growth factors, and generate toxic molecules, including NO, oxygen-free radicals, AA derivatives, and cytokines. Additionally, microglia produce TGF-β1 and plasminogen, which are also involved in neuronal repair *(223)*. Nevertheless, the exact function of microglia in contributing to neuronal ischemic injury from ischemia and reperfusion still remains speculative.

Nitric Oxide

Endothelium-derived NO release, which is important in sepsis, may also have a function following ischemic damage *(224)*. NO is a free radical generated from the conversion of amino acid L-arginine to L-citrulline by the enzyme nitric oxide synthase (NOS). Both constitutive and inducible NOS isoforms are expressed in human *(225)*. Constitutive isoforms of the enzymes are located in endothelium, perivascular nerves, and parenchymal neurons *(226)*. There are two isoforms of NOS in the brain: the neuronal isoform (nNOS) found in neurons and the endothelial isoform (eNOS) found primarily within the vascular endothelium *(227)*. eNOS and nNOS generate NO, but NO generation from these two isoforms can have opposing roles in the process of ischemic injury. Increased NO production from nNOS in neurons can lead to neuronal injury, although NO production from eNOS can decrease ischemic injury by inducing vasodilation. It is thought that NO derived from nNOS in the ischemic brain is cytotoxic because it can react with the superoxide radical forming the potent oxidant peroxynitrite *(228)*. When regional perfusion is diminished, NO generated from eNOS causes NO-mediated vasodilation that decreases regional vasculature resistance, and, in turn, improves regional blood flow *(229)*.

Large amounts of NO are also produced and released if inducible NOS is stimulated, such as by porinflammatory cytokines *(230)*. After ischemia and reperfusion, neuronal cell death is followed by microglial activation. NO, which is known to be produced by activated microglia, may participate in the process of neuronal injury following cerebral ischemia *(231)*. Direct trapping and measurement of NO by electron paramagnetic resonance (EPR) techniques have shown that NO generation is increased greatly in the brain after ischemia *(232)*. Activation of NMDA, AMPA, and metabotropic receptors are all capable of stimulating NOS *(233)*. It is postulated that overstimulation of these receptors during ischemia and reperfusion may result in an overproduction of NO, which may be toxic to the neuron *(234)*. It is feasible that NO mediates excessive vasodilation during CA, which may render successful resuscitation less likely *(235)*.

The mechanism by which increased NOS may cause neuronal injury have not been firmly established. NO can form nitrosonium cations and nitroxyl anions, interact with sulfhydryl groups on proteins, and alter the redox state of metalloproteins *(114)*. In the presence of superoxide radicals, peroxynitrite anion is created, which under acidic conditions is protonated and breaks up to form hydroxyl radicals without requirement for iron *(236)*. Peroxynitrite is able to cause lipid peroxidation and oxidation of sulfhydryl groups *(236)*. Peroxynitrite may represent a mechanism for neuronal injury during early reperfusion when both superoxide and NO concentrations are expected to be increased. It is unknown, however, if peroxynitrite is formed in sufficient quantities in vivo to cause neuronal injury.

Assessment of the Cerebral Injury

Accurate prognostic estimation of neurological recovery of CA survivors is important because medical management decisions are partly influenced by the patient's prognosis. If a given patient is considered as having no probability of survival to hospital discharge, treatments such as resuscitation may not be germane. Ideally, resuscitation should not be performed if the outcome leads to a poor quality of life with persistent severe brain damage. Conversely, it is important not to prevent these treatments for patients with a reasonably good outcome. Therefore, research in methods of improving cerebral resuscitation should continue to include studies on how to accurately estimate neurological outcome after a CA.

Many CA victims are hospitalized unconscious after a resuscitation from a CA, with an uncertain prognosis. More than 75% of initially comatose patients die during their hospitalization *(237)*. The pattern of injury and subsequent neurological impairment may be quite different among individual victims of CA as a result of differences in cerebral circulation, preexisting medical conditions, and severity of the ischemic insult. Some patients after CA will awaken rapidly and recover normal or near-normal pre-arrest neurological function. Others, usually resuscitated after an extended period of global ischemia will never awaken from coma and persist with no meaningful quality of life. Still others will awaken after some length of coma but only to incur permanent neurological disability ranging from mild memory impairment to severe deficits and complete dependence on others for all activities of daily living.

Counseling families of patients sustaining a CA about the prognosis for neurological recovery is an important element of management. Central to this is awareness about the basic approach to and limitations of neurological estimation after CA. The neurological evaluation performed shortly after a CA, however, is an unreliable indicator of the ultimate recovery of neurological function because some patients initially in coma recover without neurological sequellae *(238)*. Additionally, when estimating a patient's prognosis, an important aspect is the specificity of the examination used. In other words, it is important for that test to be as accurate as possible when it estimates poor neurological outcome, otherwise the patient could be denied treatment when his or her prospect of survival is not indeed hopeless. The sensitivity of a test is less important because no prognostic test can accurately identify all patients who will die in the hospital, because death occurs from many etiologies, such as cerebral hypoxia, arrhythmias, heart failure, infections, and other causes. Many methods have been evaluated for estimating the neurological prognosis after a CA. These include, but are not limited to, clinical algorithms, neurophysiological tests, tests that quantify structural brain injury, and laboratory evaluations.

Furthermore, what constitutes an "acceptable" neurological outcome highly varies between individuals and may not coincide with what the physician believes. Although it would be inappropriate to apply a single standard to all patients, one can use a number of outcome scales to estimate outcomes in terms of cerebral performance and requirements for assistance in living that are meaningful and potentially helpful in making management decisions.

Neurological Scales

The Glascow Coma Score (GCS) and the Glascow-Pittsburgh Coma Scale (GPCS), which measures the depth of coma plus brain stem function have been used to estimate neurological prognosis after CA (237,238). The GCS is an assessment of motor and sensory function, speech, and the ability to follow verbal commands (239). The GPCS is based on the GCS but also assesses the integrative abilities of a patient, such as ability to lead an independent life or living with partial or complete dependence on others (240). Although a low initial GCS connotes patients at increased risk of in-hospital mortality, high specificity is only obtained when the GCS is measured 3 to 5 days after hospitalization. Change, or lack of change in the GCS score over time is more accurate in estimating neurological outcome than a single initial assessment. Patients who awaken rapidly after brief coma generally perform well (241). Continuation of coma, on the other hand, bodes poorly. Coma of 48 hours or greater duration following a CA predicts poor outcome (242). At 72 hours after a CA, a GCS of 5 or less, absent motor response to pain, or absent pupillary response predicts a persistent vegetative state in all patients (243). An ability to respond after verbal commands was correlated with recovery of moderate-to-good cerebral function. The utility of these scoring system, however, is limited in artificially ventilated patients and in patients requiring sedation and neuromuscular blockade.

Assessment of brain-stem function is useful for predicting neurological outcome (241). A more sophisticated scoring system utilizing variables such as pupil response, doll's eyes reflex, blink reflex, and presence or absence of seizures has been developed (241). From these data, a flowchart algorithm has been produced to estimate prognosis at different time points following a CA. In particular, persistent absence of the pupillary reflex estimated either mortality or severe neurological function with reasonable specificity, even early after CA. Once again, this examination scores is limited in patients requiring sedation and neuromuscular blockade.

Another commonly used scale after CA is the Cerebral Performance Category (CPC), which stratifies outcome based on levels of living dependence and cerebral performance (244). Using this scoring system, good or favorable outcome is predicted for patients independent in activities of daily living (CPC 1 or 2), and bad, poor, or unfavorable outcome is predicted for patients who are dependent on others, vegetative, or dead (CPC 3, 4, or 5).

Electrophysiological Measures

The EEG measures cerebral activity at rest and can be valuable in estimating neurological outcome after CA (245). Specific EEG findings, such as dominant, monomorphic, and nonreactive α activity (α coma); δ activity of low voltage; θ-δ activity without α activity; burst suppression; and a flat-to-isoelectric patterns have been markers of poor prognosis *(246)*. However some patients survive despite having these findings. Recent animal studies demonstrated that early EEG bursting patterns during the first 30 to 40 minutes after resuscitation correlated with good outcome *(247)*. In patients who have no detectable cortical activity on the EEG immediately after resuscitation from CA, those who recover have burst suppression occurring within 3.3 hours and continuous EEG activity within 10.5 hours *(248)*. The presence of generalized myoclonic activity correlates with burst suppression on EEG, cerebral edema or infarcts on computed tomography (CT), and with extremely poor prognosis *(249)*.

Visual, brain stem, event-related, and somatosensory-evoked potentials (SSEPs) have been tested for usefulness in estimating neurological outcome. Of these, SSEPs have been shown the most accurate. Cerebral SSEPs assess the integrity of the sensory pathways by stimulating a peripheral sensory nerve distally and recording the expected cortical electrical activity over the sensory cortex in response to defined stimuli. Cortical response to median nerve stimulation can reliably identify subgroups with a poor prognosis with a specificity that is superior to clinical scoring algorithm or EEG. Bilateral absence of the initial cortical response connotes poor prognosis *(250)*.

Neuroimaging

Evaluation of the magnitude of the cerebral injury caused by CA may also be helpful in estimating prognosis.CT and magnetic resonance imaging (MRI) are, however of limited use, and can usually only detect gross abnormalities, such as watershed infarcts, swelling, or intracranial hemorrhage *(251,252)*. Nevertheless, a reversal of the normal gray and white matter densities indicates a severe hypoxic-ischemic insult and is correlated with a poor prognosis. MRI is superior to CT in delineating deep cerebral infarctions, however these findings were not predictive of long-term neurological prognosis *(252)*. Hence, the role of neuroimaging in estimating neurological recovery remains speculative.

Cerebral Blood Flow

The absence of CBF on cerebral angiography is pathognomonic of brain death. Normal CBF measured by xenon-133 washout with multiple detectors 6 to 46 hours after ROSC was associated with good recovery *(253)*. Whereas increased blood flow or a late decline in CBF correlated with lack of recovery and an isoelectric EEG.

Single-photon emission computed tomography used 24 hours after a CA usually detects persistent frontal hypoperfusion in most patients *(254)*. Perfusion defects greater than 50% of the supratentorial brain were associated with coma and death, but perfusion defects as large as 42% were found to be compatible with good neurological function.

Biochemical Studies

Brain injury can also be detected by using biochemical markers in a manner analogous to that of cardiac enzymes in myocardial infarction. Two markers appear most promising, neuron-specific enolase (NSE) and astroglial protein S-100. A serum NSE concentration greater than 22 μg/L measured within 1 week of CA has a sensitivity of 80% and a specificity of 100% for persistent coma *(255)*. Serum S-100 concentration greater than 0.7 μg/L as early as 24 hours after CA identifies a subgroup with poor prognosis *(256)*.

These findings are based on small cohorts and require confirmation in a larger scale before they can be applied to clinical decision making.

Brain-specific isozyme of creatinine phosphokinase in cerebrospinal fluid are elevated after CA in comatose patients. High levels correlate with poor outcomes, but there is lack of agreement among studies regarding absolute serum levels that separate good from poor neurological outcome *(257)*.

THERAPEUTIC AGENTS DIRECTED AGAINST SPECIFIC PATHOPHYSIOLOGICAL MECHANISMS OF CEREBRAL INJURY

Knowledge about the mechanism for cerebral dysfunction caused by ischemia and reperfusion may provide a fundamental basis for a rational approach to cerebral resuscitation that in the future will allow substantial amelioration of the often dismal neurological outcome now associated with resuscitation form CA. Treatment options include the following: (a) barbiturates, (b) calcium channel entry blockers, (c) excitatory amino acid blockers (NMDA and AMPA receptor blocker), (d) oxygen-free radical inhibitors, (e) protein synthesis inhibitors and antiapoptotic therapy, (f) ATP-magnesium chloride (ATP-MgCl$_2$), (g) endothelin type-A antagonist, (h) growth hormone and insulin, (i) tissue-type plasminogen activator, (j) phenytoin, (k) metabolic substrates, and (l) selective NOS inhibitors.

With advanced cerebral-oriented resuscitation, CA much longer than 5 minutes on occasion may be reverted to normal neurological function *(15,258)*. However, despite the growing understanding of the mechanism of neuronal injury after cerebral ischemia and reperfusion, effective therapy has remained at best disappointing *(15,259)*. The failure of therapeutic approaches directed at blockade of different mechanisms indicates that these hypotheses do not yet adequately explain the underlying mechanisms involved in the injured neurons. Not until very recently, however, has there been a therapeutic modality that has shown significant improvement in neurological and survival outcomes after CA in a subset of humans. This treatment is the induction of mild hypothermia, which will be discussed later in the chapter.

Barbiturates

Barbiturates afford some protection against damage from focal ischemia and global ischemia *(260)*. The exact mechanism by which barbiturates may ameliorate cerebral dysfunction after ischemia and reperfusion is not well understood. Actions beneficial from barbiturates administration have included reduction of cerebral metabolic rate and cerebral O$_2$ consumption, enhanced restoration of cerebral energy state, decreased formation of cerebral edema, reduced ICP and blood volume, reduced free fatty acid and cyclic adenosine monophosphate (cAMP), scavanger-free radicals, suppressed seizure activity, and shift metabolism to synthesizing pathways *(261–263)*.

Large and moderate doses of thiopental and pentobarbital, given before or after experimental focal ischemia, reduce the size of the infarct *(264)*. In patients, administration of thiopental before cardiac or neurosurgical procedures has been shown to reduce neurological deficits from incomplete multifocal ischemic emboli *(265)*. Although barbiturates decrease ICP in experimental animal models, this effect has not been noted in humans after head trauma *(266)*.

In the global brain ischemia monkey model, thiopental loading (90 mg/kg) immediately after reperfusion, and after 7 days of intensive care, reduced neurological deficit scores and showed less cerebral histological damage *(267)*. More recent experimental animal studies showed no difference with barbiturate therapy *(262,267,268)*. The original global ischemic model had major flaws in its methodology. These included a small sample size, most control animals were experimented prior to the treatment group, use of historical controls, use of a large number of excluded animals, and uncontrolled differences in the intensive care between groups *(269)*.

Despite the majority of animal data suggesting little or no effectiveness from barbiturate administration, the first multi-institutional international randomized clinical trial of cardiopulmonary-cerebral resuscitation using thiopental loading (30 mg/kg) after human CA was conducted. It showed no statistically overall difference in the proportion of patients with good cerebral outcome, however, there was a numerically higher proportion of good outcomes after thiopental administration in patients with the severest insults *(4,258,270)*. Unfavorable cardiovascular side effects from the high-dose thiopental may have contributed to the overall disappointing results of human trials by placing cerebral perfusion at risk. In a recent dog model with mild post-arrest induced hypothermia there was some mitigation in the brain damage when a lower dose of thiopental (30 mg/kg), dexamethasone, and phenytoin was given after 12.5 minutes of VF arrest *(271)*. Therefore, future research may be focused on using lower doses of barbiturates in order to prevent decreases in cerebral perfusion and excessive use of vasopressor therapy, both implicated in the unfavorable results associated with barbiturate therapy.

Calcium Channel Entry Blockers

To counteract the proposed detrimental actions of calcium influx during ischemia, calcium channel blockers have been recommended as therapy following CA *(272)*. Agents that block calcium entry may decrease further calcium loading of neuronal cells after CA and suppress cascades from noxious mediators within blood elements, thereby attenuating neuronal injury *(4,273,274)*. Calcium channel blockers may have an additional effect, which is to improve CBF during the hypoperfusion phase of reperfusion following global ischemia. Diminished CBF during reperfusion may be improved through amelioration of cerebral vasospasm and redistribution of regional flow. Nimodipine appears to be the most selective cerebral vasodilator and in some studies showed increased CBF without a concomitant increase in cerebral oxygen consumption *(275)*.

Studies evaluating the therapeutic efficacy of calcium channel anatgonists in experimental models of global cerebral ischemia have yielded mixed results. Improvements in neurological outcome have been reported in some animal models, whereas others report worsening outcomes and in some models, no difference was seen between those treated with calcium channel blockers and those with no treatment *(43,272,274,276–280)*. The rationale for inconsistent findings from experimental models may stem from the fact that there are different voltage-sensitive calcium channels and that calcium channel blockers may only affect one of these channels.

Nevertheless, despite a logical rationale for the use of calcium channel blockers, a well-designed prospective clinical trial in comatose survival of CA did not demonstrate a benefit in neurological prognosis with the use of the calcium channel blocker lidoflazine *(4,281)*. As with barbiturate therapy, the results may have been confounded as a result of the detrimental hemodynamic effects of the drug *(282)*. The group receiving lidoflazine had more hypotension and recurrent VF, which could significantly affect cerebral perfusion. Among a subgroup of patients without postresuscitation hypotension, however, a significantly higher proportion had better cerebral outcome in the lidoflazine group *(283)*. A similar study using nimodipine also failed to show significant cerebral improvement *(284)*. Therefore, the use of calcium channel antagonist following CA still requires evaluation to further clarify its potential role in ameliorating neuronal injury.

Excitatory Amino Acid Receptor Blockers (NMDA and AMPA Receptor Blockers)

Drugs that block the excitatory amino acids have not shown any difference in neurological outcome or improvement in the neuropathologic examinations after CA *(285)*. The administration of NMDA anatgonists has been limited by the fact that the BBB prevents the penetration of most of these compounds into the brain in sufficient quantities to obtain an adequate concentrations of agent needed to be effective *(286)*. Additionally, most NMDA receptor antagonist have been limited clinically because of their untoward side effects, such as hypertension and behavioral effect as psychosis and hyperlocomotion *(287)*. However, these side effects can be avoided by the administration of the modulatory site antagonists of the NMDA receptors. These modulatory sites include glucine, Mg^{2+}, and polyamines.

Pretreatment therapy with the NMDA glutamate receptor blocker MK-810 prevents excitatory neurotransmitter release and has been shown to ameliorate neuronal injury following focal or incomplete ischemia *(288)*. It has been demonstrated to attenuate *c-fos* and *c-jun* expression in rat neuronal cell cultures *(289)*. MK-801 was shown to reduce hippocampal damage after ischemia, however the drug inadvertently also caused hypothermia *(290)*. When brain temperature was controlled, MK-801 did not show improved neurological outcomes in an animal model of VF *(291)*. Administration of MK-801 in a VF CA model followed by reperfusion with cardiopulmonary bypass (CPB) did not show neurological improvement, even if the drug was administered prior to the induction of CA *(292)*.

Another competitive NMDA receptor antagonist, GPI-3000, has been shown to improve short-term physiological recovery after incomplete global cerebral ischemia, however mortality also increased *(293)*. In another animal model it worsened neurological damage following CA *(293)*. Therefore, it seems that drugs that block NMDA receptors have been largely ineffective in neuronal preservation after complete ischemia. They, however, appear to be more promising in neuronal salvage in the penumbral zone surrounding the area of severe ischemia following focal ischemia as seen with ischemic stoke models. The effectiveness of NMDA receptor antagonists in the penumbral zone is thought to result from ongoing occurrence of periodic depolarization in the penumbra.

In contrast to NMDA receptor anatagonist, AMPA receptors antagonists have been shown to ameliorate neuronal injury in some models of global ischemia. Treatment with NBQX during early reperfusion after 10 minutes of ischemia decreased neuronal loss in the CA1 hippocampal cells *(61,294)*. This neuronal protection has even seen when the drug is administered up to 12 hours after ischemia *(128)*. Hence, drugs that block AMPA receptor show some promise in the amelioration of neurological injury when administered after global ischemia and further studies are warranted. However, not every AMPA receptor antagonist affords protection. In a recent study of CP-465,022, a potent, and selective noncompetitive AMPA receptor antagonist, demonstrated no prevention of neuronal loss after global ischemia *(295)*. The absence of neuroprotective action of this compound call into question the neuroprotective efficacy of AMPA receptor inhibition after ischemia and careful evaluation of each agent is required prior to any implementation.

Oxygen-Free Radical Inhibitors

Drugs directed at inhibiting oxygen-derived free radical reactions either by inactivating the iron with an iron-chelating agent or by directly inactivating the radical species do not appear to reduce biochemical evidence of neuronal injury following ischemia and reperfusion but demonstrate only marginal improvement neuronal function *(296,297)*. Indomethacin, a cyclooxygenase inhibitor can prevent oxygen-free radicals by blocking the protaglandin H synthesase pathway. Indomethacin has been shown to inhibit superoxide anion generation during reperfusion in asphyxiated piglets *(90)*. No studies exists on its efficacy in preventing neurological injury following CA.

The 21-aminosteroids constitute a family of antioxidants capable of inhibiting lipid peroxidation by performing as a radical chain reaction terminator *(298)*. The most frequently evaluated 21-aminosteroid is tirilazad mesylate (U74006F), a lipid-soluble free radical inhibitor, has been shown to have stabilizing effects on cell membranes, because it can localize within the hydrophobic core of the cell membrane and cause increase in lipid ordering of the phospholipid bilayer *(299)*. Tirilazad mesylate, an antioxidant and inhibitor of lipid peroxidation, is also a steroid that mimics the pharmacological actions of high-dose methyl prednisolone. Pretreatment with U74006F improved neurological outcome after global ischemia in some animal models, however, this effect was not confirmed in subsequent studies *(198,300–302)*. In an animal model of ischemia, high-dose (20 mg/kg) desmethyl tirilazad was shown to improve the neurofunctional outcome, however there was no improvement in the pathologic examination of the brains *(303)*. Additionally, it has been shown not to ameliorate cerebral hypoperfusion following CA nor improve outcome after VF in dogs *(302)*.

Evidence also exists that superoxide dismutase, an endogenous free radical scavenger, improves cerebral cortical blood flow and metabolism following a focal cerebral ischemic injury *(304)*. Treatment with SOD reduces production of O_2^- and catalase, which prevents production of free radicals, H_2O_2 and OH•. This beneficial effect is augmented when SOD is linked to polyethylene glycol to enhance transmission across the BBB *(23)*. The beneficial effects of SOD, as measured by improved cortical evoked potentials and amelioration of the delayed postischemic cerebral hypoperfusion, may also be increased when combined with deferoxamine *(44)*. Improved neurological outcome with deferoxamine may involve the ability of deferoxamine to inhibit generation of oxygen radicals by inhibiting the conversion of hydrogen peroxide to the hydroxyl radical by the Haber-Weiss reaction. In various models of cerebral ischemia, deferoxamine has also been shown to reduce the amount of damage caused by oxygen-free radicals. Deferoxamine can help the recovery of cerebral pH, ATP, and phosphocreatine after incomplete cerebral ischemia and decrease morphologic damage following ischemia in neonatal rats *(305)*. Hydroxyethyl starch-conjugated deferoxamine has been demonstrated to decrease neurological damage and the accumulation of lipoperoxidation products *(306)*. Deferoxamine administered 5 minutes prior to resuscitation in a prolonged (17 minutes) asphyxial arrest rat model showed significantly improved cerebral perfusion and survival with less neurological injury *(307)*.

Catalase, another agent that inhibits the production of superoxide radicals, when linked to polyethylene glycol has also been shown to decrease the size of the infarct in rats exposed to focal ischemia *(308)*. The use of allopurinol, if given prior to global ischemia, has been shown to improve neurological outcome and to decrease biochemical markers of brain injury *(309)*. The mechanism is believed to be related to the ability of allopurinol to inhibit XO-generated synthesis of free radicals, which occur during oxidative metabolism of adenosine by-products.

Various antireoxygenation injury cocktails have been shown to improve postresuscitation CBF or EEG recovery but as of yet has not been shown to improve outcome *(296,310,311)*. These pharmacologic approaches have been directed toward specific mechanisms of injury with disappointing results. Explanations for such poor outcomes may include too severe ischemic insult model or the fact that most of these agents, such as deferoxamine and SOD cross the BBB poorly *(312)*. Whether any of these agents by themselves or in combination with other drugs afford long-term neuronal protection after CA remains unknown.

The net result of all these studies is an intense interest in oxygen-free radical inhibitors. To date, however, no human data are available and animal experiments can best be described as stimulating. Further research, however, must be performed prior to the recommendation for the use of a specific or a combination of superoxide radical scavenger following CA.

Protein Synthesis Inhibitors and Anti-Apoptotic Therapy

Based on the knowledge that apoptosis has a function in promoting neurological injury following CA, a variety of new neuroprotective therapeutic strategies have emerged. These novel therapeutic agents have included caspase inhibitors, viral anti-apoptotic proteins, modulation of systemic anti- and pro-apoptotic protein expression, and death receptor antagonisms.

It has become increasingly clear that some of the genes induced during cerebral ischemia may actually serve to rescue the cell from death. However, the injured neuron may not be capable of expressing protein at levels high enough to be protective. One of the most exciting arenas of such interventions is the use of viral vectors to deliver potentially neuroprotective genes at high levels. Neurotrophic herpes simplex virus strains have been employed because of their natural ability to invade the brain. By using bipromoter vectors one is capable of transferring various genes to neurons. It has been possible to enhance neuron survival against cerebral ischemia by overexpressing genes that target various phases of injury. These include energy restoration by the glucose transporter (GLUT-1), buffering calcium excess by calbindin, preventing protein malfolding or aggregation by stress proteins and inhibiting apoptotic death by *Bcl-2*. In the future with more investigations, gene therapy may offer new therapeutic avenues for ameliorating neuronal damage in patients after a CA.

The neurological protective effect of protein synthesis inhibitors on delayed neuronal death has been reported *(313)*. *Bcl-2*, a member of the *Bcl-2* gene family, has been shown to have an anti-apoptotic action in many cell types *(314)*. After cerebral ischemia, *Bcl-2* could be induced in surviving neurons, suggesting its protective effect on ischemic brain injury *(315)*. Overexpression of *Bcl-2* by gene transfer or in transgenic mice decrease infarction size and was shown to be protective against selective vulnerability after transient global ischemia *(316)*. Additionally, *Bcl-X$_L$*, an anti-apoptotic protein has also shown positive results after global ischemia *(317)*.

Viral caspase inhibitors have been utilized after global ischemia *(317,318)*. Ventricular infusion of Z-DEVD-FMK, a caspase-3 inhibitor has been shown to decrease caspase-

3 activity in vulnerable neurons and reduced neuronal injury after ischemia *(317)*. A transgenic rat-line expressing baculovirus p35, a broad-spectrum caspase inhibitor in neurons has been developed *(318)*. Following CA and resuscitation transgenic rats showed improved survival, however there was no improvement seen in the selectively vulnerable neurons *(318)*.

This new data is exciting and should foster further research in attempting to ameliorate neuronal damage after CA by using a different mechanism than that which was employed previously. However, to date, no human data are available and the strategy cannot be recommended for use after CA.

ATP Magnesium Chloride

ATP-MgCl$_2$, a compound able to restore depleted energy stores and improve function in heart, kidney, and liver after ischemia, sepsis, and hemorrhagic shock *(319)*. However, a major limiting factor in administering ATP-MgCl$_2$ is that fact that it causes significant vasodilation and hypotension, a factor not conducive to increasing cerebral blood flow in the postresuscitation phase. Co-administration of norepinephrine will ameliorate the vasodilation and prevent hypotension *(320)*. Preliminary studies have shown better preservation of hippocampal CA1 neurons and significantly improved protein synthesis after administration of ATP-MgCl$_2$ in a rat CA model *(321)*. However, caution should be used when evaluating this data because the researches did not control for a possible role of increased CBF by norepinephrine and subsequently improved neuronal survival. Further research must be performed to determine the effects on protein synthesis and improved neuronal survival after CA by ATP-MgCl$_2$.

Endothelin Type-A Antagonist

Successful recovery of neurons following CA requires unimpaired microcirculatory reperfusion. One of the mechanisms of postischemic cerebral hypoperfusion presumably is mediated through activation of endothelin type-A receptors. Antagonists of endothelin type-A receptor, with BQ123, has been shown to improve postischemic hypoperfusion and neurological outcome after 12 minutes of VF arrest in a rat model *(322,323)*. It was also shown to improve postarrest hemodynamics and early electrophysiologic recovery. Not until further studies are available, the use of endothelial type-A receptor antagonism to ameliorate postischemic neuronal injury cannot be endorsed.

Tissue-Type Plasminogen Activator

Tissue-type plasminogen activator (rt-PA) combined with heparin significantly diminishes the cerebral no-reflow phenomenon of the forebrain in cats *(324)*. In accordance with this finding, heparin and fibrinolytic agents, or both are associated with an immediate improvement in cerebral microcirculatory reperfusion; an improvement of myocardial contractility, and an increase in the survival rate after experimentally induced CA *(325,326)*. In humans, fibrinolytic therapy and heparin have been shown to improve the rate of ROSC *(327)*. In a study of patients suffering CA from cardiac causes in whom ROSC was not achieved after 15 minutes were randomized to receive recombinant tissue-type plasminogen activator and heparin or placebo. Fibrinolysis was repeated in 30 minutes if there was no ROSC. There were no reported significant bleeding complications in patients receiving fibrinolytics and anticoagulation. Those receiving therapy had significantly more ROSC and admissions to the hospital. Unfortunately there was not a significant number who were alive at 24 hours or were discharged home, but there was a trend for improvement. This latter finding may have resulted from early termination of the study as a result of interim analysis showing significant benefit at 24 hours from the treatment group. The benefits in this study demonstrate what others have found that fibrinolytic therapy and anticoagulation promote general improvement in microcirculatory reperfusion which may lead to improved cerebral function *(324,325)*.

Phenytoin

Few studies on phenytoin have shown amelioration of neuronal injury after cerebral ischemia *(328)*. A small uncontrolled human study showed 90% neurological recovery when phenytoin (7 mg/kg) was administered after CA during or after anesthesia *(329)*. An animal model of VF resuscitated with mild hypothermia, CPB, and the administration of thiopental, phenytoin, and methylprednisolone showed enhancement of the effects of hypothermia on neuronal survival *(330)*. The proposed mechanism of action for phenytoin is not well defined. Increased CBF or decreased CBF have been described *(331,332)*. Others have postulated that the protective effect of phenytoin resulted from decreased cerebrospinal fluid K^+ accumulation, thus modulating its harmful effect during an ischemic insult *(73)*. The decrease efflux of K^+ may be caused by an improved function of the Na^+-K^+ ATPase-dependent pump, a membrane stabilizing effect. Another possibility is that phenytoin may act via suppression of the postischemic abnormal EEG, which may represent seizure activity *(329)*. All of these preliminary investigations seem to show a beneficial effect of phenytoin on ameliorating neuronal injury from CA, however, further studies are required to evaluate its effectiveness, especially in humans.

Growth Factors and Insulin

Growth factors are involved in basic cellular regulation of protein synthesis, including transcription of the AP-1 complex and membrane synthesis and repair. It is not surprising that the administration of growth factors has been shown to improve postischemic neuronal survival *(333)*. FGF substantially inhibits glutamate receptor-mediated neuronal injury *(334)*. Both NGF and IGF-1 administered following global ischemia ameliorated damage to hippocampal CA1 neurons and cerebral cortex, respectively *(335)*. There is now substantial evidence that the insulin-class growth factors have neuron-sparing effects against neuronal damage by ischemia and reperfusion when administered within 2 hours after reperfusion *(333)*. Insulin given before or after ischemia in rats has also been shown to reduce cortical and striatal neuronal necrosis *(336,337)*. In the case of insulin, the beneficial effect on neurons is independent of blood glucose reduction a predictable consequence of the fact that neuronal glucose transport is insulin independent *(336)*.

In a rat asphyxia model, infusion of insulin with glucose lessened the neurological injury when compared with insulin alone *(338)*. Insulin as compared to IGF-1 and NGF may have the greatest potential for clinical application because the capillary endothelium has a dedicated transport mechanism to move insulin across the BBB. Both IGF-1 and NGF do not have similar transport mechanisms and can only be introduced into the brain by direct injection limiting their usefulness clinically. The addition of antioxidants and antagonists of proteolysis may enhance the effectiveness of insulin. This particular approach, however, has not yet been investigated in the laboratory setting but has significant theoretical appeal.

The actions of insulin are mediated by a membrane receptor tyrosine kinase that shares homology with other growth factor receptors *(339)*. After insulin receptor activation, the initial effect of insulin is autophosphorylation of tyrosine and activation of the intrinsic tyrosine kinase. Other proteins are either phosphorylated by activated kinases or dephosphorylated by protein phosphatases, which lead to activation of these proteins (340). Calmodulin is phosphorylated by the insulin receptor, which decreases its ability to bind calcium, a reaction that affords antilipolytic effects (341). Selectively vulnerable neurons show marked elevation of the level of both phosphotyrosine-containing proteins and of insulin receptors (342). Furthermore, phosphotyrosine-containing proteins are found in the highest concentrations in the nuclei of these neurons, consistent with a transcriptional regulatory function for these proteins (342).

Insulin has multiple effects, including those on fundamental cell regulatory functions, well beyond the maintenance of euglycemia. Insulin has the potential to reverse phosphorylation of elF-2α, promote effective translation on the mRNA transcripts following ischemia and reperfusion. This leads to transcription of c-fos/c-jun, increase mRNA efflux from nucleus, induce enzymatic systems for de novo lipogenesis, activate the mitochondrial pyruvate dehydrogenase complex, modify the phosphatidylinositrol transcytoplasmic signaling system, and stimulate the heat shock response (339–343). Additionally, they augment neuronal defenses against radicals, and stimulate lipid synthesis vital to membrane repair. Insulin also reduces apoptosis of neurons following ischemia although hyperglycemia exacerbates apoptosis (344).

These data suggest that it is feasible to manipulate the cell's own regulatory machinery to achieve both neuronal resistance to injury and early neuronal repair of damage during reperfusion. However, the benefits may be counteracted by the current clinical use of large doses of adrenergic agents. Catecholamines, such as epinephrine, cause prompt and prolonged inhibition of insulin secretion by the pancreas (345). Epinephrine induces hepatic gluconeogenesis and glycogenolysis (346). Epinephrine may also mediate the production of hypoinsulinemia by decreasing blood perfusion of the whole pancreas including the islets of Langerhans (347). Most important, however, may be a direct effect of epinephrine on the islets that results in suppression of B-cell electrical activity and thus insulin secretion (348). Epinephrine can reduce the activity of tyrosine kinase of the insulin receptor through cAMP-mediated phosphorylation of serine and threonine residues on the receptor (349). Epinephrine may also interfere with ligand activation of glucocorticoid receptors and subsequent transcriptional activation of AP-1. Moreover, catecholamines are known to accelerate iron-mediated lipid peroxidation and neuronal death in vitro (350). Recently, a study of 762 CA patients showed an association of worsening neurological outcome with those who received larger doses of catecholamines (351). Therefore, further research on the effects of catecholamine on cerebral growth factor levels and receptor responsiveness need to be conducted in the setting of CA and resuscitation.

Metabolic Substrates

FRUCTOSE-1, 6-BIPHOSPHONATE

Fructose-1, 6-biphosphonate (FBP), an endogenous intermediate of glycolysis, may protect the brain against ischemia-reperfusion injury. It is postulated that FBP is of therapeutic benefit by entering the Embden-Meyerhof pathways distal to the action of phosphofructokinase (PFK), the rate-limiting enzyme, which is inactivated by the progressive acidosis associated with ischemia, thereby enhancing anaerobic glycolysis and allowing the cell to maintain energy ATP production despite deficits of glucose and oxygen during ischemia (352). However, as with hyperglycemia, one of the effects of increasing energy production by augmenting anaerobic glycolysis is progressive accumulation of lactic acid, which has been shown to be deleterious to the brain *(43)*. FDP also preserves glutathione intracellulary and protects cortical neurons against oxidative stress *(353)*. However, in an animal model of global cerebral ischemia, FBP did not improve neurological function as demonstrated by EEG amplitude.

SUCCINATE

Succinate is a Kreb cycle intermediate that has been shown to cross the BBB and enhance respiration and ATP production in homogenates of brain, liver, and kidney following anoxia *(354)*. In an animal model of global ischemia, succinate was shown to improve EEG amplitude when compared to controls *(354)*.

IMMUNOSUPPRESSION

Tracolimus (FK506), a potent immunosuppressive drug, has been shown to attenuate neuronal damage after global and partial ischemia and this effect is present up to 2 hours after the ischemia *(355)*. Tracolimus has been shown to downregulate protein kinase C (PKC)γ and calcium/calmodulin-dependent protein kinase II (CaMKII), which may partially explain some of its beneficial effects on cerebral ischemia *(356)*.

NITRIC OXIDE INHIBITION

During spontaneous circulation, nonspecific inhibition of constitutive NOS by N(G)-nitro-L-arginine methyl ester (L-NAME) increases systemic vascular resistance and, therefore, mean arterial pressure. In an animal model of VF arrest, administration of L-NAME vs saline demonstrated an increase in coronary pressure and resulted in significantly better initial short-term resuscitation when compared with saline infusion *(357)*. However, in this study no additional vasopressors, such as epinephrine were given. Thus, the interaction of epinephrine and L-NAME are unknown. Administration of L-NAME and 7-nitroindazole, another neuronal NOS inhibitor after global ischemia showed amelioration of ischemic damage in CA1 neurons *(358)*.

Treatments Shown to Improve Cerebral Perfusion During CA and Resuscitation

Artificial perfusion is the principal weak link in the resuscitation armamentarium. Despite the universal use of closed chest CPR for CA, this method has been shown repeatedly to suffer from lack of clinical efficacy. Although external chest CPR can clearly save lives, the inherent inefficiency of this method and the challenges related to teaching and retaining the skills needed to perform the technique have limited its overall effectiveness. Unfortunately, external chest CPR when performed exceptionally well has been shown to generate blood flow equivalent only to about 25 to 35% of normal cardiac output *(359)*. If there is any delay prior to the initiation of CPR, as commonly occurs, the progressive loss of peripheral arterial resistance substantially decreases the blood flow generated by CPR. Therefore, one of the greatest challenges in the development of improved resuscitative interventions is to develop more effective methods of artificial perfusion or drug administration that can be initiated within the critical time frame allowing for an increased ROSC with good neurological outcome.

CPR Techniques

Much of the research in CPR during the last decade has centered on finding newer techniques to improve both cerebral and coronary perfusion. The best guide to monitor the adequacy of CPR is the coronary perfusion pressure (end-diastolic aortic pressure minus end-diastolic central venous pressure *(360)*. Coronary perfusion pressure greater than 15 mmHg has been shown to correlate with increased cardiac resuscitation and thus ROSC, which impact on the degree of neurological damage. A number of alternative techniques of CPR have been invented and evaluated to accomplish these goals and those only shown to improve cerebral blood or outcome are discussed below.

Increasing Compression to Ventilation Ratio

The optimal ratio of chest compression to ventilation during standard CPR is unknown. In a swine model of CA with 3-minute VF duration, various forms of CPR for 12 minutes were compared: (a) standard CPR with a ratio of 15:2 compressions to ventilations; (b) chest compressions alone; (c) CPR with a ratio of 50:5 compressions to ventilations; then CPR without ventilation for 4 minutes followed by a 100:2 compressions to ventilations ratio (100:2 CPR *[361]*). The technique using a ratio of 100:2 compressions to ventilations achieved significantly better neurological scores at 4 hours when compared to the other techniques *(361)*. Therefore, it seems that a higher compression to ventilation ratio may allow a greater CPP to be generated, which may translate into an improvement in neurological outcome.

Interposed Abdominal Compression CPR

Interposed abdominal compression (IAC)-CPR is another revised technique of standard CPR that has been proposed as a technique to improve cerebral and coronary blood flow. IAC-CPR requires another rescuer positioned alongside or opposite the rescuer applying chest compressions in the standard fashion. This additional rescuer places his or her hands on the abdomen, usually near the umbilicus, and compresses the abdomen during the relaxation phase of chest compressions. The ratio of chest compressions to abdominal compressions is one to one, so that the rate of abdominal compression is also 80 to 100 per minute. Some researchers place a blood pressure cuff or another measuring device between the hands of the resuer and the abdominal wall in order to measure and perhaps limit the amount of force applied to the abdomen. The amount of pressure applied has ranged from 20 to 150 mmHg. With IAC-CPR, abdominal counterpulsations aim to increase intrathoracic and aortic pressure, provide retrograde aortic flow and thereby improve blood flow to the brain and heart, and increase venous return. IAC-CPR improves both cerebral and coronary blood flow *(362,363)*.

Several human trials have shown higher MABP with IAC-CPR when performed after failure of resuscitation with conventional CPR *(364,365)*. A large prehospital trial of IAC-CPR showed, however, no difference in success of initial resuscitation, however the use of IAC-CPR was interrupted when the patient was driven to the hospital because of lack of personnel *(366)*. Although there has been a human trial showing improved resuscitation rates, improved neurological outcome in patients at discharge could not be demonstrated *(366,367)*. One randomized in-hospital trial of IAC-CPR showed improvements in ROSC, discharge from hospital and specifically neurological outcome *(367)*. In another follow-up study, IAC-CPR was applied to patients with electrocardiograms displaying only asystole or pulseless electrical activity and showed improved ROSC, however, none of the survivals were neurologically intact *(368)*. In settings of out-of-hospital CA, however, there is as yet no persuasive proof that IAC-CPR improves neurological function after a CA *(364,369)*. Nevertheless, IAC-CPR may be used for in-hospital resuscitation when sufficient personnel trained in the technique are available.

Open-Chest Cardiac Massage

The superiority of open-chest compressions has long been recognized, although its advantages with respect to preservation of the brain and heart have been recently investigated. Initial animal studies demonstrated that open-chest CPR produced greater aortic pressure and cardiac output *(370)*. In humans, open-chest CPR also generates greater cardiac index, stroke index, perfusion pressure, and aortic diastolic and mean pressure *(371,372)*. Additionally, open-chest CPR has been shown to improve both cerebral and myocardial blood flow *(373)*. Open-chest CPR has been shown experimentally to sustain EEG activity during prolonged resuscitation, and to lead to improved cerebral and cardiac recovery *(371,372,374)*. Moreover, open-chest CPR produces nearly normal CBF when compared to external chest compressions *(371,372,375)*. Limited data on humans exist with open-chest CPR. However, most reported cases in which open-chest CPR has been applied is after failed closed-chest CPR, usually greater than 20 minutes, in which the success of resuscitation dwindles *(177)*. Therefore, if this technique is to improve survival and cerebral function following CA it must be applied and evaluated early in the resuscitation *(376)*.

Vest CPR

Vest CPR is another innovative technique that has been shown to improve cerebral and coronary perfusion pressure. During vest CPR, a bladder-containing vest, analogous to a large blood pressure cuff, is placed circumferentially around the patient's chest and cyclically inflated and deflated by an automated pneumatic system. The device allows one to regulate the rate of and compression duration, and inflation pressure. It can also be connected to a defibrillator and cardiopulmonary monitoring system. The vest maintains a small amount of positive pressure on the chest between compressions, except when ventilations are given in which the vest completely deflates. The vest is generally inflated in adults to a pressure of approx 250 mmHg, 60 to 80 times a minute. Vest CPR increases IAP fluctuations by circumferential changes in the dimensions of the thorax and thereby improves venous return and forward aortic flow. By encircling the chest, force can be applied evenly, thus resulting in a large decrement in the volume of the chest with minimal displacement of the chest wall itself.

Initial animal studies utilizing vest CPR showed increases in cerebral and myocardial perfusion pressures, blood flows, and survival outcomes *(277)*. They were able to demonstrate myocardial blood flow 40% of pre-arrest values, and CBF almost equal to pre-arrest blood flow. Institution of CPR with pneumatic thoracic vest CPR and epinephrine infusion after 6 minutes of induced VF arrest was capable of generating cerebral perfusion pressure of approx 80 mmHg and a CBF of 57 mL per minute per 100 g *(179)*. Cerebral ATP recovered to 86 ± 7% of control by 6 minutes of vest CPR and cerebral pH recovered to 6.88 ± 0.05 by 12 minutes of vest CPR. An initial human trial, however, in 10 patients showed no improvement in CPP *(376)*. Another small human study, utilizing an improved version of the pneumatic vest CPR compared to standard external CPR resulted in greater CPP, more ROSC but there was no difference in survival between the two techniques *(378)*.

Active-Decompression CPR

The case of the patient resuscitated with a plunger led rapidly to the development of a hand-held suction cup device *(379)*. This new form of CPR, active-decompression CPR

(ACD-CPR) has been touted as improving cerebral and coronary perfusion pressure above that achieved with standard CPR. The device includes a handle, a suction cup, and a force gauge. ACD-CPR (Cardio-Pump™ device) operates by the same principle as vest CPR with increased intrathoracic pressure fluctuations and enhanced cardiac compression and forward aortic flow. Venous return is increased with a greater generated negative IAP during decompression. The ACD device is placed over the midsternum and provides active manual compression of the chest as well as active chest decompression. It utilizes a suction-cup device to pull up on the chest during chest relaxation. Additionally, the device may give the rescuer a mechanical advantage in performing chest compression, which results in substantially higher sternal forces being applied than with standard external CPR.

Animal studies have shown increased cerebral and coronary blood flow, cardiac output, and CPP when compared to standard CPR *(380)*. In an effort to enhance the efficiency of ACD-CPR, a new inspiratory impedance threshold valve (Resuscitator valve™ or Resusci-Valve™) has been developed to increase venous return during chest relaxation *(381)*. The impedance threshold valve is a small (35 mL) disposable valve that is attached in between the endotracheal tube and the ventilator interface. It allows the rescuer to ventilate the patient as usual. When the rescuer is not actively ventilating the patient, the valve impedes inspiratory airflow during the relaxation of the chest. This creates a small vacuum and increases negative pressure within the chest that results in increased venous return and leads to improved vital organ perfusion *(382)*. In animals, use of the impedance valve with active-decompression CPR resulted in a 300% increase CBF and a 400% increase in myocardial blood flow when evaluated against conventional CPR *(383)*. Additionally, 24-hour survival rates and neurological outcomes were significantly improved with the use of the impedance device and standard CPR *(384)*.

A study with 400 patients showed that the combination of ACD-CPR and the impedance threshold valve results in near normal blood pressures during prolonged CA and doubling of 24-hour survival in patients with out-of-hospital arrest *(385)*. The neurological function in the survivors was significantly better at hospital discharge in patients treated with ACD-CPR and the impedance valve. Another study showed a 100% increase in 24-hour survival in patients with a witnessed CA treated with the impedance valve and ACD-CPR when compared to standard CPR *(386)*.

The first human trial of ACD-CPR showed improved rates of ROSC but no improvement in hospital discharge *(387)*. Additional clinical studies in humans were disappointing, because no difference in hospital survival or improved neurological outcome could be demonstrated *(387–390)*. However, recently long-term survival rates, including 1-year survival have been reported to increase by more than 100% with the ACD device *(391)*. There are many potential reasons for the discrepancies between earlier and more recent studies, but training and competency in using the device have been major concerns *(392)*. In the study showing improved long-term survival, the personnel involved in the study had been utilizing ACD-CPR for several years prior to the study and had ample experience with the use of the device. Other study differences included differences in the overall efficiency of the emergency medical services systems, fatigue associated with the technique, concurrent use of drug therapies, and the duration of CPR during clinical trials *(391,392)*. At present, the ACD-CPR method is widely used in France, some Asian countries, and parts of Canada.

Phased Chest and Abdominal Compression–Decompression CPR

Phased chest and abdominal compression–decompression CPR (Lifestick™-CPR) is a combination of the potential benefits of ACD-CPR and IAC. The Lifestick device resembles a seesaw and contains a rigid frame attached to two piston suction cups (pads). The smaller pad (20 × 17 cm) is placed on the mid-sternum, the larger pad (37 × 25 cm) on the epigastrium. The pads are fixed to the Lifestick before placement on the patient. Chest compression is coincident with abdominal decompression, followed by chest decompression plus abdominal compression. Thoracic decompression during abdominal compression leads to an increased venous return from increased negative intrathoracic pressure. Moreover, abdominal decompression during chest compression may lead to an increased blood flow because afterload is decreased *(393)*. In animal models, improved coronary perfusion, ROSC, end-tidal CO_2, survival and neurological outcome was demonstrated compared to standard CPR *(394)*. A small humans trial with CA refractory to conventional CPR showed improved CPP *(394,395)*. However, a recent clinical trial in 50 patients randomized to either phased thoraco-abdominal compression–decompression CPR or closed chest manual CPR found no difference in survival *(396)*.

Whole-Body Periodic Acceleration Aloang the Spinal Axis

A novel CPR technique known as the whole-body periodic acceleration along the spinal axis (pGz-CPR) has been shown to improve neurological outcome in a VF model in animals *(397,398)*. The technique involves securing the subject on a horizontal wooden platform. This platform is driven with a linear-displacement motor powered by an amplifier that is controlled by a sine wave controller. The platform is directly driven by the motor and articulates across the frame on stainless steel tracks and nylon wheels at a frequency between 0.5 and 10 Hz as force of 0.1-1.5g. The platform moves sinusoidally in a headword-to-footward direction. A disadvantage is that there is currently a weight limit of 30 kg for animals, thus usefulness in larger animal and adults may not be inferred.

Mechanical Devices

New mechanical devices have also been developed to improve blood flow during CA and some of these have shown improvement in cerebral and coronary perfusion pressures.

Cardiopulmonary Bypass

The use of CPB for the treatment of CA was intensively evaluated in the late 1980s. CPB can generate much higher cerebral and coronary blood flows than traditional external chest compression *(399)*. During the use of peripheral CPB for VF, there is retrograde perfusion of the aorta from the femoral arteries and antegrade perfusion of the coronary and cerebral arteries *(400)*. Organ blood flow pattern are altered when CPB is instituted after global ischemia following CA. An early hyperemic phase is seen in some organs, especially the brain and heart, and is thought to occur from ischemic vasodilation with loss of vascular autoregulation *(401)*. However, coronary and cerebral perfusion pressures are lower than normal. With the addition of epinephrine, these perfusion pressures become normal or even supranormal with a fibrillating heart *(402)*. CPB permits the control of flow, pressure, temperature, oxygenation, and composition of blood *(403)*. Another advantage is the ability to provide continued systemic perfusion during the postresuscitation phase when intrinsic cardiac function is usually inadequate and the risk of recurrent cardiac failure or arrest is high. The ability to gradually withdraw perfusion support facilitates cardiovascular stability. CPB has been shown to be even more efficacious than open-chest CPR in generating blood flow. Disadvantages include placement of the catheters during CPR making its utility usually only for in-hospital arrest. The major obstacle to implementation of this technique is the time required to get the equipment and skilled personnel needed to the patient. Even under good conditions, the time required to perform vascular access and initiate perfusion is generally 10–15 minutes.

In canine CA models, CPB has shown improved ROSC rates when compared to standard CPR with advanced life support after nonperfused normothermic VF ranging from 10 to 12.5 minutes *(404,405)*. Survivors of CPB in these studies showed improved neurological outcome at 72 hours, when compared to survivors of CPR and advanced life support. In dog studies using CPB, it has been possible to reverse normothermic CA without neurological deficit of up to 11 minutes without blood flow *(406)*. Similar results have been seen in the swine model of 10 minute VF and 5 minutes failed conventional CPR *(402)*. CBP showed better ROSC when compared with open-chest CPR and closed-chest CPR in a canine model of VF *(404)*. However, all of these animal studies were previously instrumented with a large cannulae required for operation of the peripheral CPB prior to the induction of CA. Hence, their results may not be truly clinically relevant, because when the decision is made to use CBP, one of the limiting issues for success is attaining cannulation of the vessels during CA. To improve on the success of cannulation a portable ultrasound may be utilized to assist in the location of the femoral artery prior to cannulation.

Limited case reports in humans exist with the use of CPB after CA, which showed effectiveness in restoring circulation *(407)*. Utilizing femorofemoral bypass a report of five patients who failed conventional therapy, all had ROSC and three survived to hospital dischrage *(408)*. However, those that survived usually had the CPB placed within the first 5 to 7 minutes following the arrest *(409)*.

EXTRACORPOREAL MEMBRANE OXYGENATION

The use of extracorporeal circulation has been shown to improve neurological outcome in animals, even after 30 minutes of CA, however a major disadvantage is that it is not universally available *(410)*. In pediatric patients, venoarterial extracorporeal membrane oxygenation (ECMO) has been used successfully for resuscitation from shock and CA. Although analogous to CPB, generally lower flows are used to assist the intact, but dysfunctional circulatory system. A study of 11 CA victims after open-heart surgery were placed on ECMO after unsuccessful CPR, there were 7/11 early survivors, 6 whom were long-term survivors *(411)*. Unfortunately, it takes an average of 20 to 30 minutes to set up the circuit and a perfusion team must be on call at all times for it to be effective, thus limiting its widespread use.

MINIMALLY INVASIVE DIRECT CARDIAC MASSAGE

Minimally invasive direct cardiac massage (MID-CM) utilizes a plunger-like device inserted through a small intercostal incision over the apex of the heart. Without opening the pericardium, the device is placed directly on the ventricles. It produces an artificial circulation by cyclic cardiac compression and relaxation. The device uses a padded plate connected to a handle. A defibrillator can be attached and has been effective in converting VF *(412)*. In a swine model of CA this technique generated cerebral and coronary perfusion pressure, cardiac output, and systemic blood pressure similar to that produced by conventional open-chest cardiac massage *(413)*. However, there was no difference in 24-hour survival when compared to standard CPR in a model of prolonged VF *(414)*.

AORTIC BALLOON OCCLUSION CATHETERS

There is a growing interest in the use of thoracic aortic balloon occlusion catheters to provide vital organ perfusion during CA. Intra-aortic balloon occlusion of the descending aorta is a new and promising technique in CPR. It resembles the aortic cross-clamping technique previously used in combination with open-chest cardiac massage. The technique utilizes a balloon catheter that is advanced into the ascending aorta. The balloon is inflated for 30 seconds during each minute of thoracic compression. It effectively diverts blood flow toward the coronary and cerebral circulation. Additionally, placement of an aortic balloon catheter provides unique access to the coronary and cerebral vascular beds during CPR and permits infusion of resuscitation solutions selectively to the heart and brain. This type of catheter opens a new field of possible resuscitative interventions during and after CPR.

A recent animal VF study using a balloon occlusion of the descending aorta showed improvement of cortical CBF *(415)*. Fluid infusion resulted in further increases in coronary artery perfusion that promoted ROSC. These findings are even better than with the use of high-dose epinephrine infusion. Despite the remarkable coronary perfusion generated by this technique, rapid insertion of the catheter to the ascending aortic arch during CA poses a significant challenge for successful use of these techniques. Additionally, an imaging study would almost be certainly required to confirm proper placement of the catheter tip before initiation of therapy. Another study in piglets with aortic occlusion and the infusion of vasopressin into the aorta above the site of occlusion, demonstrated improved cerebral blood flow and oxygenation *(416)*. Recently, a combination of aortic balloon occlusion, vasopressin, hypertonic saline dextran, free radical scavenger α-phenyl-*N*-tert-butyl-nitrone and cyclosporine-A alleviated neuronal damage after 8 minutes of global ishemia in piglets *(417)*.

The use of intra-aortic balloon occlusion with hypertonic saline hyperoncotic dextran solution (HSD) has been shown to increase CBF and brain oxygen supply during open-chest CPR but these effects vanish once there is return of spontaneous circulation *(418)*. Improving the rheological properties of blood flow in the postresuscitation phase may augment flow to ischemic organs. The clinical significance of the increased blood flow during CPR is unknown and remains to be investigated. HSD has direct beneficial effects on organ perfusion by expanding the intravascular volume, but is also theorized to attenuate cerebral noreflow by decreasing intracranial pressure, reducing the endothelial swelling and platelet aggregation, and the postischemic leukocyte-endothelial interaction *(419–421)*.

DRUG THERAPY TO IMPROVE CEREBRAL PERFUSION

Several experimental studies performed over the past 20 years have demonstrated that alpha adrenergic agonists improve the outcome of resuscitation from CA. α-Adrenergic agonists cause vasoconstriction of peripheral arterioles and have been shown to increase CPP by raising aortic diastolic pressure above increases in right atrial diastolic pressure *(422)*. Although adrenergic agonists increase CPP, their effect on myocardial oxygen consumption is more controversial and in fact, it is the β-adrenergic activity that increase oxygen consumption *(423)*. Epinephrine, for example, has prominent β-adrenoreceptor actions by which it increases the myocardial oxygen requirements during CA *(424)*. The increases in oxygen demand exceed increases in oxygen delivery produced by augmentation of CPP and myocardial blood flow *(424)*. Additionally, β-adrenergic stimulation during CA has also been shown to worsen the severity of postresuscitation myocardial dysfunction. Recent laboratory data indicate that β-blockade may actually be beneficial *(425)*. In a rat model of CA, administration of epinephrine in combination with the β-blocking agent esmolol during chest compression ameliorated the severity of postresuscitation myocardial dysfunction *(426)*. These results have been reproduced in large-animal models of CA *(425)*. Epinephrine has also been shown to improve cerebral perfusion and may improve neurological outcome, but the latter may only be a secondary effect of epinephrine because it increases the chance of ROSC and shortens the duration of arrest *(427)*. However, some preliminary results from animals indicate that adrenergic agents may actually have a direct neuroprotective effect *(428)*.

The optimal dose of adrenergic agonists required to increase cerebral and coronary perfusion pressures during CPR remains speculative. Numerous studies in animals have shown that epinephrine in doses of 0.2 mg/kg, so-called high-dose epinephrine, produces substantially higher cerebral and coronary perfusion pressure and greater myocardial blood flow than standard-dose epinephrine (0.01–0.02 mg/kg) *(429,430)*. However, higher doses can lead to excessive stimulation β-adrenergic adrenergic receptors and increase morbidity. This toxicity is obviously only an issue in survivors and may be prevented with β–blockade *(431)*.

Higher than the normal recommended doses of epinephrine have been shown in animals to increase both cerebral and coronary blood flow, but fail to improve overall outcomes in humans *(432–434)*. High-dose epinephrine, did significantly improve the rate of return of spontaneous circulation, but did not improve hospital discharge or neurological outcome when compared to standard dose epinephrine. These findings were confirmed in a meta-analysis of five randomized trials, which established that high-dose epinephrine was associated with a higher ROSC, but no beneficial effect on hospital discharge *(435)*. In a recent animal trial, higher doses of epinephrine (200 μg/kg vs 20 μg/kg) may actually worsen cerebral cortical blood flow measured by laser Doppler flowmetry, which may explain the failure of high-dose epinephrine on neuronal recovery in human trials *(436)*. Previous studies supporting an increased cerebral blood flow in CPR by using high-dose epinephrine measured blood flow with the microsphere technique which has a limitation of being a spot measurement of flow and not continuous *(433)*.

The best adrenergic agonist for increasing cerebral and coronary pressures is likewise controversial. Agents used during CPR have included epinephrine, methoxamine, norepinephrine, phenylephrine, and α-methylnorepinephrine (α-MNE) and varying results have been achieved *(423,437)*. Thus, no consensus yet exists concerning the best adrenergic agonists for raising cerebral and coronary pressure during CPR. A preliminary animal study showed comparable increases in coronary perfusion pressure and resuscibility for α-MNE, epinephrine, and vasopressin *(438)*. However, only α-MNE demonstrated the best postresuscitation myocardial function and survival than did vasopressin or epinephrine. This may be partially explained because α-MNE is predominantly an α-1 adrenoceptor agonist. Additionally, both vasopressin and epinephrine decreases $ETCO_2$ and presumably pulmonary blood flow, therefore, cardiac output during CPR *(439)*. However, not until more research especially in humans can α-MNE be recommended as an agent for CA.

Recently, attention has been given to vasopressin. Some investigators have shown in an animal model of prolonged arrest that vasopressin, but not epinephrine had better neurological outcomes *(440)*. Vasopressin when compared with epinephrine not only increases cerebral blood flow but also improves cerebral oxygenation and decreases cerebral venous hypercarbia when administered during CA *(441)*. In a pediatric porcine model of asphyxial arrest, however, epinephrine resulted in better cerebral and coronary blood flow and ROSC than did vasopressin *(442)*. Although in a pediatric porcine model of VF, the combination of epinephrine with vasopressin during CPR resulted in significantly higher levels of left ventricular (LV) myocardial blood flow than either vasopressin alone or epinephrine alone *(443)*. Both vasopressin alone and the combination with epinephrine with vasopressin, but not epinephrine alone, improved total CBF during CPR. In stark contrast to the pediatric asphyxial CA model, vasopressin alone or in combination with epinephrine affords a better outcome after VF. It is postulated that the improved CBF with the addition of vasopressin to epinephrine may be as a result of the unique vasopressin effect on nitric oxide release in the cerebral vasculature. However, significant side effects were noted with the epinephrine–vasopressin combination, which included decreases renal blood flow, hyperadrenergic state with the occurrence of VT, and an increase acidosis postresuscitation.

The addition of nitroglycerin to epinephrine and vasopressin in a porcine model of VF showed greater cerebral and myocardial blood flow and ROSC than epinephrine alone *(444)*. Another porcine model of VF arrest confirmed the findings of improved neurological outcomes with the combination of epinephrine and vasopressin when compared to epinephrine alone or saline *(445)*. Additionally, this model showed less complications in the postresuscitation period that may be attributed to the small dose of epinephrine used (45 vs 200 µg/kg). In a human trial of epinephrine vs vasopressin there was no difference between hospital discharge rates *(446)*. However, another human trial showed vasopressin, not epinephrine with an increased ROSC, survival at 24 hours and a trend toward better survival on hospital discharge.

Postresuscitation Management

GENERAL SUPPORTIVE MEASURES

Resuscitation of the CA patient does not terminate when there is ROSC. A significant amount of patients sustain neurological injury, which imply that there is room for improvement in achieving a better neurological outcome during the post-ROSC phase of resuscitation. The fundamental goal of cardiopulmonary-cerebral resuscitation is to improve the proportion of people stricken with an unexpected impaired neurological state to pre-arrest functional neurological recovery. Cerebral-oriented intensive care therapy is of utmost importance if the best possible outcome is to be expected. An important therapy for patients with reduced CBF should include measures to optimize cerebral perfusion pressure by maintaining a normal or even a slightly higher MABP although at the same time maintaining a normal ICP *(447)*. Additionally, it is clear from many other studies evaluating other forms of shock that patients may remain underresuscitated for days following the ischemic insult. This may be worsened in CA victims in whom aggressive treatment may be delayed because of concerns for neurological viability. Vital measurements such as heart rate, blood pressure, and urine output are poor indicators of the adequacy of resuscitation *(448)*.

After ROSC, many resuscitated CA victims may be clinically unstable for several reasons. Nearly half require mechanical ventilation, and aspiration of gastric contents during the arrest or resuscitation may exacerbate respiratory compromise. Peri-arrest arrhythmias are common and may lead to further episodes of poor perfusion or CA.

Hypotension can also result from the process that leads to CA, such as MI and from postresuscitation myocardial stunning, requiring the administration of inotropic agents or mechanical circulatory support, or both. Many resuscitated patients are elderly and in addition have serious underlying cormobid conditions that may increase morbidity or mortality following CA.

One of the other initial management priorities of a CA victim should include a basic diagnostic work-up aimed at determining the etiology of the CA, an assessment of respiratory and hemodynamic function, and an identification of extracardiac issues that may affect organ function. In the adult population, 80% are as a result of coronary syndromes. Accordingly, other causes of CA in the adult may include dysrhythmias, dilated cardiomyopathy, myocarditis, aortic stenosis, cardiac tamponade, aortic dissection, pulmonary hypertension, and electrolyte abnormalities. Other noncardiac conditions include hypoxemic respiratory failure, massive pulmonary embolism, tension pneumothorax, and exsanguinating traumatic hemorrhage. In the pediatric population, sudden infant death syndrome, asphyxial-related arrest, and near-drowning are the predominant medical causes of CA *(449)*. A primary cardiac event is less common and is usually associated with congenital heart disease, congenital coronary abnormality, hypertrophic cardiomyopathy, and myocarditis *(450)*. Once the cause is found, accordingly, efforts should be made to institute specific medical treatments.

Primary Assessment (Airway, Breathing, and Circulation)

Intensive postresuscitation care has changed very little in the last few decades but general recommendation based on recent evidence for general support can be made (Table 1; *15*). Thorough reassessment of the airway, breathing, and circulation should be performed. The airway should be evaluated for patency, looking for any evidence of obstruction. Tracheal intubation is the most reliable method for securing and maintaining a patient's airway in a patient suffering from a CA. Although direct visualization of the vocal cords as the tube is advanced into the trachea using a laryngoscope is reassuring, the tube may become dislodged following placement owing to head movement or positioning of the patient. Unintentional esophageal intubation, however, occurs in up to 8% of the attempts, and the consequences are catostrophic if misplacement of the endotracheal tube (ET) is not recognized. Confirmation of the ET should be performed. Therefore, various methods for verifying tracheal intubation and distinguishing it from esophageal intubation have been developed. Among clinical signs, auscultation of the chest is the most common method, and direct visualization of the ET between the vocal cords is one of the most dependable signs of correct tracheal intubation *(451)*.

However, these methods are not perfect. Detection of the end-tidal CO_2 concentration has become the most reliable method for verifying proper placement *(451,452)*. Carbon dioxide (CO_2) can be measured by inexpensive chemical indicators that provide semiquantitative estimates of the end-tidal CO_2 or by portable infrared CO_2 analyzers that provide quantitative estimates and displays of waveforms. A chest radiograph serves as the confirmatory method to verify the position of the ET relative to the carina.

Evaluation of breathing entails listening for equal and bilateral breath sounds and looking for equal excursion of the chest. The neck should be inspected for jugular venous distention and the trachea should be in the midline position. Evidence for rib fracture or pneumothorax should be sought. If there is decreased breath sounds on one side and it is not as a result of erroneous ET placement, then a needle thoracostomy followed by a chest thoracostomy tube should be placed for suspected pneumothorax.

Table 1
Postresuscitation and Cerebral Resuscitation Recommendations

Prehospital phase	Teach basic life support (BLS) to lay public
	Early automated external defibrillation (AED) response
	Airway support, including supplemental oxygen, bag-valve-mask (BVM) ventilation and endotracheal tube intubation
	Early administration of resuscitative drugs as recommended by advanced cardiac life support (ACLS) and pediatric advanced life support (PALS)
	Increase perfusion pressure with early administration of epinephrine
	Use of other mechanical devices, such as ACD-CPR or IAC-CPR
	Check blood glucose and maintain between 100—and 200 mg/dL
Hospital phase	Primary assessment of the airway, breathing, and circulation
	Confirmation of tracheal intubation (CXR, $ETCO_2$)
	Hypertensive bout (MABP <150 mmHg) for 15–30 minutes, afterward control normotension, normoxia, and normocarbia (avoid hypotension, hypercarbia and hyperoxia)
	Conduct hemodynamic monitoring as feasible to guide administration of drugs and fluids
	Optimize myocardial function and systemic perfusion (inotropes, vasopressors, vasodilators or mechanical devices).
	Cool brain to 32–34°C (treat hyperthermia aggressively)
	Control seizure aggressively with benzodiazepines or standard anticonvulsants
	Measures to decrease ICP (elevate head 30°, midline position).
	Diagnostic work-up aimed at determining the etiology of the CA
	Correct acidemia (fluids ± buffer therapy)
	Treat electrolyte disorders
	Maintain glucose between 100–200 mg/dL
	12-lead EKG
	Insert gastric tube to decompress stomach (allow diaphragmatic excursion)
	Keep hematocrit 30–35%, electrolytes normal

After the airway and breathing is assessed, circulatory function follows. An assessment of perfusion status includes comparison of peripheral vs central pulses, a visual assessment of the color of the extremities, and palpation of the extremities for temperature. Abnormal color such as pale, ashen, mottled, or cyanosis and a colder than normal extremity are all indications of decreased perfusion to that extremity. Bilateral femoral and carotid pulses should be assessed for rate and quality. Capillary refill time should be determined. The patient's rhythm should be monitored and a minimum of two working intravenous catheters should be established.

Secondary Assessment

In patients whose CA is caused by pump failure secondary to acute myocardial infarction, emergent cardiac catheterization with angioplasty or stenting should be considered

(453). These patients may develop profound myocardial dysfunction and require circulatory assistance with inotropic drug administration, aortic balloon counterpulsation, or both. In situations in which cardiac cathetrization is not available, fibrinolytic therapy should be administered if the CPR time was generally less than 10 minutes and no other absolute contraindications exist *(454).* If the initial arrest rhythm was VF or ventricular tachycardia or anti-arrhythmic therapy was required for successful resuscitation consider an anti-arrhythmic infusion, such as amiodarone or lidocaine. If hemodynamically significant bradycardia is present, initiate therapy to increase the heart rate, including atropine sulphate or pacemaker. At the same time, if hemodynamically significant tachycardia exists, initiate therapy to decrease the heart rate, such as adenosine, amiodarone, β-blockers, or calcium channel blockers.

CNS Assessment

In the comatose patient, the brain responds to external stimuli such as a simple physical examination or airway suctioning with increases in cerebral metabolism and ICP. This increased regional brain metabolism requires increased regional CBF at a time when the balance between oxygen supply and demand are precariously threatened. Protection from afferent sensory stimuli with administration of titrated doses of sedation and muscle relaxants may protect this balance and improve the chance for neuronal recovery.

Seizures are not a common sequella following an ischemic injury. When they occur, they should be treated with anticonvulsant therapy. If seizures occur, search for any correctable metabolic causes, such as hypoglycemia or other electrolyte disorders. Seizures can increase brain metabolism by 300 to 400%. This extreme increase in metabolic demand may tip the tissue oxygen supply–demand balance, causing devastating neurological consequences. Seizures must be treated aggressively with anticonvulsant medication. A benzodiazepine such as lorazepam, diazepam, or midazolam is often effective. No clinical evidence supports the routine administration of an antiepileptic drug to prevent post-arrest seizures, therefore are not recommended routinely. Postanoxic myoclonus is a more common problem, can interfere with nursing care and mechanical ventilation, and may be quite distressful to families. When it is generalized and repetitive it is associated with extensive brain damage *(455).* It is usually refractory to treatment and may persist past the acute setting in patients who otherwise have made a good recovery. Administration of sedatives may be useful, but it may be necessary to resort to neuromusclar paralysis in order to care for these patients.

Measures to lower ICP should be instituted. The head should be elevated to approx 30° and maintained in a midline position to aid in cerebral venous drainage if there is no evidence of suspected cervical spinal injury. Care should be observed during tracheal suctioning because of the increase in ICP during this procedure and should be limited to no more than 15 to 20 seconds. Preoxygenation with 100% oxygen helps prevent hypoxemia during suctioning.

Although there is exciting experimental data on preserving CNS function, no treatment except induced hypothermia is established sufficiently at present to warrant its routine use for cerebral resuscitation. Nonetheless, vigilant attention to the details of oxygenation and perfusion of the brain after resuscitation can significantly reduce the possibility of secondary neurological injury and maximize the chances of full neurological recovery.

Laboratory Assessment

Laboratory investigations after CA should include determination of arterial blood gases, electrolytes, glucose, serum creatinine, blood urea nitrogen, magnesium, calcium, and cardiac enzyme levels. Other laboratory analyses should be dictated by the clinical situation. Disturbances in potassium and magnesium levels in patients resuscitated from CA have been seen in 30 and 42%, respectively, and may be responsible for postresuscitation dysrrhythmias *(456)*. Accordingly, treat abnormalities in electrolytes aggressively, which may lead to improved outcome.

Acid–Base Assessment

Metabolic acidemia should be corrected, as proper acid–base balances has been shown to improve cerebral and cardiovascular recovery *(54,457)*. The single most important approach to correcting increases in tissue CO_2 and lactate accumulation is to improve perfusion and ventilation. With adequate ventilation and reperfusion, the acidemia following CA will normally resolve without the need of buffer administration. Once coronary and cerebral perfusion are optimized, however, correction of profound acidosis is warranted. This can be accomplished with bicarbonate therapy with the understanding that overshoot alkalosis may be detrimental.

The use of arterial blood gases to guide therapy may be problematic after resuscitation. Although arterial PCO_2 and PO_2 are useful for monitoring pulmonary ventilation, there is increasing evidence that arterial blood may not reliably reflect tissue acid–base conditions during low perfusion states, and that central venous blood more accurately reflects conditions at the tissue level *(458)*. The reason for this is that blood in the arterial system that remains stagnant does not reflect ongoing intracellular metabolism until some perfusion is restored, so that arterial blood gas values remain constant for up to 13 minutes in a low-flow state *(459)*. Additionally, mixed venous blood gases are more useful than arterial blood gases for assessing blood flow during CPR, because they are much less affected than arterial gases by changes in minute ventilation *(460)*. Therefore, the metabolic derangements during CA is characterized not only by venous and tissue hypercapnic and metabolic acidemia but also by hypocapnic arterial alkalemia and has been termed the arteriovenous paradox *(461)*.

The use of sodium bicarbonate during or after a CA is discouraged because of its theoretical disadvantages, which may include metabolic alkalosis, hypernatremia, and the generation of CO_2 which produces a paradoxical cerebral acidosis, thereby potentially worsening the neuronal ischemia by oxygen-free radicals *(461)*. Besides other potential side effects, the additional hypercarbic load may theoretically depress myocardial resuscitability. However, the use of a buffer during reperfusion from CA has recently been shown to have no harm effects and in fact may have a beneficial effect on the cardiovascular function that can positively influence cerebral outcome *(462)*. In an animal model, after prolong VF of 10 minutes, administration of bicarbonate has been shown to improve ROSC with less defibrillation attempts and to improve CPP *(462)*.

Other agents have also been administered during or following CA. Carbicarb is a formulation of sodium bicarbonate ($NaHCO_3$) and sodium carbonate (Na_2CO_3) designed to neutralized systemic and tissue acidosis without producing CO_2 *(463)*. Carbicarb effectively neutralizes cerebral acidosis during CA without producing a paradoxical acidosis as seen with sodium bicarbonate administration *(464)*. Recent data has shown in an animal model of CA that administration of low dose Carbicarb (3 mL/kg) was associated with an attenuation of the acidosis, improved resuscitation, and reduced neurological deficits and neuronal cell death in the hippocampus *(465)*. However, high-dose Carbicarb (6 mL/kg) resulted in the opposite result with increase neuronal damage and worsening neurological deficits. A recent study showed that the administration of Tris buffer mixture, which is a mixture of Tris buffer (tromethamine), acetate, sodium bicarbonate and phosphate, mitigated postresuscitation cerebral acidosis *(466)*. However, earlier studies using the Tris buffer mixture or THAM (tromethamine) showed no change in resuscitation survival or markedly decrease resuscitation rates, respectively, despite effectively lowering the CO_2 content of the blood *(467)*. This may be explained because THAM induces arterial vasodilation and reduces systemic resistance with consequent decreases in MABP and CPP *(468)*. Therefore, the use of buffer agents in CA requires careful scrutiny before its administration can be fully recommended.

Glucose Assessment

Experimental data suggest that postischemic blood glucose concentration plays a vital role in modulating both cerebral ischemia and selective neuronal necrosis. Prolonged hypoglycemia (blood glucose <50 mg/dL in adults; <30 mg/dL in neonates) is deleterious to the brain *(43)*. Depending on its severity, hypoglycemia has three important effects on the CNS: (a) it invokes a counterregulatory stress response that is characterized by increases in plasma norepinephrine, epinephrine, glucagon, growth hormone, and cortisol levels; (b) it causes CBF impairment; and (c) it alters cerebral metabolism, ultimately leading to energy depletion and permanent brain injury *(469,470)*.

Increases in blood glucose concentration can impair neuronal recovery following ischemia. Severe hyperglycemia before and during global cerebral ischemia in animal models worsens neurological outcomes by increasing brain lactic acidosis and decreasing pH *(16,471,472)*. Hyperglycemia after ischemia impairs recovery of high-energy phosphates and causes greater delayed hypoperfusion *(471)*. In fact, an animal model of asphyxial arrest demonstrated that glucose and insulin administration may improve cerebral outcome *(473)*. High blood glucose concentrations occurring over the first 24 hours after CA in humans have been correlated with worsening functional neurological recovery *(474)*. Hyperglycemia increases progressively with duration of resuscitation. Because the duration of resuscitation is a well-known prognostic factor for outcome, it is unknown whether the hyperglycemia is just an epiphenomenon of prolonged resuscitation and not the cause of a poor outcome *(475)*. One study controlled for duration of resuscitation after witnessed arrest and still found a correlation between high glucose levels and deleterious neurological recovery *(474)*.

The cause of hyperglycemia after a CA in a nondiabetic patient or a patient not receiving exogenous glucose remains speculative. Hyperglycemia can generally occur from either elevated endogenous hormones release during CA or from exogenous administration of epinephrine *(476)*. Hyperglycemia enhances the translocation of PKC to cell membranes and this might contribute to the detrimental effects on neuronal injury following ischemia *(477)*. There is evidence that following a CA there is progressive decline in plasma insulin levels despite the presence of marked hyperglycemia *(478)*. Others have shown that glucose administration prior to ischemia induces mitochondrial dysfunction with mitochondrial release of cytochrome *c* to the cytoplasm, which leads to activation of caspase-3 and apoptosis *(479)*. Another proposed mechanism whereby hyperglycemia accentuates ischemic brain damage relates to an excessive production of tissue lactic acid or to an associated derangements in pH homeostasis *(480)*. With sufficient intracellular lactate accumulation, intracellular pH decreases, and this decrease may lead to compromised cellular function and cell death *(481)*. Cerebral lactic acidosis during brain ischemia and reperfusion may promote oxygen-free radical reactions *(482)*. Others have suggested the mechanism to be an increased BBB permeability or postischemic seizures *(483)*.

Presumably, excessive lactate production during hyperglycemic cerebral ischemia is caused by a greater acceleration of anaerobic glycolytic flux than that which occurs when the circulating glucose concentration is not increased. A recent report contradicts this mechanism. Rats given glucose infusion 120 minutes prior to arrest had neurological damage similar to control, but when glucose is administered 5 minutes prior to arrest, neurological damage was significantly higher *(484)*. Additionally, rats pretreated with glucose 120 minutes prior to arrest and also given α-cyano-4-hydroxycinnamate (4-CIN), an agent used to inhibit utilization of lactate, showed dramatic increases in neurological damage. These data stipulate that brain oxidative lactate utilization post-ischemia reduces the degree of delayed CA1 neuronal damage in the hippocampus. It can be further explained, that under aerobic conditions and in the absence of glucose during reperfusion and reoxygenation, lactate can easily enter the tricarboxylic acid cycle via pyruvate to maintain ATP reproduction as efficiently as glucose does. Hence, the very process aimed at supplying ATP to oxygen-deprived tissue has been promoted to be the one that causes the demise of that very tissue.

The "glucose paradox" of cerebral ischemia in which the aggravation of ischemic damage by post-ischemic hyperglycemia has been described, may not be actually the reason for hyperglycemic-induced neuronal damage *(485)*. Administration of metyrapone, a steroid biosynthesis inhibitor, has been shown to prevent the glucose-induced aggravation of cerebral injury and unmask the ability of glucose to protect against ischemic damage even when administered shortly pre-ischemia *(485)*. Pretreatment of hyperglycemic rats with the corticosterone synthesis inhibitor metyparone or the corticosterone receptor antagonist, RU38486, prevents hyperglycemic aggravation of ischemic neuronal damage *(486)*. Therefore, it seems that glucose-induced corticosterone release may be the culprit behind the glucose paradox. It also seems that glucose may have some neuroprotective effects because the glucose level in metyrapone-treated, glucose-loaded rats was as high as those rats loaded with glucose but not treated with metyrapone. Therefore, for the patient suffering a CA post-arrest monitoring and titration of blood glucose levels between 100 and 200 mg/dL seems reasonable. Not until further evaluation in humans can other recommendations be made safely.

Respiratory Support

In the postresuscitation phase, patients may experience various degrees of respiratory dysfunction. The lung is generally not considered to be a primary target of the ischemic and reperfusion injury following CA. Patients undergoing cardiopulmonary resuscitation, however, are liable to pulmonary complications stemming from attempts to establish an artificial airway, chest compression with potential injury to the ribs and intrathoracic viscera, and aspiration of gastric contents with subsequent development of pneumonia *(487)*. Pulmonary edema evident immediately after successful resuscitation has been reported in up to 30% of patients *(488)*. A clinical examination and review of the chest radiograph is essential. Meticulous attention should be made to discover complications of resuscitation, such as pneumothorax, pneumomediatinum, rib fractures, and dislodgement of the ET. Proper placement of an ET should be verified during the post-resuscitation phase.

Some patients (especially those who have depressed neurological function) will require mechanical ventilation and supplemental oxygen. Controlled ventilation for the comatose patient for at least 12 hours is favorable to prevent the development of cardiovascular-pulmonary failure. Ventilation should also be supported if there is evidence of significant respiratory distress with agitation, poor air exchange, cyanosis, hypercarbia, or hypoxemia. The level of ventilatory support, such inspiratory oxygen concentration, positive-end expiratory pressure (PEEP), and minute ventilation is determined by the blood gas analysis, respiratory rate, and perceived work of breathing. An arterial catheter may be required in patients requiring prolonged mechanical ventilation and to facilitate repeated arterial blood sampling. Additionally, systemic blood pressure can be accurately and continuously monitored from the arterial catheter. As spontaneous ventilation becomes more efficient, the level of ventilatory support can be weaned until respiration is entirely spontaneous.

Oxygenation

The amount of oxygenation required for a postresuscitation victim is unknown. Supplemental oxygen should be provided until it can be confirmed that oxygenation and oxygen-carrying capacity are satisfactory. Recent evidence suggests that neurological outcome after ischemia and reperfusion may be influenced greatly by the concentration of oxygen inspired immediately following ROSC. Even short periods of postresuscitative hyperoxia may contribute to delayed neuronal death and worsening neurological outcome after global cerebral ischemia. This has led to reconsideration of the prolonged use of 100% oxygen following resuscitation from CA *(489)*. The production of oxygen-derived free radicals may be proportional to PO_2 and the inspired fractions of O_2 (FiO_2) during the hyperemic phase of the postresuscitation period. In contrast, deficient or too low O_2 supply during resuscitation may cause cellular energy failure with further neuronal loss *(490)*. Therefore, it seems that a gradual reintroduction of oxygen during early resuscitation may reduce the neuronal postischemic reoxygenation injury *(491)*.

There is no evidence that arterial hyperoxia (PaO_2 >80–120 mmHg) is helpful for survival of the selectively vulnerable neurons. Oxygenation with 21% oxygen after recovery from CA has been shown to be equal to 100% oxygen *(492)*. In fact, reoxygenation with 100% was not superior to 21% oxygen in restoring tissue metabolism after critical hypoxia *(493)*. Reoxygenation, although essential and effective in restoring energy charge, also might provoke chemical cascades, especially the formation of free radicals and free iron that result in lipid peroxidation of membranes *(89,105,494)*. Because formation of reactive oxygen species (ROS) requires delivery of molecular oxygen to ischemic tissue, restricting inspired oxygen during reperfusion may decrease reperfusion lipid peroxidation and neurological damage *(489)*. In a recent animal model of global ischemia, hypoxemic reperfusion (PaO_2 = 35 mmHg) vs hyperoxemic reperfusion (PaO_2 >300 mmHg) showed significantly fewer histological changes in the brain *(495)*. In a neonatal animal model subjected to severe hypoxic insult reoxygenation with 100% oxygen showed increased arterial and venous hydrogen peroxide (H_2O_2) concentration in leukocytes and near normal levels when reoxygentaed with 21% oxygen *(496)*. Therefore, resuscitation with 100% oxygen after CA exacerbates neurological dysfunction when compared to normoxic (FiO_2 = 0.21) resuscitation *(497)*.

There is, however, one rat asphyxial model that did not show benefit from reducing the oxygen content during resuscitation from 100 to 21% *(498)*. The difference in this study was that the rat brains were examined at a longer time interval of 72 hours and it is well established that neuronal injury may develop over days after reperfusion *(32,499)*. In another neonatal animal model, the use of a hypoxemic resuscitation with an average oxygen concentration of 12 to 18%, was found to be more detrimental with increasing levels of extracellular aspartate and glutamate, when compared to the use of either 21 or 100% oxygen *(500)*. In a dog model, it was again shown that hypoxic resuscitation showed reduced overall survival and greater neurological deficit when compared to normoxic resuscitated dogs *(497)*. It seems appropriate to reduce the arterial oxygen concentrations to normal level, avoiding excessive oxygenation, immediately after resuscitation and to direct clinically intense effort toward maintaining normal arterial oxygenation throughout the hours and days following resuscitation. However, one must not lower the level below normal, which may actually worsen neurological damage *(497)*.

Rate of Ventilation

The rate of ventilation for the resuscitated patient has been a matter of controversy over the years. Hyperventilation was used originally as a procedure to reduce cerebral edema from head injury or global cerebral ischemia. It was shown in early studies to ameliorate neuronal damage from ischemia *(501)*. However, recent evidence supports the theory that sustained hypocapnea (low $PaCO_2$) may worsen cerebral ischemia *(502)*. Hyperventilation has been shown in animal models to correlate with worsening neurological outcomes *(503)*. After CA, restoration of blood flow results in an initial hyperemic blood flow response that lasts 5 to 40 minutes. This hyperemic phase is followed by a prolonged period of diminished blood flow. During this period of delayed hypoperfusion, a mismatch between oxygen demand and supply may occur. If the patient is hyperventilated at this stage, the additional cerebral vasoconstriction resulting from hypocapnea may further decrease CBF and worsen cerebral ischemia. The potential risk for cerebral ischemia is real and has been observed in traumatic head injuries *(504)*. Additionally, hyperventilation may generate airway pressures and auto-PEEP, leading to an increase in cerebral venous blood flow and ICPs *(505)*. The increase in cerebral vascular pressure results in a further decrease in CBF and a further worsening of cerebral ischemia. This mechanism has been shown to be independent of its effects on $PaCO_2$ or pH on cerebral vessel reactivity. Hyperventilation should be avoided after CA except in the rare circumstance when it may be used to treat acute herniation syndromes.

Hyperbaric Oxygenation

Despite growing evidence showing worsening neurological outcome with hyperoxia during postresuscitation after a CA, paradoxically there is limited evidence that hyperbaric oxygen (HBO) despite greatly elevating tissue oxygen can ameliorate reperfusion injury after global ischemia induced by vascular occlusion *(506)*. HBO therapy has been advocated as a method to improve tissue oxygen delivery, especially to areas of diminished blood flow, as seen in the postresuscitation phase *(507)*. It has been suggested that HBO can enhance neuronal viability by its ability to increase the amount of dissolved oxygen in the blood without significantly altering blood viscosity.

Postischemic hypoperfusion causes a mismatch between cerebral oxygen supply and demand. An increase in the cerebral extraction ratio occurs, which leads to a decrease in oxygenation in the brain's venous outflow. When cerebral oxygen extraction reaches a critical point, cerebral consumption decreases causing more ischemic damage. HBO has the potential to increase post-ischemic oxygen delivery, theoretically overcoming postresuscitative delivery-dependent cerebral ischemia.

The ability of HBO to improve neurological recovery after cerebral injury is controversial, as studies in animals and humans have yielded conflicting results *(507,508)*. Some of the discrepancy in the results of these studies is as a result of the fact that the investigators vary in the time after insult at which HBO was given, many depths and duration of exposure have been used, and most studies have not had adequate controls. In several models of ischemia and reperfusion, HBO has been shown to reduce cerebral edema, decrease neutrophil adherence to the endothelium, decrease lipid peroxidation, maintain the BBB integrity, and cause increased activity of SOD *(509–511)*. However, the role of inflammation after global ischemia is not understood well and the importance of HBO-mediated prevention of leukocyte migration into the brain after ischemia and reperfusion remains unclear. HBO may also alter gene expression that may be neuroprotective. HBO prior to ischemia causes elevation of brain levels of *Bcl-2*, an anti-apoptotic protein, and Mn-SOD, an enzyme that detoxifies ROS *(512)*. Additionally, HBO downregulates the expression of cyclooxygenase-2, a potential source of toxic ROS that has been implicated in post-ischemic oxidative stress *(513)*.

Others investigators have shown that hyperbaric therapy after ischemia does not ameliorate the morphological or functional recovery of neurons *(514)*. Additionally, a human trial of HBO therapy for stroke had a worsened outcome *(515)*. In stark contrast, a recent trial of HBO after VF arrest in a beagle model showed for the first time improved neurological function and reduction in neuronal cell death *(516)*. This was the first CA model as opposed to using vessel occlusion to simulate global ischemia. Neuroprotection in this model does not seem to result from increased cerebral oxygen delivery or oxygen consumption. In fact, normalization of cerebral oxygen extraction with HBO occurred without an increase in oxygen consumption. This suggests, as others have seen, that there may not be ongoing ischemia during post-ischemic hypoperfusion *(517)*. After global ischemia, therefore, energy metabolism may not be limited by oxygen delivery but rather by the activity of aerobic metabolic enzymes *(518)*.

Cardiovascular Support

After ROSC, as stated earlier it is important to determine whether the patient is suffering from a myocardial infarction. Standard 12-lead and right-sided electrocardiograms (ECGs) should be obtained as soon as possible to search for ongoing ischemia. Without an appropriate history, it may be difficult to determine whether evidence of ischemia on the ECG is the cause or result of the CA. Treatment for the post-arrest patient suffering from a myocardial infarction is obviously optimized if a well-thought out multidisciplinary approach is already established. Patients who have had less than 10 minutes of CPR without evidence of significant CPR-induced trauma and who are not in cardiogenic shock should be considered for fibrinolytic therapy (519). Patients who have had more than 10 minutes of CPR or sustained significant CPR trauma or are in cardiogenic shock should be considered for immediate angioplasty or stenting. Without effective revascularization strategies, myocardial dysfunction is likely to worsen and lead to hypoperfusion of many organs, including the brain. Heparin and aspirin may be given if there is no evidence of hemorrhage or profound hypertension. Nitrates and β-blockers as an adjunctive therapy in the hypotensive patient are best administered when guided by invasive hemodynamic monitoring.

Initial cardiovascular evaluation must include a complete heart and vascular examination with continual monitoring of vital signs and urine output. The clinical signs of
circulatory dysfunction include tachycardia, hypotension, delayed distal perfusion, cool
extremities, and abnormal extremity color. If the patient's hemodynamic condition is
unstable, assess both circulating fluid volume and ventricular function. Avoid even mild
hypotension because it can impair recovery of cerebral function. Noninvasive assessment of blood pressure may be inaccurate in patients with poor cardiac output and concomitant peripheral vasoconstriction. Intra-arterial assessment of blood pressure is
usually more accurate in these patients and allows better titration of catecholamine infusions. In the presence of severe vasoconstriction, blood pressure measurement from
radial artery may be inaccurate, and a femoral artery catheter may be required.

Persistent circulatory dysfunction is observed often after resuscitation from CA (6,7).
In fact, most patients in the postresuscitation state suffer from some degree of shock
(520). This phenomenon represents a form of global myocardial stunning in which varying degrees of reversible systolic and diastolic dysfunction develop following resuscitation from CA. Restoration of prearrest myocardial function may take hours, days, or even
weeks. Studies in animals and in humans have shown that mortality after CA may be
partly as a result of persistent heart failure or dysrhythmias (521). A low perfusion state
could also be linked, however, to the precipitating etiology of the CA. Despite achieving
normalization of blood pressure, central venous pressure, and heart rate, some patients
will have continued myocardial dysfunction and exhibit poor oxygenation or perfusion.
Persistent myocardial dysfunction occurring after restoration of perfusion is contingent
on the severity and duration of the ischemic insult (522). During CA and resuscitation,
severity of cardiac injury depends on the interval between arrest and the start of CPR and
the efficacy of the resuscitation efforts. Prevention of the postresuscitation myocardial
dysfunction is contingent on decreasing the downtime and increasing blood flow to the
myocardium during CPR. Early identification of the postresuscitation myocardial dysfunction is a critical issue for its management and secondarily improvement cerebral
outcome.

In the initial evaluation and treatment of a critically ill resuscitated patient, in addition
to monitoring the blood pressure, heart rate, and urine output; central venous pressure
helps guide resuscitative efforts. Despite normalization of these variables, some patients
will have persistent global tissue hypoxia, which has been implicated in the development
of multiorgan failure and increased mortality. Derangements in oxygen transport are best
detected and managed by appropriate hemodynamic monitoring. All patients with successful resuscitation should have adequate oxygenation and tissue perfusion assured,
with use of volume expansion and vasopressor therapy as required. Therapy in these cases
should be guided by right heart catheterization, central venous oximetry, and lactate
levels. Additionally, calculations of the shock index (heart rate/systolic arterial pressure)
can be used to assess the adequacy of tissue oxygenation and cardiac function (523).
Echocardiogram can aid in determining abnormalities in wall motion and cardiac output.
In recent years, transthoracic echocardiography (TTE) has emerged as a noninvasive
technique for assessing LV function. In most critically ill patients, however, TTE is too
time consuming or provides inadequate images because of limitations imposed by
mechanical ventilation, lung disease, and positioning. By contrast, transesophageal
echocardiography (TEE) provides excellent images of the heart in critically ill patients
by monitoring from a retrocardiac location in the distal esophagus and proximal stomach.

TEE offers an accurate and reliable assessment of cardiac preload, global and regional right and left ventricular wall motion and the pericardium. Although TEE is not totally without risk, it is minimally invasive and is probably associated with fewer complications than pulmonary arterial catheterization *(524)*.

During CPR a high-oxygen extraction ratio has been demonstrated, which is consistent with the low delivery state during external chest compressions *(525)*. During the postresuscitation period after CA, a decline in oxygen extraction has been demonstrated with corresponding increases in central venous oxygen saturation *(526)*. Postresuscitation venous hyperoxia is associated with poor outcome and reflects a postresusciation extraction defect and a phenomenon well explained in patients with septic shock and acute respiratory distress syndrome *(527)*. During the postresuscitation period, the goal is to provide an environment conducive to repaying the oxygen debt incurred following the global hypoperfusion of CA.

In critically ill patients, invasive hemodynamic monitoring is often undertaken with a pulmonary artery catheter. The use of these devices is controversial, however, these catheters permit measurements of the pulmonary circulation and cardiac output *(528)*. If both cardiac output and pulmonary artery occlusive pressures are low, fluid challenge with reassessment of pressures and cardiac output is indicated. In patients with myocardial infarction, ventricular compliance may be reduced and ventricular filling pressure increased. Evidence of both systolic and diastolic dysfunction is present after CA. Higher than normal filling pressures may be necessary to optimize LV preload. If optimization of preload does not result in a physiologically adequate cardiac output and systemic oxygen delivery, administration of pharmacologic agents to increase contractility are indicated. If hypotension or hypoperfusion persists after filling pressure is optimized, inotropic (dobutamine), vasopressor (dopamine or norepinephrine), vasodilator (nitroprusside or nitroglycerin), or combinaton inotropic/vasodilator (amrinone, milrinone) therapy may be indicated *(529)*. To prevent mesenteric or renal ischemia from using vasopressin or other vasopressors, low-dose dopamine has been shown to increase splanchnic blood flow and renal function *(530)*. Vasodilators may be required in the postresuscitation state to control excessive hypertension or improve flow by reducing afterload. Because hypertension may occur in the presence of volume depletion, preload should be optimized before vasodilator therapy is instituted *(531)*.

If hypotension is persistent, administration of vasopressors to maintain perfusion pressures may actually increase myocardial oxygen demand above supply, which might result in extension of the infarct or promote dysrhythmias and lead to further complications including rearrest. Other hemodynamic supporting measures such as mechanical support techniques for the heart should be considered in patients with low-flow states to increase oxygen delivery and utilization without placing a further burden on the ischemic heart with the use of vasopressors. The purpose is to restore hemodynamic stability when less invasive methods and especially pharmacologic interventions fail. These may be performed with the IABP, CPB, Hemopump, or ventricular assist devices *(406,532)*.

In addition to thermodilution pulmonary arterial catheter (PAC) and echocardiographic methods, many other methods have been developed to monitor cardiac output. Non-invasive techniques include thoracic bioelectrical impedance (TBI), aortic continuous wave Doppler, partial CO_2 rebreathing, and MRI. However, the use of these techniques still requires further evaluation in patients after CA.

Dysrhythmias are common in the postresuscitation phase and some may require therapy. Sinus tachycardia with increased supraventricular and ventricular ectopic activity is frequent encountered during the early postresuscitation phase. Unless these abnormalities compromise hemodynamic stability, they should not be treated because they usually subside after the myocardial ischemia and after the effects of endogenous and exogenous catecholamines recede. Ventricular dysrhythmias can be treated with either amiodarone or lidocaine and prophylaxis with these agents should be considered when ventricular tachycardia and VF is the precipitating cause of CA or if anti-arrhythmic administration was required to successfully convert the patient (533). Adenosine has become the drug of choice for treatment of atrial tachydysrhythmias (534). Accordingly, other forms of tachycardia may require therapy to decrease the heart rate, such as amiodarone, β-blockers, or calcium channel blockers. If hemodynamically significant bradycardia is present, initiate therapy to improve the heart rate, including atropine sulphate, dobutamine, or pacemaker, either transcutaneous or transvenous.

Cerebral Blood Flow Promotion and Hypertension

There has been keen interest in maintaining a brief period of immediate postarrest hypertension (535). Most patients will undergo a brief period postarrest hypertension secondary to the circulation of adrenergic agents given during the CA, especially if high-dose epinephrine was administered. Elevated arterial blood pressure has been shown to open up blood vessels and overcome the no-reflow phenomenon during reperfusion (57,531,536,537). The immediate post-arrest no-reflow is most likely caused by blood sludging or thrombosis (324,538). The no-reflow phenomenon seems to be accentuated only with hypotensive reperfusion. It is unknown if it actually occurs in scattered areas of the brain with normotensive reperfusion and seem to be abolished with hypertensive reperfusion (57). Additionally, hypertension has been shown to delay the onset of apoptosis (539).

In a cat model, after 1 hour of global ischemia, elevated reperfusion pressure (MABP >140 mmHg) correlated with recovery of EEG activity (540). In a dog study, a brief hypertensive period (MABP 150–200 mmHg for 1–5 minutes) followed by controlled normotension abolished evidence of immediate no-reflow and correlated with improved neurological outcome (57,536). The addition of mild hypothermia (34°C) with a 1-hour induced hypertension after resuscitation in an animal model improved survival up to 4 weeks (541).

A strategy known as cerebral blood promotion, which includes the use of induced moderate hypertension, mild hemodilution, and normocapnia plus resuscitative hypothermia, has been shown to improve cerebral outcome (24). This technique has been shown to increase reperfusion pressure by hypertension and reduce blood cerebral viscosity by hemodilution, which results in improved CBF and less cerebral dysfunction (24,57). In a dog model of VF with 12 minutes of no-flow and external CPR, followed by an immediate post-CPR combination of norepinephrine-induced hypertension, intracarotid hemodilutaion with dextran 40, and heparinization, improved neurological outcomes (24). Besides the anticoagulatory effect of heparin, dextran decreases platelet adhesiveness and promotes endogenous fibrinolysis (542). The rationale for hemodilution after CA is that blood flow is inversely proportional to blood viscosity, which increases in the microcirculation during cerebral ischemia. Hematocrit is the primary element influencing blood viscosity. Hemodilution reduces the viscosity of blood, which varies directly with the third power of the hematocrit and the square of the fibrinogen concentration.

Additionally, it has been shown to reduce the release of troponin I and cerebral protein s-100 after CA in a porcine model *(543)*. Reperfusion accompanied by hypertension plus hemodilution for several hours normalizes the local, multifocal, cerebral hypoperfusion post-arrest, but without mild hypothermia, by itself shows inconsistent improved cerebral outcome *(57,544)*.

A drawback to hemodilution is that if the hematocrit is lowered too much, the oxygen-carrying capacity of the blood is diminished, which may increase cerebral ischemic damage. Additional drawbacks is that the globally impaired myocardium cannot generally tolerate it and this technique may theoretically increase the development of vasogenic edema *(545,546)*. Additionally, severe hypertension (MABP >150 mmHg) correlates with worsening neurological recovery after global brain ischemia *(546)*. Although induced hypertension has not been formally tested in a clinical trial in humans, it is known that early post-arrest hypertension was an independent predictor of good cerebral outcome, whereas hypotension after ROSC correlated with poor cerebral outcome *(537)*. However, the optimal reperfusion pressure has not yet been determined. Even though systemic induced hypertension has not been formally studied, nevertheless, if immediately after ROSC there is a period of hypertension, aggressive therapy may not be indicated initially but should be instituted after 15 to 30 minutes, or if there is excessive hypertension (MABP >150 mmHg) or if there is evidence of heart failure *(537,547,548)*.

If induced postresuscitation hypertension is considered, a titrated intravenous infusion of either epinephrine or norepinephrine may be more effective than phenyephrine or dopamine. Additionally, there is some data to suggest that norepinephrine may be less arrhythmogenic *(533)*.

Temperature Regulation

Tissue temperature during and after cerebral ischemia has a major influence on cerebral outcome.

Hyperthermia

Regional cerebral metabolic rate determines the regional blood flow requirements of the brain. The cerebral metabolic rate increases approx 8% with every degree Celsius elevation of body temperature *(549)*. Because increasing metabolic demand may worsen neurological damage in a state of low blood flow, it is not surprising that the presence of hyperthermia after brain ischemia is associated with worse neurological outcomes *(550)*. Additionally, the denaturing effect of hyperthermia on proteins may exacerbate structural and biochemical damage.

Numerous experimental models demonstrate worsening brain injury if brain temperature is increased during ischemia or postresuscitation *(15,550,551)*. Furthermore, within the first 24 hours after resuscitation, hyperthermia has been shown to be damaging to neurons, but not if it occurs after 24 hours *(550,552)*.

After successful resuscitation, hyperthermia may occur spontaneously or may occur from bacteremia or pulmonary infection *(549,553)*. Hyperthermia must be treated aggressively after a successful resuscitation with active cooling to achieve a normal core temperature as soon as possible. Shivering that may occur from cooling will further increase metabolic demand and should be treated aggressively. Sedation may be adequate to control shivering, but neuromuscular blockade may be needed. If a patient requires neuromusclar blockade, a cerebral function monitor or continuous EEG to detect the possibility of seizure activity may be required.

Hypothermia

Hypothermia, in contrast, has been shown to be an effective method in suppressing cerebral metabolic activity. Mild resuscitative hypothermia currently is the only monotherapy that has been shown to ameliorate cerebral damage associated with CA in human subjects. It has been postulated to attenuate most, if not all of the mechanisms responsible for the injury associated with ischemic and reperfusion. Although previously used widely during cardiovascular surgery, hypothermia has some significant detrimental effects that have to be cautioned against its widespread use *(554)*. Side effects of hypothermia have included increased blood viscosity, coagulopathy, impaired cardiac function, dysrhythmias, shivering, abnormalities in vasopressor function, and increased susceptibility to infection *(555–557)*. As hypothermia is induced, there is the fear that an increase in blood viscosity would result in an increase in cerebral vascular resistance and potentially worsen the hypoxia state *(558)*. The prevalence and severity of these side effects is proportional to the depth and duration of hypothermia. Investigators inducing mild hypothermia (33–35°C) have not reported significant hypothermia-related side effects.

Protective-preservative hypothermia (i.e., induction of hypothermia during CA) was first evaluated in the 1940s to 1950s. Cerebral protection and preservation via induced hypothermia prevented post-ischemic brain injury following total circulatory arrest in the setting of cardiothoracic or neurological surgery. Moderate hypothermia (30°C), induced prearrest, protects the brain during no flow for up to 20 minutes *(559)*. Moderate hypothermia induced immediately after the ischemic insult yielded unconvincing results after CA in dogs and patients *(560)*. On the other hand, deep hypothermia (15°C) was detrimental with worsening cerebral and cardiac outcomes and therefore was discontinued because of its side effects *(561)*.

Interest in hypothermic research remained dormant between the 1960s and 1980s as a result of the associated side effects with moderate hypothermia. Interest in hypothermia as a treatment modality for brain injury was rekindled in the 1980–1990s after the initial studies of drug therapy for cerebral resuscitation after CA were disappointing. After carefully performed experimental animal models of brain injury and CA showed that even mild intra-ischemic hypothermia could be neuroprotective and reduce the pathological consequences of brain ischemia after CA, hypothermic research bloomed *(561–565)*. Other investigators showed that mild resuscitative hypothermia could reduce histologic damage in hippocampal and other vulnerable brain areas after global brain ischemia *(565,566)*. In fact, even cooling the brain as little as 1°C during cerebral ischemia can produce measurable neurological benefit *(567)*.

The mechanism by which hypothermia protects and preserves the brain after an ischemic and reperfusion injury is not so clear; and considered after numerous experimental models to be multifactorial *(563)*. The ability of hypothermia to reduce cerebral metabolic rate by 5 to 8°C alone is not enough explanation for its protective effects *(568)*. It is known that mild hypothermia after CA does not mitigate the post-arrest cerebral oxygen supply and demand mismatching and does not improve patterns of restricted CBF *(569,570)*. Even with mild to moderate hypothermia, the brain's small oxygen stores are rapidly depleted. Hypothermia has been shown to:

1. preserve ATP
2. improve glucose utilization
3. mitigate intraneuronal calcium mobilization

4. reduce excitatory neurotransmitter release
5. reduce production of superoxide anions and attenuate free-radical reactions
6. inhibit the accumulation of lipid peroxidation products
7. reduce production of NO
8. reduce lactate production and tissue acidosis
9. attenuate post-ischemic CBF disturbances
10. reduce ICP
11. reduce amount of neutrophil migration into ischemic areas
12. reduce post-ischemic cytotoxic and vasogenic edema
13. decrease expression of heat shock proteins (i.e., *hsp-70*)
14. accelerate expression of early genes hypothesized to participate in neuronal recovery from damage
15. attenuate injury of microtubule-associated protein 2 needed for cross-linking of the neuronal cytoskeleton
16. protect fluidity of the plasma lipoprotein membranes *(15,55,565,571–580)*.

Recently, hypothermia has been shown to increase the levels of brain-derived neurotrophic factor (BDNF), a growth factor known to mitigate neuronal injury after both focal and global ischemia *(581)*. Mild hypothermia also inhibits apoptosis, although more severe hypothermia may actually induce apoptosis *(582)*.

The ability to improve neurological outcomes by cooling brain-injured humans was first shown when a randomized, controlled trial comparing the effects of moderate hypothermia (23–33°C) for 24 hours with normothermia in 82 patients with severe closed-head injuries *(583)*. A study of 22 adults who were cooled to 33°C by surface cooling with ice packs after ROSC for 12 hours. These patients were compared with historical normothermic patients, which demonstrated improvement in neurological outcome (50 vs 13%) and reduction in mortality rate *(584)*. Following this preliminary study, a prospective, randomized trial of induced hypothermia in comatose survivors of out-of-hospital CA was performed *(585)*. There were 43 patients randomized to hypothermia (33°C for 12 hours) compared to 34 patients in the normothermic group. Once again, better outcomes was seen in the hypothermic group (49 vs 26%, $p = 0.046$) which correlated with an odds ratio for good outcome of 5.25 (95% confidence interval [CI] 1.47–18.76). Patients in the hypothermic, however, had more episodes of decreased cardiac output.

Two prospective randomized trials compared mild hypothermia with normothermia in comatose survivors of out-of-hospital CA in Europe and Australia *(585,586)*. In the European multicenter randomized trial of successfully resuscitated patients from VF, 136 patients were randomly assigned to undergo therapeutic hypothermia (32–34°C) over a period of 24 hours and 137 patients received standard treatment with normothermia *(586)*. Cooling was initiated at a median of 105 minutes after ROSC, and the target temperature of 32–34°C was not achieved until an average of 8 hours after ROSC. The results clearly showed that therapeutic mild hypothermia increased the rate of favorable neurological outcome and reduced mortality. Hypothermic patients also had a lower 6-month mortality rate, with 41% in the hypothermic group vs 55% in the normothermic group (relative risk [RR] 0.74, 95% CI 0.58–0.95). Additionally, 55% in the hypothermia group had a favorable neurological outcome at 6 months compared to 39% in the normothermic group (RR 1.40, 95% CI 1.08–1.81).

Patients in the Australian trial were randomized to even vs odd days after being successfully resuscitated in the prehospital setting. In this study, surface cooling was begun in the field and the target temperature was reached with 2 hours of ROSC. It again showed similar findings of improved neurological outcomes and survival with therapeutic hypothermia (33°C for 12 hours) *(585)*. In this study, 49% treated with hypothermia has good neurological function at discharge compared with 26% in the normothermic group (RR 1.85, 95% CI 0.97–3.34). Mortality at discharge was 51% in the hypothermia group and 68% in the normothermic group (RR 0.76, 95% CI 0.52–1.10). Importantly, in neither study was hypothermia associated with deleterious side effects such as sepsis, bleeding, severe electrolyte disturbances or myocardial dysfunction. One finding that may be of concern is that hypothermic patients had more hyperglycemia than normothermic patients *(585,586)*. If hypothermia is used, careful monitoring should be performed to prevent hyperglycemia.

Both of these studies included a highly selected group of patients, excluding up to 92% of patients with out-of-hospital CA. Those excluded included persistent hypotension, and other causes of coma other than CA, such as head injury, drug overdose, or stroke. Other limitations included that the health care providers could not be blinded to treatment with hypothermia. After a period of hypothermia, patients are slowly rewarmed by active methods such as heated air blankets, which may produce shivering. Sedation and paralytic agents are routinely used for prevention of shivering and subsequent heat production, which may potentially lead to respiratory infection if used for a prolonged period, especially in pediatric patients *(587)*. Also during induction of hypothermia there may be mild shivering, which generally responds to sedation, but on occasion may require paralytic agents.

These human trials from a clinical perspective should be considered landmark research in the field of cerebral resuscitation because to date no resuscitative therapy has ever been proven to be effective in ameliorating cerebral ischemic injury. However, although these results are encouraging, one cannot assume that similar neurological improvement of mild resuscitative hypothermia can be achieved for all other types of CA. These studies only included patients with CA after dysrhythmia. Thus, patients with other causes of arrest such as sepsis, cardiogenic shock, trauma, or asphyxia may not respond as well and deserve to be evaluated.

Despite a wealth of animal models and limited human data on the effectiveness of hypothermia in cerebral outcome, therapeutic cooling has not yet achieved widespread use during human resuscitation. This may be explained partly by questions about its feasibility and time to reach therapeutic hypothermia, especially when most deaths occur outside of the hospital setting. Also, there is a belief that profound or prolonged cooling is necessary for therapeutic benefit. There have been recent studies showing the feasibility of controlled cooling with the use of numerous techniques, including ice bags, helmet, or blanket and a mattress *(588,589)*. Systemic surface cooling with a water-circulating blanket is the most widely used method. Although it is simple and feasible, it is unreliable and several hours usually elapse before temperatures reach the desired level of hypothermia, and obese patients are often refractory to this technique of cooling *(590)*. Selective head cooling, using ice bags applied to the head and neck or a specialized cooling helmet, although free of the adverse effects associated with systemic surface cooling, does not effectively lower cerebral temperature in adult population but is effective in newborns. This may be as a result of the smaller body surface area of neonates *(591)*. Cooling from inside the body, through either the intravenous or intra-arterial route, is an alternative method that has the potential to induce hypothermia more rapidly than surface cooling. Infusion of a 40 mL kg ice-cold saline solution (4°C) over a 30-minute period through a central venous catheter decreased core temperature by 2.5°C in healthy volunteers

(592). Although the method is simple, it remains unclear whether administration of a large volume of cold saline solution over a 30-minute period can be tolerated by critically ill patients when compromised cardiac functions exists. However, recently a report of a clinical trial using rapid infusion of large-volume (30 mL/kg), ice-cold (4°C) lactated Ringer's solution in comatose survivors of out-of-hospital CA resulted in a decreased core temperature by 1.6°C over 25 minutes *(593).* It was also associated with improved MABP, renal function, and acid–base. Extracorporeal cooling is a complicated method that necessitates the use of an extracorporeal pump and circuit, and routine use may not be readily available. Nevertheless, it has been demonstrated to improve survival after prolonged CA in dogs and its ability to restore circulation can be helpful in patients resuscitated after out-of-hospital CA. Newer techniques that may be promising include ice water nasal lavage, direct carotid infusion of cold fluids, and peritoneal cooling *(594).*

If these techniques are used, core temperature monitoring must be used to avoid excessive hypothermia. External auditory canal temperature could provide an approximation to brain temperature. The most accurate method that reflects brain temperature, however is by a thermocouple imbedded in a ventriculostomy catheter, a central pulmonary artery thermistor probe or jugular vein temperature, but these techniques are more invasive *(595).* Although many experimental studies measured brain temperature, most clinical studies measure core (bladder or rectal) temperature instead of brain temperature because of fear of infection and additional brain damage resulting from insertion of a thermosensor. Although the core temperature is simple to measure, it should be noted that it is usually 0.3 to 1.1°C lower than brain temperature, and this difference may widen during hypothermia *(596).*

The therapeutic time window or optimal duration for resuscitative hypothermia is yet unknown. The earliest possible time for induction of mild hypothermia following a CA seems desirable. Animal data suggest that the sooner cooling is initiated after reperfusion from CA, the better the outcome, although an impressive therapeutic benefit was also demonstrated in clinical studies when cooling was delayed for several hours *(594).* In rats with induced partial ischemic injury, histologic brain damage was mitigated when cooling was initiated within 5 minutes *(597).* Others have, however, shown improved outcome after temporary global brain ischemia even after hypothermia was induced at 2 hours in rats or 6 hours in gerbils *(573,597).* Therefore, different types of ischemic insults and animal species used have an effect on the therapeutic window for hypothermia, making it more difficult to translate to humans. Additionally, the optimal duration of mild hypothermia is also quite controversial. Hypothermia has been shown to be better if performed for greater than 12 hours then for only 1–2 hours *(561,563,564).* Rat studies suggested that 4 hours of mild hypothermia may only delay the loss of neurons; but 24 hours seems to afford permanent benefit *(598,599).* Patients can tolerate therapeutic mild to moderate hypothermia of 24 hours *(600).* Dogs or monkeys have developed complications, such as pulmonary infection or coagulopathy with moderate hypothermia of greater than 24 hours duration *(601,602).* It is not clear whether mild hypothermia can also cause these complications. Further research is needed to determine optimal duration of therapeutic hypothermia, optimum target temperature, and rates of cooling and rewarming.

The Advanced Life Support Task Force of the International Liaison Committee on Resuscitation has recently recommended that unconscious adult patients with spontaneous circulation after out-of-hospital CA be cooled to 32–34°C for 12 to 24 hours when the initial rhythm is VF *(603).* These recommendations do not include infants or children.

However, it seems reasonable if the infant or child has mild hypothermia post-ROSC not to try to raise the temperature with radiant lights. A considerable body of evidence suggests that even a mild elevation in temperature after a CA is detrimental *(550,552)*. On the contrary, mild hypothermia may be beneficial and using only mild hypothermia should not be associated with significant adverse effects. Those with more moderate hypothermia (<33°C) should have passive rewarming until temperature is above 33°C.

SUMMARY

Cerebral dysfunction occurs after global ischemia and reperfusion, such as with CA and resuscitation. Ischemia results in rapid loss of high-energy phosphates and generalized depolarization. Selectively vulnerable neurons are vulnerable to both voltage-dependent calcium channels and glutamate-regulated calcium channels. Activation of these channels allow a massive increase in intracellular calcium to occur. This leads to the initiation of lipolysis, a process that occurs more intensely in the selectively vulnerable neurons. Early during reperfusion, a burst of excess production of oxygen-free radicals occur, and iron is released from storage proteins by reduction. The availability of this transition metal allows initiation of lipid peroxidation of the plasmalemma, which is once again localized to the selectively vulnerable neurons. The vulnerable neurons respond with transcription products for heat shock proteins and immediate-early genes, a response that is directed at enhancing the competence of antioxidant effects and membrane repair. However, translation initiation is deeply suppressed by alterations in regulatory phosphorylation of initiation factors, and therefore the transcriptional response does not result in translation of the appropriate protein products. Activation of caspases leads to apoptosis and under these circumstances the process of membrane damage during reperfusion proceed unchecked, leading to neuronal death.

Artificial perfusion is the principal weak link in the resuscitation armamentarium. Methods of newer lifesaving CPR techniques and devices must be developed to improve the likelihood of successful resuscitation. Some of these techniques have shown some improvement in neurological outcome and should be used more extensively such as ACD-CPR, IAC-CPR, and CPB. Cerebral dysfunction following a CA is contingent on the severity and duration of the ischemic insult. The shorter the interval between onset of CA and restoration of systemic and therefore CBF, the greater is the success of resuscitation and hospital discharge with a better neurological outcome. Accordingly, the prevention of the postresuscitation cerebral dysfunction is dependent on decreasing the downtime and increasing the perfusion to the brain and heart during CPR. To achieve these goals there should be an early activation of the emergency medical services, early basic CPR, early defibrillation, and early advanced life support.

With a better understanding of the pathophysiologic processes involved in neuronal damage from ischemia and reperfusion, it should be possible in the near future to design effective clinical strategies to improve neurological outcome significantly after CA and resuscitation. It is evident that the mechanisms for neuronal damage after a CA are multifactorial. Monotherapy toward a single mechanism that has characterized the numerous research approaches in the past is unlikely going to ameliorate the damage. A logistical approach should include a multi-drug therapeutic approach. This approach may include the use of: EAA receptor blockers, barbiturates, calcium channel antagonists, oxygen-free radical inhibitors, protein synthesis modulators, peptide growth factors, inhibition of calpain, caspase inhibition, inhibitors of neuronal apoptosis, inhibitors of vasoconstrictive mediators, leukocytes, and coagulation factors, and CBF promotion techniques (hypertension, hemodilution, normocapnia). Such a multifactorial therapeutic approach to the molecular injury mechanisms now appears essential for the development of substantially improved clinical treatment for brain ischemia and reperfusion. Thus far, only mild hypothermia has been shown to be the most promising method, which by itself attacks many of the mechanisms implicated in neuronal damage. This method should be instituted as soon as possible. Future CPR research is needed to focus on finding methods that are feasible not only in the hospital but also in the prehospital setting.

REFERENCES

1. White BC, Grossman LI, O'Neil BJ, et al. Global brain ischemia and reperfusion. Ann Emerg Med 1996; 27:588–594.
2. Singh NC, Kochanek PM, Schiding JK, Melick JA, Nemoto EM: Uncoupled cerebral blood flow and metabolism after severe global ischemia in rats. J Cereb Blood Flow Metab 1992; 12:802–808.
3. Safar P. Brain resuscitation. Special symposium issue. Crit Care Med 1978; 6:199–214.
4. Abramson NS, Sutton-Tyrell K, Safar P. A randomized clinical study of a calcium-entry blocker (lidoflazine) in the treatment of comatose survivors of cardiac arrest. Brain Resuscitation Clinical Trial II Study Group. N Engl J Med 1991; 324:1225–1231.
5. Eisenberg MS, Horwood BT, Cummins RO, Reynolds-Haertle TR. Cardiac arrest and resuscitation: a tale of 29 cities. Ann Emerg Med 1990; 19:179–186.
6. Lucking SE, Pollack MM, Fields AI. Shock following generalized hypoxic-ischemic injury in previously healthy infants and children. J Pediatr 1986; 108:359–364.
7. Kern KB, Hilwig RW, Berg RA, et al. Postresuscitaion left ventricular dysfunction systolic and diastolic dysfunction: treatment with dobutamine. Circulation 1997; 95:2610–2613.
8. ACCP-SCCM Consensus Conference Definitions for sepsis and organ failure and guidelines for the use of innovative therapies in sepsis. Chest 1992; 101:1644–1655.
9. Oppert M, Gleiter CH, Müller C, et al. Kinetics and characteristics of an acute phase response following cardiac arrest. Intensive Care Med 1999; 25:1386–1394.
10. Shapiro HM: Intracranial hypertension, therapeutic and anesthetic considerations. Anesthesiology 1975; 43:445–471.
11. Cantu RC, Ames A, DiGancinto G, et al: Hypotension: a major factor limiting recovery from cerebral ischemia. J Surg Res 1969; 9:525–529.
12. Enna B, Wenzel V, Schocke M, et al. Excellent coronary perfusion pressure during cardiopulmonary resuscitation is not good enough to ensure long-term survival with good neurological outcome: a porcine case report. Resuscitation 2000; 47:41–49.
13. Homer-Vanniasinkam S, Crinnion JN, Gough MJ. Post-ischemic organ dysfunction: a review. Eur J Vasc Endovasc Surg 1997; 14:195–203.
14. Nielsen VG, Tan S, Baird MS, McCammon AT, Parks DA. Gastric intramucosal pH and multiple organ injury: impact of ischemia-reperfusion and xanthine oxidase. Crit Care Med 1996; 24:1339–1344.
15. Safar P. Cerebral resuscitation after cardiac arrest: A review. Circulation 1986; 74(Suppl):IV138–IV153.
16. Charlat MI, O'Neill PG, Hartley CJ, Roberts R, Bolli R. Prolonged abnormalities of the left ventricular diastolic wall thinning in the "stunned" myocardium in conscious dogs: time course and relation to systolic function. J Am Coll Cardiol 1989; 13:185–194.
17. Eisenberg MS, Bergner L, Hallstrom AP. Out-of-hospital cardiac arrest: improved survival with paramedics services. Lancet 1980; 1:812–815.
18. AHA medical/scientific statement: improving survival from sudden cardiac arrest: the "chain of survival" concept. Circulation 1991; 83:1832–1847.
19. Lee SK, Vaagenes P, Safar P, Stezoski SW, Scanlon M. Effect of cardiac arrest time on cortical cerebral blood flow during subsequent standard external cardiopulmonary resuscitation in rabbits. Resuscitation 1989; 17:105–117.
20. Bircher N, Safar P, Stewart R. A comparison of standard, "MAST"-augmented and open chest CPR in dogs. A preliminary investigation. Crit Care Med 1980; 8:147–152.
21. Safar P. Cerebral resuscitation after cardiac arrest: research initiatives and future direction. Ann Emerg Med 1993; 22:324–349.
22. Negovsky VA. Postresuscitation disease. Crit Care Med 1988; 16:942–946.

23. Beckman JS, Minor RL Jr, White CW, Repine JE, Rosen GM, Freeman BA. Superoxide dismutase and catalase conjugated to polyethylene glycol increases endothelial enzyme activity and oxidant resistance. J Biol Chem 1988; 263:6884–6892.
24. Safar P, Stezoski W, Nemoto EM. Amelioration of brain damage after 12 minutes of cardiac arrest in dogs. Arch Neurol 1976; 33:91–95.
25. Siesjö BK. Mechanisms of ischemic brain damage. Crit Care Med 1988; 16:954–963.
26. Safar P. Effects of the postresuscitation syndrome on cerebral recovery from cardiac arrest. Crit Care Med 1985; 13:932–935.
27. White BC, Sullivan JM, DeGarcia DJ, et al. Brain ischemia and reperfusion: molecular mechanism of neuronal injury. J Neurol Sci 2000; 179:1–33.
28. Kumar K, Goosmann M, Krause GS, et al. Ultrastructural and ionic changes in global ischemic dog brain. Acta Neuropathol 1987; 73:393–399.
29. Sato M, Hashimoto H, Kosaka F. Histological changes of neuronal damage in vegetative dogs induced by 18 minutes of complete global brain ischemia: two-phase damage of Purkinje cells and hippocampal CA_1 pyramidal cells. Acta Neuropathol 1990; 80:527–534.
30. Garcia JH, Lossinsky AS, Kauffman FC, Conger KA. Neuronal ischemic injury: light microscopy, ultrastructure and biochemistry. Acta Neuropathol 1978; 43:85–95.
31. Martin LJ. Neuronal cell death in nervous system development, disease, and injury. Int J Mol Med 2001; 7:455–778.
32. Pulsinelli W, Brierley JB, Plum F. Temporal profile of neuronal damage in a model of transient forebrain ischemia. Ann Neurol 1982; 11:491–498.
33. Lind B, Snyder J, Safar P. Total brain ischemia in dogs: cerebral physiologic and metabolic changes after 15 minutes of circulatory arrest. Resuscitation 1975; 4:97–113.
34. Morimoto Y, Yamamura T, Kemmotsu O. Influence of hypoxic and hypercapnic acidosis on brain water content after forebrain ischemic in the rat. Crit Care Med 1993; 21:907–913.
35. Chan PH. Role of oxidants in ischemic brain damage. Stroke 1996; 27:1124–1129.
36. Rosenberg GA. Ischemia brain edema. Prog Cardiovasc Dis 1999; 42:209–216.
37. Taniguchi M, Yamashita T, Kumura E, et al. Induction of aquaporin-4 water channel mRNA after focal cerebral ischemia in rat. Brain Res Mol Brain Res 2000; 78:131–137.
38. Fujimura M, Gasche Y, Morita-Fujimura Y, Massengale J, Kawase M, Chan PH. Early appearance of activated matrix metalloproteinase-9 and blood- brain barrier disruption in mice after focal cerebral ischemia and reperfusion. Brain Res 1999; 842:92–100.
39. Heo JH, Lucero J, Abumiya T, Koziol JA, et al. Matrix metalloproteinases increase very early during experimental focal cerebral ischemia. J Cereb Blood Flow Metab 1999; 19:624–633.
40. Ereci¬Ωska M, Silver IA: ATP and brain function. J Cereb Blood Flow Metab 1989; 9:2–19.
41. Koehler RC, Backofen JE, McPherson RW, Jones MD Jr, Rogers MC, Traystman RJ. Cerebral blood flow and evoked potentials during Cushing response in sheep. Am J Physiol 1989; 256:H779–H788.
42. Symon L. Flow thresholds in brain ischemia and the effects of drugs. Br J Anesth 1985; 57:34–43.
43. Siesjö BK: Cell damage in the brain: A speculative synthesis. J Cereb Blood Flow Metab 1981; 1:155–185.
44. Cerchiari EL, Hoel TM, Safar P, Sclabassi RJ. Protective effects of combined superoxide dismutase and deferoxamine on recovery of cerebral blood flow and function after cardiac arrest in dogs. Stroke 1987; 18:869–878.
45. Sundgreen C, Larsen FS, Herzog TM, Knudsen GM,Boesgaard S, Aldershvile J. Autoregulation of cerebral blood flow in patients resuscitated from cardiac arrest. Stroke 2001; 32:128–132.
46. Shaffner DH, Eleff SM, Brambrink AM, et al. Effect of arrest time and cerebral perfusion pressure during cardiopulmonary resuscitation on cerebral blood flow, metabolism, adenosine triphosphate recovery, and pH in dogs. Crit Care Med 1999; 27:1335–1342.
47. Hossman KA, Ophoff BG. Recovery of monkey brain after prolonged ischemia. I. Electrophysiology and brain electrolytes. J Cereb Blood Flow Metab 1986; 6:15–21.
48. Opie LH. Effects of regional ischemia on metabolism of glucose and fatty acids. Cir Res 1978; 38(Suppl): 52–74.
49. Cole SL, Corday E. Four-minute limit for cardiac resuscitation. JAMA 1956; 161:1454–1458.
50. Eleff SM, Schleien CL, Koehler RC, et al. Brain bioenergetics during cardiopulmonary resuscitation in dogs. Anesthesiology 1992; 76:77–84.
51. Kompala SD, Babbs CF, Blaho KE. Effect of deferoxamine on late deaths following CPR in rats. Ann Emerg Med 1986; 15:405–407.
52. Fleischer JE, Lanier WL, Milde JH, Michenfelder JD. Failure of deferoxamine, an iron chelator, to improve neurological outcome following complete ischemia in dogs. Stroke 1987; 18:124–127.

53. Schanne FA, Kane AB, Young EE, Farber JL. Calcium dependence of toxic cell death: a final common pathway. Science 1979; 206:700–702.
54. Rehncrona S, Rosen I, Siesjö BK. Excessive cellular acidosis: an important mechanism of neuronal damage in the brain? Acta Physiol Scand 1980; 110:435–437.
55. Benveniste H. The excitotoxin hypothesis in relation to cerebral ischemia. Cerebrovasc Brain Metab Rev 1991; 3:213–245.
56. Petito CK, Feldmann E, Pulsinelli WA, Plum F. Delayed hippocampal damage in humans following cardiorespiratory arrest. Neurology 1987; 37:1281–1286.
57. Leonov Y, Sterz F, Safar P, Johnson DW, Tisherman SA, Oku K. Hypertension with hemodilution prevents multifocal cerebral hypoperfusion after cardiac arrest in dogs. Stroke 1992; 23:45–53.
58. Cohan SL, Mun SK, Petite J, et al. Cerebral blood flow in humans following resuscitation from cardiac arrest. Stroke 1989; 20:761–765.
59. Todd NV, Picozzi P, Crockard HA, Russell RR. Reperfusion after cerebral ischemia: influence of duration of ischemia. Stroke 1986; 17:460–466.
60. Nishijima MK, Koehler RC, Hurn PD, et al. Postischemic recovery rate of cerebral ATP, phosphocreatine, pH, and evoked potentials. Am J Physiol 1989; 257:H1860–H1870.
61. Buchan AM, Li H, Cho S, Pulsinelli WA. Blockade of the AMPA receptor prevents CA1 hippocampal injury following severe but transient forebrain ischemia in adult rats. Neurosci Letter 1991; 132:255–258.
62. Wolfson SK Jr, Safar P, Reich H, et al. Dynamic heterogenicity of cerebral hypoperfusion after prolonged cardiac arrest in dogs measured by the stable xenon/CT technique: a preliminary study. Resuscitation 1992; 23:1–20.
63. Sterz F, Leonov Y, Safar P, et al. Multifocal Cerbral blood flow Xe-CT and global cerebral metabolism after prolonged cardiac arrest in dogs. Reperfusion with open-chest CPR or cardiopulmonary bypasss. Resuscitation 1992; 24:27–47.
64. Barone FC, Globus MY, Price WJ, et al. Endothelin levels increase in rat focal and global ischemia. J Cereb Blood Flow Metab 1994; 14:337–342.
65. Kågström E, Smith ML, Siesjö BK. Cerebral circulatory responses to hypercapnia and hypoxia in the recovery period following complete and incomplete cerebral ischemia in the rat. Acta Physiol Scand 1983; 118:281–291.
66. Obrenovitch TP, Hallenbeck JM. Platelet accumulation in regions of low blood flow during the postischemic period. Stroke 1985; 16:224–234.
67. Artru AA, Michenfelder JD. Anoxic cerebral potassium accumulation reduced by phenytoin : Mechanism of cerebral protection? Anesth Analg 1981; 60:41.
68. Hossmann KA, Kleihues P. Reversibility of ischemic brain damage. Arch Neurol 1973; 29:375–384.
69. Hossmann KA. Treatment of experimental cerebral ischemia. J Cereb Blood Flow Metab 1982; 2: 275–297.
70. Kleber AG. Resting membrane potential, extracellular potassium activity, and intracellular sodium activity during acute global ischemia in isolated perfused guinea pig hearts. Cir Res 1983; 52:442–450.
71. Siesjö BK. Pathophysiology and treatment of focal cerebral ischemia. I. Pathophysiology. J Neurosurgery 1992; 77:169–184.
72. Wahl P, Schousboe A, Honoré T, Drejer J. Glutamate-induced increase in intracellular $Ca^{2}+$ in cerebral cortex neurons is transient in immature cells but permanent in mature cells. J Neurochem 1989; 53:1316–1319.
73. Eisner DA, Lederer WJ. Na-Ca exchange: stoichiometry and electrogenecity. Am J Physiol 1985; 248:C189–C202.
74. Fagg GE. L-glutamate, excitatory amino acid receptors and brain function. Trends Neuro Sciences 1985; 8:207–210.
75. Olson JE, Evers JA. Correlations between energy metabolism, ion transport, and water content in astrocytes. Can J Physiol Pharmacol 1992; 70:S350–S355.
76. Kleber AG. Resting membrane potential, extracellular potassium activity, and intracellular sodium activity during acute global ischemia in isolated perfused guinea pig hearts. Cir Res 1983; 52:442–450.
77. Krause GS, White BC, Aust SD, Nayini NR, Kumar K. Brain cell death following ischemia and reperfusion: a proposed biochemical sequance. Crit Care Med 1988; 16:714–726.
78. Tosaki A, Hellegouarch A, Braquet P. Cicletanine and reperfusion injury: is there any correlation between arrhythmias, 6-keto-PGF1alpha, thromboxane B2, and myocardial ion shifts (Na+, K+, Ca2+, and Mg2+) induced by ischemia/reperfusion in isolated rat hearts. J Cardiovasc Pharmacol 1991; 17:551–559.

79. Blaustein MP, Goldman WF, Fontana G, et al. Physiological roles of the sodium-calcium exchanger in nerve and muscle. Ann N Y Acad Sci 1991; 639:254–274.

80. Benveniste H, Jørgensen MB, Diemer NH, Hansen AJ. Calcium accumulation by glutamate receptor activation is involved in hippocampal cell damage after ischemia. Acta Neurol Scand 1988; 78: 529–536.

81. Mayer ML, Westbrook GL. Cellular mechanisms underlying excitotoxicity. Trends Neurosci 1987; 10:59–61.

82. Chan PH, Kerlan R, Fishman RA. Reductions of gamma-aminobutyric acid and glutamate and (Na^++K^+)-ATPase activity in brain slices and synaptosomes by arachidonic acid. J Neurochem 1983; 40:309–315.

83. Drejer J, Benveniste H, Diemer NH, Schousboe A. Cellular origin of ischemic-induced glutamate release from brain tissue in vivo and in vitro. J Neurochem 1985; 45:145–150.

84. Pin JP, Duvoisin R. Neurotransmitter receptors I: The metabotropic glutamate receptors: Structure and functions. Neuropharmacol 1995; 34:1–26.

85. Samoilov MO, Semenov DG, Tulkova EI, Lazarewicz JW. Early postanoxic changes of polyphosphoinositides and bound Ca2+ content in relation to neuronal activity in brain cortex. Resuscitation 1992; 23:33–43.

86. Yasuda H, Kishiro K, Izumi N, Nakanishi M. Biphasic liberation of arachidonic and stearic acids during cerebral ischemia. J Neurochem 1985; 45:168–172.

87. Irvine RF. How is the level of free arachidonic acid controlled in mammalian cells? Biochem J 1982; 204:3–16.

88. Umemura A. Regional differences in free fatty acid release and the action of phospholipase during ischemia in rat brain. No To Shinkei 1990; 42:979–986.

89. McCord JM, Oxygen-derived free radicals in postischemic tissue injury. N Engl J Med 1985; 312: 159–163.

90. Pourcyrous M, Leffler CW, Bada HS, Korones SB, Busiji DW. Brain superoxide anion generation in asphyxiated piglets and effect of indomethacin at therapeutic dose. Pediatr Res 1993; 34:366–369.

91. Farber JL. The role of calcium in cell death. Life Sci 1981; 29:1289–1295.

92. Siesjö BK, Bengtsson F. Calcium fluxes, calcium antagonists, and calcium-related pathology in brain ischemia, hypoglycemia, and spreading depression: a unifying hypothesis. J Cereb Blood Flow Metab 1989; 9:127–140.

93. Erecinska M, Silver IA. Relationship between ions and energy metabolism: cerebral calcium movements during ischaemia and subsequent recovery. Can J Physiol Pharmacol 1992; 70:S190–S193.

94. Boening JA, Kass IS, Cottrell JE, Chambers G. The effect of blocking sodium influx on anoxic damage in the rat hippocampal slice. Neuroscience 1989; 33:263–268.

95. Berger JR, Busto R, Ginsberg MD. Verapamil: failure of metabolic amelioration following global forebrain ischemia in the rat. Stroke 1984; 15:1029–1032.

96. Taguchi J, Graf R, Rosner G, Heiss WD. Prolonged transient ischemia results in impaired CBF recovery and secondary glutamate accumulation in cats. J Cereb Blood Flow Metab 1996; 16:271–279.

97. Cheung JY, Bonventre JV, Malis CD, Leaf A. Calcium and ischemic injury. N Engl J Med 1986; 314: 1670–1676.

98. Yoshida S, Ikeda M, Busto R, Santiso M, Martinez E, Ginsberg MD. Cerebral phosphoinositide, triacylglycerol, and energy metabolism in reversible ischemia: origin and fate of free fatty acids. J Neurochem 1986; 47:744.

99. Ernster L. Oxygen as an environmental poison. Chemica Scripta 1986; 26:525–527.

100. Bulkley GB. The role of oxygen free radicals in human disease processes. Surgery 1983; 94:407–411.

101. Krause GS, Nayini NR, White BC, et al. Natural course of iron delocalization and lipid peroxidation following a 15 minute cardiac arrest in dogs. Ann Emerg Med 1987; 16:1200–1205.

102. Halliwell B, Gutteridge JM. Oxygen toxicity, oxygen radicals, transition metals and disease. Biochem J 1984; 219:1–14.

103. Okada D. Two pathways of cyclic GMP production through glutamate receptor-mediated nitric oxide synthesis. J Neurochem 1992; 59:1203–1210.

104. Fridovich I. Superoxide radical: an endogenous toxicant. Ann Rev Pharmacol Toxicol 1983; 23: 239–257.

105. White BC, Aust SD, Arfros KE, Aronson LD. Brain injury by ischemic anoxia-hypothesis. A tale of two ions? Ann Emerg Med 1984; 13:862–867.

106. Samdani AF, Dawson TM, Dawson VL. Nitric oxide synthase in models of focal ischemia. Stroke 1997; 28:1283–1288.

107. Ambrosio G, Weisfeldt ML, Jacobus WE, Flaherty JT. Evidence for a reversible oxygen radical-mediated component of reperfusion injury: reduction by recombinant human superoxide dismutase administered at the time of reflow. Circulation 1987; 75:282–291.

108. Hall ED, Yonkers PA. Attenuation of postischemic cerebral hypoperfusion by the 21-aminosteroid U74006F. Stroke 1988; 10:340–344.

109. Hillered L, Ernster L. Respiratory activity of isolated rat brain mitochondria following in vitro exposure to oxygen radicals. J Cereb Blood Flow Metab 1983; 3:207–214.

110 Weissmann G, Smolen JE, Korchak HM. Release of inflammatory mediators from stimulated neutrophils. N Engl J Med 1980; 303:27–34.

111. Au AM, Chan PH, Fishman RA. Stimulation of phospholipase A2 activity by oxygen-derived free radicals in isolated brain capillaries. J Cell Biochem 1985; 27:449–453.

112. Zaleska MM, Wilson DF. Lipid hydroperoxides inhibit reacylation of phospholipids in neuronal membranes. J Neurochem 1989; 52:255–260.

113. Beckman JS. The double-edged role of nitric oxide in brain function and superoxide-mediated injury. J Vevelopmental Physiol 1991; 15:53–59.

114. Stamler JS, Singel DJ, Loscalzo J. Biochemistry of nitric oxide and its redox-activated forms. Science 1992; 258:1898–1902.

115. Bodsch W, Takahashi K, Barbier A, Ophoff B, Hossmann KA. Cerebral protein synthesis and ischemia. Prog Brain Res 1985; 63:197–210.

116. Nowak TS Jr, Fried RL, Lust D, Passonneau JV. Changes in brain energy metabolism and protein synthesis following transient bilateral ischemia in the gerbil. J Neurochem 1985; 44:487–494.

117. Dienel GA, Pulsinelli WA, Duffy TE. Regional protein synthesis in rat brain following acute hemispheric ischemia. J Neurochem 1980; 35:1216–1226.

118. Morimoto K, Yanagihara T. Cerebral ischemia in gerbils: polyribosomal function during progression and recovery. Stroke 1981; 12:105–110.

119. DeGarcia DJ, O'Neil BJ, Frisch C, et al. Studies of the protein synthesis system in the brain cortex during global ischemia and reperfusion. Resuscitation 1993; 21:161–170.

120. White BC, Grossman LI, Krause GS. Brain injury by global ischemia and reperfusion: a theoretical perspective on membrane damage and repair. Neurology 1993; 43:1656–1665.

121. de Haro C, Manne V, de Herreros AG, Ochoa S. Heat-stable inhibitor of translation in reticulocyte lysates. Proc Natl Acad Sci USA 1982; 79:3134–3137.

122. Merrick WC: Mechanism and regulation of eukaryotic protein synthesis. Microbiol Rev 1992; 56: 291–315.

123. Burda J, Martín ME, García A, Alcázar A, Fando JL, Salinas M. Phosphorylation of the " subunit of initiation factor 2 correlates with the inhibition of translation following transient cerebral ischaemia in the rat. Biochem J 1994; 302:335–338.

124. DeGarcia DJ, Neumar RW, White BC, Krause GS. Global brain ischemia and reperfusion: modifications in eukaryotic initiation factors associated with inhibition of translation initiation. J Neurochem 1996; 67:2005–2012.

125. Rotman EI, Brostrom MA, Brostrom CO. Inhibition of protein synthesis in intact mammalian cells by arachidonic acid. Biochem J 1992; 282:487–494.

126. Gaitero F, Limas GG, Mendez E, de Haro C. Purification of a novel heat-stable translational inhibitor from rabbit reticulocyte lysates. FEBS Lett 1988; 236:479–483.

127. Kleihues P, Hossmann KA, Pegg AE, Kobayashi K, Zimmermann V. Resuscitation of the monkey brain after one hour complete ischemia. III. Indications of metabolic recovery. Brain Res 1975; 95:61–73.

128. Bodsch W, Barbier A, Oehmichen M, Grosse Ophoff BG, Hossmann KA. Recovery of monkey brain after prolonged ischemia. II. Protein synthesis and morphologic alterations. J Cereb Blood Flow Metab 1986; 6:22–33.

129. Widmann R, Kuroiwa T, Bonnekoh P, Hossman KA. [^{14}C] Leucine incorporation into brain proteins in gerbils after transient ischemia: relationship to selective vulnerability of hippocampus. J Neurochem 1991; 56:789–796.

130. Dienel GA, Cruz NF, Rosenfeld SJ. Temporal profiles of proteins responsive to transient ischemia. J Neurochem 1985; 44:600–610.

131. Cattaneo E, McKay R. Proliferation and differentiation of neuronal stem cells regulated by nerve growth factor. Nature 1990; 347:762–765.

132. Werther GA, Hogg A, Oldfield BJ, et al. Localization and characterization of insulin receptors in rat brain and pituitary gland in vitro autoradiography and computerized densitometry. Endocrinology 1987; 121:1562–1570.

133. Wanaka A, Jonhson EM Jr, Milbrandt J. Localization of FGF receptor mRNA in the adult rat central nervous system by in situ hybridization. Neuron 1990; 5:267–281.
134. Koh S, Oyler GA, Higgins GA. Localization of nerve growth factor receptor messenger RNA and protein in the adult rat brain. Exp Neurol 1989; 106:209–221.
135. Lauterio TJ. Regulation and physiological function of insulin-like growth factors in the central nervous system. Adv Exp Med Biol 1991; 293:419–430.
136. Plata-Salaman CR. Epidermal growth factor and the nervous system. Peptides 1991; 12:653–663.
137. DeGarcia DJ, O'Neil BJ, White BC, et al. Insulin induces tyrosine phosphorylation of a 90-kDa protein during postischemic brain reperfusion. Exp Neurol 1993; 124:351–356.
138. Jørgensen MB, Deckert J, Wright DC, Gehlert DR. Delayed c-fos proto-oncogene expression in the rat brain following transient forebrain ischemia. Brain Res 1989; 484:393–398.
139. Schiaffonati L, Rappocciolo E, Tacchini L, Cairo G, Bernelli-Zazzera A. Reprogramming of gene expression in post-ischemic rat liver: Induction of protooncogenes and hsp-70 gene family. J Cell Physiol 1990; 143:79–87.
140. Beckmann RP, Mizzen LE, Welch WJ. Interaction of HSP-70 with newly synthesized proteins: implications for protein folding and assembly. Science 1990; 248:850–854.
141. Nowak TS Jr. Synthesis of a stress protein following transient ischemia in the gerbil. J Neurochem 1985; 45:1635–1641.
142. Kanduc D, Mittleman A, Serpico R, et al. Cell death: apoptosis versus necrosis. Int J Oncol 2002; 21: 165–170.
143. Davis JN, Antonawich FJ. Role of apoptotic proteins in ischemic hippocampal damage. Ann N Y Acad Sci 1997; 835:309–320.
144. Bredesen DE. Keeping neurons alive: the molecular control of apoptosis. Neuroscientist 1996; 2: 211–216.
145. Yuan J, Yankner BA. Apoptosis in the nervous system. Nature 2000; 407:802–809.
146. Nitatori T, Sato N, Waguri S, et al. Delayed neuronal death in the CA1 pyramidal cell layer of the gerbil hippocampus following transient ischemia is apoptosis. J Neurosci 1995; 15:1001–1011.
147. Vexler ZS, Roberts TP, Bollen AW, Derugin N, Arieff AI. Transient cerebral ischemia. Association of apoptosis induction with hypoperfusion. J Clin Invest 1997; 99:1453–1459.
148. Wyllie AH, Beattie GJ, Hargreaves AD. Chromatin changes in apoptosis. Histochem J 1981; 13: 681–692.
149. Wyllie AH. Glucocorticoid-induced thymocyte apoptosis is associated with endogenous endonuclease activation. Nature 1980; 284:555,556.
150. Hengartner MO. The biochemistry of apoptosis. Nature 2000; 407:770–776.
151. MacManus JP, Buchan AM, Hill IE, Rasquinha I, Prrston E. Global ischemia can cause DNA fragmentation indicative of apoptosis in rat brain. Neurosci Lett 1993; 164:89–92.
152. Schutz JB, Weller M, Moskowitz MA. Caspases as treatment targets in stroke and neurodegenerative diseases. Ann Neurol 1999; 45:421–429.
153. Bredesen DE. Neuronal apoptosis. Ann Neurol 1995; 38:839–851.
154. Miuai M, Zhu H, Rotello R, Hartwieg EA, Yuan J. Induction of apoptosis in fibroblasts by IL-1 beta-converting enzyme, a mammalian homolg of the C. elegans cell death gene ced-3. Cell 1993; 75: 653–660.
155. Chen J, Nagayama T, Jin K, et al. Induction of caspase-3-like protease may mediate delayed neuronal death in the hippocampus after transient cerebral ischemia. J Neurosci 1998; 18:4914–4928.
156. Strasser A, O'Connor L, Dixit VM. Apoptosis signaling. Annu Rev Biochem 2000; 69:217–245.
157. Hu WH, Johnson H, Shu HB. Tumor necrosis factor-related apoptosis-inducing ligand receptors signal NF-κB and JNK activation and apoptosis through distinct pathways. J Biol Chem 1999; 274: 30,603–30,610.
158. Ahmad M, Srinivasula SM, Wang L, et al. CRADD, a novel human apoptotic adaptor molecule for caspase-2 and FasL/tumor necrosis factor receptor-interacting protein RIP. Cancer Res 1997; 57: 615–619.
159. Antonsson B: Bax and other pro-apoptotic Bcl-2 family "killer-proteins" and their victim the mitochondrion. Cell Tissue Res 2001; 306:347–361.
160. Chopp M, Li Y. Apoptosis in focal cerebral ischemia. Acta Neurochir Suppl 1996; 66:21–26.
161. Hara H, Friedlander RM, Gagliardini V, et al. Inhibition of interleukin 1 beta converting enxyme family proteaes reduces ischemic and excitotoxic neuronal damage. Proc Natl Acad Sci USA 1997; 94:2007–2012.
162. Satoh MS, Lindahl T. Role of poly (ADP-ribose) formation in DNA repair. Nature 1992; 356:356–358.

163. Lindahl T, Satoh MS, Poirier GG, Klungland. Post-translational modification of ploy(ADP-ribose) polymerase induced by DNA strand breaks. Trends Biochem Sci 1995; 20:405–411.
164. Nicholson DW, Ali A, Thornberry NA, Vaillancourt JP, Dang CK, Gallant M, Gareau Y, Griffin PR, Labelle M, Lazebnik YA. Identification and inhibition of the ICE/CED-3 protease necessary for mammalian apoptosis. Nature 1995; 376:37–43.
165. Patel T, Gores GJ, Kaufmann SH. The role of proteases during apoptosis. FASEB 1996; 10:587–597.
166. Eliasson MJL, Sampei K, Mandir AS, et al. Poly (ADP-ribose) polymerase gene disruption renders mice resistant to cerebral ischemia. Nat Med 1997; 3:1089–1095.
167. Cole KK, Perez-Polo JR. Poly (ADP-ribose) polymerase inhibition prevents both apoptotic-like delayed neuronal death and necrosis after H_2O_2 injury. J Neurochem 2002; 82; 19–29.
168. Enari M, Sakahira H, Yokoyama H, Okawa K, Iwanatsu A, Nagata S. A caspase-activated DNase that degrades DNA during apoptosis, and its inhibitor ICAD. Nature 1998; 391:43–50, Erratum in: Nature 1998; 28:393–396.
169. Daugas E, Nochy D, Ravagnan L, Loeffler M, Susin SA, Zamzami N, Kroemer G. Apoptosis-inducing factor (AIF): a ubiquitous mitochondrial oxidoreductase involved in apoptosis. FEBS Lett 2000; 476: 118–123.
170. Li LY, Luo X, Wang X. Endonuclease G is an apoptotic DNase when released from mitochondria. Nature 2001; 412:95–99.
171. Cao G, Pei W, Lan J, et al. Caspase-activated DNase/DNA fragmentation factor 40 mediates apoptotic DNA fragmentation in transient cerebral ischemia and in neuronal cultures. J Neurosci 2001; 21: 4678–4690.
172. Chesler M. The regulation and modulation of pH in the nervous system. Prog Neurobiol 1990; 34: 401–427.
173. Eleff SM, Schleien CL, Koehler RC, et al. Brain bioenergetics during cardiopulmonary resuscitation in dogs. Anesthesiology 1992; 76:77–84. Erratum in anesthesiology 1992; 76:666.
174. Johnson BA, Weil MH. Redefining ischemia due to circulatory failure as dual defects of oxygen deficit and of carbon dioxide excesses. Crit Care Med 1991; 19:1432–1438.
175. Duggal C, Weil MH, Gazmuri RJ, et al. Regional blood flow during closed-chest cardiac resuscitation in rats. J Appl Physiol 1993; 74:147–152.
176. von Planta M, Weil MH, Gazmuri RJ, Bisera J, Rackow EC. Myocardial acidosis associated with CO2 production during cardiac arrest and resuscitation. Circulation 1989; 80:684–692.
177. Sanders AB, Kern KB, Atlas M, Bragg S, Ewy GA. Importance of the duration of inadequate coronary perfusion pressure on resuscitation from cardiac arrest. J Am Coll Cardiol 1985; 6:113–118.
178. Hurn PD, Koehler RC, Norris SE, Blizard KK, Traystman RJ. Dependence of cerebral energy phosphate and evoked potential recovery on end-ischemic pH. Am J Physiol 1991; 260:H532–H541.
179. Maruki Y, Koehler RC, Eleff SM, Traystman RJ. Intracellular pH during reperfusion influences evoked potential recovery after complete cerebral ischemia. Stroke 1993; 24:697–704.
180. Martin GB, Nowak RM, Paradis N, et al. Characterization of cerebral energetics and brain pH by ^{31}P spectroscopy after graded canine cardiac arrest and bypass reperfusion. J Cereb Blood Flow Metab 1990; 10:221–226.
181. Welsh FA, Ginsberg MD, Rieder W, Budd WW. Deleterious effect of glucose pretreatment on recovery from diffuse cerebral ischemia in the cat. II. Regional metabolic levels. Stroke 1980; 11:355–363.
182. Pulsinelli WA, Waldman S, Rawlinson D, Plum F. Moderate hyperglycemia augments ischemic brain damage: a neuropathologic study in the rat. Neurology 1982; 32:1239–1246.
183. Warner DS, Gionet TX, Todd MM, McAllister AM. Insulin-induced normoglycemia improves ischemic outcome in hyperglycemic rats. Stroke 1992; 23:1775–1781.
184. Tyson R, Peeling J, Sutherland G. Metabolic changes associated with altering blood glucose levels in short duration forebrain ischemia. Brain Res 1993; 608:288–298.
185. O'Donnell BR, Bickler PE. Influence of pH on calcium influx during hypoxia in rat cortical brain slices. Stroke 1994; 25:171–177.
186. Rehncrona S, Hauge HN, Siesjö BK. Enhancement of iron-catalyzed free radical formation by acidosis in brain homogenates: difference in effect by lactic acid and CO2. J Cereb Blood Flow Metab 1989; 9:65–70.
187. Halliwell B. Reactive oxygen species and the central nervous system. J Neurochem 1992; 59:1609–1623.
188. Siesjö BK, Bendek G, Koide T, Westerberg E, Weiloch T. Influence of acidosis on lipid peroxidation in brain tissues in vitro. J Cereb Blood Flow Metab 1985; 5:253–258.
189. Hossmann KA, Hossmann V. Coagulopathy following experimental cerebral ischemia. Stroke 1977; 8:249–253.

190. Hekmatpanah J. Cerebral blood flow dynamics in hypotension and cardiac arrest. Neurology 1973; 23:174–180.
191. Böttiger BW, Martin E. Thrombolytic therapy during cardiopulmonary resuscitation and the role of coagulation activation after cardiac arrest. Curr Opin Crit Care 2001; 7:176–183.
192. Böttiger BW, Motsch J, Böhrer H, et al. Activation of blood coagulation after cardiac arrest is not balanced adequately by activation of endogenous fibrinolysis. Circulation 1995; 92:2573–2578.
193. Fischer M, Hossmann K. No-reflow after cardiac arrest. Intensive Care Med 1995; 21:132–141.
194. Lin SR, O'Connor MJ, Fischer HW, King A. The effect of combined dextran and streptokinase on cerebral function and blood flow after cardiac arrest: an experimental study on the dog Invest Radiol 1978; 13:490–498.
195. Love S, Barber R. Expression of P-seletin and intracellular adhesion molecule-1 in human brain after focal infarction or cardiac arrest. Neuropathol Appl Neurobiol 2001; 27:465–473.
196. Danton GH, Dietrich WD. Inflammatory mechanisms after ischemia and stroke. J Neuropathol Exp Neurol 2003; 62:127–136.
197. Schott RJ, Natale JE, Ressler SW, Burney RE, D'Alect LG. Neutrophil depletion fails to improve neurological outcome after cardiac arrest in dogs. Ann Emerg Med 1989; 18:517–522.
198. Buchan AM, Bruederlin B, Heinicke E, Li H. Failure of the lipid peroxidation inhibitor, U7400GF, to prevent postischemic selective neuronal injury J Cereb Blood Flow Metab 1992; 12:250–256.
199. Hallenbeck JM, Dutka AJ, Tanishimi T, et al. Polymorphonuclear leukocyte accumulation in brain regions with low blood flow during the early postischemic period. Stroke 1986; 17:246–253.
200. Dutka AJ, Kochanek P, Francis TJ, Hallenbeck JM. Leukopenia ameliorates multifocal brain ischemia. Neurology [Abstract] 1987; 37(Suppl):249.
201. Bednar M, Smith B, Pinto A, Mullane KM. Nafazatrom-induced salvage of ischemic myocardium in anesthetized dogs is mediated through inhibition of neutrophil function. Cir Res 1985; 57:131–141.
202. Crawford MH, Grover FL, Kolb WP, et al. Complement and neutrophil activation in the pathogenesis of ischemic myocardial injury. Circulation 1988; 78:1449–1458.
203. Kirschfink M: Controlling the complement system in inflammation. Immunopharmacol 1997; 38: 51–62.
204. Foreman KE, Vaporciyan AA, Borish BK, et al. C5a-induced expression of P-selectin in endothelial cells. J Clin Invest 1994; 94:1147–1155.
205. Butcher EC. Leukocyte-endothelial cell adhesion recognition: Three (or more) steps to specificity and diversity. Cell 1991; 67:1033–1036.
206. Czurko A, Nishino H. Appearance of immunoglobulin G and complement factor C3 in the striatum after transient focal ischemia in the rat. Neurosci Lett 1994; 166:51–54.
207. Nathan C, Sporn M. Cytokines in context. J Cell Biol 1991; 113:981–986.
208. Kishimoto TK. A dynamic model for neutrophil localization to inflammatory sites. J NIH Res 1991; 3:75–77.
209. McEver RP. Selectins: novel adhesion receptors that mediate leukocyte adhesion during inflammation. Thromb Haematol 1991; 65:223–229.
210. Tilton RG, Berens KL. Functional role for selectins in the pathogenesis of cerebral ischemia. Drugs News Perspect 2002; 15:351–357.
211. Bevilacqua MP, Nelson RM. Selectins J Clin Invest 1993; 91:379–387.
212. Ghezzi P, Dinarello CA, Bianchi M, Rosandich ME, Repine JE, White CW. Hypoxia increases production of interleukin-1 and tumor-necrosis-factor by mononuclear cells. Cytokine 1991; 3:189–194.
213. Patel KD, Zimmerman GA, Prescott SM, McEver RP, McIntyre TM. Oxygen radicals induce human endothelial cells to express GMP-140 and bind neutrophils. J Cell Biol 1991; 112:749–759.
214. Clark WM, Lauten JD, Lessov N, Woodward W, Coull BM. Time course of ICAM-1 expression and leukocyte subset infiltration in rat forebrain ischemia. Mol Chem Neuropathol 1995; 26:213–230.
215. Springer T. Adhesion receptors of the immune system. Nature 1990; 346:425–434.
216. Howard EF, Chen Q, Cheng C, Caroll JE, Hess D. NF-ŒfB and ICAM-1 gene expression is upregulated during reoxygentaion of human brain endothelial cells. Neurosci Lett 1998; 248:199–203.
217. Lindsberg PJ, Yue TL, Frerichs KU, Hallenbeck JM, Feuerstein G. Evidence for platelet-activating factor as anovel mediator in expiremental stroke in rabbits. Stroke 1990; 21:1452–1457.
218. Kubes P, Ibbotson G, Russell J, Wallace JL, Granger DN. Role of platelet-activating factor in ischemia/reperfusion-induced leukocyte adherence. Am J Physiol 1990; 259; G300–G305.
219. Susuki M, Asako H, Kubes P, Jennings S, Grisham MB, Granger DN. Neutrophil-derived oxidants promote leukocyte adherence in postcapillary venules. Microvasc Res 1991; 42:125–138.
220. Weiss SJ. Tissue destruction by neutrophils. N Engl J Med 1989; 320:365–376.

221. Ma XL, Lefer DJ, Lefer AM, Rothelein R. Coronary endothelial and cardiac protective effects of a monoclonal antibody to intercellular adhesion molecule-1 in myocardial ischemia and reperfusion. Circulation 1992; 86:937–946.
222. Dreyer WJ, Michael LH, West MS, DC, Entman ML. Neutrophil accumulation in ischemic myocardium: insights into time course, distribution, and mechanism of localization during early reperfusion. Circulation 1991; 84:400,411.
223. Lees GJ. The possible contribution of microglia and macrophages to delayed neuronal death after ischemia. J Neurol Sci 1993; 114:119–122.
224. Wei G, Dawson VL, Zweier JL. Role of neuronal and endothelial nitric oxide synthase in nitric oxide generation in the brain following cerebral ischemia. Biochim Biophys Acta 1999; 1455:23,34.
225. De Belder AJ, Radomski MW, Why HJ, et al. Nitric oxide synthase activities in human myocardium. Lancet 1993; 341:84,85.
226. Nozaki K, Moskowitz MA, Maynard KI, et al. Possible origins and distribution of immunoreactive nitric oxide synthase-containing nerve fibers in cerebral arteries. J Cereb Blood Flow Metab 1993; 13:70–79.
227. Bredt DS, Snyder SH. Isolation of nitric oxide synthase, a calmodulin-requiring enzyme. Proc Natl Acad Sci, USA 1990; 87:682–685.
228. Fukuyama N, Takizawa S, Ishida H, Hoshiai K, Shinohara Y, Nakazawa H. Peroxynitrite formation in focal cerebral ischemia-reperfusion in rats occurs predominantly in the peri-infarct region. J Cereb Blood Flow Metab 1996; 18:123–129.
229. Bolanos JP, Almeida A. Roles of nitric oxide in brain hypoxia-ischemia. Biochim Biophys Acta 1999; 1411:415–436.
230. Ungureanu-Longrois D, Balligand JL, Simmons WW, et al. Induction of nitric oxide synthase activity by cytokines in ventricular myocytes is necessary but not sufficient to decrease contractile responsiveness to $-adrenergic agonists. Circ Res 1995; 77:494–502.
231. Park SY, Lee H, Hur J, et al. Hypoxia induces nitric oxide production in mouse microglia via p38 mitogen-activated protein kinase pathway. Brain Res Mol Brain Res 2002; 107:9–16.
232. Tominaga T, Stao S, Ohnishi T, Ohnishi ST. Electron paramagnetic resonance (EPR) detection of nitric oxide produced during focal ischemia in the rat. J Cereb Blood Flow Metab 1994; 14:715–722.
233. Southam E, East SJ, Garthwaite J. Excitatory amino acid receptors coupled to the nitric oxide/cyclic GMP pathway in rat cerebellum during development. J Neurochem 1991; 56:2072–2081.
234. Garthwaite J, Garthwaite G, Palmer RMJ, Moncada S. NMDA receptor activation induces nitric oxide synthesis from arginine in rat brain slices. Eur J Pharmacol 1989; 172:413–416.
235. Kilbourn RG, Traber DL, Szabo C. Nitric oxide and shock. Dis Mon 1997; 43:277–348.
236. Radi R, Beckman JS, Bush KM, Freeman BA. Peroxynitrite oxidation of sulfhydryls. J Biol Chem 1991; 266:4244–4250.
237. Mullie A, Verstringe P, Buylaert W, et al. Predictive value of Glascow coma score for awakening after out-of-hospital cardiac arrest. Cerebral resuscitation study group of the Belgian Society for Intensive care. Lancet 1988; 1:137–140.
238. Grubb NR, Elton RA, Fox KA. In-hospital mortality after out-of-hospital cardiac arrest. Lancet 1995; 346:417–421.
239. Teasdale G, Jennett B. Assessment of coma and impaired consciousness: a practical scale. Lancet 1974; 2:81–84.
240. Kelsey SF, Abramson NS, Detre KM, Monroe J. Brain Resuscitation Clinical Trail I Study Group. A randomized clinical study of cardiopulmonary-cerebral resuscitation: design, methods, and patient characteristics. Am J Emerg Med 1986; 4:72–86.
241. Levy DE, Caronna JJ, Singer BH, Lapinski RH, Frydman H, Plum F: Predicting outcome from hypoxic-ischemic coma. JAMA 1985; 253:1420–1426.
242. Berek K, Jeschow M, Aichner F. The prognostication of cerebral hypoxia after out-of-hospital cardiac arrest in adults. Eur Neurol 1997; 37:135–145.
243. Edgren E, Hedstrand U, Kelsey S, Sutton-Tyrrell K, Safar R. Assessment of neurological prognosis in comatose survivors of cardiac arrest. BRCT I Study Group. Lancet 1994; 343:1055–1059.
244. Fiser DH, Long N, Roberson PK, Hefley G, Zolten K, Brodie-Fowler M. Relationship of pediatric overall performance category and pediatric cerebral performance category scores at pediatric intensive care unit discharge with outcome measures collected at hospital discharge and 1- and 6-month follow-up assessments. Crit Care Med 2000; 28:2616–2620.
245. Synek VM. Value of a revised EEG coma scale for prognosis after cerebral anoxia and diffuse head injury. Clin Electroencephalogr 1990; 21:25–30.

246. Yamashita S, Morinaga T, Ohgo S, Sakamoto T, Kaku N, Sugimoto S, Matsukura S. Prognostic value of electroencephalogram (EEG) in anoxic encephalopathy after cardiopulmonary resuscitation: relationship among anoxic period, EEG grading and outcome. Intern Med 1995; 34:71–76.

247. Geocadin RG, Sherman DL, Christian Hansen H, et al. Neurological recovery by EEG bursting after resuscitation from cardiac arrest in rats. Resuscitation 2002; 55:193–200.

248. Jørgensen E, Malchow-Moller A. Natural history of global and critical brain ischemia. Part I: EEG and neurological signs during the first year after cardiopulmonary resuscitation in patients subsequently regaining consciousness. Resuscitation 1981; 9:133–153.

249. Wijdicks EF, Parisi JE, Sharborough FW. Prognostic value of myoclonus status in comatose survivors of cardiac arrest. Ann Neurol 1994; 35:239–243.

250. Rothstein TL, Thomas EM, Sumi SM. Predicting outcome in hypoxic-ischemic coma. A prospective clinical and electrophysiological study. Electroencephalogr Clin Neurophysiol 1991; 79:101–107.

251. Kjos BO, Brant-Zawadzki M, Young RG. Early CT findings of global central nervous system hypoperfusion. Am J Roentgenol 1983; 141:1227–1232.

252. Roine RO, Raininko R, Erkinjuntti T, Ylikoski A, Kaste M. Magnetic resonance imaging findings associated with cardiac arrest. Stroke 1993; 24:1005–1014.

253. Cohan SL, Mun SK, Petitie J, Correia J, Tavelra Da Silva AT, Waldhom RE. Cerebral blood flow in humans following resuscitation from cardiac arrest. Stroke 1989; 20:761–765.

254. Roine RO, Launes J, Nikkinen P, Lindroth L, Kaste M. Regional cerebral blood flow after human cardiac arrest. A hexamethylpropyleneamine oxime single photon emission computed tomographic study. Arch Neurol 1991; 48:625–629.

255. Barone FC, Clark RK, Price WJ, White RF, Feuerstein GZ, Barone FC. Neuron-specific enolase increases in cerebral and systemic circulation following focal ischaemia. Brain Res 1993; 623: 77–82.

256. Hachimi-Idrissi S, Van der Auwera M, Schiettecatte J, Ebinger G, Michotte Y, Hughens L. S-100 protein as early predictor of regaining consciousness after out of hospital arrest. Resuscitation 2002; 53:251–257.

257. Karkela J, Bock E, Kaukinen S. CSF and serum brain-specific creatine kinase isoenzyme (CK-BB), neuron-specific enolase (NSE) and neural cell adhesion molecule (NCAM) as prognostic markers for hypoxic brain injury after cardiac arrest in man. J Neurol Sci 1993; 116:100–109.

258. Abramson NA, Safar P, Detre KM, Kelsey SF, Monroe J, Reinmuth O, Snyder JV: Neurological recovery after cardiac arrest: effect of duration of ischemia. Crit Care Med 1985; 13:930–931.

259. Safar P. Resuscitation from clinical death: pathophysiologic limits and therapeutic potentials. Crit Care Med 1988; 16:923–941.

260. Selman WR, Spetzler RF, Roski RA. Barbiturate resuscitation from focal cerebral ischemia- A review. Resuscitation 1981; 9:189–196.

261. Nordstrom CH, Rehncrona S, Siesjo BK. Restitution of cerebral energy state, as well as of glycolytic metabolites, citric acid cycle intermediates and associated amino acids after 30 minutes of complete ischemia in rats anesthetized with nitrous oxide or pentobarbital. J Neurochem 1978; 30:479–486.

262. Todd MM, Chadwick HS, Shapiro HM, Dunlop BJ, Marshall LF, Dueck R. The neurological effects of thiopental therapy following experimental cardiac arrest in cats. Anesthesiology 1982; 57:76–86.

263. Safar P. Amelioration of postischemic brain damage with barbiturates. Stroke 1980; 11:34–38.

264. Smith AL, Hoff JT, Nielson SL, Larson CP. Barbiturate protection against cerebral infarction. Stroke 1974; 5:1–7.

265. Nussmeier NA, Arlund C, Slogoff S. Neuropsychiatric complications after cardiopulmonary bypass: cerebral protection by a barbiturate. Anesthesiology 1986; 64:165–170.

266. Ward JD, Becker DP, Miller DJ, et al. Failure of prophylactic barbiturate coma in the treatment of severe head trauma. J Neurosurg 1985; 62:383.

267. Bleyaert AL, Nemoto EM, Safar P, et al. Thiopental amelioration of brain damage after global ischemia in monkeys. Anesthesiology 1978; 49:390–398.

268. Snyder BD, Ramirez-Lessepas M, Sukhum P, Fryd D, Sung JH. Failure of thiopental to moderate global anoxic injury. Stroke 1979; 10:135.

269. Rogers MC, Kirsch JR. Current concepts in brain resuscitation. JAMA 261:3143–3147.

270. Safar P. Brain resuscitation. Special symposium issue. Critical care Med 1978; 6:199–214.

271. Ebmeyer U, Safar P, Radovsky A, et al. Thiopental combination treatments for cerebral resuscitation after prolonged cardiac arrest in dogs. Exploratory outcome study. Resuscitation 2000; 45:119–131.

272. Vaagenes P, Cantadore R, Safar P, et al. Amelioration of brain damage by lidoflazine after prolonged ventricular fibrillation cardiac arrest in dogs. Crit Care Med 1984; 12:846–855.

273. White BC, Winegar CD, Wilson RF, Hoehner PJ, Trombley JH Jr. Possible role of calcium blockers in cerebral resuscitation: A review of the literature and synthesis for future studies. Crit Care Med 1983; 11:202–207.

274. White BC, Gadzinski DS, Hoehner PJ, et al. Effect of flunarizine on canine cerebral cortical blood flow and vascular resistance post cardiac arrest. Ann Emerg Med 1982; 11:119–126.

275. Mohamed AA, Mendelow AD, Teasdale GM, Teasdale GM, Harper Am, McCulloch J. Effect of the calcium antagonist nimodipine on local cerebral blood flow and metabolic coupling. J Cereb Blood Flow Metab 1985; 5:26–33.

276. Steen PA, Gisvold SE, Milde JH, et al. Nimodipine improves outcome when given after complete cerebral ischemia in primates. Anesthesiology 1985; 62:406–414.

277. Fleischer JE, Lanier WL, Milde JH, Michenfelder JD. Lidoflazine does not improve neurological outcome when administered after complete cerebral ischemia in dogs. Anesthesiology 1987; 66: 304–311.

278. Calle PA, Paridaens K, De Ridder LI, Buylaert WA. Failure of nimodipine to prevent brain damage in a global brain ischemia model in the rat. Resuscitation 1993; 25:59–71.

279. Lanza RP, Cooper DK, Barnard CN. Lack of efficacy of high-dose verapamil in preventing brain damage in baboons and pigs after prolonged partial cerebral ischemia. Am J Emerg Med 1984; 2:481–485.

280. White BC, Winegar CD, Wilson RF, Krause GS. Calcium blockers in cerebral resuscitation. J Trauma 1983; 23:788–794.

281. Kelsey SF, Sutton-Tyrrell K, Abramson S, et al. A randomized clinical trial of calcium entry blocker administration to comatose survivors of cardiac arrest. Design, methods, and patient characteristics. Brain resuscitation Clinical Trial II Study Group. Control Clin trials 1991; 12:525–545.

282. Safar P. Cerebral resuscitation after cardiac arrest: research initiatives and future directions. Ann Emerg Med 1993; 2:324–349.

283. Abramson NS, Kelsey SF, Safar P, Sutton-Tyrell K. Simpson's paradox and clinical trials: what you find is not necessarily what you prove. Ann Emerg Med 1992; 21:1480–1482.

284. Roine RO, Kaste M, Kinnunen A, Nikki P, Sarna S, Kajaste S. Nimodipine after resuscitation from out-of-hospital ventricular fibrillation. A placebo-controlled, double-blind randomized trial. JAMA 1990; 264:3171–3177.

285. Fleischer JE, Tateishi A, Drummond JC, et al. MK-801, an excitatory amino acid antagonist, does not improve neurological outcome following cardiac arrest in cats. J Cereb Blood Flow Metab 1989; 9:795–804.

286. Schwarcz R, Meldrum B. Excitatory aminoacid antagonists provide a therapeutic approach to neurological disorders. Lancet 1985; 2:140–143.

287. Muir KW, Grosset DG, Lees KR. Effects of prolonged infusions of the NMDA antagonist aptiganel hydrochloride (CNS 1102) in normal volunteers. Clin Neuropharmacol 1997; 20:311–321.

288. Gill R, Foster AC, Woodruff GN: Systemic administration of MK-801 protects against ischaemia-induced hippocampal neuroregeneration in the gerbil. J Neurosci 1987; 7:3343–3349.

289. Gerlach R, Beck M, Zeitschel U, Seifert V: MK 801 attenuates c-Fos and c-Jun expression after in vitro ischemia in rat neuronal cell cultures but not in PC 12 cells. Neurol Res 2002; 24:725–729.

290. Gill R, Foster A, Woodruff GN. MK-801 is neuroprotective in gerbils when administered during the post-ischemic period. Neurosci 1988; 25:847–855.

291. Lanier WL, Perkins WJ, Karlsson BR, et al. The effects of dizocilpine melaete (MK-801) an antagonist of the N-methyl-D-aspartate receptor, on neurological recovery and histopathology following complete cerebral ischemia in primates. J Cereb Blood Flow Metab 1990; 10:252–261.

292. Sterz F, Leonov Y, Safar P, et al. Effect of excitatory amino acid receptor blocker MK-801 on overall and neurological outcome after prolonged cardiac arrest in dogs. Anesthesiology 1989; 71:907–918.

293. Helfaer MA, Ichord RN, Martin LJ, Hurn PD, Castro A, Traystman RJ. Treatment with the competitive NMDA antagonist GPI 3000 does not improve outcome after cardiac arrest in dogs. Stroke 1998; 29: 824–829.

294. Nellgård B, Wieloch T. Postischemic blockade of AMPA but not NMDA receptors mitigates neuronal damage in the rat brain following transient severe cerebral ischemia. J Cereb Blood Flow Metab 1992; 12:2–11.

295. Menniti FS, Buchan AM, Chenard BL, et al. CP-465,022, a selective noncompetitive AMPA receptor antagonist, blocks AMPA receptors but is not neuroprotective in vivo. Stroke 2003; 34:171–176.

296. Cerchiari EL, Hoel TM, Safar P, Sclabassi RJ. Protective effects of combined superoxide dismutase and deferoxamine on recovery of cerebral blood flow and function after cardiac arrest in dogs. Stroke 1987; 18:869–878.

297. Vaagenes P, Safar P, Cantadore R, et al. Outcome trails of free radical scavengers and calcium entry blockers after cardiac arrest in two dog models [abstract]. Ann Emerg Med 1986; 15:665.
298. Natale JE, Schott RJ, Hall ED, Braughler JM. The 21-aminosteroid U74006F reduces systemic lipid peroxidation, improves neurological function, and reduces mortality after cardiopulmonary arrest in dogs. Prog Clin Biol Res 1989; 308:891–896.
299. Hall ED. Lipid antioxidants in acute central nervous system injury. Ann Emerg Med 1993; 22:1022–1027.
300. Perkins WJ, Milde LN, Milde JH, Michenfelder JD. Pretreatment with U74006F improves neurological outcome following complete cerebral ischaemia in dogs. Stroke 1991; 22:902–909.
301. Beck T, Bielenberg GW. Failure of the lipid peroxidation inhibitor U74006F to improve neurological outcome after transient forebrain ischemia in the rat. Brain Res 1990; 532:336–338.
302. Sterz F, Safar P, Johnson DW, Oku K, Tisherman SA. Effects of U74006F on multifocal cerebral blood flow and metabolism after cardiac arrest in dogs. Stroke 1991; 22:889–895.
303. Feng Y, LeBlanc MH, LeBlanc EB, et al. Desmethyl tirilazad improves neurological function after hypoxic ischemic brain injury in piglets. Crit Care Med 2000; 28:1431–1438.
304. Meyer FB, Sundt TM, Yanagihara T, Anderson RE. Focal cerebral ischemia: pathophysiologic mechanisms and rationale for future avenues of treatment. Mayo Clin Proc 1987; 62:35–55.
305. Palmer C, Roberts RL, Bero C. Deferoxamine posttreatment reduces ischemic brain injury in neonatal rats. Stroke 1994; 25:1039–1045.
306. Rosenthal RE, Chanderbhan R, Marshall G, Fiskum G. Prevention of post-ischemic brain lipid conjugated diene production and neurological injury by hydroxyethyl starch-conjugated deferoxamine. Free Radic Biol Med 1992; 12:29–33.
307. Liachenko S, Tang P, Xu Y. Deferoxamine improves early postresuscitation reperfusion after prolonged cardiac arrest in rats. J Cereb Blood Flow Metab 2003; 23:574–581.
308. Liu TH, Beckman JS, Freeman BA, Hogan EL, Hsu CY. Polyethylene glycol-conjugated dismutase and catalase reduce ischemic brain injury. Am J Physiol 1989; 256:H589–H593.
309. Itoh T, Kawakami M, Yamauchi Y, Shimizu S, Nakamura M. Effecet of allopurinol on ischemia and reperfusion-induced cerebral injury in spontaneous hypertensive rats. Stroke 1986; 17:1284–1287.
310. Forsman M, Fleischer JE, Milde JH, Steen PA, Michenfelder JD. Superoxide dismutase and catalase failed to improve neurological outcome after cerebral ischemia in the dog. Acta Anaesthesiol Scand 1988; 32:152–155.
311. Reich H, Safar P, Angelos M, Basford R, ernster L. Failure of a multifaceted anti-reoxygenation injury (RI) therapy to ameliorate brain damage after ventricular fibrillation (VF) cardiac arrest (CA) of 20 minutes in dogs [abstract]. Crit Care Med 1988; 16:387.
312. Cerchiari EL, Sclabassi RJ, Safar P, Hoel TM. Effects of combined superoxide dismutase and deferoxamine on recovery of brainstem auditory evoked potentials and EEG after asphyxial cardiac arrest in dogs. Resuscitation 1990,19:25–40.
313. Shigeno T, Yamasaki Y, Kato G, et al. Reduction of delayed neuronal death by inhibition of protein synthesis. Neurosci Lett 1990; 120:117–119.
314. Davies AM. The Bcl-2 family of proteins, and the regulation of neuronal survival. Trends Neurosci 1995; 18:355–358.
315. Chen J, Graham SH, Nakayama M, Zhu RL, Jin K, Stetler RA, Simon RP. Apoptosis repressor genes Bcl-2 and Bcl-x-long are expressed in the rat brain following global ischemia. J Cereb Blood Flow Metab 1997; 17:2–10. Erratum in: J Cereb Blood Flow Metab 1998; 18:931.
316. Kitagawa K, Matsumoto M, Tsujimoto Y, et al. Amelioration of hippocampal neuronal damage after global ischemia by neuronal overexpression of Bcl-2 in transgenic mice. Stroke 1998; 29:2616–2621.
317. Chen J, Nagayama T, Jin K, Stetler RA, Zhu RL, Graham SH, Simon RP. Induction of caspase-3-like protease may mediate delayed neuronal death in the hippocampus after transient cerebral ischemia. J Neurosci 1998; 18:4914–4928.
318. Vogel P, Putten H, Popp E, Krumnikl JJ, et al. Improved resuscitation after cardiac arrest in rats expressing the baculovirus caspase inhibitor protein p35 in central neurons. Anesthesiology 2003; 99:112–121.
319. Harkema JM, Chaudry IH. Magnesium-adenosine triphosphate in the treatment of shock, ischemia and sepsis. Crit Care Med 1992; 20:263–275.
320. Fukunaga AF. Intravenous administration of large doses of adenosine or adenosine triphosphate with minimal blood pressure fluctuations. Life Sci 1995; 56:PL209–PL218.
321. Paskitti M, Reid KH. Use of an adenosine triphosphate-based 'cocktail' early in reperfusion substantially improves brain protein synthesis after global ischemia in rats. Neurosci Lett 2002; 331:147–150.

322. Krep H, Brinker G, Schwindt W, Hossmann KA. Endothelin type A-antagonist improves long-term neurological recovery after cardiac arrest in rats. Crit Care Med 2000; 28:2873–2880.

323. Krep H, Brinker G, Phillekamp F, Hossman KA. Treatment with an endothelin type A receptor-antagonist after cardiac arrest and resuscitation improves cerebral hemodynamic and functional recovery in rats. Crit Care Med 2000; 28:2866–2872.

324. Fischer Böttiger BW, Popov-Cenic S, Hossman KA. Thrombolysis using plasminogen activator and heparin reduces cerebral no-reflow after resuscitation from cardiac arrest: an experimental study in the cat. Intensive care Med 1996; 22:1214–1223.

325. Safar P, Xiao F, Radovsky A, Tanigawa K, et al. Improved cerebral resuscitation from cardiac arrest in dogs with mild hypothermia plus blood flow promotion. Stroke 1996; 27:105–113.

326. Lin SR, O'Conner MJ, Fischer HW, King A. The effects of combined dextran and streptokinase on cerebral function and blood flow after cardiac arrest: an experimental study on the dog. Invest Radiol 1978; 13:490–498.

327. Böttiger BW, Bode C, Kern S, et al. Efficacy and safety of thrombolytic therapy after initially unsuccessful cardiopulmonary resuscitation: A prospective clinical trial. Lancet 2001; 357:1583–1585.

328. Cullen JP, Aldrete JA, Janovsky L, Romo-Salas F. Protective action of phenytoin in cerebral ischemia. Anesth Analg 1979; 58:165–169.

329. Aldrete JA, Romo-Salas F, Mazzia VD, Tan SL. Phenytoin for brain resuscitation after cardiac arrest: An uncontrolled clinical trial. Crit Care Med 1981; 9:474.

330. Ebmeyer U, Safar P, Radovsky A, et al. Thiopental combination treatments for cerebral resuscitation after prolonged cardiac arrest in dogs. Exploratory outcome study. Resuscitation 2000; 45:119–131.

331. Taft WC, Clifton GL, Blair RE, DeLorenzo RJ. Phenytoin protects against ischemia-produced neuronal cell death. Brain Res 1989; 483:143–148.

332. Kennedy C, Grave GD, Jehle JW. The effect of diphenylhydantoin on local cerebral blood flow. Neurology 1972; 22:451.

333. Varon S, Hagg T, Manthorpe M. Nerve growth factor in CNS repair and regeneration. Adv Exp Med Biol 1991; 296:267–276.

334. Mattson MP, Murrain M, Gurthrie PB, Kater SB. Fibroblast growth factor and glutamate: opposing roles in the generation and degeneration of hippocampal neuroarchitecture. J Neurosci 1989; 9: 3728–3740.

335. Shigeno T, Mima T, Takakura K, Graham DI, Kato G, Hashimoto y, Furukawa S. Amelioration of delayed neuronal death in the hippocampus by nerve growth factor. J Neurosci 1991; 11:2914–2919.

336. Voll CL, Aver RN. Insulin attenuates ischemic brain damage independent of its hypoglycemic effect: J Cereb Blood Flow Metab 1991; 11:1006–1014.

337. LeMay DR, Gehua L, Zelenock GB, D'Alecy G. Insulin administration protects neurological function in cerebral ischemia in rats. Stroke 1988; 19:1411–1419.

338. Katz LM, Wang Y, Ebmeyer U, Radovsky A, Safar P. Glucose plus insulin improves cerebral outcome after asphyxial cardiac arrest. Neuroreport 1998; 9:3363–3367.

339. Yarden Y. Growth factor receptor tyrosine kinases. Annu Rev Biochem 1988; 57:443–478.

340. Pillion DJ, Kim SJ, Kim H, Meezan E. Insulin signal transduction: the role of protein phosphorylation. Am J Med 1992; 303:40–52.

341. Sacks DB, Fujita-Yamaguchi Y, Gale RD, McDonald JM. Tyrosine-specific phosphorylation of calmodulin by the insulin receptor kinase purified from human placenta. Biochem J 1989; 263:803–812.

342. Moss AM, Unger JW, Moxley RT, Livingston JN. Location of phosphotyrosine-containing proteins by immunocytochemistry in the rat forebrain corresponds to the distribution of the insulin receptor. Proc Natl Acad Sci USA 1990; 87:4453–4457.

343. Ting LP, Tu CL, Chou CK. Insulin-induced expression of human heat shock protein gene. J Biol Chem 1989; 264:3403–3408.

344. Parrizas M, Saltiel AR, LeRoith D. Insulin-like growth factor 1 inhibits apoptosis using the phophatidylinositol 3'-kinase and mitogen-activated protein kinase pathways. J Biol Chem 1997; 272:154–161.

345. Drews G, Debuyser A, Nenquin M, Henquin JC. Galanin and epinephrine act on distinct receptors to inhibit insulin release by the same mechanisms, including an increase in K+ permeability of the $-cell membrane. Endocrinology 1990; 126:1646–1653.

346. Cryer PE. Physiology and pathophysiology of the human sympathoadrenal neuroendocrine system. N Engl J Med 1980; 303:436–444.

347. Jansson L. Influence of adrenaline on blood perfusion and vascular conductance of the whole pancreas and the islets of Langerhans in the rat. Arch Int Pharmacodyn 1991; 313:90–97.

348. Rorsman P, Bokvist K, Ammala C, et al. Activation by adrenaline of a low-conductance G protein-dependent K+ channel in mouse pancreatic B cells. Nature 1991; 349:44–79.

349. Yu KT, Pessin JE, Czech MP. Regulation of insulin receptor kinase by multisite phosphorylation. Biochime 1985; 67:1081–1090.

350. Sotomatsu A, Nakano M, Hirai S. Phospholipid peroxidation induced by the catechol-Fe^{3+} (Cu^{2+}) complex: a possible mechanism of nigrostriatal cell damage. Arch Biochem Biophys 1990; 283: 334–341.

351. Callaham M, Madsen CD, Barton CW, Saunders CE, Pointer J. A randomized clinical trial of high-dose epinephrine and norepinephrine in prehospital cardiac arrest. JAMA 1992; 268:2667–2672.

352. Markov AK, Oglethorpe N, Grillis M, Neely WA, Hellems HK. Therapeutic action of fructose-1,6-diphosphate in traumatic shock. World Surg 1983; 7:430–406.

353. Vexler ZS, Wong A, Francisco C, et al. Fructose-1, 6-biphosphate preserves intracellular glutathione and protects cortical neurons against oxidative stress. Brain Res 2003; 960:90–98.

354. Woodhall B, Kramer RS, Currie WD, Sanders AP. brain energetics and neurosurgery. A review of recent studies done at Duke University. J Neurosurgery 1971; 34:3–14.

355. Furuichi Y, Katsuta K, Maeda M, et al. Neuroprotective action of tracolimus (FK506) in focal and global cerebral ischemnia in rodents: dose dependency, therapeutic time window and long-term efficacy. Brain Res 2003; 965:137–145.

356. Katsura K, Kurihara J, Hiraide T, Takahashi K, Kato H, Katayama Y. Effects of FK506 on the translocation of protein kinase C and CaM kinase II in the gerbil hippocampal CA1 neurons. Neurol Res 2003; 25:522–527.

357. Kirsmer AC, Linder KH, Wenzel V, Rainer B, Muller G, Lingnau W. Inhibition of nitric oxide improves coronary perfusion pressure and return of spontaneous circulation in a porcine cardiopulmonary resuscitation model. Crit Care Med 2001; 29:482–486.

358. Sasaki T, Hamada J, Shibata M, Araki N, Fukuuchi Y. Inhibition of nitric oxide production during global ischemia ameliorates ischemic damage of pyramidal neurons in the hippocampus. Keio J Med 2001; 50:182–187.

359. Ditchey RV, Winkler JV, Rhodes CA. Relative lack of coronary blood flow during closed-chest resuscitation in dogs. Circulation 1982; 66:297–302.

360. Paradis NA, Martin GB, Rivers EP, et al. Coronary perfusion pressure and the return of spontaneous circulation in human cardiopulmonary resuscitation. JAMA 1990; 263; 1106–1113.

361. Sanders AB, Kern KB, Berg RA, Hilwig RW, Heidenrich J, Ewy GA. Survival and neurological outcome after cardiopulmonary resuscitation with four different chest compression-ventilation ratios. Ann Emerg Med 2002; 40:553–562.

362. Ralston SH, Babbs CF, Niebauer MJ. Cardiopulmonary resuscitation with interposed abdominal compression in dogs. Anesth Analg 1982; 61:645–651.

363. Walker JW, Bruestle JC, White BC, Evans AT, Indreri R, Bialek H. Perfusion of the cerebral cortex by use of abdominal counterpulsation during cardiopulmonary resuscitation. Am J Emerg Med 1984; 2:391–393.

364. Howard M, Carruba C, Foss F, Janiak B, Hogan B, Guinness M. Interposed abdominal compression-CPR: its effects on parameters of coronary perfusion in human subjects. Ann Emerg Med 1987; 16: 253–259.

365. Berryman CR, Phillips GM. Interposed abdominal compression-CPR in human subjects. Ann Emerg Med 1984; 13:226–229.

366. Mateer J, Steuven HA, Thompson BM, Aprahamian C, Darin JC. Pre-hospital IAC-CPR versus standard CPR: Paramedic resuscitation of cardiac arrests. Am J Emerg Med 1985; 3:143–146.

367. Sack JB, Kesselbrenner MB, Bregman D. Survival from in-hospital cardiac arrest with interposed abdominal counter pulsation during cardiopulmonary resuscitation JAMA 1992; 267:379–385.

368. Sack JB, Kesselbrenner MB, Jarrad A. Interposed abdominal compression-cardiopulmonary resuscitation and resuscitation outcome during asystole and electromechanical dissociation. Circulation 1992; 86:1692–1700.

369. Mateer JR, Stueven HA, Thompson BM., et al. Interposed abdominal compression CPR versus standard CPR in prehospital cardiopulomnary arrest: preliminary results. Ann Emerg Med 1984; 13:764–766.

370. Weiser FM, Adler LN, Kuhn LA. Hemodynamic effects of closed and open chest cardiac resuscitation in normal dogs, and those with acute myocardial infarction. Am J Cardiol 1962; 10:555–561.

371. Del Guercio LR, Feins NR, Cohn JD, Coomaraswamy RP, Wollman SB, State D. Comparison of blood flow during external and internal cardiac massage in man. Circulation 1965; 31/32 (Suppl I):I-171–I-180.

372. Sanders AB, Kern K, Ewy GA, Atlas M, Bailey L. Improved resuscitation from cardiac arrest with open-chest massage. Ann Emerg Med 1984; 13:672.
373. Fleisher G, Sagy M, Swedlow DB, Belani K. Open- versus closed-chest cardiac compression in a canine model of pediatric cardiopulmonary resuscitation. Am J Emerg Med 1985; 3:305–310.
374. Kern KB, Sanders AB, Badylak SF, et al. Long-term survival with open-chest cardiac massage after ineffective closed-chest compression in a canine preparation. Circulation 1987; 75:498–503.
375. Arai T, Dote K, Tsukahara I, Nitta K, Nagaro T. Cerebral blood flow during conventional, new and open-chest cardio-pulmonary resuscitation in dogs. Resuscitation 1984; 12:147–154.
376. Geehr EC, Lewis, Auerbach PS. Failure of open heart massage to improve survival after pre-hospital non-traumatic cardiac arrest. N Engl J Med 1986; 314:1189,1190.
377. Halperin HR, Guerci AD, Chandra N, et al. Vest inflation without simultaneous ventilation during cardiac arrest in dogs: improved survival from prolonged cardiopulmonary resuscitation. Circulation 1986; 74:1407–1415.
378. Halperin HR, Tsitlik JE, Gelfand M, et al. A preliminary study of cardiopulmonary resuscitation by circumferential compression of the chest with use of a pneumatic vest. N Engl J Med 1993; 329:762–768.
379. Lurie KG. Active compression–decompression CPR: a progress report. Resuscitation 1994; 28: 115–122.
380. Lindner KH, Pfenninger EG, Lurie KG, Schürmann W, Lindner IM, Ahnefeld FW. Effects of active compression–decompression resuscitation on myocardial and cerebral blood flow in pigs. Circulation 1993; 88:1254–1263.
381. Lurie K, Zielinski T, McKnite S, Sukhum P. Improving the efficiency of cardiopulmonary resuscitation with an inspiratory impedance threshold valve. Crit Care Med 2000; 28:N207–N209.
382. Voelckel WG, Lurie KG, Zielinski T, et al. The effects of positive end-expiratory pressure during active compression decompression cardiopulmonary resuscitation with the inspiratory threshold valve. Anesth Analg 2001; 92:967–974.
383. Lurie KG, Coffeen P, Shultz J, McKnite S, et al. Improving active compression–decompression cardiopulmonary resuscitation with an inspiratory impedance valve. Circulation 1995; 91:1629–1632.
384. Lurie K, Zielinski T, McKnite S, Aufderheide T, Voelckel W. Use of an inspiratory impedance valve improves neurologically intact survival in a porcine model of ventricular fibrillation. Circulation 2002; 105:124–129.
385. Plaisance P, Lurie KG, Payen D. Inspiratory impedance during active compression -decompression cardiopulmonary resuscitation: a randomized evaluation in patients in cardiac arrest. Circulation 2000; 101:989–994.
386. Wolcke BB, Mauer DK, Schoefmann MF, et al. Standard CPR versus active compression–decompression CPR with an impedance threshold valve in patients with out of hospital cardiac arrest [Abstract]. Resuscitation 2002; 55:115.
387. Cohen TJ, Goldner BG, Maccaro PC, et al. Comparison of active compression–decompression cardiopulmonary resuscitation with standard cardiopulmonary resuscitation for cardiac arrests occurring in the hospital. N Engl J Med 1993; 329:1918–1921.
388. Lurie KG, Shultz JJ, Callaham ML, et al. Evaluation of active compression–decompression CPR in victims of out-of-hospital cardiac arrest. JAMA 1994; 271:1405–1411.
389. Schwab TM, Callaham ML, Madsen CD, Utecht TA. A randomized clinical trial of active compression–decompression CPR vs standard CPR in out-of-hospital cardiac arrest in two cities. JAMA 1995; 273:1261–1268.
390. Stiell IG, Hébert PC, Wells GA, et al. The Ontario trial of active compression–decompression cardiopulmonary resuscitation for in-hospital and prehospital cardiac arrest. JAMA 1996; 275:1417–1423.
391. Plaisance P, Lurie K, Vicaut E, et al. Comparison of standard cardiopulmonary resuscitation and active compression–decompression for out-of-hospital cardiac arrest. N Engl J Med 1999;341:569–575.
392. Mauer DK, Nolan J, Plaisance P, et al. Effect of active compression–decompression resuscitation (ACD-CPR) on survival: a combined analysis using individual patient data. Resuscitation 1999; 41:249–256.
393. Babbs CF, Weaver JC, Ralston S, Geddes LA. Cardiac, thoracic, and abdominal pump mechanisms in cardiopulmonary resuscitation: studies in an electrical model of the circulation. Am J Emerg Med 1984; 2:299–308.
394. Tang W, Weil MH, Schock RB, et al. Phased chest and abdominal compression–decompression. A new option for cardiopulmonary resuscitation. Circulation 1997; 95:1335–1340.
395. Sterz FBW, Berzanovich A. Active compression–decompression of thorax and abdomen (Lifestick CPR) in patients with cardiac arrest [Abstract]. Circulation 1996; 94:19.

396. Arntz H, Agrawal R, Richter A, et al. Phased chest and abdominal compression–decompression versus conventional cardiopulmonary resuscitation in out-of-hospital cardiac arrest. Circulation 2001; 104: 768–772.

397. Adams JA, Bassuk J, Wu D, Kurlansky P. Survival and normal neurological outcome after CPR with periodic GZ acceleration and vasopressin. Resuscitation 2003; 56:215–221.

398. Adams JA, Mangino MJ, Bassuk J, Kurlansky P, Sackner MA. Novel CPR with periodic Gz acceleration. Resuscitation 2001; 51:55–62.

399. Reich H, Angelos M, Safar P, Sterz F, Leonov Y. Cardiac resuscitability with cardiopulmonary bypass after increasing ventricular fibrillation times in dogs. Ann Emerg Med 1990; 19:887–890.

400. Angelos MG, Gaddis ML, Gaddis GM, Leasure JE. Improved survival and reduced myocardial necrosis with cardiopulmonary bypass reperfusion in a canine model of coronary occlusion and cardiac arrest. Ann Emerg Med 1990; 19:1122–1128.

401. Angelos MG, Ward KR, Hobson J, Beckley PD. Organ blood flow following cardiac arrest in a swine low flow cardiopulmonary bypass model. Resuscitation 1994; 27:245–254.

402. Gazmuri RJ, Weil MH, von Planta M, Gazmuri RR, Shah DM, Rackow EC. Cardiac resuscitation by extracorporeal circulation after failure of convention CPR. J Lab Clin Med 1991; 118:65–73.

403. Safar P, Abramson NS, Angelos M, et al. Emergency cardiopulmonary bypass for resuscitation from prolonged cardiac arrest. Am J Emerg Med 1990; 8:55–67.

404. Levine R, Gorayeb M, Safar P, Abramson N, Stezoski W, Kelsey S. Cardiopulmonary bypass after cardiac arrest in prolonged closed-chest CPR in dogs. Ann Emerg Med 1987; 16:620–627.

405. Martin GB, Nowak RM, Carden DL, Eisiminger RA, Tomlanovich MC. Cardiopulmonary bypass versus CPR as treatment for prolonged canine cardiopulmonary arrest. Ann Emerg Med 1987; 16:628–636.

406. Safar P, Abramson NS, Angelos M, et al. Emergency cardiopulmonary bypass for resuscitation from prolonged cardiac arrest. Am J Emerg Med 1990; 8:55–67.

407. Reichman RT, Joyo CI, Dembitsky WP, et al. Improved patient survival after cardiac arrest using a cardiopulmonary support system. Ann Thorac Surg 1990; 49; 101–105.

408. Phillips SJ, Zeff RH, Kongtahworn C, et al. Percutaneous cardiopulmonary bypass: application and indication for use. Ann Thorac Surg 1989; 47:121–123.

409. Martin GB, Rivers EP, Paradis NA, Goetting MG, Morris DC, Nowak RM. Emergency department cardiopulmonary bypass in the treatment of human cardiac arrest. Chest 1998; 113:743–751.

410. Iijima T, Bauer R, Hossmann KA. Brain resuscitation by extracorporeal circulation after prolonged cardiac arrest in cats. Intensive Care Med 1993; 19:82–88.

411. del Nido PJ, Dalton HJ, Thompson AE, Siewers RD. Extracorporeal membrane oxygenator rescue in children during cardiac arrest after cardiac surgery. Circulation 1992; 86(5 Suppl 2):II300–II304.

412. Walcott GP, Booker RG, Ideker RE. Defibrillation with a minimally invasive direct cardiac device. Resuscitation 2002; 55:301–307.

413. Buckman RF Jr, Badellino MM, Eynon AC, et al. Open-chest cardiac massage without major thoracotomy: metabolic indicators of coronary and cerebral perfusion. Resuscitation 1997; 34:247–253.

414. Paiva EF, Kern KB, Hilwig RW, Scalabrini A, Ewy GA. Minimally invasive direct cardiac massage versus closed-chest cardiopulmonary resuscitation in a porcine model of prolonged ventricular fibrillation cardiac arrest. Resuscitation 2000; 47: 287-299.

415. Tang W, Weil MH, Noc M, Sun S, Gazmuri RJ, Bisera J. Augmented efficacy of external CPR by intermittent occlusion of the ascending aorta. Circulation 1993; 88: 1916-1921.

416. Nozari A, Rubertsson S, Wiklund L. Improved cerebral blood supply and oxygenation by aortic balloon occlusion combined with intra-aortic vasopressin administration during experimental cardiopulmonary resuscitation. Acta Anaesthesiol Scand 2000; 44:1209–1219.

417. Liu XL, Nozari S, Basu G, Ronquist S, Rubertsson S, Wiklund L. Neurological outcome after experimental cardiopulmonary resuscitation: a result of delayed and potentially treatable neuronal injury? Acta Anaesthesiol Scand 2002; 46:537–546.

418. Nozari A, Rubertsson S, Gedeborg R, Nordgren A, Wiklund L. Maximisation of cerebral blood flow during experimental cardiopulmonary resuscitation does not ameliorate post-resuscitation hypoperfusion. Resuscitation 1999; 40:27–35.

419. Reed RL, Johnston TD, Chen Y, Fischer RP. Hypertonic saline alters plasma clotting times and platelet aggregation. J Trauma 1991; 31:8–14.

420. Nolte D, Bayer M, Lehr HA, et al. Attenuation of postischeamic microvascular disturbances in striated muscle by hyperosmolar saline dextran. Am J Physiol 1992; 263:1411–1416.

421. Steinbauer M, Harris A, Hoffman T, Messmer K. Pharmacologic effects of dextrans on the postischemic leukocyte-endothelial interaction. Prog Appl Microcirc 1996; 22:114–125.

422. Otto CW, Yakaitis RW, Blitt CD. Mechanism of action of epinephrine and resuscitation from asphyxial arrest. Crit Care Med 1981; 9:364,365.

423. Brown CG, Taylor RB, Werman HA, Luu T, Ashton J, Hamlin RL. Myocardial oxygen delivery/consumption during cardiopulmonary resuscitation: a comparison of epinephrine and phenylephrine. Ann Emerg Med 1988; 17:302–308.

424. Ditchey RV, Lindenfeld J. Failure of epinephrine to improve the balance between myocardial oxygen supply and demand during closed-chest resuscitation in dogs. Circulation 1988; 78:382–389.

425. Ditchey RV, Rubio-Perez A, Slinker BK. Beta-adrenergic blockade reduces myocardial injury during experimental cardiopulmonary resuscitation. J Am Coll Cardiol 1994; 24:804–812.

426. Midei MG, Sugiura S, Maughan, L Sagawa K, Weisfeldt ML, Guerci AD. Preservation of ventricular function by treatment of ventricular fibrillation with phenylephrine. J Am Coll Cardiol 1990; 16:489–494.

427. Michael JR, Guerci AD, Koehler RC, et al. Mechanism by which epinephrine augments cerebral and myocardial perfusion during cardiopulmonary resuscitation in dogs. Circulation 1984; 69:822–835.

428. Koide T, Wieloch TE, Siesjö BK. Circulating catecholamines modulate ischemic brain damage. J Cereb Blood Flow Metab 1986; 6:559–565.

429. Chase PB, Kern KB, Sanders AB, Otto CW, Ewy GA. Effects of greater doses of epinephrine on both non-invasive and invasive measures of myocardial perfusion in blood flow during cardiopulmonary resuscitation. Crit Care Med 1993; 21:413–419.

430. Brown CG, Werman HA, Davis EA, Hamlin R, et al. Comparative effect of graded doses of epinephrine on regional brain blood flow during CPR in a swine model. Ann Emerg Med 1986; 15:1138–1144.

431. Menegazzi JJ, Davis EA, Yealy DM, et al. An experimental algorithm versus standard advanced cardiac life support in a swine model of out-of-hospital cardiac arrest. Ann Emerg Med 1993; 22:235–239.

432. Berkowitz ID, Gervais H, Schleien CL, Koehler RC, Dean JM, Traystman RJ. Epinephrine dosage effects on cerebral and myocardial blood flow in an infant swine model of cardiopulmonary resuscitation. Anesthesiol 1991; 75:1041–1050.

433. Steill IG, Hebert MD, Weitzman BN, et al. High dose epinephrine in adult cardiac arrest. N Engl J Med 1992; 327:1045–1050.

434. Brown CG, Martin DR, Pepe PE, et al. A comparison of standard-dose and high-dose epinephrine in cardiac arrest outside the hospital. The multicenter high-dose epinephrine study group. N Engl J Med 1992; 327:1051–1055.

435. Vandycke C, Martens P. High dose versus standard dose epinephrine in a cardiac arrest- a meta-analysis. Resuscitation 2000; 45:161–166.

436. Gedeborg R, Silander HC, Ronne-Engstrom E, Rubertsson S, Wiklund L. Adverse effects of high-dose epinephrine on cerebral blood flow during experimental cardiopulmonary resuscitation. Crit Care Med 2000; 28:1423–1430.

437. Roberts D, Landolfo K, Dobson K, Light RB. The effects of methoxamine and epinephrine on survival and regional distribution of cardiac output in dogs with prolonged ventricular fibrillation. Chest 1990; 98:999–1005.

438. Klouche K, Weil MH, Sun S, Tang W, Zhao DH. A comparison of "-methylnorepinephrine, vasopressin and epinephrine for cardiac resuscitation. Resuscitation 2003; 57:93–100.

439. Weil MH, Bisera J, Trevino RP, Rackow EC. Cardiac output and end-tidal carbon-dioxide. Crit Care Med 1985; 13:907–909.

440. Wenzel V, Lindner KH, Krismer AC, et al. Survival with full neurological recovery and no cerebral pathology after prolonged cardiopulmonary resuscitation with vasopressin in pigs. J Am Coll Cardiol 2000; 35:527–533.

441. Prengel AW, Lindner KH, Keller A. Cerebral oxygenation during cardiopulmonary resuscitation with epinephrine and vasopressin in pigs. Stroke 1996; 27:1241–1248.

442. Voelckel WG, Lurie KG, McKnite S, et al. Comparison of epinephrine and vasopressin in a pediatric porcine model of asphyxial cardiac arrest. Crit Care Med 2000; 28:3777–3783.

443. Voelckel WG, Lurie KG, McKnite S, et al. Effects of epinephrine and vasopressin in a piglet model of prolonged ventricular fibrillation and cardiopulmonary resuscitation. Crit Care Med 2002; 30:957–962.

444. Lurie KG, Voelckel WG, Iskos DN, et al. Combination drug therapy with vasopressin, adrenaline (epinephrine) and nitroglycerin improves vital organ blood flow in a porcine model of ventricular fibrillation. Resuscitation 2002; 54:187–194.

445. Stadlbauer KH, Wagner-Berger HG, Wenzel V, et al. Survival with full neurological recovery after prolonged cardiopulmonary resuscitation with a combination of vasopressin and epinephrine in pigs. Anesth Analg 2003; 96:1743–1749.

446. Stiell IG, Hebert PC, Wells GA, et al. Vasopressin versus epinephrine for inhospital cardiac arrest: a randomised controlled trial. Lancet 2001; 358:105–109.

447. Koehler RC, Michael JR. Cardiopulmonary resuscitation, brain blood flow, and neurological recovery. Crit Care Clin 1985; 1:205–222.

448. Rivers EP, Rady MY, Martin GB, e H, Appelton T, Nowak RM. Venous hyperoxia after cardiac arrest: characterization of a defect in systemic oxygen utilization. Chest 1992; 102:1787–1793.

449. Kuisma M, Suominen P, Korpela R. Paediatric out-of-hospital cardiac arrests- epidemiology and outcome. Resuscitation 1995; 30:141–150.

450. Liberthson RR. Sudden death from cardiac causes in children and young adults. N Engl J Med 1996; 334:1039–1044.

451. Takeda T, Tanigawa K, Tanaka H, Hayashi Y, Goto E, Tanaka K. The assessment of three methods to verify tracheal tube placement in the emergency setting. Resuscitation 2003; 56:153–157.

452. Ornato JP, Shipley JB, Racht EM, et al. Multicenter study of a portable, hand-size, colorimetric end-tidal carbon dioxide detection device. Ann Emerg Med 1992; 21:518–523.

453. Spaulding CM, Joly LM, Rosenberg A, et al. Immediate coronary angioraphy in survivors of out-of-hospital cardiac arrest N Engl J Med 1997; 336:1629–1633.

454. Tenaglia AN, Califf RM, Candela RJ, et al. Thrombolytic therapy in patients requiring cardiopulmonary resuscitation. Am J Cardiol 1991; 68:1015–1019.

455. Wijdicks EF, Parisi JE, Sharborough FW. Prognostic value of myoclonus status in comatose survivors of cardiac arrest. Ann Neurol 1994; 35:239–243.

456. Buyleart WA, Calle PA, Houbrechts HN. Serum electrolyte disturbances in the post-resuscitation period. The Cerebral resuscitation Study Group. Resuscitation 1989; 17(Suppl):S189–S206.

457. Vukmir RB, Bircher NG, Radovsky A, Safar P. Sodium bicarbonate may improve outcome in dogs with brief or prolonged cardiac arrest. Crit care Med 1995; 23; 515–522.

458. Emerman CL, Pinchak AC Hagen JF, Hancock D. A comparison of venous blood gases during cardiac arrest. Am J Emerg Med 1988; 6:580–583.

459. Tucker KJ, Idris AH, Wenzek V, Orban DJ. Changes in arterial and mixed venous blood gases during untreated ventricular fibrillation and cardiopulmonary resuscitation. Resuscitation 1994; 28:137–141.

460. Idris AH, Staples ED, O'Brian D, et al. Effect of ventilation on acid-base balance and oxygenation during low blood flow states. Crit Care Med 1994; 22:1827–1834.

461. Weil MH, Rackow EC, Trevino R, Grundler W, Falk JL, Griffel MI. Difference in acid-base state between venous and arterial blood during cardiopulmonary resuscitation. N Engl J Med 1986; 315:153–156.

462. Leong EC, Bendall JC, Boyd AC, Einstein R. Sodium bicarbonate improves the chance of resuscitation after 10 minutes of cardiac arrest in dogs. Resuscitation 2001; 51:309–315.

463. Filley G, Kindig N: Carbicarb, an alkalizing ion generating agent of possible clinical usefulness. Trans Am Clin Climatol Assoc 1984; 96:141–153.

464. Shapiro J, Whalen M, Kucera R, Kindig N, Filley GF, Chan L. Brain pH responses to sodium bicarbonate during systemic acidosis. Am J Physiol 1989; 256:H1316–H1321.

465. Katz LM, Wang Y, Rockoff S, Bouldin TW. Low-dose Carbicarb improves cerebral outcome after asphyxial cardiac arrest in rats. Ann Emerg Med 2002; 39:359–365.

466. Liu X, Nozari A, Rubertsson S, Wiklund L. Buffer administration during CPR promotes cerebral reperfusion after return of spontaneous circulation and mitigates post-resuscitation cerebral acidosis. Resuscitation 2002; 55:45–55.

467. Wiklund L, Ronquist G, Stjernström H, Waldenström A. Effects of alkaline buffer administration on survival and myocardial energy metabolism in pigs subjected to ventricular fibrillation and closed chest CPR. Acta Anaesthesiol Scand 1990; 34:430–439.

468. von Planta M, Gudipati CV, Weil MH, Kraus LJ, Rackow EC. Effects of tromethamine and sodium bicarbonate buffers during cardiac resuscitation. J Clin Pharmacol 1988; 28:594–599.

469. De Feo P, Perriello G, De Cosmos S, et al. Comparison of glucose counterregulation during short-term and prolonged hypoglycemia in normal humans. Diabetes 1986; 35:563–569.

470. Siesjö BK, Ingvar M, Pelligrino D. Regional differences in vascular autoregulation in the rat brain in severe insulin-induced hypoglycemia. J Cereb Blood Flow Metab 1983; 3:478–485.

471. Ginsberg MD, Welsh FA, Budd WW. Deleterious effect of glucose pretreatment on recovery from diffuse cerebral ischemia in the cat. Stroke 1980; 11:347–354.

472. Nakakimura K, Fleischer JE, Drummond JC, et al. Glucose administration before cardiac arrest worsens neurological outcome in cats. Anesthesiology 1990; 72: 1005-1011.

473. Katz LM, Wang Y, Ebmeyer U, Radovsky A, Safar P. Glucose plus insulin infusion improves cerebral outcome after asphyxial cardiac arrest. Neuroreport 1998; 9:3363–3367.

474. Müllner M, Sterz F, Binder M, Schreiber W, Deimel A, Laggner AN. Blood glucose concentration after cardiopulmonary resuscitation influences functional neurological recovery in human cardiac arrest survivors. J Cereb Blood Flow Metab 1997; 17:430–436.

475. Longstreth WT Jr, Diehr P, Cobb LA, Hanson RW, Blair AD. Neurological outcome and blood glucose levels during out-of-hospital cardiopulmonary resuscitation. Neurology 1986; 36:1186–1191.

476. Schultz CH, Rivers EP, Feldkamp CS, et al. A characterization of hypothalamic-pituitary-adrenal axis function during and after human cardiac arrest. Crit Care Med 1993; 21:1339–1347.

477. Katsura K, Kurihara J, Siesjö BK, Wieloch T. Acidosis enhances translocation of protein kinase C but not Ca (2+)/calmodulin-dependent protein kinase II to cell membranes during complete cerebral ischemia. Brain Res 1999; 849:119–127.

478. Martin GB, O'Brien JF, Best R, Goldman J, Tomlanovich MC, Nowak RM. Insulin and glucose levels during CPR in the canine model. Ann Emerg Med 1985; 14:293–297.

479. Budihardjo I, Oliver H, Lutter M, Luo X, Wang X. Biochemical pathways of caspase activation during apoptosis. Annu Rev Cell Dev Biol 1999; 15:269–290.

480. Rehncrona S, Rosen I, Siesjö BK. Excessive cellular acidosis: an important mechanism of neuronal damage in the brain? Acta Physiol Scand 1980; 110:435–437.

481. Rehncrona S, Rosen I, Siesjö BK. Brain lactic acidosis and ischemic cell damage: 1. Biochemistry and neurophysiology. J Cereb Blood Flow Metab 1981; 1:297–311.

482. Rehncrona S, Hauge HN, Siesjö BK. Enhancement of iron-catalyzed free radical formation by acidosis in brain homogenates: Difference in effect by lactic acid and CO_2. J Cereb Blood Flow Metab 1989; 9:65–70.

483. Dietrich D, Alonso O, Busto R. Moderate hyperglycemia worsens acute blood-brain barrier injury after forebrain ischemia in rats. Stroke 1993; 24:111–115.

484. Schurr A, Payne RS, Tseng MT, Miller JJ, Rigor BM. The Glucose paradox in cerebral ischemia. New insights. Ann NY Acad Sci 1999; 386:386–390.

485. Schurr A, Payne RS, Miller JJ, Tseng MT. Preischemic hyperglycemia-aggravated damage: evidence that lactate utilization is beneficial and glucose-induced corticosterone is detrimental. J Neurosci Res 2001; 66:782–789.

486. Rayne RS, Teseng MT, Schurr A. The glucose paradox of cerebral ischemia: evidence for corticosterone involvement. Brain Res 2003; 971:9–17.

487. Rello J, Valles J, Jubert P, et al. Lower respiratory tract infections following cardiac arrest and cardiopulmonary resuscitation. Clin Infect Dis 1995; 21:310–314.

488. Dohi S. Postcardiopulmonary resuscitation pulmonary edema. Crit Care Med 1983; 11:434–437.

489. Liu Y, Rosenthal RE, Haywood Y, Miljkovic-Lolic M, Vanderhoek JY, Fiskum G. Normoxic ventilation after cardiac arrest reduces oxidation of brain lipids and improves neurological outcome. Stroke 1998; 29:1679–1686.

490. Zwemer CF, Whitesall SE, D'Alecy LG. Hypoxic cardiopulmonary-cerebral resuscitation fails to improve neurological outcome following cardiac arrest in dogs. Resuscitation 1995; 29:225–236.

491. Fercakova A, Marsala M, Marsala J. Influence of graded postischemic reoxygenation on reperfusion alterations in rabbit dorsal root ganglion neurons. J Hisrnforsch 1994; 35:295–302.

492. Rootwelt T, Loberg EM, Moen A, Oyasaeter S, Saugstad OD. Hypoxemia and reoxygentaion with 21% or 100% oxygen in newborn pigs: changes in blood pressure, base deficit, and hypoxanthine and brain morphology. Pediatr Res 1992; 32:107–113.

493. Klaus S, Heringlake M, Gliemroth J, Pagel H, Staubach K, Bahlmann L. Biochemical tissue monitoring during hypoxia and reoxygenation. Resuscitation 2003; 56:299–305.

494. Ernster L: Biochemistry of reoxygenation injury. Crit care Med 1988; 16:947–953.

495. Douzinas EE, Patsouris E, Kypriades EM, et al. Hypoxaemic reperfusion ameliorates the histopathological changes in the pig brain after a severe global cerebral ischaemic insult. Intensive Care Med 2001; 27:905–910.

496. Kutzsche S, Ilves P, Kirkeby OJ, Saugstad OD. Hydrogen peroxide production in leukocytes during cerebral hypoxia and reoxygenation with 100% or 21% oxygen in newborn piglets. Pediatr Res 2001; 49:834–842.

497. Zwemer CF, Whitesall SE, D'Alecy LG. Cardiopulmonary-cerebral resuscitation with 100% oxygen exacerbates neurological dysfunction following nine minutes of normothermic cardiac arrest in dogs. Resuscitation 1994; 27:159–170.

498. Lipinski CA, Hicks SD, Callaway CW. Normoxic ventilation during resuscitation and outcome from asphyxial cardiac arrest in rats. Resuscitation 1999; 42:221–229.

499. Dietrich WD. Morphological manifestations of reperfusion injury in brain. Ann N Y Acad Sci 1994; 723:15–24.

500. Feet BA, Gilland E, Groenendaal F, et al. Cerebral excitatory amino acids and Na+, K+-ATPase activity during resuscitation of severely hypoxic newborn piglets. Acta Paediatr 1998; 87:889–895.

501. Vanicky I, Marsala M, Murar J, Marsala J. Prolonged postischemic hyperventilation reduces acute neuronal damage after 15 min of cardiac arrest in the dog. Neurosci Lett 1992; 135:167–170.

502. Muizelaar JP, Marmarou A, Ward JD, Kontos HA, Choi SC, Becker DP, Gruemer H, Young HF: Adverse effects of prolonged hyperventilation in patients with severe head injury: a randomized clinical trial. J Neurosurg 1991; 75:731–739.

503. Safar P, Xiao F, Radovsky A, et al. Improved cerebral resuscitation from cardiac arrest in dogs with mild hypothermia plus blood flow promotion. Stroke 1996; 27:105–113.

504. Rosner MJ, Daughton S. Cerebral perfusion pressure management in head injury. J Trauma 1990; 30:933–941.

505. Ligas JR, Mosleshi F, Epstein MA. Occult positive end-expiratory pressure with different types of mechanical ventilators. J Crit Care 1990; 52:95–100.

506. Krakovsky M, Rogatsky G, Zarchin N, Mayevsky A. Effect of hyperbaric oxygen therapy on survival after global cerebral ischemia in rats. Surg Neurol 1998; 49:412–416.

507. Kapp JP, Phillips M, Markov A, Smith RR. Hyperbaric oxygen after circulatory arrest: modification of postischemic encephalopathy. Neurosurg 1982; 11:496–499.

508. Iwatsuki N, Takahashi M, Ono K, Tajima T. Hyperbaric oxygen combined with nicardipine administration accelerate neurological recovery after cerebral ischemia in a canine model. Crit Care Med 1992; 20:858–863.

509. Miljkovic-Lolic M, Silbergleit R, Fiskum G, Rosenthal RE. Neuroprotective effects of hyperbaric oxygen treatment in experimental focal cerebral ischemia are associated with reduced brain leukocyte myeloperoxidase activity. Brain Res 2003; 971:90–94.

510. Thom SR. Functional inhibition of leukocyte B_2 integrins by hyperbaric oxygen in carbon monoxide-mediated brain injury in rats. Toxicol Appl Pharmacol 1993; 123:248–256.

511. Mink RB, Dutka AJ. Hyperbaric oxygen after cerebral ischemia in rabbits reduces brain vascular permeability and blood flow. Stroke 1995; 26:2307–2312.

512. Wada K, Miyazawa LJ. Inflammatory cell adhesion molecules in ischemic cerebrovascular disease. Stroke 2002; 173:168–181.

513. Yin W, Badr AE, Mychaskiw G, Zhang JH. Down regulation of COX-2 is involved in hyperbaric oxygen treatment in a rat transient focal cerebral ischemia model. Brain Res 2002; 926:165–171.

514. Gunther A, Manaenko A, Franke H, Dickel T, Berrouschot J, Wagner A, Illes P, Reinhardt R. Early biochemical and histological changes during hyperbaric or normobaric reoxygenation after in vitro ischaemia in primary corticoencephalic cell cultures of rats. Brain Res 2002; 946:130–138.

515. Rusyniak DE, Kirk MA, May JD, et al. Hyperbaric oxygen therapy in acute ischemic stroke: results of the Hyperbaric Oxygen in Acute Ischemic Stroke Trial Pilot Study. Stroke 2003; 34:571–574.

516. Rosenthal RE, Silbergleit R, Hof PR, Haywood Y, Fiskum G. Hyperbaric oxygen reduces neuronal death and improves neurological outcome after canine cardiac arrest. Stroke 2003; 34:1311–1316.

517. McKinley BA, Morris WP, Parmley CL, Butler BD. Brain parenchyma P_{O2}, P_{CO2}, and pH during and after hypoxic, ischemic brain insult in dogs. Crit Care Med 1996; 24:1858–1868.

518. Bogaert YE, Sheu KF, Hof PR, et al. Neuronal subclass-selective loss of pyruvate dehydrogenase immunoreactivity following canine cardiac arrest and resuscitation. Exp Neurol 2000; 161:115–126.

519. ACC/AHA Task Force Report. Guidelines for early management of patients with acute myocardial infarction. J Am Coll Cardiol 1990; 16:249–292.

520. Rivers EP, Wortsman J, Rady M, Blake HC, McGeorge FT, Buderer NM. The effect of the total cumulative epinephrine dose administered during human CPR on hemodynamic, oxygen transport, and utilization variables in the postresuscitation period. Chest 1994; 106:1499–1507.

521. Tang W, Weil MH, Sun SJ, Gazmuri RJ, Bisera J. Progressive myocardial dysfunction after cardiac resuscitation. Crit Care Med 1993; 21:1046–1050.

522. Charlat ML, O'Neill PG, Hartley CJ, Roberts Bolli R. Prolonged abnormalities of the left ventricular diastolic wall thinning in the "stunned" myocardium in conscious dogs: time course and relation to systolic function. J Am Coll Cardiol 1989; 13:185–194.

523. Rady MY, Rivers EP, Martin GB, Smithline H, Appelton T, Nowak RM. Continuous central venous oximetry and shock index in the emergency department: use in the evaluation of clinic shock. Am J Emerg Med 1992; 10:538–541.

524. Stoddard MF, Longaker RA. The safety of transesophageal echocardiography in the elderly. Am Heart J 1993; 125:1358–1362.

525. Rivers EP, McGeorge FT, Boczar ME. A hemodynamic comparison of mechanical, standard, and active compression–decompression CPR in human cardiac arrest [Abstract]. Clin Intensive Care 1994; 5:S30.

526. Rivers EP, Rady MY, Martin BG, et al. Venous hyperoxia after cardiac arrest. Chest 1992; 102: 1787–1793.

527. Rivers EP, Wortsman J, Rady MY, Blake HC, McGeorge FT, Buderer NM. The effects of the total cumulative epinephrine dose administered during human CPR on hemodynamics, oxygen transport, and utilization in the postresuscitation period. Chest 1994; 106:1499–1507.

528. Bernard GR, Sopko G, Cerra F, et al. Pulmonary artery catheterization and clinical outcomes: National Heart, Lung, and Blood Institute and Food and Drug Administration Workshop Report. Consensus Statement. JAMA 2000; 283:2568–2572.

529. Meyer RJ, Kern KB, Berg RA, Hilwig RW, Ewy GA. Post-resuscitation right ventricular dysfunction: delineation and treatment with dobutamine. Resuscitation 2002; 55:187–191.

530. Voelckel WG, Lindner KH, Wenzel V, et al. Effect of small-dose dopamine on mesenteric blood flow and renal function in a pig model of cardiopulmonary resuscitation with vasopressin. Anesth Analg 1999; 89:1430–1436.

531. Leir CV. Regional blood flow response to vasodilators and inotropes in congestive heart failure. Am J Cardiol 1988; 25:75–83.

532. Figulla HR. Circulatory support devices in clinical cardiology. Current concepts. Cardiology 1994; 84:149–155.

533. Jaffe AS. The use of antiarrhythmics in advanced cardiac life support. Ann Emerg Med 1993; 22:307–316.

534. DiMarco JP, Miles W, Akhtar M, et al. Adenosine for paraxosmal supraventricular tachycardia: dose ranging and comparison with verapamil: assessment in placebo-controlled, multicenter trials: the Adenosine for PSVT Study Group. Ann Intern Med 1990; 113:104–110.

535. Hashimi-Idrissi S, Corne L, Huyghens L. The effect of mild hypothermia and induced hypertension on long term survival rate and neurological outcome after asphyxial cardiac arrest in rats. Resuscitation 2001; 49:73–82.

536. Sterz F, Leonov Y, Safar P, Radovsky A, Tisherman SA, Oku K. Hypertension with or without hemodilution after cardiac arrest in dogs. Stroke 1990; 21:1178–1184.

537. Spivey WH, Abramson NS, Safar P. Correlation of blood pressure with mortality and neurological recovery in comatose postresuscitation patients [abstract]. Ann Emerg Med 1991; 20:453.

538. Ames A 3rd, Wright RL, Kowada M, Thurston JM, Majno G. Cerebral ischemia. The no-reflow phenomenon. Am J Pathol 1968; 52:437–453.

539. Smrcka M, Horky M, Otevrel F, Kuchtickova S, Kotola V, Muzik J. The onset of apoptosis of neurons induced by ischemia-reperfusion injury is delayed by transient period of hypertension in rats. Physiol Res 2003; 52:117–122.

540. Hossman KA. Resuscitation potentials after proilonged global ischemia in cats. Crit Care Med 1988; 16:964–971.

541. Hashimi-Idrissi S, Corne L, Huyghens L. The effect of mild hypothermia and induced hypertension on long term survival rate and neurological outcome after asphyxial cardiac arrest in rats. Resuscitation 2001; 49:73–82.

542. Eriksson M, Saldeen T. Effect of dextran on plasma tissue plasminogen activator (t-PA) and plasminogen activator inhibitor-1 (PAI-1) during surgery. Acta Anaesthesiol Scand 1995; 39:163–166.

543. Krieter H, Denz C, Janke C, et al. Hypertonic-hyperoncotic solutions reduce the release of cardiac troponin I and s-100 after successful cardiopulmonary resuscitation in pigs. Anesth Analg 2002; 95:1031–1036.

544. Safar P, Sterz F, Leonov Y, Radovsky A, Tisherman S, Oku K. Systematic development of cerebral resuscitation after cardiac arrest. Three promising treatments: cardiopulmonary bypass, hypertensive hemodilution, and mild hypothermia. Acta Neurochir Suppl 1993; 57:110–121.

545. Klatzo I. Brain edema following brain ischaemia and the influence of therapy. Br J Anaesth 1985; 57:18–22.

546. Bleyaert AL, Sands PA, Safar P, et al. Augmentation of postischemic brain damage by severe intermittent hypertension. Crit Care Med 1980; 8:41–47.

547. Mullner M, Sterz F, Binder M, Hellwagner K, Meron G, Herkner H, Laggner AN. Arterial blood pressure after human cardiac arrest and neurological recovery. Stroke 1996; 27:59–62.

548. Sasse HC, Safar P, Kelsey SF. Arterial hypertension after cardiac arrest is associated with good cerebral outcome in patients [Abstract]. Crit Care Med 1999; 27:A29.
549. Hickey RW, Kochanek PM, Ferimer H, Graham SH, Safar P. Hypothermia and hyperthermia in children after resuscitation from cardiac arrest. Pediatrics 2000; 106:118–122.
550. Hickey RW, Kochanek PM, Ferimer H, Alexander HL, Garman RH, Graham SH. Induced hyperthermia exacerbates neuronal histologic damage after asphyxial cardiac arrest in rats. Crit Care Med 2003; 31:531–555.
551. Zeiner A, Holzer M, Sterz F, Schorkhuber W, Eisenberger P, Uray T, Behringer W. Hyperthermia after cardiac arrest is associated with an unfavorable neurological outcome. Arch Intern Med 2001; 161:2007–2012.
552. Morris MC, Nadkarni VM. Temperature regulation after cardiac arrest: Timing is everything! Crit Care Med 2003; 31:654,655.
553. Gaussorgues P, Gueugniaud PY, Vedrinne JM, Salord F, Mercatello A, Robert D. Bacteremia following cardiac arrest and cardiopulmonary resuscitation. Intensive Care Med 1988; 14:575–577.
554. Sweeney MS, Cooley DA, Reul GJ, Ott DA, Duncan JM. Hypothermic circulatory arrest for cardiovascular lesions: technical considerations and results. Ann Thorac Surg 1985; 40:498–503.
555. Weiss SJ, Muñiz AE, Ernst AA, Lippton HL, Nick TG. The Effect of Prior Hypothermia on the Physiological Response to Norepinephrine. Resuscitation 2000; 45:201–207.
556. Steen PA, Soule EH, Michenfelder JD. Detrimental effect of prolonged hypothermia in rats and monkeys with and without regional cerebral ischemia. Stroke 1979; 10:522–529.
557. Rohrer MJ, Natale AM. Effect of hypothermia on the coagulation cascade. Crit Care Med 1992; 20:1402–1405.
558. Ji Y, Lui J. Numerical studies on the effect of lowering temperature on the oxygen transport during brain hypothermia resuscitation. Comput Biol Med 2002; 32:495–514.
559. Rosomoff HL. Protective effects of hypothermia against pathological processes of the nervous system. Ann N Y Acad Sci 1959; 80:475–486.
560. Benson DW, Williams GR, Spencer FC. The use of hypothermia after cardiac arrest. Anesth Analg 1958; 38:213–245.
561. Weinrauch V, Safar P, Tisherman S, Kuboyama K, Radovsky A. Beneficial effect of mild hypothermia and detrimental effect of deep hypothermia after cardiac arrest in dogs. Stroke 1992; 23: 1454–1462.
562. Holzer M, Behringer W, Schorkhuber W, et al. Hypothermia for Cardiac Arrest (HACA) Study Group. Mild hypothermia and outcome after CPR. Acta Anaesthsiol Scand Suppl 1997; 111:55–58.
563. Leonov Y, Sterz F, Safar P, Radovsky A, Oku K, Tisherman S, Stezoski SW. Mild cerebral hypothermia during and after cardiac arrest improves neurological outcome in dogs. J Cereb Blood Flow Metab 1990; 10:57–70.
564. Sterz F, Safar P, Tisherman S, Radovsky A, Kuboyama K, Oku K. Mild hypothermic cardiopulmonary resuscitation improves outcome after prolonged arrest in dogs [see comments]. Crit Care Med 1991; 19:379–389.
565. Busto R, Dietrich WD, Globus MY, Valdes I, Scheinberg P, Ginsberg MD. Small differences in intraischemic brain temperature critically determine the extent of ischemic neuronal injury. J Cereb Blood Flow Metab 1987; 7:729–738.
566. Xiao F, Safar P, Radovsky A. Mild protective and resuscitative hypothermia for asphyxial cardiac arrest in rats. Am J Emerg Med 1998; 16:17–25.
567. Wass CT, Lanier WL, Hofer RE, Scheithauer BW, Andrews AG. temperature changes of > 1 C alter functional neurological outcome and histopathology in a canine model of complete cerebral ischemia. Anesthesiology 1995; 83:325–335.
568. Rosomoff HL, Holaday DA. Cerebral blood flow and cerebral oxygen consumption during hypothermia. Am J Physiol 1954; 179:85–88.
569. Kuboyama K, Safar P, Oku KL, et al. Mild hypothermia after cardiac arrest in dogs does not affect postarrest cerebral oxygen uptake/delivery mismatching. Resuscitation 1994; 27:231–244.
570. Oku K, Sterz F, Safar P, et al. Mild hypothermia after cardiac arrest in dogs does not affect postarrest multifocal cerebral hypoperfusion. Stroke 1993; 24:1590–1597.
571. Busto R, Globus MY, Dietrich D, Martinez E, Valdes I, Ginsberg MD. Effect of mild hypothermia on ischemic-induced release of neurotransmitters and fatty acids in rat brain. Stroke 1989; 20: 904–910.
572. Kumar K, Wu X, Evans AT, Marcoux F. The effects of hypothermia on induction of heat shock proteins (HSP)-72 in ischemic brain. Metab Brain Dis 1995; 10:283–291.

573. Kamme F, Campbell K, Wieloch T. Bipahsic expression of the fos and jun families of transcription factors following transient forebrain ischemia in the rat. Effect of hypothermia. Eur J neurosci 1995; 7:2007–2016.

574. Winfree CJ, Baker CJ, Connolly ES Jr, Fiore AJ, Solomon RA. Mild hypothermia reduces penumbal glutamate levels in the rat permanent focal cerebral ischemia model. Neurosurg 1996; 38:1216–1222.

575. Kristian T, Katsura K, Siesjö BK. The influence of moderate hypothermia on cellular calcium uptake in complete ischemia: implications for the excitotoxic hypothesis. Acta Physiol Scand 1992; 146: 531,532.

576. Kil HY, Zhang J, Piantadosi CA. Brain temperature alters hydroxyl radical production during cerebral ischemia/reperfusion in rats. J Cereb Blood Flow Metab 1996; 16:100–106.

577. Taft WC, Yang K, Dixon CE, Clifton GL, Hayes RL. Hypothermia attenuates the loss of hippocampal microtubule-associated protein 2 (MAP2) following traumatic brain injury. J Cereb Blood Flow Metab 1993; 13:796–802.

578. Hicks SD, DeFranco DB, Callaway CW. Hypothermia during reperfusion after asphyxial cardiac arrest improves functional recovery and selectively alters stress-induced protein expression. J Cereb Blood Flow Metab 2000; 20:520–530.

579. Dempsey RJ, Combs DJ, Maley ME, Cowen DE, Roy MW, Donaldson DL. Moderate hypothermia reduces postischemic edema development and leukotriene production. Surgery 1987; 21:177–181.

580. Ginsburg MD, Busto R, Castella Y. The protective effect of moderate intraischemia brain hypothermia is associated with improved postischemic glucose utilization [abstract]. J Cereb Blood Flow Metab 1989; 9:S380.

581. D'Cruz BJ, Fertig KC, Filiano A, Hicks SD, DeFranco DB. Hypothermic reperfusion after cardiac arrest augments brain-derived neurotrophic factor activation. J Cereb Blood Flow Metab 2002; 22: 843–851.

582. Shibano T, Morimoto Y, Kemmotsu O, Shikama H, Hisano K, Hua Y: Effects of mild and moderate hypothermia on apoptosis in neuronal PC12 cells. Br J Anaesth 2002; 89: 301-305.

583. Marion DW, Leonov Y, Ginsberg M, et al. Resuscitative hypothermia. Crit Care Med 1996; 24: S81–S89.

584. Bernard SA, Jones BM, Horne MK: Clinical trial of induced hypothermia in comatose survivors of out-of-hospital cardiac arrest. Ann Emerg Med 1997; 30:146–153.

585. Bernard SA, Gray TW, Buist MD, Jones BM, Silvester W, Gutteridge G, Smith K. Treatment of comatose survivors of out-of-hospital cardiac arrest with induced hypothermia. N Engl J Med 2002; 346:557–563.

586. The Hypothermia After Cardiac Arrest Study Group. Mild therapeutic hypothermia to improve the neurological outcome after cardiac arrest. N Engl J Med 2002; 346:549–556.

587. Schwab S, Schwarz S, Spranger M, Keller E, Bertram M, Hacke W. Moderate hypothermia in the treatment of patients with severe middle cerebral artery infarction. Stroke 1998; 29:2461–2466.

588. Hachimi-Idrissi S, Corne L, Ebinger G, Michotte Y, Huyghens L. Mild hypothermia induced by a helmet device: a clinical feasibility study. Resuscitation 2001; 51:275–281.

589. Zeiner A, Holzer M, Sterz, F, et al. Mild resuscitative hypothermia to improve neurological outcome after cardiac arrest. A clinical feasibility trial. Hypothermia After cardiac Arrest (HACA) Study Group. Stroke 2000; 31:86–94.

590. Felberg RA, Krieger DW, Chuang R, et al. Hypothermia after cardiac arrest: feasibility and safety of an external cooling protocol. Circulation 2001; 104:1799–1804.

591. Gunn AJ, Gluckman PD, Gunn TR. Selective head cooling in newborn infants after perinatal asphyxia: a safety study. Pediatrics 1998; 102:885–892.

592. Rajek A, Greif R, Sessler DL, Baumgardner J, Laciny S, Bastanmehr H. Core cooling by central venous infucion of ice-cold (4EC and 20EC) fluid: isolation of core and peripheral thermal compartments. Anesthesiology 2000; 93:629–637.

593. Brenard S, Buist M, Monteiro O, Smith K. Induced hypothermia using large volume, ice-cold intra-venous fluid in comatose survivors of out-of-hospital cardiac arrest: A preliminary report. Resuscitation 2000; 56:9–13.

594. Xiao F, Safar P, Alexander H. Peritoneal cooling for mild cerebral hypothermia after cardiac arrest in dogs. Resuscitation 1995; 30:51–59.

595. Ao H, Moon JK, Tanimoto H, Sakanashi Y, Terasaki H. Jugular vein temperature reflects brain temperature during hypothermia. Resuscitation 2000; 45:111–118.

596. Henker RA, Brown SD, Marion DW. Comparison of brain temperature with bladder and rectal temperatures in adults in adults with severe head injury. Neurosurgey 1998; 42:1071–1075.

597. Ao H, Tanimoto H, Yoshitake A, Moon JK, Terasaki H. Long-term mild hypothermia with extracorporeal lung and heart assist improves survival from prolonged cardiac arrest in dogs. Resuscitation 2001; 48:163–174.
598. Dietrich WD, Busto R, Alonso O, Globus MY, Ginsberg MD. Intraischemic but not postischemic brain hypothermia protects chronically following global forebrain ischemia in rats. J Cereb Blood Flow Metab 1993; 13:541–549.
599. Colubourne F, Li H, Buchan AM. Indefatigable CA1 sector neuroprotection with mild hypothermia induced 6 hours after severe forebrain ischemia in rats. J Cereb Blood Flow Metab 1999; 19:742–749.
600. Marion DW, Penrod LE, Kelsey SF, et al. Treatment of traumatic brain injury with moderate hypothermia. N Engl J Med 1997; 336:540–546.
601. Pomeranz S, Safar P, Radovsky A, Tisherman SA, Alexander H, Stezoski W. The effect of resuscitative moderate hypothermia following epidural brain compression on cerebral damage in a canine outcome model. J Neurosurg 1993; 79:241–251.
602. Ebmeyer U, Safar P, Radovsky A, Obrist W, Alexander H, Pomeranz S. Moderate hypothermia for 48 hours after temporary epidural brain compression injury in a canine outcome model. J Neurotrauma 1998; 15:323–336.
603. Nolan JP, Morley PT, Vanden Hoek TL, et al. ALS Task Force: Therapeutic hypothermia after cardiac arrest. An advisory statement by the Advanced Life Support Task Force of the International Liaison Committee on Resuscitation. Circulation 3002; 108:118–122.

31 Pediatric Cardiopulmonary Resuscitation

Robert A. Berg, MD, FAAP, FCCM
and Vinay M. Nadkarni, MD, FAAP, FCCM

INTRODUCTION

Cardiovascular disease remains the most common cause of disease-related death in the United States, resulting in approx 1 million deaths per year. It is estimated that 400,000–460,000 Americans will die from cardiac arrest (CA) each year, nearly 90% in prehospital settings *(1,2)*. Data regarding the incidence of unexpected childhood cardiopulmonary arrest (CPA) is less robust, but the best recent data suggest that approx 16,000 American children suffer a CA each year with an annual incidence of roughly 20 out of 100,000 children *(3,4)*.

Although prehospital CA in children constitute less than 10% of all cases of prehospital CA, the potential years of life lost when a child dies a preventable death is generally an order of magnitude greater than when his or her parent or grandparent dies. Therefore, the number of years of life lost from prehospital pediatric CAs rivals that for adult CAs. Moreover, the death of a child (i.e., the loss of a family's future) is much more devastating to the family and society than the expected death of an older adult. Consequently, this is a substantial public health problem, which deserves intense investigation.

In contrast to adults, children rarely suffer sudden ventricular fibrillation (VF) CA from coronary artery disease (CAD). The causes of pediatric arrests are more diverse and are usually secondary to profound hypoxia or asphyxia as a result of respiratory failure or circulatory shock *(5–7)*. Prolonged hypoxia and acidosis impair cardiac function and

From: *Contemporary Cardiology: Cardiopulmonary Resuscitation*
Edited by: J. P. Ornato and M. A. Peberdy © Humana Press Inc., Totowa, NJ

ultimately lead to CA. By the time the arrest occurs, all organs of the body have generally suffered significant hypoxic-ischemic insults. Additionally, bystander cardiopulmonary resuscitation (CPR) is only provided to approx 30% of prehospital pediatric CA victims *(4,8)*. It is therefore not surprising that the outcome from CA in children is poor.

Appropriate pediatric CPR differs from that in adults because children are anatomically and physiologically different from adults. Additionally, the pathogenesis of the CAs and the most common rhythm disturbances are different in children *(9,10)*. Moreover, children of various ages exhibit developmental changes that affect cardiac and respiratory physiology before, during, and after CA. For example, newborns undergoing transitional physiological changes during emergence from an environment of amniotic fluid to a gaseous environment certainly differ from adolescents. Similarly, newborns and infants have much less cardiac and respiratory reserve, and higher pulmonary vascular resistance compared to older children *(11)*. Additionally, many children who experience in-hospital CA have pre-existing developmental challenges and other organ dysfunction *(12-15)*. Finally, pediatrics is developmental medicine, and pediatric neurological tools that are appropriate at one age may not be accurate or valid at another age. These neurodevelopmental issues suggest that simple extrapolated use of the adult outcome scales may be inadequate. Different and more sophisticated neurodevelopmental tools may be preferable to assess long-term postresuscitation neurological outcome in children *(16)*.

Perhaps the most profound difference between children and adult CA is the devastation that the death of a child wreaks on a family. Coping with a sudden unexpected death is always difficult. When the individual is a child, the loss tends to be even more devastating. We do not expect children to die before their parents and thus are unprepared. Therefore, health care providers who are otherwise able to deal with most devastating problems, often become very emotional, and occasionally dysfunctional, when faced with a dying child. The experience for the family is naturally intense and long lasting.

THE FOUR PHASES OF CPR

CA has some common features in children and adults. One can identify four distinct phases of CA and CPR interventions: pre-arrest, no flow (untreated CA), low flow (CPR), and postresuscitation. Interventions to improve outcome from pediatric CA should optimize therapies targeted to the time and phase of CPR as suggested in Table 1.

The pre-arrest phase includes preexisting conditions (e.g., neurological, cardiac, respiratory, or metabolic problems), developmental status (e.g., premature neonate, mature neonate, infant, child, or adolescent), and precipitating events (e.g., respiratory failure or shock). It may represent a period of low, normal, or high blood flow. Interventions during the pre-arrest phase focus on prevention, with special attention to early recognition and treatment of respiratory failure and shock in children.

Interventions during the no flow phase of untreated CA focus on early recognition of CA, effective monitoring, and prompt initiation of basic (BLS) and advanced life support (ALS). Effective CPR attempts to optimize coronary perfusion pressure (CPP) and cardiac output to critical organs to support vital organ viability during the low-flow phase. As noted below, important tenets of BLS are PUSH HARD, PUSH FAST, and minimize interruptions. Optimal CPP, exhaled carbon dioxide and cardiac output during the low-flow phase of CPR is consistently associated with improved chance for return of spontaneous circulation (ROSC) and improved short- and long-term outcome. For ventricular fibrillation (VF) and pulseless ventricular tachycardia (VT), rapid determination of electrocardiographic rhythm and prompt defibrillation are most important for successful

Table 1

Phase	Interventions
Pre-arrest phase (protect)	• Optimize community education regarding child safety • Optimize patient monitoring • Prioritize interventions to avoid progression of respiratory failure and /or shock to CA
Arrest (no-flow) phase (preserve)	• Minimize interval to BLS and ALS • Organized 911/Code Blue Response system • Preserve cardiac and cerebral substrate • Minimize interval to defibrillation, when indicated
Low-flow (CPR) phase (resuscitate)	• Effective CPR to optimize myocardial blood flow and cardiac output (coronary and cerebral perfusion pressures and end-tidal CO_2) • Consider adjuncts to improve vital organ perfusion during CPR • Match oxygen delivery to oxygen demand • Consider extracorporeal CPR if standard CPR/ALS not promptly successful
Postresuscitation phase (immediate) (hours to days)	• Optimize cardiac output and cerebral perfusion • Treat arrhythmias, if indicated • Avoid hyperglycemia, hyperthermia • Consider mild resuscitative systemic hypothermia (for 24–48 hours following resuscitation) • Possible future role for antioxidants, anti-inflammatory agents, thrombolytics, mediators of hibernation, and modulation of excitatory neurotransmitters
Postresuscitation phase longer term rehabilitation (regenerate)	• Early intervention with occupational and physical therapy • Bioengineering and technology interface • Possible future role for stem cell transplantation

CA, cardiac arrest; BLS, basic life support; ALS, advanced life support; CPR, cardiopulmonary resuscitation.

resuscitation. For CAs as a result of asphyxia and/or ischemia, provision of adequate myocardial perfusion and myocardial oxygen delivery is most important.

The postresuscitation phase includes *immediate postresuscitation* management, the *next few hours to days*, and long-term *rehabilitation*. The *immediate postresuscitation* stage is a high-risk period for ventricular arrhythmias and other reperfusion injuries. Interventions during the immediate postresuscitation stage and the next few days target matching oxygen and substrate delivery to meet metabolic tissue demand in order to minimize reperfusion injury and support cellular recovery. Injured cells can hibernate, die, or partially or fully recover function. Cell death can occur as a result of necrosis or apoptosis, programmed cell death. This post-arrest phase may have the most potential for innovative advances in the understanding of cell injury and death, inflammation, apoptosis and hibernation, ultimately leading to novel interventions. Careful management of temperature, glucose, blood pressures, coagulation, and carbon dioxide *(17)* may be particularly important in this phase. The rehabilitation stage concentrates on salvage of injured cells, recruitment of hibernating cells, and reengineering of reflex and voluntary communications of these cell and organ systems to improve functional outcome.

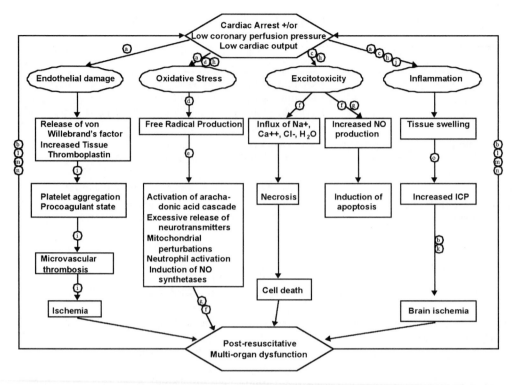

Fig. 1. A schematic of physiologic processes that result from CA and initial resuscitation, with annotation of some promising interventions, denoted by lower-case letters. Many complex interconnections and feedback loops between these processes have been omitted from the schematic in order to generate an overview of the processes and potential interventions.

a: Excellent chest compressions with
   or without adjunctive devices
b: Inotropes/vasoconstrictors
c: Intra/postresuscitative mild hypothermia
d: Avoidance of superoxia
e: Free radical scavengers
f: Modulation of neurotransmitters
g: Nitric oxide synthetase inhibitors

h: Strict avoidance of hyperthermia (fever)
i: Heparin/thombolytics
j: Steroids
k: Head at midline and 45° elevated
l: Consider ECMO
m: Optimize oxygen carrying capacity
n: Decrease oxygen demand (sedation,
   neuromuscular blockade, mild hypothermia)
o: Mannitol

The specific phase of resuscitation dictates the focus of care. Interventions that improve outcome during one phase may be deleterious during another. For instance, intense vasoconstriction during the low flow phase of CA may improve CPP and probability of ROSC (18). The same intense vasoconstriction during the postresuscitation phase may increase left ventricular (LV) afterload and worsen myocardial strain and dysfunction (18,19). Current understanding of the physiology of CA and recovery enables us to titrate blood pressure crudely, oxygen delivery and consumption, body temperature, inflammation, coagulation, and other physiologic parameters to optimize outcome. Future strategies will likely take advantage of increasing knowledge of cellular inflammation, thrombosis, reperfusion, mediator cascades, cellular markers of injury and recovery, and transplantation technology.

An overview of some of the pathophysiologic pathways perturbed by CA and resuscitation, along with potential avenues for intervention is shown in Fig. 1.

EPIDEMIOLOGY

Pediatric CAs are often secondary to respiratory arrests; the CA resulting from global asphyxia rather than from a sudden arrhythmic cardiac event. Sudden infant death syndrome is the leading cause of out-of-hospital pediatric CA, followed by trauma, airway obstruction, and drowning *(20)*.

Although sudden death from cardiac causes is unusual in children, it is estimated that approx 16,000 American children suffer a CA each year with an annual incidence of 20 out of 100,000 children. Sudden CAs caused by commotio cordis (sudden blow to the chest), acute ingestions of toxic medications (e.g., tricyclic antidepressant medications), or congenital heart disease with abnormal coronary artery anatomy are more likely to be of primary arrhythmia etiology. In children who are younger than 1 year old, sudden cardiac death is often associated with complex congenital cardiac disease. After the first year, the most common causes of sudden cardiac death in the pediatric population include myocarditis, hypertrophic cardiomyopathy, CAD, congenital coronary artery anomalies, conduction system abnormalities, mitral valve prolapse, commotio cordis, and aortic dissection.

The true incidence of pediatric pulseless arrest is difficult to estimate because of the inconsistency of terminology in the literature and difficulty in assessing pulselessness in children *(21–23)*. Approximately 5% of newborn infants require some degree of BLS in the delivery room but only 0.12% require chest compressions and/or administration of epinephrine *(24–26)*. Neonatal asphyxia accounts for 1 million deaths per year worldwide. CA occurred in 3% of children admitted to one children's hospital, in 1.8% of all children admitted to pediatric intensive care units (ICUs), and in 4% of children admitted to a pediatric cardiac (ICU) *(13,15,27,28)*. Initial ROSC occurs in 5 to 64% of pediatric CAs in different settings, and 20 to 83% of survivors suffer significant neurologic sequelae (Table 2). Survival rates differ dramatically depending on the environment in which arrest occurs, the duration of no flow prior to resuscitation, the initial electrocardiogram (EKG) rhythm detected, the quality of the BLS and ALS interventions provided, and the preexisting condition of the child. Long-term survival from pediatric out-of-hospital CA is generally less than 5%, whereas survival from arrest in a pediatric ICU is 15 to 24% *(13,14,27,28)*. Survival following CA in a specialized pediatric cardiac ICU is as high as 44% *(28–30)*, and following bradycardia requiring chest compressions in a neonatal ICU as high as 51% *(24,25)*.

Lack of uniform definitions or consistent reporting to a centralized registry of pediatric CPR impedes comparison of outcomes. A uniform style (Utstein) is recommended for reporting outcomes from CPR, with emphasis on four standard surrogate outcomes: (a) ROSC; (b) survival of event; (c) survival to hospital discharge; and (d) intact neurologic survival *(22,31)*. Future pediatric resuscitation research must focus not only on how to increase survival from CA, but how to maximize the probability that these survivors remain neurologically intact.

Several well-designed in-hospital pediatric CPR investigations with long-term follow-up have established that pediatric CPR and ALS can be remarkably effective (Table 2). Nearly two-thirds of these patients were initially successfully resuscitated (i.e., attained sustained ROSC). Survival decreased progressively with time, in large part as a result of the underlying disease processes. Most of these arrests/events occurred in pediatric ICUs as a result of progressive life-threatening illnesses that had not responded to treatment despite critical care monitoring and supportive care. The 1-year survival rates

Table 2

Summary of Representative Studies of Outcome Following Pediatric CA

Author, Year (Reference)	Setting	No. of patients	Return of spontaneous circulation (ROSC)	Survival to discharge	Intact neurological survival
Reis, 2002 (13)	In-hospital CA	129	83 (64%)	21 (16%)	19 (15%)
NRCPR, 2002 (21)	In-hospital CA	286	119 (42%)	65 (23%)	44 (15%)
Slonim, 1997 (27)	In-hospital PICU CA	205	Not reported	28 (14%)	Not reported
Zaritsky, 1987 (12)	In-hospital RA or CA RA 40	CA 53	Not reported	CA 5 (9%) RA 27 (68%)	Not reported
Channanvanak, 2000 (24)	In-hospital Intubated NICU patients who received chest compressions secondary to bradycardia	39	33/39 (85%)	20/39 (51%)	5 (13%) (6 additional patients lost to follow-up)
Extracorporeal Life Support Organization, 2002	In-hospital Resuscitation from CA via ECMO	232	Included only patients successfully resuscitated via ECMO	88 (38%)	Not reported
Parra, 2000 (28)	Pediatric cardiac ICU CA	32	24/38 arrests (63%)	14/32 patients (44%)	8/32 (25%)
Tunstall-Pedoe, 1992 (265)	In-hospital and Out-of-hospital CA	3765	1411 (38%)	706 (19%)	Not reported
Young, 1999 (4)	Meta-analysis mixed in- and out-of-hospital	Out-of-hospital CA: 1568 In-hospital CA: 544	Not reported	Out-of-hospital: 132 (8.4%) In-hospital: 129 (24%)	Not reported
Dieckmann, 1995 (33)	Out-of-hospital CA	65	3 (5%)	2 (3%)	1 (1.5%)
Gausche, 2000 (42,266)	Out-of-hospital RA	820	N/A	233 (28%)	177 (22%)
Kuisma, 1995 (14)	Out-of-hospital CA	34	10 (29%)	5 (15%)	4 (12%)
Schindler, 1996 (267)	Out-of-hospital RA or CA	101	64 (64%)	15 (15%)	0 (0%) of CA patients
Sirbaugh, 1999 (8)	Out-of-hospital CA	300	33 (11%)	6 (2%)	1 (<1%)
Suominen, 1998 (260)	Out-of-hospital CA in trauma patients	41	10 (24%)	3 (7%)	2 (5%)
Suominen, 1997 (268)	Out-of-hospital CA	50	13 (26%)	8 (16%)	6 (12%)

CA, cardiac arrest; RA, respiratory arrest; NRCPR, National Registry of Cardiopulmonary Resuscitation; PICU, pediatric intensive care unit; NICU, neonatal intensive care unit; ECMO, extracorporeal membrane oxygenation.

of 10–44% are superior to outcomes from out-of-hospital pediatric CPR, and substantially superior to the certain 0% survival rate if CPR and ALS were not provided. Most importantly, the vast majority of the survivors had good neurological outcomes (i.e., normal or no demonstrable change in their neurological status compared to pre-arrest).

The National Registry of Cardiopulmonary Resuscitation (NRCPR) is an American Heart Association (AHA)-sponsored, prospective, multisite, observational study of in-hospital resuscitation, which is currently the largest registry of its kind in the world. The NRCPR describes the first comprehensive, Utstein-based, standardized characterization of in-hospital resuscitation in the United States (32). CA etiology, intervention, and life support training emphasis differs between children and adults. Three hundred sixty-seven pediatric and 14,492 adult consecutive pulseless CA index event records using standardized consensus operational definitions and outcome measures were submitted to the NRCPR from 210 US hospitals (January 2000–June 2002). Neonatal ICU and out-of-hospital CA cases were excluded. Preliminary analysis of the NRPCR suggests that survival to hospital discharge from in-hospital pulseless CA is better for children than for adults, with reasonably good neurologic outcome in both children and adults (21). Initial shockable rhythms (VF/VT) were less common in children than in adults, but were not rare. Improved pediatric survival was likely as a result of better survival from pulseless electrical activity (PEA) and asystole. This data suggests that CPR and ALS can be effective interventions in certain resuscitation circumstances.

Is CPR in the Pre-Hospital Setting Effective for Children?

The outcomes from pediatric pre-hospital CA are dismal (4,8,33). In contrast, outcomes from in-hospital pediatric asphyxial CAs are much better (13,15,34). In Kouwenhoven et al.'s seminal report of successful resuscitation with closed-chest cardiac massage (35), the initial patients were asphyxiated children in the operating room with immediate effective resuscitation and excellent outcomes. Furthermore, our clinical experience suggests that excellent outcomes can occur after various types of bystander CPR, including mouth-to-mouth (MTM) rescue breathing alone, chest compressions (CC) alone, or standard chest compressions and mouth-to-mouth rescue breathing (CC+MTM) (36). Nevertheless, some reports question the effectiveness and advisability of pre-hospital pediatric CPR.

Pre-hospital pediatric asphyxial arrests were simulated in animal models to further delineate these issues. In the first study, asphyxia was induced by clamping of the tracheal tube of piglets until CA occurred, defined by loss of aortic pulsation. The mean time until loss of aortic pulsations was 8.9 ± 0.4 minutes. After loss of aortic pulsations, animals were randomized to simulated bystander CPR (MTM, CC, or MTM+CC) or no CPR until simulated emergency medical services (EMS) arrival 8 minutes later (37). A similar study was performed with intervention at a slightly earlier point in the asphyxial process, when the pulse was "no longer palpable," as defined by systolic pressure less than 50 mmHg. The mean tracheal tube clamp time to induce this severe hypotension was 6.8 ± 0.3 minutes, clearly a severe asphyxial insult (38). Not surprisingly, after a complete CA 24-hour survival was clearly superior in the CC+MTM group compared to the other groups Fig. 2).

When intervention was provided earlier in the process (i.e., after severe hypotension but before complete loss of aortic pulsation), even though CA would have been the clinical diagnosis, 24-hour survival was best with MTM+CC, but was better with MTM or

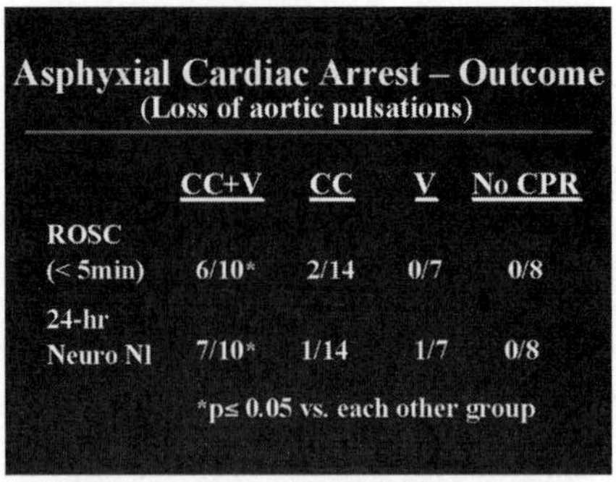

| Asphyxial Cardiac Arrest – Outcome | | | |
| (Loss of aortic pulsations) | | | |
	CC+V	CC	V	No CPR
ROSC (< 5min)	6/10*	2/14	0/7	0/8
24-hr Neuro Nl	7/10*	1/14	1/7	0/8

*p≤ 0.05 vs. each other group

Fig. 2. After prolonged experimental asphyxial cardiac arrest, 24-hour survival was superior when chest compressions (CC) and rescue breathing (V) were provided compared to no intervention, or either intervention alone *(38)*.

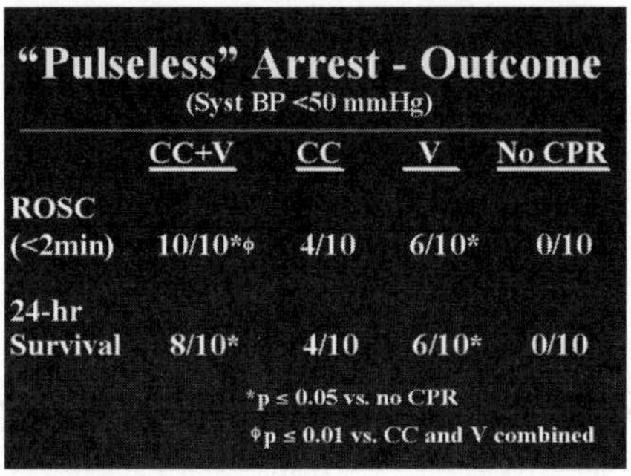

| "Pulseless" Arrest - Outcome | | | |
| (Syst BP <50 mmHg) | | | |
	CC+V	CC	V	No CPR
ROSC (<2min)	10/10*φ	4/10	6/10*	0/10
24-hr Survival	8/10*	4/10	6/10*	0/10

*p ≤ 0.05 vs. no CPR
φp ≤ 0.01 vs. CC and V combined

Fig. 3. When interventions were provided earlier during experimental, after severe hypotension and bradycardia but prior to loss of aortic pulsations, 24-hour survival was best with rescue ventilation (V) + chest compressions (CC). However, survival was better with either V or CC than with no "bystander CPR " at all *(38)*.

CC than no "bystander CPR." (Fig. 3; *38*) Interestingly, most of the animals with 24-hour survival had ROSC before the simulated EMS arrival. CPR was not futile in these models of prehospital pediatric CA. Excellent CPR was remarkably effective when provided early enough.

Sirbaugh and colleagues demonstrated that the outcomes from pediatric prehospital CAs were dismal in a large prospective study in Houston over 3 years *(8)*. Only 6 of the 300 children (2%) survived to hospital discharge, and only 1 of the 300 survived without significant neurological deficits. As in most such studies, EMS providers established the diagnosis of cardiac arrest when they arrived at the scene. Note that children in CA who attained ROSC after bystander CPR before EMS arrival were excluded from analysis. Notably, 41 children who had received bystander CPR were not in CA at the time of EMS arrival; all 41 presumably had drowning-related CAs, and all survived with good neurological outcomes (Fig. 4A and 4B). Most were quite ill when they arrived at a hospital emergency department. In contrast, none of the other 24 children with drowning-related CAs who were still in CA when the EMS personnel arrived survived with a good neurological outcome.

These data and similar data from Hickey et al. *(39)* are consistent with the animal data, reported clinical experience, and in-patient pediatric CPR data. Thus, CPR can be quite

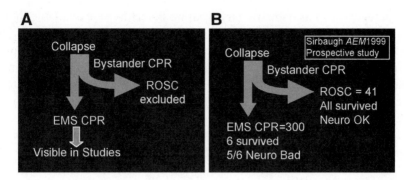

Fig. 4. Demonstrate the importance of understanding the denominator from which resuscitation reports include in their calculations. If those who collapse with absent signs of circulation assessed by rescuers at the scene and who respond to CPR interventions before arrival of EMS arrives *(8)* are eliminated, then the survival outcome reports are dramatically affected.

effective for asphyxial CAs, but timing of interventions is critically important. Recent prospective evaluation of a decade-long, population-based study of pediatric drowning-related events in Houston *(8)* demonstrated 421 children with drowning events in a population of approx 2 million total and roughly 400,000 children (annual incidence of 10per 100,000 children), and 234 required resuscitation. Of these, 193 resuscitated children (82%) received bystander CPR and 72% were long-term survivors. An astonishing 99% of the long-term survivors were neurologically intact. However, if the child was still apneic and pulseless when EMS personnel arrived, fewer than 5% were revived, and none of these subsequent survivors were ultimately neurologically intact. These data are further evidence that prehospital CPR can be quite effective for drowning-associated acute asphyxial CAs, if provided promptly. Recent adult data in out-of-hospital CA as a result of VF *(40,41)* similarly reinforces that the timing and intensity of resuscitative intervention is important, particularly when no-flow time is longer than 5 minutes.

In summary, animal and human data both indicate that CPR for children can be quite effective. Additionally, these data support the notion that BLS early is more important than ALS late. Contrary to popular opinion, prompt action by a citizen bystander in the prehospital setting or a provider in the in-patient setting is generally more effective than late heroic efforts in our ICUs.

INTERVENTIONS DURING THE LOW-FLOW PHASE: CPR

Airway and Breathing

The most common precipitating event for CAs in children is respiratory insufficiency. Therefore, providing adequate ventilation and oxygenation must remain the first priority. Effective ventilation does not necessarily require a tracheal tube. One randomized, controlled study comparing outcomes of children with out-of-hospital respiratory arrest who received bag-mask ventilation compared to bag-mask ventilation followed by tracheal intubation did not demonstrate that prehospital placement of a tracheal tube improves outcome *(42)*. However, the results of this study require interpretation in light of the fact that transport times were short and providers were trained in bag-mask ventilation extensively.

Airway adjuncts such as pediatric laryngeal mask airways are available in most hospital settings. Their use may be considered in the patient in whom tracheal intubation is not immediately feasible. Pediatric emergency, critical care and anesthesia physicians should be comfortable with their use. Emergency airway techniques such as transtracheal jet ventilation and emergency crico-thyroidotomy are rarely, if ever, required during CPR. Effective bag-mask ventilation skills remain the cornerstone of providing effective emergency ventilation.

Provision of adequate oxygen delivery to meet metabolic demand and removal of carbon dioxide is the goal of initial assisted breathing. During CPR, cardiac output and pulmonary blood flow are approx 10–25% of that during normal sinus rhythm. Consequently, much less ventilation is necessary for adequate gas exchange from the blood traversing the pulmonary circulation during CPR.

Circulation

OPTIMIZING CARDIAC OUTPUT, CORONARY, AND CEREBRAL PERFUSION PRESSURE DURING CPR

Blood is circulated during CPR by at least three different mechanisms: (a) the cardiac pump (direct compression of the heart between the sternum and the spine); (b) the thoracic pump (increases in intrathoracic pressure generating a gradient for blood to flow from the pulmonary vasculature, through the heart, and into the peripheral circulation); and (c) the abdominal pump (abdominal compression forces arterial blood from the abdomen to the periphery against a closed aortic valve and forces venous blood from the inferior vena cava back to the heart). The cardiac pump mechanism predominates in young children because of the relatively compliant thoracic wall *(43,44)*. In children from infancy through adolescence, the heart is immediately posterior to the lower third of the sternum *(44,45)*, suggesting that focusing compressions in this area may optimize the cardiac pump in pediatric CPR.

RATIO OF COMPRESSIONS TO VENTILATION

Current compression to ventilation ratios and tidal volumes recommended during CPR are based on rational conjecture, tradition, and educational retention theory. Recent physiological estimates suggest the amount of ventilation provided should match, but not exceed, perfusion and should be titrated to the phase of resuscitation (no flow, low flow, high flow) and metabolic demand of the tissues *(36)*. Current Pediatric Advanced Life Support (PALS) recommendations for the ratio of chest compressions to ventilations in an child less than 8 years old is five chest compressions to one ventilation, with a chest compression rate of 100 per minute. In children more than 8 years old, the recommended ratio is 15 chest compressions to 2 ventilations, with the chest compression rate remaining at 100 per minute *(46)*.

Although **A**irway and **B**reathing take first priority in the pediatric **ABC** algorithm, that priority has been challenged in certain circumstances. Coronary perfusion pressure, which correlates with ROSC *(47)*, rises during sequential CCs and falls during ventilation *(48,49)*. In adult CA, increasing the number of CCs to as high as 50 between ventilations, or eliminating ventilation during bystander CPR may result in better hemodynamics and increased rates of ROSC *(50,51)*. In animal models of sudden VF CA, acceptable PaO_2 and $PaCO_2$ persist with sudden CA for 4–8 minutes in the absence of any rescue breathing *(52,53)*. A randomized, controlled study of dispatcher-assisted bystander CPR in adults found a trend toward improved survival in the patients who received CCs alone compared to those who received ventilation and CCs *(54,55)*.

Because oxygenation and ventilation are clearly important for survival from fibrillatory CA, why is rescue breathing not necessary for so long in VF, yet quite important in asphyxia? Immediately after an acute VF CA, aortic oxygen and carbon dioxide concentrations do not vary from the pre-arrest state because there is no blood flow and aortic oxygen consumption is minimal. Therefore, when CCs are initiated, the blood flowing from the aorta to the coronary circulation provides adequate oxygenation at an acceptable pH. At that time, myocardial oxygen delivery is limited more by blood flow than oxygen content. Over the next several minutes, arterial oxygenation and pH become increasingly important for effective resuscitation. Adequate oxygenation and ventilation can continue without rescue breathing because of CC-induced gas exchange and spontaneous gasping ventilation during CPR. Rescue breathing is not necessary in the VF arrests for up to 12 minutes because arterial oxygenation and pH can be adequate with CCs alone. Most importantly, myocardial oxygen delivery does not differ whether rescue breathing is provided or not, in part because rescue breathing may have adverse effects on hemodynamics .

Unlike VF, during asphyxia, blood continues to flow to tissues, and arterial and venous oxygen saturation decrease although carbon dioxide and lactate continue to increase for many minutes. Additionally, continued pulmonary blood flow before the CA depletes the pulmonary oxygen reservoir. Therefore, asphyxia results in significant arterial hypoxemia and acidemia prior to resuscitation in contrast to VF.

Consequently, children with asphyxial CAs typically have a significantly higher $PaCO_2$ and lower PaO_2 at the onset of CA and following tracheal intubation during resuscitation from CA than adults *(56)*. Because respiratory arrest and asphyxia generally precede pediatric CA, foregoing ventilation in the pediatric CA patient is not prudent.

A mathematical model of oxygen delivery during CPR performed with variable ratios of CCs to ventilations revealed that with correctly delivered CCs, the optimal compression to ventilation ratio is 30:2 in adults *(51)*. When the model was adjusted using CCs as generally delivered by a lay rescuer, the optimal compression to ventilation ratio was 60:2. Mathematical models of compression–ventilation ratios suggest that matching of the amount of ventilation to the amount of reduced pulmonary blood flow during closed-chest CCs should favor a very high compression to ventilation ratio. Babbs and Kern have suggested that the best way to determine compression to ventilation ratios is to choose one that maximizes oxygen delivery to peripheral tissues (or perhaps a combination of oxygen delivery and blood flow *[51]*). Maximizing systemic oxygen delivery during single-rescuer CPR requires a tradeoff between time spent doing CCs and time spent doing MTM ventilations. Theoretically (ignoring the small amount of ventilation caused by CCs), neither compression only nor ventilation only CPR can sustain systemic oxygen delivery. Some intermediate value of the compression to ventilation ratio is needed. The best intermediate value depends on many factors including the compression rate, the tidal volume, the blood flow generated by compressions, and the time that compressions are interrupted to perform ventilations. These issues can be related in a simple mathematical formula based on classical physiology. These variables necessarily change as a function of the size of the patient. Such considerations may help refine the amount of ventilation recommended for both adults and children *(56a)*.

A CCto ventilation ratio of 15:2 delivered the same minute ventilation as CPR with a CC to ventilation ratio of 5:1 in a mannequin model of pediatric CPR, but the number of CCs delivered was 48% higher with the 15:2 ratio *(57)*. The ratio of chest compressions to ventilations during no-flow and low-flow phases of CPR remains an area of high interest, controversy, and future research. Some have suggested the potential to simplify the algorithm to 15 chest compressions and 2 ventilations in all children.

Duty Cycle

In a model of human adult CA, cardiac output and coronary blood flow are optimized when CCs last for 30% of the total cycle time (approx 1:2 ratio of time in compression to time in relaxation *[58]*). As the duration of CPR increases, the optimal duty cycle may increase to 50%. In a juvenile swine model, a relaxation period of at 250–300 ms (a duty cycle of 40–50% if 120 compressions are delivered per minute) correlates with improved cerebral perfusion pressure when compared to shorter duty cycles of 30% *(59,60)*.

Circumferential vs Focal Sternal Compressions

In adults and animal models of CA, circumferential (Vest) CPR improves CPR hemo-dynamics dramatically *(61–64)*. In smaller infants, it is often possible to encircle the chest with both hands and depress the sternum with the thumbs, while compressing the thorax circumferentially. In an infant model of CPR, this "two-thumb" method of compression resulted in higher systolic and diastolic blood pressures and a higher pulse pressure than traditional two-finger compression of the sternum *(65–68)*.

End-Tidal Carbon Dioxide Monitoring During CPR

The generation of exhaled carbon dioxide (CO_2) depends on pulmonary blood flow. Thus, circulation generated by CCs can be assessed to an extent by measuring end-tidal CO_2. Chest compressions can be titrated to exhaled CO_2 as an index of pulmonary perfusion and cardiac output. In adults with CA, an end-tidal CO_2 of greater than 10 torr is associated with ROSC and with hospital survival *(69–72)*. In an animal model, end-tidal CO_2 during CPR correlates with CPP and with ROSC.

In pediatric animal models of asphyxial CA, end-tidal CO_2 is high at the initiation of CPR (likely representing exhalation of CO_2 that accumulated in the tissues and venous system while the animals were apneic but not yet pulseless) and then falls to levels similar to those seen during adult CPR *(73,74)*. Although end-tidal CO_2 monitoring is useful during pediatric CPR, pediatric-specific data is limited.

Open-Chest CPR

Excellent standard closed-chest CPR generates a cerebral blood flow (CBF) that is approx 50% of normal. By contrast, open chest CPR can generate a CBF that approaches normal. Although open-chest massage improves CPP and increases the chance of suc-cessful defibrillation in animals and humans, performing a thoracotomy to allow open-chest CPR is impractical in many situations.

A retrospective review of 27 cases of CPR following pediatric blunt trauma (15 with open-chest CPR and 12 with closed-chest CPR) demonstrated that open-chest CPR increased hospital costs without altering rates of ROSC or survival to discharge *(75)*. However, survival in both groups was 0%, indicating that the population may have been too severely injured or too late in the process to benefit from this aggressive therapy. Earlier institution of open-chest CPR may warrant reconsideration in selected special resuscitation circumstances *(76–79)*.

Mechanical Devices to Improve CPR Hemodynamics

The goal of mechanical adjuncts to CPR is to increase cardiac output by increasing the action of the cardiac, thoracic, or abdominal pump *(80)*. Several potentially beneficial mechanical devices have been developed to improve CPR hemodynamics. A *pneumatic vest* can replace standard CCs with repetitive circumferential compression of the thorax in efforts to maximize the contribution of the thoracic pump to circulation *(61,81)*. *Active compression–decompression cardiopulmonary resuscitation* (ACD-CPR*)* uses a hand-held plunger-type suction device, applied mid-sternum, to alternately compress the chest then actively decompress the chest *(82–86)*. This technique generates negative intrathoracic pressure during "diastole," increasing venous return and cardiac output. ACD-CPR, combined with interposed abdominal compression (IAC) improves outcome from CA in animal models. Mathematical models of human physiology also suggest this ACD technique can increase cardiac output in human adult CA *(80,82,87)*. *Minimally invasive direct cardiac massage* is the use of a device that allows for open-heart massage through a 1–2 centimeter thoracotomy *(88–90)*.

Additionally, an *inspiratory impedance threshold valve* can be attached to either a tracheal tube or a face mask and serves to prevent inspiratory airflow until a preset "cracking pressure" across the valve is reached *(91–95)*. With a spontaneously breathing patient, this valve increases the magnitude of negative intrathoracic pressure necessary to initiate inspiration, increasing venous return and right ventricular (RV) preload. During CPR, patients are generally not making spontaneous respiratory efforts. Nonetheless, the use of this valve during CPR may decrease intrathoracic pressure during natural chest recoil, increasing venous return.

Although all of these mechanical adjuncts to CPR are more cumbersome than traditional CPR and require additional provider training, they hold great promise to improve hemodynamics during the low-flow cardiopulmonary-cerebral resuscitation (CPCR) phases of resuscitation, especially when prolonged CPR is necessary. In addition to increasing the probability of ROSC, these adjuncts may provide for near normal hemodynamics and adequate vital organ perfusion in a patient who cannot be resuscitated immediately, allowing for initiation of ECMO or other intermediate-term supports. These devices were developed mainly for use in adults. None of these adjuncts to CPR has yet been evaluated specifically in children.

ECMO-CPR

The use of veno-arterial extracorporeal membrane oxygenation (ECMO) to reestablish circulation and provide controlled reperfusion following CA has been reported, but prospective, controlled studies are lacking. Nevertheless, these series have reported extraordinary results with the use of a ECMO as a rescue therapy for pediatric CAs, especially from potentially reversible acute postoperative myocardial dysfunction or arrhythmias *(28–30,96,97,97a)*. In one study, 11 children who suffered CA in the pediatric ICU after cardiac surgery were placed on ECMO during CPR after 20 to 110 minutes of CPR. Prolonged CPR was continued until ECMO cannulae, circuits, and personnel were available. Of these 11 children, 6 were long-term survivors without apparent neurological sequelae. More recently, two centers have reported an additional remarkable 8 pediatric cardiac patients provided with mechanical cardiopulmonary support during CPR within 20 minutes of the initiation of CPR. All 8 survived to hospital discharge. CPR and ECMO are not curative treatments. They are simply cardiopulmonary supportive measures that may allow tissue perfusion and viability until recovery from the precipitating disease process. As such, they can be powerful tools.

Potential advantages of ECMO stem from its ability to maintain tight control of physiological parameters after resuscitation. For example, blood flow rates, oxygenation, ventilation, and body temperature can be manipulated precisely through the ECMO circuit. As more is discovered about the processes of secondary injury following CA, ECMO might enable controlled perfusion and temperature management to minimize reperfusion injury and maximize cell recovery.

Intraosseous Vascular Access

In infants and children requiring emergent access for resuscitation from CA, intraosseous (IO) vascular access should be established if reliable venous access cannot be achieved rapidly. Because of the difficulty establishing vascular access in pediatric CA victims, it may be preferable to attempt IO access immediately. A practical approach is to pursue IO and peripheral or central venous access simultaneously.

IO vascular access provides access to a noncollapsible marrow venous plexus, which serves as a rapid, safe, and reliable route for administration of drugs, crystalloids, colloids, and blood during resuscitation. IO vascular access often can be achieved in 30 to 60 seconds. Although a specially designed, IO styleted, Jamshidi-type needle is preferred to prevent obstruction of the needle with cortical bone, butterfly needles and standard hypodermic needles have been used successfully. The IO needle is typically inserted into the anterior tibial bone marrow; alternative sites include the distal femur, medial malleolus or the anterior superior iliac spine, and the distal tibia. In adult and older children, alternative sites include the distal femur, distal tibia (medial malleolus), anterior-superior iliac spine, distal radius, and distal ulna.

This IO vascular access technique can be used in all age groups, from preterm neonates to adults. The needle should be twisted into, rather than shoved through, the bone marrow. Evidence for successful entry into the bone marrow includes the following: (a) the sudden decrease in resistance after the needle passes through the bony cortex; (b) the needle remains upright without support; (c) aspiration of the bone marrow into a syringe (this is not consistently achieved); and (d) the fluid infuses freely without evidence of subcutaneous infiltration.

Resuscitation drugs, fluids, and blood products can be administered safely by the IO route. The IO route can also support continuous catecholamine infusions. Onset of action and drug levels following IO infusion during CPR are comparable to those achieved following vascular administration, including central venous administration *(98–111)*. IO vascular access can be used to also obtain blood specimens for chemistry, blood gas analysis, and type and crossmatch, although administration of sodium bicarbonate through the IO cannula eliminates the close correlation with mixed venous blood gases *(112–114)*.

Complications occur in less than 1% of patients following IO infusion. Complications include tibial fracture, lower extremity compartment syndrome, severe extravasation of drugs, and osteomyelitis *(115–125)*. Most of these complications can be avoided by careful technique. Although microscopic pulmonary fat and bone marrow emboli occur in animal models, they have never been reported clinically and appear to occur just as frequently during CA without IO drug administration. Animal data and one human follow-up study indicate that local effects of IO infusion on the bone marrow and bone growth are minimal.

Medication Use During Cardiac Arrest

VASOPRESSORS

Epinephrine (adrenaline) is an endogenous catecholamine with potent α and β stimulating properties. The α-adrenergic action (vasoconstriction) increases systemic and pulmonary vascular resistance, increasing both systolic and diastolic blood pressure. The rise in diastolic blood pressure directly increases CPP, thereby increasing coronary blood flow and increasing the likelihood of return of spontaneous circulation. Epinephrine also increases CBF during CPR because peripheral vasoconstriction directs a greater proportion of flow to the cerebral circulation. The β-adrenergic effect increases myocardial contractility and heart rate and relaxes smooth muscle in the skeletal muscle vascular bed and bronchi. Epinephrine also increases the vigor and intensity of VF, increasing the likelihood of successful defibrillation.

High-dose epinephrine (0.05–0.2 mg/kg) improves myocardial and CBF during CPR more than standard-dose epinephrine (0.01–0.02 mg/kg), and may increase the incidence of initial ROSC. Administration of high-dose epinephrine, however, can worsen a patient's postresuscitation hemodynamic condition *(126,127)*. Retrospective studies indicate that use of high-dose epinephrine in adults or children may be associated with a worse neurologic outcome *(33,128–140)*. A randomized, controlled trial of rescue high-dose epinephrine vs standard-dose epinephrine following failed initial standard-dose epinephrine in pediatric in-hospital CA demonstrated a worse 24-hour survival in the high-dose epinephrine group (1/27 vs 6/23, $p < 0.05$) *(141a)*. High-dose epinephrine cannot be recommended routinely for initial or rescue therapy.

Wide variability in catecholamine pharmacokinetics and pharmacodynamics dictate individual titration of therapy in non-CA situations. Therefore, it is likely that a lifesaving dose during CPR for one patient may be life threatening to another. Perhaps high-dose epinephrine should be considered as an alternative to standard-dose epinephrine in special circumstances of refractory pediatric CA (e.g., patient on high-dose epinephrine infusion prior to CA) and/or when continuous direct arterial blood pressure monitoring allows titration of the epinephrine dosage to diastolic (relaxation phase) arterial pressure during CPR. Nevertheless, high-dose epinephrine has not been demonstrated to improve outcome should only be used with caution.

Vasopressin is a long-acting endogenous hormone that acts at specific receptors to mediate systemic vasoconstriction (V_1 receptor) and reabsorption of water in the renal tubule (V_2 receptor). In experimental models of CA, vasopressin increases blood flow to the heart and brain and improves long-term survival compared to epinephrine *(141–162)*. Vasopressin may decrease splanchnic blood flow during and following CPR. In a small randomized trial comparing the efficacy of epinephrine to vasopressin in shock-resistant out-of-hospital VF in adults, vasopressin produced a higher rate of return of spontaneous circulation *(153)*. Effective CPR and ALS were delayed somewhat in this out of hospital study. In a study of adult in-hospital CA with rapid response of effective CPR and ALS, vasopressin produced a rate of survival to hospital discharge similar to epinephrine *(163)*.

In a pediatric porcine model of prolonged VF, the use of vasopressin and epinephrine in combination resulted in higher LV blood flow than either pressor alone, and both vasopressin alone and vasopressin plus epinephrine resulted in superior CBF than epinephrine alone *(164,165)*. By contrast, in a pediatric porcine model of *asphyxial* CA, return of spontaneous circulation was more likely in piglets treated with epinephrine than in those treated with vasopressin *(165a)*. A case series of four children who received vasopressin during six prolonged CA events suggests that the use of bolus vasopressin may result in return of spontaneous circulation when standard medications have failed *(166)*. Vasopressin has also been reported to be useful in low cardiac output states associated with sepsis syndrome and organ recovery in children *(167–169)*. Although vasopressin will not likely replace epinephrine as a first-line agent in pediatric CA, there is preliminary data to suggest that its use in conjunction with epinephrine in pediatric CA deserves further investigation.

CALCIUM

Use of calcium in CA is reported to be high, despite lack of evidence for efficacy when administered routinely in CA *(170–174)*. In the absence of hypocalcemia, the administration of calcium does not improve outcome in CA. Calcium administration is appropriate for the following known or suspected conditions: hypocalcemia, hyperkalemia, hypermagnesemia, and calcium channel blocker overdose.

BUFFER SOLUTIONS

The routine use of sodium bicarbonate for a child in CA is not recommended. Clinical trials involving critically ill adults with severe metabolic acidosis did not demonstrate a beneficial effect of sodium bicarbonate on hemodynamics despite correction of acidosis *(173,175–184)*. However, the presence of acidosis may depress the action of catecholamines, and so the use of sodium bicarbonate may be considered in an acidemic child who is refractory to catecholamine administration. Acidosis may increase the threshold for myocardial stimulation in a patient with an artificial cardiac pacemaker; therefore, administration of bicarbonate or another buffer is appropriate for management of acidosis in these children. The administration of sodium bicarbonate is also indicated in the patient with a tricyclic antidepressant overdose, hyperkalemia, hypermagnesemia, or sodium channel blocker poisoning.

The buffering action of bicarbonate occurs when a hydrogen cation and a bicarbonate anion combine to form carbon dioxide and water. If carbon dioxide is not effectively cleared through ventilation, its build-up will counterbalance the buffering effect of bicarbonate. Therefore, there is not a role for the use of bicarbonate in the management of respiratory acidosis. Unlike sodium bicarbonate, tromethamine (THAM) provides buffering action without the generation of carbon dioxide *(185–190)*. In a patient with limited potential for ventilation, THAM may be a reasonable choice when buffering is necessary. THAM undergoes renal elimination, and renal insufficiency may be a relative contraindication to its use. Carbicarb, an equimolar combination of sodium bicarbonate and sodium carbonate, is another buffering solution thought to generate less CO_2 than sodium bicarbonate. In a canine model of CA comparing animals given normal saline, sodium bicarbonate, THAM, or Carbicarb, the animals given buffer solution had a higher rate of ROSC than the animals given normal saline *(185)*. In the animals given sodium bicarbonate or Carbicarb, the interval to ROSC was significantly shorter than in animals given normal saline. However, at the end of the 6-hour study period, all resuscitated animals were in a deep coma, so no inferences regarding meaningful survival can be drawn. It is premature to recommend either THAM or Carbicarb during CPR at this time.

Ventricular Fibrillation in Children

VF has been an underappreciated pediatric problem. Two important studies demonstrated VF as the initial rhythm in 19 to 24% of out-of-hospital pediatric CA victims

(6,39). Most previous investigations had indicated an incidence of VF in the range of 6–10%, but included substantial numbers of babies with Sudden Infant Death Syndrome (SIDS). Most of these SIDS babies had been dead for some time, often with rigor mortis, and all had initial EKG evidence of asystole. Therefore, these two studies with high incidences of VF excluded SIDS patients. The provocative investigation by Mogayzel and colleagues also documented that 5 of 29 children (17%) presenting with VF in a prehospital setting survived with good neurologic outcome vs only 2 of 128 (2%) presenting with asystole/PEA (*p* < 0.01).

The incidence of VF varies by setting and age. In special circumstances, such as tricyclic antidepressant overdose, cardiomyopathy, postcardiac surgery, and prolonged QT syndromes, VF and pulseless VT are more likely. Furthermore, in one study VF/VT occurred in only 3% of children in CA from 0 to 8 years of age, but 17% of CA victims from 8 to 30 years of age.

VF can also occur secondary to asphyxia. It is well documented among near-drowning patients. In careful prospective studies of VF among asphyxiated piglets, the incidence of VF was 28% and 33% at some time during the CA *(191,192)*. However, many of the piglets had converted from VF to asystole during time intervals that are consistent with medical personnel arrival. Therefore, it is likely that continuous EKG monitoring would demonstrate that the incidence of VF is similarly more common in children with asphyxial CAs, such as submersion events. Although continuous EKG monitoring during the asphyxial episode is not practical, the important message is: VF occurs during pediatric CA events. This is supported by preliminary data from the AHA National Registry of In-Hospital CPR events from January 2000 to June 2002, which suggests that shockable rhythm is the initial rhythm seen in 7% of all in-hospital pediatric arrest events requiring chest compressions and 15% of all pulseless CA events *(13,21)*. Furthermore, as many as 25% of pulseless CA patients exhibited a shockable rhythm at some point during their CA management.

The treatment of choice for short duration VF is prompt defibrillation. VF must be identified before defibrillation can be provided. Diagnosis is by EKG. An attitude that VF is rare in children can be a self-fulfilling prophecy with a uniformly fatal outcome.

The recommended defibrillation dose is 2 J/kg, but the data supporting this recommendation is not optimal. In the mid-1970s, authoritative sources recommended starting doses of 60 to 200 J for all children *(193)*. Because of concerns for myocardial damage and animal data suggesting that generally 0.5 to 10 J/kg were adequate for defibrillation in a variety of species, Gutgesell and colleagues retrospectively evaluated the efficacy of their strategy to defibrillate with 2 J/kg *(194)*. Seventy-one transthoracic defibrillations on 27 children were evaluated. Shocks within 10 J of 2 J/kg resulted in successful defibrillation in 91% of the defibrillation attempts.

The major determinant of successful defibrillation besides duration of VF is the countershock current. This current depends on the defibrillator energy and transthoracic impedance. Studies in children indicate that the transthoracic impedance of infants and children overlap greatly. Although there is a statistically significant correlation between size and transthoracic impedence, the correlation is weak *(195,196)*. These studies provide only weak support for the present dogma that the defibrillator energy dose should vary directly with weight *(197,198)*. Nevertheless, the present recommendation of 2 J/kg has stood the test of time.

Anti-Arrhythmic Medications

Administration of anti-arrhythmic medications should never delay administration of defibrillation in a patient with VF. However, after three unsuccessful attempts at electrical defibrillation, medications to increase the effectiveness of defibrillation should be considered. In both pediatric and adult patients, the current first-line medication in VF is epinephrine. If epinephrine with or without vasopressin and a subsequent repeat attempt to defibrillate are unsuccessful, lidocaine or amiodarone should be considered.

LIDOCAINE AND AMIODARONE

Lidocaine has been recommended traditionally for shock-resistant VF in adults and children. However, the only anti-arrhythmic agent that has been prospectively determined to improve survival to hospital admission in the setting of shock-resistant VF when compared to placebo is amiodarone *(199–207)*. In another study of shock-resistant out-of-hospital VF, patients receiving amiodarone had a higher rate of survival to hospital admission than patients receiving lidocaine. Neither study included children. Because there is moderate experience with amiodarone usage as an anti-arrhythmic agent in children and because of the above-mentioned adult study, it is rational to use amiodarone similarly in children with shock-resistant VF/VT. The recommended dosage is 5 mg/kg by rapid intravenous bolus. There are no published comparisons of anti-arrhythmic medications for pediatric refractory VF. Although extrapolation of adult data and electrophysiological mechanistic information suggest that amiodarone may be preferable for pediatric shock-resistant VF, the optimal choice is not clear.

Pediatric Automated External Defibrillators

Automated external defibrillators (AEDs) have improved survival from adult VF. AEDs are recommended for use in children 8 years or older with CA. The available data suggest that some AEDs can accurately diagnose VF in children of all ages, but many AEDs are limited because the defibrillation pads and energy dosage are for adults. Adapters that have smaller defibrillation pads and that dampen the amount of energy delivered have been developed as attachments to adult AEDs to allow their use in children *(208)*.

Because lack of defibrillation (0 J/kg) is clearly lethal (i.e., an LD_{100}) for pediatric VF, it is preferable to provide a shock with an appropriate pediatric dose or even a high dose shock rather than no shock. However, it is important that the AED diagnostic algorithm is sensitive and specific for pediatric VF. The diagnostic algorithms from several AED manufactures have been tested for such sensitivity and specificity *(209– 211)*, and can, therefore, be reasonably used in younger children.

Monophasic vs Biphasic Defibrillator Waveforms (and Beyond)

In a randomized, controlled trial comparing the efficacy of a biphasic (impedance-compensated biphasic-truncated exponential) energy waveform with two different types of monophasic waveforms (monophasic-truncated exponential and monophasic-damped sine), defibrillation efficacy (i.e., termination of fibrillation) was superior for the biphasic waveform than for either of the two types of monophasic waveforms *(212–228)*. AEDs currently use biphasic waveforms to deliver energy. Although internal (implantable) pediatric defibrillators are all biphasic waveform, there is no data on the safety and efficacy of biphasic transthoracic defibrillation in children, and a study in children is not feasible. Recent data suggests that higher doses and alternative waveforms may be safe and effective in small children *(197,198,229,230)*.

Smarter AEDs

An ideal AED would be readily available, easy to operate without training, and applicable to children or adults. It would determine the presence of respiratory arrest alone or CA and respiratory arrest and would prompt the appropriate intervention. Additionally, it would be capable of identifying cardiac rhythms amenable to defibrillation and would prompt the rescuer to the optimal time to deliver a shock based on an analysis of the amplitude and frequency of fibrillation wavelets. The rhythm analysis could ideally occur during ongoing CCs or during very brief interruptions in CCs. The components of this "ideal AED" have all been studied in animal models and will likely become part of routinely available AEDs.

POSTRESUSCITATION INTERVENTIONS
Temperature Management

Fever following CA is associated with poor neurological outcome. Hyperthermia following CA is common in children *(231)*. Mild resuscitative systemic hypothermia may improve neurologic outcome in adults after resuscitation from out of hospital VF arrest *(232–237)*. Mild systemic hypothermia may benefit children resuscitated from CA, but the question demands further study. At a minimum, it is advisable to strictly avoid even mild hyperthermia in children following CPR. Scheduled administration of antipyretic medications *and* use of external cooling devices is often necessary to avoid hyperthermia in this population

Glucose Control

Hyperglycemia following adult CA is associated with worse neurological outcome after controlling for duration of arrest and presence of cardiogenic shock *(238–243)*. In an animal model of asphyxial CA, administration of insulin and glucose, but not administration of glucose alone, improved neurologic outcome compared to administration of normal saline *(244)*. Clinicians should target tight glucose control with avoidance of hyperglycemia and hypoglycemia following CA.

Blood Pressure Management

Compared to healthy volunteers, adults resuscitated from CA have impaired autoregulation of CBF. Hence, they may not maintain cerebral perfusion pressure in the face of systemic hypotension, and likewise may not be able to protect the brain from acutely increased blood flow in the face of systemic hypertension. Blood pressure variability should be minimized as much as possible following resuscitation from CA.

A brief period of hypertension following resuscitation from CA may diminish the no-reflow phenomenon *(245–247)*. In animal models, brief induced hypertension following resuscitation results in improved neurological outcome compared to normotension. In a retrospective human study, postresuscitative hypertension was associated with a better neurological outcome after controlling for age, gender, duration of CA, duration of CPR, and preexisting diseases *(248)*.

After CA or resuscitation from shock, the individual may have ongoing hemodynamic compromise secondary to a combination of inadequate cardiac pumping function, excessively increased systemic or pulmonary vascular resistance, or very low systemic vascular resistance. The last is most common in the patient with septic shock, although recent data shows that most children with *fluid-refractory* septic shock have high rather than low systemic vascular resistance and poor myocardial pumping function *(249–256)*. Children with cardiogenic shock typically have poor myocardial function and a compensatory increase in systemic and pulmonary vascular resistance as the body attempts to maintain an adequate blood pressure.

The classes of agents used to maintain circulatory function are usually characterized as inotropes, vasopressors, and vasodilators. Inotropes increase cardiac pumping function and often increase heart rate as well. Vasopressors increase systemic and pulmonary vascular resistance; they are most commonly used in children with inappropriately low systemic vascular resistance. Vasodilators are designed to reduce systemic and pulmonary vascular resistance. Although they do not directly increase pumping function, vasodilators reduce ventricular afterload, which often improves stroke volume and therefore cardiac output. They are the only class of agents that can increase cardiac output and simultaneously reduce myocardial oxygen demand.

Optimal use of these agents requires titration of medication to the patient's cardiovascular physiology. Invasive hemodynamic monitoring, including measurement of central venous pressure, pulmonary capillary wedge pressure, and cardiac output, may be appropriate. Furthermore, vasoactive agents have different hemodynamic effects at different infusion rates. For example, at low infusion rates, epinephrine is a potent inotrope and lowers systemic vascular resistance through a prominent action on vascular β-adrenergic receptors. At higher infusion rates, epinephrine remains a potent inotrope and increases systemic vascular resistance by activating vascular α-adrenergic receptors. Because the pharmacokinetic and pharmacodynamic responses are not uniform across ages and across different diseases *(257)*, careful monitoring of the patient's response to vasoactive agents is needed for optimal use.

LIMITATIONS TO UNDERSTANDING PEDIATRIC CARDIAC ARREST AND CPR

Our knowledge of the epidemiology and appropriate treatment of pediatric CA has been limited, in part, because we have lumped diverse diseases and pathophysiologies, thereby obscuring potentially important "signals" amidst all of the "noise." In contrast to CAs in adults, most pediatric arrests are secondary to profound hypoxia or asphyxia as a result of variety of diseases resulting in respiratory failure or circulatory shock. Pediatric studies tend to include all pediatric CAs, including those secondary to sudden respiratory failure (e.g., drowning, foreign body aspiration), progressive respiratory failure from infections and/or neuromuscular diseases, trauma, SIDS, septic shock, hypovolemic shock, anaphylaxis, primary cardiomyopathy, primary arrhythmia (e.g., VF or VT), drug intoxications, and so on *(4,13–15,22,33,34,258–260)*. Some pediatric studies have lumped respiratory arrests with CAs, and many have included both prehospital and in-hospital CAs in their data. Moreover, many of the CA victims in these studies had been dead for a prolonged period of time (e.g., SIDS), and, therefore, data such as initial cardiac rhythm of asystole and lack of response to therapy are not helpful in terms of understanding the etiology, pathophysiology, or appropriate therapy. When included in an interventional trial, these patients who can no longer be resuscitated are not meaningful participants in the study (i.e., they limit the ability to discriminate whether the intervention could help those who could be resuscitated). Additionally, most pediatric studies have focused on either prehospital or in-hospital data collection, often without adequate integration. As a result, important data was neither reported nor available. Finally, most pediatric arrest studies have suffered from inadequate and nonuniform data collection.

Lack of uniformity in data reporting has been a well-recognized methodological problem for both adult and pediatric CA research. In response to this issue, international resuscitation experts have established the series of Utstein-style international consensus guidelines regarding uniform reporting of CA data for adult out-of-hospital CA, adult in-hospital CA, and pediatric ALS (22,23,261,262). These guidelines have resulted in the use of more consistent terminology and data collection in CA investigations. Therefore, these efforts to standardize data collection and reporting have allowed CA research to focus on the important experimental "signals" rather than be obscured by experimental "noise."

A subtler obstacle to investigating pediatric CA and CPR is the intense emotional response to a child in CA. Parents lay persons, EMS providers, and hospital personnel are often emotionally overwhelmed during provision of CPR on a child. Providers and investigators often attempt to ameliorate the pain by avoidance, denial, and minimizing contact time. These responses discourage thorough investigations. Because of these limitations and because CAs are much more common in adults, most clinical studies on various aspects of CPR have focused on adults almost exclusively. Therefore, guidelines for CPR in children have largely been extrapolated from data obtained in adults or in animal models of VF. This results in a therapeutic orphan status that is less than optimal.

RESUSCITATION RESEARCH: MOVING THE FIELD FORWARD

The PULSE Initiative

The Postresuscitation and Initial Utility in Lifesaving (PULSE) conference (263) gathered international leaders in resuscitation research to highlight opportunities for improvement in outcomes after CPR and resuscitation from major traumatic injury. The consensus paper highlights priority topics within resuscitation research. A few of the projects that warrant immediate study include: hibernation physiology in settings of ischemia and reperfusion, hypothermia, methods for inducing hypothermia, controlled reperfusion, improved understanding of pharmacologic agents in CA, mechanisms of generating greater blood flows during CPR, biosensors for detecting critical limitations of blood flows, vascular access for reperfusion technologies, simulation and telemedicine, the development of regional, national, and international trauma and CPR registries, and the development of clinical trials networks.

Clinical Trials Network and Registry Development

Multicenter collaboration has obvious advantages over isolated single-center investigations. Pediatric CAs are uncommon events; even large single institutions do not have a volume of CAs that can allow for effective prospective resuscitation research. Such collaboration allows national experts to cooperate in the development of research protocols, and the involvement of many institutions provides a vastly larger patient population. A clinical trials network to focus on pediatric CPR and cerebral resuscitation is needed urgently and is under development.

The NRCPR (www.nrcpr.org), through the AHA, is a nationwide registry of in-hospital CPR with the capability for separate pediatric analysis. Improved awareness of, and reporting to, this registry will facilitate improved pediatric resuscitation research.

Exception to Informed Consent and Community Consultation

The physiological repercussions of whole-body hypoxia and ischemia are complex and poorly understood. There is an urgent need to reestablish circulation and interrupt the cascade of events that result in reperfusion injury. Medical research in the United States generally occurs only after a process of informed consent intended to protect the rights of research subjects and their families. However, the therapeutic window for interventions that may improve intact neurological survival following pediatric CA is very short, and this requirement limited resuscitation research in the United States for many years. In 1996, the Food and Drug Administration and the Department of Health and Human Services published parallel guidelines allowing for an exception to the traditional informed consent process for particular types of research in which the patient's condition is emergent and life threatening and it is impractical to obtain informed consent. A process of community consultation is required *(264)*. These guidelines have not yet been successfully applied to pediatric resuscitation research, but adaptation of the adult approach is likely to be required to allow for pediatric resuscitation research to proceed.

CONCLUSION

Outcomes from pediatric CA and CPR appear to be improving. Perhaps, the evolving understanding of pathophysiologic events during and after pediatric CA and the developing fields of pediatric critical care and pediatric emergency medicine have contributed to these apparent improvements. Additionally, there are exciting breakthroughs in basic and applied science laboratories that are on the immediate horizon for study in specific subpopulations of CA victims. By strategically focusing therapies to specific phases of CA and resuscitation and to evolving pathophysiology, there is great promise that critical care interventions will lead the way to more successful cardiopulmonary and cerebral resuscitation in children.

To shed the "therapeutic orphan" status of treatment for pediatric sudden CA and improve outcome for children, the following are necessary: a large pediatric sudden death registry, more and better pediatric sudden arrest and asphyxial arrest animal studies, and multicenter therapeutic trials in pediatric sudden arrest populations. Treatment of sudden death in children in the future needs to be more evidence-based and less anecdotal. Timing of therapeutic interventions to prevent arrest, and protect, preserve, and promote restoration of intact neurological survival is of high priority.

REFERENCES

1. American Heart Association in collaboration with International Liaison Committee on Resuscitation. Guidelines 2000 for Cardiopulmonary Resuscitation and Emergency Cardiovascular Care: International Consensus on Science, Part 6: Advanced Cardiovascular Life Support: 7B: Understanding the Algorithm Approach to ACLS. Circulation 2000; 102(Suppl):I140,I141.
2. American Heart Association in collaboration with International Liaison Committee on Resuscitation. Guidelines 2000 for Cardiopulmonary Resuscitation and Emergency Cardiovascular Care: International Consensus on Science, Part 12: From Science to Survival: Strengthening the Chain of Survival in Every Community. Circulation 2000; 102(Suppl):I358–I370.
3. Seidel JS, et al. Pediatric prehospital care in urban and rural areas. Pediatrics 1991; 88:681–690.

4. Young KD, Seidel JS. Pediatric cardiopulmonary resuscitation: a collective review. Ann Emerg Med 1999; 33:195–205.
5. Appleton GO, et al. CPR and the single rescuer: at what age should you "call first" rather than "call fast"? Ann Emerg Med 1995; 25:492–494.
6. Mogayzel C, et al. Out-of-hospital ventricular fibrillation in children and adolescents: causes and outcomes. Ann Emerg Med 1995; 25:484–491.
7. Hazinski MF. Is pediatric resuscitation unique? Relative merits of early CPR and ventilation versus early defibrillation for young victims of prehospital cardiac arrest. Ann Emerg Med 1995; 25:540–543.
8. Sirbaugh PE, et al. A prospective, population-based study of the demographics, epidemiology, management, and outcome of out-of-hospital pediatric cardiopulmonary arrest [published correction appears in Ann Emerg Med 1999; 33:358]. Ann Emerg Med 1999; 33:174–184.
9. Liberthson RR. Sudden death from cardiac causes in children and young adults. N Engl J Med 1996; 334:1039–1044.
10. Maron BJ, et al. Clinical profile and spectrum of commotio cordis. JAMA 2002; 287:1142–1146.
11. Part 10: pediatric advanced life support. Resuscitation 2000; 46:343–399.
12. Zaritsky A. Cardiopulmonary resuscitation in children. Clin Chest Med 1987; 8:561–571.
13. Reis AG, et al. A prospective investigation into the epidemiology of in-hospital pediatric cardiopulmonary resuscitation using the international Utstein reporting style. Pediatrics 2002; 109:200–209.
14. Kuisma M, Suominen P, Korpela R. Paediatric out-of-hospital cardiac arrests: epidemiology and outcome. Resuscitation 1995; 30:141–150.
15. Suominen P, et al. Utstein style reporting of in-hospital paediatric cardiopulmonary resuscitation. Resuscitation 2000; 45:17–25.
16. Fiser DH. Assessing the outcome of pediatric intensive care. J Pediatr 1992; 121:68–74.
17. American Heart Association in collaboration with International Liaison Committee on Resuscitation. Guidelines 2000 for Cardiopulmonary Resuscitation and Emergency Cardiovascular Care: International Consensus on Science, Part 6: Advanced Cardiovascular Life Support: Section 8: Postresuscitation Care. Circulation 2000; 102(Suppl):I166–I171.
18. Yakaitis RW, Otto CW, Blitt CD. Relative importance of alpha and beta adrenergic receptors during resuscitation. Crit Care Med 1979; 7:293–296.
19. Otto CW, Yakaitis RW, Blitt, CD. Mechanism of action of epinephrine in resuscitation from asphyxial arrest. Crit Care Med 1981; 9:364,365.
20. American Heart Association in collaboration with International Liaison Committee on Resuscitation. Guidelines 2000 for Cardiopulmonary Resuscitation and Emergency Cardiovascular Care: International Consensus on Science, Part 9: Pediatric Basic Life Support. Circulation 2000; 102(Suppl): I253–I290.
21. Nadkarni VM, et al. Survival outcome for in-hospital pulseless cardiac arrest reported to the National Registry of CPR is better for children than adults [abstract]. Crit Care Med 2003; 30(Suppl):A14.
22. Zaritsky A, et al. Recommended guidelines for uniform reporting of pediatric advanced life support: the pediatric Utstein style. A statement for healthcare professionals from the American Academy of Pediatrics, the American Heart Association, and the European Resuscitation Council. Circulation 1995; 92: 2006–2020.
23. Cummins RO, et al. Recommended guidelines for reviewing, reporting, and conducting research on in-hospital resuscitation: the in-hospital 'Utstein style'. American Heart Association. Circulation 1997; 95:2213–2239.
24. Chamnanvanakij S, Perlman JM. Outcome following cardiopulmonary resuscitation in the neonate requiring ventilatory assistance. Resuscitation 2000; 45:173–180.
25. Perlman JM, Risser R. Cardiopulmonary resuscitation in the delivery room: associated clinical events. Arch Pediatr Adolesc Med 1995; 149:20–25.
26. Wyckoff MH, Perlman J, Niermeyer S. Medications during resuscitation—what is the evidence? Semin Neonatol 2001; 6:251–259.
27. Slonim AD, et al. Cardiopulmonary resuscitation in pediatric intensive care units. Crit Care Med 1997; 25:1951–1955.
28. Parra DA, et al. Outcome of cardiopulmonary resuscitation in a pediatric cardiac intensive care unit. Crit Care Med 2000; 28:3296–3300.
29. Dalton HJ, et al. Extracorporeal membrane oxygenation for cardiac rescue in children with severe myocardial dysfunction. Crit Care Med 1993; 21:1020–1028.
30. del Nido PJ, et al. Extracorporeal membrane oxygenator rescue in children during cardiac arrest after cardiac surgery. Circulation 1992; 86(Suppl):II300–II304.

31. Nadkarni V, et al. Pediatric resuscitation: an advisory statement from the Pediatric Working Group of the International Liaison Committee on Resuscitation. Circulation 1997;95:2185–2195.

32. Peberdy MA, et al. Cardiopulmonary resuscitation of adults in the hospital: a report of 14720 cardiac arrests from the National Registry of Cardiopulmonary Resuscitation. Resuscitation 2003; 58:297–308.

33. Dieckmann RA, Vardis R. High-dose epinephrine in pediatric out-of-hospital cardiopulmonary arrest. Pediatrics 1995; 95:901–913.

34. Zaritsky A, et al. CPR in children. Ann Emerg Med 1987; 16:1107–1111.

35. Kouwenhoven WB, Jude JR, Knickerbocker GG. Closed-chest cardiac massage. JAMA 1960; 173: 1064–1067.

36. Becker, LB, et al. A reappraisal of mouth-to-mouth ventilation during bystander-initiated cardiopulmonary resuscitation. A statement for healthcare professionals from the Ventilation Working Group of the Basic Life Support and Pediatric Life Support Subcommittees, American Heart Association. Resuscitation 1997; 35:189–201.

37. Berg RA, et al. Simulated mouth-to-mouth ventilation and chest compressions (bystander cardiopulmonary resuscitation) improves outcome in a swine model of prehospital pediatric asphyxial cardiac arrest. Crit Care Med 1999; 27:1893–1899.

38. Berg RA, et al. "Bystander" chest compressions and assisted ventilation independently improve outcome from piglet asphyxial pulseless "cardiac arrest". Circulation 2000; 101:1743–1748.

39. Hickey RW, et al. Pediatric patients requiring CPR in the prehospital setting. Ann Emerg Med 1995; 25:495–501.

40. Cobb LA, et al. Influence of cardiopulmonary resuscitation prior to defibrillation in patients with out-of-hospital ventricular fibrillation. JAMA 1999; 281:1182–1188.

41. Hallstrom A, et al. Cardiopulmonary resuscitation by chest compression alone or with mouth-to-mouth ventilation. N Engl J Med 2000; 342:1546–1553.

42. Gausche M, et al. Effect of out-of-hospital pediatric endotracheal intubation on survival and neurological outcome: a controlled clinical trial. JAMA 2000:283:783–790.

43. Orlowski JP. Optimum position for external cardiac compression in infants and young children. Ann Emerg Med 1986; 15:667–673.

44. Orlowski JP. Mechanisms of blood flow during CPR. Circulation 1980; 62:1141.

45. Finholt DA, et al. The heart is under the lower third of the sternum: implications for external cardiac massage. Am J Dis Child 1986; 140:646–649.

46. Part 9: pediatric basic life support. Resuscitation 2000; 46:301–341.

47. Paradis NA, et al. Coronary perfusion pressure and the return of spontaneous circulation in human cardiopulmonary resuscitation. JAMA 1990; 263:1106–1113.

48. Berg RA, et al. Adverse hemodynamic effects of interrupting chest compressions for rescue breathing during cardiopulmonary resuscitation for ventricular fibrillation cardiac arrest. Circulation 2001; 104: 2465–2470.

49. Sanders AB, et al. Survival and neurologic outcome after cardiopulmonary resuscitation with four different chest compression-ventilation ratios. Ann Emerg Med 2002; 40:553–562.

50. Kern KB, et al. Importance of continuous chest compressions during cardiopulmonary resuscitation: improved outcome during a simulated single lay-rescuer scenario. Circulation 2002; 105:645–649.

51. Babbs CF, Kern KB. Optimum compression to ventilation ratios in CPR under realistic, practical conditions: a physiological and mathematical analysis. Resuscitation 2002; 54:147–157.

52. Berg RA, et al. Assisted ventilation does not improve outcome in a porcine model of single-rescuer bystander cardiopulmonary resuscitation. Circulation 1997; 95:1635–1641.

53. Berg RA, et al. Assisted ventilation during 'bystander' CPR in a swine acute myocardial infarction model does not improve outcome. Circulation 1997; 96:4364–4371.

54. Rea TD, et al. Dispatcher-assisted cardiopulmonary resuscitation and survival in cardiac arrest. Circulation 2001; 104:2513–2516.

55. Hallstrom AP. Dispatcher-assisted "phone" cardiopulmonary resuscitation by chest compression alone or with mouth-to-mouth ventilation. Crit Care Med 2000; 28(Suppl):N190–N192.

56. Berg RA, et al. Initial end-tidal CO_2 is markedly elevated during cardiopulmonary resuscitation after asphyxial cardiac arrest. Pediatr Emerg Care 1996; 12:245–248.

56a. Babbs CF, Nadkarni V. Optimizing chest compression to rescue ventilation ratios during one-rescuer CPR by professionals and lay persons: children are not just little adults. Resuscitation 2004; 61:173–181

57. Kinney SB, Tibballs J. An analysis of the efficacy of bag-valve-mask ventilation and chest compression during different compression-ventilation ratios in manikin-simulated paediatric resuscitation. Resuscitation 2000; 43:115–120.

58. Halperin HR, et al. Determinants of blood flow to vital organs during cardiopulmonary resuscitation in dogs. Circulation 1986; 73:539–550.
59. Dean JM, et al.Improved blood flow during prolonged cardiopulmonary resuscitation with 30% duty cycle in infant pigs. Circulation 1991; 84:896–904.
60. Dean JM, et al. Age-related changes in chest geometry during cardiopulmonary resuscitation. J Appl Physiol 1987; 62:2212–2219.
61. Halperin H, et al. Cardiopulmonary resuscitation with a hydraulic-pneumatic band. Crit Care Med 2000; 28(Suppl):N203–N206.
62. Halperin HR, et al. Vest inflation without simultaneous ventilation during cardiac arrest in dogs: improved survival from prolonged cardiopulmonary resuscitation. Circulation 1986; 74:1407–1415.
63. Halperin HR, et al. A preliminary study of cardiopulmonary resuscitation by circumferential compression of the chest with use of a pneumatic vest. N Engl J Med 1993; 329:762–768.
64. Halperin HR, Weisfeldt ML. New approaches to CPR. Four hands, a plunger, or a vest [editorial]. JAMA 1992; 267:2940,2941.
65. David R. Closed chest cardiac massage in the newborn infant. Pediatrics 1988; 81:552–554.
66. Menegazzi JJ, et al. Two-thumb versus two-finger chest compression during CPR in a swine infant model of cardiac arrest. Ann Emerg Med 1993; 22:240–243.
67. Thaler MM, Stobie GH. An improved technique of external cardiac compression in infants and young children. N Engl J Med 1963; 269:606–610.
68. Whitelaw CC, Slywka B, Goldsmith LJ. Comparison of a two-finger versus two-thumb method for chest compressions by healthcare providers in an infant mechanical model. Resuscitation 2000; 43: 213–216.
69. Sanders A, et al. Expired pCO2 as an index of coronary perfusion pressure. Am J Emerg Med 1985; 3: 147–149.
70. Sanders A, Ewy G, Taft T. Prognostic and therapeutic importance of the aortic diastolic pressure in resuscitation from cardiac arrest. Crit Care Med 1984; 12:871–873.
71. Kern KB, et al. Changes in expired end-tidal carbon dioxide during cardiopulmonary resuscitation in dogs: a prognostic guide for resuscitation efforts. J Am Coll Cardiol 1989:13:1184–1189.
72. Sanders AB, et al. Expired PCO_2 as a prognostic indicator of successful resuscitation from cardiac arrest. Ann Emerg Med 1985; 14:948–952.
73. Bhende MS, Karasic DG, Karasic RB. End-tidal carbon dioxide changes during cardiopulmonary resuscitation after experimental asphyxial cardiac arrest. Am J Emerg Med 1996; 14:349,350.
74. Bhende MS, Thompson AE. Evaluation of an end-tidal CO_2 detector during pediatric cardiopulmonary resuscitation. Pediatrics 1995; 95:395–399.
75. Sheikh A, Brogan T. Outcome and cost of open- and closed-chest cardiopulmonary resuscitation in pediatric cardiac arrests. Pediatrics 1994; 93:392–398.
76. Beaver BL, et al. Efficacy of emergency room thoracotomy in pediatric trauma. J Pediatr Surg 1987; 22:19–23.
77. Calkins CM, et al. A critical analysis of outcome for children sustaining cardiac arrest after blunt trauma. J Pediatr Surg 2002; 37:180–184.
78. Fisher B, Worthen M. Cardiac arrest induced by blunt trauma in children. Pediatr Emerg Care 1999; 15:274–276.
79. Li G, et al. Cardiopulmonary resuscitation in pediatric trauma patients: survival and functional outcome. J Trauma 1999; 47:1–7.
80. Babbs CF. CPR techniques that combine chest and abdominal compression and decompression: hemodynamic insights from a spreadsheet model. Circulation 1999; 100:2146–2152.
81. Beattie C, et al. Mechanisms of blood flow during pneumatic vest cardiopulmonary resuscitation. J Appl Physiol 1991; 70:454–465.
82. Babbs CF. Circulatory adjuncts. Newer methods of cardiopulmonary resuscitation. Cardiol Clin 2002; 20:37–59.
83. Chang MW, et al. Active compression-decompression CPR improves vital organ perfusion in a dog model of ventricular fibrillation. Chest 1994; 106:1250–1259.
84. Cohen T, et al. A comparison of active compression-decompression cardiopulmonary resuscitation with standard cardiopulmonary resuscitation for cardiac arrests occurring in the hospital. N Engl K Med 1993; 329:1918–1921.
85. Lindner KH, Wenzel V. New mechanical methods for cardiopulmonary resuscitation (CPR): literature study and analysis of effectiveness [in German]. Anaesthesist 1997; 46:220–230.
86. Lurie K. Bringing back the nearly dead. The hope and the challenge. Minn Med 2002; 85:39–42.

87. Babbs CF. Efficacy of interposed abdominal compression-cardiopulmonary resuscitation (CPR), active compression and decompression-CPR and Lifestick CPR: basic physiology in a spreadsheet model. Crit Care Med 2000; 28(Suppl):N199–N202.

88. Hanouz JL, et al. Insertion of the minimally invasive direct cardiac massage device (MIDCM): training on human cadavers. Resuscitation 2002; 52:49–53.

89. Paiva EF, et al. Minimally invasive direct cardiac massage versus closed-chest cardiopulmonary resuscitation in a porcine model of prolonged ventricular fibrillation cardiac arrest. Resuscitation 2000; 47:287–299.

90. Smith T. Alternative cardiopulmonary resuscitation devices. Curr Opin Crit Care, 2002; 8:219–223.

91. Langhelle A, et al. Inspiratory impedance threshold valve during CPR. Resuscitation 2002; 52:39–48.

92. Lurie K, et al. Use of an inspiratory impedance threshold valve during cardiopulmonary resuscitation: a progress report. Resuscitation 2000; 44:219–230.

93. Lurie K, et al. Improving the efficiency of cardiopulmonary resuscitation with an inspiratory impedance threshold valve. Crit Care Med 2000; 28(Suppl):N207–N209.

94. Lurie KG, et al. Improving standard cardiopulmonary resuscitation with an inspiratory impedance threshold valve in a porcine model of cardiac arrest. Anesth Analg 2001; 93:649–655.

95. Lurie KG, et al. Use of an inspiratory impedance valve improves neurologically intact survival in a porcine model of ventricular fibrillation. Circulation 2002; 105:124–129.

96. Tecklenburg FW, et al. Pediatric ECMO for severe quinidine cardiotoxicity. Pediatr Emerg Care 1997; 13:111–113.

97. Thalmann M, et al. Resuscitation in near drowning with extracorporeal membrane oxygenation. Ann Thorac Surg 2001; 72:607.608.

97a. Morris MC, Nadkarni VM. Pediatric cardiopulmonary-cerebral resuscitation: an overview and future directions. Crit Care Clin 2003; 19:337–364.

98. Andropoulos DB, Soifer SJ, Schreiber MD. Plasma epinephrine concentrations after intraosseous and central venous injection during cardiopulmonary resuscitation in the lamb. J Pediatr 1990; 116: 312–315.

99. Banerjee S, et al. The intraosseous route is a suitable alternative to intravenous route for fluid resuscitation in severely dehydrated children. Indian Pediatr 1994; 31:1511–1520.

100. Cameron JL, Fontanarosa PB, Passalaqua AM. A comparative study of peripheral to central circulation delivery times between intraosseous and intravenous injection using a radionuclide technique in normovolemic and hypovolemic canines. J Emerg Med 1989; 7:123–127.

101. Friedman FD. Intraosseous adenosine for the termination of supraventricular tachycardia in an infant. Ann Emerg Med 1996; 28:356–358.

102. Getschman SJ, et al. Intraosseous adenosine. As effective as peripheral or central venous administration? Arch Pediatr Adolesc Med 1994; 148:616–619.

103. Glaeser PW, et al. Five-year experience in prehospital intraosseous infusions in children and adults. Ann Emerg Med 1993; 22:1119–1124.

104. Herman MI, et al. Methylene blue by intraosseous infusion for methemoglobinemia. Ann Emerg Med 1999; 33:111–113.

105. Katan BS, Olshaker JS, Dickerson SE. Intraosseous infusion of muscle relaxants. Am J Emerg Med 1988; 6:353–354.

106. Kramer GC, et al. Resuscitation of hemorrhage with intraosseous infusion of hypertonic saline/dextran. Braz J Med Biol Res 1989; 22:283–286.

107. Kruse JA, Vyskocil JJ, Haupt MT. Intraosseous infusions: a flexible option for the adult or child with delayed, difficult, or impossible conventional vascular access [editorial]. Crit Care Med 1994; 22: 728,729.

108. Orlowski JP, et al. Comparison study of intraosseous, central intravenous, and peripheral intravenous infusions of emergency drugs. Am J Dis Child 1990; 144:112–117.

109. Prete MR, Hannan CJJ, and Burkle FMJ. Plasma atropine concentrations via intravenous, endotracheal, and intraosseous administration. Am J Emerg Med 1987; 5:101–104.

110. Voelckel WG, et al. Comparison of epinephrine with vasopressin on bone marrow blood flow in an animal model of hypovolemic shock and subsequent cardiac arrest. Crit Care Med 2001; 29:1587–1592.

111. Warren DW, et al. Pharmacokinetics from multiple intraosseous and peripheral intravenous site injections in normovolemic and hypovolemic pigs. Crit Care Med 1994; 22:838–843.

112. Abdelmoneim T, et al. Acid-base status of blood from intraosseous and mixed venous sites during prolonged cardiopulmonary resuscitation and drug infusions. Crit Care Med 1999; 27:1923–1928.

113. Brickman KR, et al. Typing and screening of blood from intraosseous access. Ann Emerg Med 1992; 21:414–417.
114. Voelckel WG, et al. Intraosseous blood gases during hypothermia: correlation with arterial, mixed venous, and sagittal sinus blood. Crit Care Med 2000; 28:2915–2920.
115. Christensen DW, et al. Skin necrosis complicating intraosseous infusion. Pediatr Emerg Care 1991; 7: 289,290.
116. Dedrick DK, et al. The effects of intraosseous infusion on the growth plate in a nestling rabbit model. Ann Emerg Med 1992; 21:494–497.
117. Fiallos M, et al. Fat embolism with the use of intraosseous infusion during cardiopulmonary resuscitation. Am J Med Sci 1997; 314:73–79.
118. Fiser RT, et al. Tibial length following intraosseous infusion: a prospective, radiographic analysis. Pediatr Emerg Care 1997; 13:186–188.
119. Galpin RD, et al. Bilateral lower extremity compartment syndromes secondary to intraosseous fluid resuscitation. J Pediatr Orthop 1991; 11:773–776.
120. Katz DS, Wojtowycz AR. Tibial fracture: a complication of intraosseous infusion. Am J Emerg Med 1994; 12:258,259.
121. LaSpada J, et al. Extravasation rates and complications of intraosseous needles during gravity and pressure infusion. Crit Care Med 1995; 23:2023–2028.
122. Moscati R, Moore GP. Compartment syndrome with resultant amputation following intraosseous infusion [letter]. Am J Emerg Med 1990; 8:470–471.
123. Rosovsky M, et al. Bilateral osteomyelitis due to intraosseous infusion: case report and review of the English-language literature. Pediatr Radiol 1994; 24:72,73.
124. Simmons CM, et al. Intraosseous extravasation complication reports. Ann Emerg Med 1994; 23: 363–366.
125. Vidal R, Kissoon N, Gayle M. Compartment syndrome following intraosseous infusion. Pediatrics 1993; 91:1201,1202.
126. Berg RA, et al. A randomized, blinded trial of high-dose epinephrine versus standard-dose epinephrine in a swine model of pediatric asphyxial cardiac arrest. Crit Care Med 1996; 24:1695–1700.
127. Berg RA, et al. High-dose epinephrine results in greater early mortality after resuscitation from prolonged cardiac arrest in pigs: a prospective, randomized study. Crit Care Med 1994; 22:282–290.
128. Callaham M, et al. A randomized clinical trial of high-dose epinephrine and norepinephrine vs standard-dose epinephrine in prehospital cardiac arrest. JAMA 1992; 268:2667–2672.
129. Brown C, et al. A comparison of standard-dose and high-dose epinephrine in cardiac arrest outside the hospital. New Engl J Med 1992; 327:151–155.
130. Callaham M, Barton CW, Kayser S. Potential complications of high-dose epinephrine therapy in patients resuscitated from cardiac arrest. JAMA 1991; 265:1117–1122.
131. Callaham M, et al. A randomized clinical trial of high-dose epinephrine and norepinephrine versus standard-dose epinephrine in prehospital cardiac arrest. JAMA 1992; 268:2667–2672.
132. Carpenter TC, Stenmark KR. High-dose epinephrine is not superior to standard-dose epinephrine in pediatric in-hospital cardiopulmonary arrest. Pediatrics 1997; 99:403–408.
133. Goetting MG, Paradis NA. High-dose epinephrine improves outcome from pediatric cardiac arrest. Ann Emerg Med 1991; 20:22–26.
134. Gueugniaud PY, et al. A comparison of repeated high doses and repeated standard doses of epinephrine for cardiac arrest outside the hospital. European Epinephrine Study Group. N Engl J Med 1998; 339: 1595–1601.
135. Lindner KH, Ahnefeld FW, Prengel AW. Comparison of standard and high-dose adrenaline in the resuscitation of asystole and electromechanical dissociation. Acta Anaesthesiol Scand 1991; 35:253–256.
136. Lipman J, et al. High-dose adrenaline in adult in-hospital asystolic cardiopulmonary resuscitation: a double-blind randomised trial. Anaesth Intensive Care 1993; 21:192–196.
137. Niemann J, et al. Treatment of prolonged ventricular fibrillation: immediate countershock versus high-dose epinephrine and CPR preceding countershock. Circulation 1992; 85:281–287.
138. Paradis NA, et al. The effect of standard- and high-dose epinephrine on coronary perfusion pressure during prolonged cardiopulmonary resuscitation. JAMA 1991; 265:1139–1144.
139. Sherman BW, et al. High-dose versus standard-dose epinephrine treatment of cardiac arrest after failure of standard therapy. Pharmacotherapy 1997; 17:242–247.
140. Stiell IG, et al. High-dose epinephrine in adult cardiac arrest. N Engl J Med 1992; 327:1045–1050.
141. Achleitner U, et al. The effects of repeated doses of vasopressin or epinephrine on ventricular fibrillation in a porcine model of prolonged cardiopulmonary resuscitation. Anesth Analg 2000; 90:1067–1075.

141a. Perondi MB, Reis AG, Paiva EF, Nadkarni VM, Berg RA. A comparison of high-dose and standard-dose epinephrine in children with cardiac arrest. N Engl J Med 2004; 350:1722–1730.

142. Argenziano M, et al. Arginine vasopressin in the management of vasodilatory hypotension after cardiac transplantation. J Heart Lung Transplant 1999; 18:814–817.

143. Babar SI, et al. Vasopressin versus epinephrine during cardiopulmonary resuscitation: a randomized swine outcome study. Resuscitation 1999; 41:185–192.

144. Babbs CF, et al. Use of pressors in the treatment of cardiac arrest. Ann Emerg Med 2001; 37(Suppl): S152–S162.

145. Chugh SS, Lurie KG, Lindner KH. Pressor with promise: using vasopressin in cardiopulmonary arrest. Circulation 1997; 96:2453,2454.

146. Kern KB, Halperin HR, Field J. New guidelines for cardiopulmonary resuscitation and emergency cardiac care: changes in the management of cardiac arrest. JAMA 2001; 285:1267–1269.

147. Kono S, et al. Vasopressin and epinephrine are equally effective for CPR in a rat asphyxia model. Resuscitation 2002; 52:215–219.

148. Krismer AC, et al. The efficacy of epinephrine or vasopressin for resuscitation during epidural anesthesia. Anesth Analg 2001; 93:734–742.

149. Krismer AC, et al. Cardiopulmonary resuscitation during severe hypothermia in pigs: does epinephrine or vasopressin increase coronary perfusion pressure? Anesth Analg 2000;90:69–73.

150. Krismer AC, et al. The effects of endogenous and exogenous vasopressin during experimental cardiopulmonary resuscitation. Anesth Analg 2001; 92:1499–1504.

151. Krismer AC, et al. Arginine vasopressin during cardiopulmonary resuscitation and vasodilatory shock: current experience and future perspectives. Curr Opin Crit Care 2001; 7:157–169.

152. Lindner KH, et al. Effect of vasopressin on hemodynamic variables, organ blood flow, and acid-base status in a pig model of cardiopulmonary resuscitation. Anesth Analg 1993; 77:427–435.

153. Lindner KH, et al. Randomised comparison of epinephrine and vasopressin in patients with out-of-hospital ventricular fibrillation. Lancet 1997; 349:535–537.

154. Lindner KH, et al. Release of endogenous vasopressors during and after cardiopulmonary resuscitation. Heart 1996; 75:145–150.

155. Lindner KH, et al. Vasopressin administration in refractory cardiac arrest. Ann Intern Med 1996; 124:1061–1064.

156. Lindner KH, et al. Vasopressin improves vital organ blood flow during closed-chest cardiopulmonary resuscitation in pigs. Circulation 1995; 91:215–221.

157. Mayr VD, et al. Developing a vasopressor combination in a pig model of adult asphyxial cardiac arrest. Circulation 2001; 104:1651–1656.

158. Morley P. Vasopressin or epinephrine: which initial vasopressor for cardiac arrests? Lancet 2001; 358: 85,86.

159. Morris DC, et al. Vasopressin can increase coronary perfusion pressure during human cardiopulmonary resuscitation. Acad Emerg Med 1997; 4:878–883.

160. Nozari A, Rubertsson S, Wiklund L. Differences in the pharmacodynamics of epinephrine and vasopressin during and after experimental cardiopulmonary resuscitation. Resuscitation 2001; 49:59–72.

161. Prengel AW, et al. Splanchnic and renal blood flow after cardiopulmonary resuscitation with epinephrine and vasopressin in pigs. Resuscitation 1998; 38:19–24.

162. Raedler C, et al. Vasopressor response in a porcine model of hypothermic cardiac arrest is improved with active compression-decompression cardiopulmonary resuscitation using the inspiratory impedance threshold valve. Anesth Analg 2002; 95:1496–1502, table of contents.

163. Stiell IG, et al. Vasopressin versus epinephrine for inhospital cardiac arrest: a randomised controlled trial. Lancet 2001; 358:105–109.

164. Voelckel WG, et al. Effects of vasopressin and epinephrine on splanchnic blood flow and renal function during and after cardiopulmonary resuscitation in pigs. Crit Care Med 2000; 28:1083–1088.

165. Voelckel WG, et al. Comparison of epinephrine and vasopressin in a pediatric porcine model of asphyxial cardiac arrest. Circulation 1999; 36:1115–1118.

165a. Voelckel WG, Lurie KG, McKnite S, et al. Comparison of epinephrine and vasopressin in a pediatric porcine model of asphyxial cardiac arrest. Crit Care Med. 2000; 28:3777–3783.

166. Mann K, Berg RA, Nadkarni V. Beneficial effects of vasopressin in prolonged pediatric cardiac arrest: a case series. Resuscitation 2002; 52:149–156.

167. Katz K, et al. Vasopressin pressor effects in critically ill children during evaluation for brain death and organ recovery. Resuscitation 2000; 47:33–40.

168. Butt W. Septic shock. Pediatr Clin North Am 2001; 48:601–625.

169. Rosenzweig EB, et al. Intravenous arginine-vasopressin in children with vasodilatory shock after cardiac surgery. Circulation 1999; 100(Suppl):II182–II186.

170. Dembo DH. Calcium in advanced life support. Crit Care Med 1981; 9:358,359.

171. Harrison EE, Amey BD. The use of calcium in cardiac resuscitation. Am J Emerg Med 1983; 1: 267–273.

172. Urban P, et al. Cardiac arrest and blood ionized calcium levels. Ann Intern Med 1988; 109:110–113.

173. van Walraven C, et al. Do advanced cardiac life support drugs increase resuscitation rates from in-hospital cardiac arrest? The OTAC Study Group. Ann Emerg Med 1998; 32:544–553.

174. Yusuf S, et al. Routine medical management of acute myocardial infarction: lessons from overviews of recent randomized controlled trials. Circulation 1990; 82(Suppl):II117–II134.

175. Ammari AN, Schulze KF. Uses and abuses of sodium bicarbonate in the neonatal intensive care unit. Curr Opin Pediatr 2002; 14:151–156.

176. Bar-Joseph G. Is sodium bicarbonate therapy during cardiopulmonary resuscitation really detrimental? [letter]. Crit Care Med 2000; 28:1693,1694.

177. Bar-Joseph G, et al. Clinical use of sodium bicarbonate during cardiopulmonary resuscitation—is it used sensibly? Resuscitation 2002; 54:47–55.

178. Cooper DJ, et al. Bicarbonate does not improve hemodynamics in critically ill patients who have lactic acidosis: a prospective, controlled clinical study. Ann Intern Med 1990; 112:492–498.

179. Federiuk CS, et al. The effect of bicarbonate on resuscitation from cardiac arrest. Ann Emerg Med 1991; 20:1173–1177.

180. Graf H, Leach W, Arieff AI. Evidence for a detrimental effect of bicarbonate therapy in hypoxic lactic acidosis. Science 1985; 227:754–756.

181. Kette F, Weil MH, Gazmuri RJ. Buffer solutions may compromise cardiac resuscitation by reducing coronary perfusion presssure [published correction appears in JAMA 1991; 266:3286]. JAMA 1991; 266:2121–2126.

182. Sanders AB, et al. The role of bicarbonate and fluid loading in improving resuscitation from prolonged cardiac arrest with rapid manual chest compression CPR. Ann Emerg Med 1990:19:1–7.

183. von Planta M, et al. Pathophysiologic and therapeutic implications of acid-base changes during CPR. Ann Emerg Med 1993; 22(Pt 2):404–410.

184. Weil MH, et al. Difference in acid-base state between venous and arterial blood during cardiopulmonary resuscitation. N Engl J Med 1986; 315:153–156.

185. Bar-Joseph G, et al. Comparison of sodium bicarbonate, Carbicarb, and THAM during cardiopulmonary resuscitation in dogs. Crit Care Med 1998; 26:1397–1408.

186. Minuck M, Sharma GP. Comparison of THAM and sodium bicarbonate in resuscitation of the heart after ventricular fibrillation in dogs. Anesth Analg 1977; 56:38–45.

187. von Planta M, et al. Effects of tromethamine and sodium bicarbonate buffers during cardiac resuscitation. J Clin Pharmacol 1988; 28:594–599.

188. Wiklund L, et al. Effects of alkaline buffer administration on survival and myocardial energy metabolism in pigs subjected to ventricular fibrillation and closed chest CPR. Acta Anaesthesiol Scand 1990; 34:430–439.

189. Rubertsson S, Wiklund L. Hemodynamic effects of epinephrine in combination with different alkaline buffers during experimental, open-chest, cardiopulmonary resuscitation. Crit Care Med 1993; 21: 1051–1057.

190. Zaritsky A. Pediatric resuscitation pharmacology. Members of the Medications in Pediatric Resuscitation Panel. Ann Emerg Med 1993; 22(Pt 2): 445–455.

191. Berg RA, et al. Ventricular fibrillation in a swine model of acute pediatric asphyxial cardiac arrest. Resuscitation 1996; 33:147–53.

192. Nadkarni V. Ventricular fibrillation in the asphyxiated piglet model, in Ventricular Fibrillation: a Pediatric Problem. Quan L, Franklin WH, eds. Armonk, NY: Futura Publishers, 2000, pp. 43–54.

193. Standards and guidelines for cardiopulmonary resuscitation (CPR) and emergency cardiac care (ECC). JAMA 1980; 244:453–509.

194. Gutgesell HP, et al. Energy dose for ventricular defibrillation of children. Pediatrics 1976; 58:898–901.

195. Atkins DL, et al. Pediatric defibrillation: importance of paddle size in determining transthoracic impedance. Pediatrics 1988; 82:914–918.

196. Atkins DL, Kerber RE. Pediatric defibrillation: current flow is improved by using "adult" electrode paddles. Pediatrics 1994; 94:90–93.

197. Tang W, et al. Fixed-energy biphasic waveform defibrillation in a pediatric model of cardiac arrest and resuscitation. Crit Care Med 2002; 30:2736–2741.

198. Berg RA, et al. Comparison of weight-based monophasic and fixed sequence biphasic defibrillation dosing for resuscitation in a model of pediatric prolonged cardiac arrest. J Am Coll Cardiol 2003; 41(Suppl):350.

199. Anastasiou-Nana MI, et al. Effects of amiodarone on refractory ventricular fibrillation in acute myocardial infarction: experimental study. J Am Coll Cardiol 1994; 23:253–258.

200. Connolly SJ. Meta-analysis of antiarrhythmic drug trials. Am J Cardiol 1999; 84:90R–93R.

201. Dorian P, et al. Amiodarone as compared with lidocaine for shock-resistant ventricular fibrillation. N Engl J Med 2002; 346:884–890.

202. Figa FH, et al. Clinical efficacy and safety of intravenous Amiodarone in infants and children. Am J Cardiol 1994l; 74:573–577.

203. Helmy I, et al. Use of intravenous amiodarone for emergency treatment of life-threatening ventricular arrhythmias. J Am Coll Cardiol 1988; 12:1015–1022.

204. Kowey PR, et al. Randomized, double-blind comparison of intravenous amiodarone and bretylium in the treatment of patients with recurrent, hemodynamically destabilizing ventricular tachycardia or fibrillation. The Intravenous Amiodarone Multicenter Investigators Group. Circulation 1995; 92: 3255–3263.

205. Kudenchuk PJ. Intravenous antiarrhythmic drug therapy in the resuscitation from refractory ventricular arrhythmias. Am J Cardiol 1999; 84:52R–55R.

206. Kudenchuk, PJ, et al. Amiodarone for resuscitation after out-of-hospital cardiac arrest due to ventricular fibrillation. N Engl J Med 1999; 341:871–878.

207. Perry JC, et al. Intravenous amiodarone for life-threatening tachyarrhythmias in children and young adults. J Am Coll Cardiol 1993; 22:95–98.

208. Samson RA, et al. Use of automated external defibrillators for children: an update: an advisory statement from the pediatric advanced life support task force, International Liaison Committee on Resuscitation. Circulation 2003; 107:3250–3255.

209. Atkinson E, et al. Specificity and sensitivity of automated external defibrillator rhythm analysis in infants and children. Ann Emerg Med 2003; 42:185–196.

210. White RD, Hankins DG, Atkinson EJ. Patient outcomes following defibrillation with a low energy biphasic truncated exponential waveform in out-of-hospital cardiac arrest. Resuscitation 2001; 49:9–14.

211. Atkins DL, Hartley LL, York DK. Accurate recognition and effective treatment of ventricular fibrillation by automated external defibrillators in adolescents. Pediatrics 1998; 101(Pt 1):393–397.

212. Bain AC, et al. Multicenter study of principles-based waveforms for external defibrillation. Ann Emerg Med 2001; 37:5–12.

213. Bardy G, et al. Truncated biphasic pulses for transthoracic defibrillation. Circulation 1995; 91: 1768–1774.

214. Bardy GH, et al. A prospective randomized evaluation of biphasic versus monophasic waveform pulses on defibrillation efficacy in humans. J Am Coll Cardiol 1989:14:728–733.

215. Bardy GH, et al. Multicenter comparison of truncated biphasic shocks and standard damped sine wave monophasic shocks for transthoracic ventricular defibrillation. Transthoracic Investigators. Circulation 1996; 94:2507–2514.

216. Cummins RO, et al. Low-energy biphasic waveform defibrillation: evidence-based review applied to emergency cardiovascular care guidelines: a statement for healthcare professionals from the American Heart Association Committee on Emergency Cardiovascular Care and the Subcommittees on Basic Life Support, Advanced Cardiac Life Support, and Pediatric Resuscitation. Circulation, 1998; 97:1654–1667.

217. Gliner BE, et al. Treatment of out-of-hospital cardiac arrest with a low-energy impedance-compensating biphasic waveform automatic external defibrillator. The LIFE Investigators. Biomed Instrum Technol 1998; 32:631–644.

218. Gliner BE, et al. Transthoracic defibrillation of swine with monophasic and biphasic waveforms. Circulation 1995; 92:1634–1643.

219. Greene HL, et al. Comparison of monophasic and biphasic defibrillating pulse waveforms for transthoracic cardioversion. Biphasic Waveform Defibrillation Investigators. Am J Cardiol 1995; 75: 1135–1139.

220. Higgins SL, et al. A comparison of biphasic and monophasic shocks for external defibrillation. Physio-Control Biphasic Investigators. Prehosp Emerg Care 2000; 4:305–313.

221. Killingsworth CR, et al. Defibrillation threshold and cardiac responses using an external biphasic defibrillator with pediatric and adult adhesive patches in pediatric-sized piglets. Resuscitation 2002; 55:177–85.

222. Martens PR, et al. Optimal Response to Cardiac Arrest study: defibrillation waveform effects. Resuscitation 2001; 49:233–243.
223. Walcott GP, et al. Mechanisms of defibrillation for monophasic and biphasic waveforms. Pacing Clin Electrophysiol 1994; 17(Pt 2):478–498.
224. Walker RG, et al. Comparison of a biphasic truncated exponential waveform to two standard monophasic waveforms for external defibrillation. J Am Col Cardiol 2000; 35(Suppl):400A.
225. White RD. Early out-of-hospital experience with an impedance-compensating low-energy biphasic waveform automatic external defibrillator. J Interv Card Electrophysiol 1997; 1:203–208.
226. van Alem AP, et al. A prospective, randomised and blinded comparison of first shock success of monophasic and biphasic waveforms in out-of-hospital cardiac arrest. Resuscitation, 2003; 58:17–24.
227. van Alem AP, Sanou BT, Koster RW. Interruption of cardiopulmonary resuscitation with the use of the automated external defibrillator in out-of-hospital cardiac arrest. Ann Emerg Med 2003; 42:449–457.
228. van Alem AP, et al. Use of automated external defibrillator by first responders in out of hospital cardiac arrest: prospective controlled trial. BMJ 2003; 327:1312.
229. Tang W, et al. Pediatric fixed energy biphasic waveform defibrillation using a standard AED and special pediatric electrodes [abstract]. Circulation 2001; 104(Suppl):Abstract no. 41222.
230. Berg RA, et al. Automated external defibrillation versus manual defibrillation for prolonged ventricular fibrillation: lethal delays of chest compressions before and after countershocks. Ann Emerg Med 2003; 42:458–467.
231. Hickey RW, et al. Hypothermia and hyperthermia in children after resuscitation from cardiac arrest. Pediatrics 2000; 106(Pt 1):118–122.
232. Sterz F, et al. Mild resuscitative hypothermia and outcome after cardiopulmonary resuscitation. J Neurosurg Anesthesiol 1996; 8:88–96.
233. Holzer M, et al. Mild hypothermia and outcome after CPR. Hypothermia for Cardiac Arrest (HACA) Study Group. Acta Anaesthesiol Scand Suppl 1997; 111:55–58.
234. Zeiner A, et al. Mild resuscitative hypothermia to improve neurological outcome after cardiac arrest. A clinical feasibility trial. Hypothermia After Cardiac Arrest (HACA) Study Group. Stroke 2000; 31: 86–94.
235. Bernard S, et al. Induced hypothermia using large volume, ice-cold intravenous fluid in comatose survivors of out-of-hospital cardiac arrest: a preliminary report. Resuscitation 2003; 56:9–13.
236. Bernard SA, et al. Treatment of comatose survivors of out-of-hospital cardiac arrest with induced hypothermia. N Engl J Med 2002; 346:557–563.
237. Hypothermia After Cardiac Arrest Study Group. Mild therapeutic hypothermia to improve the neurologic outcome after cardiac arrest. N Engl J Med 2002; 346:549–556.
238. Broderick JP, et al. Hyperglycemia and hemorrhagic transformation of cerebral infarcts. Stroke 1995; 26:484–487.
239. Cherian L, Goodman JC, Robertson CS. Hyperglycemia increases brain injury caused by secondary ischemia after cortical impact injury in rats. Crit Care Med 1997; 25:1378–1383.
240. Pulsinelli WA, et al. Moderate hyperglycemia augments ischemic brain damage: a neuropathologic study in the rat. Neurology 1982; 32:1239–1246.
241. Van den Berghe G, et al. Intensive insulin therapy in critically ill patients. N Engl J Med 2001; 345: 1359–1367.
242. Yip PK, et al. Effect of plasma glucose on infarct size in focal cerebral ischemia-reperfusion. Neurology 1991; 41:899–905.
243. Mullner M, et al. Blood glucose concentration after cardiopulmonary resuscitation influences functional neurological recovery in human cardiac arrest survivors. J Cereb Blood Flow Metab 1997; 17: 430–436.
244. Krukenkamp I, et al. Direct effect of high-dose insulin on the depressed heart after beta- blockade or ischemia. Thorac Cardiovasc Surg 1986; 34:305–309.
245. Safar P, et al. Systematic development of cerebral resuscitation after cardiac arrest. Three promising treatments: cardiopulmonary bypass, hypertensive hemodilution, and mild hypothermia. Acta Neurochir Suppl (Wien) 1993; 57:110–121.
246. Safar P, et al. Improved cerebral resuscitation from cardiac arrest in dogs with mild hypothermia plus blood flow promotion. Stroke 1996; 27:105–113.
247. Sterz F, et al. Hypertension with or without hemodilution after cardiac arrest in dogs. Stroke 1990; 21: 1178–1184.
248. Mullner M, et al. Arterial blood pressure after human cardiac arrest and neurological recovery. Stroke 1996; 27:59–62.

249. Carcillo JA, Davis AL, Zaritsky A. Role of early fluid resuscitation in pediatric septic shock. JAMA 1991; 266:1242–1245.
250. Ceneviva G, et al. Hemodynamic support in fluid-refractory pediatric septic shock. Pediatrics 1998; 102:19.
251. Angus DC, et al. Epidemiology of severe sepsis in the United States: analysis of incidence, outcome, and associated costs of care. Crit Care Med 2001; 29:1303–1310.
252. Carcillo JA. Pediatric septic shock and multiple organ failure. Crit Care Clin 2003; 19:413–440, viii.
253. Carcillo JA, Fields AI. [Clinical practice parameters for hemodynamic support of pediatric and neonatal patients in septic shock]. J Pediatr (Rio J) 2002; 78:449–466.
254. Despond O, et al. Pediatric sepsis and multiple organ dysfunction syndrome. Curr Opin Pediatr 2001; 13:247–253.
255. Han YY, et al. Early reversal of pediatric-neonatal septic shock by community physicians is associated with improved outcome. Pediatrics 2003; 112:793–799.
256. Watson RS, et al. The epidemiology of severe sepsis in children in the United States. Am J Respir Crit Care Med 2003; 167:695–701.
257. Berg RA, Padbury JF. Sulfoconjugation and renal excretion contribute to the interpatient variation of exogenous catecholamine clearance in critically ill children. Crit Care Med 1997; 25:1247–1251.
258. Suominen P, et al. Prehospital care and survival of pediatric patients with blunt trauma. J Pediatr Surg 1998; 33:1388–1392.
259. Suominen P, et al. Impact of age, submersion time and water temperature on outcome in near-drowning. Resuscitation 2002; 52:247–254.
260. Suominen P, Rasanen J, Kivioja A. Efficacy of cardiopulmonary resuscitation in pulseless paediatric trauma patients. Resuscitation 1998; 36:9–13.
261. Cummins RO, Chamberlain DA. AHA Medical/Scientific Statement. Recommended Guidelines for Uniform Reporting Data From Out-of-Hospital Cardiac Arrest: The Utstein Style. 1991.
262. Idris AH, et al. Utstein-style guidelines for uniform reporting of laboratory CPR research. A statement for healthcare professionals from a Task Force of the American Heart Association, the American College of Emergency Physicians, the American College of Cardiology, the European Resuscitation Council, the Heart and Stroke Foundation of Canada, the Institute of Critical Care Medicine, the Safar Center for Resuscitation Research, and the Society for Academic Emergency Medicine. Resuscitation 1996; 33:69–84.
263. Becker LB, et al. The PULSE initiative: scientific priorities and strategic planning for resuscitation research and life saving therapies. Circulation 2002; 105:2562–2570.
264. Baren JM, et al. An approach to community consultation prior to initiating an emergency research study incorporating a waiver of informed consent. Acad Emerg Med 1999; 6:1210–1215.
265. Tunstall-Pedoe H, et al. Survey of 3765 cardiopulmonary resuscitations in British hospitals (the BRESUS Study): methods and overall results. BMJ 1992; 304:1347–1351.
266. Gausche M, et al. A prospective, randomized study of the effect of out-of-hospital pediatric intubation on patient outcome. Acad Emerg Med 1998; 5:428.
267. Schindler MB, et al. Outcome of out-of-hospital cardiac or respiratory arrest in children. N Engl J Med 1996; 335:1473–1479.
268. Suominen P, et al. Paediatric cardiac arrest and resuscitation provided by physician-staffed emergency care units. Acta Anaesthesiol Scand 1997; 41:260–265.

32   In-Hospital Resuscitation

Mary Ann Peberdy, MD, FACC

CONTENTS

INTRODUCTION
THE IN-HOSPITAL CHAIN OF SURVIVAL
THE NATIONAL REGISTRY OF CARDIOPULMONARY RESUSCITATION
REFERENCES

INTRODUCTION

Resuscitation began in the hospital setting nearly 40 years ago and little has been done since that time to provide a critical evaluation of the process by which resuscitation is performed. Recent regulatory and federal guidelines are forcing hospitals to assess both process and outcome variables to improve the care given to victims of cardiac arrest (CA). The purpose of this chapter is to review process evaluation issues for hospital-based resuscitation programs and to describe the National Registry of Cardiopulmonary Resuscitation (NRCPR) as a tool for enhancing quality improvement and resuscitation science in the hospital.

THE IN-HOSPITAL CHAIN OF SURVIVAL

The American Heart Association (AHA) first developed the Chain of Survival concept in 1991 to facilitate a timely and appropriate response to victims of a CA *(1)*. The now familiar chain consists of the four links of early access, early basic life support (BLS), early defibrillation, and early advanced cardiac life support (ACLS). Pre-hospital emergency medical services (EMS) systems have paid meticulous attention to strengthening each link in the chain of survival, specifically with respect to early defibrillation, and communities have been rewarded with improved survival over the past decade. Hospitals, however, have been rather reluctant to critically evaluate their process of providing resuscitation efforts in order to assure that all the links in the chain are optimized and occurring in a timely manner. Some of this may be the belief that because hospitals are filled with health care providers, they automatically have an optimized response. Many people familiar with hospital-based resuscitation would disagree because many physicians and nurses have minimal advanced life support (ALS) training and use these skills very infrequently. Another possibility may be that resuscitation practices are often "orphaned" within a hospital system. Providing an

From: *Contemporary Cardiology: Cardiopulmonary Resuscitation*
Edited by: J. P. Ornato and M. A. Peberdy © Humana Press Inc., Totowa, NJ

adequate response is a hospital-wide effort and requires hospital wide support. Although many hospitals have a few champions for the cause, most lack overt organizational backing for critical process evaluation and enhancement. The last few years have seen the beginning of a shift toward process and outcome improvements for in-hospital resuscitation but the trend is slow to take hold and is complicated by what appears to be reluctance to use strategies that have been successful in the pre-hospital setting, such as first responder automatic external defibrillator (AED) use to deliver early defibrillation. Overall survival from cardiopulmonary arrest in the hospital setting has remained constant over the past 30 years with reports quoting a range from 3 to 27%, depending on the criteria and definitions used for inclusion criteria and outcomes *(2–4)*.

Although one could argue the impact of acute comorbidities in the hospital population, it is concerning that survival has never improved in this setting despite significant advances in technology that have translated into improved survival in out-of-hospital CA populations. This fact alone, independent of the need for quality review, should prompt hospitals to critically evaluate the process by which they perform resuscitation. Specific attention should be paid to both the process and clinical issues in order to identify issues that could potentially impact survival.

The AHA published its Recommended Guidelines for Reviewing, Reporting, and Conducting Research on In-Hospital Resuscitation: The In-Hospital Utstein Style in 1997 *(5)*. This scientific statement defined a set of data elements deemed as essential or desirable for documenting in-hospital CA responses. It was developed as a mechanism for international standardization of process evaluation and reporting for in-hospital resuscitation. By encouraging hospitals to use uniform definitions and methodology, the Utstein template provides greater accuracy in comparing and contrasting data from individual hospitals as well as across multiple studies. This document was the first widespread effort to encourage hospitals to systematically evaluate resuscitation efforts and outcomes

The Joint Commission for the Accreditation of Healthcare Organizations (JCAHO) placed further emphasis on hospital resuscitation practices with the publication of new regulations in 1998. As of January 1, 2000 the JCAHO required all accredited hospitals in the United States to have effective resuscitation services available throughout the hospital and to collect outcomes data. The JCAHO regulation Tx.8 states the following:

1. Appropriate policies, protocols, procedures, and processes governing the provision of resuscitation services
2. Appropriate equipment placed strategically throughout the hospital close to areas where patients are likely to require resuscitation services
3. Appropriate staff trained and competent to recognize the need to and use of designated equipment in resuscitation efforts
4. Appropriate data collection related to the process and outcomes of resuscitation
5. Ongoing review and outcomes related to resuscitation in the aggregate to identify opportunities for improvement in resuscitation efforts

This new set of standards provides an opportunity for hospitals to pay specific attention to the process of resuscitation and re-enforces the fact that resuscitation responses are a system-wide effort. By evaluating policy, protocols, and procedure hospitals are forced to review the way resuscitation efforts are carried out, specifically with respect to making sure that all populations are covered (inpatient, outpatient, visitor, adult, and pediatric) and that the response process chosen does everything that it can to strengthen the chain of survival in the hospital community. The second standard mandates that appropriate equipment be placed throughout the hospital and should stimulate an analytical approach by individual institutions to assure they have the most appropriate equipment for providing prompt, first responder, BLS with early defibrillation followed by ALS. The equipment must be appropriate for the population at potential risk for CA. The third regulation involves documenting competency for persons responding to CA. This is the fist time that hospitals have been held accountable for assuring skills retention in this area. There are many approaches toward training and competency testing, ranging from traditional classroom educational models to computer-based scenario testing that can be done on the practitioners own time schedule at the convenience of their own computer. Training and skills documentation can be uniquely designed to fit the needs and resources of individual institutions. Hospitals are now required to collect data related to both the process and outcomes of resuscitation. Never before have hospitals been mandated to perform periodic quality review of the entire process of resuscitation efforts. If done honestly and correctly, hospitals should critically evaluate every link in the chain of the resuscitation process. Examples of questions to be asked include the following:

- Is there a team response? Who should be on that team?
- Are the right people responding?
- How are responders trained to handle medical emergencies?
- How can we best provide early defibrillation?
- How does the team get summoned?
- How is the telepage operator involved?
- If a pager system is used, is there a lag time?
- How far does the team have to travel to cover the resuscitation area?
- What are the response-time intervals to the arrival of key personnel and interventions?
- How is time documented and is time documentation accurate?
- Is event documentation accurate?
- Are proper BSL and ALS guidelines being followed?
- What policies are in place regarding the "do not attempt resuscitation" (DNAR) decision pre-, or even postarrest?

Each area of the hospital that participates in the resuscitation process, such as nursing, pharmacy, anesthesia, respiratory therapy, central supply, medicine, surgery, professional education, and telepage, needs to evaluate the role it plays and develop the strongest process possible. For this to be done effectively and efficiently, a multidisciplinary committee should be formed to provide oversight and direction to this entire process. Because resuscitation services are used by everyone in the hospital and typically owned by no one, it is important that the committee have the resources and authority to do its job well.

THE NATIONAL REGISTRY OF CARDIOPULMONARY RESUSCITATION

The AHA's NRCPR is a prospective, multisite registry of in-hospital resuscitation. The registry was developed by AHA volunteers with expertise in cardiology, emergency medicine, adult and pediatric critical care medicine, nursing administration, and nursing education, and is based on the in-hospital Utstein guidelines for data collection. One of the unique features of the NRCPR is that it provides explicit definitions for every data element. This not only allows for interfacility comparison, but also permits data from numerous facilities to be combined and evaluated for trends in process, treatment, and outcomes. The goals of the NRCPR are to provide a standardized mechanism for quality data collection and review, to give local hospitals a mechanism to critically evaluate resuscitation process issues, treatment patterns, and outcomes, and to provide an ongoing data source for the development of evidence-based guidelines for resuscitation practices. Participating hospitals join the NRCPR voluntarily and have specially trained coordinators to enter information about each CA into a computer database. Data is submitted by either diskette or encrypted internet transfer to the central data repository. Each patient is assigned a unique code and no specific patient identifiers are transferred. Hospitals receive extensive quarterly reports on their own facility data along with comparisons to the national dataset. These reports provide hospitals with a comprehensive mechanism to meet JCAHO requirements for hospital-based resuscitation review.

The data set contains the following six major categories of variables:
1. facility data.
2. patient demographic data.
3. pre-event data.
4. event data.
5. outcome data.
6. quality improvement data.

Inclusion criteria are any adult (>18 years) or pediatric (<18 years) patient, visitor, employee, or staff who experience a resuscitation event that requires chest compression and/or defibrillation, elicits an emergency response by facility personnel, and has a resuscitation record completed for review. Events that begin outside of the hospital, in the neonatal intensive care unit (ICU), or occur in newborns in the delivery room are excluded.

Peberdy et al. *(6)* recently published the largest descriptive report of in-hospital resuscitation events in adults from the NRCPR data set. The report includes 14,720 CAs from 207 hospitals over a 2.5-year period. Demographic data of adults experiencing a CA in the hospital are 57% male with a mean age of 67.6 + 15.4 years. Eighty percent of arrests occurred on the medical services, being equally divided between cardiac and noncardiac. Forty-eight percent of arrests occurred in the ICU, 32% on general inpatient wards, 11% in the emergency department (ED), 4% in diagnostic areas, and 2% in the operating room. Less than 1% occurred in ambulatory care or visitors areas, although hospitals are required to have adequate responses for resuscitation in these populations. Knowledge of the likely service and location could have significant impact on staffing, training, and equipment placement.

The most common pre-existing conditions for adults experiencing CA in the hospital are myocardial infarction (36%), respiratory insufficiency (35%), congestive heart failure (34%), arrhythmia (29%), renal insufficiency (29%), diabetes mellitus (28%), and pneumonia (24%). Eighty-six percent of CA events are witnessed and/or monitored with 66% being both witnessed and monitored, 11% witnessed and not monitored, and 9% monitored and not witnessed.

The three most common nonexclusive precipitating issues present in the hour before the arrest are cardiac arrhythmia (49%), respiratory insufficiency (37%), and hypotension (32%). Although cardiac arrhythmias may occur suddenly without much warning, they are often the result of prolonged respiratory insufficiency or hypotension. More than two-thirds of adult CAs in the hospital are precipitated by disturbances that, if identified and intervened on promptly, may prevent the CA from occurring. This stresses the importance of having nurses and physicians trained to recognize and intercede in the pre-arrest period to prevent the occurrence of a full CA. Some hospitals have employed medical emergency teams specifically trained in the pre-arrest crisis intervention to be summoned to assist with the care of a patient before the code team is needed *(7–11)*. Some of these teams have been able to actually decrease the number of CAs that occurred and have also improved survival.

The first pulseless rhythm documented for adult CA is ventricular fibrillation/ventricular tachycardia (VF/VT) in 25%, pulseless electrical activity (PEA) in 30%, and asystole in 36%. The prevalence of VF as an initial rhythm is surprisingly low in the hospital setting. This is in contrast to the majority of out-of-hospital CAs that occur with a continuous monitor in place, in monitored cardiac rehab, and in some public access defibrillation programs such as the casinos *(12,13)*. Although the occurrence of VF as a presenting rhythm diminishes over time, the fact that 86% of events were monitored or witnessed in the hospital suggests that a delay in rhythm recognition does not solely account for the infrequent presence of VF as the initial arrest rhythm. In-hospital CA may have different mechanisms and pathophysiology than prehospital arrest. This may account for the predominance of asystole and PEA in this population compared to prehospital arrests.

Overall return of spontaneous circulation was 44% with overall survival-to-hospital discharge of 17%. Broken down by presenting rhythm, VF/VT carries a 35% survival rate to hospital discharge, in which survival from asystole and PEA are 10% each. The higher percent of asystole and PEA patients having a lower survival further dilutes the better survival in the comparatively smaller VF group. Of those patients that survived their initial arrest but died in the hospital, 63% were declared DNAR status after their index event, and 43% of these had life support actively withdrawn. The aggressiveness with which an individual hospital withholds resuscitation efforts and withdraws care can significantly impact survival and have tremendous influence on the outcomes of clinical trials requiring survival-to-hospital discharge as an endpoint. The average hospital length of stay is nearly 2 weeks for survivors and less than 2 days for those who die in the hospital. The majority of those being declared DNAR are being done so very early after their index event, perhaps even before meaningful recovery could be expected. Further investigation is needed to determine DNAR practice patterns and to identify accurate predictors of nonsurvival after initial CA.

Fifty-one percent of patients surviving a pulseless index arrest were discharged to home. More than 30% of survivors were discharged to a rehabilitation facility or a skilled nursing facility when less than 6% had lived in such a facility prior to their arrest. It is reassuring however, that 86% of patients with a Cerebral Performance Category-1 (CPC-1) at the time of admission had a CPC-1 at the time of discharge.

AEDs in the Hospital

Despite the fact that only 25% of pulseless CAs in the hospital are caused by VF, survival in this group is much better than when asystole or PEA are the presenting rhythms (35 vs 10% respectively). Hospitals must assure that defibrillation can be delivered promptly in order to appropriately treat the small group of arrest patients who have the best chance of survival. Survival from VF arrest is inversely related to the time to shock. This is true for both pre-hospital and in-hospital settings. Data from witnessed arrests during cardiac rehabilitation *(14)* or induced in the electrophysiology laboratory *(15)* report survival rates of more than 90% and nearly 100%, respectively. Valunzuela et al. *(13)* reported a 74% survival-to-hospital discharge from out-of-hospital CA when on-site lay first responders provide defibrillation in less than 3 minutes.

Caffrey et al. *(16)* found an overall survival rate of 66% in victims of VF arrests in the Chicago airport public access defibrillation (PAD) system. Data from NRCPR has correlated improved survival with shorter time to shock intervals. The survival rate was 38% when the first shock was delivered within 3 minutes, compared to only 21% when delivery was reported as more than 3 minutes. Even though many communities and public venues have markedly improved survival from CA by using AED technology and implementing PAD systems, hospitals have been slow to adopt the concept of having hospital first responders deliver lifesaving defibrillation. Inside the ICU, nurses often initiate CPR and provide defibrillation based on rhythm recognition and standing order. Outside of the ICU, nurses and other first responders perform CPR but typically must await the arrival of a physician to provide defibrillation. In-hospital use of AEDs by non-ICU nurses and other first responders was first described in 1995 *(17,18)* and 8 years later only 33% of NRCPR-participating hospitals reported having AED capability anywhere in their institutions. Critical evaluation of timing documentation, process issues, outcomes, and a willingness to explore different approaches to enhance early defibrillation are necessary for hospitals to begin to improve survival from VF arrest.

Outpatient Facilities

Medical practice in the United States is experiencing a continuous shift toward outpatient care. Both the volume and acuity of patients seen in the ambulatory care setting has increased dramatically since the 1990s. Numerous diagnostic and therapeutic procedures performed previously on in-patients are now occurring routinely on outpatients. Because of the use of conscious and deep sedation and increasing numbers of invasive and interventional procedures, outpatient facilities are faced with higher risk patients than in the past. The JCAHO mandates that a similar standard of care must be provided throughout all areas of the hospital, including ambulatory care facilities. This does not mean that the exact process for responding to CA be the same throughout but rather that a similar level of care be provided in all areas. The mechanism to achieve that level of care may differ by location. This is extremely important when designing a resuscitation response for hospital-affiliated outpatient centers.

Many hospital-affiliated outpatient facilities consist of several distinct buildings that may or may not be physically connected to the in-patient hospital complex or the ED. Providing a timely, appropriate, and consistent response to victims of CA or other medical emergencies can be challenging. Emergency response options for these areas include calling the in-patient code team, having an on-site response team in the ambulatory care areas, calling 911, or a combination of these. There are also growing numbers of satellite offices in remote locations not in close proximity to the main hospital. The only viable response to emergencies in these areas is to have an on-site response team and/or to call 911. Healthcare Finance Administration regulations state that hospitals must be able to respond to all persons experiencing a medical emergency on the premises. This requires a prompt and proper response for pediatric and adult patients, visitors, and staff. Suitable training and equipment are necessary to respond appropriately to cardiorespiratory arrest and other potentially life-threatening medical emergencies. Immediate, advanced life support capable transportation also needs to be available to relocate the patient to the ED or appropriate in-patient facility.

Consistent physician staff in ambulatory facilities is uncommon. Physicians provide only a transient source of emergency medical care because they are often only present when they have a specific clinic or procedure scheduled. Although the typical "knee-jerk" reaction might be to have them as the backbone of the response team, this may not always be the most prompt and efficient response. Patients often come to clinic early in the morning to register or stay later in the evening awaiting rides, picking up prescriptions, etc. It is highly unlikely that a physician would be available on site at these times to respond to a medical emergency. This inconsistent presence coupled with the fact that many staff physicians are not current on basic or ACLS practices makes them less than ideal candidates for a reliable first response to a CA in this setting. A physician-led first response would also require training and recurrent competency testing for all potential physician responders. Using physicians in this setting can be costly, constraining, and may potentially interfere with care of other patients of the physician is in the middle of a procedure, test, or consultation.

The nursing staff in most outpatient facilities has a much more consistent presence throughout the day. Most nurses are already trained in BLS, and many have undergone training with the AHA's Healthcare Provider BLS course (BLS-D) that includes early defibrillation training with an AED. In many facilities, the nursing staff may provide an ideal first response for CA.

Many hospitals routinely have their in-patient code teams respond to episodes of cardiorespiratory arrest that occur in the outpatient areas. Response time intervals may be excessive given the travel distance required to reach many ambulatory care buildings. If the in-patient team is used, full resuscitation equipment and immediate transportation to the ED or appropriate inpatient facility must be readily available to all outpatient areas. In-hospital code teams are trained to respond to victims of cardiorespiratory arrest but are often not trained to respond to other medical emergencies, such as falls or injuries that require immobilization. Pulling the in-patient team to a remote outpatient building may significantly delay the response to a simultaneous inpatient arrest. Hospitals must critically evaluate their ambulatory care facility layout with specific attention to staffing and available resources and realize that a hospital-wide standard of care for responding to victims of CA consisting of BLS with early defibrillation followed by ALs may be achieved by very different mechanisms in in-patient vs outpatient areas. An example of how a large academic medical center with several on- and off-site ambulatory care areas chose to provide a prompt, consistent, and appropriate response to CA and other medical emergencies in their outpatient facilities was described by Peberdy et al. *(19)*. The Virginia Commonwealth University Health System developed a Medical Emergency Response Team (MERT) to respond to medical emergencies in its outpatient areas. The team is designed as a two-tiered system. The first tier response is on-site BLS-D provided by a cohort of nurses working full time in the ambulatory care areas that underwent training in BLS, early defibrillation with AEDs, and first aid. Outpatient clinics and diagnostic areas are equipped with AEDs and a BLS bag containing barrier, noninvasive airway, and first aid equipment. The second tier of the response is provided by the local EMS system. The Richmond Ambulance Authority is an all ALS system with a median response time interval of 4.2 minutes to any location within the city. This is as fast or faster than it would take for the in-patient code team to respond. The paramedics provide adult and pediatric ALS, including all ALS equipment, and prompt transport to the ED. They are capable of performing coordinated resuscitation efforts during the entire transport, very unlike most in-hospital transportation systems. The MERT system does not prohibit the participation of any on-site physician trained to respond to CA but is not dependent on it. A portable bag containing intravenous setups, airway equipment, and resuscitation medications is available in each building if an on-site physician is ready to start ALS resuscitation efforts prior to arrival of the paramedics. A cost analysis done on the development and maintenance of this program over a 10-year period found that it added only an additional 5 cents per outpatient visit. This strategy is one example of how a hospital-affiliated ambulatory care system developed a fiscally responsible, prompt, and appropriate response for medical emergencies.

REFERENCES

1. Cummins RO, Ornato JP, Thies WH, Pepe PE. Improving survival from sudden cardiac arrest: the "chain of survival" concept. A statement for health professionals from the Advanced Cardiac Life Support Subcommittee and the Emergency Cardiac Care Committee, American Heart Association. Circulation 1991; 83:1832–1847.
2. McGrath RB. In-house cardiopulmonary resuscitation—after a quarter of a century. Ann Emerg Med 1987; 16:1365–1368.
3. DeBard ML. Cardiopulmonary resuscitation: analysis of six years' experience and review of the literature. Ann Emerg Med 1981; 10:408–416.
4. Jastremski MS. In-hospital cardiac arrest. Ann Emerg Med 1993; 22:113–117.
5. Cummins RO, Chamberlain D, Hazinski MF, et al. Recommended guidelines for reviewing, reporting, and conducting research on in-hospital resuscitation: the in-hospital 'Utstein style'. American Heart Association. Circulation 1997; 95:2213–2239.
6. Peberdy MA, Kaye W, Ornato JP, et al. Cardiopulmonary resuscitation of adults in the hospital: a report of 14720 cardiac arrests from the National Registry of Cardiopulmonary Resuscitation. Resuscitation 2003; 58:297–308.
7. Buist MD, Moore GE, Bernard SA, Waxman BP, Anderson JN, Nguyen TV. Effects of a medical emergency team on reduction of incidence of and mortality from unexpected cardiac arrests in hospital: preliminary study. BMJ 2002; 324:387–390.
8. Bellomo R, Goldsmith D, Uchino S, et al. A prospective before-and-after trial of a medical emergency team. Med J Aust 2003; 179:283–287.
9. Salamonson Y, Kariyawasam A, van Heere B, O'Connor C. The evolutionary process of Medical Emergency Team (MET) implementation: reduction in unanticipated ICU transfers. Resuscitation 2001; 49:135–141.
10. Franklin C, Mathew J. Developing strategies to prevent inhospital cardiac arrest: analyzing responses of physicians and nurses in the hours before the event. Crit Care Med 1994; 22:244–247.
11. Smith AF, Wood J. Can some in-hospital cardio-respiratory arrests be prevented? A prospective survey. Resuscitation 1998; 37:133–137.
12. Bayes de Luna A, Coumel P, Leclercq JF. Ambulatory sudden cardiac death: mechanisms of production of fatal arrhythmia on the basis of data from 157 cases. Am Heart J 1989; 117:151–159.
13. Valenzuela TD, Roe DJ, Nichol G, Clark LL, Spaite DW, Hardman RG. Outcomes of rapid defibrillation by security officers after cardiac arrest in casinos. N Engl J Med 2000; 343:1206–1209.
14. Fletcher GF, Cantwell JD. Ventricular fibrillation in a medically supervised cardiac exercise program. Clinical, angiographic, and surgical correlations. JAMA 1977; 238:2627–2629.
15. Horowitz LN. Drug therapy for survivors of sudden cardiac death. Pacing Clin Electrophysiol 1988; 11(Pt 2):1960–1967.
16. Caffrey S. Feasibility of public access to defibrillation. Curr Opin Crit Care 2002; 8:195–198.
17. Kaye W, Mancini ME, Giuliano KK, et al. Strengthening the in-hospital chain of survival with rapid defibrillation by first responders using automated external defibrillators: training and retention issues. Ann Emerg Med 1995; 25:163–168.
18. Kaye W, Mancini ME, Richards N. Organizing and implementing a hospital-wide first-responder automated external defibrillation program: strengthening the in-hospital chain of survival. Resuscitation 1995; 30:151–156.
19. Peberdy MA, Boze CM, Ornato JP. Strategy for developing a hospital affiliated ambulatory care medical emergency response team: Is it worth a nickel to save a life? Critical Pathways in Cardiology 2002; 1:209–217.

33

Successful Systems
for Out-of-Hospital Resuscitation

Paul E. Pepe, MD, FACEP, FACP, FCCM,
Lynn P. Roppolo, MD,
and Leonard A. Cobb, MD, FACP

CONTENTS

INTRODUCTION

A patient with out-of-hospital cardiac arrest (CA) stands little chance for survival without prior organization and preparations for immediate resuscitation. Fortunately, many communities have achieved relative success with resuscitation since the 1970s. In the 1970s, cities such as Seattle and Milwaukee achieved overall survival-to-hospital discharge rates for the subgroup of patients with out-of-hospital ventricular fibrillation (VF) that exceeded 20 to 30% *(1,2)*. Both of these communities used a classic deployment system for out-of-hospital CA that sent a three- to four-member firefighter crew as a neighborhood "first-responder" (FR) followed by a two- (or more) member paramedic ambulance crew. In cases of witnessed collapse in which the patient received immediate basic cardiopulmonary resuscitation (BCPR) by bystanders and presented to paramedics with VF, survival rates in these systems exceeded 40%. This finding was duplicated in several other communities, including the City of Houston Emergency Medical Services (EMS) system after a major restructuring in the 1980s *(3)*.

One of the key variables associated with successful out-of-hospital resuscitation and survival-to-hospital discharge found in these systems was a relatively short paramedic response-time interval *(4)*. The inverse time relationship between outcome and para-

From: *Contemporary Cardiology: Cardiopulmonary Resuscitation*
Edited by: J. P. Ornato and M. A. Peberdy © Humana Press Inc., Totowa, NJ

medic arrival time may have only reflected the time it took to defibrillate the patient with VF *(5)*. The inability to demonstrate the efficacy of individual pharmacological interventions such as high-dose epinephrine in the late 1980s to early 1990s *(6–8)*, supported the common notion that early defibrillation is the main therapeutic action provided by EMS systems. In some communities, all ambulances became staffed by paramedics in order to provide faster defibrillation. In turn, this led to the introduction of FR firefighter and police defibrillation programs with the introduction of the automated external defibrillator (AED) in the 1980s *(5,9–12)*. Using this new tool, communities with previously low survival rates began to achieve modest improvements in outcomes, particularly with the incorporation of bystander BCPR programs. However, in some cases, the successes were profound.

By the 1990s, a police patrol car FR defibrillation program appeared in Rochester, Minnesota, rapid-responding paramedic crews were preceded by police in patrol cars equipped with an AEDs. Over the first 7 years, overall VF survival rates exceeded 40%, and, in witnessed VF cases in which there was BCPR by bystanders, a frequent occurence in Rochester, survival exceeded 60% *(5,10,11)*.

On the surface, one might assume that high survival rates were simply a result of rapid paramedic or police car responses coupled with bystander CPR. However, regardless of the EMS system employed, most of these statistics have been forged by multiple factors that are often difficult to quantify. First of all, 70 to 80% of out-of-hospital CAs occur in residences and not public settings. Because there is no way that a professional 911 responder can reach a person's side reliably within 4 to 5 minutes *after the time of collapse*, it is incumbent on bystanders to perform BCPR to achieve optimal survival. BCPR is most effective when started immediately (usually by family members), within moments after the time of collapse. If BCPR is performed but is not started soon after the onset of CA (in which case it is often provided by a nonfamily member who has to be summoned to the scene, i.e., "retrieved persons"), the delay leads to a loss of peripheral vascular tone as a result of hypoxia in the vascular musculature. In turn, this leads to a diminished aortic pressure and thus less flow into the coronary arteries as compared to BCPR that is provided immediately *(13)*. A frequency of bystander actions at less than 15% probably reflects a low prevalence of training throughout the community with a lesser likelihood of immediate (i.e., family member) CPR. Conversely, successes in communities like Seattle and Rochester, Minnesota also reflect, in part, the level of community-wide CPR training and the frequency of truly "immediate BCPR."

Beyond the issues of bystander-performed BCPR, there is also evidence that advanced life support (ALS) techniques performed by paramedics have a lifesaving effect. Although survival rates are relatively low for patients who do not have VF as their initial rhythm, there are still a number of "no shock" survivors *(14,15)*. Although it is unknown what intervention or interventions make the difference, ALS interventions (collectively) obviously work. Paramedic skills (and speed at performing them) are likely factors as well *(2,16)*.

Although these considerations have received traditional recognition *(12)*, a number of subtle factors affect the performance of an EMS system, as well. These include the logistical procedures of dispatch centers and related dispatch medical protocols. It also includes the intense involvement of expert EMS medical directors. Some of the factors for success may be counterintuitive. For example, certain paramedic-deployment strategies that utilize fewer paramedics can improve both skills and outcomes *(16,17)*. There are also some evolving data indicating that traditional FR defibrillation approaches may not be as optimal as first thought *(18,19)*. In fact, some of the FR programs, under certain circumstances, may even be detrimental *(18,19)*. Also, local geography, logistics, and population bases can have significant effects on outcomes.

All of these issues are discussed subsequently in detail, but the key concept is the need to think multidimensionally (many factors to consider at once) and also to drill down on individual aspects of the so-called "chain of survival" *(12)*. Meticulous attention to seemingly trivial items, such as having the endotracheal tube (ET) placed at the top of the paramedic's equipment bag and having partially unrolled adhesive tape nearby so that it is ready to secure an inserted airway, often make the difference between successful and unsuccessful systems by saving precious seconds that can make the difference between life and death. The quality of basic training and the opportunity to practice lifesaving techniques are also key elements in a successful EMS system *(2,16,17)*. This chapter focuses on these concepts and traces their development from ideas to effective functional units. Additionally, practical details for providing the most efficient, timely treatment for cardiac arrest victims are also presented.

UNDERSTANDING THE TRADITIONAL CHAIN OF SURVIVAL

The Chain of Survival in Perspective

The concept of the "chain of survival" is an educational metaphor used to explain the simple principle that a series of multiple and distinct (but interlinking) actions must be taken to optimize survival from cardiac arrest *(12)*. The American Heart Association (AHA) has promulgated a four-link chain comprising the following *(12)*:

1. the *access link* (e.g., in the United States, the 911 telephone call or equivalent)
2. the *early CPR link* (e.g., bystander-initiated CPR)
3. the *early defibrillation link* (e.g., FR automated defibrillation procedures)
4. the *ALS link* (e.g., paramedic, nurse, or physician ALS interventions).

Any weak link can result in a poor outcome, even if all of the other links are strong. However, there is more to an EMS system organization than this simple educational concept.

Understanding Elements Within Each Link

It is important to understand of all of the intrinsic components within each link when using the chain of survival concept as a model for improving resuscitation rates. As an example, the "access link" is not just having a well-publicized emergency telephone number in place (e.g., 911 in the United States or 113 or 114 in Europe or "triple 9" in Australia). To ensure more rapid defibrillation, one must also ensure that the medical dispatch system is directly linked and authorized to dispatch the fire or police FR unit simultaneously with EMS. With computerized, enhanced 911 systems that display the caller's address automatically, both paramedics and fire department/police crews can be dispatched within 30–45 seconds of the time that the 911 call is received.

Historically, in some systems (particularly large cities with high volumes) that utilized private, health department or "third-service" ambulance programs, the dispatch of the FR crews often was delayed. Firefighters or police officers equipped with AEDs were sent as FRs in these systems, but the call for help was first relayed to the EMS (medical) dispatchers who in turn had to contact the fire or police dispatcher. Therefore, system managers needed to integrate EMS and fire dispatch processes, at least electronically. Not surprisingly, simultaneous FR dispatches were always part of the protocol *(1,2)* for many of the original, effective EMS systems (e.g., Seattle, Houston, and Milwaukee). Other cities operating health department or third-service programs discovered this principle when implementing FR-AED programs. For example, in the 1980s, San Francisco improved both response intervals and outcomes by integrating fire FR dispatch with the EMS dispatch.

Effective access links also require supervision and regular medical review and research of dispatchers' protocols to ensure that the time interval from the first 911 ring to dispatch is not delayed significantly and that CAs are identified rapidly. Recognizing that agonal breathing might be interpreted as "Yes, my husband is still breathing," some EMS systems now simply ask if the patient is responsive and "breathing normally" *(20)*. If the reply to both is negative, research shows that the yield for CA is high. More importantly, the capture of patients with a higher chance for successful resuscitation (those still having agonal breaths) is much higher and does not impose significant risk to the low percentage of patients who are picked up as false-positives (treated as a CA when it's not). In systems that only ask the traditional question, "Is the patient breathing?", only those who have deteriorated into apnea (and less likely to survive) will receive CPR instructions from dispatchers prior to EMS arrival.

In addition to these issues, successful EMS systems continue to research better ways of providing service. In a recent controlled, clinical trial of "pre-arrival" instructions (instructions given to the callers at the site by the dispatchers prior to arrival of the EMS responders), it was found that, contrary to traditional beliefs, "chest compressions-only" CPR was more effective than standard CPR that includes pauses for rescue breathing *(20)*.

Dynamics of the Individual Links

Linkages must also be provided in a timely sequential manner. Simply having a bystander or advanced cardiac life support (ACLS) link in place does not ensure success if they are provided too late to be of value. For example, an EMS system may have both rapid dispatch and a high frequency of bystander-initiated CPR always available, but if the defibrillator arrives too late, survival rates will remain low.

Increasing the number of people trained and performing CPR in a community not only increases the survival rate by increasing the frequency of bystander CPR, but it also ensures a more rapid (and therefore more physiologically effective) provision of CPR. Although CPR performed by retrieved persons will be classified as "bystander CPR" and may even be performed better (technically speaking), it is more likely to be performed relatively too late and therefore less effectively (physiologically speaking) *(13)*. So there is a dynamic related to widespread CPR training and one must understand that subgroup statistical analysis of the binary code of "bystander CPR: yes or no?" will not reflect a defect in the links or the true value of BCPR.

Sublime and Nonintuitive Issues to Success

Less quanifiable factors such as the *organization* of EMS systems and *intensity of medical direction* may be the most significant keys to success in resuscitation *(3,16,17)*. Some of the most successful large city EMS systems operate two-tiered ambulance systems in which basic EMT ambulances are dispatched for minor injuries, and ALS/paramedic ambulances are reserved for major cases by virtue of a well-tested dispatch priority dispatch protocol (1,2,16,17). In such systems, fewer ALS ambulances are needed and consequently a smaller number of paramedics are needed to staff them. Not only does this relieve the more highly trained paramedics from dealing with and transporting patients with minor injuries and illness, but it also provides the individual paramedic with more frequent experience in using ALS techniques such as invasive airway and intravenous access (2,16,17). Ultimately, this enhances their capabilities and even survival rates (21,22). Some systems will have the primary service make the immediate responses and then turn the more minor cases over to either BLS or private transport units. In some cases, the ALS providers can respond in either transport units or response cars without transport capabilities.

The use of two highly skilled, experienced paramedics who can work together efficiently may be more effective than a larger cadre of paramedics, even those who can arrive a minute or two earlier. Completion of skills and medical tasks on-scene is the critical end-point, not the surrogate variable of arrival on-scene. In large city EMS systems with two-tiered (ALS–BLS) ambulance deployment, a team of two or more highly skilled paramedics may provide definitive care more quickly than colleagues in other cities who are lesser skilled and may take longer to perform their tasks, even if they arrive on scene sooner. Paradoxically, running such tiered systems with fewer paramedics may even improve response-time intervals because paramedic ambulances are not continually occupied transporting the more minor cases to the hospital. Instead, they become much more available for ALS responses that require a more rapid response (16,17,21,23).

Therefore, although putting more paramedics into the system would seem to make sense, the opposite is often true. Obviously, there is a finite lower limit in terms of the number of paramedics needed to respond. Also, the tiered ambulance deployment approach would not be appropriate in a smaller city with less than 50,000 residents in which only two or three ambulances are needed. Nevertheless, cities like Seattle operate their successful EMS systems with very few paramedic units. Accompanied by a cadre of BLS (basic EMT-operated) ambulances and some private ambulance transport services, the Seattle Medic One program operated the EMS system for their 500,000 residents during the 1970s with only four paramedic ambulances and still had the best published survival rates for out-of-hospital VF in the United States (exceeding 30% for all cases, witnessed or unwitnessed, bystander CPR or not).

More recently, research has shown the feasibility of sending only FR crews alone as initial responders to triage low risk 911 calls such as automated alerts, motor vehicle incidents in which there is no information transmitted about the situation, and so-called 911 hang-ups in which a call is made but the caller hangs up prior to talking to dispatchers (23). Such a practice is relatively safe yet spares ambulances, and particularly paramedics, from unnecessary responses.

Above all, the key factor in an EMS systems is a knowledgeable, "street-wise," and empowered physician who is not only expert in providing care in the out-of-hospital setting, but also intensely involved around the clock in all aspects of the EMS system (3). Although this factor is often difficult to prove scientifically or to analyze methodically, it may be the strongest correlation with success (3). From Seattle, Washington to Boston, Massachusetts or Rochester, Minnesota to Houston, Texas, public satisfaction and survival rates can be correlated with the reputation and intensity of the EMS medical direction (24).

Highly skilled paramedics may have their greatest impact in terms of their expertise in postresuscitative monitoring and the titration of resuscitative care. Dr. Peter Safar, often referred to as "the father of cardio-cerebral resuscitation," has always emphasized that the greatest success in resuscitation is achieved with a focus on the postresuscitative (titration) phase of care, particularly when the physician's hands are locked on the pulse of the patient in anticipation of any potential deterioration. For most paramedics, it has not been typical to have them focus on meticulous maintenance of restored spontaneous circulation. Without on-scene expert physician mentoring and role-modeling, the art of maintaining and supporting cardiovascular stability may be lost. Although it is difficult to measure objectively, it can be inferred from several studies that postresuscitative care is just as critical as other links in the chain of survival.

For example, postresuscitative systolic blood pressure is associated directly with neurological outcome. There is a clear indication that patients whose blood pressures remain low (<90 mmHg) have poor neurological outcomes *(25)*. Although a higher systolic blood pressure may simply be a marker for shorter ischemic intervals, reflected by a more intact peripheral vascular tone at the time of return of spontaneous circulation (ROSC; leading to rapidly improved cerebral perfusion and outcome), studies suggest that postresuscitative titration of blood pressure can affect neurological outcome *(25)*. Experienced physicians (and, in turn, well-trained and highly skilled paramedics) appreciate that initially high blood pressures (at the first return of pulses) may suddenly decrease as the effect of previously infused catecholamines wear off. Anticipating this, experienced clinicians will have pressors or other catecholamines ready to maintain the postresuscitative "hyperperfusion" state during the critical first 15 to 20 minutes after resuscitation.

Other Potential Variables

Although meta-analyses and surveys have indicated the traditional tiered ALS–BLS systems can be more effective than all paramedic ALS systems *(24)*, there are numerous confounding variables that preclude assurance of these conclusions. Many large urban EMS systems have very poor survival rates even though they use ALS–BLS systems.

To account for the discrepancies in survival rates, it has been suggested that the size of the city or demographics might play a role. Recent reports from some urban centers suggest that racial and sex differences can affect the resuscitation survival rate *(26)*. Seattle, where some of the highest survival rates are found, has a population that is largely white middle or upper class. It is possible that this population has less chronic left ventricular (LV) injury from chronic hypertension or other comorbidities. Nevertheless, other large cities like Houston and Milwaukee, with very large non-white populations, have also achieved high salvage rates *(2,3,21)*. Seattle, Milwaukee, and Houston have also enjoyed excellent survival rates in injury management as well *(2,27,28)*. Therefore, it is clear that appropriate training, medical supervision, and system organization are factors that are likely more influential in terms of success in resuscitation.

Distances and other logistics may make many of these recommendations impractical in some rural or remote areas. Beyond the issues of limited resources for deployment is the issue of limited skills performance. Because EMS personnel in low-volume areas use their skills infrequently, there is a vicious cycle of lack of successful performance. Even if one allows for occasional patient care service in busier urban settings or provides more operating room or emergency department experience for ET and intravenous access placement, it is no replacement for actual in-field experience.

More recently, it has become evident that overzealous assisted ventilation may have been an unrecognized detrimental variable that may have confounded prehospital clinical trials and even resulted in negative results and worse outcomes on a day-to-day basis *(6–8,19,20,29–33)*.

It has been observed that circulatory arrest patients are more apt to survive in EMS programs utilizing slow ventilatory rates *(1,3,27,28,31,33)*. Therefore, something as subtle as a ventilatory rate can have major impact on success. Other factors, such as the interval from interruption of chest compressions to application of shock, may have similar dramatic effects *(34–37)*.

Melding the Links Together

AEDs are easy to operate and are becoming more available to the public. The recent experience at two Chicago airports demonstrates that random bystanders at the scene of a CA are not only capable, but also willing to use an AED with outstanding results *(9)*. The majority of patients who were defibrillated within the first few minutes after arrest were not only resuscitated but also were awakening before traditional EMS responders arrived on scene. In essence, these "public responders" melded the first three elements of the chain of survival together by providing the access to care, bystander CPR, and early defibrillation.

Although widespread public access to defibrillation, including eventual widespread in-home storage and use of AEDs, seems feasible and has the potential to yield dramatically better results, there are limitations to this as a single solution to the care of out-of-hospital CAs. First of all, in most locales, the number of witnessed collapses following VF is only about 60%, so a large percentage of cases do not receive immediate access to the system and prompt CPR *(13,14)*. In many cases, the patients do not even present with VF (i.e., asystole or organized rhythms) and do not require defibrillation. Other mechanisms of CA such as predisposing respiratory arrest, drowning, choking, electrocution, and even trauma will require alternatives to the typical chain of survival. Therefore, although training all school children in BCPR (which today includes AED use) is a rationale public health strategy along with the promotion of both public and home AED placement, it will only solve a certain fraction of the problem of out-of-hospital CA.

Summary Recommendations Based on Current Knowledge

If one were to design a system for a large US city today, this chapter's authors would recommend the following arrangements:

- Employ a highly qualified, academically oriented, "street-wise" physician medical director (and assistant medical directors in systems over a half million population) who has/have line authority over medical operations (e.g., EMS supervisors) and who is/are intensely involved in all aspects of the EMS system around the clock.
- Train all schoolchildren in BCPR techniques including AED use, promulgate workplace CPR-AED training and promote public access defibrillation programs along with Good Samaritan laws and develop short (30-minute) validated courses to better appeal to employers to promulgate"on-the-job" training for all lay people.
- Utilize an enhanced 911 system that is preferably linked to computerized dispatch protocols that can quickly identify an inclusive group of potential CA victims and also simultaneously dispatches FR units equipped with AEDs.
- Continuous quality assurance, re-evaluation and research of dispatch protocols that can conserve utilization of resources, enhance availability of paramedics, improve

response intervals for all applicable responders, improve paramedic skills and enhance the efficacy of pre-arrival instructions.

- Establish a cadre of 911 FR crews (fire, police or both) and promote CPR-AED training among security personnel and other employees in the private and public sectors, especially in highly trafficked areas.
- Train ALS providers not only in practical "street-oriented" techniques and patient care strategies, but also in postresuscitative "titration" of reperfusion and logistical efficiencies.
- Provide continuous quality improvement of CA management through maintenance of a comprehensive database, in-field supervision of EMS personnel, and continuous initiation of research protocols.

EVOLVING PARADIGMS

Focusing Away From Traditional Paramedic Ambulances

Recent cost-containment pressures have led to questions about the cost-effectiveness of ALS procedures in the prehospital setting *(22)*. It has been suggested that lesser trained, lower paid BLS personnel could be provided with equipment and procedures that require much less in terms of ongoing training and supervision. For example, they could be equipped with AEDs, adjunct airways, and perhaps even glucose infusions to handle the clear majority of cases in which timeliness of treatment might be a factor.

Some studies confirm the value of pre-hospital ALS independent of defibrillation in some mature EMS systems *(14,15,38)*. However, this incremental lifesaving effect may not be achievable routinely in many locales *(22)*. It is possible that, in their political judgment, governmental leaders would take the position that the cost of saving only a few lives is not worth the increased expense necessary to provide paramedic services (e.g., training, recertification, staffing, etc). Such a political judgment does not seem likely at the present time, especially with the typical patient's desire to always have the highest level of health care. In fact, this societal philosophy has driven the concept of all-paramedic ambulance staffing in many venues in the United States and Europe.

Regardless of the path chosen, the deployment of FR firefighter or police crews (who use AEDs as well as other BLS skills) comes the closest to universal acceptance among all of the EMS deployment strategies in the United States and many other countries as well. The additional cost and resource utilization of such a service is almost negligible *(23)*. Indeed, the FR fire truck is often considered to be the *backbone* of the EMS program and fire crews routinely accompany paramedic responses for the majority of ALS responses. Although further research is encouraged to define the most effective training level and response schedule for this deployment strategy, the neighborhood FR team is now receiving more of a focus than even the traditional paramedic ambulance in some locales. In areas covered by only volunteer fire services, the routine use of on-duty police patrol officers to provide early defibrillation should be considered to shorten the time to treatment for patients with out-of-hospital VF.

First Responder Advanced Life Support

A growing trend is the use of paramedics on fire trucks and even in police teams. Union leaders and fire administrators help to protect or even strengthen their position with such a strategy when competing with the threat of privatization of the EMS service or the decommissioning of fire apparatus. Although this approach seems logical, it conflicts with the experience cited by tiered ALS–BLS ambulance deployment systems that fewer paramedics in a system leads to better skills and outcomes *(16,17,21,24)*. Staffing each FR fire apparatus with even one paramedic may dilute the ALS experience for others staffing the ambulances.

Having stated that position, evolving evidence may possibly help to support the concept of providing ALS as early as possible, even before defibrillation. Recent laboratory and clinical data have begun to suggest that the current standard of *immediately providing countershock may be detrimental* when VF has been prolonged beyond several minutes *(39,40)*. Several studies now suggest that when myocardial energy supplies and oxygenation begin to dwindle with prolonged VF, *improvements in coronary artery perfusion must first be achieved* to prime the heart for successful ROSC after defibrillation *(15,18–20,39)*. Along with this supportive clinical evidence, histological and physiological studies have created an evolving hypothesis that delivery of an electrical countershock to an ischemic heart may be more damaging than when it is delivered immediately (within the first 2–3 minutes of VF *[40]*).

In Seattle, there was a marked improvement in outcome when FR firefighter crews provided 90 seconds of BCPR (chest compressions) prior to defibrillation attempts *(19)*. Although this study used a historical control (2 years of no preshock CPR vs a subsequent period using 90 seconds CPR first), survival rates were improved, when patients received 90 seconds of CPR first when EMS response intervals were greater than 4 minutes. When EMS responded in less than 4 minutes, there was little difference in outcome, but clearly not worse with the 90 seconds of CPR first. However, it should be understood that even in witnessed cases, there is a finite amount of time before EMS is called following the collapse and another minute or two required to reach the patient's side and deliver the shock after EMS on-scene arrival. Therefore, this "4-minute response interval" may translate into a 7 or 8 minute period of VF.

Similarly, Wik and colleagues in Oslo, Norway, reported almost identical results in a controlled clinical trial *(18)*. Patients were randomized to either 3 minutes of chest compressions first vs shock first. Patients receiving BCPR first did much better, particularly those with more than 5-minute EMS response intervals (i.e., presumed 8–9 minutes of VF). ROSC occurred in the group with 3 minutes of CPR first when response intervals exceeded 5 minutes (62 vs 39%; $p < 0.02$) and return of circulation was similar in the groups for whom the response was less than 5 minutes. The authors concluded that because the former patients do no worse, 3 minutes of CPR prior to defibrillation is indicated unless the patient collapses in the presence of EMS.

Preshock interventions may explain the lack of success for previous clinical studies of so-called high-dose epinephrine (i.e., >1 mg/kg doses) and other ACLS procedures *(6,8,39,40)*. In keeping with international guidelines, these study protocols called for the use of the test intervention following multiple countershocks (in VF cases). In contrast, the successful preclinical studies had used the drugs prior to countershock. This explanation has been substantiated by canine experiments that subsequently tested the resuscitation effects of high-dose epinephrine administered before and after countershocks *(39)*. In such studies, ROSC was improved by first administering the high-dose epinephrine following only 7.5 minutes of VF. Several other animal models now strongly corroborate this concept of "drugs first" in prolonged VF *(40)*. Using a "cocktail" (multiple-drug) regimen, including high-dose epinephrine, anti-arrhythmics and antioxidants, investigators have demonstrated similar effects in terms of resuscitation and short-term survival in swine that experienced 8 minutes of VF prior to interventions *(41)*.

In recent clinical trials, the first resuscitation drugs were usually given, on average, as late as 17 to 21 minutes following notification of the CA event *(6,29,30)*. Some of the cities in these studies had excellent response time intervals and higher than average survival rates indicating a "best case" scenario. Therefore, FR ALS providers may eventually prove to be of untapped value in terms of drug effectiveness.

Pros and Cons of Predefibrillatory Interventions

The pre-shock intervention approach poses problems for current resuscitation policies and the use of AEDs (whose protocols traditionally recommend immediate rhythm analysis rather than CPR). However, technology exists to help to define the "shockability" of the heart using power spectrum analysis of the VF waveform on the electrocardiograph such as median frequency or scaling exponent analysis *(42–45)*. In the future, there may be a need for responders to at least provide chest compressions first if not intravenous drug infusions. This may not require full-fledged paramedic support, but it does imply a change in philosophy in terms of training FR crews. Other systems might be put into place to enhance endotracheal intubation (ETI) skills using a second tier of responders or paramedic supervisors. Even in the recent study of PAD at the Chicago airports in which three-quarters of the patients were resuscitated and achieved full neurological recovery when shocked within 5 minutes of collapse, all survivors received some period of chest compressions and other BCPR techniques, even if briefly, while awaiting defibrillatory attempts *(9)*. The authors of this chapter feel that rapid defibrillation should be a priority in the first few minutes after arrest although basic CPR may be provided if it does not delay the shocks. However, after several minutes of arrest (perhaps 4 or 5 minutes), BCPR and perhaps other ACLS interventions may need to be provided prior to the shocks *(40)*.

Counterarguments to Assigning Paramedics to First-Responder Units

In considering the optimal level of training of FR personnel, the presence of a paramedic with ALS skills in the neighborhood fire truck may provide a potential survival advantage, particularly in the more timely administration of drugs. However, the downside to such an arrangement is that, with paramedics on board, FR firefighters might have less opportunity to practice their own skills and other paramedics have less opportunities to maintain skills, such as ETI.

Therefore some considerations around this issue include:

1. Prove that ALS skills before defibrillation are useful;
2. If certain intravenous drug infusions are all that is needed, then perhaps an "IV EMT" is all that is needed and the intubation can come later with a small cadre of advanced ALS providers who frequently perform this skill (tiered ALS unit or EMS supervisor);
3. In a fire department-based system, run a tiered ALS–BLS transport system and occasionally rotate the paramedics from the busiest ALS ambulance/ALS units (e.g., those that respond to more than 450–500 incidents a month in a large city) onto fire trucks, thus maintaining both ALS and firefighter skills.

ROOTS AND APPROPRIATE PHILOSOPHY FOR EFFECTING OUT-OF-HOSPITAL ON-SCENE RESUSCITATIONS

Seminal EMS Systems: Doctors and Public Safety Officers Cross Paths

In 1967, Dr. Leonard Cobb in Seattle and several other academics across the nation became interested in the experiences of Dr. Frank Pantridge and his mobile intensive care unit in Belfast, Northern Ireland *(1)*. Dr. Pantridge originally had intended to reach patients with evolving myocardial infarction (patients with chest pain) very early after onset of symptoms, so that oxygen, rest, and other supportive care could limit myocardial damage. Although many victims died within hours after the onset of pain, presumably from severe myocardial damage, Pantridge found that several of these people simply needed to be defibrillated after sudden onset of VF. This observation prompted Dr. Cobb and physicians in other venues, to patrol their city streets in a systematic attempt to treat VF as a primary process. These enterprising physicians soon learned, however, that the provision of emergency resuscitative care was entirely different from in-hospital care.

Apart from the logistical challenges of distance and traffic, they had to learn to control the adrenaline rush that accompanied emergency response. They learned that it was virtually impossible to manage a patient single-handedly in a timely manner, particularly to provide simultaneously defibrillation, endotracheal intubation, intravenous access, and drug administration. They had also to develop strategies and priorities for delivering emergency care in this unique setting, in front of family members or crowds of bystanders. What evolved was a new practice of medicine rooted in experimental resuscitative care, but delivered in the unique out-of-hospital setting.

This unique experience provided the foundation of the Seattle experience as well as that of many other cities such as Miami, Los Angeles, Columbus, and others. Although the doctors believed that their response to the scene could alter patient outcomes positively, they also recognized that their responses throughout the entire breadth of the city from their base hospital meant delays to some areas. The concept of having a simultaneous response from someone in closer proximity to the incident was created, not only to provide earlier BLS, but also to help at the scene.

For Seattle, the involvement of the fire department became a logical step in building and effective EMS system *(1)*. A first aid apparatus ("aid car") was a service already in place in the Seattle Fire Department (SFD) for rehabilitation and first aid at fire scenes. They even responded to citizen requests for assistance. Philosophically, involvement of SFD in Dr. Cobb's activities was consistent with the stated mission of the fire service at large ("to save lives and protect property"). When Dr. Cobb and associates approached the fire chief to send crews out with the doctors to provide BLS, they received a very positive response. Eventually, neighborhood fire truck crews were sent to ensure coverage rapidly throughout the city and to also provide more logistical backup and on-scene medical support.

Subsequent studies have demonstrated the cost-effectiveness and safety of this approach. Because the apparatus are already purchased and maintained, and because the fire crews staffing them are already in place (and receiving salary), and because they generally respond only in their own station house's immediate territory, the entire additional cost (equipment, fuel, additional maintenance, training, etc.,) of sending fire apparatus to tens of thousands of annual EMS calls in a large city has been shown to be less expensive than commissioning just one new ambulance and staffing it around the clock *(23)*. Even the busiest fire trucks may be away from their station for about only one-twentieth of a 24-hour period just for EMS responses and responses to major fires are not missed. Because they are not occupied with transporting patients to the hospital and thus remain readily available in their own territory, today, the FR response not only allows for faster and more reliable delivery of medical interventions (e.g., CPR and defibrillation), but it also enhances public satisfaction in terms of system responsiveness.

The original SFD crews also had other special advantages. There were about 30 fire stations to cover 90 square miles. This resulted in a relatively dense coverage with fire apparatus allowing for an average response interval (leaving the station to the front door) of about 2 minutes. Even considering the processing time to receive the call and dispatch the fire crews, those first responders could still get to the scene and to the patient's side within 4 to 6 minutes in the majority of cases *(1)*.

Rapid response time and performance of CPR were the original contributions of the SFD, but as the system developed, Cobb's group of physicians turned to firefighters to assist with other procedures, including on-scene defibrillation, as a means of expediting delivery of care under the physician's supervision. They realized that because many of the on-scene activities for resuscitation involved coordination of multiple simultaneous skills—countershock, intubation, intravenous access—they thought that it might he feasible to train a selected number of firefighters in these skills and deploy them strategically throughout the city to achieve even earlier resuscitative care.

Accordingly, in the late 1960s, about a dozen trainees joined their physician mentors on responses for about 1 year, gleaning from them the experience and hands-on approach that the mentors themselves had learned as they developed the new found practice of out-of-hospital resuscitative medicine. The student paramedics *learned* not only practical resuscitation techniques, but they also received extensive role-modeling from their mentors, which helped them achieve a professional and compassionate demeanor at all times. It even instilled a sense of on-going scientific inquiry.

The Pivotal Role of the Apprenticeship

After the year of intense apprenticeship, the physician mentors knew their protégés so well that they could tell state legislators that they would readily let these specially trained lay persons treat their own family members. This strong vote of confidence resulted in authorization for these paramedics to respond on their own and perform medical functions, provided that their physician mentors would not only be *responsible,* but also be held *accountable* for the activities of these trainees.

The value of this original intensive apprenticeship cannot be overemphasized. To this day, the Seattle Medic I founders state that the historical and current success of the Seattle EMS system could not have been realized without the original physician leadership and apprenticeship. Yet, unfortunately, this kind of training is not found in most EMS systems today. Unlike medical student and resident clinical training, paramedic training is not provided by physician mentors and if it is, it is seldom conducted in the actual patient care.

Even when the SFD paramedics were allowed to respond "solo" without their physician mentors, they were in constant radio contact with them. The closeness of the apprenticeship permitted the mentor to sense a problem, even from the tone of the paramedic's voice over the radio transmission. It also allowed them to focus on any particular idiosyncrasy or weakness in a given paramedic. Over the first few years of the Medic One program, survival rates for out-of-hospital patients presenting with VF in Seattle soon exceeded 20%, translating to more than 100 annual resuscitations and more than 50 surviving-to-hospital discharge *(1)*. These numbers later improved even further, as the number and frequency of lay bystanders performing CPR increased to nearly half of the cases by the first decade of operation *(4)*.

Institutionalization of Intensive Medical Supervision

In 1973, Dr. Michael Copass assumed the post of deputy medical director of the Seattle paramedic program and director of paramedic training under Dr. Cobb. In this capacity, he reasserted and centralized the authoritative component of on-line supervision 24 hours a day by physician mentors, and amplified it by making it his personal charge. Philosophically, he viewed each 911 phone call for medical emergencies to be a personal consult to him from the medical community at large to provide the best possible care for their patients in the out-of-hospital setting. Thus, every citizen of Seattle was potentially one of his patients. As a result, Dr. Copass developed a keen sense of public trust that any person calling 911 would receive the same level of care as if he had been there in person. He personally trained and intensively monitored the firefighters, EMTs, paramedics, and physicians assisting him (nearly round the clock, 7 days a week). Each morning he would also personally review all fire department records from the previous day. Accordingly, he also became a role model for many of the physicians who trained with him and who later assumed similar roles in other cities (3). In turn, these habits were passed on to several next generation medical directors, meaning that his meticulous and compulsive oversight significantly influenced the development of successful EMS systems in many other cities, such as Tucson and Houston. In fact, introduction of such medical director behaviors and philosophical approaches have been demonstrated in published studies to dramatically improve survival rates (3,24).

Backbone of the EMS System: Orchestrated Management by First-Responders

As stated previously, in reviewing the published successes of lifesaving pioneer EMS systems, the neighborhood fire truck has always been a key element (e.g., Milwaukee and Seattle). Dispatch of a FR unit seems logical from a response interval point of view. Following suit, beginning in 1985, firefighter crews in Houston were sent to assist with cardiac arrest cases using a specified task-oriented management approach. FR crews, in many EMS systems, may simply stand by waiting for instructions from an lone EMT crew member (such as help with lifting or other directed assistance) while the individual EMT tends to the patient single-handedly. However, in successful EMS systems, each member of the FR crews, including the officer in charge, has a specific duty.

One task-oriented approach mimics the day-to-day assignments given to crew members for fire responses such as, "plug man," "first line man," and "engineer." For the medical responses, each of the four-crew members, including the apparatus officer, is trained by the medical director to perform specific tasks in an A-B-C-D-E assignment approach. The first crew member (the "A–B" firefighter for "Airway–Breathing") applies oxygen and marks the respiratory rate and any signs of distress while auscultating for equal breath sounds. In cases of CA or respiratory arrests, the A–B person correctly performs bag-valve mask ventilations. The second crew member (the "C" firefighter for "Circulation") is responsible for preserving circulation. This person stops any overt bleeding and checks the blood pressure and pulses. In pulseless patients, the "C" person provides basic chest compressions as necessary. The third crew member (the "D" person for "Disability") is responsible, in essence, for assessing the current degree of disability and preventing further disability. This responsibility includes ensuring spinal immobilization as needed and checking motor activity, pupillary response, and mental status. In a CA case, the D crew member assists the A–B crew member with proper two-person bag-valve mask application and ventilation, After paramedics arrive, this person sets up medications and intravenous drips as necessary, allowing paramedics to perform ALS actions and monitor the patient more closely (e.g., fingers constantly on the femoral pulse). A current or former paramedic may be best suited for the "D" position.

The officer or lead firefighter is the "E" person *(for "Executive" or "Emergency Team Leader")*. This officer who ensures that all of the other members are performing their tasks properly. In a CA case, the officer often sets up the AED around the C crew member to ensure its rapid application and use without interrupting chest compressions. The officer also assesses the scene for hazards, both environmental and sociological and keeps records of the interventions provided as well as the time at which they are provided. The officer also maintains (or delegates) communications with dispatchers and in-coming crews and also interacts with family members or bystanders (or both). If feasible, the "E" person obtains the patient's medical history and a list of all recent and current medications.

Even when firefighters and paramedics are dispatched from the same station, firefighters should perform these basic functions, allowing the paramedics to provide more advanced procedures, such as intravenous access, drug administration, and ETI. Studies have shown that, as a result, these three critical procedures can be performed in a significantly shorter time. In successful EMS systems, the FR crew is not thought of as simply a supplemental crew for faster response, but rather as the basic response supplemented by transport or ALS specialists in the 10 to 15% of cases that may involve ALS monitoring or active interventions (<5% of most EMS incidents). Therefore, the fire apparatus and its crew are considered to be the primary EMS responders in their EMS systems, and paramedics are thought of as responders who are specially trained as ALS specialists for the uncommon case requiring such services. The analogy is similar to a hazardous material (haz-mat) response. The fire truck crew is still the primary responder, but if haz-mat specialists are needed, they respond and manage that aspect of the fire as the basic firefighters continue with their basic responsibilities. If, because of the specific situation, the haz-mat providers need to take over the scene, then they may proceed to redirect the basic crews accordingly. The same would be true for paramedics who are "specialized" in ALS procedures, but the basic concept of the FR being the backbone of the EMS response should not be lost when there is a so-called "higher level of care."

PRACTICAL APPROACHES TO CARDIAC ARREST MANAGEMENT IN THE OUT-OF-HOSPITAL SETTING

A Cardiac Arrest is a Cardiac Arrest

One practical approach to successful resuscitation of the CA patient in the out-of-hospital setting is to maintain an organized, yet simplified methodology that will accomplish the appropriate interventions as rapidly as possible with little interruption. Although there are many different pathophysiologies and, accordingly, resultant outcomes for CAs, the management can be simplified under "one roof." In essence, the approach to all cases is *rapid* restoration of brisk coronary artery perfusion with oxygenated blood. Therefore, the uniform avenues to achieve this goal are as follows:

1. *Adequately inflate the lungs bilaterally* (on an intermittent basis, to ensure adequate O_2 saturation of red cells);
2. *Adequately circulate the oxygenated red cells* with basic CPR (chest compressions or other alternative CPR devices/methodolgies);
3. *As necessary, enhance basic CPR with potent vasopressors* (e.g., epinephrine, norepinephrine, vasopressin) for pulselessness or persistent hypotension to enhance coronary perfusion pressure;

4. *When there is VF or ventricular tachycardia (VT), one must apply the "bookends" of* clearing the VF/VT; and then helping to maintain electrical stability with anti-arrhythmics (e.g., lidocaine, amiodarone).

Following this simple, four-step approach, almost every case of cardiac arrest can be managed appropriately.

Use of other traditional drugs like atropine sulfate and sodium bicarbonate should be considered supplemental (in certain cases) to the basic strategies used to restore strong perfusion of the coronary arteries. The key to success then becomes the training issues in terms of understanding the critical caveats of the descriptors, "adequately" and "as necessary." Nevertheless, the often confusing multiple algorithm approach to CA (i.e., one for VF, one for "asystole," one for "pulseless electrical activity," (PEA) one for "bradycardia," and one for "respiratory arrest," etc.,) can be simplified for the out-of-hospital resuscitator.

For example, once the left "bookend" of defibrillation for a patient with unmonitored VF results in a post-conversion electrocardiographic (ECG) rhythm with wide QRS complexes and a rate of 40 per minute, the treatment of the patient is going to be the same as if the patient originally presented with pulselessness and wide QRS complexes at a rate of 40 per minute. It does not necessarily require a special VF algorithm. Likewise, defibrillation resulting in asystole is treated the same as a case in which the person presents with an ECG flat line.

On another front, a common reaction in many venues is to administer atropine to a patient with a rate of 40 per minute because of the "bradycardia protocol." Although this drug may actually be helpful in some patients, in the pulseless state, the bradycardia is most likely to be secondary to myocardial hypoxia (no energy supplies) or some form of myocardial "stunning" (e.g., electroporation), and not from an overactive vagal nerve. Simply put, it is difficult to "stimulate" a heart with no oxygenation.

Therefore, most successful drug actions and mechanical methodologies during CPR conditions will usually result from indirect "stimulation" of the heart by helping to better restore adequate aortic "diastolic pressure" and, in turn, better coronary artery perfusion. Therefore, atropine would be more of afterthought to the priorities of basic CPR, ETI, and vasopressor.

Table 1 presents an "ABCDEF" checklist that can be applied almost universally to nontraumatic out-of-hospital CA management in which other factors such as hypovolemia, tension pneumothorax, pericardial tamponade, and other reversible processes have at least been considered and tentatively ruled out. The following sections analyze each part of this practical and simplified approach and explain the meanings of "adequate" and "as necessary" using current knowledge about such issues.

Monitored (Provider-Witnessed) Arrest

If the strategy for CA management could be summarized into a single phrase, it would be that "the sooner a strong spontaneous circulation is restored, the better the outcome." Consequently, for the most "treatable" presentation of primary CA, namely that resulting from sudden VF of short duration, spontaneous circulation will not occur until the VF is terminated. Therefore, the priority in most VF- or VT-associated circulatory arrest of short duration (<4 or 5 minutes) is to *terminate the ventricular dysrhythmia* with defibrillatory countershocks. Whereas it may be argued that, after more prolonged VF, "successful" defibrillation (conversion into electrical rhythm that leads to spontaneous circulation)

Table 1
General Approach to Nontraumatic Cardiac Arrest Management

I. Prepare to clear out VF/VT, while considering spinal injury/immobilization and follow the "ABCs" checklist below. In a monitored arrest, shock as soon as possible, otherwise provide 2–3 minutes of uninterrupted chest compressions first (and occasional breaths).

II. Follow the ABCs checklist:

    A. Adequate, Slow, Lung Inflations, slowly and Bilaterally with O_2? (check endotracheal tube centimeter mark, stomach/breaths sounds and symmetry, bite block, respiratory rate and end-tidal CO_2 level).

    B. Blood Pressure or Chest Compressions; adequate?
(check compression force/depth, ensure uninterrupted performance and maintain rate at 100 per minute; feel for femoral pulses, monitor end-tidal CO_2 level).

    C. Catheter(s); drips, rate and patency? (use multiple large bore catheters in antecubital sites if possible).

    D. Drugs—Drug Check list: "4A—BCD" Consider each one and go back again.

        A. Anti-Arrthythmic—e.g., Amiodarone or Lidocaine: in VF/VT (except with wide, slow QRS on electrocardiogram not "driven" by P wave). Remember to load (e.g., Lidocaine IV 3 mg/kg or second dose for amiodarone).

        Adrenergic—e.g. epinephrine or vasopressin: pulseless despite good O_2 and CPR or pulseless with definite long interval of time post-arrest.

        Atropine—*(a)* hypotensive *and (b)* heart rate less than 60 per minute or less (or atrioventricular block).

        Altered mental status considerations (e.g., glucose test; naloxone).

        B. Bicarbonate: no significant response to initial "rounds" of therapy or known/highly suspected hyperkalemia or tricyclic overdose.

        C. Chemical imbalances (Mg^{++}, Ca^{++}, K^+, etc.).

        D. Drips of Pressors—e.g., pressors like levarterenol, dopamine, epinephrine; pulses present, but hypotensive (or epinephrine, vasopressin soon to be wearing off). Set up ahead of time in anticipation of need.

    E. Electrial functions ("GAMES") and pacemaker trial.
        Gain?
        Attached Leads?
        Mode (paddles vs chest leads)?
        EGG Vector (check several leads)?
        Strip (document with a "hard copy")?

    F. Further History and Physical (e.g., medications, recent symptoms/injury, asymmetry, auto-positive end-expiratory pressure, etc.).

III. Repeat above steps over and over.

may not occur until a better myocardial environment (restoration of reasonable myocardial oxygenation) is first created, clearing of VF must eventually be accomplished to restore "a strong spontaneous circulation" *(40)*.

Rapid defibrillation, such as that done within 1 minute of a monitored collapse, will allow the heart to beat spontaneously and thus restore circulation. It may then also result in stronger spontaneous respiration and rapid wakening. In turn, very early defibrillation might even obviate the need for these other ALS procedures. In the recent study of public access to defibrillation at the Chicago airports, most of the patients shocked within the first 4 to 5 minutes were awakening and almost all were awake prior to hospital admission *(9)*. Therefore, in monitored VF/VT-associated arrest, the patient should first receive one or two successive countershocks until the VF/VT clears, be it done with a manual defibrillator or an AED.

Unmonitored Arrest: The Classic Response

The approach may be different for patients with unmonitored arrest who must await traditional EMS responders, even in EMS systems providing relatively short response intervals *(40)*. Given the classic correlation of time to defibrillation with outcome, the "defibrillate-first" approach has traditionally been well accepted for all patients presenting with VF/VT. However, as discussed previously, recent animal and clinical data also suggest that improved coronary perfusion should be accomplished first if CA has exceeded 4–5 minutes, especially without rapid performance of bystander-initiated BCPR *(40)*. In those studies, lower rates of conversion occurred with the "shock first" approach. Although "CPR-first" was most useful for those patients with longer response intervals, Wik et al. have argued that "CPR-first" should always be the approach by arriving responders because, in their controlled study, it did not significantly diminish the chances of a favorable outcome for patients as compared to those receiving countershock first *(18)*.

Therefore, it seems logical to perform chest compressions, with as little interruption as possible, for 2–3 minutes, followed by immediate countershock *(18,19)*.

Defibrillation efficiency has dramatically improved at lower energies using improved ("biphasic" or "rectilinear") waveforms. More than 90% of out-of-hospital VF patients can be cleared of VF successfully using three shocks (or less) at 200 J, even with the historic use of dampened sinusoidal monophasic waveforms. Today, many patients are cleared of VF with equal efficiency using 150 J or less of biphasic energy within one or two shocks. This approach may be preferable because many lower energies are less injurious to myocardial cells. In the future, multiphasic defibrillators may lower energy requirements even further.

However, others believe that in certain patients with larger hearts (larger mass of fibrillating myocardium) or with chest walls with higher transthoracic resistance, there may be a need for escalating "doses" of energies. Also, the repeated application of shocks could also be detrimental. Therefore, it is believed by some that rapid escalation to higher energies in such cases should be considered. At the time of publication, this still remained an open-ended issue.

Likewise, in children, the heart size and mass of fibrillating myocardium are obviously much smaller. Therefore, the starting "dose" of 2 J/kg has been recommended as a rough guideline, but the most appropriate level of defibrillation energy has not yet been clearly established for the pediatric population, especially with the evolution of newer waveforms. Experts agree that most AEDs used in adults could be used in children 8 years of age or older.

Step A: Adequate Lung Inflation Slowly and Bilaterally With Oxygen

Persons with sudden CA do not stop breathing suddenly. Most will have agonal gasping respirations, which may even be more efficient than assisted breathing. Because of the specific interdependent architecture of the lungs, spontaneous respirations (largely diaphragmatic contractions) generally open up those dependent lung zones that tend to collapse during expiration. In fact, at first, these breaths are usually larger than "normal" (5–7 mL/kg) respirations, thus they are more efficient, not in terms of inflating those lung zones, but also in terms of removing carbon dioxide (proportionately less dead space per breath). They also enhance venous return.

In contrast, positive pressure (assisted) breaths act by "pushing" the lungs open and not "pulling" them open. As a result, the specific dependent lung zones may not be as affected by a positive pressure breath. In fact, positive pressure breaths coming from the upper airways will, at first, distribute gases to areas of less resistance and not necessarily those dependent lung zones that need to be inflated. Even with a protected airway (i.e., ETI), it will often take tidal volumes twice the normal tidal volume size (i.e., 10–12 mL/kg) to effect adequate lung inflation. Therefore, during the first few minutes of a sudden CA, the patient's spontaneous respirations may be more effective than mouth-to-mouth assisted ventilations by a bystander, particularly considering the accompanying risks for gastric insufflation and the lower than normal inspired oxygen fractions (0.16–0.17) in an assisted breath *(31)*.

Nevertheless, without adequate circulation, gasping respirations eventually dissipate as a result of loss of adequate oxygenation of those respiratory muscles and the brainstem. Also, with a loss of smooth muscle tone at the gastroesophageal junction, there is a greater risk of gastric insufflation, of regurgitation and subsequent aspiration of gastric contents. Therefore, the early placement of an endotracheal tube is strongly advised. ETI not only helps protect the airway from aspiration of gastric contents, but it also definitively helps to restore adequate lung inflation to reverse the critical hypoxemia that will eventually ensue after cardiopulmonary arrest. Particularly with the force of chest compressions, it may be difficult to reinflate the lungs with a bag-valve mask system alone. The use of ETI helps to guarantees the 10–12 mL/kg positive pressure breathing that may be required to reverse most of the intrapulmonary shunt that results from the associated collapse of gas-exchange units, particularly in dependent lung zones. If the patient receives a correctly placed ET, accompanied by the delivery of 10–12 mL/kg tidal volumes and 100% inspired oxygen, inadequate PaO_2 levels leading to significant red blood (hemoglobin) desaturation rarely occurs, even in time presence of significant lung disease.

In the best of hands, bag-valve devices may be used without significant gastric insufflation, but, in general, there are concerns that bag-valve devices will lead to too much gastric inflation. Recent recommendations have been to use smaller tidal volumes in such circumstances of unprotected airways if supplemental oxygen is available. Nevertheless, without supplemental oxygen, tidal volumes of 10 mL/kg are still recommended even though the proportionate risk for gastric insufflation increases. Therefore, rapid performance of ETI is strongly encouraged.

Although persons with cardiopulmonary arrest usually need assistance with lung inflation to ensure oxygenation, persons in circulatory arrest have unusually low total body oxygen consumption, subsequent low CO_2 production, and low flow back to the lungs. In turn, they require much less ventilation. In fact, because twice normal tidal volumes need to be used to ensure adequate oxygenation, those breaths can remove more than twice the amount of CO_2 removed by normal breaths. Therefore, low ventilatory rates (8 per minute or less in adults) may be much more than adequate.

Also, moderate (or even "normal") rates of positive pressure ventilation may lead to compromised cardiac output. Spontaneous respirations work by creating intermittent negative intrathoracic pressures (vacuum effect) that suck air into the chest. Likewise, these negative intrathoracic pressure swings help to enhance venous return. In contrast, assisted positive pressure breaths, transiently inhibit venous return. Although recoil from chest compressions can create some negative intrathoracic pressures, frequent positive pressure breaths inhibit this process, particularly if one interrupts chest compressions to perform the breaths. Until spontaneous circulation is restored, lower respiratory rates are recommended (i.e., 5–8 breaths per minute). Again, this assumes that 10–12 mL/kg are being used and, with a protected airway (ETI), compressions should not be interrupted to provide those breaths.

After spontaneous respirations return, rates of breathing can be increased. Two key cautions to this return to faster rates (i.e., >10 per minute) would be patients with severe expiratory flow limitation (i.e., asthma, chronic obstructive pulmonary disease) and patients with hypovolemia who are most susceptible to the hemodynamic effects of positive pressure breaths on venous return *(31)*. Hypovolemia is a problem because of already diminished preload, whereas expiratory flow obstruction maintains positive pressure in the chest through most of the respiratory cycle, thus inhibiting venous return. Many cases of PEA or the more classical term of "electromechanical dissociation" are probably the result of inadvertent cardiac output compromise from assisted positive pressure breaths *(31–33)*. A brief interruption of breaths to see if spontaneous pulses return will occasionally help to unmask such a problem. Obviously, fluid resuscitation and/or treatment of the underlying expiratory flow obstruction may also help. The easiest action is to slow the respiratory rate. As long as adequate size breaths are provided five to six times a minute, oxygenation generally will be maintained, particularly with expiratory flow obstruction *(33)*.

Step B: Blood Pressure or CPR Adequacy

The "B" in this mnemonic is not "breathing" as in BLS, but rather "blood pressure" (BP). If adequate lung inflation bilaterally with O_2 guarantees red cell saturation in virtually all cases, the next endpoint is brisk perfusion of the coronaries with those oxygenated cells by restoring a *strong* coronary artery perfusion pressure. If the BP is less than 110 to 120 mmHg systolic, the coronary artery perfusion pressure may not be adequate, especially when the end-diastolic pressure typically is not even clinically detectable. Although chest compressions may be less important in a patient primarily presenting with hypotension, in the post-CPR situation when the myocardium has been underperfused for a while, chest compressions may still augment ROSC in the hypotensive state. Even though pulses have returned, if the BP remains lower than 90–100 mmHg (e.g., absence of radial pulse or *strong* femoral pulses), this may be insufficient for adequate restoration of the O_2 debt to the "stunned myocardium" and may not supply the steady-state circulation required to support coronary perfusion. Moreover, chest compressions should be deep and quick (rate = 100/min) and, most importantly, rarely interrupted.

It has been demonstrated that when compressions are transiently held to deliver breaths, coronary perfusion falls off dramatically and, in turn, it takes as many as 10 or 15 compressions to restore the perfusion pressure to the previous pressure *(34–37)*. Therefore, once an endotracheal tube is placed, breathing and chest compressions do not need to be synchronized, meaning that compressions can be provided continuously. *With unprotected airways* (e.g., mouth-to-mouth or bag-valve-mask ventilation), however, assisted breathing does need to be synchronized (i.e., compressions held transiently to deliver a breath without impediment from back-pressure during compression down-strokes). Nevertheless, growing evidence suggests that those interruptions should be less frequent *(31–33)*. As noted previously, during cardiac arrest, the need to ventilate (to clear CO_2) is markedly reduced and one may only need to provide 30 to 50 compressions to two ventilations for adults and bigger children and perhaps 15 to 20 compressions to two breaths for smaller children, and again with negligible pauses to deliver the breaths *(46)*.

With the endotracheal tube in place, compressions should be continuous. However, certain pauses will be required to switch compressors or to deliver shocks or to assess the cardiac rhythm or check for the presence of pulses. In fact, continuous end-tidal CO_2 monitoring will often demonstrate diminishing levels of CO_2 output as the chest compressor begins to fatigue, indicating a good reason to substitute personnel. Nevertheless, all of these reasons to transiently halt chest compressions should be coordinated. If it is anticipated that a pulse and ECG assessment will needed at three minute mark, then that may be a good time to switch off personnel. And just prior to that interruption of compressions, the assessing rescuers should have their fingers already poised at the femoral pulse site (or whatever pulse they are checking) while watching the monitor. Only then should they command a halt to assisted ventilations followed immediately by the extremely brief interruption of chest compressions with a ready command to resume compressions (and ventilation).

Anecdotally, one can often observe rescuers giving a "hold CPR" directive, followed by a lengthy stare at a monitor. Discovering that ventilation is still going on, they then ask for those actions to be halted as well. Then re-staring at the monitor, the question arises, "Does 'that' (the abnormal rhythm on the monitor) have a pulse?," followed by several searches at the groin and neck. To make matters worse, the chest compressor will await orders to "resume CPR" and simply stand by while orders for additional adrenaline doses (or whatever additional therapies) are provided. The interruption of CPR can become significant and, most likely, lethal if continually repeated.

The other issue that is important to consider is the "compression to shock interval." Studies have shown a rapid drop-off in survival rates when the delivery of the shock occurs more than 5 or 10 seconds after compressions are halted to provide the counter-shock *(34–37)*. Long pauses should not occur. Methods should be employed to prepare to have the defibrillator charged and ready to fire as soon as the command to "halt compressions" is given and the compressing rescuer clears body contact.

Step C: Catheters

Although endotracheal administration of drugs such as epinephrine can be an alternative approach in adults in whom intravenous access is not available, this method is a poor choice in the absence of adequate circulation, particularly for lidocaine and atropine, which are not absorbed very well even in the patient with normal circulation. Therefore, intravenous catheters with large bore cannulaes (e.g., no. 14 or no. 16 French gauge) should be placed as quickly as possible. Placement is best accomplished either at the antecubital, forearm, or external jugular sites. As drugs are administered during CPR conditions, they should subsequently be flushed in vigorously. For example, in an antecubital site, the intravenous solution (e.g., D_5W) can be squeezed in under pressure with the arm elevated well above heart level. In this situation, a 20- to 30-second flush is probably adequate.

Theoretically, one might hold compressions and positive pressure breaths during the last 5 seconds of the flush in order to help overcome obstruction to flow into the chest from elevated intra-thoracic pressures. For external jugular or direct central venous access, a shorter flush with immediate halting of breaths and compressions would seem reasonable.

Multiple cannulations would be preferred eventually, as long as other key interventions are not delayed. This not only permits multiple therapies (e.g., anti-arrhythmic drips in one site and pressor drips in another), but it also better ensures constant IV access in case of inadvertent dislodgement or site infiltration.

Although seemingly a straightforward issue, care should be taken to ensure that bubbles have been removed from the intravenous fluid tubing as well as the injectable medications, especially in children. Although a "few air bubbles" are generally not considered to be harmful by most clinicians, they may accumulate with multiple rapid drug dosings, especially if the IV fluid (flush) is infused under pressure as previously recommended. Intuitively, a small visible bubble in IV tubing may be as large as an infant or small child's inflow/outflow track in the central and pulmonary circulation. Therefore, one should pay attention to this under-appreciated detail. Likewise, the injectable medication should be pointed upward before infusion with flicking of bubbles upward and the plunger gently elevated until all air is expelled and the bubble-less drops begin to flow from the injection needle/outlet.

While IV access at the femoral site (or other lower extremity placement) may be better than no IV access at all, it may not be as effective as upper extremity placement in view of the low flow, distance to the heart, and intermittent intra-thoracic pressure elevations. The same is true for endotracheal infusions where drugs are poorly absorbed in the absence of circulation and thus depot in the pulmonary track, later to be absorbed, unpredictably, if and when circulation is restored.

Step D: Drugs

To date, no single drug has been shown to improve survival *definitively* in the clinical setting. However, there are excellent animal studies as well as preliminary results of small clinical trials and other inferential data that support their efficacy *(14,15,29,38,47)*. The appropriate use and timing of drugs need to be definitively characterized and therefore Table 1 (and the following discussion) should serve more as a general template that can guide the protocol choices based on current available data (e.g., amiodarone versus lidocaine for the anti-arrhythmic therapy or noradrenaline vs vasopressin-epinephrine for the vasopressor). Patients who present with ventricular fibrillation can re-fibrillate and, therefore, though not yet explicitly proven to increase long-term survival, the use of anti-arrhythmics is theoretically of benefit, especially after re-establishment of pulses *(29,30)*.

More broadly, the concept of restoration of pulses by re-perfusing the coronaries (and maintaining brisk perfusion) is the key factor in resuscitation *(34–37,46)*. Use of drugs that can enhance back flow into the coronary arteries can be one reasonable strategy for establishing restoration of spontaneous circulation *(6,47)*. Because cardiac arrest patients develop peripheral vascular relaxation *(13)*, administration of vasopressor agents, particularly ones that may have mostly vasopressive actions and less β activity (i.e., less arrhythmogenic), may be of benefit. Although results of clinical studies to date have not yet provided confirmatory evidence, the laboratory evidence for this strategy is very strong *(6,47)*. Also, as stated previously, the timing of these drugs (e.g., before or after shocks) has yet to be addressed definitively, but it is clear that something about resuscitative drugs does work *(14,15)*.

Also, although initial boluses of drugs (e.g., epinephrine) may help to restore resuscitation, their effects may wear off and so the early establishment of pressor drips (even prior to blood pressure deterioration) may be a worthwhile strategy. In fact, one problem in resuscitation practices is the timing of all repeat medications. For example, a protocol may call for "1 mg. IV q 3 to 5 min." Instead of a routine schedule of administration, what generally happens in actual practice is that someone will ask, "When did we give the last epi?" Recognizing that more than 5 minutes may have passed, an epinephrine is ordered, but that then requires a search into the drug box, the unwrapping of the packaging and often a screwing of an injector into the vial. This would then be followed by ejection of the air bubble, and finally intravenous administration after double-checking for absence of pulse and the ECG rhythm. In other words, another minute or even two may pass after there is recognition that a drug needs to be administered (well beyond the proscribed schedule).

Rescuers and their trainers should therefore pay attention to such details and focus more how meet that "schedule." If a q 3 min schedule is the protocol, then rescuers should not have to ask when the last epi was given. Specifically, at the moment, one is ready to administer the drug, the person administering it should examine the vial to confirm that it is the correct drug and announce out loud, "I am now giving 1 mg of 1:10,000 epinephrine IV" to provide the actual time of administration (not ordering of the drug) for those documenting the medical record and also to double check the appropriateness of the dosing at that moment among all of the fellow team members (another error-reducing, quality assurance tactic). As the drug is pushed into the IV site, the "3 min" (180 second) clock begins. Assuming the drug is pushed over 10 to 15 seconds and then flushed for another 15 to 25 seconds, nearly 20% of the schedule is already exhausted. If the reaction of the drug is gauged 2 minutes later (typical time frame), and another dose needs to be given, then it is already time to give that repeat infusion. Therefore, the subsequent (repeat) drug administration needs to be anticipated, including its acquisition and preparation, right at the time of any current infusion. Although this strategy may lead to a concern over a potential waste of an opened vial if pulses return, the cost of epinephrine (in this case) is relatively low compared to the entire cost of the resuscitation effort, successful or not, let alone the cost of the life. More importantly, one must always still anticipate deterioration of the original epinephrine effect and having a "quick fix" available is wise and potentially lifesaving.

Atropine is probably of little value in a circumstance of no flow, but has theoretical potential in certain cases, particularly those in which vagal tone, insecticides or toxic "nerve agents" may have played a role, and especially if it involves low but spontaneous flow states involving supra-ventricular complexes occurring at bradycardic rates.

Sodium bicarbonate remains controversial as a routine drug to administer, but it has theoretical advantages in tricyclic overdoses and known (or highly suspected) hyperkalemia such as a dialysis patient who has not been dialyzed for quite a while. It should theoretically be avoided in carbon monoxide poisoning because it causes additional left shift in the hemoglobin-dissociation curve, thus further diminishing oxygen unloading at the tissues. Hypothetically, a relatively acidotic state should be beneficial in shock conditions to facilitate oxygen unloading. In fact, previous trends and teachings to compensate for metabolic acidosis by "hyperventilation" through positive pressure ventilation is clearly a concern because of the concomitant effects on intrathoracic pressure and the resulting inhibition of venous return and subsequent reduction in cardiac output *(31,32)*. It is even possible that, in the future, permissive hypercapnea, balanced by some titration of extreme acidosis with some alkalinizer, may prove to be a preferred tactic. Even better, devices that create enhanced negative intrathoracic pressure for breathing (and enhanced venous return) may be the best method to control extreme acidosis just as an acidotic sprinter normally does after the race or a grand mal seizure patient does in the post-ictal period.

One should consider other potential problems predisposing to the arrest (e.g., a severe ion deficiency such as hypomagnesemia or hypokalemia—or both) and other factors that may lead to or exacerbate a cardiac arrest such as drug overdose or hypoglycemia which are reversible with medications such as naloxone or dextrose (glucose) administration. Since the major concern with narcotics is postural hypotension and respiratory depression, one could argue that the narcotic antagonist would not be a critical consideration if respirations are controlled and the patient is supine. The main indication would be for the patient for whom the airway is not secured and control of breathing is limited or in the case of the resuscitated person who has not awoken quickly. In the case of dextrose administration, considering that there has been some theoretical concern over high glucose levels in terms of neurological recovery, dextrose should not be administered capriciously and just because a person is reportedly "diabetic." Therefore, glucose levels should be checked if there is a suspicion of hypoglycemia (actually a rare event in cardiac arrest) such as in the case of person using insulin or hypoglycemia agents and β-blockers.

Step E: Electrical Functions and Pacemaker Trial

Regardless of the rhythm, perfusion of the coronary arteries with oxygen is a priority in pulseless states. However, the electrical and ECG functions may provide some assistance in resuscitation. First of all, it is important to confirm the actual cardiac rhythm. One mnemonic to help in this analysis is the word "GAMES" (Table 1). One should check the machine's "Gain" to see if it is dampened or could be used to better identify the rhythm when physiologic factors might obscure the electrical activity (e.g., obesity, chronic bullous lung disease or pericardial fluid). One should always confirm that the ECG leads are "Attached" because they may have a tendency to fall off a wet person or after a shock or after aggressive chest compressions. Likewise, rescuers should confirm the "Mode" (e.g., paddle vs lead II or lead I) on the monitor, particularly if switching leads to view different vectors. In that respect, it may very well be helpful to actively search various "ECG Vectors" to confirm asystole (in multiple leads) or to better delineate the ECG complex width in different views. It must be reinforced that asystole is not a "flatline," it is a physiologic state of no heartbeat evidenced by absence of auscultated heartsounds (insensitive) or ultrasound demonstration of no heartbeat, no pulses, and no detectable electrical activity anywhere in the heart. Documentation of the rhythm with a printed "Strip" can be helpful, not only in terms of the medical record, but also in terms of immediately showing what has transpired to subsequent caretakers (e.g., arriving supervisors or the emergency department doctors). Even when the longitudinal ECG information is stored electronically by today's built-in computers, having a hard copy of the initial presentation can help with immediate record-keeping and on-line quality assurance during transfer of care to the hospital personnel.

Pacemaker trials are usually ineffective if myocardial energy supplies have dwindled, but may be useful in extremely hypotensive patients with slow rates who have not yet progressed into a state of extreme circulatory compromise. It may also be of value once spontaneous pulses have returned. To some extent, a pacemaker, a device which can be shut off or better controlled, might be more useful than atropine considering that it the drug may unpredictably predispose the patient to a sustained tachycardic effect once resuscitation has occurred. Still, the earlier the intervention, the better the result and so atropine would be preferred if would take too long to set up a pacemaker in targeted patients.

Step F: Further History and Physical Factors

Whether or not a patient responds to initial interventions, it is important to consider additional historical and physical factors. Historical factors such as medications used, potential drug abuse, chronic lung disease or a circumstance leading to profound hypovolemia should be considered. Likewise, one should evaluate for physical signs such as asymmetric breath sounds (e.g., potential pneumothorax), prolonged expiratory phase (i.e., Auto-PEEP), nitroglycerin (or other) patches (which should be removed), signs of hypovolemia, internal or external bleeding, aberration in core temperature, and other physical signs that may alter interventions.

For example, a prolonged expiratory phase, particularly in circumstances that have inexplicable pulselessness in the face of well-organized ECG complexes may actually reflect an "auto-PEEP" effect in which the person with chronic obstructive pulmonary disease (COPD) or severe asthma has trouble exhaling the entire positive pressure breath before the next breath is delivered, resulting in persistent positive intrathoracic pressure throughout the respiratory cycle (i.e., positive end-expiratory pressure because of the person's obstructive lung disease and relatively overzealous positive pressure ventilation). As discussed previously, an auto-PEEP effect (or any prolonged phase of positive pressure in the chest) leads to severely impaired venous return and subsequent impairment of cardiac output. Whereas COPD and asthma patients are at greatest risk, this phenomenon can occur in persons with normal lungs, especially in the face of severe hypovolemia or hemorrhage. Sometimes a brief pause in assisted breathing (e.g, 10–15 seconds) may be enough to allow return of palpable pulses and uncover a situation of "pseudo-EMD" caused by unnecessarily high respiratory rates. In these cases, attempted treatment of bronchospasm with intra-tracheally administered epinephrine may have theoretical benefit, but intentionally slower ventilation is still the key therapeutic intervention. In the absence of applied PEEP, a relatively larger breath (e.g., 10–12 mL/kg) may be more efficient in terms of removing carbon dioxide and also result in faster recoil of the lungs allowing much slower rates (e.g., five breaths per minute if necessary). Again, longstanding COPD patients, even those resuscitated with strong pulses (and particularly those known to be chronic carbon dioxide retainers), may fare very well with high end-tidal carbon dioxide values.

As discussed previously, hypoglycemia and toxic overdose should be considered in historical analysis and the medication history should be put into context (e.g., β-blockers causing less effective response to catecholamine or tricyclic antidepressants indicating the potential use of sodium bicarbonate). A history of digoxin and loop diuretic use may prompt considerations of hypomagnesemia and/or hypokalemia, especially with persistent ventricular fibrillation or ventricular tachycardia (indicating potential use of magnesium infusion). A history of delayed dialysis may raise the issue of hyperkalemia (indicating sodium bicarbonate or calcium chloride use). In addition, one should also think about the classical considerations of occult (or obvious) trauma, pericardial tamponade and hypothermia/hypothermia.

LOGISTICS OF RESUSCITATION

The management of time and logistical considerations may the most critical "therapies" that rescuers can provide for cardiac arrest. As stated before, placement of an endotracheal tube at the top of resuscitation kit or alternating chest compressors at the same time one wishes to examine the ECG monitor, are all strategies that may actually help to save a life. It is likely that a life is probably saved by a rescuer who has used the toilet before laying down for a 3 AM. nap at the station than one who has memorized the dosing of some new anti-arrhythmic. The point being, if a rescuer significantly delays a response to a subsequent 4 AM. sudden death event because he has to urgently use the toilet on the way out the door, the impact may be greater than some (often arbitrary) dosing of a drug. Although this analogy seems somewhat crude, it serves to emphasize the concept that time efficiencies are paramount in cardiac arrest.

At the same time, two highly skilled and coordinated medics arriving on scene 8 minutes after an arrest may be more successful than two lesser trained medics who arrive at 6 minutes. The two coordinated and highly skilled medics may get the defibrillation, intubation and drug infusion all finished minutes before the lesser trained team because they understand the logistics and efficiencies that get the job done faster. Likewise, understanding relative priorities (e.g., once IV access is obtained, injecting and flushing the drug even before taping in the catheter and tubing) is paramount. Appreciating that intubation or IV access does not need to be delayed just to check a pulse post-defibrillation is appropriate judgment.

In the following sections, certain tricks of the trade will be detailed as considerations to facilitate rapid patient care. although these suggestions may be helpful, they are not the "definitive" methods. It is eventually up to all rescuers to find ways to make themselves more efficient, more coordinated and more skilled at rapid interventions.

Coordination of Personnel, Both Professional and Laypersons

Drilling and continually providing coordinated training with FR teams and ALS crews is a key to success. If the FR fire apparatus crew provides the previously described ABCDE approach while the medics simultaneously provide ETI and IV access, the coordinated response will enhance efficiency and rapid completion of necessary tasks. This response should be drilled before (and reviewed after) a given incident by supervisors to ensure improved performance at the next resuscitative event.

But other factors are involved. If arriving at a high rise or corporate complex maze, first responders being led by security officers to the scene should take action to ensure that ensuing rescuers (e.g., ambulance crews, supervisors) will also be guided to the site of the collapsed patient just as rapidly. For that matter, local EMS agencies should establish a coordinated response with such facilities long before the event. In fact, in some communities, such activities can be coordinated with corporate CPR training and AED placement in these facilities along with education and planned coordination regarding likely dispatch interrogation and procedures. Also, the CPR instruction should address likely scenarios and what to expect to see (e.g., cyanosis, anoxic seizure, agonal breaths) and they should encourage would-be bystanders to act rapidly and not to hesitate to use rescue procedures because of potential social mores or code of conduct implications (e.g., removal of a co-worker's blouse to apply AED pads). As applicable, actions should also include statements like "Call 9-1-1—and tell them we're going to be doing CPR." This second phrase should help to markedly expedite the dispatch process, especially in priority dispatch systems (16,17).

Anticipation of what rescuers are likely to encounter and what bystanders are likely to experience is crucial to a well-designed EMS system. Case reviews, follow-up interviews and on-scene response by system designers are important activities to learn about these factors and to enhance expedited responses to cardiac arrest in the community. Mass CPR education should not only be sought across the community (with required school training and workplace initiatives serving as the nucleus), but that education should provide expectations of what to anticipate in such events, including the logistical issues. Such training might even involve role-playing with likely scenarios that involve anoxic fits, regurgitation and lone or multiple rescuer situations.

This approach coupled with shorter (e.g., 30-minute) CPR practice-based training might be preferable to current multihour (mostly didactic) approaches. This strategy may also lead to more persons taking courses because of the more manageable time allotment, particularly for employees, and it may also permit more frequent re-training. It is not only likely that more people would know CPR but that the retention of skills would then be better as well. Therefore, logistical issues for life-saving apply in terms of preparation across the entire community, just as much as they do in an individual cardiac scenario.

Quality Assurance is Key: Some On-Line and Off-Line Examples

One potential advantage to police FR programs or private ambulance services that deploy roving, "stationless" systems, is that the rescuers are dressed, in their vehicles and ready to respond as compared to colleagues in a fire station who may have lain down to nap on the night shift and still need to awaken, pull up their pants, "slide down the fire pole," start the ignition and look both ways before coming out of the fire station's garage. To diminish such time-consuming problems, some EMS agencies have established systems that light up the station and automatically open station doors with a microwave signal while also delivering a voice or electronic alarm. Perhaps boots are in place on the truck and a comfortable (but presentable) jump suit (that can also be slept in) is worn. Whatever it takes to crop off seconds in the response, those suggestions should be entertained. Added up, 5 seconds here and 5 seconds there can mean a 10 or 20% reduction for the cardiac arrest patient's chance of surviving and returning to their families.

One suggestion to reduce wasted time is that one should always consider each call a "worst-case scenario." By not announcing the dispatch type until the crews are in active response to the initially dispatched location, one removes bias about the urgency. This may also backfire considering that cardiac arrests are only about 1% of all EMS responses and that most responses are not as time-dependent. Therefore, intensive quality assurance should track the time intervals from dispatch to actual response and do so not only at each station, but also according to each shift at each station. This helps to eliminate (or, in some cases, prove) the claim that there is something unique about the particular station that causes a crew's frequent tardiness or delays. Feedback and emphasis on the concept of "seconds count" should ensue and friendly competitions encouraged.

Likewise, at the other end of the response, one may find an unusually long inter-shift or inter-station differential in terms of arrival at the street address location to arrival at the patient's side or from arrival at the patient's side to delivery of the first shock. In a classic "Hawthorne effect," some EMS systems have demonstrated a marked reduction in time and even increased survival rates by a simple quality assurance intervention such as having the crews announce over the radio when they have arrived at the scene, when they are at the patient's side and then again when they have delivered the first shock. Therefore, the quality assurance can be done both "off-line" in follow-up review of electronic records, or by "on-line" with "real-time" actions. In both cases, positive feedback and comparison to others—with objective data—are all key components of risk management and EMS system success in resuscitation.

Of course, there are a multitude of quality improvement techniques, some involving hard data, some more clinical and experience-based. For example, the use of on-scene supervisors, discussed in a subsequent section, can be a key quality assurance factor, especially during scene activities, that can go far beyond the findings in a chart or database. Again, each system needs to employ multiple layers of such quality assurances.

Paying Attention to Details: Airway Techniques as an Example

Certain things may seem straightforward to the experienced and knowledgeable clinician-educator such as defibrillator electrode placement or the way a breath is delivered through a bag-valve device. However, in under-scrutinized EMS systems, particularly those without on-scene supervision of EMS personnel, one may find a defibrillator-monitor pad placed over the left upper quadrant of the abdomen (or even lower) or a breath delivered rapidly and the manual squeeze sustained instead of a steady squeeze over 2 to 3 seconds with a quick release to allow the bag to quickly re-inflate with oxygen. Accordingly, as discussed in the following sections, attention to every detail is important in successful EMS systems.

Although seemingly a noncritical issue, oxygen flow may be either too low or too high. If an 800 mL tidal volume is being delivered at a rate of six per minute (4.8 L per minute volume), then at least five liters per minute flow of oxygen flow should be provided. On the other hand, if, in that circumstance, 20 L per minute flow is provided, the small portable tank will soon deplete unnecessarily. This will cause a premature break in oxygenation to change out bottles (even assuming that the depletion is anticipated and recognized immediately). Conversely, when strong pulses are returned and sustained and minute volume needs to be increased accordingly, the flow should be re-titrated to the new level of delivery.

As an aside, there are situations in which rescuers may be faced with the resuscitation of an infant (or anyone for that matter) without the applicable ventilatory adjuncts but with availability of supplemental oxygen. In such circumstances, rescuers can themselves breathe the oxygen in and raise their own inspired oxygen fraction. Since expired oxygen fraction is usually about 4 to 5% less than the inspired, a 40% inspired mixture can lead to delivery of about 35% with the mouth-to-mouth breath, a level much better than the usual 16 to 17% breath usually provided by inspiring only ambient air.

Attention to details in many other airway and breathing aspects of the resuscitation can improve patient care. Immediately after the performance of endotracheal intubation, very typically a ritual typically ensues among inexperienced resuscitators in which someone shouts, "Check the breathsounds!" and a scramble for a stethoscope ensues followed by auscultation of the chest, right and left, up and down and then the epigastric area. In the meantime, 10 L or more of gas may have been pumped into the stomach if there was an inadvertent esophageal placement of the tube. Even with immediate end-tidal carbon dioxide monitoring, it may take a few breaths or more to confirm pulmonary carbon dioxide excretion. Instead, as part of a more appropriate intubation ritual, a stethoscope worn by a second rescuer should be poised for auscultation over the left epigastrium at the costal margin (and not the supra-umbilical area!) before the first breath is delivered. Also, as that first "test breath" is provided, the chest wall should be observed for concomitant rise and if a loud "breathsound" is heard over the stomach and the chest wall does not rise, one can avoid the inappropriate delivery of any more gas into the esophagus. Conversely, if the chest wall rises and the epigastrium is quiet except for a slight "swoosh" sound that is clearly heard much better on the next breath over the right upper chest (and then the left), one can feel more confident that additional breaths can be given without gastric insufflation. Efficiencies and details are important to successful systems of resuscitation and logistics (e.g., stethoscope in place before the first breath) are paramount.

Along these same lines, in both adults and children, a properly placed endotracheal tube can become an iatrogenic airway obstruction if the patient awakens and begins to bite down on the tube. The cardiac sequelae (bradycardia/asystole) can be insidious and dramatic, especially in children. Key monitoring actions include continuously feeling for resistance on the bag device or closely checking the automated ventilator and the end-tidal carbon dioxide output as well as constantly recycling through the steps in Table 1. But even if the obstruction is immediately recognized, it could be hard to un-do once a patient is beginning to bite down. Therefore, (anticipated) use of a bite block or gap in the teeth should be part of the routine and a detail that should not be ignored.

Although endotracheal tubes can be secured by specialized devices or additional spinal immobilization techniques, particularly for transport, one should not waste significant time doing this if the resuscitation is still in progress and other advanced tasks need to be performed. A simple roll of one inch white bandaging adhesive tape can serve as a rapid and strong device for anchoring the tube. Without tearing the tape, a 2 to 3 cm. piece can be extended out from the roll and taped around the tube right at the level of the front teeth, in turn, serving as an additional marker for tube depth. Specifically, the tape's lower lateral edge is secured snugly at the marker on the endotracheal tube (e.g., 21 cm) that denotes the distance between the front teeth and the point at which the endotracheal tube cuff has just past the vocal cords. The tape is then pulled out a foot or so and quickly wrapped around the back of the head snugly with the tape lying just above the ear, across the occiput, above the other ear and cheek, and then re-wrapped around the tube at the same level of the original marker point—and, most importantly, it is tightened snugly without any slack. Therefore, one should also avoid taping around the neck where the tight tape would compress main arteries and veins, but also not placed too high around the head that it could predispose the tape to slip off, especially with dampness and vomit at the taping sites (that can lubricate the tape and diminish adhesiveness). This entire procedure can take less than 10 seconds in experienced hands and, if done properly, will almost always prevent self-extubation in a awakening, combative patient.

The act of endotracheal intubation may be difficult outdoors in daylight because of glare and the rescuers pupils not adjusted to look down a poorly lit throat. Therefore, one logistical trick is to have a jacket or opaque cloth that can be placed well over the rescuer's and patient's heads to blot out light (like an old-time photographer's camera cloak). This technique should be considered immediately under such circumstances to facilitate the intubation in order to get the intubator's eyes more accustomed to less light.

Table 2
Recommendations for Optimal Bag-Valve-Mask (BVM) Device Use

C	*Consider C-spine Injury* (e.g., consider potential for post-incident or accompanying fall; or motor vehicle collision, etc., and position accordingly).
O	*Oral Airway* (properly sized to push the tongue up and out of the way).
P	*Position the head* (neutral position if there is a risk of cervical spine injury; or sniffing position—tilted back and elevated off the ground—if no suspicion of cervical spine risk).
E	*Elevate the Jaw* (usually with the tips of the fourth and fifth fingers, bilaterally, placed at the angle of the jaw, lifting it directly upward and perpendicularly to the ground).
S	*Seal the mask* with two hands (forming two opposite "C-shaped clamps," by placing the thumbs on the bridge of the nose and the index fingers over the chin).
S	*Slow, steady squeeze* (a second person provides a full 10 mL/kg squeeze of the bag without supplemental oxygen—or lesser volume with oxygen—but at a deliberate steady rate of delivery over a 2- to 3-second period, followed by a quick release to allow the bag and reservoir bag to fill with O_2 before the next breath).
O	*Oxygen* (delivered at a titrated rate to maintain full reservoir bag inflation—if applicable—just prior to the next breath; depletion of the tank is anticipated).
S	*Sellick's maneuver* (moderate cricothyroid pressure; best done by a third person if available).

Reducing Error Through Team Work

The intubating paramedic should take steps to decrease the chance of critical error and even an (inappropriate) accusation of not having placed an endotracheal tube correctly by a physician who quickly pulls out the tube in the emergency department when breath sounds appear markedly diminished bilaterally due to a patient's individual chronic physiology (e.g., COPD) or acute pathophysiology (e.g., bilateral hemothorax). Specifically, in addition to end-tidal monitoring, one should also have a colleague also take a confirmatory direct visualization to reassure that the tube is passing right between the vocal cords. Direct visualization by two different rescuers *as part of the routine expectation* diminishes the risks of error from an arrogant clinician ("You don't need to check me—it's in"). This approach also makes a stronger case, for example, when it is a physician's word against one medic's. Nevertheless, use of end-tidal monitors and additional monitoring (continually rechecking tube position), particularly on transfer from the ambulance to the emergency department stretcher, and especially in children, is critical.

If the intubation is delayed or unsuccessful on the initial attempt, one may use bag-valve-mask (BVM) devices. In such circumstances, the airway is unprotected and there is risk for inadequate lung inflation and gastric insufflation, particularly with on-going chest compressions and subsequent decreases in thoracic compliance. In turn, there is risk for hypoxemia, regurgitation and potential aspiration of gastric contents. The frequency of these complications can be decreased, however, by techniques that will lower the rise in airway pressure as well as those that optimize airway opening. As much as it uses up resources, these techniques are best accomplished with two to three rescuers, one to position the head, place oral airways, elevate the jaw and seal the mask and another to deliver the gas in a slow steady way with a quick release (and perhaps a third rescuer to provide cricothyroid cartilage pressure. This approach can be organized according to the mnemonic, "COPES SOS" (Table 2). If there is no concern about a spinal injury, elevation of the head 2 to 3 inches above the floor with a towel or jacket in order to create a better "sniffing position" and thus optimize the airway opening. In addition, an appropriate oral airway and a concomitant jaw thrust with the fourth and fifth fingers on each side of the rear angle of the mandible can create improved airway opening, while a Sellick's maneuver would compress the esophagus and diminish risks for regurgitation and gastric insufflation. Recent studies have emphasized that, with an unprotected airway, lower and slowly delivered tidal volumes are preferable to diminish gastric insufflation, specifically, 10 mL/kg without supplemental oxygen and lower tidal volumes with oxygen supplementation. Therefore, a reasonable recommendation is to provide that estimated tidal volume with a very deliberate steady squeeze over 2 to 3 seconds (followed by a quick release) in order to allow the bag to fill itself with supplemental oxygen.

Supervisor System

Although a cardiac arrest can often be managed fairly efficiently by two highly skilled paramedics who are supported by first responders using the organized "ABCDE" approach, there are advantages to EMS supervisory systems. Supervisory systems can include the use of experienced EMS physicians and/or veteran paramedic officers who respond (preferably in separate response vehicles) to all cardiac arrests in their assigned territory (48). Without taking away primary skills performance from the front-line paramedics, they double-check actions taken (per understood routine) and they also offer back-up assistance. They tend more to monitor the overall situation and evolving strategy and reinforce adherence to the cycle in Table 1. They also perform procedures whenever the front-line medics encounter a difficult situation, but generally they tend to step back and think ahead to the next move (e.g., preparing pressor drips early) and adhere to infusion schedules. They also interact with family members and/or bystanders.

In some EMS systems, certain supervisors may attend 25 to 30 cardiac arrests a month giving them more exposure to difficult cases, sociologically and physiologically, as well as more overall frequent experience with cardiac arrest management. In turn, both their skills and judgment are honed by longtime experience. This experience also makes such EMS supervisors an ideal subject to implement a pilot procedure or investigatory drug procedure, especially if the supervisor maintains close relationships and on-line contact with their designated medical director (49). In Houston, for example, supervisors have received close monitoring and routine field interaction with intensely involved medical directors (3,48) who maintain extremely close 24/7 radio/cell-phone contact.

In progressive EMS systems, supervisors usually rove in assigned territories and make announced and unannounced responses. They are routinely notified for certain key incidents such as "child shot," "CPR in progress," or "major explosion." The supervisor also ensures that interactions with the "environment" are controlled. This not only includes recognition of potential hazards, but also paying attention to family members and other bystanders, before and after the resuscitation effort. In most EMS systems, the majority of out-of-hospital cardiac arrest patients will not have their pulses restored at all, let alone restored immediately. Therefore, one of the supervisor's roles can be to assure the family and bystanders that the patient is receiving all of the most appropriate interventions right there at the scene. Even if pulses are not returned (or the patient eventually dies), the resuscitation *effort* can still be considered successful if the rescuers have truly provided the best interventions that medicine can offer in the most timely and optimal manner and the family is satisfied with the way things were handled.

This "success" is particularly true if the observing family members feel confident in the rescuers and if they believe that "everything possible was done" for their loved one. As soon as the supervisor checks that the endotracheal tube is in place and other actions are well underway, he or she can begin to interact and gain the confidence of the bystanders assuring them that everything that could be done at the hospital is being done right at that moment. The supervisor, recognizing that there is no immediate response to treatment, also can begin to prepare the family and bystanders for the eventuality that the outcome will be negative. To gain confidence, statements such as the following can be one early tactic, "Please forgive me and let me know if I'm too blunt with you, but I personally believe that you should know about everything that is going on—and as soon as possible" followed later by "You need to understand that his heart stopped and that is obviously very bad—if we ever get a heart re-started it's usually right away—and so far it doesn't look good—but we're going to keep trying—at least for now—let me get back to him now—but don't hesitate to ask me anything." Although there are many other approaches, and this particular example may even be a bad one in some circumstances, the concept is to gain confidence, provide a confident, calm demeanor and to exude professionalism and compassion, especially in the face of emotion, be it anger, grief, guilt, anxiety, or disbelief.

Another role for the supervisor can also be to gain more historical details, preferred physician or hospital destinations, and also initiate discussions about on-scene termination of efforts and begin to finesse that sensitive concept *(50)*. Also, veteran supervisors can bring along tricks of the trade from years of "trial and error." As an example, in a tight elevator space, the supervisor might remember a previous resolution and ask that the back board be removed and that the patient be turned around on the stretcher so that the patient's feet and legs are at the "head" of the stretcher which, in turn, can be lifted up, still allowing the head and thorax to lay flat while the legs are elevated, making just enough room to fit the stretcher in the cramped space.

Above all, EMS supervisors can provide invaluable insight to re-thinking system design and the way we provide interventions. Be they "street-wise" and creative physicians or wise, veteran medics, or both, we need to continually pay attention to details, focus on logistics and re-evaluate our interventions. The simplistic uni-dimensional approaches that have often led to ineffective EMS systems in the past will always have a tendency to re-surface. The future will therefore lie in our ability to continually "re-search" what we do and our ability to be nurturing mentors who provide expert role models for future medics and EMS physicians in successful systems for out-of-hospital resuscitation.

REFERENCES

1. Cobb LA, Alvarez H, Copass MK. A rapid response system for out-of- hospital cardiac emergencies. Med Clin North Am 1976; 60:283–290.
2. McManus WF, Tresch DD, Darin JC. An effective prehospital emergency system. J Trauma 1977; 17: 304–310.
3. Pepe PE, Mattox KL, Duke JH. Effect of full-time specialized physician supervision on the success of a large, urban emergency medical services system. Crit Care Med 1993; 21:1279–1286.
4. Eisenberg M, Bergner L, Hallstrom A. Paramedic programs and out-of-hospital cardiac arrest: I factors associated with successful resuscitation. Am J Public Health 1979; 69:30–38.

5. White RD, Vukov FL, Bugliosi TF. Early defibrillation by police: Initial experience with measurement of critical time intervals and patient outcome. Ann Emerg Med 1995; 23:1009–1013.

6. Brown CG, Martin DR, Pepe PE, et al. A comparison of standard-dose and high dose epinephrine in cardiac arrest outside the hospital. The Multicenter High-Dose Epinephrine Study Group. N Engl J Med 1992; 327:1051–1055.

7. Callaham M, Madsen CD, Barton CW, Saunders CE, Pointer J. A randomized clinical trial of high dose epinephrine and norepinephrine vs. standard-dose epinephrine in prehospital cardiac arrest. JAMA 1992; 268:2667–2672.

8. Stiell IG, Hebert PC, Weitzman Bnea. A study of high–dose epinephrine in human CPR. N Engl J Med 1992; 237:1047–1050.

9. Caffrey SL, Willoughby PJ, Pepe PE, Becker LB. Public use of automated external defibrillators. N Engl J Med 2002; 347(16):1242–1247.

10. White RD. Early out-of-hospital experience with an impedance-compensating low-energy biphasic waveform automatic external defibrillator. J Interv Card Electrophysiol 1997; 1:203–208.

11. White RD, Hankins DG, Bugliosi TF. Seven years' experience with early defibrillation by police paramedics in an emergency medical services system. Resuscitation 1998; 39:145–151.

12. Cummins RO, Ornato JP, Thies WH, Pepe PE. Improving survival from sudden cardiac arrest: the "chain of survival" concept. A statement for health professionals from the Advanced Cardiac Life Support Subcommittee and the Emergency Cardiac Care Committee, American Heart Association. Circulation 1991; 83:1832–1847.

13. Lee SK, Vaaganes P, Safar P, Stezoski SW, Scanlon M. Effect of cardiac arrest time on cortical cerebral blood flow during subsequent standard external cardiopulmonary resuscitation in rabbits. Resuscitation 1989; 17:105–117.

14. Pepe PE, Levine RL, Fromm RE, Curka PA, Clark PS, Zachariah BS. Cardiac arrest presenting with rhythms other than ventricular fibrillation: Contribution of resuscitation efforts toward total survivorship. Crit Care Med 1994; 21:1838–1843.

15. Pepe PE. ACLS systems and training programs—do they make a difference? Respir Care 1995; 30:427–433.

16. Stout J, Pepe PE, Mosesso VN Jr. All-advances life support vs. tiered-response ambulance systems. Prehosp Emerg Care 2000; 4:1–6.

17. Curka PA, Pepe PE, Ginger VF, Sherrard RD, Ivy MV, Zachariah BS. Emergency medical services priority dispatch. Ann Emerg Med 1993; 22:1688–1695.

18. Wik L, Hansen TB, Fylling F, et al. Delaying defibrillation to give basic cardiopulmonary resuscitation to patients with out-of-hospital ventricular fibrillation: a randomized trial. JAMA 2003; 289:1389–1395.

19. Cobb LA, Fahrenbruch CE, Walsh TR, et al. Influence of cardiopulmonary resuscitation prior to defibrillation in patients with out-of-hospital ventricular fibrillation. JAMA 1999; 281:1182–1188.

20. Hallstrom A, Cobb L, Johnson E, Copass M. Cardiopulmonary resuscitation by chest compression alone or with mount-to-mouth ventilation. N Engl J Med 2000; 342:1546–1533.

21. Persse DE, Key CB, Bradley RN, Miller CC, Dhingra A. Cardiac arrest survival as a function of ambulance deployment strategy in a large urban emergency medical services system. Resuscitation 2003; 59: 97–104.

22. Stiell IG, Wells GA, Field B, et al. Advanced cardiac life support in out-of-hospital cardiac arrest. N Engl J Med 2004; 351:647–656.

23. Key CB, Pepe PE, Persse DE, Calderon D. Can first responders be sent to selected 9-1-1 emergency medical services calls without an ambulance? Acad Emerg Med 2003; 10:339–346.

24. Davis R. Six minutes to live or die. USA Today July 2003; 28–30, pp. A1–D7.

25. Sasser HC, Safar P, and the Brain Resuscitation Clinical Trial Study Group. Arterial hypertension after cardiac arrest is associated with good cerebral outcome in patients. Crit Car Med Suppl 1999; 27:A29.

26. Wigginton JG, Pepe PE, Bedolla JP, DeTamble LA, Atkins JA. Sex-related differences in the presentation and outcome of out-of-hospital cardiopulmonary arrest: A multiyear, prospective population-based study. Crit Care Med 2002; 30(Suppl): S1–S6.

27. Copass MK, Oreskovich MR, Bladergroen MR, Carrico CJ. Prehospital cardiopulmonary resuscitation of the critically injured patient. Am J Surgery 1984; 148:20–26.

28. Durham LA, Richardson RJ, Wall MJ, Pepe PE, Mattox KL. Emergency center thoracotomy: impact of prehospital resuscitation. J Trauma 1992; 32:775–779.

29. Kudenchuk PJ, Cobb LA, Copass MK, et al. Amiodarone for resuscitation after out-of-hospital cardiac arrest due to ventricular fibrillation. N Engl J Med 1999; 341:871–878.

30. Dorian P, Cass D, Schwartz B, Cooper R, Gelaznikas R, Barr A. Amiodarone as compared with lidocaine for shock-resistant ventricular fibrillation. N Engl J Med 2002; 346:884–890.
31. Roppolo LP, Wigginton JA, Pepe PE. Emergency ventilatory management as a detrimental factor in resuscitation practices and clinical research efforts. In: Vincent J-L, ed. 2004 Yearbook of Intensive Care and Emergency Medicine. Berlin: Springer; 2004:139–151.
32. Aufderheide TP, Sigurdsson G, Pirrallo RG, et al. Hyperventilation-induced hypotension during cardiopulmonary resuscitation. Circulation 2004; 109:1960–1965.
33. Pepe PE, Raedler C, Lurie K, Wigginton JG. Emergency ventilatory management in hemorrhagic states: elemental or detrimental? J Trauma 2003; 54:1048–1057.
34. Yu T, Weil MH, Tang W, et al. Adverse outcomes of interrupted precordial compression during automated defibrillation. Circulation 2002; 106(3):368–372.
35. Koster RW. Limiting 'hands-off' periods during resuscitation. Resuscitation 2003; 58(3):275–276.
36. Eftestol T, Sunde K, Steen PA. Effects of interrupting precordial compressions on the calculated probability of defibrillation success during out-of-hospital cardiac arrest. Circulation 2002; 105(19): 2270–2273.
37. Berg RA, Sanders AB, Kern KB, Hilwig RW, Heidenreich JW, Porter ME, Ewy GA. Adverse hemodynamic effects of interrupting chest compressions for rescue breathing during cardiopulmonary resuscitation for ventricular fibrillation cardiac arrest. Circulation 2001; 104:2465–70.
38. Niemann JT, Stratton SJ, Cruz B, et al. Outcome of out-of-hospital postcountershock asystole and pulseless electrical activity versus primary asystole and pulseless electrical activity. Crit Care Med 2001; 29:2366–2370.
39. Niemann J, Cairns C, Sharma J, Lewis R. Treatment of prolonged ventricular fibrillation. Immediate countershock versus high-dose epinephrine and CPR preceding countershock. Circulation 1992; 85(1): 281–287.
40. Pepe PE, Fowler R, Roppolo L, Wigginton J. Re-appraising the concept of immediate defibrillatory attempts for out-of-hospital ventricular fibrillation. Crit Care 2004; 8:41–45.
41. Menegazzi J, Seaberg D, Yealy D, Davis E, MacLeod B. Combination pharmacotherapy with delayed countershock vs. standard advanced cardiac life support after prolonged ventricular fibrillation. Prehosp Emerg Care 2000; 4(1):31–37.
42. Strohmenger HU, Lindner KJ, Keller A, Lindner IM, Pfenninger EG. Spectral analysis of ventricular fibrillation and closed-chest cardiopulmonary resuscitation. Resuscitation 1996; 33:155–161.
43. Strohmenger HU, Lindner KJ, Brown CG. Analysis of the ventricular fibrillation ECG signal amplitude and frequency parameters as predictors of counter shock success in humans. Chest 1997; 111:584–589.
44. Strohmenger JU, Lindner KH, Keller A. Lindner IM, Pfenninger E, Bothner U. Effects of graded doses of vasopressin on median fibrillation frequency in a porcine model of cardiopulmonary resuscitation: Results of a prospective, randomized, controlled trial. Crit Care Med 1996; 24:1360–1365.
45. Angelos MG, Menegazzi JJ, Callaway CW. Bench to bedside: Resuscitation from prolonged ventricular fibrillation. Acad Emerg Med 2001; 8(9):909–924.
46. Babbs CF, Nadkarni V. Optimizing chest compression to rescue ventilation ratios during one-rescuer CPR by professionals and lay persons: children are not just little adults. Resuscitation 2004; 61(2): 173–181.
47. Wenzel V, Krismer AC, Arntz HR, et al. A comparison of vasopressin and epinephrine for out-of-hospital cardiopulmonary resuscitation. N Engl J Med 2004; 350(2):105–113.
48. Benitez FL, Pepe PE. On-scene supervision. EMS Medical Director's Handbook. Kuehl E. ed. St. Louis, MO: Mosby, 2002, pp. 330–339.
49. Pepe PE. Out-of-hospital resuscitation research: Rationale and strategies for controlled clinical trials. Ann Emerg Med 1993; 22:17–23.
50. Pepe PE, Swor RA, Ornato JP, et al. Resuscitation in the out-of-hospital setting: medical futility criteria for on-scene pronouncement of death. Prehosp Emerg Care 2001; 5:79–87.

34 Animal Models of Resuscitation

Kevin R. Ward, MD
and R. Wayne Barbee, PhD

CONTENTS

INTRODUCTION
UNIQUENESS OF PROBLEMS AND QUESTIONS ASKED IN CA RESEARCH
MODELING VARIABLE
SUMMARY
REFERENCES

INTRODUCTION

The ultimate goal of cardiopulmonary resuscitation (CPR) is the total reanimation of the cardiac arrest (CA) victim back to their pre-arrest status. Much of what we know and do regarding human CPR is based on animal modeling of the many components of CA and its treatment. Ideally, hypotheses regarding mechanisms of injury caused by arrest and treatments to improve outcome should first be tested in robust preclinical models of this disease followed by clinical testing. Although some aspects of the disease and treatment lend themselves to computational, cell culture, and isolated organ modeling, whole animal experimentation remains the standard for preclinical testing *(1–4)*. To this end, the proper design and use of the preclinical model is crucial to ensure that clinical trials are warranted and optimally designed for ultimate validation of the hypotheses.

It is not the purpose of this chapter to review all known animal models of CPR but rather to provide an overview of the principles and challenges of animal modeling of CA and CPR. An understanding of these principles will assist the reader in the interpretation of past, current, and future preclinical literature and in the design of future clinically relevant preclinical models.

UNIQUENESS OF PROBLEMS AND QUESTIONS ASKED IN CA RESEARCH

Similar to other shock states such as hemorrhagic, cardiogenic, and septic shock, the major pathophysiologic challenge that the body faces from CA hinges on the processes associated with ischemia and reperfusion. However, unlike other shock states, the ischemia of CA is absolute and affects each major organ system, especially the heart and

From: *Contemporary Cardiology: Cardiopulmonary Resuscitation*
Edited by: J. P. Ornato and M. A. Peberdy © Humana Press Inc., Totowa, NJ

brain immediately. Thus, there is no active compensatory redistribution of blood flow to the heart and brain during the arrest period. The tissue blood flow produced by CPR is not sufficient to restore oxidative metabolism and membrane potentials to cells routinely and this period of intervention can be viewed as additional ischemia. This degree of total body ischemia is unique to the shock state of CA and the resulting challenges in regards to achieving return of spontaneous circulation (ROSC) and neurological recovery are similarly unique.

It is difficult to draw conclusions from studies of isolated organ ischemia and apply or mix them with those of CA. For example, global brain ischemia is studied widely using non-CA models. These results are applied frequently to CA because it is by far the entity most responsible for producing global brain ischemia (5). On the surface, results from models of isolated global brain ischemia might seem to be fully relevant to the global brain ischemia of CA. However, there may be significant confounding variables (e.g., ischemia to the brain itself), which might negate the major similarity between the two models. CA is associated with total body ischemia, which will drastically change the postresuscitation biochemical milieu that will reperfuse the brain. This includes a tremendous difference in the acid–base status of the blood, creation of other circulating mediators (e.g., cytokines produced by remote organ ischemia), immune and stress regulating events triggered by the arrest, and additional cerebral hypoperfusion that might be caused in the postresuscitation phase from a stunned and dysfunctional heart (6–8). Similar arguments can be made in the case of isolated ischemia-reperfusion models of the heart, which are not routinely perfused or reperfused with acidotic blood returning from ischemic organs. In such models, the heart does not contain the important component of neutrophil and endothelial interactions, which may impact on the final damage caused by the arrest (1,9).

The lack of models that incorporate causative conditions of CA such as coronary artery stenosis and myocardial ischemia or important comorbid conditions such as hypertension, congestive heart failure (CHF), or diabetes also severely hamper to ability to apply results of animal models to clinical CA. As with other models, issues of anesthesia, preparatory surgery, and monitoring are debated to their effects on clinically relevant outcomes or pathophysiologic processes that are being studied. If, for example, brain protein synthesis is believed to be a vitally important cellular process adversely affected by ischemia and reperfusion, the effects of various anesthetics should be considered first (10,11). Ketamine, which is a popular anesthetic used in CA models examining neuronal protein synthesis, depresses protein synthesis severely compared to other anesthetics such as sodium pentobarbital (12). Even what might be deemed minor or inconsequential preparatory issues such as anticoagulation to keep monitoring catheters patent are potentially controversial. The effects of heparin provide significant protection against endothelial cell dysfunction (not simply from its anticoagulant effects) in the ischemia-reperfusion injury of trauma (13,14). It is likely to effect microvascular function in the setting of CA as well and will need further study. Even postsurgical antibiotics such as tetracycline may have downstream protective effects on tissue injury not related to their antimicrobial actions (15).

Researchers must remain cognizant of the unique features of CA and how the downstream effects of other organ systems or model preparation will influence the results. There is perhaps no other experimental model containing as many unknowns as CA.

MODELING VARIABLES

The goal of all animal research is to measure an end-point (dependent variable). The two major end-points in CPR animal research are process and outcome variables *(16)*. Process variables in CPR research are innumerable and measure or describe events at the subcellular, cellular, organ, organ system, or whole-body level. Specific examples of these might include effects of CA on production of reactive oxygen species, the role of protein synthesis in contributing to neuronal necrosis or apoptosis, and the effects of CPR on coronary perfusion pressure (CPP), acid–base chemistry, and regional organ blood flow. Data obtained on process variables helps in solving the puzzle of CA and CPR in terms of pathophysiology and treatment mechanisms. In terms of their effects on human trials, process variables are used infrequently to support human trials examining outcomes. Process variables in animal experimentation are used to refine mechanistic hypotheses, which can be tested in humans to substantiate mechanisms. For example, sampling tissue or hemodynamic parameters during arrest, CPR, or the postresuscitation period may confirm in humans a proposed mechanism of injury or potential benefits of a technique demonstrated in animals.

Outcome variables in resuscitation research usually describe an organism's function after resuscitation with the most common variables being actual ROSC and neurologic outcome. Although debate exists, an argument can be made that human outcome trials are warranted when properly designed animal trials demonstrate an improvement in ROSC even if neurologic outcome is not improved because improvements in the rate of ROSC in humans is the first step toward improving neurologic function after CA resuscitation.

Species

Not all aspects of CA, CPR, and postresuscitation care need to be modeled simultaneously when asking certain questions. However, it would be nice if the same model could be used by all so that questions asked and studied would come as close as possible to the clinically relevant. Ideally, animal models used to study process or outcome variables would be amenable to modeling all aspects of the disease including the ischemia of the arrest itself (down time), the period of low flow produced by CPR, and the postresuscitation period after ROSC. This means that if the cause of the arrest could be incorporated in the model, the model would have the same metabolic profile allowing clinically relevant durations of arrest and resuscitation to be performed. Clearly defined end-points such as neurological outcome could be used if desired. Additionally, the models would incorporate important underlying conditions such as coronary heart disease or comorbid conditions such as hypertension and/or CHF if adult CA is being modeled. Finally, the ability to manipulate the model genetically to assist in identifying and understanding various pathophysiologic mechanisms would greatly add to the science of CA research. Unfortunately, no such model exists and is unlikely to exist for some time to come. When it is finally developed, it is likely to be quite expensive. Despite this, it is incumbent that researchers balance issues of realism and cost to match the importance of the question asked with the most appropriate model.

Models of CA and CPR have included rodents, rabbits, cats, canines, swine, and primates. Each has its advantages and disadvantages ranging from price to complexity. Of these, the models using rodents, canines, and swine predominate. A brief overview of each of these species along with primates follows.

RODENTS

Although rodents are the most commonly studied animal species in biomedical research, their use in CA research is relatively new *(17,18)*. Rats have been used most frequently for CA research. The use of mice has been reported only recently *(19)*. The most obvious advantages of using rodents for CA research are their relatively low cost and maintenance, the controlled genetic variability, and most recently the potential to examine cellular mechanisms of pathophysiology and treatment through the use of genetic knock-out strains in mice and soon for rats.

Rodents are valuable for testing of interventions expected to produce small but important changes in outcome thus necessitating the study of a greater number of animals. They are also valuable for hypothesis testing of process variables at the cellular level. There are, however, very important limitations in the use of rodents for CA research. The anatomy and physiology of rodents are, markedly different from humans. For example, rodents defibrillate themselves spontaneously, and thus are difficult to use if ventricular fibrillation (VF) is the mode of arrest. Another major potential difference that has not been adequately studied is the issue of metabolism and individual organ tolerance to ischemia. Fundamental questions of basal oxygen delivery and consumption of individual organs and the level of oxygen delivery that results in ischemia and accumulation of oxygen debt have not been well defined *(20)*. This lack of information prevents basic comparisons of the effect of arrest times on process and outcome variables between rodents, larger animals, and humans. Is a 4-minute arrest in a rat or mouse equivalent to a 10-minute arrest in humans? Can anything but basic process variables at a cellular level be compared to humans? These are basic questions that should be asked and studied if rodents are to become an important link in the chain of CA research.

Neurological outcome studies in rodents is appealing because they can be trained easily (compared to large animals) to perform tasks requiring memory prior to the arrest and then be tested postarrest. However, provision of postresuscitation care to rodents is difficult in terms of providing clinically relevant ventilation and cardiovascular support. This is an important but often overlooked issue when examining neurological outcome several days after the arrest. Similar to other species, postresuscitation process and outcome variables may be misinterpreted if animals are left to their own resuscitation after CA. For example, something as simple as postresuscitation hypoxemia that occurs from tracheal or bronchial secretions might result in death or a worsened neurologic outcome and negate any positive findings proposed as the result of an experimental intervention.

Rodents can be obtained that are bred to have important comorbid conditions associated with CA such as hypertension and age *(21,22)*. Although tempting, the use of genetic knock-out strains of rodents to study cellular processes associated with CA and CPR should be viewed with caution. Nature will have a tendency to compensate for removal of a gene. Good examples of this are (a) the upregulation of various isoforms of nitric oxide synthase when the gene for the endothelial form of the synthase to maintain microvascular vasodilation is removed, or (b) the increase in capillary density that occurs in response to removal of the gene responsible for making myoglobin to maintain oxygen delivery *(23)*.

In terms of animal husbandry, there are differences between inbred and outbred species of rodents. Viruses and bacterial pathogens such as rat respiratory virus or *Myocplasma*, may produce adverse and unintended experimental outcomes even when clinical signs are not present *(24)*. Thus, attempts should be made to assure that animals are *pathogen-free*. Even what might be minor pre-experimental events such as cold or transport stress should be taken into account when planning experiments examining both process and outcome variables as these events may significantly alter the animals' immune system and response to the stress of surgery.

CANINES

Until the mid-1980s, canines were the favored large animal model used in CA research. Although canine cardiovascular function in general is similar to humans, the canine heart contains extensive collateral circulation. Additionally, the thoracic dimensions of most canines (which are keel chested) are substantially different from humans, making comparison of chest compression techniques to humans difficult. Between breeds there is significant difference in the size and shape of the chest, heart, and brain that may potentially affect outcome. Additionally, some feel that the cardiac output and regional blood flow in canines are higher before and during resuscitation compared to humans *(25)*.

Despite these shortcomings, canines remain a valuable model and there exists extensive neurologic and histopathologic outcome data for the species in the setting of CA and CPR. Specific neurological outcome scores have been developed for canines, which appear to correlate well with histopathology *(26)*. Canines can also be "engineered" (nongenetically) to develop via diet and other means to have clinically relevant causal or comorbid conditions such as atherosclerosis and CHF.

Canines can be obtained from colonies that are *purpose-bred*, which indicates that animals were bred specifically for research in a regulated facility. Such animals are conditioned and should thus be free of clinical disease and vaccinated from such entities as heartworms. Use of canines from local sources such as shelters or pounds is discouraged because uniform health and size among animals cannot be guaranteed.

SWINE

Swine use in CA research has greatly increased and appears to be currently favored over canines for a variety reasons. They are generally less expensive than canines and can be obtained in more uniform sizes and ages for experiments modeling infants, children, and adults. From an anatomical standpoint, the swine thorax has more similarities to humans and the swine heart has less collateral circulation than canines. Humans and swine are also very similar in terms of metabolism and cardiovascular function. The electrophysiology of the heart and the central hemodynamic and organ-specific blood flow of the swine in response to CPR and pharmacology appear to be more similar to humans and may allow for better preclinical studies on techniques and interventions, which take place during the period of CPR than with rodents and canines *(27)*. Similar to canines, the size of swine allows for easier measurement of central hemodyanics such as cardiac output and organ-specific hemodynamics such as regional blood flow than rodents. As with canines, this is especially important in the postresuscitation phase in which a level of critical care similar to humans can be provided to examine longer term variables such as neurological outcome and histopathology or shorter term variables such as myocardial function *(28,29)*.

Similar to canines, swine also allow for the potential advantage of imputing other important variables into a model of CA including coronary atherosclerosis and CHF*(30–33)*. It is also likely that swine will be the first large animal to have its genome sequenced and to undergo knock-out experimentation although the same compensatory caveats will exists with swine as exists with rodents.

Swine can be obtained from herds accredited by a national agency and can be indicated as such by the term *specific-pathogen-free*. However, even in such circumstances, such pre-existing disease states as pneumonia can be present and are difficult to diagnoses unless animals are radiographed prior to use. Use of swine that are contracted out from local farms is discouraged because it will be more difficult to ensure uniform health among animals prior to experimentation.

NONHUMAN PRIMATES

Despite their similarity to humans and ability to be bred to have human cardiac disease, primates have not been used frequently for CA research *(34–36)*. The ability to observe and test for functional neurological changes produced by the arrest and treatment and their extrapolation to humans is enticing. However, the expense of purchase and upkeep of these animals are major deterrents. Additionally, among animal models, primates will have the greatest degree of genetic variability that may or may not be valuable when looking for an initial treatment effect. Many CA clinical trials have been based on data obtained from species other than nonhuman primates *(37–40)*. It is unclear what benefit or changes would have occurred if nonhuman primates had been used prior to human trials in these instances.

Lessons and Examples From the Literature

Following are a number of studies that have been performed in CA research, which serve to stress the importance of clinical relevance and the sometimes counterintuitive results of clinical studies that were not supported by animal studies.

Perhaps one of the greatest stumbling blocks in CA research is the clinical relevance of the model chosen. If outcome variables of an animal model such as ROSC and neurologic outcome are chosen to mimic out-of-hospital CA as a prelude to clinical studies, as many clinical variables should be incorporated as possible that mimic the clinical scenario so that any improvement in the outcome variable is more likely to be observed in a clinical study.

This is not specific to CA research but permeates research in other shock states. For example, models of hemorrhagic shock examining the effects of a treatment on outcome can be criticized because none contains all of the common clinical elements of severe soft tissue injury, pain, hypoxemia, resuscitation with stored packed cells, prolonged mechanical ventilation, and potentially intra-abdominal hypertension in addition to volume hemorrhage leading to severe oxygen debt. In this situation, events concomitant to hemorrhage that occur in the individual of multisystem trauma as a result of both injury and treatment have the potential to effect outcome profoundly. For instance, stored packed red cells (commonly used in the clinical setting) have been demonstrated to adversely effect microcirculatory tissue oxygen delivery adversely compared to citrated or heparinized fresh whole blood (never clinically used *[41]*). Pain from sever soft tissue injury has been demonstrated to significantly increase oxygen consumption and decrease splanchnic blood flow, both of which have the potential to potentiate cumulative oxygen debt *(42,43)*. This can be compounded by increases in intra-abdominal pressure, which further decreases splanchnic perfusion and cardiac output *(44)*. Prolonged (>24 hours) mechanical ventilation is injurious to the lungs, increasing the chance of acute lung injury after hemorrhage *(45)*. It is easy to envision how a model designed to test the ability of a new blood substitute vs crystalloid fluid and fresh hemorrhaged whole blood on 24 to 48 hours survival could significantly underestimate the severity of injury and illness if the model was one of simple pressure hemorrhage. Significant benefits of the blood substitute found in such a simple experiment may not be present when applied to the more complex everyday clinical scenario. Failure to model all of the above entities is also likely to be responsible for why there are no animal models of trauma-induced multisystem organ failure.

Similar disparities exist when modeling out-of-hospital CA. Epinephrine dosing is a prime example. The original recommendation by the American Heart Association (AHA) that epinephrine be administered to adults at a dose of 1 mg was based on the studies of Redding who used 1 mg of epinephrine on 10-kg weight dogs (46). Without critical evaluation, this dose was accepted before realizing that the human dose may not have been properly extrapolated from animal data. This in turn led to a large number of animal studies that examined the effects of much higher doses of epinephrine. The results of these animal studies demonstrated higher doses of epinephrine significantly improved variables such as CPP, which are associated with increases in ROSC (47,48). However, when tested in humans, high-dose epinephrine failed to improve outcome (37). Close examination of the clinical studies revealed several important issues that may not have been taken into account in animal studies (49). Chief among these was the timing of administration. Whereas most animal studies examined the use of the drug approx 10 minutes after onset of CA, analysis of human trails found that the time to first drug administration averaged 18 to 20 minutes, a time almost double that of animals. Additionally, postresuscitation care of humans after CA is not standardized and indeed had not been studied at that point in animals to understand what affects high doses of catecholamines would have on postresuscitation myocardial function and microcirculatory blood flow (50). Clinicians were ill prepared to treat the postresuscitation systemic effects of massive catecholamine dosing that were found to produce significant tissue oxygen defects (51,52).

Another major issue not taken into account was whether higher doses of epinephrine would be able to increase myocardial blood flow in the face of significant coronary artery stenosis. This is an important question because the majority of adult arrest victims will have significant coronary artery disease (CAD) and a very important segment of these victims will have had a myocardial infarction (MI) as a cause of their arrest (53). In a remarkable series of studies performed by Kern and colleagues, coronary artery lesions of 50% or less were shown to drastically reduce distal myocardial blood flow during CPR for a given perfusion pressure (54–56). Although the effect of high-dose epinephrine was not examined in these studies, a distinct possibility exists that the benefits demonstrated in previous animal models of CPR without coronary lesions would have been less impressive and may not have reached significance if they had been studied in models incorporating coronary artery stenosis. Additionally, MI-induced VF is rarely modeled (57). Instead, VF is induced electrically. The ability to obtain ROSC in an infarcted heart with significant CAD and a prolonged post-arrest predrug administration time of 20 minutes will be much more difficult than that of a nondiseased, noninjured pre-arrest heart with a post-arrest predrug administration time of 10 minutes. Therapies that significantly improve ROSC and neurological outcome in the former model should have much less chance of failure in a clinical trial.

Use of asphyxial models that correspond to the clinical experience presents similar challenges and pitfalls in attempting not to underestimate the severity of the insult.

Rodent models of asphyxia have used asphyxia times of 8 to 10 minutes to produce actual CA times of only 4 to 8 minutes (18,58,59). With the exception of drowning, asphyxia (at least in adults) is likely to be much more prolonged and produced by more insidious processes as exacerbations of acute airway diseases such as asthma or emphysema in which the individual fatigues and finally becomes hypoxemic enough to arrest. In these settings, the accumulated oxygen debts of the individuals will be significantly higher than the short durations of total asphyxia and arrest produced in current preclinical models. Additionally, arrest times prior to interventions such as drug therapy will be prolonged much more clinically (49).

Using vasoactive agents again as an example, animal studies can be designed in such as way as not to see an affect at all or to see something artificial. Both human and animal studies have demonstrated the need to create a minimum CPP for ROSC to occur. In order to demonstrate that the new agent is helpful in achieving critical CPP, baseline chest compressions should be performed to create the suboptimal range of CPP that occurs clinically (60–62). If, however, chest compressions are performed in the animal model and in of themselves produce a CPP above the critical threshold for ROSC and produce ROSC without the need for exogenous vasoactive agents, it becomes less likely that the vasoactive agent(s) being tested will be demonstrated to superior over each other (63). In fact, it might be possible in this model to find detrimental effects of one agent over another that would not be found ordinarily because administration of the agent such as high-dose epinephrine in this model would be similar to producing a model of simple catecholamine overdose.

A much overlooked part of animal models of CA is the issue and importance of modeling the postresuscitation phase of care. For as much emphasis as has been placed on demonstrating the ability of experimental agents or techniques to improve neurological outcome, it is amazing how much this aspect of modeling has been neglected because neurologic outcome cannot be predicted immediately upon ROSC but instead takes several days to determine. The postresuscitation care of animals has ranged from literally extubating comatose animals within several hours of ROSC and placing them into cages to providing clinically relevant intensive care from the onset of ROSC and lasting 96 hours (26,63–65). Failure to provide aggressive postresuscitation care to animals may lead to the inability to observe the ability of an intervention delivered during CPR to improve ROSC and long-term outcome because poor postresuscitation care may increases mortality or morbidity as a result of cardiovascular or respiratory events that would have ordinarily been avoided with proper monitoring in the clinical setting. Conversely, aggressive postresuscitation care from a cardiovascular standpoint immediately after ROSC my also lead to the inability to observe differences in outcome because in the clinical environment, it may take several hours to instrument patients properly and optimize cardiovascular performance and cerebral blood flow.

Finally, there are animal models demonstrating benefit of an intervention on outcome that have also significantly underestimated the benefit of the intervention in humans. A prime example of this has been in the large animal studies of hypothermia to improve neurological outcome after CA. A significant body of work examining the effects of postresuscitation hypothermia in canines demonstrated that in order to be effective in improving neurological outcome, hypothermia had to be instituted in less than 15 minutes after ROSC (65). This would present many challenges in applying hypothermia as a clinical postresuscitation treatment. Despite these findings, several large clinical trials demonstrated a significant improvement in neurological outcome when hypothermia was instituted in the postresuscitation phase, even when the therapy could not be immediately instituted and the time to reach target temperature was several hours longer than animal studies suggested would be effective *(39,66,67)*. It was also demonstrated that delays in instituting hypothermia in rat models of CA did not negate its effectiveness *(68)*. These findings appear to violate the hierarchical approach to clinical trials in which one would originally screen a therapy in rodents followed by movement to a higher species such as canines or swine, and then finally move to a clinical trial. Why canines demonstrated little improvement in neurological outcome after delayed cooling remains a mystery but again points out that there is no perfect preclinical model.

Utstein Guidelines

Historically, it has been difficult to compare the results of clinical studies with each other, the results of laboratory studies with each other and the results of clinical and laboratory studies to each other. One of the major reasons for this difficulty is the lack of standardization and the use of nonuniform terminology. In 1990, an international conference on the topic of out of hospital resuscitation was held at the Utstein Abbey in Norway to discuss the lack of standardized nomenclature and language in clinical research reports. That same year, an additional meeting was held to develop a consensus. This resulted in development of a uniform style of reporting and definitions of clinical resuscitation research and was termed the *Utstein Style (69)*. That same year, the European Academy of Anaesthesiology developed a similar approach for animal models that led to a series of conferences and workshops culminating in 1996 with an Utstein-Style guidelines for uniform reporting of laboratory CPR research *(70,71)*. In a survey performed by Idris and colleagues, it had been noted that lack of simple uniform definitions and item reporting made comparison between studies difficult. These included failure to define and report such basic but important issues as minute ventilation, CPP and ROSC *(72)*. The aim of Utstein-type guidelines for laboratory study were not to encourage or discourage one species or model over another but simply to include enough uniform reporting information concerning aspects of the laboratory study to allow its comparison with other published studies. The guidelines are centered around nine templates and include the following:

- Study design
- Subjects
- Preparation of animals
- Methods for monitoring
- Experimental protocol
- Outcome variables
- Analytical approach
- Results
- Discussion and conclusions *(71)*

These templates cover almost every conceivable aspect of a laboratory CPR experiment using animals and ranges form living conditions of the animals prior to the experiment to mode of ventilation to comparing the statistical and biologic significance of results. However, despite being published in 1996, the extent of adherence to these guidelines remains unclear.

SUMMARY

In the quest to develop successful treatments for CA, animal research will remain an invaluable asset. However, researchers must critically evaluate the appropriateness of the model used based on the clinical relevance of the question asked as it relates to process vs outcome variables to be assessed. When placed in the greater context of the actual clinical experience, more robust animal models are likely to be created. Clinical trials based on such data will hopefully be at less risk of failure.

REFERENCES

1. Angelos MG, Murray HN, Gorsline RT, Klawitter PF. Glucose, insulin and potassium (GIK) during reperfusion mediates improved myocardial bioenergetics. Resuscitation 2002; 55:329–336.
2. O'Neil BJ, Alousi SS, White BC, Rafols JA. Ultrastructural consequences of radical damage before and after differentiation of neuroblastoma B-104 cells. Acta Neuropathol (Berl) 1996; 92:75–89.
3. Babbs CF, Thelander K. Theoretically optimal duty cycles for chest and abdominal compression during external cardiopulmonary resuscitation. Acad Emerg Med 1995; 2:698–707.
4. Babbs CF, Ralston SH, Geddes LA. Theoretical advantages of abdominal counterpulsation in CPR as demonstrated in a simple electrical model of the circulation. Ann Emerg Med 1984; 13(Pt 1):660–671.
5. Traystman RJ. Animal models of focal and global cerebral ischemia. Ilar J 2003; 44:85–95.
6. Schultz CH, Rivers EP, Feldkamp CS, Goad EG, Smithline HA, Martin GB, et al. A characterization of hypothalamic-pituitary-adrenal axis function during and after human cardiac arrest. Crit Care Med 1993; 21:1339–1347.
7. Basha MA, Meyer GS, Kunkel SL, Strieter RM, Rivers EP, Popovich J. Presence of tumor necrosis factor in humans undergoing cardiopulmonary resuscitation with return of spontaneous circulation. J Crit Care 1991; 6:185–189.
8. Feuerstein GZ, Liu T, Barone FC. Cytokines, inflammation, and brain injury: role of tumor necrosis factor-alpha. Cerebrovasc Brain Metab Rev 1994; 6:341–360.
9. Frangogiannis NG, Smith CW, Entman ML. The inflammatory response in myocardial infarction. Cardiovasc Res 2002; 53:31–47.
10. Sullivan JM, Alousi SS, Hikade KR, et al. Insulin induces dephosphorylation of eukaryotic initiation factor 2alpha and restores protein synthesis in vulnerable hippocampal neurons after transient brain ischemia. J Cereb Blood Flow Metab 1999; 19:1010–1019.
11. Krause GS, Tiffany BR. Suppression of protein synthesis in the reperfused brain. Stroke 1993; 24:747–755; discussion 55,56.
12. Reid KH, Paskitti M, Guo SZ, Schmelzer T, Iyer V. Experience with ketamine and sodium pentobarbital as anesthetics in a rat model of cardiac arrest and resuscitation. Resuscitation 2003; 57:201–210.
13. Rana MW, Singh G, Wang P, Ayala A, Zhou M, Chaudry IH. Protective effects of preheparinization on the microvasculature during and after hemorrhagic shock. J Trauma 1992; 32:420–426.
14. Wang P, Ba ZF, Chaudry IH. Endothelial cell dysfunction occurs after hemorrhage in nonheparinized but not in preheparinized models. J Surg Res 1993; 54:499–506.
15. Tikka TM, Koistinaho JE. Minocycline provides neuroprotection against N-methyl-D-aspartate neurotoxicity by inhibiting microglia. J Immunol 2001; 166:7527–7533.
16. Yealy DM. How much "significance" is significant? The transition from animal models to human trials in resuscitation research. Ann Emerg Med 1993; 22:11–16.
17. von Planta I, Weil MH, von Planta M, Bisera J, et al. Cardiopulmonary resuscitation in the rat. J Appl Physiol 1988; 65:2641–2647.
18. Katz L, Ebmeyer U, Safar P, Radovsky A, Neumar R. Outcome model of asphyxial cardiac arrest in rats. J Cereb Blood Flow Metab 1995; 15:1032–1039.
19. Song L, Weil MH, Tang W, Sun S, Pellis T. Cardiopulmonary resuscitation in the mouse. J Appl Physiol 2002; 93:1222–1226.
20. Dawson TH. Engineering design of the cardiovascular system of mammals. Englewood Cliffs, NJ: Prentice Hall, 1991.
21. Takiguchi Y, Wada K, Nakashima M. Hemodynamic effects on thrombogenesis and platelet aggregation in spontaneously hypertensive rats. Clin Exp Hypertens 1993; 15:197–208.
22. Akiyama K, Tanaka R, Sato M, Takeda N. Cognitive dysfunction and histological findings in adult rats one year after whole brain irradiation. Neurol Med Chir (Tokyo) 2001; 41:590–598.

23. Godecke A, Schrader J. Adaptive mechanisms of the cardiovascular system in transgenic mice—lessons from eNOS and myoglobin knockout mice. Basic Res Cardiol 2000; 95:492–498.

24. Damy SB, de Lourdes Higuchi M, et al. Coinfection of laboratory rats with Mycoplasma pulmonis and Chlamydia pneumoniae. Contemp Top Lab Anim Sci 2003; 42:52–56.

25. Halperin HR, Tsitlik JE, Guerci AD, et al. Determinants of blood flow to vital organs during cardiopulmonary resuscitation in dogs. Circulation 1986; 73:539–550.

26. Leonov Y, Sterz F, Safar P, Radovsky A. Moderate hypothermia after cardiac arrest of 17 minutes in dogs. Effect on cerebral and cardiac outcome. Stroke 1990; 21:1600–1606.

27. Gross DR. Animal Models in Cardiovascular Research. Boston, MA: Kluwer Academic Publishers, 1985.

28. Kern KB, Hilwig RW, Rhee KH, Berg RA. Myocardial dysfunction after resuscitation from cardiac arrest: an example of global myocardial stunning. J Am Coll Cardiol 1996; 28:232–240.

29. Wenzel V, Lindner KH, Krismer AC, et al. Survival with full neurologic recovery and no cerebral pathology after prolonged cardiopulmonary resuscitation with vasopressin in pigs. J Am Coll Cardiol 2000; 35:527–533.

30. Bocan TM. Animal models of atherosclerosis and interpretation of drug intervention studies. Curr Pharm Des 1998; 4:37–52.

31. King MK, Coker ML, Goldberg A, et al. Selective matrix metalloproteinase inhibition with developing heart failure: effects on left ventricular function and structure. Circ Res 2003; 92:177–185.

32. Argenziano M, Dean DA, Moazami N, et al. Inhaled nitric oxide is not a myocardial depressant in a porcine model of heart failure. J Thorac Cardiovasc Surg 1998; 115:700–708.

33. Yarbrough WM, Spinale FG. Large animal models of congestive heart failure: A critical step in translating basic observations into clinical applications. J Nucl Cardiol 2003; 10:77–86.

34. Gilroy BA, Rockoff MA, Dunlop BJ, Shapiro HM. Cardiopulmonary resuscitation in the nonhuman primate. J Am Vet Med Assoc 1980; 177:867–869.

35. Eshel G, Safar P, Radovsky A, Stezoski SW. Hyperthermia-induced cardiac arrest in monkeys: limited efficacy of standard CPR. Aviat Space Environ Med 1997; 68:415–420.

36. Malinow MR. The role of nonhuman primates in research on atherosclerosis regression- hypothetical mechanisms implicated in regression. Artery 1981; 9:2–11.

37. Brown CG, Martin DR, Pepe PE, et al. A comparison of standard-dose and high-dose epinephrine in cardiac arrest outside the hospital. The Multicenter High-Dose Epinephrine Study Group. N Engl J Med 1992; 327:1051–1055.

38. Randomized clinical study of thiopental loading in comatose survivors of cardiac arrest. Brain Resuscitation Clinical Trial I Study Group. N Engl J Med 1986; 314:397–403.

39. Mild therapeutic hypothermia to improve the neurologic outcome after cardiac arrest. N Engl J Med 2002; 346:549–556.

40. Halperin HR, Tsitlik JE, Gelfand M, et al. A preliminary study of cardiopulmonary resuscitation by circumferential compression of the chest with use of a pneumatic vest. N Engl J Med 1993; 329:762–768.

41. van Bommel J, de Korte D, Lind A, et al. The effect of the transfusion of stored RBCs on intestinal microvascular oxygenation in the rat. Transfusion 2001; 41:1515–1523.

42. Mackway-Jones K, Foex BA, Kirkman E, Little RA. Modification of the cardiovascular response to hemorrhage by somatic afferent nerve stimulation with special reference to gut and skeletal muscle blood flow. J Trauma 1999; 47:481–485.

43. Rady MY, Little RA, Edwards JD, Kirkman E, Faithful S. The effect of nociceptive stimulation on the changes in hemodynamics and oxygen transport induced by hemorrhage in anesthetized pigs. J Trauma 1991; 31:617–621; discussion 21–22.

44. Saggi BH, Sugerman HJ, Ivatury RR, Bloomfield GL. Abdominal compartment syndrome. J Trauma 1998; 45:597–609.

45. Slutsky AS. Lung injury caused by mechanical ventilation. Chest 1999; 116(Suppl):9S–15S.

46. Redding JS, Pearson JW. Evaluation of drugs for cardiac resuscitation. Anesthesiology 1963; 24:203–207.

47. Hoekstra JW, Rinnert K, Van Ligten P, Neumar R, Werman HA, Brown CG. The effectiveness of bystander CPR in an animal model [see comments]. Ann Emerg Med 1990; 19:881–886.

48. Brown CG, Werman HA, Davis EA, Hobson J, Hamlin RL. The effects of graded doses of epinephrine on regional myocardial blood flow during cardiopulmonary resuscitation in swine. Circulation 1987; 75:491–497.

49. Hoekstra JW, Banks JR, Martin DR, et al. Effect of first-responder automated defibrillation on time to therapeutic interventions during out-of-hospital cardiac arrest. The Multicenter High Dose Epinephrine Study Group. Ann Emerg Med 1993; 22:1247–1253.

50. Tang W, Weil MH, Sun S, Noc M, Yang L, Gazmuri RJ. Epinephrine increases the severity of postresuscitation myocardial dysfunction. Circulation 1995; 92:3089–3093.

51. Rivers EP, Wortsman J, Rady MY, Blake HC, McGeorge FT, Buderer NM. The effect of the total cumulative epinephrine dose administered during human CPR on hemodynamic, oxygen transport, and use variables in the postresuscitation period. Chest 1994; 106:1499–1507.

52. Rivers EP, Rady MY, Martin GB, et al. Venous hyperoxia after cardiac arrest. Characterization of a defect in systemic oxygen use. Chest 1992; 102:1787–1793.

53. Zahger D. Immediate coronary angiography in survivors of out-of-hospital cardiac arrest. N Engl J Med 1997; 337:1321,1322.

54. Kern KB, Lancaster L, Goldman S, Ewy GA. The effect of coronary artery lesions on the relationship between coronary perfusion pressure and myocardial blood flow during cardiopulmonary resuscitation in pigs. Am Heart J 1990; 120:324–333.

55. Kern KB, Ewy GA. Minimal coronary stenoses and left ventricular blood flow during CPR. Ann Emerg Med 1992; 21:1066–1072.

56. Kern KB, de la Guardia B, Ewy GA. Myocardial perfusion during cardiopulmonary resuscitation (CPR): effects of 10, 25 and 50% coronary stenoses. Resuscitation 1998; 38:107–111.

57. Angelos MG, Gaddis ML, Gaddis GM, Leasure JE. Improved survival and reduced myocardial necrosis with cardiopulmonary bypass reperfusion in a canine model of coronary occlusion and cardiac arrest. Ann Emerg Med 1990; 19:1122–1128.

58. Neumar RW, Bircher NG, Sim KM, et al. Epinephrine and sodium bicarbonate during CPR following asphyxial cardiac arrest in rats. Resuscitation 1995; 29:249–263.

59. Mayr VD, Wenzel V, Voelckel WG, et al. Developing a vasopressor combination in a pig model of adult asphyxial cardiac arrest. Circulation 2001; 104:1651–1656.

60. Paradis NA, Martin GB, Goetting MG, et al. Simultaneous aortic, jugular bulb, and right atrial pressures during cardiopulmonary resuscitation in humans. Insights into mechanisms [see comments]. Circulation 1989; 80:361–368.

61. Paradis NA, Martin GB, Rivers EP, et al. Coronary perfusion pressure and the return of spontaneous circulation in human cardiopulmonary resuscitation. JAMA 1990; 263:1106–1113.

62. Paradis NA, Martin GB, Rosenberg J, et al. The effect of standard- and high-dose epinephrine on coronary perfusion pressure during prolonged cardiopulmonary resuscitation. JAMA 1991; 265:1139–1144.

63. Berg RA, Otto CW, Kern KB, et al. A randomized, blinded trial of high-dose epinephrine versus standard-dose epinephrine in a swine model of pediatric asphyxial cardiac arrest. Crit Care Med 1996; 24:1695–1700.

64. Kern KB, Carter AB, Showen RL, et al. Comparison of mechanical techniques of cardiopulmonary resuscitation: survival and neurologic outcome in dogs. Am J Emerg Med 1987; 5:190–195.

65. Kuboyama K, Safar P, Radovsky A, Tisherman SA, Stezoski SW, Alexander H. Delay in cooling negates the beneficial effect of mild resuscitative cerebral hypothermia after cardiac arrest in dogs: a prospective, randomized study. Crit Care Med 1993; 21:1348–1358.

66. Bernard SA, Jones BM, Horne MK. Clinical trial of induced hypothermia in comatose survivors of out-of- hospital cardiac arrest. Ann Emerg Med 1997; 30:146–153.

67. Bernard SA, Gray TW, Buist MD, et al. Treatment of comatose survivors of out-of-hospital cardiac arrest with induced hypothermia. N Engl J Med 2002; 346:557–563.

68. Hickey RW, Ferimer H, Alexander HL, et al. Delayed, spontaneous hypothermia reduces neuronal damage after asphyxial cardiac arrest in rats. Crit Care Med 2000; 28:3511,3516.

69. Cummins RO, Chamberlain D, Hazinski MF, et al. Recommended guidelines for reviewing, reporting, and conducting research on in-hospital resuscitation: the in-hospital 'Utstein style'. American Heart Association. Circulation 1997; 95:2213–2239.

70. Aitkenhead AR, Bahr SJ, Cavaliere F, et.al. Animal research in cardiopulmonary resuscation: revised recommendations of a working party of the European Academy of Anaesthesiology. Eur J Anaestheiol 1990; 7:83–87.

71. Idris AH, Becker LB, Ornato JP, et al. Utstein-style guidelines for uniform reporting of laboratory CPR research. A statement for healthcare professionals from a task force of the American Heart Association, the American College of Emergency Physicians, the American College of Cardiology, the European Resuscitation Council, the Heart and Stroke Foundation of Canada, the Institute of Critical Care Medicine, the Safar Center for Resuscitation Research, and the Society for Academic Emergency Medicine. Writing Group. Circulation 1996; 94:2324–2336.

72. Idris AH, Becker LB, Wenzel V, Fuerst RS, Gravenstein N. Lack of uniform definitions and reporting in laboratory models of cardiac arrest: a review of the literature and a proposal for guidelines. Ann Emerg Med 1994; 23:9–16.

35 Design of Clinical Trials Relating to Medical Emergencies

Alfred Hallstrom, PhD

INTRODUCTION

The purpose of any clinical trial is to evaluate treatment(s) in an at-risk population. Clinical trial design principles are the same regardless of the setting. Three very readable books that cover fundamentals and specifics of clinical trial design are those by Friedman, Furberg, and DeMets *(1);* Meinert *(2)*; and Pocock *(3)*. Clinical trial design is much more than inclusion/exclusion criteria, sample size, randomization to treatment arm, and counting endpoints. Defining and monitoring data collection, monitoring and maintaining compliance, and monitoring and reporting potential adverse events are often the most demanding design aspects.

The details of clinical trial design follow from three general concerns: ethics, believability, and cost. Details that are partially or entirely driven by ethics include the following:

- Consent
- Randomization schemes (one-to-one, many-to-one, play the winner)
- Monitoring (Data and Safety Monitoring Boards, stopping rules)
- One-sided vs two-sided test of the null hypothesis (H_0)
- Control arm (placebo, standard of care)
- Sampling

Believability is largely based on sufficient evidence and a probabilistic foundation for making conclusions. Aspects of design that follow from the requirement of a probabilistic foundation include the following:

- Sampling (registry)
- Randomization (blocking, weighted allocation)

From: *Contemporary Cardiology: Cardiopulmonary Resuscitation*
Edited by: J. P. Ornato and M. A. Peberdy © Humana Press Inc., Totowa, NJ

- Intention to treat
- Unbiased outcome measurement (blinding)

The need for adequate evidence will influence design issues such as:

- Sample size
- Type 1 error (finding a treatment effect when there is none) – α-level
- Type 2 error (not finding a treatment effect when there is one) – β-level (or power = $1-\beta$)
  - § Compliance
  - § Efficacy analysis (analysis based on therapy received)
- Data (type, extent, accuracy)

Unfortunately, substantial resources are needed to conduct a clinical trial. No trial should be begun without an estimate of the cost, if for no other reason than to ensure that the trial can be completed. Details that may be largely dictated by cost include the following:

- Selection (inclusion/exclusion criteria)
- Length of trial
- Choice of primary endpoint (surrogate, composite)
- Secondary endpoints (cost, quality of life)
- Basic design (crossover, matched-pairs, two-sample, many-sample, groups)
- Covariate ascertainment (what, how, quality)
- Subgroups
- Mechanisms

GENERAL COMMENTS ON TRIAL DESIGN
Ethics

CONTROL ARM

In the emergency setting, there is little time or opportunity for a placebo effect on the patient. Use of a placebo would be solely to blind study personnel so to avoid biased use of concomitant therapy and bias in outcome assessment. Thus, in the emergency setting, use of a placebo must not reduce the efficacy of standard of care, because there is no potential for an offsetting placebo effect.

RANDOMIZATION SCHEMES

Clinical trials should be completed as quickly as possible and at the same time should protect the safety of the trial participants. In the emergency setting, outcomes are essentially immediate and one-to-one randomization will usually be most efficient, that is, will result in the shortest trial. Play-the-winner strategies (which weight the randomization toward the therapy that is currently winning) result in more patients being placed on the superior arm, generally at the expense of extending the duration of the trial with only modest reduction in the number of bad outcomes in the inferior treatment arm. Many-to-one allocation schemes cannot be based on ethical arguments because such use would actually suggest lack of equipoise on the part of the investigators. However, if a new therapy is to be compared to a well-known standard therapy, enrolling two or three patients to the new therapy per patient enrolled to standard may be desirable to obtain more precise information about secondary and adverse endpoints of the new therapy.

DATA AND SAFETY MONITORING

Trials with mortality or serious morbid outcomes must be monitored on an ongoing basis for safety and efficacy of the therapies *(4–9)*. To preserve objectivity, the Data

Safety Monitoring Board (DSMB) should consist of persons not vested in the conduct or outcome of the trial *(5)*. At minimum, the DSMB should include a statistician with clinical trials experience, a generalist with clinical trial experience, and a person with special expertise in the specific subject matter of the study *(4)*. Because frequent assessment of the efficacy of the treatments increases the likelihood of observing a large but chance difference (Fig. 1), formal stopping rules are usually employed to maintain the Type I error rate or α-level *(10–12)*. The effect of these rules is, on average, to terminate trials early when there is, in fact, a substantial treatment difference at little cost in terms of the total length of the trial should the rules not come into play. From the perspective of minimizing trial subject exposure to the inferior therapy, these rules will tend to be much more efficacious than play-the-winner allocation strategies. A simple monitoring rule and its consequences are shown in Table 1. So-called futility rules based on conditional power (the probability of observing a difference if the alternative is true given the data observed to date) may also be used *(13,14)*. These rules tend to stop the trial if the conditional power becomes quite low. Although futility rules increase the type II error rate, the increase is very small compared with the savings in cost and participant time that can accrue in a study that is unlikely to impact future therapies. A simple futility rule and its consequences are shown in Table 2.

SAMPLING

Certain groups (e.g., minorities, rural dwellers, or older persons) can be oversampled to maximize the ability to determine whether the study results can be extrapolated to the entire population.

Believability—Probabilistic Function

SAMPLING

It is desirable for results of a completed trial to be applicable to the population at large. Generalizability is usually valid if the study participants were selected randomly from the at-risk population. Generally, this cannot be done and even if it can, nonconsenting patients may be quite distinct from consenting patients. Generalizability of trial results can be evaluated to the extent that the population screened can be defined clearly and a simple registry maintained of eligible consenting and nonconsenting patients. Fortunately, in the emergency setting, exemption of consent will result in almost full sampling in a, hopefully, representative sample of communities. Thus, for trials of emergency care, the key sampling issue is selection of which communities should participate.

RANDOMIZATION

The fundamental basis for inference is the process of randomization. The hundreds of millions of dollars spent on epidemiologic studies of the relationship between smoking and cancer and smoking and heart disease were necessary because of the lack of randomization, creating a milieu in which results could be challenged easily. A few simple, moderately sized, randomized trials would have provided unassailable evidence and in a much shorter time frame.

Even with randomization, one might, by chance, encounter unequal allocation of risk in the randomized groups. This can be partially controlled through a technique called blocking to ensure that in certain "natural" strata, approximately equal numbers of participants are randomized to both arms. For example, if there are several centers participating in the study, blocking on center will ensure that each center has patients participating in both arms. If the enrollment will occur over a substantial number of years,

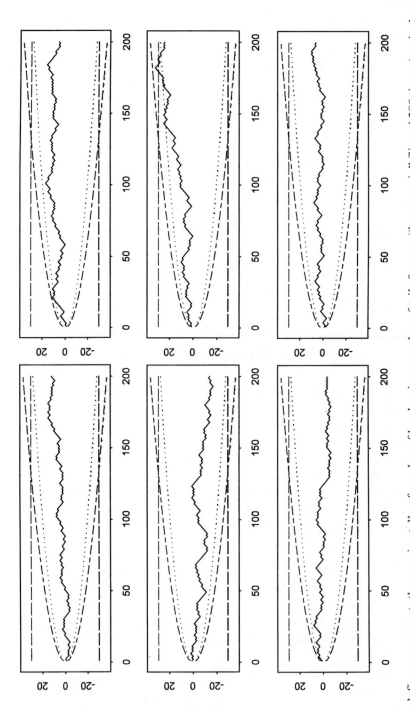

Fig. 1. Each figure represents the ongoing tally of number of heads minus number of tails from an "honest coin" flipped 200 times (equivalent to a "no difference" trial enrolling 200 patients). The dotted curve represents the "nominal" 0.05 boundary for chance. For example, if the tally was only "looked at" at, say, the 100th flip, the tally would fall outside that curve only 1 in 20 times (in this case it is 0 out of 6). The other curves represent boundaries (liberal, and conservative) that adjust for looking at the tally after every flip. Notice that the nominal boundary is exceeded in three of the six trials, although the liberal boundary is just attained (rather early) in one of the six trials and the conservative boundary is exceeded (rather late) in one of the six trials.

Table 1
Effect of Sequential Monitoring on Sample Size
for a Conservative and a Liberal Monitoring Boundary

Monitoring Plan (equally spaced looks)

Number of looks	Boundary[a]	Maximum sample size	Actual treatment effect		
			0.3	0.4	0.5
			Expected sample enrollment		
1	1.96	707	707	707	707
2[b]	2.8, 1.98	712	670	638	577
2[c]	2.18, 2.18	785	687	600	592
3[b]	3.47, 2.45, 2.00	719	662	607	569
3[c]	2.29, 2.29, 2.29	824	691	571	564

Binomial outcome: Control rate = 0.3, Hypothesized alternative rate = 0.4, α = 0.05, power = 0.8, two-sided, sequential monitoring for rejecting null only

[a] If absolute value of Z statistic exceeds value, stop for difference.

[b] Conservative boundary (i.e., requires substantial difference to stop early).

[c] Liberal boundary (i.e., requires moderate difference to stop early).

Table 2
Effect of Futility Monitoring on Sample Size
for a Conservative and a Liberal Monitoring Boundary

Monitoring Plan (equally spaced looks)

Number of looks	Futility boundary[a]	Maximum sample size	Actual treatment effect		
			0.2	0.3	0.4
			Expected sample enrollment		
2[b]	0.1 (300)	600	309	429	492
2[c]	0.4 (300)	600	303	401	483
3[b]	−0.5 (200), 0.1 (400)	700	237	458	491
3[c]	−0.2 (200), 0.5 (400)	700	224	391	476

Binomial outcome, Control rate = .3, Hypothesized alternative rate = .4, α = 0.05, power = 0.8, 1-sided, sequential monitoring for rejecting null using conservative boundary, sequential monitoring for futility (little chance of rejecting the null by end of study).

[a] If Z statistic is less than value, stop for futility; value in ( ) is when (in terms of number of enrolled patients) look is made.

[b] Conservative boundary (i.e., requires trend in opposite direction or very close to null to stop early).

[c] Liberal boundary (i.e., requires trend moderately close to null to stop early).

blocking on year of entry will ensure that approximately equal numbers of patients are randomized to each arm in each time period. In the emergency setting, blocking on season and/or weekend may be relevant. Blocking is also sometimes done within important clinical confounders. One must be careful not to block randomization on too many strata as this can lead to a higher likelihood of imbalance in total numbers between the two arms *(15)*. Weighting the randomization allocation according to the accumulated risk factors in the two treatment arms has also been advocated. This approach is generally unsuitable for the emergency setting because it requires time to process. Moreover, imbalance in measured risk factors can be at least partially addressed through analytic techniques.

INTENTION TO TREAT

Although virtually everyone accepts randomization as a keystone to inference, not everyone accepts intention to treat (analysis according to which arm the patient was randomized to as opposed to the actual treatment that the patient received) as the appropriate method of analysis *(16,17)*. For example, it is difficult to understand why a patient who dies after randomization but prior to any treatment being instituted should be counted as an endpoint in the arm to which the patient was randomized; or if a patient was randomized to therapy A but inadvertently was given therapy B why that patient should not be analyzed in treatment arm B. However, not receiving the randomized therapy is almost never a haphazard proposition, but instead is as a result of very specific biases. For example, if therapy A takes three times as long to initiate as therapy B, one might expect three times as many patients to die prior to initiation of therapy A than prior to initiation of therapy B, thus eliminating more of the high-risk patients from the therapy A arm if one does not include such patients in the analysis.

UNBIASED OUTCOME MEASUREMENT

Unfortunately, if there is any subjectivity at all possible in the outcome measurement, humans seem by nature inclined to measure what they want to see. As noted earlier, there is no time for a placebo effect in the emergency setting. However, there may well be a need for a placebo to mask study personnel to the therapy assignment, thus preventing biased outcome measurement. Death, but not mode of death, is a nonsubjective endpoint, but an outcome measure based on death can still be biased if outcome ascertainment is not complete. Because death—or rather its opposite—survival, is the important measure in most emergency trials, substantial effort must be devoted to ensure complete ascertainment.

Believability—Adequate Evidence

SAMPLE SIZE

The cornerstone of adequate evidence is sufficient sample size. *P* values that are viewed with some credulity (0.1, 0.075, 0.05) would achieve levels that are seldom questioned (0.035, 0.021, 0.01) if the study had been twice as large.

TYPE I ERROR

For good or evil, an α-level of 0.05 has been adopted as the appropriate level for adequate evidence for most clinical trials. Occasionally, perhaps because the control therapy is very inexpensive or the alternative therapy is very expensive, type I error rates less than 0.05 may be desired.

TYPE II ERROR

If the trial does not result in a rejection of the null hypothesis, then believing that the alternative hypothesis is not true will increase according as the type II error is small. Generally, type II error rates less than 0.2 are acceptable, but rates less than 0.1 are preferred. Type II error rates are increased by noncompliance to the randomized therapy. For this reason, studies must be designed to monitor and maintain compliance. Efforts spent on maintaining good compliance will provide a much greater return in believability than attempting to do efficacy analyses because of poor compliance. Sufficient conditions for an efficacy analysis to have validity (shown in Table 3a) cannot usually be verified. Verifiable necessary, but not sufficient, conditions are listed in Table 3b.

Table 3
Efficacy "On Treatment" Analysis

Must be able to define "on and off treatment."

(a) If "off treatment" is

1) independent of treatment assignment and outcome
then efficacy analysis is valid and unbiased
2) independent of treatment assignment but not outcome
then efficacy analysis is valid but biased

(b) Verifiable necessary, but not sufficient, conditions for an efficacy
analysis to be valid are that both study arms must have the same

1) "off treatment" rates (overall and over time)
2) outcome rates in "off treatment" groups
3) baseline characteristics in "off treatment" groups

DATA

Extensive accurate data can enhance believability by allowing rigorous comparisons of characteristics in the two randomized groups. Ascertainment of nonrandomized therapies and process indicators showing equal exposure to the study during follow-up and, as well, ancillary outcomes can be used to support and/or help explain the trial primary outcome.

Cost

SELECTION

Screening requires study coordinator time but also can be expensive if special tests are required to evaluate inclusion and exclusion criteria. Thus, costs will be reduced if inclusion/exclusion criteria are few and easily determined. However, more extensive screening may be cost effective, for example, to ensure that a high risk population is enrolled (a 20% relative reduction in a control rate of 10% will require almost three times as many patients as a 20% relative reduction in a control rate of 50%), or to enroll patients who will comply with therapy and follow-up (a 25% crossover from control would affect the design in such a way to require almost twice as many patients to achieve the same power).

LENGTH OF TRIAL

Infrastructure costs are a substantial portion of the costs of multicenter trials and are directly related to the number of participating centers. A longer trial at fewer centers will generally cost less.

CHOICE OF PRIMARY ENDPOINT

A good surrogate is an endpoint that occurs sooner than the real endpoint and for which the therapies being compared will have an effect similar to the effect that they would have on the real endpoint *(18–20)*. For example, blood pressure is sometimes thought to be a reasonable surrogate for mortality and morbidity outcomes in hypertensive studies.

There are no good surrogates for the endpoint of death in the emergency setting because the primary endpoint occurs almost immediately. Return of spontaneous circulation or hospital admission occur in essentially the same time frame as death so that they cannot actually be cost-saving surrogates. In some settings, composite endpoints may be both appropriate and reduce sample size. For example, a composite of death and infarct size, for those who did not die, may be useful for evaluating treatment of acute myocardial infarction (MI). The choice of such endpoints must however, be made with extreme caution. How, for example, would one interpret the results if the composite endpoint indicated therapy A was superior but there were actually more deaths on therapy A?

SECONDARY ENDPOINTS

Every secondary endpoint adds to the expense of the trial. Two endpoints that are particularly expensive to collect are cost and quality of life. Cost data requires, first of all, knowledge that a health care utilization has occurred and then access to the billing information for that utilization, neither of which is readily available except in certain closed health care systems such as the Veterans Administration. Quality of life, if not self-administered, is time-consuming and expensive although if self-administered, is often missing. Consideration should be given to restricting ascertainment of secondary endpoints to a (random) subsample.

BASIC DESIGN

Designers of a trial conducted in an emergency setting should give careful consideration to whether individuals can be randomized or whether groups should be randomized *(21,22)*. Because of the emergency setting, randomization of individuals will not allow efficient designs such as crossover or matched pairs to be employed. Randomization of groups, for example, communities, shifts, ambulances, could utilize crossover and matched pair designs. The choice of individual vs group randomization will have many ramifications including defining the outcome measure and can have a decided impact on the cost of the trial. However, if individual randomization is possible, randomizing individuals is preferable unless there are compelling cost savings.

COVARIATE ASCERTAINMENT

Ascertainment of baseline covariates is important for defining subgroups and ascertainment of covariates during follow-up may be important for eliciting mechanisms. However, coordinator time spent both in baseline and follow-up is directly related to the number of data items collected. Cost can be substantially curtailed if subgroup and mechanistic analyses are carefully thought through and only those considered of fundamental importance pursued. Some "attractive" data items (e.g., time from collapse to 911 call), may not be cost-effective generally *(23)*.

CASE EXAMPLES OF RECENT CLINICAL TRIALS CONDUCTED IN AN EMERGENCY SETTING

This section reviews four clinical trials that were conducted in the emergency setting and some of the design issues that were encountered.

Myocardial Infarction Triage Intervention Trial (24)

The Myocardial Infarction Triage Intervention (MITI) trial was initiated shortly after use of fibrinolytics in the hospital had demonstrated benefit in the setting of acute ST-segment elevation myocardial infarction (STEMI). The hypothesis was that providing fibrinolytics in the field would shorten the time to fibrinolytic therapy and result in less insult to the myocardium. Inclusion criteria included a finding on emergency medical services (EMS) arrival of chest pain consistent with acute MI, patient consent, and after consent, a 12-lead electrocardiogram (EKG) transmitted to a baseline hospital showing ST elevation or depression. The primary exclusion was contraindication to fibrinolytic therapy. A patient was randomized if the fibrinolytic kit was opened. The kit contained either fibrinolytics and an infusion pump or dummy materials of size and weight to make the control kit indistinguishable without being opened.

This trial was conducted before the current regulations concerning investigations in emergency settings were formulated. Initially, investigators felt that informed consent was not feasible. However, the institutional review board insisted on consent and ultimately agreed on a one-paragraph verbal consent being read by the paramedics to the patient. It is unclear whether this provided informed consent. Very few persons refused consent. It is also unclear whether such a trial would require individual consent today or whether exemption from consent would apply.

In the initial design that was considered, fibrinolytic therapy was to be offered every other day (i.e., the unit of randomization was the day). A fundamental argument against this was the question of whether the paramedics would screen for chest pain consistent with acute MI with the same level of intensity if they knew that fibrinolytic therapy was not available. Of less concern was the question of how to compute sample size. How would one treat a day in which no patients present with chest pain? How would one treat the day in which several patients present with chest pain? The issue here is how to define the outcome measure. If days are randomized, the outcome measure would have to be some average measure of the endpoint across all of the eligible patients for that day.

Finally, the investigators faced the concern of whether it was ethical to obtain consent and transmit a 12-lead EKG to the baseline hospital when the kit contained dummy materials, possibly lengthening the time before transport for those patients who ended up in the control arm. The solution employed was to provide the potential for better care of the control patient because the hospital could anticipate arrival of a patient having an acute MI and included having a fibrinolytic kit available in the emergency room. However, this solution resulted in serious problems with interpretation of the trial result, which was that there was no significant difference in the primary endpoint for those treated in the field vs those treated in the hospital. Unfortunately, the time to treatment in the hospital fell from more than 1 hour prior to study implementation to a fraction of an hour during study implementation, presumably because the hospital was tipped off to the imminent arrival of a patient with acute MI and because of the availability of the fibrinolytic kit in the emergency department. The magnitude of the Hawthorne (study) effect in the control arm was so great as to make it impossible to interpret failure to reject the null hypothesis (i.e., no difference in outcome) as rejection of the alternative (i.e., fibrinolytics in the field resulting in better outcome).

TeleCPR

The dispatcher-assisted cardiopulmonary resuscitation (TeleCPR) trial randomized episodes of presumed out-of-hospital cardiac arrest (CA) to dispatcher instruction in CPR with the randomization being between the type of instructions that the dispatcher provided, standard American Heart Association (AHA) airway breathing and compression instructions vs instructions just involving chest compressions *(25)*. Inclusion criteria for this trial were the absence of a positive response to the following questions:

- Is the patient awake or conscious?
- Is the patient breathing normally?
- Is the patient an infant or child?
- Is anyone there doing or intending to do CPR?

  And a positive response to the question

- Would you like me to give you CPR instructions?

Exclusion criteria included such things as relayed calls, patients in inaccessible locations, patients beyond the possibility of treatment (dead on arrival), and arrests as a result of overdoses or other noncardiac causes such as trauma.

This study was begun before the current consent procedures were formulated. Who exactly was consenting? It was agreed that the patient could not possibly give consent. It was felt that time could not be spent explaining the study to the caller. Consent for the caller consisted essentially of asking the question for those eligible patients of whether the caller would be willing to do CPR following dispatcher instructions (follow-up data for the patient if they were admitted to the hospital and follow-up telephone interviews with callers did require formal consent).

A major difficulty with the teleCPR trial had to do with the issue of intention-to-treat analysis. Because of the emergency setting, it was not ethical for the dispatcher to pursue each of the exclusionary criteria exhaustively. In fact, unless they were mentioned incidentally during the interrogation protocol, they were not explicitly determined. Consequently, many excluded episodes were randomized, including a substantial number in which no out-of-hospital CA occurred, a substantial number whose arrest was as a result of overdose, and a substantial number who were beyond the potential for treatment. Because the nonarrest cases would all survive and most of the overdose patients would survive, including these survivors in the intention-to-treat analysis would overwhelm the numerators in comparison to the number of eligible episode survivors. It is possible to exclude randomized patients from the analysis without destroying the basis (i.e., the randomized basis) for inference. The exclusions must be based on the following: (a) data available at the time of randomization, (b) absence of any knowledge of what the randomization was, and (c) verifiable by an independent party. Importantly, if such an exclusion process is to take place, *all randomized cases must be subjected to the same rigorous review*, not just those that are "convenient" or "come to light."

The telephone CPR study was a single-center study and took 10 years to accumulate sufficient episodes. Additionally, prior to the randomized trial, a quasi-experimental design had been conducted for 3 years in which no dispatcher instruction, chest compression-only instruction, or the AHA ABC instruction had been given in consecutive 3-month periods. This quasi-experimental phase pointed out the inherent biases of the dispatchers in that compliance to the interrogation protocol was lowest in the control phase and highest in the ABC phase. Even in the randomized phase, dispatcher bias reduced power somewhat because they administered ABC instructions 2% of the time when the randomized assignment was chest compressions and administered chest compression instructions only 1% of the time when ABC was assigned. Could the study have been completed in a shorter length of time if multiple centers participated? In theory, the answer is yes. However, when a second "experienced" center was considered, it had to be abandoned because dispatcher compliance was close to 0. The point is that in the emergency setting, compliance is extremely difficult to enforce. It cannot be done at the time of therapy administration. It must be accomplished through extensive pretraining and education and through ongoing extensive quality control and corrective action. Compliance is inherently much more difficult in multicenter than in single-center trials.

Finally, because of the difficulty in determining inclusion and exclusion criteria, could a design in which dispatch centers, rather than individual episodes, were randomized have been possible? Again theoretically, the answer is yes, but such a design would create issues regarding the outcome measure. Only a minority of episodes would be expected to benefit (knowledgeable bystanders would be available in perhaps 50% of episodes) and because the impact of this differential CPR instruction could not be expected to be huge, the contribution to the numerator (survivors of out-of-hospital CA) could not be large, although the denominator (all out-of-hospital CAs) might be difficult to standardize across centers. Thus, a large number of centers would probably be necessary to achieve reasonable power, leading to an extremely costly study.

Amiodarone for Resuscitation After Out-of-Hospital CA as a Result of Ventricular Fibrillation (ARREST) Trial

The ARREST trial sought to determine whether intravenous amiodarone would improve the rate of successful resuscitation in patients who remained in ventricular fibrillation (VF) after receiving three or more precordial shocks (26). Prepackaged identical kits were used, one containing amiodarone, the other containing a placebo solution. This study was conducted under current regulations with an exception from informed consent. The study endpoint was admission to the hospital with a spontaneously perfusing rhythm. The study demonstrated a significant increase in the proportion of patients admitted to the hospital. One issue that this study faced was inclusion criteria, which were so stringent to include only patients with a very low likelihood of survival to hospital admission. This was driven by the ethical concern that devoting resources and time to an untested therapy (or placebo) potentially delayed the advent of more useful therapies, including transport to the hospital. The placebo was deemed necessary to blind the paramedics and avoid the potential of substantial imbalance in concomitant medications because of knowledge of the study therapy (in particular, the use of nonstudy amiodarone or other anti-arrhythmics). The other issue that this study faced was that it used an endpoint, which, at best, might be a surrogate for survival. Unfortunately, although the study found an increase in the rates of admission to the hospital, no effect on survival-to-hospital discharge was observed. At face value, this study is a negative study in that it adds cost to the resuscitation effort without any benefit. The study had such low power for the secondary endpoint of survival that failure to reject the null did not result in rejection of the alternative. The study needs to be repeated with at least two substantive changes. It should include patients with a higher likelihood of survival (e.g., perhaps including patients who have failed only one precordial shock) and the sample size must be increased so that the important endpoint, survival, can be evaluated adequately.

Public Access Defibrillation (PAD) Trial

The PAD trial seeks to determine whether survival rates will improve if automated external defibrillators are made available for use by trained laypersons in public settings (27). The general concept in PAD is to identify community units such as office buildings, high-rise apartment buildings, and so on in which there is a sufficient density of at-risk persons to provide a reasonable likelihood of a CA occurring over a period of several years. The unit should not have persons already responsible for responding to medical emergencies. Thus, nursing homes for example are excluded. After a unit is identified, individuals within the unit who are willing (consent is required) are provided with standard CPR training. Some, or perhaps all, could then be trained to use automatic external defibrillators (AEDs) and AEDs would be installed in appropriate locations. Suggestions for how individual episodes could be randomized included that the AEDs would be enclosed in a box and when that box was opened, the layperson would find either an AED or CPR-assist devices such as a face mask and pictorial reminder of how to do CPR. The reason for wanting all units to be treated the same regarding training and installation of devices was because of concern about an Hawthorne effect. It was thought that the presence of the AED might act as a widget stimulating more rapid and aggressive response and hence, without a "placebo" to blind the lay responder, any difference in outcome might not be able to be attributed to the actual action of the AED.

It was agreed ultimately that it would be impossible to randomize individual episodes and that if the device worked because it was a "widget," that was still an appropriate, although ostensibly expensive, objective. Accordingly, the PAD design involved randomization of community units. After units were identified and certified as eligible (sufficient risk of a CA occurring and no traditional responders) the unit was randomized to control arm (lay persons were taught traditional CPR) or treatment arm (lay persons were taught traditional CPR and use of an AED and AEDs were installed). The endpoint of interest in PAD is survival from an out-of-hospital CA. The problem facing PAD was defining an outcome measure. The numerator would be the "saves." The denominator ideally would be all of the out-of-hospital CAs that occurred in the unit.

The concern was whether out-of-hospital CAs could be enumerated in each unit without bias created by the differential treatments in the control and treatment arms. For example, where does a person discovered dead fit in? Where does a "do not resuscitate" patient fit in? Where does a person with chest pain who goes into CA seconds after being loaded into an ambulance and subsequently dies or survives fit in? Would more out-of-hospital CA be identified properly in the AED arms because the presence of an AED could provide a recording demonstrating VF?

Other denominators were found to be equally problematic. One conceivable denominator is the sum of all successes and all deaths that occur in the community unit, irrespective of cause. However, the EMS system has no natural link with deaths that are not associated with a call to 911. Depending on the nature of the community unit, capturing all deaths that occur in the unit might be extremely difficult and time consuming.

Another potential denominator is the population size of the unit. However, such populations are highly variable, particularly in public units, as a result of fluctuations related to time of day, day of the week, month, season, and so on. Randomizing communities instead of individuals makes the definition of the outcome measure an extremely difficult and critical part of the design.

The principal problem is that unbiased ascertainment of the components of the outcome measure may be very difficult. The second issue, which is touched on a bit later under sample size, is that variability between communities must be included in sample size calculations in addition to variability in individual response to treatment. The PAD design team ultimately chose to ignore a denominator and simply used the count of saves as the outcome measure. Simulations showed that there would be virtually no loss of power using this outcome measure and a substantial protection against biased ascertainment. Although initially surprising that there was no loss of power by ignoring the denominator, the fact that a substantial number of units (1000) were randomized essentially assured that whatever denominator could have been used would be equally distributed between the two treatment arms. If, as is more common in community-based randomized trials, only 20 to 40 communities had been randomized, there would undoubtedly have been a substantial loss of power.

Because PAD randomized community units, design considerations such as matched pairs and crossover designs were available. The initial PAD design required field centers to identify matched pairs of community units and also contemplated a crossover midway through follow-up between the matched pairs. The matched pair design would provide greater efficiency and the crossover design would help eliminate any *widget* effect. However, the PAD investigators were very concerned about compliance to study therapy, particularly in the control arm, because AEDs were readily available and there was substantial advocacy on the part of the AHA as well as on the part of manufacturers to install AEDs. It was felt that to control the crossover rate, the duration of the trial needed to be reduced from 2.5 years to 1.25 years (which would not allow sufficient time for crossover). It was also thought that it would be easier to recruit a sufficient number of unmatched units to achieve the same power as would be provided by a design involving matched units.

SAMPLE SIZE

Sample size is a critical component in trial design. To determine sample size, two quantitative estimates must be obtained and the importance of these to pursuing the trial cannot be overstated: (a) how variable, σ, is the endpoint in the population of interest?; and (b) how much better, Δ, than therapy B can therapy A reasonably be expected to be, i.e., $\mu_A = \mu_B + \Delta$? Here, μ is the outcome measure (e.g., mean or proportion). These two quantities determine the so-called "effect size," $e = \Delta/\sigma$. These estimates must come from an extensive review of relevant literature and/or from pilot studies. Some typical effect sizes are given in Table 4. A rough but useful estimate of total sample size (assuming one-to-one allocation) is then given by (*see also* Fig. 2)

$$N = 2n = 4 (Z_\alpha + Z_\beta)^2 / e^2$$

in which $Z_\alpha = 1.96$ if $\alpha = 0.05$ and the test is two-sided, $Z_\alpha = 1.96$ if $\alpha = 0.025$ and the test is one-sided, $Z_\beta = 0.84$ if $\beta = 0.2$, $Z_\beta = 1.28$ if $\beta = 0.1$

At this point, careful thought must go into formulating the appropriate null, H_0, and alternative, H_a, hypotheses and whether the test should be one- or two-sided. There is not uniform agreement on the latter (28–33). I believe that the appropriate decision follows from the answer to: What will be the consequences on use of therapies A and B depending on the outcome of the trial? The most likely scenarios are tabulated in Table 5. The major dilemma with a one-sided test is that if the data support the opposite effect (say $p < 0.05$), the correct conclusion, and the conclusion that should be published, is simply that the null cannot be rejected. This may be difficult to accept. If sequential monitoring is to be employed, there is a simple solution to this conundrum; namely, if, based on the consequences criteria, a one-sided test seems appropriate, it should be not only appropriate, but desirable to have a futility boundary, as well as the efficacy boundary, for the alternative

Table 4
Typical Effect Sizes

For Proportions

Control Rate	% Reduction				
	5%	20%	40%	60%	80%
.02	.007	.029	.057	.086	.11
.05	.011	.046	.092	.14	.18
.1	.017	.067	.13	.20	.27
.15	.021	.084	.17	.25	.34
.25	.029	.12	.23	.35	.46
.5	.05	.20	.40	.60	.80
.75	.087	.35	.69	1.04	1.39
.99	.50	1.98	3.96	5.97	7.96

Magnitude of sample size

- 100,000 s
- 10,000 s
- 1,000 s
- 100 s
- 10 s

For Continuous variables (based on a post-MI population with asymptomatic ectopic [VPCs] beats)

	Uncertainty (σ)	Control value	Δ/effect size		
LVEF	.13	~.45	.02/.15	.05/.38	.1/.77
Serum Cholesterol	1.3	~5.5	.2/.15	.5/.38	1.5/1.2
Infarct Size	.16	~.25	.05/.31	.1/.62	.15/.94
ln (VPC/hr)	.25	~2	.2/.42	.4/.85	1/2.8
Cost-effectiveness ($/yr)	30,000	~50,000	5,000/.17	10,000/.33	25,000/.83
Trait Anxiety Scale	10	~35	.7/.07	(Note: .7 was difference observed between survivors and non-survivors.)	
Beck Depression Scale	7	~9	4/.57	(Note: 4 was difference observed between survivors and non-survivors.)	
SF-36	.6	~.3	.2/.33	(Note: .2 was difference corresponding to difference of 1 heart failure class.)	

708

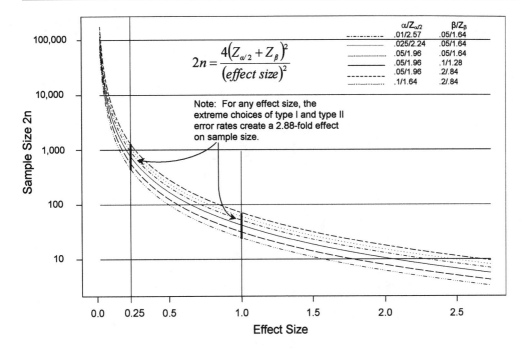

Fig. 2. The formula is technically correct only in the case when the underlying distributions are normal with the same variance. However, other distributional assumptions will have little impact, particularly for effect sizes less than 0.5.

of interest. Then, if the data are trending toward the "wrong" side, the trial will be stopped by the futility boundary long before the trend in the data can reach nominal significance. If that occurs, and if there are good reasons to do so, a new trial with a one-sided test of the other side can be quickly mounted with the unspent resources and the trial mechanism that is in place.

An example of what monitoring boundaries might look like for monitoring efficacy in a two-sided (0.05) level trial and for monitoring efficacy and futility in a one-sided (0.05) level trial is shown in Fig. 3. Note the smaller sample size required for the one-sided test. If the "wrong" side actually represented the particular true effect, the expected "time" this particular trial would be stopped by the futility boundary is at 205 patients enrolled.

When groups are randomized, the outcome measure must be defined at the group level. For example, if the endpoint is death, the outcome measure might be the number of deaths in the group during the course of the study divided by the number of persons in the group. To determine an effect size in this setting, one must estimate the variance, σ^2, of this outcome measure. That variance will have two components: σ_B^2, the variance between groups, and the chance variation within each group, σ_w^2 *(21)*. The latter is the ratio of the intrinsic variation in the endpoint, τ^2, [e.g., if θ = probability of death, $\tau^2 = \theta(1-\theta)$]

$$\sigma^2 = \sigma_B^2 + \sigma_w^2 = \sigma_B^2 + \frac{\tau^2}{n}$$

Table 5
Some Scenarios That Would Suggest a One- or Two-Sided Design

Consequence	H_0	H_a	Test	Example
A not used if μ_A not $> \mu_B$	$\mu_A \leq \mu_B$	$\mu_A \geq \mu_B + \Delta$	one-sided	1) A = std, B = placebo 2) A = new, B = std and A cost[a] more than B
A will be used if $\mu_A \geq \mu_B$	$\mu_A \leq \mu_B - D$	$\mu_A \geq \mu_B$	one-sided	A = new (or available), B = std and A cost $\leq$ B
No change in use if μ_A not $> \mu_B$ and μ_B not $> \mu_A$	$\mu_A = \mu_B$	$\|(\mu_A - \mu_B)\| > \Delta$	two-sided	A = std (or available), B = std and A cost same as B

[a] Cost can be in terms of dollars or quality of life

710

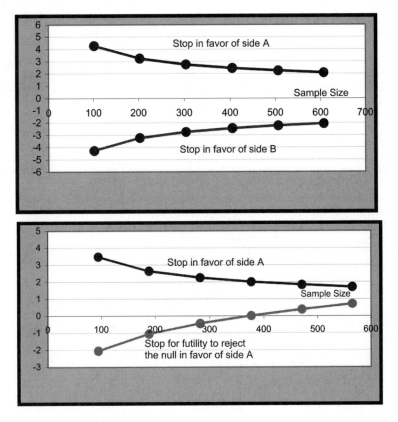

Fig. 3. Efficacy monitoring boundaries for a two-sided design (upper panel) and efficacy and futility boundaries for a one-sided design (lower panel).

Thus, large groups will reduce the within-group contribution, but only increasing the number of groups can offset a large between-group variance. Once the effect size is determined, the sample size obtained from Fig. 2 represents the number of groups needed, not the total number of individuals.

REFERENCES

1. Friedman L, Furberg C, DeMets D. Fundamentals of Clinical Trials, 3rd ed. Springer Verlag, 1998.
2. Meinert CL. Clinical Trials: Design, Conduct and Analysis. Oxford University Press, 1986.
3. Pocock SJ. Clinical Trials: A Practical Approach. John Wiley & Sons, 1984.
4. Cairns JA, Hallstrom A, Held P. Should all trials have a data safety and monitoring committee? Am Heart J 2001; 141:156–163.
5. Packer M, Wittes J, Stump D. Terms of reference for Data and Safety Monitoring Committees. Am Heart J 2001; 141:542–547.
6. Pocock S, Furberg CD. Procedures of data and safety monitoring committees. Am Heart J 2001; 141: 289–294.
7. Califf RM, Ellenberg SS. Statistical approaches and policies for the operations of Data and Safety Monitoring Committees. Am Heart J. 2001; 141:301–305.
8. Fisher L, Klibaner M. Regulatory issues for Data and Safety Monitoring Committees. Am Heart J 2001; 141:536–541.

9. Weaver WD, Greenberg S. Making changes in clinical trials. Am Heart J. 2001; 141:295–300.
10. Whitehead J. The Design and Analysis of Sequential Clinical Trials. Chichester: Ellis Horwood, 1983.
11. O'Brien PC, Fleming TR. A multiple testing procedure for clinical trials. Biometrics 1979; 35:549–556.
12. Pocock SJ. Group sequential methods in the design and analysis of sequential clinical trials. Biometrika 1977; 64:191–199.
13. Lin DY. A General Theory on Stochastic Curtailment for Censored Survival Data. Journal of the American Statistical Association 1999; 94:510–521.
14. Fisher LD. Self-designing clinical trials. Stat Med 1998; 17:1551–1562.
15. Gould AL, Pecore VJ. Group sequential methods for clinical trials allowing early acceptance of H_0 and incorporating costs. Biometrika 1982; 69:75–80.
16. Begg CB. Ruminations on the intent-to-treat principle. Control Clin Trials 2000; 21:241–243.
17. Gibaldi M, Sullivan S. Intention-to-treat analysis in randomized trials: who gets counted? J Clin Pharmacol 1997; 37:667–672.
18. Prentice RL. Surrogate endpoints in clinical trials: definition and operational criteria. Stat Med 1989; 8:431–440.
19. Hughes MD, DeGruttola V, Welles SL. Evaluating surrogate markers. J Acquir Immune Defic Syndr Hum Retrovirol 1995; 10(Suppl 2):S1–S8.
20. Hallstrom AP, Greene HL, Wilkoff BL, et al. Relationship between rehospitalization and future death in patients treated for potentially lethal arrhythmia. J Cardiovasc Electrophysiol 2001; 12:990–995.
21. Koepsell TD, Wagner EH, Cheadle AC, et al. Selected methodological issues in evaluating community-based health promotion and disease prevention programs. Annu Rev Public Health 1992; 13:31–57.
22. Koepsell TD, Martin DC, Diehr PH, et al. Data analysis and sample size issues in evaluations of community-based health promotion and disease prevention programs: a mixed-model analysis of variance approach. J Clin Epidemiol 1991; 44:701–713.
23. Hallstrom AP. Should time from cardiac arrest until call to emergency medical services (EMS) be collected in EMS research? Crit Care Med 2002; 30:S127–S130.
24. Weaver WD, Cerqueira M, Hallstrom AP, et al. Prehospital-initiated vs hospital-initiated thrombolytic therapy. The Myocardial Infarction Triage and Intervention Trial. JAMA 1993; 270:1211–1216.
25. Hallstrom A, Cobb L, Johnson E, et al. Cardiopulmonary resuscitation by chest compression alone or with mouth-to-mouth ventilation. N Engl J Med 2000; 342:1546–1553.
26. Kudenchuk PJ, Cobb LA, Copass MK, et al. Amiodarone for resuscitation after out-of-hospital cardiac arrest due to ventricular fibrillation. N Engl J Med 1999; 341:871–878.
27. PAD Trial Investigators. The Public Access Defibrillation (PAD) Trial study design and rationale. Resuscitation 2003; 56:135–147.
28. Enkin MW. One and two sided tests of significance. One sided tests should be used more often. BMJ 1994; 309:874.
29. Dunnett CW, Gent M. An alternative to the use of two-sided tests in clinical trials. Stat Med 1996; 15:1729–1738.
30. Bland JM, Altman DG. One and two sided tests of significance. BMJ 1994; 309:248.
31. Knottnerus JA, Bouter LM. The ethics of sample size: two-sided testing and one-sided thinking. J Clin Epidemiol 2001; 54:109,110.
32. Fisher LD. The use of one-sided tests in drug trials: an FDA advisory committee member's perspective. J Biopharm Stat 1991; 1:151–156.
33. Moye LA, Tita AT. Defending the rationale for the two-tailed test in clinical research. Circulation 2002; 105:3062–3065.

36 Ethics in Resuscitation

Antonio E. Muñiz, MD, FACEP, FAAP, FAAEM

CONTENTS

INTRODUCTION

Seriously ill patients often face tragically difficult choices. Commonly, an advanced resuscitative intervention offers a chance of longer life, with a chance, too, of profound suffering. In a given day, all over the world, thousands undergo the procedure of cardiopulmonary resuscitation (CPR), whereas others are placed on a "do not attempt resuscitation" (DNAR) status. In the United States, it has been estimated that approx 100,000 lives may be saved with advanced resuscitation [1]. The performance of CPR, however, may conflict with the patient's own desires and may not be in his or her best interest, especially if suffering from a terminally ill condition. It has also been shown that up to 20% of individuals do not wish to be resuscitated [2,3]. Decisions concerning CPR are complicated by the fact that often the decision to initiate CPR must be made within seconds by health care providers who generally have very little knowledge about the patient's illness or of any existing advance directives.

The indications for CPR, as for any medical therapy, depend on its efficacy. There is a general presumption by many laypersons that health care professionals will make all reasonable endeavors to resuscitate any patient who suffers a cardiac arrest (CA). When introduced approx 40 years ago, CPR was meant to avert premature death in a previously healthy individual, who sustained a sudden respiratory or CA. The primary intention of CPR was to provide artificial respiration and circulation with the hope of attaining spontaneous ventilation and heart function. Over the last 40 years, attempts at resuscitation began to occur after any person suffered a CA, regardless of the associated comorbidities, illness severity, or etiology for the CA. CPR was not intended to be a procedure performed in every potential death encounter, and yet it has been initiated in many irreversible illnesses in which, not surprisingly, it has been shown to be of little benefit [4]. Additionally, CPR is considered futile if restoration of breathing and heart rate is achieved without satisfactory quality of life. Therefore, the ultimate goal of resuscitation must be to restore patients to their pre-arrest function.

From: *Contemporary Cardiology: Cardiopulmonary Resuscitation*
Edited by: J. P. Ornato and M. A. Peberdy © Humana Press Inc., Totowa, NJ

Patients participate in decisions about their medical care today as never before. As the physician–patient relationship has evolved into a collaborative one, patients are expected to understand and evaluate complex information, often at a time of great emotional hardship. This is especially true when it comes to decisions about resuscitation. In general, the patient as a person should decide the course taken at the end of his or her own life. But, even more importantly, sometimes what a patient really wants is to be kept comfortable and not to be resuscitated.

In general, advanced resuscitation techniques may be lifesaving in patients with a previously good performance status who suffer a sudden, unexpected event. It will almost certainly not work and should not be attempted in patients with advanced terminal illnesses and those with extensive and irreversible underlying disease whose general condition is deteriorating. Stated another way, resuscitation attempts to counter sudden, unexpected CA in an otherwise reasonably healthy individual rather than to prolong the dying process in those who are terminally ill or injured.

ETHICAL PRINCIPLES

Ethical issues are an integral part of any medical decision-making process, especially those associated with resuscitation because of the close relationship between CA and death. The decision to issue an order not to initiate resuscitation in an individual patient has profound ethical implications. However, this is not the only ethical issue involved in resuscitation *(5,6)*. Initiation and termination of resuscitation are guided by complex ethical, sociologic, religious, and cultural norms, which can be profoundly dissimilar in different societies.

There are four broad ethical principals that apply to health care provider responsibilities to others and are generally accepted as guiding principles of ethical conduct. These include *beneficence*, *nonmaleficence*, *justice*, and *autonomy*. Although these ethical principles may be accepted across different cultures, the priority of these principles, once again may vary greatly among cultures. For example, in the United States, the greatest emphasis is placed on the autonomy of the patient although in other countries (in which financial resources may be scarce) the benefit to society at large outweigh the patient's autonomy .

CPR is no different from any other medical or surgical procedure, and the basic ethical considerations are the same for all procedures. Applying these principles to resuscitation, the principle of beneficence dictates that we have a moral responsibility to "do good" to others. This implies that health care providers should act in the best interest of their patients. Doing what is right for the patient, however, often involves serious risks. Resuscitation should, therefore, be initiated only when likely to be effective.

The principle of nonmaleficence dictates that health care professionals have a moral responsibility to avoid harming others. Resuscitation should not be attempted when it is neither indicated clinically, nor wished by the patient and is more likely to be of harm than benefit. Inappropriate CPR is considered maleficent. Ethical dilemmas may arise between nonmaleficence and autonomy when patients request interventions, which are without benefit and are harmful or dangerous. A physician is required to only provide medical therapy that has benefit to patients. No ethical principle ever requires doctors to do what is of no net medical benefit to the patient. Thus, withholding an ineffective intervention is sound ethically. Justice demands that effective medical intervention should be available universally to those who require it. Resources should be allocated fairly to ensure that resuscitation is available to all persons. Ineffective CPR fails justice criteria.

Prior to 1970, patients as well as physicians, believed that medical decisions should be made by the physician without input from the patient. Physicians attempted to make the best medical decisions possible, sparing the patient and family from the burdens associated with difficult choices. This paternalism emphasized beneficence to the exclusion of other ethical principles, especially patient autonomy. Unfortunately, physicians are not always able to determine or actually know what is in their patients' best interests, and personal biases are unavoidable *(7)*.

By the mid-1980s, the concept of paternalistic physician beneficence was replaced by an overwhelming emphasis on patient autonomy. Respect for patient autonomy is the driving fundamental ethical principle involved in the current medical decision-making process of medicine in most countries and in some countries has legal implications *(8,9)*. Physicians have recognized the right of the patient to participate in medical decision making for the last 20 years. The responsibilities of physicians and other health care professional have changed, and now include facilitating informed medical decisions *(10)*. Essential to this decision-making process is an understanding of the patients' preferences for medical care, and factors that affect these preferences. Patients have the right to choose actions consistent with their values, goals, and life plan, even if their decisions are not in concordance with the wishes of family members or the recommendations of their physician. Patients who might benefit from resuscitation have the right to state in advance that they do not wish it, even if it is appropriate medically. Choices should be free from interference and control by others. The right to refuse medical treatment does not depend on the presence or absence of terminal illness, the agreement of family members, or the approval of physicians. This, however, requires that a patient is competent and able to communicate and can consent to or refuse an intervention. In many countries, adult patients are presumed to have the right for decision-making capacity unless a court of law has declared that individual incompetent to make such decisions.

Because preservation of life is generally assumed to be a legitimate interest to the patient, the refusal of lifesaving procedures creates the potential for ethical conflict. This conflict between autonomy and beneficence forms the basis of most ethical dilemmas involving resuscitation. Allowing the patient to die may be viewed by some as a violation of beneficence, although forcing the patient to undergo resuscitation is a violation of his or her autonomy.

On the other hand, an overemphasis on patient's autonomy can also be dangerous. As the physician–patient relationship has evolved into a collaborative one, patients are expected to understand and evaluate complex medical information, often at a time of great emotional stress. Patients and family members are often made to feel that they have to "make the decision" regarding whether to perform any resuscitation. Patients, families, and surrogates should not be in a position to determine whether an intervention is appropriate medically. It is more opportune that patients decide whether an offered procedure from their physician is acceptable to them. Far too often, physicians blur this distinction and mistakenly ask patients and families to make medical decisions. Physicians, additionally, may not give advice so as not to seem paternalistic, although patients or family members are often confronted with an open-ended request to inform the medical team what "they want to have done." Often their response is to "have everything done" and amazingly, this is accepted by the patient's physician as a request for advanced resuscitation when the physician, in fact, believes that this would be a great mistake. In this scenario, the physician abandons his or her traditional responsibility to protect the patient against inappropriate procedures, rejecting beneficience in favor of preserving complete autonomy. In reality, this approach diminishes autonomy by depriving patients of expert advice. Often, patients chose medical procedures based on unrealistic beliefs and interpreted silence by the physicians as tacit approval for these decisions.

The better thing for the physician to do is to decide whether the medical intervention can be successful in prolonging quality of life and then, inform the patient and families of this determination and the rationale. If CPR is considered futile, it should not be offered as an option. If CPR is appropriate, patients and families should be given the option to accept or refuse it. What constitutes a successful resuscitation depends on the goal of therapy, which must confirm to the patient's best wishes.

In recent years, the pendulum has begun to swing back from an absolute autonomy paradigm toward a more balanced approach. These models have been termed enhanced autonomy or the fiduciary role, but in reality they are a realization that a model based solely on one ethical principle, such as autonomy, is no better than one based solely on another, such as beneficence *(11,12)*. There are certain situations in which advanced resuscitation, including CPR should not be offered, and the physician should bestow his or her medical judgment and experience regarding the appropriateness of these therapies in the same regard as any other medical procedure.

The basis for deciding to forego resuscitation is generally that the burdens of the resuscitation outweigh the potential benefits *(9)*. Burdens can include suffering and pain from the treatment itself or impaired cognitive functioning after the resuscitation is completed. Benefits may include life propagation. Balancing the burdens and benefits depends on both a statistical assessment of their likelihood and a weighing of their importance by the patient.

Before patient preferences can be accepted to direct future medical care, physicians have an obligation to determine whether these preferences are based on a good understanding of resuscitation and its outcomes. Appropriate decision making rests on a good understanding of the real outcomes from resuscitation. This goal, however, can be complicated by physician misconceptions. Many physicians cannot predict accurately the chances of survival from a cardiac arrest and quality of life. Additionally, many laypersons have only a vague understanding of resuscitation and its consequences. The public and some health care professionals have an unrealistic expectation of the benefit of CPR and these beliefs have been reinforced by television *(13)*. Many television shows portray a much better positive outcome after resuscitation and generally ignore the real risk of permanent neurological disabilities. Thus, giving truly informed consent for resuscitation continues to be a challenge for most health care professionals.

For a patient to make a medical decision he or she must also receive and comprehend accurately the nature of the illness and prognosis, the nature of the proposed interventions, the alternatives for therapy, the implications of these options, and ultimately understand the consequences of their decisions. It is up to the physician to determine the patient's decision-making capacity before concluding that a patient cannot represent him or herself. The physician has a legal responsibility to provide all necessary information in a manner that is understandable, provide professional advice, and finally administer or withhold therapy based on the patient's decision. A useful technique to assess understanding is to ask the patient to summarize what has just been discussed and to correct any incongruencies. When the patient understands all of these facets, then a sound decision can be made.

Unfortunately, almost 50% of individuals older than 85 years have dementia, which usually precludes their awareness of many complex issues involved in choosing among treatment options for end-of-life preferences *(14)*. There are other situations when decision-making capacity is also impaired, such as with concurrent illness, pain, medications or psychiatric diseases. Some cognitively intact patients are delirious during an acute illness and are incapable of complex discussions about their care at just the time that important decisions must be performed. Patients who are depressed may represent a unique situation. Depressed patients can meet the criteria for decision capacity, but their choices are clouded by their mood disorder *(15)*. In these cases, the decision for resuscitation must be made very carefully *(16)*. The incompetent patient's participation in decision making is, by definition, inappropriate. Thus, establishing competency is of paramount importance. This determination can usually be made by the patient's physician, although the physician may occasionally petition assistance by psychiatric consultation. In rare cases, the estimation of competence becomes a legal matter, as when there is lack of agreement between physicians and patient, or amongst family members, or when the life of a child is considered.

In most cases, determining the patient's decision capacity for a specific medical procedure requires neither legal intervention nor psychiatric expertise. There is, however, no known accurate medical testing that will determine effectively the medical decision capacity of a person. The mini-mental status examination does not predict the capacity of an individual to make medical decisions, except in cases in which there is extreme mental impairment *(17)*. A physician can be satisfied that a patient is capable of making decisions if he or she has the ability to communicate, can comprehend the proposed therapy and alternative interventions, is able to to grasp the consequences of accepting or rejecting the treatment plans, and has the ability to reason *(18)*.

If the patient is felt to be mentally incompetent, it is necessary to designate an individual who will represent the patient, and therefore become involved in all aspects of the decision-making process *(19)*. Patients do not lose their autonomy once declared incompetent. Physicians have traditionally acted paternalistically on behalf of their patients. However, contemporary biomedical ethics suggest that physicians should not take on this function because they usually do not know what their patients want done in the event of serious illness *(20)*. Additionally, physicians systematically underestimate the quality of life of their patients and are thereby less likely than their patients to favor life-sustaining treatments *(93)*.

The appointment of a patient surrogate is customarily the responsibility of the physician who usually relies on the spouse or another immediate relative for this role. Ideally, the surrogate should be chosen by the patient when he or she is able to make such a decision. Competent patients in anticipation of incapacity to render decisions later can designate a surrogate decision maker or grant a durable power of attorney for health care *(22)*. Durable power of attorney for health care allows an individual to make medical decisions for the patient when his or her decision-making capacity is not available.

The surrogate is the patient's legal representative and is entitled to the same knowledge that the patient would receive concerning the diagnosis, treatment modalities, risks, and prognosis. In the best of circumstances, the surrogate has access to the patient's advance directives or living will, and is guided by the patient's own wishes. Surrogates should base their decision on the patient's previously expressed choices, or should make decisions based on the patient's best interests. The accuracy of substituted opinion is correlated directly with prior patients and proxies communications *(23)*. There is some evidence, however, that even surrogates do not consistently reflect the patients' preferences *(23)*. This may be based on the fact that patients and surrogate decision makers often do not discuss medical care preferences. This issue is even further confused by the finding that up to 31% of patients report that they would prefer to have their physicians follow the decision of their surrogate even if the surrogate's decision conflicts with their own expressed preferences *(24)*. When there is (a) an emergency, (b) no competent family member present, and (c) the preferences of the patient are unknown, it would be prudent to provide standard medical care. If the surrogate cannot ascertain what the patient would choose, then the decision should be based on the best interests of the patient, which is defined as what most people in that situation would want *(25)*. In the event that there is dissension among family members, if it is unclear who should represent the patient, or if there are no immediate family members available, a court appointment of a surrogate may become necessary *(26)*.

Ethical issues near the end of life arise almost exclusively because of concerns about how much care and how aggressive that care should be. There is often conflict between physicians, other health care providers, or family members about what comprises appropriate care. Many of these controversies can be avoided by clarifying who makes the difficult decisions for resuscitation or to limit care. Health care workers should be sensitive to such family concerns, but in the end, it is the patient's wishes that must prevail. Even with this in mind, there are occasions when the decision to render CPR is controversial. A frank and open discussion of the ostensible burdens and benefits associated with CPR is the cornerstone of conflict resolution in these situations. If the conflict cannot be resolved, the physician has other alternatives such as consultation with another colleague or an ethics committee. Consultation helps to ensure that all viewpoints and alternatives are considered carefully and in this situation can be instrumental in achieving conflict resolution.

ADVANCE DIRECTIVES

Advance directives is a term applied to preferences of a person's end-of-life care *(27)*. They help patients control health care decisions when they may be unable to direct their medical care. Such directives provide careful instructions on limitations of care, including resuscitation from CA. Advance directives can include dialogue, written directives, living wills, or durable powers of attorney for health care. Conversations the patient had with family members, friends, or physicians, while considered competent, are generally the most common form of directives employed today. In many countries, the courts consider written advance directives to be more reliable than individuals recollections of preceding conversations. Abiding by the advance directives of patients when the decision-making capacity are lost respects their autonomy, as well as in many countries, the law *(9,28)*. They have also been sanctioned as a way to lessen the high cost of end-of-life health care *(29)*.

The living will is the most widely employed written advance directive *(22)*. Living wills constitute clear and convincing evidence of patient's wishes. Living wills are legal in most states. In living wills, patients direct their physicians in the provision of medical care, especially in circumstances in which they become terminally ill with no chance of recovery and are incompetent to make their own decisions. Living wills can be modified to include provisions for specific procedures, such as CPR, ventilators, fluid and antibiotic administration, or enteral feedings. Nonetheless, living wills have significant drawbacks. First, a will drafted in specific language cannot give guidance for occurrences that were not anticipated when the will was written. If, on the other hand, the will was written in general language to cover a broad range of possible events, then its terms may be ambiguous in specific situations. They usually do not specify what interventions are to be avoided and are generally applicable only to a "terminal condition," which is generally defined as an irreversible condition that makes death inevitable. Again, many statutes limit the kinds of provisions that can be included in a living will.

The durable power of attorney for health care or a health care proxy allows competent patients to designate a surrogate, typically a family member or friend, to make the medical decisions if the patient once again becomes incompetent. This can be accomplished by completing a simple form and does not require involvement of an attorney. Durable powers of attorney for health care have important advantages over living wills. Although living wills are often limited to treatments in the setting of a terminal illness in which death is inevitable, durable power of attorney for health care can predominantly be used to delegate health care decisions in all cases of patient incompetence.

There is no legal requirement that an individual choose a proxy. The next of kin can function in that role even without a formal designation from the patient (30). Nevertheless, choosing a surrogate helps clarify the identity of the patient's representative when there is a significant difference of opinion amongst different family members regarding consent for treatment (31).

Both patients and physicians deem that advance directives are important and should be discussed (32). Yet, in modern society, most adults do not prepare advance directives or discuss resuscitation with their physicians (33,34). Physicians frequently attend to their patients without knowledge of their preferences with regards to end-of-life issues (35). Patients often believe it is their physician's responsibility to initiate an advance care dialogue, although physicians believe the subject should be raised by their patient (36). Sadly, most patients, even those who are terminally ill, are never asked by a physician if they desire to be resuscitated (37). Although several surveys illustrate that most physicians desire patient participation in the decision-making process, many physicians feel uncomfortable discussing the possibility of resuscitation with patients except in special circumstances, such as when the patient is terminally ill (38–40). Some physicians are reluctant to discuss these issues with patients for a variety of reasons, including time constraints, communications issues, and the possibility that patients may have distress and react negatively to the discussion. Although some physicians may perceive death as medical failure others do not want to ruin patients' hopes, need time to develop a relationship with their patients, and feel discussions about advance directives should occur late in the course of a patient's illness (41,42). Physicians may be uncomfortable with managing the dying patient and may lack the appropriate communication skills to sufficiently discuss death with the patient as well as their family. This may originate from the fact that most medical training programs provide limited or no formal training in dealing with the dying patient (43,44).

Elderly patients who have chronic medical illnesses are more content with their physicians when advance directives are discussed (45). Patients desire to be more involved in the decision-making process regarding their end-of-life care choices (46–48). Physicians and patients may not have the same ideal goals or perception of quality of life after resuscitation when dealing with end-of-life care decisions (49). A survey of physicians demonstrated that they would not want resuscitation to be performed on themselves and would want life-sustaining therapy withdrawn should the prognosis for meaningful survival be poor *(50)*. In stark contrast to most physicians' beliefs, most elderly patients want to be resuscitated in the case of a CA *(51,52)*. In fact, data from the SUPPORT (Study to Understand Prognoses and Preferences for Outcomes and Risks of Treatment) project show that two-thirds of those older than 70 years opted for resuscitation *(53)*.

Advance directives must also be re-evaluated periodically. Patients inevitably change their perceptions about the quality of their life in about living longer as they get older or have a significant alteration in their health status. In the SUPPORT project, patients who chose a DNAR order initially changed their decision more often than those who wanted resuscitation in case of a CA *(35,54,55)*. Most patients have a deep desire to live, and health care providers tend to underestimate that desire *(56)*. Every patient should have the right to decree their end-of-life care, but this decision must be reevaluated at regular intervals.

As of 1991, the Patient Self-Determination Act requires health care institutions in the United States to inquire whether patients have advance directives at the time of admission *(48)*. They must inform the patient that they have the right to accept or refuse any kind of medical intervention, including CPR *(29)*. In 1990, the US Supreme Court ruled that patients have the right to determine what is done with their bodies and therefore have the right to refuse treatment of whatever kind *(57)*. Additionally, institutions must assist patients in completing their advance directives if they desire them. This act applies to hospitals, home health agencies, skilled nursing facilities, hospices, and health maintenance organizations that participate in Medicare and Medicaid. Despite this law and numerous public education efforts, advance directives have had minimal impact on actual resuscitation decisions in patients. Once again, in the SUPPORT project only 20% of the seriously ill patients had prepared advance directives *(35)*.

In the United States, an advance directive cannot be used to withhold life-sustaining treatment unless certain criteria are fulfilled. These include permission to withhold treatment by a surrogate authorized in name by the directive, and a terminal condition that is confirmed by two physicians, including the attending physician or a physician with expertise in evaluating cognitive function, who certifies that the patient is in persistent vegetative state.

Children

Respect for autonomy and self-determination requires involvement of children in decision making. However, such involvement should be consistent with their level of maturity. They should be asked to consent to procedures when able. Conflicts of interest may lead parents to make choices that are not in the best interests of their children. Outside consultation should be obtained if patients, surrogates, or parents cannot agree with physicians on the care of children. In these cases, consultation with another physician, ethics committee, or governmental child protection agency may be required. Consultation, once again, ensures that all viewpoints and alternatives are attentively considered.

Do Not Attempt Resuscitation

The discussion to limit life support is a difficult task for physicians who have been taught that preservation of life is the ultimate goal, but it is a significant responsibility that cannot be disregarded. There may be occasions when the physician's own values differ drastically from the patient's, particularly when a terminally ill patient wants no further aggressive treatment. The physician has an ethical responsibility to honor the resuscitation preferences expressed by the patient. In this situation, physicians should not permit their personal value judgments about quality of life to hinder the implementation of a patient's preferences regarding the use of resuscitation. Before a DNAR order is evoked, the physician has some very important responsibilities to fulfill. First, it is fundamental for the diagnosis to be firmly established. If there is any uncertainly, the physician should be aggressive with life-support therapies until a potentially reversible illness is excluded. Secondly, the physician must have a thorough understanding of the pathophysiology and prognosis so this information can be used in determining available treatment choices.

Before instituting DNAR orders, it is prudent to consider whether any of these two conditions exist: (a) resuscitation is proven to be of no benefit and will not prolong life; (b) the individual will suffer poor quality of life after resuscitation *(58)*. In the first instance, in which there is no proof of benefit, the goal of communication with the patient should be to create an awareness that resuscitation is not a treatment option. Herein lies one of the most difficult burdens a physician must master: the task of compassionately informing a patient that he or she has an irreversible illness, for which there is no reasonable opportunity of quality survival. There is a precarious balance between leaving the patient with no hope, and giving false hope. By raising the option of resuscitation, the physician implies that it may be of benefit, when in fact it will never be. In the second instance, when the quality of life is the impetus for foregoing resuscitation, the choice must rest with the patient. The physician cannot depend on his or her own personal values in an attempt to persuade the patient. Under ideal situations, the patient–physician relationship should be amply established. Years of caring for a patient may provide some insight into the patient's own system of beliefs.

The decision to limit life-sustaining support should probably occur as early in the course of the illness as possible. Clearly, it is a responsibility that physicians tend to ignore, as only 19% of patients in one study had these issues discussed prior to a CA *(42)*. However, the appropriate time for this discussion is yet to be defined. Whether it should be done on admission or when the patient deteriorates is a matter of controversy *(59)*. A discussion of code status at the time of deterioration is the most common time that this is performed. Targeting sicker patients reinforces the belief that discussion of a DNAR order equates with a poor outcome. One major drawback, however, is that waiting until there is deterioration may render that patient incompetent and unable to partake in the decision-making process.

Prior to the development of modern medical therapy, medicine had four primary goals: to do no harm, to relieve suffering, to attenuate disease, and to refrain from treating those who are hopelessly ill. Patients with a terminal illness were assured a rapid demise. In this situation, the physician served as a source of comfort and compassion, and to allay pain and suffering. However, advances in resuscitation techniques within the last 40 years have drastically reduced the mortality of life-threatening illnesses previously considered hopeless. Unfortunately, there also exists the potential to abuse medical advancements and prolong the process of dying without having much effect on actual patient outcome. Perhaps this occurs because the physician takes a professional oath to sustain life, or the physician has strong personal beliefs on the value of life, or fears possible litigation. Regardless, it is clear that, although the terminally ill patient always deserves close medical attention to relieve pain and suffering, the use of aggressive therapies, such as resuscitation, may not always be required in all situations and may not be what the patient desires.

Failure to understand and communicate the potential for harm and absence of benefit associated with some "life-sustaining" therapies in certain circumstances has produced a climate of misunderstanding among physicians and patients. In the United States, families often equate limiting care as "not caring" for their loved ones. Others believe that not providing resuscitation may stem from limited financial resources. Additionally, a DNAR order is not the same as withholding medical treatment. It does not preclude therapies such as administration of parenteral fluids, oxygen, analgesics, sedation, antibiotics, antiarrhythmics or vasopressors, unless specifically stated. Some patients may want defibrillation and chest compression but not endotracheal intubation and mechanical ventilation. An informed patient, family member, or surrogate may choose only limited resuscitative efforts, but must have the understanding that the chances of successful resuscitation are markedly decreased.

Orders to not attempt resuscitation should not lead to abandonment of patients or denial of appropriate and indicated medical and nursing interventions. DNAR orders should never convey a sense of giving up to the patient, family members, or surrogate and most importantly to the rest of the health care staff. One of the greatest fears that patients and family have is that this order will somehow influence the attention, care, support, and comfort they need. The patient should know that he or she will receive care that ensures comfort and dignity. Many patients fear pain and abandonment more than death. Effective management of physical symptoms can allay patients' fears and enable them to address the psychosocial and spiritual tasks that they face as they prepare for death *(60,61)*. However, in one study, a discordance between patient and physician rating of pain predicted insufficient pain control *(62)*. The realization that terminally ill patients deserve a unique management approach prompted several major hospitals to develop protocols for the care of these patients *(63)*. There are several different levels of support that must be considered whenever there is a decision to limit advanced resuscitation therapies. Some patients receive comfort measures only, whereas others receive general medical therapies such as intravenous fluids, antibiotics, or oxygen. Comfort care is provided to minimize pain, dyspnea, delirium, convulsions, or other terminal complications. Additionally a patient requiring intensive care treatment should be allowed these therapies regardless if they have DNAR order.

In the United States, the Joint Commission on the Accreditation of Health care Organizations (JCAHO) requires hospitals to have written policies for limitation-of-treatment orders (such as DNARs). Once the decision has been made, the DNAR order is placed in the patient's chart with a note explaining the rationale for the order and any specific limitations of care. However, this order must be communicated and interpreted correctly by everyone involved in the patient's care. Such discussion ensures that the hospital staff is informed about the wishes of the patient and gives time to resolve any conflicts that may arise. Other countries require that these orders be signed by two attending physicians. As with advance directives, the DNAR order should be reviewed and reevaluated at regular intervals because changes are common, especially if the patient's prognosis changes.

In situations were the medical staff believed that resuscitation would not be beneficial, in the past it became a common practice to not call for a "code blue" or to perform a less than full resuscitation. Knowingly providing ineffective resuscitation, such as what may be referred to as a "slow code" or "show codes," is inappropriate to say the least. This practice compromises the ethical integrity of health care professionals and undermines the health care worker–patient relationship. This type of resuscitation should never be considered or performed.

Principle of Medical Futility

Based on the ethical principles of beneficence and nonmaleficence that underlie the practice of medicine and define its goals, the intention of a life-sustaining procedure should be to restore or maintain a patient's well-being and it should not have as its sole goal the unqualified extension of a patient's biological life. On this basis, a medical treatment is considered futile when it cannot establish any meaningful survival, specifically length of life and quality of life, both of which would have value to that patient as an individual. Survival in a state with permanent loss of consciousness and completely lacking cognitive and sentient capacity, should be regarded as having no values for such a patient. A careful estimation of the patient's prognosis for both length and quality of life will establish whether resuscitation is appropriate for that situation.

From a medical point of view, when survival is not anticipated or if the patient's quality of life is low, resuscitation is considered ineffective and health care providers have no obligation to provide such intervention because there are no health benefits *(64,65)*. Likewise, this is true if the family or surrogate wishes for the intervention to be performed. A patient does not have an unqualified right to demand medical treatment that offers no benefit. Physicians also are not mandated to provide care that violates their own ethical principles. In these cases, care may need to be transferred to another physician. There is no medical or ethical justification for treatment that is clearly futile, offering no hope of any medical benefit.

The moral foundation of the physician–patient relationship is the commitment of the physician for beneficence. Actions that do not subscribe to this end are not morally mandated *(66)*. To coerce physicians to provide medical interventions that are incisively futile would undermine the ethical integrity of the medical profession. If a physician resolves to withhold such an intervention, he or she has a responsibility to inform the patient, family, or surrogate decision maker of that decision and to explain the decision's rationale and the medical facts that support the decision *(58)*. Additionally, the patient should be reassured that he or she will continue to receive all other care that is medically indicated within the context of the overall medical treatment plan. If there is disagreement over restricting interventions under these circumstances, the family should be allowed to relocate the patient's care to another physician or institution; if this is not possible, then the patient's health care providers with their institution's support should consider petitioning judicial review to resolve the differences.

The major predicament in making choices about the futility of resuscitation centers on the patient's estimation of meaningful survival. To judge that a life-sustaining intervention would lack medical efficacy requires the capacity to estimate the outcome of that intervention with a high degree of confidence. Although a growing body of scientific knowledge is available to guide physicians in estimating the outcome of some life-threatening conditions, meaningful prognosis remains an inexact science when applied to an individual patient *(67)*. Even for patients who have conditions for which survival with resuscitation is unprecedented, the prediction that the next patient also will not survive is only the assertion of a high probability, not a logical certainty. Physicians can consult other physicians to try to lessen the likelihood of error in choices based on prognosis. However, most physicians are poor at estimating survival from resuscitation (68). One study demonstrated patients with cancer had similar outcomes of survival from resuscitation when compared to the rest of the hospital population (69). Consequently, it is impossible to know beforehand the outcome of a given resuscitation intervention. Physicians can only provide probabilities for a given outcome. This uncertainty is greatly augmented when the available information about the patient is incomplete. Such is usually the case when resuscitating a patient in the emergency department (ED) or when a cardiac arrest occurs in a hospital during the night.

It is reasonable that health care providers most often choose to err on the side of overtreatment and preservation of life because failure to provide resuscitation in this circumstance is an irreversible decision. However, this bias toward resuscitation should not extend to situations in which clear judgment to withhold resuscitation has already been established. When the effectiveness of an intervention is still questionable, a time-limited trial of the intervention may increase the certainly of the prognosis.

Oppositionists to medical futility argue that a robust role of futility judgments in medical decision making would undermine patient autonomy and lead to paternalistic physician–patient relationships. The reverse, however, may be actually true. The reason for physician authority over the use of futile treatment is actually the protection of patient autonomy. If the patient takes the physician–patient relationship to be a fiduciary one, the physician who offers a choice of futile resuscitation sends a misleading message that is very difficult to untangle sufficiently to ensure an informed and autonomous decision by the patient. In offering to perform a resuscitation, the physician implies that the procedure offers a benefit reasonably worth pursuing. Otherwise, why would a conscientious physician acting on his or her fiduciary obligations feel a duty to make such an offer? When resuscitation is clearly ineffective, physicians should not be required to discuss it as an option. Respect for patient autonomy does not require that the physician initiate discussion of medically senseless procedures. Moreover, most patients and families are not accustomed to being offered a treatment with the suggestion that it be refused. Some will assume that if medical care is offered it must have some benefit and will interpret refusal as giving up or abandoning the patient.

To summarize, there is no duty to provide futile treatments, patients, or families have no right to demand them, and physician integrity may forbid offering them; patient autonomy does not mandate discussion of senseless procedures, and compassion for struggling families may in some cases argue against it.

Noninitiation of CPR

No scientific data exists on which to base a clear-cut standard for estimating the medical futility or outcome of resuscitation accurately (70,71). Even patients with metastatic cancer may be in relatively good health when they have an incidental arrhythmic CA and go on to survive the event. The prognosis in this situation is similar in patients with or without metastatic disease, as shown in a recent study that reported a 10% survival to hospital discharge rate for patients with metastatic disease (69). Of these survivors, 4% lived for 1 year (33,34,49). There are no available scoring systems, severity of symptoms, medical diseases, or initial rhythms that have an acceptable level of sensitivity for accurately estimating a universally poor outcome. No one can predict when the rate of survival is so low that resuscitation should not be offered to a patient who requires it. Also, physician's predictions of outcome after CPR tend to be inaccurate (70).

With this in mind, some have suggested attempting resuscitation in all patients who develop CA unexpectedly unless the patient has a valid DNAR order, or the patient has signs of irreversible death, such as, rigor mortis, decapitation, or dependent lividity. If there is no expected survival from maximal therapy for septic or cardiogenic shock, it is prudent not to attempt resuscitation. In the newly born, attempts to resuscitate may be withheld in cases in which resuscitation is known to be futile. These include known gestational age of less than 23 weeks, weight less than 400 g, anencephaly, or confirmed trisomy 13 or 18.

Termination of Resuscitation

Numerous determinants affect the decision to withdraw resuscitative efforts. These may include but are not limited to time from CA to initiation of CPR, time to defibrillation, comorbid disease states, pre-arrest medical status, initial arrest rhythm, and time of current resuscitation. None of these factors alone or in combination is exclusively predictive of outcome *(71)*. Of these, the best predictor of poor outcome is the elapsed time of the ongoing resuscitation *(72–74)*. The possibility of hospital discharge with no neurological disability decreases as the time for resuscitation increases *(75–77)*. Resuscitative efforts should be terminated when the chance for meaningful survival is unlikely. In the absence of mitigating issues, prolonged resuscitation is unlikely to be successful if there is no return of spontaneous circulation (ROSC) at any time after 30 minutes of advanced cardiac life support (ACLS *[78]*). For the newborn, termination of resuscitative efforts may be appropriate if ROSC has not occurred after 15 minutes or if asystole is present for greater than 10 minutes *(54,55,79)*. If ROSC of any duration occurs at any time during the resuscitation, it may be worthwhile considering an extended period of resuscitation. Additionally, there should be the absence of persistently recurring or refractory ventricular fibrillation (VF) or ventricular tachycardia (VT). Other extenuating issues that may play a role in deciding the duration of resuscitation may include pre-arrest hypothermia or the presence of drug intoxications that may mask recovery from the central nervous system (CNS).

Pre-Hospital Setting

Except in certain extenuating circumstances, pre-hospital responders are urged and expected to attempt resuscitation. Exceptions to this rule include the patient who has signs of irreversible death (e.g., rigor mortis, decapitation, or dependent lividity); cases in which attempts at resuscitation would place the rescuer at risk of significant harm, or cases in which a valid DNAR order exists. Most emergency medical services (EMS) protocols have provisions to identify adult or children with DNAR orders *(80,81)*. This could be through an order form, identification card, or bracelets.

In certain circumstances, it may be difficult to establish whether resuscitation should be initiated. Another awkward situation for prehospital personnel may include when family members, surrogates, or the patient's physician request resuscitation despite the presence of a valid DNAR order. In the case of an out-of-hospital resuscitation in which there is no definite DNAR order, living will, or advance directive, EMS personnel should initiate resuscitation. It is ethical for the ED health care providers to terminate resuscitative efforts initiated by EMS personnel if a valid DNAR is found later. This includes removal of the endotracheal tube and intravenous catheters and halting the infusion of medications and solutions, provided such actions are not prohibited by a medical examiner's investigation.

Rescuers who initiate resuscitation should continue until one of the following occurs: (a) effective spontaneous ventilation and circulation have been reestablished; (b) care is transferred to another trained person who continues resuscitation; (c) care is transferred more advanced trained health care providers; (d) a physician terminates the resuscitation efforts; (e) reliable evidence of irreversible death are recognized; (f) the rescuer is too exhausted to continue resuscitation; (g) environmental hazards endanger the scene, or continued resuscitation would endanger the lives of others; or (h) a valid DNAR order is presented to the rescuers.

Out-of-hospital emergency resuscitation affects not only the patient but may have strong impact on family members present at the scene. Emergency personnel are entrusted with the responsibility of managing not the patient and the surviving family members *(82)*. Prolonged resuscitative efforts are unlikely to be successful if there is no ROSC at any time after 30 minutes of ACLS *(78)*. There should also be the absence of persistently recurring or refractory VF or VT or any continued neurological activity, such as spontaneous respiration, eye opening, or motor response *(70)*. There is a growing body of evidence that ED resuscitation of patients who arrive pulseless, despite out-of-hospital ACLS, is futile *(83–85)*. Consequently, criteria for field termination of unsuccessful out-of-hospital CA resuscitations have been widely developed *(86)*. Some rescuers (especially in remote areas) have prolonged transport time intervals before reaching a definitive care facility. The risk of vehicular accidents during high-speed emergency transport must be weighed against the likelihood of successful resuscitation *(83,87,88)*. A study showed that 96% of family members were satisfied with terminating resuscitative efforts in the field *(89)*. Furthermore, family members of patients for whom resuscitation efforts are terminated in the field, compared with those of patients who were first transported to an ED, showed similar satisfaction regarding the manner in which they were informed about the death and the overall care provided by the EMS system.

State and local EMS authorities should be encouraged to develop protocols for the initiation and withdrawal of resuscitation in the prehospital setting. Physicians, EMS, and medical directors remain ultimately responsible for determination of death, and pronouncement of death in the prehospital setting and should have the concurrence of on-line medical control *(90)*. ROSC for even a brief period of time is a positive prognostic signs and warrants consideration of transport to a hospital. Other patients who may benefit from a transport to the hospital include those with pre-arrest hypothermia or the presence of drug intoxications that may mask recovery from the CNS.

Withdrawal of Life Support

Withdrawal of life support in any patient is an emotionally complex decision for a family and medical staff. Because preservation of life is a legitimate interest of the patient, the refusal of life-prolonging treatments creates the potential for conflict. The conflict between beneficence and autonomy constitutes the basis of most ethical dilemmas involving life-sustaining treatment. Allowing the patient to die can be viewed as a violation of beneficence, although pressuring the patient to undergo heroic supportive measures is a potential violation of his or her autonomy.

Physicians and other health care providers have a responsibility to respect autonomy by withholding or withdrawing any life-sustaining treatments as requested by an informed and capable patient, family member, or surrogate. In this regard, withholding and withdrawing life support are considered ethically equivalent. Helping a patient to forgo life support under these situations is regarded as distinct from participating in assisted suicide or active euthanasia. Patients, families, and physicians often struggle with the question of whether withdrawing treatment is the same as "killing" the patient. A decision to withdraw life support is justifiable if the physician and the patient or surrogate agree that additional treatment would not be beneficial to the patient. The stimulus for withdrawal of therapy should be eliminating a burdensome intervention, not causing the patient's death.

The patient's physician and other health care providers also have a responsibility for carrying out the patient's wishes in a humane and compassionate manner. To this end, the patient's pain and other suffering, including dyspnea, should be relieved by administration of sedatives and analgesics.

Brain death criteria cannot be established during an emergency resuscitation attempt. Determination of brain death criteria must conform to nationally accepted guidelines. In the case of a patient who meets brain death criteria, life-sustaining medical treatment is withdrawn unless consent for organ donation has been given. If such consent has been given, previous DNAR orders are replaced with standard cadaver-care transplant protocols until the organs have been procured.

Family Presence During Resuscitation

The presence of family members during resuscitations or other advanced medical procedures has usually not been accepted by the health care community because of the assumption that this experience would have an undesirable effect. This premise is more common as the invasiveness of the procedure increases and is especially true for resuscitations. Other explanations for excluding family members may be based on the fear that family members will interfere with the resuscitation or that their observations may reveal weaknesses and failures of medical care. There are, however, no data to support any of these contentions. In fact, studies have shown that there is a growing interest in family members being present during the resuscitation or during procedures being performed on their loved ones (91–97). Such participation has been demonstrated to ease the family members' own grieving process and some have felt a sense of helping (91). A large proportion of parents indicated that they would want to be present during procedures performed on their children (94,98). This is especially true with parents of chronically ill children. These mothers are often more knowledgeable about their child's condition and are comfortable around medical equipment and emergencies. Of family members who were present during attempted resuscitation of an adult relative in CA, 97% said they would want to be present again and 76% felt it helped them to grieve their relative's death. Others have shown that family presence during procedures was beneficial for both the family and the ED personnel (99).

Certainly, the decision for parents or family members to be present during a procedure or resuscitation needs to be individualized. The relationship between the family member and the patient, the desire of the family to stay or leave, and the need for the physician to maintain control in difficult situations must all be considered when determining family presence during procedures or resuscitations.

Parents or family members seldom ask if they can be present unless they have been encouraged to do so (94–97). In one study, only 11% of family members were asked if they could go into the resuscitation room and the majority of those interviewed wished that they had been offered the opportunity (93). Families want to be given the option to remain during procedures, and when given the option, often choose to remain *(100)*. Health care providers should offer the opportunity for family members to be present whenever possible *(92,101)*. Resuscitation team members should be sensitive to the presence of family members during resuscitative efforts. Furthermore, during any major resuscitation, special preparation of family members and a dedicated staff member to accompany them may be necessary to minimize confusion and fear in this emotionally difficult situation. This team member can be a chaplain, social worker, patient advocate or nurse and should be able to answer questions, clarify information, and be willing to perform other comfort measures *(101)*.

Notification of Death

Despite all the medical treatments currently available, the majority of patients undergoing resuscitation will die. Notifying family members of the death of their loved one is an important aspect of the resuscitation continuum and is one of the most difficult tasks that a physician or health care provider must fulfill.

Health care providers are frequently unaware of the enormous impact that they have on the family and the unique position that the they are in to affect the families' grief reaction. Health care providers must be honest and sensitive to the needs of the families by using appropriate words and body language, displaying professional and caring attitudes, being knowledgeable, responding to questions about the care that was provided, and explaining what procedures will be followed after the patient's death. Additionally, there must be a mechanism provided for future questions to be answered and arrangements for a follow-up for the surviving family *(102,103)*.

If the death occurs in the ED, it usually involves a sudden medical event or traumatic injury, and is, consequently unexpected. The family has not had time to evolve through the stages of accepting death *(104)*. The surviving family members are often thrown into an acute grief reaction and are at increased risk for morbid, prolonged, or complicated grief. Additionally, the physician is shouldered with the task of informing the family of their relative's death without the benefit of establishing any prior relationship with the family.

After resuscitation is terminated, the physician must be able to shift quickly from the intense attempts to preserve life to support the family members who must cope with the death of relative. Emotions must be suppressed during resuscitation to avoid distraction. In contrast, communication with family members requires resounding sensitivity and is often charged emotionally. Some physicians develop a defensive measure to protect themselves from the stress of this situation. At times, physicians may attempt to decrease their own stress by delaying the notification process, which in turn raises the family's anxiety; or by rushing in unprepared and delivering the news in a disorganized manner. Although there is no painless way of informing family members of their relative's death, certain key elements in the delivery that may help prevent undue emotional distress to both the family and physician.

Contacting the Family

If family members were not present when the patient died, they must be located and notified. Family members are often notified by an unknown person and, additionally, may be unfamiliar with the hospital. Therefore, the caller should identify himself or herself and establish their relationship to the deceased. In most cases, it is preferable not to communicate the death over the telephone. Alternatively, they can be told that their relative is seriously ill or injured and that they should come directly to hospital *(105)*. The caller should encourage the relative to travel to the hospital with a close friend or relative, and to let that person drive the car *(105)*. It must be emphasized that rushing to the hospital will not change the patient's condition. In certain situations, however, such as a long travel time or inability to arrive at the hospital, it may be essential to notify them of the patient's death over the telephone.

Arrival of Family Members

Family members should be greeted immediately by a knowledgeable member of the hospital staff, preferably a chaplain, patient advocate or social worker. Even a short delay can be perceived as disturbingly long for the family waiting impatiently *(82)*. The family should be taken into a quiet room in which they can have privacy without interruption. In a private place the family will be free to express their grief. The room should be near a bathroom and contain facial tissue, drinking water, and a telephone. If the patient is still alive, a staff member should provide periodic updates. It should ideally be the same staff member so that the family does not have deal with a large number of strangers. The family's need to be informed must not be taken as an aggravation, but should be respected *(95)*.

Preparation Prior to the Notification of Death

The physician taking care of the patient should be the one who informs the family. Informing a family of the loss of a loved one is a difficult task and is more difficult in the ED because the physician usually has no relationship with the relatives prior to the death of the patient. Prior to talking with the family, the physician should take a moment in time and concede to any strong personal feelings surrounding the case. A sudden unexpected death may produce a state of mind of disappointment and animosity. The health care provider can sometimes perceive a "failed" resuscitation attempt as a personal and professional failure. Such perceptions lead to feelings of guilt and remorse even if the medical treatment was quite within acceptable standards of care. Events surrounding the resuscitation, especially if it was difficult, can impart emotions that can misunderstood by family members as not caring. Some health care providers may look for acceptance and support from family members instead of providing support to the family. Such emotions should be set aside for later resolution rather than carried into the room in which the family is situated.

Before meeting the relatives it may be useful to review the medical treatment and responses that occurred during the resuscitation. This will allow the physician to order their thoughts and help identify or foresee areas that might be difficult to elucidate. This preparation can prevent unexpected verbal stumbling blocks during an inevitable stressful situation.

It is valuable to enlist the assistance of a nurse, chaplain, patient advocate, or social worker who is willing and able to provide added support to the family, particularly if the physician is not comfortable with this task *(106)*. It is always helpful to share the emotional demands of the encounter with someone. Additionally, find out as much as possible about the relatives. Obtain knowledge about the family member present, what there relationship is, was the death unexpected, what they have been told about the patient's condition thus far, and how they have reacted to this information. Obtaining this information attenuates the surprise potential and can better enable you to prepare for special problems. Find out if any of the relatives may be at high risk for pathological grief. Finally, ask that close friends wait outside until the news is communicated; the family then may resolve how to notify these people *(107)*.

Notification of Death

When entering the room, introduce yourself as the patient's physician and establish the identity of the family members present. Assume the same posture as the family, recognizing that sitting is better than standing. The physician often is tempted to remain standing, however, this may lead to the impression that he or she cannot stay long or cannot join the family in this moment of grief. Unless the situation is hostile, move away from the door and physically join the group *(108)*.

Give a chronological history of the events leading up to the patient's death using common sense and terminology the family can understand and avoiding medical jargon or vague descriptions. Inform them of the events prior to arriving and during the resuscitation and the results to such interventions. Presenting the actual facts of the event will help the family acknowledge death intellectually and reassure them that everything possible was done. When given the full account of what happened, many family members are surprised at the actual labor involved, much more than after hearing the more common and vague cliché "we did all that we could." Additionally, it allows the family to have a more firm cognitive basis from which to react with normal grief. Allow time for reactions and questions of the family members. Communication is only as good as what is heard and understood by the listener. Then, most significantly, state clearly that the patient "died" or "was pronounced dead." Everyone understands this word and it is exact. Avoid euphemistic language, such as "passed on," "did not make it," "succumbed," "taken a turn for the worst," "expired," or "given up." Because an announcement of death causes some degree of shock, it may be wise to say "died" at least twice during the announcement.

An expression of compassion is important, but there is no need to sound apologetic, such as "I'm sorry," when informing the family. These statements, in an attempt to sound sympathetic may be understood by the angry family as an effort to conceal something. Sympathy can be clearly expressed by stating, "you certainly have my sympathy." Relatives need only to be acknowledged for their loss with sympathy.

Allow Grief Response

With any death, particularly if unexpected, the family is unprepared and the initial grief response may be exaggerated. It is important that the family begin to grapple with the reality of death and be encouraged to release their initial emotional response. Allow a short period of time for the immediate grief response. If comfortable doing so, give support to the family members. Touching or holding the survivor when appropriate will be appreciated. The expression of grief is determined by many issues including cultural, social and religious beliefs. Family members may cope with crisis by being histrionic, with loud crying and sobbing; others will be stoic, with little visible signs of emotion. Do not move away from them, unless there is a real threat to be harmed *(109)*. Family members will be in severe emotional shock. Be prepared to weather their initial unrest of anger or denial without inhibiting their expression of grief or responding to accusations.

Facilitate Grief Effectively

After their immediate grief response has subsided, talk with the family members about their perceptions of the event and try to establish how they feel. If they are upset with the health care providers, their anger should be understood as displaced emotion covering up unresolved internal conflicts. Do not answer to accusations but instead bring out their feelings on the senselessness and unfairness of their relative's demise *(108)*. Reassure them that the patient had no pain, unless this was not a fact *(109)*. Endorse the actions of the prehospital workers and the health care providers involved in the resuscitation. Do not address any issues that occurred during the resuscitation at this point *(109)*. Alleviate any feelings of guilt by reassuring that they did everything possible, that their actions were appropriate, and that the actions they omitted would have not changed the result. In nearly all cases, the use of sedation is discouraged because they tend to extend the grieving process *(105,108,110)*.

As the physician assesses the grief response, the predisposition to and symptoms of pathological grief must be identified and therapy begun immediately. Examples of pathological grief may include death of a spouse of many years in which thoughts of suicide may arise. These patients should have arrangements made with a relative or friend to remain with them over the next few days. Another is when a family member threatens actual suicide or has active psychotic features in which psychiatric consultation and small doses of sedation may be required. The death of one parent that leaves the other parent with an enormous burden caring for their children may lead to grief being postponed indefinitely. Finally, cases in which the survivor may have actually caused the patient's death may be a setup for pathological grief.

Seeing the Body

For most people, seeing the body seems to help in the grieving process, although this may not always be the case *(104,111)*. Viewing the body should be encouraged because this act validates that the death has occurred and helps the family overcome denial. Failure to see the body may prolong the grief process because the survivor cannot acknowledge that the person is really dead. However, if a relative does not want to see the body, by no means should they feel forced to do so or guilty for not choosing to see the body. If at first they refuse to see the body, they should be offered another chance later when they have had time to collect their thoughts. It is important to remember to refer to the body by their name or "him" or "her" and not as "it" because this may make the encounter more personal to family members.

Prior to viewing the body, it is wise to clean any blood or debris that may make the viewing unpleasant to the family (provided this does not interfere with a medical examiner's forensic evaluation). The family should be warned of what to expect prior to seeing the body. Prepare them for the presence of injuries, intravenous lines, and endotracheal tubes if present. If there are deformed or mutilated body parts, it preferable for them to be covered with a sheet.

If possible the body should be moved to a quiet room, which allow grievers both privacy and a more pleasant setting for this indelible event. The family should be accompanied by either a chaplain, social worker, or nurse although seeing the body to give support, answer questions, or simply stand quietly nearby.

Children

Family members always should be encouraged to talk to children about the death. An honest discussion can be a positive emotional experience and may help diminish the misconceptions that children may fantasize about death. No one should lie or alter of the facts. Family members should be encouraged to discuss their feelings openly with the child and not to change the child's feelings about the death. Adults should be encouraged to disclose their grief openly rather than privately. This establishes a model that the child can learn that open expression of feelings is acceptable. This form of expression will allow the child to accept death as reality.

When the deceased is a parent, young children often need constant reassurance that the surviving parent will not vanish and will continue the same role as before and maintain the family together. When adults avoid talking about death with children, they create an atmosphere of fear and anxiety for children who are sensitive to evasion and family stress levels.

Concluding Process

Once the body is viewed, the family's visit to the ED or hospital should be formally concluded in a manner that covers the remaining necessary details. The physician has the responsibility to answer any final questions, to request an autopsy, or ask the family about organ and tissue donation as indicated, and to provide follow-up. Asking for a postmortem examination, especially if mandated by the coroner's office, may be especially anxiety provoking. It is helpful for the physician to communicate that this is an operative procedure done by a skilled professional to determine possibly the cause of death. Transfer of the body to the coroner's office or mortuary should be addressed. A packet of materials containing information on transportation of the body from the hospital, death certification, autopsy and medical examiner requirements, and organ and tissue donation is useful.

Relatives should be taught about the symptoms of grief and what to expect in the weeks to come. Some of the common symptoms include depression, sleep disturbances, difficulty concentrating, anorexia, and preoccupation with the deceased *(112)*. They should be reassured that all of these symptoms are normal and may have them for up to 1 or 2 months *(105)*. Finally, family members should be told that there is nothing else to do and they may leave the ED or the hospital. When possible, escorting the family and explaining to them that there is nothing more that they can do helps bring their visit to a formal close.

Follow-Up

Relatives of patients requiring resuscitation should have a follow-up phone call or letter. Especially in cases of sudden death, these relatives are commonly so stunned that they forget to ask important questions. A follow-up not only eases grief by resolving these important questions, but can alert the physician to possible pathologic grief and need for psychiatric consultation and therapy.

Health Care Providers' Emotional Needs

Unfortunately, health care providers, especially those involved in the resuscitation are not expected to grieve when their patients die. Health care providers are considered support figures who should be resistant to the emotional impact of death. Outwardly, health care providers meet those expectations at work. They rarely display their feelings, continue to manage other patient problems in an objective fashion and do not discuss their emotions, even with unexpected death.

Certainly the justification why health care providers seem less affected by death are complex, but may include the need to satisfy assumed professional and personal expectations. Still, there is every reason to expect that death adversely affects the health care providers' sense of accomplishment and satisfaction, and incites feelings of guilt and failure. They often experience emotional reactions similar to those of family members. To neglect these feelings or to allow them to go unaddressed is not acceptable. It is important for health care providers to identify their feelings, whether they be relief, sadness, guilt, or failure. Health care providers must understand and accept these emotions as natural consequences of interacting with a patient who dies. Emotions concerning a patient's death are experienced by all individual involved in a resuscitation, and that they are important for our personal and professional growth and maturity. Having health care providers discuss their feelings openly with other coworkers or a chaplain eases the bereavement process.

Organ and Tissue Donations

Recent advances in surgical techniques, organ preservation, immunosuppressive therapy, and life-supporting technologies have allowed organ and tissue transplantation to play a major role in the treatment of patients with end-organ failure. Consequently, the demand for transplantable organs is increasing rapidly. The major obstacle to organ procurement is the limited organ supply *(94)*.

Health care providers should support efforts to procure organs and tissues for the increasing number of patients who may benefit from these procedures. In the United States, permission for organ and tissue donations must be obtained from the patient's relatives.

Research and Training on Newly Dead

Patients demand and count on safe and effective medical treatments when faced with an acute illness. Also, the public expects the health care community to continually improve the efficacy and safety of available medical technology. Public expectation for advances in acute medical technologies necessitates research into the etiology and treatments of acute illness. Research into emergency procedures is essential to society to achieve these stated goals. The current standards used in the resuscitation of patients have been created from research performed in unconscious patients who were unable to give informed consent.

An enormous amount of research is performed in the area of resuscitation. Research topics have included techniques to maximize cardiac and cerebral perfusion and drug therapy to prevent damage from resuscitation and reperfusion. However, virtually all this research is occurring in animal models. There is a significant paucity of studies corroborating preliminary animal data in humans. Even though some researchers are performing limited studies on humans, many questions cannot be conducted in humans because of ethical reasons *(113)*. Therefore advancement in resuscitation research is difficult as a result of this obstacle.

The use of a newly dead patient for research or training has raised important ethical, and at times, legal issues. The ethics of biomedical research involving human subjects are based on well established principles. The principle of beneficence entails promoting the well-being of research subjects although protecting them from harm or nonmaleficence. This has always been ensured by having independent committees review the research protocols, although maintaining the subjects' rights. The ethical principle of autonomy, which allows individuals to control any procedures done on their bodies, and the legal requirements set by the federal agencies that supervise human research dictate, that, in general, a competent patient must give informed consent for any research *(90)*. However, prospective informed consent for resuscitation research in the emergency setting is nearly impossible to obtain *(114–116)*.

The consent from a family member is ideal and respects the autonomy of the newly dead. However, this is often not possible in the case of a CA. Resuscitation for cardiopulmonary events is usually unanticipated and requires immediate intervention. Because of this, identifying populations prior to such occurrence is impractical, and obtaining informed consent after such events is impractical at best, and often impossible. The infeasibility of obtaining consent for resuscitation cannot be the absolute barrier in preventing emergency research. Advocates of research on the newly dead maintain that a greater good is accomplished, which benefits the living. Enrollment of a patient into an emergency research protocol without consent has been shown to be not only acceptable to but also appreciated by family members who, in most cases, consented to the research protocol *(115)*.

Some researches have attempted to overcome the problem with informed consent was the use of deferred or presumed consent *(117)*. The investigators deducted that participants would want to enter the trial because prognosis from resuscitation is poor and experimental treatment may be better than the standard treatment. It was believed that patients would want to enroll, or at least want to initially "preserve their option" to participate. These patients received initial therapy provided that family or surrogate could be contacted and informed consent obtained within a reasonable time. Patients whose family or surrogates refused to give consent were withdrawn from the study at that time. Objection to deferred consent is that no one can quantify the risk or benefit from an experimental protocol accurately, and in this circumstance it is unreasonable to assume that most patients would choose to participate. Additionally, this belief goes against the principle of autonomy, because patients have a right to do what they want to do with their bodies, which includes enrolling in a research study. Therefore, presumed consent, even if it saves the option to participate, still abrogates the principle of autonomy and informed consent. It is interesting that deferred consent is an approved standard for providing resuscitation but has been considered to be inappropriate in the research of resuscitation.

The problem with presumed consent is the assumption that a reasonable person would consent under the same circumstances. In many countries, deferred consent is the premise for procurement of organs and tissues. Extrapolation of this philosophy to include medical training and research is unfounded. In a Norwegian study, 60% of parents who had recently lost an infant were opposed to deferred consent for procedures *(118)*. Deferred consent for medical training and research with the newly dead should demands a well-informed public with allowance for discussion so that individuals have the right to refuse consent.

In the United States, unlike most other countries, the topic of informed consent for resuscitation research has become one of the most vital impediments for future progress in resuscitation. Research in victims of cardiac arrest has been restricted severely because prospective informed consent cannot usually be obtained. Research on such patients has captivated much public attention because of the possibility of unethical research. However, most research done in this field has consisted of well-designed, carefully monitored studies that have led to significant advances for society in general. After much public debate with the Food and Drug Administration and the National Institutes of Health, a new regulation that allows an initial exception of informed consent in certain very strict circumstances has been adopted *(119)*. Research can be performed in emergency situations if prospective subjects are in a life-threatening situation and prospective informed consent is not practical. Additionally, present therapy is unproven or unsatisfactory, research is required to determine what intervention is best, and the risk and benefits are reasonable without undue risks from entering the protocol. Moreover, there are stringent pretrial requirements for consultation with experts, as well as lay persons who might be study patients, and full public disclosure of the details and results of the study are required if this waiver is to be invoked.

The process of obtaining consent to perform procedures or research on the newly dead places a considerable strain on both the family, who must consent in this stressful circumstance, and the health care provider, who must ask for it. In the same Norwegian study, 8% of parents would have been angry if they were asked to use their newly dead infant for practice of endotracheal tube intubation *(118)*. However, 73 to 78% of parents reported that they would have agreed if they had been asked *(118,120)*.

Patients deserve and expect modern, safe, and effective medical therapies when they are acutely ill. The public desires advances in acute resuscitation procedures in order to improve outcomes. The benefits of emergency research include potential improvement in survival and quality of life from CA, threatening condition that otherwise would have a dismal outcome.

CONCLUSIONS

The therapeutic advancements in the last half of the century have allowed health care providers to change the natural history of many diseases. For certain patients, the treatments have been a remarkable achievement resulting in reversal of an acute illness, and in some cases near certain death. Although for others, the effort of resuscitation has been futile and resulted in a prolongation of an inevitable death. Physicians have the responsibility to recognize their limitations. Patients should not bear the inappropriate use of medical technology.

The principles of medical ethics are intimately involved when patients exercise informed consent to have or to forgo a medical procedure. Neither autonomy or beneficence are fostered when physicians do not provide reasonable estimations and prognosis with benefits and burdens that the patient will incur with any medical intervention, especially with resuscitation. It is even worse if the physician offers treatments that are known to be inappropriate or futile for that patient. The principle of patient autonomy does not shift the responsibility for medical choices onto patients, families, or surrogates. Rather it demands that this information be provided as honestly as possible and, if possible, recommend which treatment may be most beneficial to the patient. Moreover, the physician should explain why certain procedures, such as resuscitation may not be offered.

Failure to convey and understand the potential for harm and absence of benefit from resuscitation have produced a climate of mistrust among health care providers and patients. Families often wonder whether limiting care to a patient is the same as not caring for that patient and are frequently unaware of any possible reason other than financial why certain treatments are withheld from the patient. It must be explained clearly that certain procedures may not only produce a worse outcome but may actually prolong death. On the other hand, some physicians are not willing to discuss the withholding of resuscitation with patients and families. This may be explained by either the physician thinking that he or she has given up for the patient or that they feel inadequate that they cannot save the patient or are uncomfortable with medical uncertainty. Frank discussions with patients and their families about the benefits and burdens of the medical treatments are necessary to provide patients with the best opportunity to make informed decisions.

Once a decision is made, respect should be given for that decision. Patients not wanting resuscitation should be given all the comfort care and other necessary medical therapies that are medically indicated and should never be abandoned.

REFERENCES

1. Standards and guidelines for cardiopulmonary resuscitation (CPR) and emergency cardiac care (ECC)-Part I: Introduction. JAMA 1986; 255:2905–2914.
2. Skerrit U, Pitt B. 'Do not resuscitate': How? When? Why? Int J Geriatr Psychiatry 1997; 12:667–670.
3. Evans AL, Brody BA. The do-not-resuscitate order in teaching hospitals. JAMA 1985; 253:2236–2239.
4. Tunstall-Pedoe H. Do not resuscitate decisions. Resuscitation should not be part of every death. Br Med J 2001; 322:102–103.
5. Baskett PJ. ABC of resuscitation. The ethics of resuscitation. Br Med J 1986; 293:189,190.
6. Hilberman M, Kutner J, Parsons D, Murphy DJ. Marginally effective medical care: ethical analysis of issues in cardiopulmonary resuscitation (CPR). J Med Ethics 1997; 23:361–367.
7. Schneiderman LJ, Kaplan RM, Pearlman RA, Teetzel H. Do physicians' own preferences for life-sustaining treatment influence their perceptions of patients' preferences? J Clin Ethics 1993; 4:28–33.
8. President's Commission for the Study of Ethical Problems in medicine and Biomedical and Behavioral research. Making Health care decisions: the legal and ethical implications of informed consent in the patient-practitioner relationship. Washington DC: United States Government Printing Office, 1982.
9. President's Commission for the study of ethical problems in medicine and biomedical and behavioral research. Deciding to forgo life-sustaining treatment: ethical, medical and legal issues in treatment decisions. Washington DC: United States Government Printing Office, 1983.
10. Perkins HS. Ethics at the end of life: practical principles for making resuscitation decisions. J Gen Intern Med 1986; 1:170–176.
11. Quill TE, Brody H. Physician recommendations and patient autonomy: finding a balance between physician power and patient choice. Ann Intern Med 1996; 125:763–769.
12. Prendergast TJ. Resolving conflicts surrounding end-of-life care. New Horiz 1997; 5:62–71.
13. Diem SJ, Lantos JD, Tulsky JA. Cardiopulmonary resuscitation on television. Miracles and misinformation. N Engl J Med 1996; 334:1578–1582.
14. Evans DA, Funkenstein HH, Albert MS, et al. Prevalence of Alzheimer's disease in a community population of older persons. Higher than previously reported. JAMA 1989; 262:2551–2556.
15. Blank K, Robison J, Doherty E, Prigerson H, Duffy J, Schwartz HI: Life-sustaining treatment and assisted death choices in depressed older patients. J Am Geriatr Soc 2001; 49:153–161.
16. Jackson DL, Youngner S. Patient autonomy and "death with dignity": some clinical caveats. N Engl J Med 1979; 301:404–408.
17. Marson DC, Hawkins L, McInturff B, Harrell LE. Cognitive models that predict physician judgements of capacity to consent in mild Alzheimer's disease. J Am Geriatr Soc 1997; 45:458–464.
18. Appelbaum PS, Roth LH. Clinical issues in the assessment of competency. Am J Psychiatry 1981; 138:1462–1467.
19. Brock DW. Surrogate decision-making for incompetent adults: an ethical framework. Mt Sinai J Med 1991; 58:388–392.
20. Seckler AB, Meier DE, Mulvihill M, Paris BE. Substituted judgement: how accurate are proxy predictions. Ann Intern Med 1991; 115:92–98.

21. Uhlmann RF, Pearlman RA. Perceived quality of life and preferences for life- sustaining treatment in older adults. Arch Intern Med 1991; 151:495–497.

22. Bok S. Personal directions for care at the end of life. N Engl J Med 1976; 295:367–369.

23. Sulmasy DP, Terry PB, Weisman CS, et al. The accuracy of substituted judgements in patients with terminal diagnoses. Ann Intern Med 1998; 128:621–629.

24. Sehgal A, Galbraith A, Chesney M, Schdenfeld P, Charles G, Lo B. How strictly do dialysis patients want their advance directives followed? JAMA 1992; 267:59–63.

25. Emanuel EJ, Emanuel LL. Proxy decision-making for incompetent patients: An ethical and empirical analysis. JAMA 1992; 267:2067–2071.

26. Lynn J. Conflicts of interest in medical decision-making. J Am Geriatr Soc 1988; 36:945–950.

27. Annas GJ. The health care proxy and the living will. N Eng J Med 1991; 324:1210–1213.

28. Weir RF, Gostin L. Decisions to abate life-sustaining treatment for nonautonomous patients: ethical standards and legal liability for physicians after Cruzan. JAMA 1990; 264:1846–1853.

29. Gillick M. The high costs of dying: a way out. Arch Intern Med 1994; 154:2134–2137.

30. Menikoff JA, Sachs GA, Siegler M. Beyond advance directives-health care surrogate laws. N Engl J Med 1992; 327:1165–1169.

31. Lo B, Rouse F, Dornbrand L. Family decision-making on trial. Who decides for incompetent patients? N Engl J Med 1990; 322:1228–1232.

32. Lurie N, Pheley AM, Miles SH, Bannick-Mohrland S: Attitudes toward discussing life-sustaining treatments in extended care facitlity patients. J Am Geriatr Soc 1992; 40:1205–1208.

33. Hofmann JC, Wenger NS, Davis EB et al. Patient preferences for communication with physicians about end-of-life decisions. SUPPORT investigators. Study to Understand Prognoses and Preferences for Outcomes and Risks of Treatments. Ann Intern Med 1997; 127:1–12.

34. Kennedy BJ. Communicating with patients about advanced cancer. JAMA 1998; 280: 1403,1404.

35. The SUPPORT Principal Investigators. A controlled trial to improve care for seriously ill hospital patients: the study to understand prognoses and preferences for outcomes and risks of treatment (SUP-PORT). JAMA 1995; 274:1591–1598.

36. Emanuel LL, Barry MJ, Stoeckle JD, Ettelson LM, Emanuel EJ: Advance directives for medical care—a case for greater use. N Engl J Med 1991; 324:889–895.

37. Krumholz H, Philips RS, Hamel MB, et al. Resuscitation preferences among patients with severe congestive heart failure: results from the SUPPORT project. Study to Understand Prognoses and Preferences for Outcomes and Risks of Treatments. Circulation 1998; 98:648–655.

38. Ebell MH Doukas DJ, Smith MA. The do-not-resuscitate order: a comparison of physician and patient preferences and decision-making. Am J Med 1991; 91:255–260.

39. Brunetti LL, Carperos SD, Westlund RE. Physicians' attitudes toward living wills and cardiopulmonary resuscitation. J Gen Intern Med 1991; 6:323–329.

40. Bedell S, Delbanco T. Choices about cardiopulmonary resuscitation in the hospital: When do physicians talk with patients? New Engl J Med 1984; 310:1089–1093.

41. Johnston SC, Pfeifer MP. End-of-Life Study Group. Patient and physician roles in end-of-life decision-making. J Gen Intern Med 1998; 13:43–45.

42. Johnson SC, Pfeifer MP, McNutt R. The discussion about advance directives. Patient and physician opinions regarding when and how it should be conducted. End-of-Life Study Group. Arch Intern Med 1995; 155:1025–1030.

43. Billings JA, Block S. Palliative care in undergraduate medical education. Status report and future directions. JAMA 1997; 278:733–738.

44. Hill TP. Treating the dying patient. The challenge for medical education. Arch Intern Med 1995; 155:1265–1269.

45. Tierney WM, Dexter PR, Gramelspacher GP, Perkins AJ, Zhou XH, Wolinsky FD. The effect of discussions about advance directives on patients' satisfaction with primary care. J Gen Intern Med 2001; 16:32–40.

46. Sowden AJ, Forbes C, Entwistle V, Watt I. Informing, communicating and sharing decisions with people who have cancer. Qual Health Care 2001; 10:193–196.

47. Layson RT, Adelman HM, Wallach PM, Pfeifer MP, Johnstons S, McNutt RA. Discussions about the use of life-sustaining treatments: a literature review of physicians' and patient' attitudes and practices. End of Life Study Group. J Clin Ethics 1994; 5:195–203.

48. Hill M, MacQuillan G, Forsyth M, Heath DA. Cardiopulmonary resuscitation: who makes the decision? Br Med J 1994; 308:1677.

49. De Vos R, Haes HC, Koster RW, de Haan RJ. Quality of survival after cardiopulmonary resuscitation. Arch Intern Med 1999; 159:249–254.
50. Marik PE, Varon J, Lisbon A, Reich HS. Physicians' own preferences to the limitation and withdrawal of life-sustaining therapy. Resuscitation 1999; 42:197–201.
51. Phillips R, Wenger N, Teno J, et al. Choices of seriously ill patients about cardiopulmonary resuscitation: correlates and outcome. SUPPORT Investigators. Study to Understand Prognoses and Preferences for Outcomes and Risks of Treatments. Am J Med 1996; 100:128–137.
52. Schonwetter RS, Walker RM, Solomon M, Indurkhya A, Robinson BE. Life values, resuscitation preferences, and the applicability of living wills in older population. J Am Geriatr Soc 1996; 44:954–958.
53. Hamel MB, Lynn J, Teno JM, et al. Age-related differences in care preferences, treatment decisions, and clinical outcomes of seriously ill hospitalized adults: lessons from SUPPORT. J Am Geriatr Soc 2000; 48(Suppl):S176–S182.
54. Yeo CL, Tudehope DI. Outcome of resuscitated apparently stillborn infants: a ten year review. J Paediatr Child Health 1994; 30:129–133.
55. Casalaz DM, Marlow N, Speidel BD. Outcome of resuscitation following unexpected apparent stillbirth. Arch Dis Child Fetal Neonatal Ed 1998; 78:F112–F115.
56. Slevin ML, Stubbs L, Plant HJ, et al. Attitudes to chemotherapy: comparing views of patients with cancer with those of doctors, nurses, and general public. BMJ 1990; 300:1458–1460.
57. Cruzan v Missouri Department of Health. 497 U.S. 111 L.Ed.2d, 110 S Ct. 2841 (1990).
58. Tomlinson T, Brody H. Ethics and communication and do not resuscitate orders. N Engl J Med 1988; 318:43–46.
59. Charlson ME, Sax FL, MacKenzie CR, Fields SP, Braham RL, Douglas RG Jr. Resuscitation: how do we decide? A prospective study of physicians' preferences and the clinical course of hospitalized patients. JAMA 1986; 255:1316–1322.
60. Stewart AL, Teno J, Patrick DL, Lynn J. The concept of life of dying persons in the context of health care. J Pain Symptom Management 1999; 17:93–108.
61. Singer PA, Martin DK, Kelner M. Quality end-of-life care: patients' perspective. JAMA 1999; 281: 163–168.
62. Cleeland CS, Gonin R, Hatfield AK, et al. Pain and its treatment in outpatients with metastatic cancer. N Engl J Med 1994; 330:592–596.
63. Rabkin MT, Gillerman G, Rice NR. Orders not to resuscitate. N Engl J Med 1976; 295:364–366.
64. Youngner SJ. Who defines futility? JAMA 1988; 260:2094,2095.
65. Tomlinson T, Brody H. Futility and the ethics of resuscitation. JAMA 1990; 264:1276–1280.
66. Brett AS, McCullough LB. When patients request specific interventions: defining the limits of the physician's obligation. N Engl J Med 1986; 315:1347–1351.
67. Bedell SE, Delbanco TL, Cook EF, Epstein FH. Survival after cardiopulmonary resuscitation in the hospital. N Engl J Med 1983; 309:569–576.
68. Ebell MH, Bergus GR, Warbasse L, Bloomer R. The inability of physicians to predict the outcome of in-hospital resuscitation. J Gen Intern Med 1996; 11:16–22.
69. Vitelli CE, Cooper K, Rogatko A, Brennan MF. Cardiopulmonary resuscitation and the patient with cancer. J Clin Oncol 1991; 9:111–115.
70. Bonnin MJ, Pepe PE, Kimball KT, Clark PS Jr. Distinct criteria for termination of resuscitation in the out-of-hospital setting. JAMA 1993; 270:1457–1462.
71. Sirbaugh PE, Pepe P, Shook JE, Kimball KT, Goldman MJ, Ward MA, Mann DM. A prospective, population-based study of the demographics, epidemiology, management, and outcome of out-of-hospital pediatric cardiopulmonary arrest [see comments] [published erratum appears in Ann Emerg Med 1999; 33: 358]. Ann Emerg Med 1999; 33:174–184.
72. Barzilay Z, Somekh M, Sagy M, Boichis H. Pediatric cardiopulmonary resuscitation outcome. J Med 1998; 19:229–241.
73. Zaritsky A, Nadkarni V, Getson P, Kuehl K. CPR in children. Ann Emerg Med 1987; 16:1107–1111.
74. Kuisma M, Suominen P, Korpela R. Paediatric out-of-hospital cardiac arrest: epidemiology and outcome. Resuscitation 1995; 30:141–150.
75. Torphy DE, Minter MG, Thompson BM. Cardiorespiratory arrest and resuscitation in children. Am J Dis Child 1984; 138:1099–1102.
76. O'Rourke PP. Outcome of children who are apneic and pulseless in the emergency room. Crit Care Med 1986; 14:466–468.
77. Schindler MB, Bohn D, Cox PN, et al. Outcome of out-of-hospital cardiac or respiratory arrest in children [see comments]. N Engl J Med 1996; 335:1473–1479.

78. Ebell MH, Bergus GR, Warbasse L, Bloomer R. The inability of physicians to predict the outcome of in-hospital resuscitation. J Gen Intern Med 1996; 11:16–22.

79. Davis DJ. How aggressive should delivery room cardiopulmonary resuscitation be for extremely low birth weight neonates? [see comments]. Pediatr 1993; 92:447–450.

80. American College of Emergency Physicians. Guidelines for 'do not resuscitate orders' in the prehospital setting. Ann Emerg Med 1988; 17:1106–1108.

81. Miles SH, Crimmins TJ. Orders to limit emergency treatment for ambulance service in a large metropolitan area. JAMA 1985; 254:525–527.

82. Parrish GA, Holdren KS, Skiendzielewski JJ, Lumpkin OA. Emergency department experience with sudden death: a survey of survivors. Ann Emerg Med 1987; 16:792–796.

83. Kellermann AI, Staves DR, Hackman BB. In-hospital resuscitation following unsuccessful prehospital advanced cardiac life support. "heroic efforts" or an exercise in futility? Ann Emerg Med 1988; 17:589–594.

84. Gray WA, Capone RJ, Most AS. Unsuccessful emergency medical resuscitation are continued efforts in the emergency department justified? N Engl J Med 1991; 325:1393–1398.

85. Bonnin MJ, Swor RA. Outcomes in unsuccessful field resuscitation attempts. Ann Emerg Med 1989; 18:507–512.

86. Bonnin MJ, Pepe PE, Kimball KT, Clark PS Jr. Distinct criteria for termination of resuscitation in the out-of-hospital setting. JAMA 1993; 270:1457–1462.

87. Weaver WD. Resuscitation outside the hospital: what's lacking? N Engl J Med 1991; 325:1437–1439.

88. Gray WA, Capone RJ, Most AS. Unsuccessful emergency medical resuscitations: are continued efforts in the emergency department justified? N Engl J Med 1991; 325:1393–1398.

89. Delbridge TR, Fosnocht DE, Garrison HG, Auble TE. Field termination of unsuccessful out-of-hospital cardiac arrest resuscitations: acceptance by family members. Ann Emerg Med 1996; 27:649–654.

90. Iserson KV. Foregoing prehospital care: should ambulance staff always resuscitate? J Med Ethics 1991:17:19–24.

91. Hanson C, Strawser D. Family presence during cardiopulmonary resuscitation: Foote Hospital emergency department's nine-year perspective. J Emerg Nurs 1992; 18:104–106.

92. Meyers TA, Eichhorn DJ, Guzzetta CE. Do families want to be present during CPR? A retrospective survey. J Emerg Nurs 1998; 24:400–405.

93. Barrat F, Wallis DN. Relatives in the resuscitation room: their point of view [see comments]. J Accid Emerg Med 1998; 15:109–111.

94. Boie ET, Moore GP, Brummett C, Nelson DR. Do parents want to be present during invasive procedures performed on their children in the emergency department? A survey of 400 parents. Ann Emerg Med 1999; 34:70–74.

95. Doyle CJ, Post H, Burney RE, Maino J, Kee FE, Rhee KJ. Family participation during resuscitation: an option. Ann Emerg Med 1987; 16:673–675.

96. Robinson SM, Mackenzie-Ross S, Campbell Hewson GL, Egleston CV, Prevost AT. Psychological effect of witnessed resuscitation on bereaved relatives. Lancet 1998; 352:614–617.

97. Offord RJ. Should relatives of patients with cardiac arrest by invited to be present during cardiopulmonary resuscitation? Intensive Crit Care Nurs 1998; 14:288–293.

98. Bouchner H, Vinci R, Waring C. Pediatric procedures: do parents want to watch? Pediatrics 1989; 84:907–909.

99. Sacchetti A, Lichenstein R, Carraccio CA, Harris RH. Family member presence during pediatric emergency department procedures. Pediatr Emerg Care 1996; 12:268–271.

100. Boudreaux ED, Francis JL, Loyacano T. Family presence during invasive procedures and resuscitations in the emergency department: a critical review and suggestions for future research. Ann Emerg Med 2002; 40:193–205.

101. Eichhorn DJ, Meyers TA, Mitchell TG, Guzzetta CE. Opening the doors: family presence during resuscitation. J Cardiovas Nurs 1996; 10:59–70.

102. Walters DT, Tupin JP. Family grief in the emergency department. Emerg Med Clin North Am 1991; 9:189–206.

103. Jones WH. Emergency room sudden death: What can be done for the survivors? Death Education 1978; 2:231–245.

104. Kubler-Ross E. On death and dying. JAMA 1972; 221:174–179.

105. Dubin WR, Sarnoff JR. Sudden unexpected death: intervention with survivors. Ann Emerg Med 1986; 15:54–57.

106. Robinson MA. Informing the family of sudden death. Am Fam Physician 1981; 23:115–118.

107. O'Keeffe KM. Death and dying. J Am College Emerg Physicians (JACEP) 1979; 8:275–279.
108. Creek LV. How to tell the family that the patient has died. Postgrad Med 1980; 68:207–209.
109. Hamilton GC. Sudden death in the ED: telling the living. Ann Emerg Med 1988; 17:382.
110. Willis RW. Bereavement management in the emergency department. J Emerg Nurs 1977; 3:35–39.
111. Cathcart F. Seeing the body after death. Br Med J 1988; 297:997,998.
112. Lindemann E. Symptomatology and management of acute grief. Am J Psychiatry 1994; 151(Suppl): 155–160.
113. Biros MH, Lewis RJ, Olson CM, Ronge JW, Cummins RO, Fost N. Informed consent in emergency research. Consensus statement from the Coalition Conference of Acute Resuscitation and Critical Care Researchers. JAMA 1995; 273:1283–1287.
114. Wolf SM, Boyle P, Callahan D, et al. Sources of concern about the Patient Self-Determination Act. N Engl J Med 325:1666–1671.
115. Abramson NS, Meisel A, Safar P. Informed consent in resuscitation research. JAMA 1981; 246: 2828–2830.
116. Abramson NS, Meisel A, Safar P. Deferred consent. A new approach for resuscitation research on comatose patients. JAMA 1986; 255:2466–2471.
117. Abramson NS, Safar P. Deferred consent: use in clinical resuscitation. Brain Resuscitation Clinical Trial II Study Group. Ann Emerg Med 1990; 19:781–784.
118. Garns MK, Vassbo K, Forde R. Intubation training on the deceased newborn: parents' opinion? Tidsskr Nor Laegenforen 1999; 119:39–41.
119. Department of Health and Human Services, US Food and Drug Administration. Protection of human subjects: informed consent and waiver of informed consent requirements in certain emergency research. 61 Federal Register. 51528 (1996) (codified at 21 CFR §50.24 and §46.408).
120. Benfield DG, Flaksman RJ, Lin TH, Kantak AD, Kokomoor FW, Vollman JH. Teaching intubation skills using newly deceased infants. JAMA 1991; 265:2360–2363.

The Future
of Cardiopulmonary Resuscitation
Combination Therapy

Joseph P. Ornato, MD, FACP, FACC, FACEP

CONTENTS

INTRODUCTION
DRUG COMBINATIONS
DEVICE COMBINATIONS
HYPOTHERMIA COMBINED WITH OTHER RESUSCITATION TECHNIQUES
CONCLUSIONS
REFERENCES

INTRODUCTION

The physiology of cardiopulmonary resuscitation (CPR) is complex and changes over time. Becker and Weisfeldt defined three time-sensitive phases of resuscitation: electrical, circulatory, and metabolic *(1)*. Each of these phases is characterized by multiple physiological abnormalities to become more profound and difficult to reverse over time. Beyond the first phase, which can often be corrected by a single intervention (e.g., prompt defibrillation for ventricular fibrillation [VF] or pulseless ventricular tachycardia, and increasing host of challenges develop (e.g., maintaining coronary and cerebral blood flow and pressure, counteracting vasodilatation, cerebral protection, minimize and postresuscitation left ventricular dysfunction).

Attempts to improve resuscitation outcome have traditionally focused on improving one intervention (or variable) at a time. Experimental models and clinical trials have, thus, attempted to keep all variables constant (either by design or randomization) except for one intervention that could be divided into a control and experimental group. Although such a design is optimal from a scientific standpoint, it handicaps the process of finding dramatic enhancements in clinical resuscitation practice because solitary interventions can only address one of the many physiological derangements that are present at a time. The situation is analogous to the search for cancer cures. Major breakthroughs, such as have been seen in the treatment of childhood leukemia or certain forms of lymphoma, have occurred because multiple intervention strategies were tested against conventional therapy. Combination therapeutic techniques have been employed with equal success in the management of patients with acquired immunodeficiency syndrome (AIDS).

From: *Contemporary Cardiology: Cardiopulmonary Resuscitation*
Edited by: J. P. Ornato and M. A. Peberdy © Humana Press Inc., Totowa, NJ

The purpose of this chapter is to review a few examples of the combination resuscitation strategies (both successful and unsuccessful) that have begun to appear in both the experimental and clinical trial literature.

DRUG COMBINATIONS

Catecholamines and Buffer Therapy

There continues to be controversy regarding whether the use of buffer therapy during CPR enhances the actions of catecholamines *(2)*. Recent evidence suggests that routine addition of buffer therapy to catecholamines *early* in resuscitation is not only unnecessary, but may actually be harmful *(3,4)*. Sun et al. induced VF in Sprague-Dawley rats. Precordial compression and mechanical ventilation were initiated after 8 minutes of untreated VF. Animals were then randomized to receive either sodium bicarbonate, tromethamine, or saline placebo. Two minutes later, epinephrine was injected intravenously. In another subgroup, epinephrine was given first followed (2 minutes later) by either buffer or placebo. Electrical defibrillation was attempted after 8 minutes of precordial compression. Both bicarbonate and tromethamine significantly decreased coronary perfusion pressure (CPP) can reduce the magnitude of the vasopressor effect of the adrenergic agents. When the vasopressor preceded the buffer, the decline in CPP after buffer administration was prevented. These results may help to explain why a randomized clinical trial involving 502 randomized, adult cardiac arrest (CA) victims had no better outcome when they received buffer therapy as opposed to placebo *(4)*.

In contrast, one recent experimental study in a canine VF model suggests that, in a prolonged resuscitation, bicarbonate therapy and a period of perfusion prior to attempted defibrillation may increase survival *(5)*. The experiment was designed to determine whether administration of sodium bicarbonate and/or epinephrine in combination with a brief period of CPR prior to defibrillation would improve the outcome of prolonged CA in dogs. After 10 minutes of VF, animals received either immediate defibrillation (followed by treatment with bicarbonate or control) or immediate treatment with bicarbonate or saline (followed by defibrillation). Treatment with bicarbonate was associated with increased rates of restoration of spontaneous circulation. This was achieved with fewer shocks and in a shorter time. CPP was significantly higher in bicarbonate-treated animals. The best outcome in this study was achieved when defibrillation was delayed for approx 2 minutes, during which time sodium bicarbonate and epinephrine were administered with ongoing CPR.

Catecholamines and β-Blockers

Redding and Pearson were the first to show the importance of maintaining peripheral vascular resistance to maximize coronary and cerebral blood flow during resuscitation *(6,7)*. Epinephrine has been the principal adrenergic agent used in resuscitation for more than 30 years, primarily because of its α-adrenergic action, which increases CPP and favors an initial return of spontaneous circulation (ROSC). However, its β-adrenergic action may have detrimental effects on postresuscitation myocardial function by increasing myocardial oxygen consumption during and, immediately following, ROSC.

In experimental rodent model optimized to study postresuscitation cardiovascular events, epinephrine increased the severity of postresuscitation myocardial dysfunction and decreased duration of survival significantly *(8)*. The researchers concluded that more selective α-adrenergic agents or use of nonselective adrenergic agents (e.g., epinephrine) with β-1 adrenergic blockade deserve further investigation. Even use of a relatively pure α-adrenergic vasoconstrictor such as phenylephrine in combination with a β-blocker (propanolol) appears to improve to balance between myocardial oxygen supply and demand during ongoing resuscitation compared to that which is seen when epinephrine is used *(9)*.

Vasopressin and Epinephrine

Another approach to creating systemic vasoconstriction without β-adrenergic stimulation during resuscitation has been the use of arginine vasopressin *(10–12)*. It was relatively easy to show that administration of vasopressin in a VF pig model leads to a significantly higher CPP and myocardial blood flow than epinephrine during closed-chest CPR *(10)*. However, in a large, well-controlled, Canadian randomized clinical trial, survival-to-hospital discharge did not differ for patients receiving either epinephrine or vasopressin during resuscitation in the emergency department, intensive care unit, or hospital in-patient units *(13)*.

This finding has been explained by some to possibly represent the lack of difference between the two vasoconstrictors early in resuscitation. This leaves open the possibility that vasopressin might be superior to epinephrine later in resuscitation when adrenergic agents typically become less effective as a result of down-regulation of receptors. Further study will be needed to determine whether vasopressin has advantages over epinephrine late in resuscitation.

In the meantime, a number of recent studies have focused on whether the combination of vasopressin and epinephrine offers advantages over the use of either agent alone *(14–18)*. The combination appears capable of maximizing both coronary and CPP. An even more novel "cocktail" involves the combination of vasopressin, epinephrine, and nitroglycerin during resuscitation. Nitroglycerin is added to offset the coronary vasoconstriction effects of vasopressin. This "cocktail" has been shown to improve survival in a rodent asphyxial CA model *(19)* and improved vital organ perfusion in a porcine model *(20)*.

DEVICE COMBINATIONS

A variety of new closed-chest compression techniques and devices have been developed and studied experimentally and clinically in the last two decades *(21–44)*. Each of these methods are designed to exploit either or both of the cardiac or thoracic pump mechanisms of blood flow. Some of the new techniques and devices are being studied with each other in various combinations, attempting to create a syngeristic physiological effect.

Impedance Threshold Valve

One of the most promising techniques is the use of an impedance threshold valve (ITV) to improve venous return in combination with other resuscitation techniques. For example, Samniah et al. *(45)* tested the feasibility of transcutaneous phrenic nerve stimulation used in conjunction with an inspiratory ITV on hemodynamic variables during hemorrhagic shock. Anesthetized pigs were subjected to profound hemorrhagic shock by withdrawal of 55% of estimated blood volume over 20 minutes. After a 10-minute recovery period, the diaphragm was stimulated with a transcutaneous phrenic nerve stimulator at 10 times per minute as the airway was occluded intermittently with the ITV between positive pressure ventilations. Hemodynamic variables were monitored for 30 minutes. Phrenic nerve stimulation in combination with the ITV ($p < 0.001$) improved right and left ventricular diameter significantly compared with hypovolemic shock values by $34 \pm 2.5\%$ and $20 \pm 2.5\%$, respectively. Phrenic nerve stimulation together with the ITV also increased transaortic, transpulmonary, and transmitral valve blood flow by $48 \pm 6.6\%$, 67 ± 13.3, and $43 \pm 8.2\%$, respectively ($p < 0.001$ for comparisons within group). Mean $\pm$ standard error of the mean (SEM) coronary perfusion and systolic aortic blood pressures were also significantly ($p < 0.001$) higher compared with values before stimulation (30 ± 2 vs 20 ± 2 mmHg, and 37 ± 2 vs 32 ± 3 mmHg, respectively). This feasibility study suggests that phrenic nerve stimulation with an ITV can improve cardiac preload and, subsequently, key hemodynamic variables in a porcine model of severe hemorrhagic shock.

The ITV is also synergistic with closed-chest compression (both standard CPR and several of the newer enhanced techniques. Voelckel et al. *(44)* evaluated the combination of active compression–decompression (ACD) CPR and ITV in a young porcine model of CA. After 10 minutes of VF, and 8 minutes of standard CPR, ACD + ITV CPR was performed in seven 4- to 6-week old pigs (8–12 kg); defibrillation was attempted 8 minutes later. Within 2 minutes after initiation of ACD + ITV CPR, mean ($\pm$ SEM) CPP increased from 18 ± 2 to 24 ± 3 mmHg ($p = 0.018$). During standard vs ACD + ITV CPR, mean left ventricular myocardial and total cerebral blood flow was 59 ± 21 vs 126 ± 32 mL per minute per 100 g, and 36 ± 7 vs 60 ± 15 mL per minute per 100 g, respectively ($p = 0.028$). Six of seven animals were defibrillated successfully and survived longer than 15 minutes. Thus, the combination of ACD + ITV CPR increased both CPP and vital organ blood flow significantly after prolonged standard CPR in a young porcine VF model.

HYPOTHERMIA COMBINED WITH OTHER RESUSCITATION TECHNIQUES

Dr. Peter Safar was the first to recognize the importance of cardiopulmonary cerebral resuscitation in effecting meaningful survival from CA. Although promising when given pre-arrest in animal models, a variety of single pharmaceutical agents have been administered postresuscitation in humans without benefit *(46)*. The most promising techniques appear to be the use of mild to moderate hypothermia begun early (within 3–4 hours) post-ROSC. Two recent multicenter, randomized clinical trials showed a clear survival advantage for comatose adult CA survivors whose core body temperature was maintained at mild hypothermic levels for 24 to 48 hours postresuscitation.

The ultimate combination will likely involve adding novel resuscitation devices to new pharmacological interventions. One such example is a recent report from Raedler et al. *(47)* who documented hemodynamic and vital organ flow benefit from the use of ACD-CPR, ITV, vasopressin, and hypothermia during resuscitation in a porcine CA model. Pigs were surface-cooled until their body core temperature was 26°C. After 10 minutes of untreated VF, 14 animals were assigned randomly to either ACD CPR with the ITV ($N = 7$) or to standard (STD) CPR ($N = 7$). After 8 minutes of CPR, all animals received 0.4 U/kg vasopressin intravenously, and CPR was maintained for an additional 10 minutes in each group; defibrillation was attempted after 28 minutes of CA, including 18 minutes of CPR. Before the administration of vasopressin, mean $\pm$ SEM common carotid blood flow was significantly higher in the ACD + ITV group compared with STD CPR (67 ± 13 vs 26 ± 5 mL per minute, respectively; $p < 0.025$). After vasopressin was given at minute 8 during CPR, mean ± SEM CPP was significantly higher in the ACD + ITV group, but did not increase in the STD group (29 ± 3 vs 15 ± 2 mmHg, and 25 ± 1 vs 14 ± 1 mmHg at minutes 12 and 18, respectively; $p < 0.001$); mean ± SEM common carotid blood flow remained higher at respective time points (33 ± 8 vs 10 ± 3 mL per minute, and 31 ± 7 vs 7 ± 3 mL per minute, respectively; $p < 0.01$). Without active rewarming, spontaneous circulation was restored and maintained for 1 hour in three of seven animals in the ACD + ITV group vs none of seven animals in the STD CPR group (NS). During hypothermic CA, ACD-CPR with the ITV improved common carotid blood flow compared with STD CPR alone. After the administration of vasopressin, CPP was significantly higher during ACD + ITV CPR, but not during STD CPR. Thus, ACD-CPR with the ITV can improve carotid blood flow (and CPP with vasopressin) compared with STD CPR.

CONCLUSIONS

Resuscitation science is continuing to progress as new discoveries unlock the secrets of the human body during catastrophic medical and traumatic events. Improvement in the rate of neurologically intact survival following resuscitation will likely come from evolutionary steps rather than a single, major breakthrough. At present, the most promising hope seems to be a multifaceted approach targeting the many physiological derangements that are present during CA.

REFERENCES

1. Weisfeldt ML, Becker LB. Resuscitation after cardiac arrest: a 3-phase time-sensitive model. JAMA 2002; 288:3035–3038.
2. Vukmir RB, Bircher N, Safar P. Sodium bicarbonate in cardiac arrest: A reappraisal. Am J Emerg Med 1996; 14:192–206.
3. Sun S, Weil MH, Tang W, Povoas HP, Mason E. Combined effects of buffer and adrenergic agents on postresuscitation myocardial function. J Pharmacol Exp Ther 1999; 291:773–777.
4. Dybvik T, Strand T, Steen PA. Buffer therapy during out-of-hospital cardiopulmonary resuscitation Resuscitation 1995; 29:89–95.
5. Leong EC, Bendall JC, Boyd AC, Einstein R. Sodium bicarbonate improves the chance of resuscitation after 10 minutes of cardiac arrest in dogs. Resuscitation 2001; 51:309–315.
6. Pearson JW, Redding JS. Peripheral vascular tone in cardiac resuscitation. Anesth Analg 1965; 44: 746–762.
7. Pearson JW, Redding JS. Influence of peripheral vascular tone on cardiac resuscitation. Anesth Analg 1967; 46:746–752.
8. Tang W, Weil MH, Sun S, Noc M, Yang L, Gazmuri RJ. Epinephrine increases the severity of postresuscitation myocardial dysfunction. Circulation 1995; 92:3089–3093.
9. Ditchey RV, Rubio-Perez A, Slinker BK. Beta-adrenergic blockade reduces myocardial injury during experimental cardiopulmonary resuscitation. J Am Coll Cardiol 1994; 24:804–812.
10. Lindner KH, Prengel AW, Pfenninger EG, et al. Vasopressin improves vital organ blood flow during closed-chest cardiopulmonary resuscitation in pigs. Circulation 1995; 91:215–221.
11. Lindner KH, Prengel AW, Brinkmann A, Strohmenger HU, Lindner IM, Lurie KG. Vasopressin administration in refractory cardiac arrest. Ann Intern Med 1996; 124:1061–1064.
12. Lindner KH, Haak T, Keller A, Bothner U, Lurie KG. Release of endogenous vasopressors during and after cardiopulmonary resuscitation. Heart 1996; 75:145–150.
13. Stiell IG, Hebert PC, Wells GA, et al. Vasopressin versus epinephrine for inhospital cardiac arrest: a randomised controlled trial. Lancet 2001; 358:105–109.
14. Mulligan KA, McKnite SH, Lindner KH, Lindstrom PJ, Detloff B, Lurie KG. Synergistic effects of vasopressin plus epinephrine during cardiopulmonary resuscitation. Resuscitation 1997; 35:265–271.

15. Wenzel V, Linder KH, Augenstein S, Prengel AW, Strohmenger HU. Vasopressin combined with epinephrine decreases cerebral perfusion compared with vasopressin alone during cardiopulmonary resuscitation in pigs. Stroke 1998; 29:1462–1467; discussion 7,8.

16. Voelckel WG, Lindner KH, Wenzel V, et al. Effects of vasopressin and epinephrine on splanchnic blood flow and renal function during and after cardiopulmonary resuscitation in pigs. Crit Care Med 2000; 28:1083–1088.

17. Mayr VD, Wenzel V, Voelckel WG, et al. Developing a vasopressor combination in a pig model of adult asphyxial cardiac arrest. Circulation 2001; 104:1651–1656.

18. Voelckel WG, Lurie KG, McKnite S, et al. Effects of epinephrine and vasopressin in a piglet model of prolonged ventricular fibrillation and cardiopulmonary resuscitation. Crit Care Med 2002; 30:957–962.

19. Kono S, Suzuki A, Obata Y, Igarashi H, Bito H, Sato S. Vasopressin with delayed combination of nitroglycerin increases survival rate in asphyxia rat model. Resuscitation 2002; 54:297–301.

20. Lurie KG, Voelckel WG, Iskos DN, et al. Combination drug therapy with vasopressin, adrenaline (epinephrine) and nitroglycerin improves vital organ blood flow in a porcine model of ventricular fibrillation. Resuscitation 2002; 54:187–194.

21. Schultz DD, Olivas GS. The use of cough cardiopulmonary resuscitation in clinical practice. Heart Lung 1986; 15:273–282.

22. Krischer JP, Fine EG, Weisfeldt ML, Guerci AD, Nagel E, Chandra N. Comparison of prehospital conventional and simultaneous compression-ventilation cardiopulmonary resuscitation. Crit Care Med 1989; 17:1263–1269.

23. Barranco F, Lesmes A, Irles JA, et al. Cardiopulmonary resuscitation with simultaneous chest and abdominal compression: comparative study in humans. Resuscitation 1990; 20:67–77.

24. Gazmuri RJ, Weil MH, von Planta M, Gazmuri RR, Shah DM, Rackow EC. Cardiac resuscitation by extracorporeal circulation after failure of conventional CPR. J Lab Clin Med 1991; 118:65–73.

25. Gazmuri RJ, Weil MH, Terwilliger K, Shah DM, Duggal C, Tang W. Extracorporeal circulation as an alternative to open-chest cardiac compression for cardiac resuscitation. Chest 1992; 102:1846–1852.

26. Cohen TJ, Tucker KJ, Redberg RF, et al. Active compression-decompression resuscitation: a novel method of cardiopulmonary resuscitation. Am Heart J 1992; 124:1145–1150.

27. Cohen TJ, Tucker KJ, Lurie KG, et al. Active compression-decompression. A new method of cardiopulmonary resuscitation. JAMA 1992; 267:2916–2923.

28. Cohen TJ, Goldner BG, Maccaro PC, et al. A comparison of active compression-decompression cardiopulmonary resuscitation with standard cardiopulmonary resuscitation for cardiac arrests occurring in the hospital. N Engl J Med 1993; 329:1918–1921.

29. Tucker KJ, Idris A. Clinical and laboratory investigations of active compression- decompression cardiopulmonary resuscitation [editorial]. Resuscitation 1994; 28:1–7.

30. Wik L, Naess PA, Ilebekk A, Steen PA. Simultaneous active compression-decompression and abdominal binding increase carotid blood flow additively during cardiopulmonary resuscitation (CPR) in pigs. Resuscitation 1994; 28:55–64.

31. Wik L, Mauer D, Robertson C. The first European pre-hospital active compression-decompression (ACD) cardiopulmonary resuscitation workshop: A report and a review of ACD-CPR. Resuscitation 1995; 30:191–202.

32. Wik L, Naess PA, Ilebekk A, Nicolaysen G, Steen PA. Effects of various degrees of compression and active decompression on haemodynamics, end-tidal CO2, and ventilation during cardiopulmonary resuscitation of pigs. Resuscitation 1996; 31:45–57.

33. Wik L, Schneider T, Baubin M, et al. Active compression-decompression cardiopulmonary resuscitation— instructor and student manual for teaching and training. Part II: A student and instructor manual. Resuscitation 1996; 32:206–212.

34. Hoekstra OS, Van Lambalgen AA, Groeneveld ABJ, Van den Bos GC, Thijs LG. Abdominal compressions increase vital organ perfusion during CPR in dogs: Relation with efficacy of thoracic compressions. Ann Emerg Med 1995; 25:375–385.

35. Lurie KG, Coffeen P, Shultz J, McKnite S, Detloff B, Mulligan K. Improving active compression-decompression cardiopulmonary resuscitation with an inspiratory impedance valve. Circulation 1995; 91:1629–1632.

36. Lurie KG. Active compression-decompression CPR: a progress report. Resuscitation 1994; 28:115–22.

37. Lurie KG, Shultz JJ, Callaham ML, et al. Evaluation of active compression-decompression CPR in victims of out-of- hospital cardiac arrest. JAMA 1994; 271:1405–1411.

38. Lurie K, Voelckel W, Plaisance P, et al. Use of an inspiratory impedance threshold valve during cardiopulmonary resuscitation: a progress report. Resuscitation 2000; 44:219–230.

39. Lurie KG, Mulligan KA, McKnite S, Detloff B, Lindstrom P, Lindner KH. Optimizing standard cardiopulmonary resuscitation with an inspiratory impedance threshold valve. Chest 1998; 113:1084–1090.

40. Lurie KG. Recent advances in mechanical methods of cardiopulmonary resuscitation. Acta Anaesthesiol Scand Suppl 1997; 111:49–52.

41. Plaisance P, Lurie KG, Vicaut E, et al. A comparison of standard cardiopulmonary resuscitation and active compression-decompression resuscitation for out-of-hospital cardiac arrest. French Active Compression-Decompression Cardiopulmonary Resuscitation Study Group. N Engl J Med 1999; 341: 569–575.

42. Plaisance P, Lurie KG, Payen D. Inspiratory impedance during active compression-decompression cardiopulmonary resuscitation: a randomized evaluation in patients in cardiac arrest. Circulation 2000; 101:989–994.

43. Shultz JJ, Lurie KG. Variations in cardiopulmonary resuscitation techniques: Past, present and future. Can J Cardiol 1995; 11:873–880.

44. Voelckel WG, Lurie KG, Sweeney M, et al. Effects of active compression-decompression cardiopulmonary resuscitation with the inspiratory threshold valve in a young porcine model of cardiac arrest. Pediatr Res 2002; 51:523–527.

45. Samniah N, Voelckel WG, Zielinski TM, et al. Feasibility and effects of transcutaneous phrenic nerve stimulation combined with an inspiratory impedance threshold in a pig model of hemorrhagic shock. Crit Care Med 2003; 31:1197–1202.

46. Gisvold SE, Sterz F, Abramson NS, et al. Cerebral resuscitation from cardiac arrest: Treatment potentials. Crit Care Med 1996; 24(Suppl):S69–S80.

47. Raedler C, Voelckel WG, Wenzel V, et al. Vasopressor response in a porcine model of hypothermic cardiac arrest is improved with active compression-decompression cardiopulmonary resuscitation using the inspiratory impedance threshold valve. Anesth Analg 2002; 95:1496–1502, table of contents.

Index